The Ophthalmic Assistant
A Text for Allied and Associated Ophthalmic Personnel

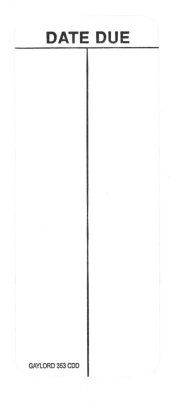

DATE DUE

GAYLORD 353 CDD

The Ophthalmic Assistant

A Text for Allied and Associated Ophthalmic Personnel

Tenth Edition

Harold A. Stein, MD MSC(Ophth) FRCS(C) DOMS(London)

Professor of Ophthalmology, University of Toronto, Toronto, Ontario, Canada; Emeritus and Past Chairman, Department of Ophthalmology, Scarborough General Hospital, Scarborough, Ontario, Canada; Emeritus, Mount Sinai Hospital, Toronto, Ontario, Canada; Past Secretary General, International Contact Lens Society of Ophthalmologists, Denver, Colorado; Past President, Joint Commission on Allied Health Personnel in Ophthalmology, St Paul, Minnesota; Past President, Contact Lens Association of Ophthalmologists, New Orleans, Louisiana; Past President, Canadian Ophthalmological Society, Ottawa, Canada; Co-director, Bochner Eye Institute, Toronto, Ontario, Canada

Raymond M. Stein, MD FRCS(C)

Co-director, Bochner Eye Institute, Toronto, Ontario, Canada; Associate Professor of Ophthalmology, University of Toronto, Ontario, Canada; Board of Directors, Foundation Fighting Blindness, Toronto, Ontario, Canada; Attending Ophthalmologist, Scarborough Hospital, Scarborough, Ontario, Canada; Attending Ophthalmologist, Mount Sinai Hospital, Toronto, Ontario, Canada; Editor, Clinical and Surgical Ophthalmology, Medicopea, Montreal, Quebec, Canada; Editor, Eye Care Update, Digital Journal, Toronto, Ontario Past President, Canadian Society of Cataract and Refractive Surgery, Montreal, Quebec, Canada; Past Commissioner, Joint Commission on Allied Health Personnel in Ophthalmology, St Paul, Minnesota, USA

Melvin I. Freeman, MD FACS

Clinical Professor of Ophthalmology, Emeritus, University of Washington School of Medicine, Seattle, Washington; Affiliate Clinical Investigator, Benaroya Research Institute at Virginia Mason, Seattle, Washington; Past Head, Section of Ophthalmology, Virginia Mason Clinic and Medical Center, Seattle, Washington; Medical Director, Emeritus, Department of Continuing Medical Education, Virginia Mason Medical Center, Seattle, Washington; Former Vice President, International Contact Lens Council, Osaka, Japan; Past President, Alliance for Continuing Medical Education, Birmingham, Alabama; Past President, Contact Lens Association of Ophthalmologists, New Orleans, Louisiana; Past President, Joint Commission on Allied Health Personnel in Ophthalmology, St Paul, Minnesota; Chair, Joint Commission on Allied Health Personnel in Ophthalmology Education and Research Foundation, St Paul, Minnesota, USA

For additional online content visit ExpertConsult.com

ELSEVIER

ELSEVIER

ELSEVIER your source for books, journals and multimedia in the health sciences

www.elsevierhealth.com

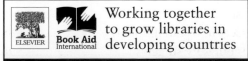

Contents

Section One: Basic Sciences

Section Two: Clinical Practice

Section Three: Common Clinical Eye Problems

Section Four: Surgical Techniques

Contents

Foreword:
An all purpose resource

The Ophthalmic Assistant, first published in 1968, has become the classic text for ophthalmic assistants and associated personnel over the past 50 years. The material presented is a mini-textbook of ophthalmology and eye care covering basic sciences, new testing procedures, new equipment, and the involvement of associated allied health personnel in the community.

In this tenth edition, Harold Stein and Raymond Stein of Toronto, Canada, are again joined by Melvin Freeman of Seattle, Washington and several new contributors in vision function and impairment and uveitis. The new chapters on the Dry Eye and an Atlas of Clinical Disorders is of particular importance. This text is well illustrated and written in a style that is easy to read and understand. Associated personnel can learn comfortably and easily. *The Ophthalmic Assistant* contains basic information on everything from testing vision and glaucoma to common surgical procedures, both minor and major, with an emphasis throughout on technical considerations. Refractive surgery is given special emphasis and the newer diagnostic modalities of ocular imaging are included. The authors' knowledge of the variety of information ophthalmic assistants need to know to perform their tasks comfortably, capably, and appropriately is obvious and impressive.

This text is of value to all ophthalmic personnel and associated health personnel who work with patients. By reviewing, discussing, and understanding the material in this book, they will be able to apply the valuable information contained in this text to their responsibilities in the best interest of patient care. Complete ophthalmologic care can best be provided when all team members are secure in their knowledge of ocular problems and clear in their roles and responsibilities. The delivery of care by teams is of increasing importance as the aging population is growing more rapidly than the capacity of existing ophthalmologists to provide care for it alone.

Previous editions of *The Ophthalmic Assistant* have been used as the standard text by ophthalmic assistants the world over, and this enhanced edition, with new and updated information and color illustrations and photographs, will continue this tradition.

Bruce E. Spivey, MD
Immediate Past President, International Council of Ophthalmology;
Founding CEO, American Academy of Ophthalmology;
Chairman Emeritus of Ophthalmology, California Pacific Medical Center, CA, USA;
Past President, American Ophthalmology Society;
Past President, American Board of Medical Specialties;
Past President, Council of Medical Specialty Societies

The Ophthalmic Assistant was originally written in 1968. Over the past nine editions and 50 years it has expanded to cover all the newer areas of eye care delivery. This updated edition includes new tests, illustrations, and photographs, as well as a diversity of new information. There are excellent illustrations throughout the tenth edition, as well as both color and black-and-white photographs interspersed throughout each chapter. It is essentially a mini-textbook in eye care delivery. It can benefit both paraoptometric assistants and optometry students. It can also benefit optometrists who are interested in the latest information on refractive surgery, wavefront technology, glaucoma, and surgical techniques that are used in the current practice of ophthalmology. This volume includes chapters devoted to cross-linking and optical coherence tomography. The text is easy to read, with excellent artwork and information interspersed throughout all the chapters.

The authors, Dr. Harold Stein, Dr. Raymond Stein, and Dr. Melvin Freeman, are well known to their peers in the educational field. While the book is mainly written by these three authors, there are many chapters contributed by specialists in various fields of eye care. The text includes close to 1000 pages of high-quality illustrations, many of which are original. This is an excellent vehicle for dissemination of information.

The text is divided into nine sections: (1) basic sciences, (2) clinical practice, (3) Common Clinical Eye Problems, (4) surgical techniques, (5) ocular imaging, (6) special procedures, (7) community ocular programs, (8) expanded roles in eye care delivery, (9) role of assistants in eye care, and (10) a newly added color atlas of eye disease and disorders. In addition, there is an extensive appendix with some material and tables not found in other textbooks.

The basic sciences section includes anatomy, physiology, optics, pharmacology, and microbiology related to the eye. The pharmacology chapter gives a considerable amount of information on newer medications that are used today.

The clinical practice section includes chapters on history taking and office efficiency as well as preliminary ocular examination. It introduces refractive errors and how to correct them along with automated refractors and their use in clinical practice. There are chapters on the basic principles of spectacles. There are three chapters devoted to rigid and soft contact lenses and advanced techniques in rigid and soft contact lens fittings. Visual fields, along with automated visual field testing, have been included, as well as chapters applied to clinical practice.

Section Three focuses on common clinical eye problems, such as ocular injuries, urgent cases, and common eye and retinal disorders and diseases. Glaucoma has a special chapter and there is a chapter on examination of children.

Section Four covers surgical technique, which includes management of the operative patient and highlights of major ocular surgery, management of laser surgery, ambulatory surgery, and refractive surgery. Those chapters related to ocular surgery and refractive surgery are of value to optometrists in comanagement situations of cataracts and refractive surgery, providing a basic text on understanding what problems may occur.

Section Five deals with ocular imaging, including ocular coherence tomography, computerized corneal topography, specular microscopy, and diagnostic ultrasound.

The special procedures described in Section Six include ocular motility and binocular vision, as well as an excellent chapter on ophthalmic photography and a chapter on low vision aids.

In Section Seven, there is a chapter on the latest techniques in cardiopulmonary resuscitation.

This textbook is a condensed version of all aspects of eye care and eye care delivery. The authors have provided both a reference book for those using the index to find some special disease or disorder and also a training book for those needing to identify areas of special concerns. In addition to individual educational benefits, the book serves as a valuable library purchase to have available on the latest in ophthalmic practice and diagnostic testing.

Desmond Fonn DipOptom MOptom FAAO
Distinguished Professor Emeritus
School of Optometry and Vision Science
University of Waterloo
Waterloo, ON, Canada

Foreword:
challenges for opticianry

Developments in ophthalmology continue apace, and the authors, Drs. Harold Stein and Raymond Stein of Canada and Dr. Melvin Freeman of the United States, are authorities in providing easy-to-read information and illustration for allied health personnel. The book is used in many teaching programs and has one of the largest worldwide text sales in ophthalmology.

Opticians are part of an allied health group that is allied to ophthalmology. They provide service in the eye care field by being end distributors of spectacles and contact lenses for the public. Part of their responsibility is the understanding, in general, of what is being achieved today in the field of ophthalmology.

The field of ophthalmology is truly amazing. Tremendous outcomes in patient care are being achieved on a daily basis in offices, clinics, and operating rooms throughout the world. The results have a very important and positive impact on the lives of the patients and their quality of life.

Members of the public often question opticians about eye care and what can be achieved today in the eye care field. Some are looking for recommendations and some are looking for positive answers to some of their symptoms and concerns. They often regard the optician as someone who can spend more time with them than their surgeon and be helpful in answering questions.

Some of these accomplishments in ophthalmology are in the area of refraction; some are in the area of medical treatment of such diseases as acanthamoeba, conjunctivitis and glaucoma. Some are in the new surgical techniques of cataract surgery, glaucoma and lasers. Sophisticated measurements such as A-scans, imaging, wavefront aberrometers, and topography are presented clearly. Other opticians may be interested in the areas of contact lenses and the problems that occur in their management.

This text is intended to fill a role for ophthalmic assistants, optometrists, and opticians in providing clinical, scientific information on the vast smorgasbord of concerns that occur in the eye care field. It is essentially a mini-textbook of ophthalmology in a single soft-cover volume. The book is well illustrated with original illustrations and color photographs of disease processes. There are sections devoted to common eye and retinal disorders that occur. Numerous surgical techniques are illustrated, covering strabismus and cataracts, as well as refractive surgery.

The impact of refractive surgery in this decade has been enormous. It is therefore important to understand how it works, including LASIK, PRK, LASEK, lensectomies, and the phakic intraocular contact lens. New bifocal implants that will correct presbyopia have become a new threshold of surgical expertise. The chapters will reveal both complications and positive results that occur.

There are special chapters devoted to low-vision aids and managing the blind patient. There are excellent chapters on photography for those who are interested in this field. There is a chapter devoted to ethics that is applicable to all those who deal with the public.

Four chapters are devoted to rigid contact lenses, soft contact lenses, advanced contact lens fitting, and the management of a contact lens practice. These cover complications and managing the dry eye patient. Although this does not compare with *Fitting Guide for Hard and Soft Contact Lenses*, written by the same authors, it does provide a basis for management of a contact lens practice.

The appendix is outstanding, with materials gleaned from many areas of research which will serve the optician well.

The well-designed illustrations and photographs that are provided throughout the text are of great help in assimilation of the information and thus contribute greatly to the usefulness of the text.

Foreword: challenges for opticianry

Opticians who are knowledgeable about the expanding testing, imaging, and surgical outcomes of ophthalmology will be better able to understand the concerns of some members of the public encountered in day-to-day practice. They will understand complications of contact lenses as well as complications that may follow surgery. They will understand the expanding role of refractive surgery in today's environment and use of the sophisticated testing instrumentation required. This information will help in binding the optician to the public.

Mo Jalie, SMSA FBDO (Hons) Hon FCGI Hon FCOptom MCMI
Visiting Professor in Optometry
School of Biomedical Sciences
Ulster University, Coleraine
Northern Ireland

Foreword:
How this textbook can be a valuable tool for physician assistants

Since the first program was established in 1965, physician assistants (PAs) have assumed an increasingly important role in the delivery of health care in the United States. According to the Physician Assistant History Society, there are currently 210 PA programs in the United States and more than 108,000 individuals who have earned certification through the National Commission on Certification of Physician Assistants (NCCPA).

PAs are employed in a wide variety of health care settings including primary care offices, emergency departments, hospitals, and in nearly every medical and surgical specialty. Although only a small number of PAs are working in ophthalmic practices, every PA who treats patients encounters refractive errors and ocular disorders.

The scope of practice for PAs varies from state to state; however, PAs are able to perform many functions traditionally performed by physicians. In ophthalmic practices, besides addressing patients' presurgical medical needs, PAs assist in surgery, administer intravitreal injections, provide pre-and postop surgical care, and manage many aspects of comprehensive ophthalmology.

Historically the curriculum in PA programs has given little attention to ocular disorders and treatments, with the main message being to refer to a specialist. However, awareness of the ocular implications of systemic diseases is vital to a holistic approach to patient care. For example, understanding the implications of a patient's 12-year history of diabetes on his or her retinal vasculature is imperative for the PA who is addressing the patient's overall health.

Since 1968 *The Ophthalmic Assistant* has been an excellent resource for those working in the field of eye care at all levels. Over the course of multiple editions, the textbook has been revised and expanded to remain relevant in a field that has seen exponential growth over the past several decades. Earlier editions of the textbook have included information on basic sciences, clinical practice, surgical techniques, ocular imaging, special procedures, community ocular programs, expanded roles in eye care delivery, and the role of assistants in eye care. There is a very detailed appendix that contains valuable reference materials. The tenth edition includes chapters with case studies of ophthalmic disorders and an atlas of common ocular conditions.

This text is laid out in a logical fashion and written in language that is understandable to those with limited knowledge about the eye. It has been the main textbook for nearly 20 years in our clinical ophthalmic assistant program. Students find it easy to understand and keep it well after graduation as the foundation for their professional library. It will make an excellent addition to the reference library of the practicing PA.

Barbara T. Harris, PA MBA COT OSC
Director, Ophthalmic Medical Assistant Program
Department Chair Health Sciences
Caldwell Community College and Technical Institute;

Past President, Consortium of Ophthalmic Training Programs (COTP)
Past Chair, PA Section North Carolina Medical Society (NCMS)
Past Board Member Joint Commission on Allied Health Personnel in
Ophthalmology (JCAHPO)

Preface

Many ophthalmic assistants and technicians have no opportunity for formal training and learn their duties on the job. Experience and repetition alone may become excellent teachers. To paraphrase Sir William Osler, experience without knowledge is to sail an uncharted course, but knowledge without experience is never to go to sea at all. *The Ophthalmic Assistant* was written expressly for ancillary ophthalmic workers who assist eye doctors in the day-to-day care of eye patients. This book was designed to fill a vacuum in our community by providing a training basis for eye care personnel and meeting their needs for a reference source. The textbook has become a textbook of practical ophthalmology.

Originally published over 50 years ago in 1968, *The Ophthalmic Assistant* has grown in size by over 300%. It became necessary to continually expand the textbook to reflect the explosive growth of opthalmic knowledge and ophthalmic technology. Over the years we broadened the scope of the textbook to provide not only practical technical information but also background information on ophthalmic disease processes and surgical procedures. In this tenth edition, we attempted to keep pace with the ever-expanding new developments in the field of eye care by updating each chapter. At the same time, we have tried to retain the original concept: to provide a concise, up-to-date review of the field of eye care that is easily readable, interesting, and illustrated.

The Ophthalmic Assistant provides reliable and competent information on eye care before and after regular visits to offices, clinics, and hospitals. Ophthalmic assistants must be familiar with sterile procedures, types of emergencies, and many technical aspects of eye care. This knowledge can increase the ophthalmic assistant's efficiency, ensuring that all details of diagnostic work-up and regimen are understood and carried out. Although *The Ophthalmic Assistant* emphasizes the paramedical functions of the ophthalmic assistant and not the secretarial duties, we recognize that both positions in a small office may have to be carried out by the same individual.

We purposely avoided controversial subjects and highly specialized technical areas because of the varying degrees of training of eye assistants throughout the world. Rather, the emphasis is placed on illustrations and photographs that illuminate and clarify ophthalmic technology and foster interest wherever possible.

While the main thrust of this book is toward the ophthalmic assistant, we hope the clarity, organization, and readability of the book will attract others in the ophthalmic community. To accommodate these readers, we included sections for the hospital ophthalmic assistant who aids in surgery, for the nurse who aids in the surgical and postoperative care of patients after surgery, and for the optometrist and their assistants who should have knowledge in recognizing diseases and disorders, particularly glaucoma and retinal disorders. We also include material of interest to those individuals working for optical and associated pharmaceutical companies. We have added and updated material for contact lens technicians, with a more detailed review to be found in our companion book, *Fitting Guide for Hard and Soft Contact Lenses*, fourth edition, published by Mosby. A companion book, *Ophthalmic Terminology*, third edition, published by Mosby, serves to expand the glossary and is designed for learning vocabulary and the origins of words. An additional publication, *Ophthalmic Dictionary and Vocabulary Builder for Eye Care Professionals*, fourth edition, authored by H.A. Stein, R.M. Stein, M.I. Freeman, and J.S. Massare and published by Jaypee-Highlights Medical Publishers, is also available for learning vocabulary and original words.

Refractive surgery and computerized corneal topography are two areas of eye care delivery that generate great clinical interest. The tenth edition expands on the chapter on refractive surgery with new emphasis on invasive surgery, as well as the section on computerized corneal topography. This edition also includes many color photographs as well as replacements in color of many black-and-white photographs.

We miss the influence and contributions of our previous coauthor, Dr. Bernard Slatt, whose premature passing away came shortly after the seventh edition was published. His memory gave us input, motivation, and direction in continuing this work.

The authors are indebted to Bruce E. Spivey, Desmond Fonn, Mo Jalie, and Barbara T. Harris for their forewords to ophthalmologists, optometrists, opticians, and physician assistants, respectively. We gratefully acknowledge new, invited chapters by Bernard R. Blais, Thellea K. Leveque and Russell N. van Gelder. Our appreciation is again extended to our invited ongoing chapter authors and coauthors for their continuing updates to their chapters: Lynn D. Anderson, Michael S. Berlin, Arielle R. Brickman, William H. Ehlers, Daniel Epstein, Peter Y. Evans, Eleanor E. Faye, Joseph D. Freeman, Michael L. Gilbert, Richard E. Hackel, Melissa A. Jones, Alex V. Levin, Shoshana (Sue) M. Levine. Efrem D. Mandelcorn, Csaba L. Mártonyi, Lynn D. Maund, Gerald E. Meltzer, Edyie G. Miller-Ellis, Richard P. Mills, Rod A. Morgan, Korosh Nikeghbal, Penny Pilliar, Phyllis L. Rakow, Hans-Walter Roth, A. Ghani Salim, Ernest R. Simpson, Rebecca L. Stein (the fourth generation of Bochner/Stein's to contribute to ophthalmic allied and associates health care education), Gwen K. Sterns, and Michael A. Ward.

New chapters have been added for the tenth edition on dry eyes, uveitis, visual impairment and disabilities, and an atlas of common ocular conditions.

Harold A. Stein
Raymond M. Stein
Melvin I. Freeman

Acknowledgements

For aid and support for the tenth edition we thank Russell Gabbedy, Joanne Scott, John Leonard, Umarani Natarajan, and the contributors and reviewers.

Acknowledgments for aid as reviewers or contributors in previous editions:

Bud Appleton[†]	David L. Guyton	Kenneth Ogle[†]
Richard Augustine	G. Peter Halberg[†]	Thomas D Padrick
Howard S. Barneby	Keith Harrison	John Parker
Joseph T. Barr	William Hunter[†]	Thomas Pashby[†]
Tony Benson	John Hymers	Charles J. Pavlin[†]
Bernard R. Blais	Anne Jackson	Scot M Peterson
Maxwell K. Bochner[†]	Jerome Kazdan	Penny Cook Pilliar
Albert Cheskes	Edna Kelly	Karen Quam
Jordan Cheskes	D'Arcy Kingsmill[†]	Paula Quigley
John Crawford[†]	Jill Klintworth	Robert Rosen
Norman Deer[†]	Steven Kraft	Barnet Sakler[†]
Katherine Delmer	Laurette LaRocque	Abraham Schlossman[†]
William Ehlers	Les Landecker	Anne Skrypznik
Saul Fainstein[†]	John Lloyd	Laurie Stein
Zoraida Fiol-Silva	Sze Kong Luke	Kenneth Swanson[†]
John Fowler	Bernice Mandelcorn	Spencer Thornton
Therese Fredette	Theodore Martens	Alyssa Tipple
Ivan Gareau	Lynn D. Maund	Len Waldbaum
Alice Gelinas	Gerald E. Meltzer	Becky Walsh
Paul Graczyk	Richard P. Mills	E. Edward Wilson, Jr.
Desmond Grant	Donald Morin[†]	Sheffield Wo
Mark Grieve	Korosh Nikeghbal	Kenneth Woodward
Darrell Guthmiller	Sherrine Nunes	

[†]Deceased

List of Contributors

The editor(s) would like to acknowledge and offer grateful thanks for the input of all previous editions' contributors without whom this new edition would not have been possible.

Lynn D. Anderson, PhD
Chief Executive Officer
Joint Commission on Allied Health Personnel in Ophthalmology
St. Paul, MN, USA
(Chapters 53 and 54)

Michael S. Berlin, MD MS
Director, Glaucoma Institute of Beverly Hills;
Professor of Clinical Ophthalmology,
Jules Stein Eye Institute, UCLA;
President, Finnish American Chamber of
Commerce on the Pacific Coast;
Los Angeles, CA, USA
(Chapter 25)

Bernard R. Blais, MD
Clinical Professor
Albany Medical College
Albany, New York, NY, USA
(Chapter 9)

Arielle R. Brickman
York University
Toronto, ON, Canada
(Chapter 24)

William H. Ehlers, MD
Associate Professor of Surgery
Division of Ophthalmology, UCONN Health
Farmington, CT, USA
(Chapter 53)

Daniel Epstein, MD PhD FARVO
Professor
Department of Ophthalmology
Spitalgasse
Bern, Switzerland
(Chapter 38)

Peter Y. Evans, MD
Professor Emeritus
Department of Ophthalmology
Georgetown University
Washington, DC, USA
(Chapter 56)

Eleanor E. Faye, MD
Formerly Ophthalmic Surgeon
Manhattan Eye, Ear and Throat Hospital, New York;
Ophthalmic Consultant, Lighthouse International
Continuing Education
New York, NY, USA
(Chapters 45 and 46)

Tina Felfeli, BSc
University of Toronto
Toronto, ON, Canada
(Chapter 24)

Joseph D. Freeman, MD FACEP
Emergency Medicine Physician
Department of Emergency Medicine
Cottage Health System
Santa Barbara, CA, USA
(Chapter 49)

Michael L. Gilbert, MD
Past Medical Editor
Eye Care Technology Magazine;
Past President
Washington Academy of Eye Physicians
Bellevue, WA, USA
(Chapter 50)

Richard E. Hackel, MA CRA FOPS
Formerly Assistant Professor
Director of Ophthalmic Photography
WK Kellogg Eye Center
Department of Ophthalmology
University of Michigan
Ann Arbor, MI, USA
(Chapter 44)

Melissa A. Jones, MEd COE OCS
Formerly Director
Department of Ophthalmology
Virginia Mason Medical Center
Seattle, WA, USA
(Chapter 6)

Thellea K. Leveque, MD MPH
Clinical Associate Professor
Department of Ophthalmology
University of Washington Medicine
Seattle, WA, USA
(Chapter 26)

Alex V. Levin, MD MHSc FAAP FAAO FRCSC
Chief, Pediatric Ophthalmology and Ocular Genetics
Wills Eye Institute;
Professor, Departments of Ophthalmology and Pediatrics
Jefferson Medical College
Thomas Jefferson University
Philadelphia, PA, USA
(Chapters 27 and 52)

Shoshana (Sue) M. Levine, LDO ABO NCLE FNAO
Visual Effects Supervisor Optical and Contact Lens Dispensary
Virginia Mason Medical Center
Seattle, WA, USA
(Chapter 13)

Efrem D. Mandelcorn, MD FRCSC DBO
Assistant Professor
Department of Ophthalmology and Vision Sciences
University of Toronto
Toronto, ON, Canada
(Chapter 24)

Csaba L. Mártonyi, CRA FOPS
Emeritus Associate Professor
Department of Ophthalmology and
Visual Sciences
University of Michigan Medical School
Ann Arbor, MI, USA
(Chapter 44)

Lynn D. Maund, BA SC CLS
Contact Lens Specialty
Manager, Laser Eye Surgery Division
Maxwell K. Bochner Eye Institute
Toronto, ON, Canada
(Chapter 18)

Gerald E. Meltzer, MD MSHA
Accreditation Surveyor
Accreditation Association for Ambulatory Health Care
Denver, CO, USA
(Chapter 50)

Edyie G. Miller-Ellis, MD
Professor of Clinical Ophthalmology
Hospitals of the University of Pennsylvania
Scheie Eye Institute
Philadelphia, PA, USA
(Chapter 54)

Richard P. Mills, MD MPH
Clinical Professor
Department of Ophthalmology
University of Washington
Past President American Academy of Ophthalmology
Seattle, WA, USA
(Chapter 20)

Rod A. Morgan, MD FRCSC Dipl. ABO FAAO LMCC
Clinical Professor, Ophthalmology
Department of Ophthalmology and Visual Sciences
University of Alberta
Edmonton, AB, Canada
(Chapter 51)

Korosh Nikeghbal
Refracting Optician
Instructor, Seneca College
Toronto, ON, Canada
(Chapter 18)

Penny Pilliar
Optician (Retired)
Maxwell K. Bochner Eye Institute
Toronto, ON, Canada
(Chapter 18)

Carol J. Pollack-Rundle, BS COMT
Technician Education and Compliance Coordinator
University of Michigan
W.K. Kellogg Eye Center
Ann Arbor, Michigan, USA
(Chapter 7)

Phyllis L. Rakow, COMT FCLSA(H) NCLEM
Director, Contact Lens Services
Princeton Eye Group
Princeton, NJ, USA
(Chapter 47)

Hans-Walter Roth, MD
Visiting Professor
The Institute of Contact Lens Optics
Ulm, Germany
(Chapter 12)

A. Ghani Salim, MD
Clinical and Research Director
Bochner Eye Institute
Toronto, ON, Canada
(Chapter 40)

Craig Simms, BSc ROUB CDOS
Director of Education
Joint Commission on Allied Health Personnel in Ophthalmology
St. Paul, MN, USA
(Chapter 53)

Ernest R. Simpson, MD (FRCSC)
Department of Ophthalmology
Mount Sinai Hospital;
Director, Ocular Oncology Service
Princess Margaret Hospital
Toronto, ON, Canada
(Chapter 34)

Rebecca L. Stein, BSc (Medicine) MBChB
Ophthalmology Resident
University of Toronto
Toronto, ON, Canada
(Chapters 32, 36, 37, 39 and 57)

Gwen K. Sterns, MD
Chief, Department of Ophthalmology
Rochester General Hospital;
Medical Director
Association for the Blind and Visually Impaired–Goodwill
Clinical Professor of Ophthalmology
University of Rochester School of Medicine and Dentistry
Rochester, NY, USA
(Chapters 45 and 46)

Russell N. van Gelder, MD PhD
Professor and Chair
Department of Ophthalmology
University of Washington Medicine
Past President American Academy of Ophthalmology
Seattle, WA, USA
(Chapter 26)

Michael A. Ward, MMSc COMT FAAO
Director, Emory Contact Lens Service and
Instructor in Ophthalmology
Emory University School of Medicine
Atlanta, GA, USA
(Chapter 5)

Peng Yan, MD FRCSC
Retinal Specialist
Department of Ophthalmology and Vision Sciences
University of Toronto
Toronto, ON, Canada
(Chapter 24)

List of Reviewers

Chiara Cino, OD (Chapter 11)

Catherine M. Magsambol, MD (Chapter 31)

John S. Massare, PhD (Chapters 14-15, and 18)

Katy Murphy, COA (Chapter 13)

Carol J. Pollack-Rundle, BS, COMT
(Overall Text)

Vinci Yan, MD (Chapters 30, 31 and 36)

Dedication

IN MEMORY OF

Dr. Maxwell K. Bochner

A master ophthalmic clinician whose skillful guidance and use of ancillary personnel in ophthalmology permitted the delivery of quality eye care to a large number of visually disabled individuals. A caring and concerned physician who developed a strong bond with each and every patient.

and

Dr. Bernard J. Slatt

A brilliant ophthalmologist whose untimely passing was a great loss to ophthalmology. He was a major contributor in all previous editions of this textbook. An accomplished ophthalmologist, writer, father, and grandfather who contributed greatly in advancing the role of allied health personnel in ophthalmology.

IN APPRECIATION

We would like to thank our spouses Anne, Nancy, and Nanette, and our children and their families for graciously allowing us the time to spend on this project.

Chapter | 1 |

Anatomy of the eye

Although the eye is commonly referred to as the *globe,* it is not really a true sphere. It is composed of two spheres with different radii, one set into the other (Figures 1.1 and 1.2). The front, or anterior, sphere, which is the smaller and more curved of the two, is called the *cornea.* The cornea is the window of the eye because it is a completely transparent structure. It is the more curved of the two spheres and sets into the other as a watch glass sets into the frame of a watch. The posterior sphere is a white opaque fibrous shell called the *sclera.* The cornea and the sclera are relatively nondistensible structures that encase the eye and form a protective covering for all the delicate structures within.

In terms of size, the eye measures approximately 24 mm in all its main diameters in the normal adult.

SURFACE ANATOMY

The eye itself is covered externally by the *eyelids,* which are movable folds protecting the eye from injury and excessive light. The lids serve to swab the eye and spread a film of tears over the cornea, thereby preventing evaporation from the surface of the eye. The upper eyelid extends to the *eyebrow,* which separates it from the forehead, whereas the lower eyelid usually passes without any line of demarcation into the skin of the cheek. The upper eyelid is the more mobile of the two and when it is open it covers about 1 mm of the cornea. A muscle that elevates the lid, the *levator palpebrae superioris,* is always active, contracting to keep the eyelid open. During sleep the eyelid closes by relaxation of this muscle. The lower lid lies at the lower border of the cornea when the eye is open and rises slightly when it shuts.

Normally, when the eyes are open, a triangular space is visible on either side of the cornea. These triangular spaces, formed by the junction of the upper and lower lids, are called the *canthi* (Figure 1.3). These canthi are denoted by the terms *medial* and *lateral,* the former being closer to the nasal bridge. Most eyes are practically the same size; therefore, when we speak of the eyes appearing large or small, we usually refer not to the actual size but to the portion of the eyeball visible on external examination, which in turn depends on the size of the *palpebral fissure.* The shape of the fissure also determines its appearance. In Asians, a fold of skin extends from the upper lid to the lower lid and covers the medial fissure, giving the eye its characteristic obliquity. In the medial fissure there are two fleshy mounds: the deeper one, called the *plica semilunaris,* and the superficial one, called the *caruncle* (Figure 1.4). The caruncle is modified skin that contains sweat and oil glands. Occasionally it also contains fine cilia

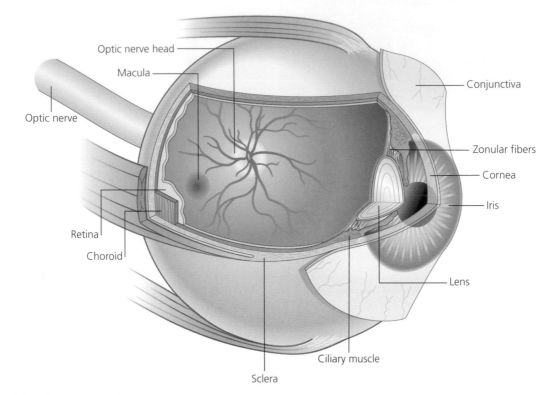

Figure 1.1 Cutaway section of the eye.

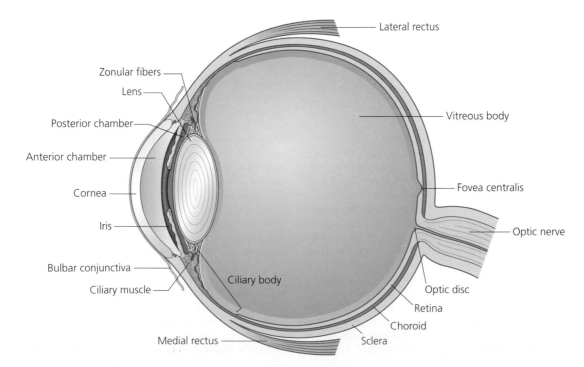

Figure 1.2 The eye cut in horizontal section.

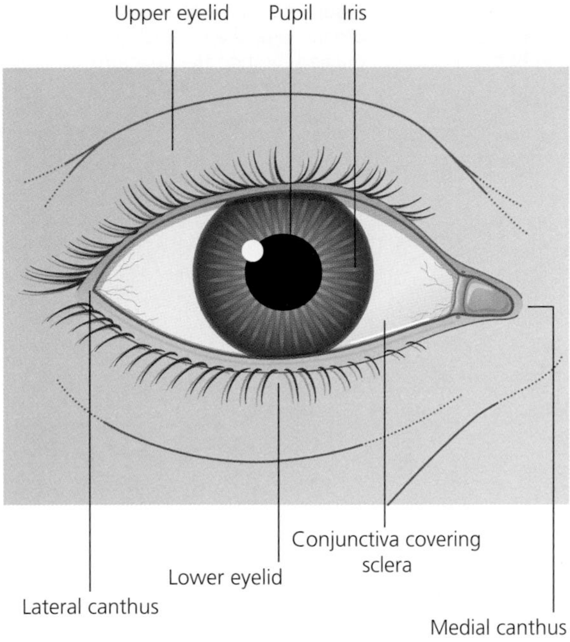

Upper eyelid   Pupil   Iris

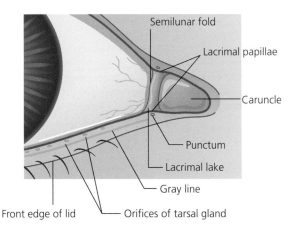

Conjunctiva covering sclera

Lower eyelid

Lateral canthus

Medial canthus

Figure 1.3 Surface anatomy of the eye.

Semilunar fold

Lacrimal papillae

Caruncle

Punctum

Lacrimal lake

Gray line

Front edge of lid   Orifices of tarsal gland

Figure 1.4 Inner canthus, showing the semilunar fold and the caruncle. Normally the punctum is not visible unless the lower lid is depressed.

or hairs. When the eyes are open, the palpebral fissures measure about 30 mm in width and 15 mm in height.

The free margin of each lid is about 2 mm thick and has an anterior and a posterior border. From the anterior, or front, border rise the *eyelashes*, which are hairs arranged in two or three rows. The upper eyelid lashes are longer and more numerous than the lower ones and they tend to curl upward. The lashes are longest and most curled in childhood. The posterior border of the lid margin is sharp and tightly abuts against the front surface of the globe. By depressing the lower lid, one can see the thin *gray line* that separates the two borders of the lid. This gray line is used in many surgical procedures to split the upper and lower lids into two portions. Also visible on both lids are the tiny openings that are the orifices of the sweat- and oil-secreting glands.

The largest oil-secreting glands, which are embedded in the posterior connective tissue substance of the lids (called the *tarsus*), are called the *meibomian glands*. The *lacrimal gland* is located above and lateral to the globe. Tears are produced by the lacrimal gland and travel through fine channels, referred to as *ducts*, to empty onto the conjunctival surface.

On the medial aspect of the lower lid where the lashes cease is a small *papilla*. At the apex of this papilla is a tiny opening called the *punctum* (see Figure 1.4). The punctum leads, by means of a small canal, through the lower lid to the *lacrimal sac* (Figure 1.5), which eventually drains into the nose. Tears are carried to the punctum by the pumping action of the lids and there they are drained effectively from the eye by means of tiny channels. A similar but smaller opening is found in the upper lid almost directly above it. The punctum normally cannot be seen by looking directly at the eye. It can be seen only by depressing the lower lid or everting the upper lid. The muscle underlying the eyelid skin is the *orbicularis oculi*, which is roughly circular. When it contracts, it closes the eye.

The portions of the eye that are normally visible in the palpebral fissures are the *cornea* and *sclera*. Because the cornea is transparent, what is seen on looking at the cornea is the underlying *iris* and the black opening in the center of the iris, called the *pupil*. The sclera forms the white of the eye and is covered by a mucous membrane called the *conjunctiva*. The conjunctiva extends from the junction of the cornea and sclera and terminates at the inner portion of the lid margin (Figure 1.6). The conjunctiva that covers the eye itself is referred to as the *bulbar conjunctiva*, whereas the portion that lines the inner surface of the upper and lower lids is called the *palpebral conjunctiva*. The junctional bay created when the two portions of the conjunctiva meet is referred to as the *fornix*. The lower fornix easily can be viewed by depressing the lower lid.

The role of the conjunctiva is to defend and repair the cornea in the event of scratches, wounds, or infections. The almost invisible blood vessels that are present dilate and leak nutrients, antibodies, and leukocytes into the tears that then wash over the avascular corneal surface. The conjunctiva also secretes mucus and oil, both of which help to keep the cornea moist and clean and to reduce friction when the lids blink over the cornea. The conjunctival mucous film over the ocular surface catches microorganisms. This mucous net then condenses into a ball and is carried to the nasal canthus where it dries and rolls onto the

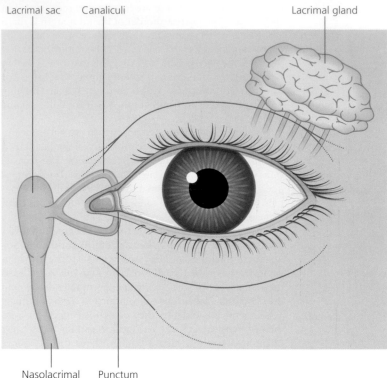

Lacrimal sac   Canaliculi

Lacrimal gland

Nasolacrimal duct   Punctum

Figure 1.5 Lacrimal apparatus. Tears produced by the lacrimal gland are drained through the punctum, lacrimal sac, and nasolacrimal duct into the nose.

skin. The conjunctiva also helps to resurface the cornea with epithelial cells if the entire corneal surface is scraped or burned.

Under the conjunctiva is a fibrous layer that overlies the sclera and rectus muscles. This is *Tenon's capsule,* a common surgical landmark.

TEAR FILM

The tear film is composed of three layers (Figure 1.7). The outermost layer consists of a lipid or fatty layer, mostly cholesterol esters, and is extremely thin. This layer is secreted by the meibomian glands and acts to prevent evaporation of the underlying aqueous layer. The central layer is chiefly aqueous, with some dissolved salts as well as glucose, urea, proteins, and lysozyme. This layer is secreted by the lacrimal glands. The third layer is a very thin mucous layer lying over the surface of the conjunctiva and cornea. This layer is secreted by specific cells of the conjunctiva referred to as *goblet cells* and is important in the stability of the tear film. Tear film abnormalities may arise in association with a number of clinical problems in older adults and in particular problems related to contact lenses.

The precorneal tear film layer serves several functions.

1. It forms a smooth refractive surface on the epithelium.
2. It maintains a moist environment for the epithelium.
3. It carries oxygen to the eye.

CORNEA

The cornea is a clear, transparent structure with a brilliant, shiny surface. It has a convex surface that acts as a powerful lens. Most of the refraction of the eye takes place not through the crystalline lens of the eye but through the cornea.

The cornea is relatively large at birth and almost attains its adult size during the first and second years. Although the eyeball as a whole increases a little less than three times in volume from birth to maturity, the corneal segment plays a small role in this part, being fully developed by 2 years of age.

The cornea is thicker at its periphery (1 mm) than at the center (0.5 mm). It can be divided into five distinct portions (Figure 1.8): the epithelium, Bowman's membrane, the stroma, Descemet's membrane, and the endothelium.

The *epithelium* is the part of the cornea usually injured by superficial abrasions or small foreign bodies. It is 5 to 7 cells

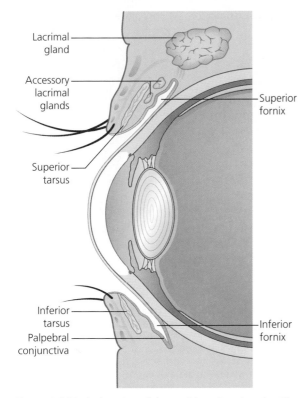

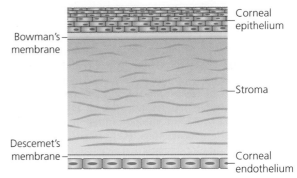

Figure 1.8 The cornea in cross-section showing the position and sequence of the layers (illustration not to scale).

Figure 1.6 Vertical section of the eyelids and conjunctiva. The lids act as a protective curtain for the eye. Only a small portion of the eye is actually exposed.

thick (50 μm) and is composed of nonkeratinized stratified squamous cells. The epithelium functions as a barrier and as an important refractive optical surface. It regenerates rapidly and heals without leaving a scar. Injury to the deeper structures usually results in formation of an opacity in the cornea.

Bowman's membrane consists of randomly oriented collagen fibrils of greater periodicity than the underlying stroma. This acellular layer, which is 10 μm thick, has no regenerative capabilities. Its function is unclear.

The layer just under Bowman's membrane is the *stroma*. This structure is 950 μm at the periphery and about 450 μm centrally; it accounts for 90% of the corneal thickness. The stroma consists of 200 to 250 evenly spaced type I collagen lamellae, which are oriented at right angles to their adjacent lamellae. It is composed of 78% water.

Descemet's membrane is 3 μm thick at birth, and 10 to 12 μm thick in older adults. It is composed of type III collagen. This very elastic layer retracts if cut. It forms the basement membrane of the epithelial cells.

The *endothelium* is a 4 to 6 μm monolayer of 500,000 cells. There is no known mechanism of attachment between the endothelium and Descemet's membrane. The endothelium is responsible for maintaining deturgescence of the cornea. No regeneration of this layer has been shown in humans. Corneal edema (swelling) can occur when contact lens materials, overwear, improper cleaning, or improper fit does not allow sufficient oxygen to reach the cornea.

The junction of the cornea and sclera is demarcated by a gray, semitransparent area referred to as the *limbus*. This transitional zone is only 1 mm wide and marks the point of insertion of the conjunctiva. The cornea, which contains no blood vessels, is completely nourished by three sources: a plexus of fine capillaries at the limbus, the tear film, and the aqueous humor.

In a paper published in *Ophthalmology* in 2013, by Dua et al., the existence of a newly described pre-Descemet's layer, hypothetically 15 μm thick, was suggested. Time will be needed to see if others can confirm the existence of this new layer and its potential significance.

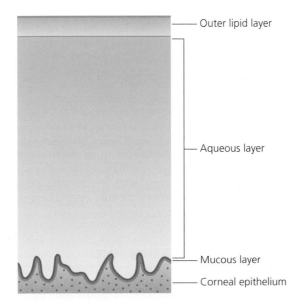

Figure 1.7 Three-layer structure of the tear film.

SCLERA

The opaque sclera forms the posterior five-sixths of the eye's protective coat. Its anterior portion is visible and constitutes the white of the eye. In children the sclera is thin, and therefore it appears bluish because the underlying pigmented structures are visible through it. In old age it may become yellowish because of the deposition of fat. Attached to the sclera are all the extraocular muscles. Through the sclera pass the nerves and the blood vessels that penetrate the interior of the eye. At its most posterior portion, the site of attachment of the *optic nerve*, the sclera becomes a thin, sieve-like structure called the *lamina cribrosa*, through which the retinal fibers leave the eye to form the optic nerve. The episcleral tissue is a loose connective and elastic tissue that covers the sclera and unites it with the conjunctiva above. Unlike the sclera, the episcleral tissue is highly vascular.

UVEA

The *uveal* tract consists of three structures: the *iris, ciliary body,* and *choroid.*

Iris

The *iris* is the most anterior structure of the uveal tract. It is perforated at its center by a circular aperture called the *pupil.* The iris has many ridges and furrows on its anterior surface. Contraction of the iris, which occurs in response to bright light, is accomplished by the activity of a flat, washer-like muscle called the *sphincter pupillae,* buried in its substance just surrounding the pupillary opening. Expansion or dilation of the pupil is facilitated by relaxation of the sphincter muscle and by activation of the radially oriented dilator muscle of the iris found at its peripheral circumference. Expansion and contraction of the iris, like an accordion, form circular pleat lines or furrows visible on its surface. In addition to these ridges and furrows, numerous white zigzag lines are formed by the blood vessels of the iris. Between the iris and the cornea is a clear fluid called the *aqueous humor.* This fluid occupies the space called the *anterior chamber* of the eye.

Ciliary body

The *ciliary body* (Figure 1.9) is in direct continuity with the iris and is adherent to the underlying sclera. Directly posterior to the iris, the ciliary body is plump and thrown into numerous folds referred to as the *ciliary processes.* This portion of the ciliary body is only about 2.5 mm in length and is responsible for the major production of aqueous fluid. The equator of the lens is only 0.5 mm from the ciliary processes and is suspended by fine, ligamentous fibers known

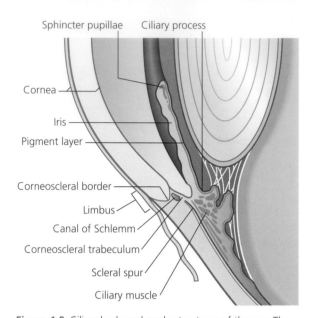

Figure 1.9 Ciliary body and angle structures of the eye. The angle is formed between the iris and the back surface of the cornea, with the aqueous humor of the anterior chamber interposed. The angle structures include the corneoscleral trabeculum, Schlemm's canal, scleral spur, a small extension of the ciliary muscle, and the root of the iris.

as the *zonular fibers* of the lens. The posterior portion of the ciliary body is flat. Most of the zonular fibers of the lens originate from the ciliary body. The ciliary body in general is triangular, with its shortest side anterior. The anterior side of the triangle in its inner part enters the formation of the angle of the anterior chamber. The iris takes root from its middle portion.

On the outer side of the triangle is the ciliary muscle, which lies against the sclera. Contraction of the ciliary muscle releases the tension of the zonular fibers, controlling the size and shape of the lens. This in turn allows the anterior surface of the lens to bulge forward and increase its power. Therefore, the ciliary muscle directly controls the focusing ability of the eye. In children this muscle is extremely active and the lens is easily deformed, which accounts for its powerful range of accommodation, or focusing abilities. The ciliary muscle declines with age; after the age of 40 its power becomes weaker and the lens is less able to change shape, so that focusing at near point, or accommodating, becomes difficult. This condition is commonly referred to as *presbyopia.*

Choroid

The choroid is in direct continuity with the iris and ciliary body and lies between the retina and sclera (see Figure 1.2). The choroid is primarily a vascular structure. Its primary function is to provide nourishment for the outer layers of the retina.

ANGLE STRUCTURES

The angle structures are formed by the tissues posterior to the cornea and anterior to the iris, with the aqueous humor intervening (see Figure 1.9). Included in the angle structures are (1) the root of the iris, (2) a portion of the anterior surface of the ciliary body, (3) a *spur* from the sclera, (4) the *canal of Schlemm*, and (5) the *corneoscleral trabeculum*.

Aqueous humor leaves the eye by filtering through the crevices of the *trabecular meshwork*. The trabecular meshwork consists of tiny pores through which aqueous humor travels until it reaches *Schlemm's canal*. From Schlemm's canal the aqueous humor leaves the eye through the aqueous veins that penetrate the sclera. Obstruction within the trabecular meshwork or the angle structures, by iris or scar tissue, results in raised intraocular pressure and glaucoma.

LENS

The lens of the eye is a transparent biconvex structure situated between the iris and the vitreous (Figure 1.10). Only that portion of the lens not covered by iris tissue (that is, only that portion directly behind the pupillary space) is visible. The center of the anterior surface of the lens, known as its anterior pole, is only about 3 mm from the back surface of the cornea. The diameter of the lens is about 9 to 10 mm. Its peripheral margin, called the *equator*, lies about 0.5 mm from the ciliary processes. It is attached to the ciliary processes and to the posterior portion of the ciliary body by means of fine suspensory ligaments referred to as the *zonular fibers* (Figure 1.11).

The lens is surrounded by a capsule, which is a transparent, highly elastic envelope. The lens material within this elastic bag is rather soft and putty-like in infants. With age it tends to grow harder, especially toward the center

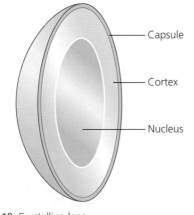

Figure 1.10 Crystalline lens.

Capsule

Cortex

Nucleus

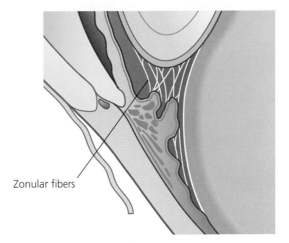

Figure 1.11 Distribution of zonular fibers. Zonular lamella forms the external layer of the lens capsule, consisting of the anterior insertion 1 mm from the equator and the posterior insertion 1.5 mm from the equator.
(Adapted from Jaffe NS: The vitreous in clinical ophthalmology. St Louis: Mosby, 1969.)

Zonular fibers

of the lens. The harder central portion of the lens found in adults 30 years of age or older is called the *nucleus* of the lens, and the outer lens fibers form the lens *cortex*. The harder nucleus is a product of the normal developmental growth of the lens. As new lens fibers are produced, the older fibers are pushed more toward the center and are compressed in a concentric fashion. It is this constant lamination of lens fibers over a period of years that eventually produces the nucleus.

VITREOUS

The vitreous is a jelly-like structure, thick and viscous, that occupies the vitreous chamber in the posterior concavity of the globe. Actually, it fills the largest cavity of the eye, occupying two-thirds of its volume. It is surrounded mainly by retina. Anteriorly it forms a slight depression behind the lens and is attached to it around the circumference of this depression. Normally the vitreous is quite transparent.

The vitreous is not simply an inert jelly. Within the body of the vitreous, fine collagen fibers crisscross in a scaffolding manner. The resulting matrix is filled with a viscous mucopolysaccharide, called hyaluronic acid. Vitreous is almost 99% water. Hyaluronic acid is a great shock absorber and can compress slowly and rebound slowly. This is important in injuries to the eye from such things as a fast-moving squash ball.

The envelope that surrounds the vitreous is primarily a condensate of the gel and is anchored to the more forward part of the retina, the *ora serrata*, and at the head of the optic nerve along the major retinal blood vessels. If the vitreous shrinks, the resulting tension on its anchors can produce a tear in the retina. This may permit the adjacent vitreous to enter between the choroid and retina and produce a retinal detachment.

With age, some of the collagen fibers of the vitreous often break away from the main structure. These may condense into strands and float freely in the watery sections of the vitreous. Patients often see floating specks or webs that move as their eyes move and that are mildly annoying but usually harmless. These often disappear in time.

RETINA

The retina, which contains all the sensory receptors for the transmission of light, is really part of the brain. The retinal receptors are divided into two main populations: the *rods* and the *cones*. The rods function best in dim light; the cones function best under daylight conditions. The cones number only about 6 million, whereas the rods number 125 million. Cones enable us to see small visual angles with great acuity. Vision with rods is relatively poor. Color vision is totally dependent on the integrity of the cones. The cones form a concentrated area in the retina known as the fovea, which lies in the center of the *macula lutea.* Damage to this area can severely reduce the ability to see directly ahead. The rods are distributed in the periphery of the retina (not in the macula). Damage to these structures results in night blindness but with retention of good visual acuity for objects straight ahead.

The junction of the periphery of the retina and the ciliary body is called the *ora serrata.* In the extreme periphery of the retina there are no cones and only a few rods. The retina is firmly attached to the choroid at the ora serrata. This is the reason that retinal detachments never extend beyond the ora serrata. The other site of firm attachment of the retina is at the circumference of the optic nerve. The posterior layer of the retina, called the *pigment epithelium,* is firmly secured to the choroid. Retinal detachment occurs as a result of cleavage between its anterior layers and the posterior pigment layer.

OPTIC NERVE

The optic nerve is located at the posterior portion of the globe and transmits visual impulses from the retina to the brain itself. Only the head of the optic nerve, called the *optic disc,* can be seen by ophthalmoscopic examination (Figure 1.12). The optic nerve contains no sensory receptors itself and therefore its position corresponds to the normal blind spot of the eye. Branching out from the surface of the optic disc are the *retinal arterioles* and *veins,* which divide soon after leaving the optic disc and extend out

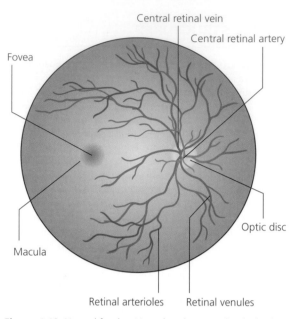

Figure 1.12 Normal fundus. Note that the central retinal vein emerges from the optic disc lateral to the central retinal artery.

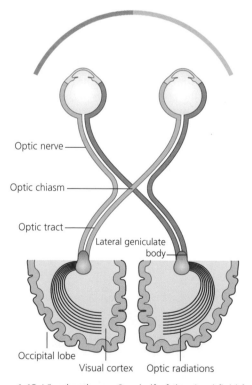

Figure 1.13 Visual pathway. One-half of the visual field from each eye is projected to one side of the brain. Thus visual impulses from the right visual field of each eye will be transmitted to the left occipital lobe.

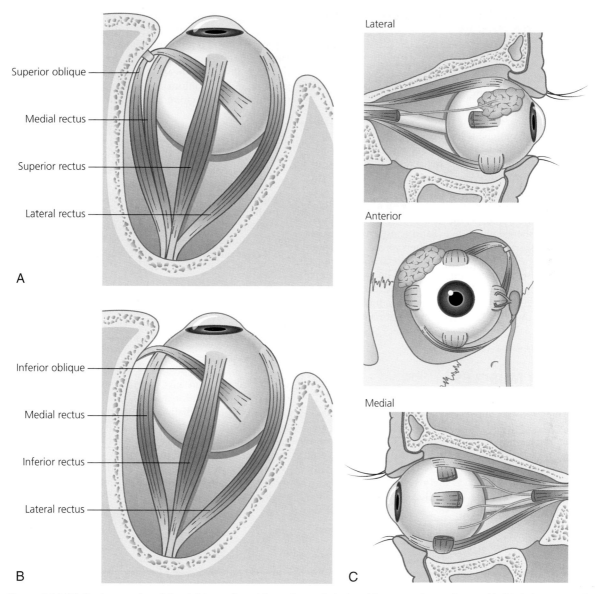

Figure 1.14 (A) Ocular muscles of the right eye viewed from above. Only the oblique muscles are inserted behind the center of rotation of the eye. All the rectus muscles are inserted in front of the center of rotation of the eye near the limbus, where they are easily accessible for muscle surgery. (B) Ocular muscles of the right eye viewed from below. (C) The right eye viewed laterally, anteriorly, and medially.

on the surface of the retina to supply the inner one-third with nutrients.

As the optic disc enters the globe, it goes through a fibrous, sieve-like structure, visible on ophthalmoscopic examination, called the *lamina cribrosa*. When the lamina cribrosa is prominent, it forms the base of a depression in the disc called the *physiologic cup*.

The optic nerve consists of 1 million axons arising from the ganglion cells of the retina. The nerve emerges from the back of the eye through a small circular opening. It extends for 25 to 30 mm and travels within the muscle cone to enter the bony optic foramen. From there it travels another 4 to 9 mm to pass into the intracranial cavity and joins its fellow optic nerve to form the optic chiasm.

VISUAL PATHWAY

As the retinal fibers leave the optic nerves, half of them cross to the opposite side (Figure 1.13). The fibers that cross are derived from the retinal receptors nasal to the macula. The structure so formed by the mutual crossing of nasal fibers by both optic nerves is the *optic chiasm*. From the optic chiasm, the nasal fibers emanating from the nasal half of the retina of one eye intermingle with the fibers derived from the temporal sector of the retina of the opposite eye, forming a band called the *optic tract*.

Fibers in the optic tract continue toward a cell station in the brain called the *lateral geniculate body*, so named because it is shaped like a knee (Latin *genu*). The geniculate body is a relay station from which fibers spread out in a fan-shaped manner and extend to the parietal and temporal lobes of the brain. They continue to their final destination, the posterior portion of the brain called the "occipital" lobe in an area denoted as the *visual striate area*. It is in this area of the brain that conscious recognition of visual impulses takes place.

OCULAR MUSCLES

Six ocular muscles move the globe: the *medial, lateral, superior*, and *inferior rectus muscles* and the *superior* and *inferior oblique muscles* (Figure 1.14). The medial rectus muscle moves the eye toward the nose or *adducts* the eye. The lateral rectus muscle moves the eye horizontally to the outer side or *abducts* the eye. The superior rectus muscle elevates the eye primarily, whereas the inferior rectus muscle depresses the eye. The rectus muscles are inserted very close to the limbus, the medial rectus lying approximately 5.5 mm and the lateral rectus approximately 7 mm from the limbus. The rectus muscles are not normally visible because they are covered with conjunctiva and subconjunctival tissue. Because they lie on the surface of the globe, they are readily accessible for muscle surgery.

The superior oblique muscle functions primarily as an intorter by rotating the vertical and horizontal axis of the eye toward the nose; it also functions to depress the eye. The inferior oblique muscle acts to extort and elevate the eye. The oblique muscles are inserted behind the equator of the globe.

In the lid the *levator palpebrae superioris* muscle serves to elevate the lid, whereas the *orbicularis oculi* muscle closes the eye during winking, blinking, or forced lid closure. If the levator muscle is weak or absent, the lid droops and *ptosis* results.

SUMMARY

A brief sketch of the anatomy of the eye and its surrounding structures has been presented. Each of these structures, when diseased, can give rise to problems, depending on its anatomic location and function. Because many diagnoses made in ophthalmology are formulated from anatomic terminology, familiarity with these structures is essential before any understanding of patients' problems can be realized. The foundation of any course in medicine is based on anatomy. The ophthalmic assistant is advised to learn this section well and use it as a foundation for further reading.

Questions for review and thought

The questions that follow, as well as those following the chapters in the rest of this book, are designed for review of the material. They are intended to sharpen your understanding by testing your knowledge of the material and stimulating you to think. Answers to some of the questions at the end of each chapter may be found in other parts of this book or, in some cases, only in other sources.

1. Draw a horizontal section of the eye with attached muscles and label as many parts as you can without referring to the text.
2. Outline the production and flow of tears.
3. Name the five layers of the cornea.
4. How does the iris contract and expand?
5. Discuss the functions of the rods and cones.
6. Draw the pathway of fibers from the optic nerve to the visual cortex.
7. What is the limbus?
8. How many ocular muscles are attached to the eye? Name them.
9. Describe the muscles that open and close the eye.
10. Describe the macula.
11. What is the ora serrata?
12. At what age is the cornea fully formed? At what age is the rest of the eyeball fully formed?
13. Describe the vitreous.

Self-evaluation questions

True–false statements

Directions: Indicate whether the statement is true **(T)** or false **(F).**

1. The main function of the sclera is to keep out light. **T** or **F**
2. If the epithelium of the cornea is damaged, a fine scar will appear. **T** or **F**
3. Aqueous humor leaves the eye by filtering through the trabecular meshwork. **T** or **F**

Missing words

Directions: Write in the missing word(s) in the following sentences.

4. The transparent lens of the eye is attached to the ciliary body by fine suspensory ligaments called _____.
5. The retina consists of rods and cones. The _____ function best in daylight.
6. The head of the optic nerve is called the _____.

Choice-completion questions

Directions: Select the one best answer in each case.

7. The meibomian glands are:
   a. in the ciliary body.
   b. in the tarsus.
   c. in the hair follicles.
   d. associated with the lacrimal glands.
   e. in the conjunctiva.
8. The vitreous body comprises:
   a. the pigment structure of the eye.
   b. the aqueous-forming part of the eye.
   c. the sensory structure of the eye.
   d. two-thirds of the volume of the eye.
   e. the heat-absorbing portion of the eye.
9. The orbicularis oculi is the muscle that:
   a. dilates the pupil.
   b. affects accommodation.
   c. closes the eyelids.
   d. opens the lids.
   e. constricts the pupil.

A **Answers, notes, and explanations**

1. **False.** The main function of the sclera is protective. The sclera is a firm fibrous coat that prevents injury from outside the eye and prevents rupture when there is increased intraocular pressure to the globe. The sclera has an opaque white appearance, in contrast to the transparent cornea, because of the greater water content of the sclera and the fact that the collagen fibers are not as uniformly oriented. In some situations, however, the sclera may become exposed and dehydrated and it can become transparent.

2. **False.** The epithelium may be removed partially or completely from the cornea and it has an amazing ability to regenerate completely and cover the other layers of the cornea without leaving a scar. Only if the injury involves the deeper layers of the cornea, such as Bowman's membrane, stroma, or through-and-through lacerations of the cornea, will an opacity form because of scar formation.

3. **True.** Water, electrolytes, and nonelectrolytes enter and leave the eye by diffusion from the ciliary body and by secretion from the epithelium of the ciliary process. From the posterior chamber, the fluid then passes through the pupil into the anterior chamber and out through the filtering trabecular meshwork. From here it passes into Schlemm's canal where about 30 collector channels conduct the fluid to about 12 aqueous veins out into the venous system.

4. **Zonular fibers.** These fine suspensory ligaments are composed of numerous fibrils arising from the surface of the ciliary body and inserting into the lens equator. Normally the ciliary muscle is relaxed and consequently the zonular fibers are taut, which reduces the anteroposterior diameter of the lens to its minimal dimension. However, when the ciliary muscle contracts to focus light from a near object, the tension is released on the zonular fibers and the lens of the eye assumes a thicker shape, with a correspondingly greater refractive power. This is what occurs during accommodation.

5. **Cones.** The cones are used during daylight to allow detailed vision and color perception. They predominate in the macular area and receive visual images, partially analyze them, and submit this modified information to the brain. If these cones are damaged, the central vision is affected and the patient will have difficulty in reading and discerning small objects in the distance.

6. **Optic disc.** The optic disc is seen with an ophthalmoscope and represents the head of the optic nerve as the nerve bundle fibers pass from the eye back toward the brain. The optic disc corresponds to the normal blind spot of the eye and represents about 1 million axons, which arise from the ganglion cells of the retina. The optic nerve then travels about 25–30 mm in the orbit within the muscle

A | Continued

cone to enter the bony optic foramen and then the cranial cavity.

7. **b. In the tarsus.** The meibomian glands lie in the tarsus and secrete sebaceous material, which creates an oily layer on the surface of the tear film. This oily layer helps prevent evaporation of the normal tear layer. When these glands become obstructed, they give rise to a condition known as meibomianitis and produce internal hordeolum or chalazion.

8. **d. Two-thirds of the volume of the eye.** The vitreous is a structure that occupies the largest cavity of the eye, over two-thirds of its volume. Normally the vitreous is transparent and jelly-like. However, it changes with age and becomes more fluid-like and less jelly-like in high degrees of myopia.

9. **c. Closes the eyelids.** The main function of the orbicularis oculi muscle is to close the eyelid. An accessory function is to evacuate the tear sac so as to continue the pumping action and removal of tears from the conjunctival sac. This muscle is innervated by the seventh cranial nerve so that when this nerve is paralyzed, the eye will fail to close. During intraocular surgery a facial block is often given to paralyze this nerve.

Chapter | 2 |

Physiology of the eye

Physiology of the eye deals with the function of the eye, its capacities, and its limitations. The actual perception of light takes place in a well-delineated area called the *field of vision*. What is not seen beyond these boundaries is cataloged and stored in our visual memory center, so that we are not uncomfortable or handicapped by this imposition. Most eyes cannot form a sharp image on the retina without an internal adjustment made by focusing or by some external appliance such as lenses placed before them. There is a limit to how much detail the eye can resolve, its magnifying abilities being only $15\times$, considerably less than most microscopes. The spectrum of light to which our retinal receptors are sensitive is confined to specific wavelengths of light; the world of ultraviolet and infrared is invisible to ordinary perception.

Despite these limitations the human eye is an extremely versatile instrument capable of seeing both in daylight and in dim light, registering colors, appreciating depth, and exercising rapid focusing adjustments. This chapter deals with the mechanisms that enable the eye to carry out these tasks.

ALIGNMENT OF THE EYES

In human beings the two eyes work as though they were one, both projecting to the same point in space and fusing their images so that a single mental impression is obtained by this collaboration. Without this delicate balance we would "see double" because two images would be formed by the independent action of each eye. In other words, stereopsis would be lost because this faculty is totally dependent on the eyes seeing in unison. The ability of the eyes to fuse two images into a single one is called *binocular vision*.

Binocular vision depends on an exquisite balance of motor and sensory function. The eyes must be parallel when looking straight ahead and they must be able to maintain this alignment when gazing in other positions. Each impulse that directs an eye to move in one direction must be equally received by the other eye. Further, the contraction of an eye muscle pulling the eye in one direction must be accompanied by an equivalent amount of relaxation of its opponent muscle. Without perfectly harmonious eye movement, binocular vision would be impossible because eyes that do not move together do not see together.

Each eye must have good vision because a clear image and a fuzzy image cannot be fused. The brain usually ignores the fuzzy image (suppression). Each macula must have its projection straight ahead, so that the line of vision from each eye intersects at one point in space. Also the field

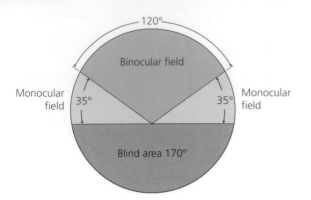

Figure 2.1 Field of vision. Binocular field of vision (120 degrees) represents the overlapping field of vision from each eye.

of vision from each eye must overlap (Figure 2.1). Although we can see more with two eyes than with one, this difference is not great (about 35 degrees) because most of the field of vision from one eye overlaps the field from the other eye. Overlapping visual fields act as a locking device, forging our peripheral vision in place and thereby ensuring central fusion.

LOOKING STRAIGHT AHEAD (FIXATION)

Fixation involves the simple task of looking straight ahead toward an object in space. Fixation requires stability of the eyes and good monocular function. If the eyes are constantly moving, such as occurs with congenital nystagmus (a shaking of the eyes), the eyes can make only scanning motions around an object and never adequately see it in detail. Needless to say, if the ability to fixate becomes compromised by constant eye movements, then the visual acuity of the affected eyes is reduced. If the macula is damaged, then fixation is difficult because anything viewed directly ahead becomes enshrouded in relative darkness.

Fixation can be reduced without organic changes in the eye. Children with strabismus often are found to have poor vision in the turned eye. If a child has crossed eyes, we would think that double vision would occur because the two eyes would not be directed to the same point in space (Figure 2.2). Children, however, have a wonderful faculty for completely ignoring the image in the turned eye to avoid confusion. It is this constant habit of actively suppressing the image in the turned eye that eventually leads to loss of vision or amblyopia. In some of these children, in whom the suppression mechanism has become profound and the resultant vision very poor,

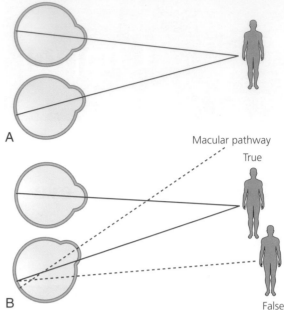

Figure 2.2 (A) Binocular vision (both eyes looking at the same figure). (B) One eye is turned in, resulting in double vision. In this case the figure is received by the macula of one eye and a point nasal to the macula of the turned eye. The projection of this nasal point results in the person seeing two images instead of one of the same figure. This is an example of uncrossed diplopia, as seen in esodeviations.

foveal function becomes so depressed that a new point just outside the fovea is used. Such an eye can no longer see straight ahead and the fixation pattern is described as *eccentric*.

LOCKING IMAGES (FUSION)

Fusion is the power exerted by both eyes to keep the position of the eyes aligned so that both foveae project to the same point in space. Because fusion is a binocular act, it is easily disrupted by covering one eye. The eye under cover drifts to its fusion-free position. The amount of movement that the eye makes is a measure of the latent muscular imbalance kept in check by fusion, or the amount of heterophoria. *Heterophoria*, then, may be defined as the position the eyes assume when fusion is disrupted. The eye under cover may drift in, called *esophoria*, or drift out, called *exophoria*. The eye also may drift up and down; this position is called *hyperphoria*. Fusion also may be disrupted by placing a Maddox rod before one eye. The Maddox rod changes

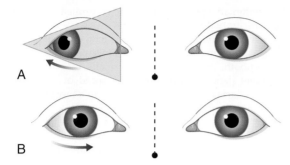

Figure 2.3 (A) The prism displaces the image toward its apex and the eye moves outward because of the fusional reflex. (B) When the prism is removed, the eye returns to its original position because of the fusional reflex.

the size and shape of the image presented to the eye under cover so that fusion becomes impossible.

The power of fusion is measurable by prisms (see Chapter 3). For example, a 4-diopter prism is placed with the base toward the nose of an observer looking at a small letter placed 16 inches (40 cm) from the eye. The prism will displace the image before that eye in a direction toward its apex and the eye moves outward to follow it because of the power exerted by the fusional reflex (Figure 2.3A). Now the prism is removed and the uncovered eye returns to its original position in response to the fusional reflex (Figure 2.3B). Normally, 20 to 40 prism diopters can be exercised by fusional convergence. The amount of fusion exercised with respect to divergence is less, being only 10 to 20 prism diopters. This is measured by using base-out prisms. Vertical imbalances are difficult to overcome because our eyes can overcome only about 2 to 4 prism diopters.

EYE MOVEMENTS

The *primary* position of the eyes is the straight-ahead position as they look at a point just below the horizon with the head held erect. Movement of the eye from the primary position to a secondary position occurs when the eyes are moved either horizontally or vertically. If the eyes are directed in an oblique position (up and in or down and in), they are said to be in a tertiary position.

The movement of one eye from one position to another in one direction is called a *duction*. In duction the fellow eye is either covered or patched. The movement of two eyes in the same direction is called a *version* (dextro-, levo-, sursum , and deorsumversion) (Figure 2.4).

- Eyes right: dextroversion
- Eyes left: levoversion
- Eyes up: sursumversion
- Eyes down: deorsumversion

An outline of the functions of the extraocular muscles is given in Table 2.1. The medial and lateral rectus muscles have only one action: to move the eye horizontally. The other four muscles of the eye have auxiliary functions. When these secondary roles are used, assisting the lateral or medial rectus muscles to abduct or adduct, these muscles are called synergists (Figure 2.5).

The main function of the oblique muscles is to rotate the globe either inward *(intorsion)* or outward *(extorsion)*. Intorsion occurs when the eye rotates on its long axis so that the 12 o'clock position on the cornea moves toward the nose. For example, if a point on the cornea of the right eye moves inward from 12 to 1 o'clock, then intorsion is said to occur because of the primary action of the right superior oblique muscle or secondary action of the

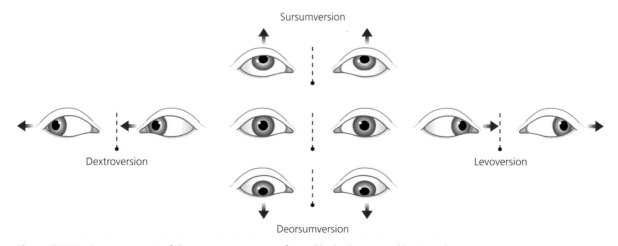

Figure 2.4 Version movements of the eyes or movements formed by both eyes working together.

Table 2.1 Actions of extraocular muscles

Muscle	Prime action	Secondary action
Medial rectus	Turns eye inward toward nose or adducts eye	None
Lateral rectus	Turns eye outward toward temples or abducts eye	None
Superior rectus	Elevates eye	Intorsion Adduction
Inferior rectus	Depresses eye	Extorsion Adduction
Superior oblique	Intorts eye	Depression Abduction
Inferior oblique	Extorts eye	Elevation Abduction

right superior rectus muscle. Similarly, if the point on the right cornea moves outward from 12 to 11 o'clock, then extorsion is said to occur because of the primary action of the right inferior oblique muscle or secondary action of the right inferior rectus muscle.

Control centers for eye movements

The eyes move in response to our own volition or in a passive manner, such as in following a slow-moving target. Volitional eye movements usually are rapid, starting at high speeds and ending just as abruptly. Such movements occur with reading, when words or phrases are quickly scanned, with an abrupt halt coming at the end of a section or a line.

These voluntary eye movements are controlled from centers in the frontal lobe of the brain.

Whereas voluntary eye movements tend to be short and choppy, following or pursuit eye movements are rather slow, smooth, and gliding. The velocity of a following movement depends entirely on the speed of the object the eye is tracking. If the fovea is fixed on a moving target with an angular velocity (less than 30 degrees per second), the eye follows the target almost exactly. With greater speeds, following movement becomes difficult and the smooth, gliding movement is replaced with an irregular, jerky movement. Pursuit movements are controlled from centers in the occipital lobe of the brain.

LOOKING TOWARD A CLOSE OBJECT

Vergence is the term applied to simultaneous ocular movements in which the eyes are directed to an object in the midline in front of the face. The term usually is applied to *convergence*, in which the eyes rotate inward toward each other, or to *divergence*, in which they rotate outward simultaneously (Figure 2.6).

Convergence is invariably accompanied by narrowing, or constriction, of the pupils and by accommodation. The triad of convergence, pupillary constriction, and accommodation is often called the *accommodative reflex*, although in the true sense these movements are merely associated reactions (a synkinesis) rather than a true reflex. Each component of the triad facilitates fixation at near. The constriction of the pupil is the attempt by the eye to form a pinhole camera device so that a clearer image is seen. Accommodation enables the object to be focused on the retina; convergence brings the eye inward toward the object of regard.

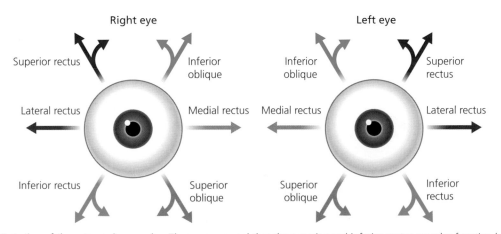

Figure 2.5 Action of the extraocular muscles. The arrows reveal that the superior and inferior rectus muscles function best as an elevator and a depressor, respectively, when the eye is abducted. The inferior and superior oblique muscles function best as an elevator and depressor, respectively, when the eye is adducted.

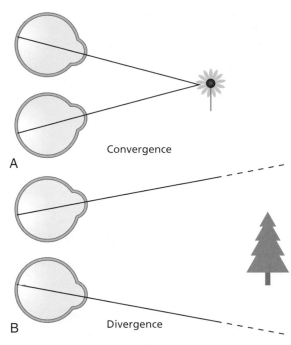

Figure 2.6 (A) Convergence. The eye is turned in toward the midline plane. (B) Divergence. The eye is turned out, away from the midline plane.

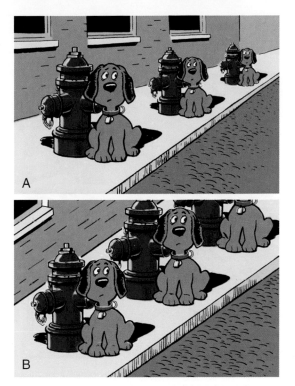

Figure 2.7 (A) Artist has drawn the picture with proper depth perspective. Monocular clues include decrease in size of dogs and confluence of lines toward a point. (B) Artist has ignored the usual monocular clues so that our appreciation of depth and size is erroneous. The second dog appears larger than the first, although both are the same size.

SEEING IN DEPTH

The ability to see in depth enables us to travel comfortably in space. Without it, we could not judge distances, estimate the size of objects beyond us, or avoid bumping into things. Without depth perception, even the simplest of tasks would be difficult. We would be unable to reach accurately for our morning coffee, and passing a car on the highway would be tantamount to suicide. Fortunately, everyone has some depth perception, whether the person has one eye or two. Those with only one eye learn to estimate depth with monocular clues (Figures 2.7 and 2.8). They know that the speck in the distance that becomes a huge train standing beside them in the station has not grown larger but has merely come closer. There are other clues in addition to changes in object size. The train tracks spread from a point and become parallel, the color of the train changes from a misty blue-gray to dark green, the sound increases, and when the train is alongside, one can feel the heat.

There are many monocular clues that facilitate depth perception, including the following:

- Magnification: well-recognized objects, if they become larger, are deemed to be nearer

- Confluence of parallel lines to a point, for example railway tracks
- Interposition of shadows
- Blue-gray mistiness of objects at a great distance
- Parallax: If two objects situated at different points in space are aligned and the head of the observer is moved in one direction, the nearer object will appear to move in the opposite direction

A monocular person, however, if removed from familiar surroundings, would have great difficulty in judging distances because of a lack of any intrinsic depth-perception mechanism. For example, a one-eyed pilot would create a hazard because of the difficulty he or she would experience in maneuvering in space without the normal monocular clues.

Stereopsis is a higher quality of binocular vision. Each eye views an object at a slightly different angle, so that fusion of images occurs by combining slightly dissimilar images. It is the combination of these angular views that yields stereopsis. The same method is used in photography in

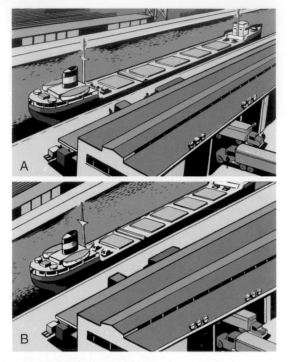

Figure 2.8 (A) The scene is drawn using normal monocular clues of distance, thereby giving it perspective. (B) The same scene is drawn without regard to the normal impressions of distance. Therefore, the scene loses its perspective.

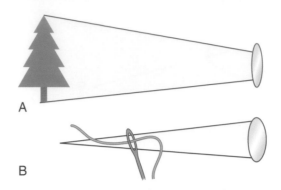

Figure 2.9 (A) Crystalline lens of the eye is thin for distant objects. (B) Crystalline lens accommodates for near objects by becoming thicker. This increases its effective power.

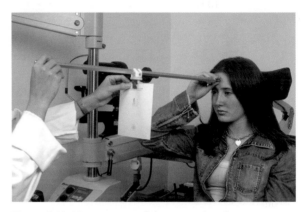

Figure 2.10 Measurement of the near point of accommodation.

making three-dimensional pictures. The stereoscopic picture is taken at slightly different angles and later viewed that way.

FOCUSING AT NEAR (ACCOMMODATION)

Any object can be moved from a distance to about 20 feet in front of an observer and still be seen clearly without accommodation. This distance is called the *range of focus*. As the object is brought closer than 20 feet, however, the eye must continuously readjust to keep the image of the object clearly focused on the retina. This readjustment requires an increase in the power of the eye and is brought about by an automatic change in the shape of the lens in response to a blurred image (Figure 2.9). This zoom-lens mechanism in the eye is very active in children; they are able to see a small letter in clear focus only 7 cm from the eye, whereas an adult of 55 years can focus no closer than 55 cm. The *range of accommodation* is the distance in which an object can be carried toward an eye and be kept in focus. The power of accommodation of an eye is the

dioptric equivalent of this distance. By age 75 years this power is zero.

Both the range and the power of accommodation are measured quite easily (Figure 2.10). When the full spectacle correction is worn, it is merely the closest point at which an accommodative target (such as a small letter) can be seen clearly. It usually is equal in both eyes. The range of accommodation is measured in centimeters, whereas the power is converted to diopters (Table 2.2).

This stimulus for accommodation is a blurred image on the retina. As an object is moved closer to the eye, the rays of light entering the pupil must be continuously converged. This change in focusing power of the eyes is brought about by active contraction of the ciliary muscle. The contraction of this muscle causes the zonular fibers of the lens to relax, which in turn allows the lens of the eye to change its shape (Figure 2.11). In the child and the young adult, the lens can be molded, and it increases its power by becoming thicker and increasing the curvature of its anterior space. In an adult the ability of the

Table 2.2 Accommodation and near point of the normal eye

Age	Near point in centimeters	Available accommodation in diopters
10	7	14
20	9	11
30	12	8
40	22	4.5
45	28	3.5
50	40	2.5
55	55	1.75
60	100	1
65	133	0.75
70	400	0.25
75	Infinity	0

ciliary muscle to effectively contract declines with age and the lens becomes harder and less malleable with advancing years.

The decline in accommodation with age, called *presbyopia*, is remedied with reading glasses or bifocals. It usually becomes apparent by the age of 45 years.

Figure 2.11 Adjustment of the crystalline lens by accommodation. When the zonular ligaments are relaxed, the inherent elasticity of the lens causes it to increase in thickness and therefore increase in power. *(Redrawn from Krug WFS: Functional neuro-anatomy. New York: The Blakiston Co., 1953.)*

TRANSPARENT PATHWAY FOR LIGHT

For light to effectively stimulate retinal receptors, clear media for transmission are necessary. One of the prime functions of the eye is maintenance of the transparent pathway for light (Figure 2.12).

The *cornea* is the window through which light rays pass on their way to the retina. It is a five-layered transparent structure whose cells and collagen fibers are arranged so that light can pass through it with a minimum of diffraction and internal reflection. The cornea is transparent because its fibrils are arranged in a parallel manner and are tightly packed and separated by less than a wavelength of light. When the cornea is swollen, this arrangement is distorted and the cornea becomes hazy. The cornea contains no opaque substances, such as blood vessels, that would mar its clarity. It receives its nourishment from perilimbal vessels, the tear film, and the aqueous humor. The cornea is kept shiny and lubricated by tears that keep its surface moist and fill out any irregularities in its superficial epithelium.

The *tears* are composed of three main layers. The outermost *oily*, or *lipid*, layer comes from the meibomian gland and retards evaporation of the aqueous or watery layer. *Aqueous water* makes up the middle layer and arises from the main lacrimal and the accessory lacrimal glands in the conjunctiva. It is filled with inorganic matter, salts, and varying amounts of mucin. This functions to keep the cornea moist. The innermost layer of the tears is *mucin*, which arises from the goblet cells of the conjunctiva and fills in the tiny irregularities of the corneal epithelium, thereby producing a mirror-like finish to the cornea.

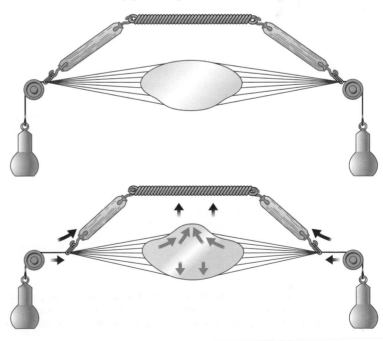

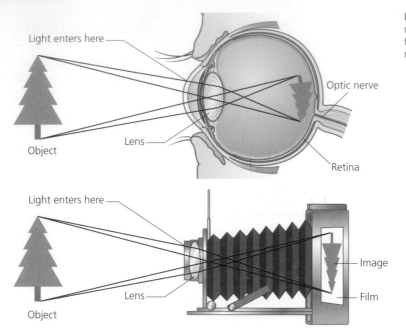

Light enters here

Object

Lens

Optic nerve

Retina

Light enters here

Object

Lens

Image

Film

Figure 2.12 The eye is like a camera. Light must have a clear pathway to be clearly focused on the sensory receptors of the retina or the film of a camera.

The most important factor in maintaining corneal transparency is the ability of the cornea to keep itself relatively dehydrated. If a section of cornea is placed in isotonic saline solution, it becomes hydrated, opaque, and edematous. However, if the sclera is dehydrated, it becomes transparent.

The cornea has an active, pump-like mechanism located in the corneal epithelium and endothelium that enables it to keep itself relatively dehydrated. Damage to the corneal epithelium or endothelium results in the cornea's becoming hydrated and swollen. Swelling of the cornea, be it localized or diffuse, always results in a loss of transparency. If the swelling (that is, corneal edema) is located centrally, then vision will be blurred. In acute angle-closure glaucoma (see Chapter 25), the sudden rise in intraocular pressure causes epithelial edema. The individual droplets in the epithelium break up white light to its colored spectral components and the patient complains of seeing colored halos around lights. The rainbow we see after a storm is similarly explained. It is merely the effect of suspended water droplets in air breaking up white light.

Transparency also is aided by the ability of the corneal epithelium to rapidly regenerate. The corneal epithelium, by sliding over defects and regenerating its cells, can cover a large abrasion within 24 hours and without leaving a scar. If Bowman's membrane or the corneal stroma is damaged, however, repair takes much longer and a permanent scar forms.

The *aqueous humor* found between the lens and the cornea is a clear, colorless, watery fluid. It is formed by active secretion from the ciliary processes and to a lesser extent by diffusion from the vessels of the iris. The aqueous humor is in constant circulation, flowing from the posterior chamber through the pupil to the anterior chamber, where it leaves the inner eye proper through the trabecular meshwork, Schlemm's canal, and the aqueous veins (Figure 2.13). If the exit of aqueous humor from the eye is blocked, the volume of fluid within the eye increases; because the coats of the eye are relatively nondistensible, the pressure within the eye also increases.

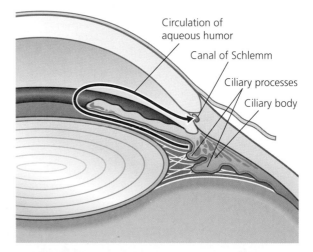

Circulation of aqueous humor

Canal of Schlemm

Ciliary processes

Ciliary body

Figure 2.13 Flow of aqueous humor. Aqueous humor is produced largely by the ciliary processes in the posterior chamber; it flows into the anterior chamber and leaves the eye through Schlemm's canal.

As light travels through the eye, the next structure it encounters is the *iris*, with its central round opening called the *pupil*. The iris is the shutter mechanism of the eye, controlling the amount of light entering the eye in the interest of clear vision. If the amount of available light is excessive, the pupil constricts by the action of the sphincter muscle of the iris to reduce excessive light or glare. If the illumination is poor, then the pupil dilates to increase the amount of light entering the eye. Other factors also control the size of the pupil. Emotional arousal (for example, fear, anxiety, or erotic stimulation) tends to dilate the pupils. Pain in the body dilates the pupil. The pupils generally are large in the young, the blue-eyed, and the myopic and they tend to be smaller in the brown-eyed and in older adults. The pupils are normally round and equal in size. If a light is directed to one eye, both pupils constrict. The constriction of the pupil on the side toward which light is directed is called the *direct light reflex*, whereas the pupillary response in the fellow eye is called the *consensual light reflex*.

As light passes through the pupil, the next structure it encounters is the *lens*. The lens of the eye is a biconvex structure, completely surrounded by a capsule. It has only a single layer of epithelial cells under its anterior capsule, which does not significantly interfere with its transparency. Like the cornea, it contains no opaque tissue such as blood vessels, nerve fibers, or connective tissue. It is nourished solely by the aqueous humor that bathes it.

Lens material in a child is very soft and putty-like in consistency. With age, however, the lens becomes harder, especially centrally. As new lens fibers form, they envelop the previously existing fibers, compressing them and pushing them into a compact unit toward the center. Thus growth of the lens is not accompanied by an increase in size after puberty but by a compression and tight lamination of the older fibers. The central hard portion, called the *nucleus*, usually becomes well formed by the age of 30 years.

There are two main parts of the lens: the dense center, or nucleus, and the surrounding cortex. This arrangement offers an optical advantage in making the total refractive power of the lens greater than if the index of refraction were uniform throughout.

The *vitreous body* is located directly behind the lens and occupies two-thirds of the entire volume of the eye. It is a transparent gel; that is, a viscous fluid midway in composition between a solid and a liquid. Functionally and metabolically the vitreous is relatively inactive. If the lens and cornea are compared with the lenses of a camera, the vitreous body is the space before the film. Frequently with age the gel breaks down in part, becoming liquid. This degeneration of the vitreous gives rise to the often-heard complaint of seeing spots before the eyes.

Once light has left the vitreous, the last great transparent structure of the eye, it finally strikes the retina, which contains all the receptors sensitive to light.

The *retinal receptors* are divided into two different populations of cells: the *rods* and the *cones* (Figure 2.14). The rods are far more numerous (approximately 125 million) than the cones (approximately 6 million) and function best in dim illumination *(scotopic vision)*.

Figure 2.14 Rods and cones of the retina.

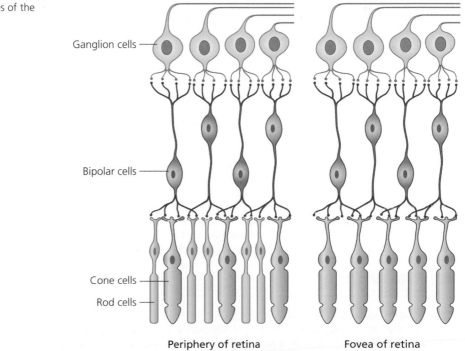

Ganglion cells

Bipolar cells

Cone cells

Rod cells

Periphery of retina   Fovea of retina

Without rods, night blindness occurs. Individuals affected by a disorder involving a selective loss of rod cells can see very well during the day as long as the illumination is high; however, under conditions of poor illumination, as in movie theaters or darkrooms, they are totally unable to adapt and behave as though blind. The cones function best in daylight (*photopic vision*) and mediate straight-ahead vision and color vision. A selective loss of cone cells results in a loss of visual acuity and an inability to perceive colors.

This difference of function among the retinal receptors is easily demonstrated by entering a darkroom illuminated only by a red light. The rods are relatively insensitive to red and therefore do not lose their function with this type of lighting. At first everything appears quite dark, then hazy, and finally the definite shapes of objects at the sides come into view as the rods begin to function. The total duration for dark adaptation to be completed is about 30 minutes. Darkrooms (for example, photography darkrooms and x-ray rooms) are usually equipped with a red light because it allows the cones to function and straight-ahead vision to be preserved while enabling the rods to become adapted to the dark.

The process of dark adaptation requires a rapid neural change in the rod cells and a slow (at least 30 minutes) chemical change in the outer segments of the rod cells. The chemical change is a complex process that requires the synthesis of the rod pigment called *rhodopsin*. Rhodopsin, or visual purple, forms under conditions of dark adaptation and is destroyed by light. Therefore, it is continuously being used and restored. One of the main components of rhodopsin is vitamin A, found in carrots and other vegetables. Vitamin A deficiency causes night blindness, but the corollary that an excess of vitamin A will help the eyes is not true. The cones also contain a pigment called *iodopsin*.

Because the fovea contains no rods but only a concentration of specialized cones, it is found that when the eye is fully dark adapted there is a central loss of vision. Although visual acuity is not as good in this state, the perception of light is enhanced because the rods have a lower threshold for light sensitivity than do the cones. Visual information in the form of light strikes the photoreceptors and this sets off a chain of events that leads to the process of seeing. Impulses from the photoreceptors are carried to the bipolar cells and then in turn to the ganglion cells. The site of connections between cells is called the *synaptic zone*. The information from the ganglion cells then travels via axons through the optic nerves, the chiasm, and the optic tract to synapse with cells in the lateral geniculate body. Impulses are then carried by axons to the occipital cortex for the processing of the information.

RETINAL IMAGES

Retinal images, once formed, persist for a very short time. They are called *positive afterimages*. Normally one is not aware of this persistence of retinal images because the eyes take up a new gaze that obliterates the former afterimage. In making movies, sensation of motion or flow is produced only when the film speed of the camera is sufficiently fast to enable fusion of the images produced by the moving frames on the film. If the camera is slowed, flickering occurs because there is a time gap between the afterimage of the first sequence and that of the next.

Negative afterimages also occur. This is commonly witnessed as a dark spot appearing before the eyes after one has been photographed with the use of a flashbulb. The high-intensity light exhausts the retinal receptors and they become unresponsive to further light stimulation for seconds after. Negative afterimages are used in a test for strabismus to determine the direction of fixation. High-intensity flashes placed in a vertical or horizontal position will produce a dark line of the same dimension as a flash. This line can be drawn by the patient. If fixation is central and straight ahead, the reproduction is exact. If the fixation pattern is eccentric, then the picture drawn will be off-centered by an amount equal to the degree of eccentric fixation.

INTRAOCULAR PRESSURE

Normal intraocular pressure is between 13 and 20 mm Hg. These numbers are derived from measurements obtained with a tonometer and indicate the pressure in the eye that will not normally cause damage to the intraocular contents. Individual eyes respond to intraocular pressures differently. Some can tolerate pressures in the high 20s (ocular hypertension) and some will have damage to the optic nerve with lower pressures (low-tension glaucoma).

Transient and physiologic variations occur in the intraocular pressure. With respiration, these variations in intraocular pressure can amount to 4 mm Hg, whereas changes of 1 to 2 mm Hg occur with each pulsation of the central retinal artery. The changes with pulse beat are nicely demonstrated on tonographic recordings, which always show a sawtooth type of graph in rhythm with the beats of the pulse. Throughout the day the intraocular pressure can vary by as much as 2 to 3 mm Hg, with the maximum pressure being found around 6 a.m. In a glaucomatous eye the fluctuations in diurnal pressures can be 6 to 8 mm Hg per day or even greater.

The pressure in the eye depends largely on the amount of aqueous humor secreted into the eye (1–3 mm^3 per minute) and the ease by which it leaves. The flow of aqueous into the eye varies with the general hydration of the body. In dehydrated states, the amount of aqueous produced decreases and so does the pressure within the eye. However, if large quantities of fluid are quickly ingested, the amount of aqueous secreted increases. Forced hydration is used in the water-drinking test: a rise of 8 mm Hg or more 45 minutes after drinking 1 L of water is suggestive of glaucoma. The drug acetazolamide (Diamox), used in the treatment of glaucoma, acts by reducing the volume of aqueous produced.

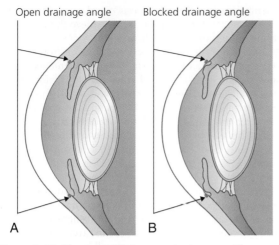

Open drainage angle   Blocked drainage angle

A   B

Figure 2.15 Glaucoma. (A) Open-angle glaucoma. The obstruction to aqueous flow lies in the trabecular meshwork. (B) Closed-angle glaucoma. The trabecular meshwork is covered by the root of the iris.

The rate of fluid exit from the eye, or its facility of outflow, is the most important single factor regulating the intraocular pressure. Glaucoma rarely or never results from an increase in aqueous production but invariably is linked to a decrease in the facility of outflow.

There are three primary methods of occluding the outflow channels of the eye. In *open-angle glaucoma* (the most common type), the diameter of the openings of the trabecular meshwork becomes narrowed, thereby increasing the resistance to fluid flow (Figure 2.15). This situation is analogous to a drainage system in which the final common drain tube is suddenly reduced to only half its diameter at the very end. The amount of water leaving the system would be very small and the pressure in the tube in front of the narrowing would be very high.

In *secondary glaucoma* the trabecular meshwork becomes blocked. The obstructing matter can be in the meshwork and may consist of red blood cells with hyphemas, tumor cells, pigment, and debris. In addition, the obstructing matter may cover the meshwork itself in the form of scar tissue or anterior synechiae between the iris and the angle structures. These adhesions, which are commonly formed after a severe iritis, an episode of angle-closure glaucoma, or a central retinal vein occlusion, produce a severe and intractable glaucomatous state.

Another method of occluding the outflow channels occurs with *pupillary block,* as typified in *primary angle-closure glaucoma.* In eyes predisposed to this condition, the angle formed by the root of the iris and the angle structures is narrow. If the pupil in such an eye is dilated, the iris tissue, which folds up like an accordion on dilation, abuts against the angle structures and partially blocks them. In addition, the aqueous humor in the posterior chamber has difficulty circulating through the anterior chamber. Therefore, the pressure in the posterior chamber increases

and bows the iris to a more forward position, obstructing even further the already compromised exit channels of the eye. This process occurs suddenly and the eye does not have the chance to accommodate itself to the high intraocular pressures reached. As a result the eye becomes red, the cornea edematous, and the pupil fixed and dilated and the patient complains of considerable pain. Angle-closure glaucoma constitutes an ocular emergency. It is relieved by a peripheral iridectomy, where a small portion of the peripheral iris is removed to facilitate transfer of fluid between chambers. This procedure can be performed in the operating room; it is more commonly performed in the office with the use of argon or neodymium YAG lasers.

TEARS

The surface of the eye is kept moist by tears formed by the lacrimal gland and the accessory lacrimal glands located in the superior and inferior fornices. Evaporation is minimized by a thin film of oil secreted by the meibomian glands over the layer of tears. Tears function to keep the globes moist and to fill in the interstices between the corneal epithelial cells, thus providing a smooth, regular corneal refractive surface.

Only 0.5 to 1 mL of tears is produced during the day; minimal tears are produced at night. About 50% of the tears are lost through evaporation; the rest are carried to the superior and inferior meatus of the nose located under the inferior turbinate (Figure 2.16).

Tears contain an antibacterial enzyme, called *lysozyme,* which is mainly effective against nonpathogenic bacteria by dissolving their outer coating.

Tear formation occurs as a result of psychic stimuli and reflex stimuli. Reflex stimuli involve uncomfortable retinal stimulation by bright lights or irritation of the cornea, conjunctiva, and nasal mucosa. The amount of tear production is measured by the *Schirmer test.* This test is performed by simply placing a strip of filter paper 5 mm wide into the lower fornix for 5 minutes; more than 10 mm of wetting indicates normal function.

COLOR VISION

The cones of the human eye are believed to contain three different photosensitive pigments in their outer segments. These pigments act by absorbing light of certain definite wavelengths according to their period of vibration. The pigments of the cones are sensitive to red, green, and blue, the three primary colors of light. (This is not to be confused with the three primary colors of red, blue, and yellow, as found in the paint-mixing field and used by artists.) Other colors are formed by mixtures of these pigments.

Color depends on *hue, saturation,* and *brightness.* An object will have a particular hue because it reflects or

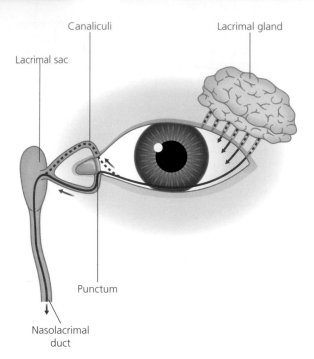

Canaliculi

Lacrimal gland

Lacrimal sac

Punctum

Nasolacrimal duct

Figure 2.16 Flow of tears. Note that most of the tears flow out through the lower punctum. Tears produced by the lacrimal gland are drained through the punctum, lacrimal sac, and nasolacrimal duct into the nose.

transmits light of a certain wavelength. The addition of black to a given hue produces the various *shades*. Saturation is an index of the purity of a hue. The brightness of an object depends on the light intensity. Today we can experiment with all these aspects of color by altering the settings on a color television set to achieve the variations of hue, saturation, and brightness.

Color vision defects are believed to arise from a deficiency or absence of one or more visual pigments. Clinically, people with abnormal color vision fall into three major categories. The *trichromat* possesses all three cone pigments and has normal color vision. Those of us who have been tested and found to be normal belong to this category. The *anomalous trichromat* has a partial deficiency of one of the three cone pigments. This person may have (1) *protanomaly*, which is deficiency in sensitivity to the first color (red), as well as poor red–green and blue–green discrimination; (2) *deuteranomaly*, which is deficiency of one pigment mediating green, as well as poor green–purple and red–purple discrimination; or (3) *tritanomaly*, which is deficiency of the cone pigment for blue, as well as blue–green and yellow–green insensitivity. The *dichromat* has a complete deficiency in one cone pigment but preserves the remaining two cone pigments. This person may have (1) *protanopia*, in which red is absent; (2) *deuteranopia*, in which green is absent; or (3) *tritanopia*, in which blue is absent. The *monochromat* has only one cone pigment.

The degree of color deficiency is determined by a series of plates or charts. The most common test used is the *Ishihara color plate test*, in which the ability to trace patterns on a multicolored chart is measured.

The milder deficiencies (*anomalous trichromacy*) are by far the most common, with red and green deficiency predominating. This type of color deficiency has a sex-linked recessive mode of inheritance and affects approximately 8% to 10% of all males and less than 1% of females.

Questions for review and thought

1. What keeps the cornea transparent?
2. What are the fixation and following reflexes?
3. What is amblyopia? What are the causes of amblyopia?
4. What muscles are involved in torsions? In the case of paralysis of the muscles that pull the eye horizontally and vertically, how do you test the function of the superior oblique muscle?
5. What is the accommodation reflex?
6. What are the clues that give a one-eyed person some appreciation of depth?
7. What structures in the human eye have no blood supply?
8. Describe the composition of the aqueous humor.
9. What would the visual acuity be in a person (a) with rods only, and (b) with cones only?
10. What are positive and negative afterimages? Why are surgical sheets in operating rooms green?
11. Why is the intraocular pressure higher than the pressure in the surrounding orbital tissue? What happens to the ocular structures when the pressure is too high and when it is too low?
12. What are the functions of tears?
13. What is the composition of the tear film?
14. What happens to an eye in which tear production is absent?
15. What are the primary colors?
16. Can a person who is totally color blind see?
17. The intraocular pressure varies during the day. What are the usual high and low periods in the normal person?
18. What visual functions are necessary to have binocular depth perception?
19. What happens to vision when the pupil is artificially dilated? Why?
20. What is the purpose of a normal pupillary response that involves constriction?
21. What is the function of blinking?

Q Self-evaluation questions

True–false statements

Directions: Indicate whether the statement is true **(T)** or false **(F)**.

1. Color vision should be tested binocularly. **T** or **F**
2. Loss of accommodation is due to failure of the ciliary muscle. **T** or **F**
3. Tear production is increased during the night. **T** or **F**

Missing words

Directions: Write in the missing word(s) in the following sentences.

4. When an object is viewed up close, three reactions occur. The eyes converge, the eye accommodates, and the pupils _____ .
5. The muscle that moves the eye up and in is called the _____ .
6. The rod pigment _____ , or visual purple, has vitamin A as its main component.

Choice-completion questions

Directions: Select the one best answer in each case.

7. The pupil is not affected by which one of the following?
   a. Pain
   b. Light
   c. Accommodation
   d. Mydriatics
   e. Congenital color blindness
8. Night vision originates in the:
   a. rods.
   b. cones.
   c. choroid.
   d. macula.
   e. fovea.
9. The most powerful refracting surface of the eye is the:
   a. front surface of the cornea.
   b. back surface of the cornea.
   c. front surface of the lens.
   d. back surface of the lens.
   e. combined refractive index of the aqueous and vitreous.

A Answers, notes, and explanations

1. **False.** Color vision should be tested separately with each eye. Although sex-linked color defects are present binocularly, certain acquired defects can occur with color vision that will produce color deficiencies in one eye only. Such conditions as optic neuritis may be responsible for a monocular type of acquired color defect and this would be missed if the examiner were testing binocular color vision.
2. **False.** Loss of accommodation is due to a gradual hardening of the lens substance, beginning with the nucleus, so that it is more resistant to changes in shape. Stimulus for accommodation is due to a blurred image, which causes the individual to contract the ciliary muscle and so relax the tension of the zonular fibers. This in turn allows the normal lens to assume a more spherical shape and increase its dioptric power. As the lens nucleus hardens with age, however, the lens is no longer as moldable and consequently is not able to bring the rays of light from a near object to focus onto the retina.
3. **False.** Tear production is decreased during the night and becomes almost nonexistent. There is, however, a compensatory lack of evaporation of tears during the sleep mechanism when the eyelids are closed. This provides adequate moisture for the cornea. The absence of tear production at night has important physiologic consequences in the development of an extended-wear

contact lens of the soft variety, which is dependent on hydration.

4. **Constrict.** The pupils constrict during this triad in an effort to form a pinhole camera device so that a clear image is seen. This triad of pupillary constriction, convergence, and accommodation is often called the accommodative reflex.
5. **Inferior oblique.** The inferior oblique muscle moves the eye up and in. The other action is a torsional action in turning the eye outward, or extorsion.
6. **Rhodopsin.** Rhodopsin, or visual purple, forms with dark adaptation and is destroyed by light. It is continually being used and restored. Its main component is vitamin A, found in carrots and other vegetables.
7. **e. Congenital color blindness.** Pain causes dilation of the pupil. Light produces a constriction of the pupil. Accommodation produces a synkinesis of convergence and pupillary constriction along with accommodation. Mydriatics are drops that produce dilation of the pupil. Color blindness, however, does not result in pupillary abnormalities.
8. **a. Rods.** There are approximately 125 million rods present in the extramacular area of the retina. These rods function best in dim light and are responsible for what is called scotopic vision. It is the adjustment after we enter a dark movie theater that permits us to walk up

A | Continued

the aisles with some degree of accuracy. Pilots during World War II soon learned they had to become dark adapted for bombing missions at night. Rods are relatively insensitive to red and therefore do not lose their function with this type of lighting. Thus red goggles were the chosen method for airline pilots and those in a number of other occupations that require rod adaptation for night vision. About 30 minutes are required for dark adaptation to occur. The use of red glasses, darkrooms, and x-ray rooms permits individuals to maintain full cone function while the rods become dark adapted.

9. **a. Front surface of the cornea.** This surface contributes about two-thirds of the refracting power to bend the rays of light coming from a distant object. The lens of the eye contributes to the remaining one-third of the refracting power of the eye. The refracting power of the cornea is equivalent to a 43.00 diopter lens.

Optics

The study of optics can be divided into three parts: *physical, geometric,* and *physiologic.* Physical optics is primarily concerned with the nature and properties of light itself. Geometric optics is that branch of optics in which the laws of geometry can be used to design lenses that include spectacles, optical instruments, telescopes, microscopes, cameras, and so forth. Physiologic optics deals with the mechanism of vision and the physiology and psychology of seeing. We deal here primarily with physical and geometric optics.

PHYSICAL OPTICS

What is light?

Our ancestors pondered and theorized about the nature of light. One theory proposed that light was wavelike and spread like ripples across a still pond (Figure 3.1). Another theory held that light was a flight of particles similar to the shooting out of droplets of water from the nozzle of a hose

(Figure 3.2). In more recent times scientists have believed that there is truth in both theories: that light can be transmitted both as particles and as waves.

How does light travel?

Light, which is basically that aspect of radiant energy to which the eye responds as a visual experience, is called *luminous radiation.* The light waves travel in a specific direction. The movement of these waves is in an up-and-down motion perpendicular to the direction in which they travel (Figure 3.3). These same light waves are capable of producing vision in human beings and lower animals by stimulating the very sensitive photoreceptors in the retina.

Nature of the world visible to humans

Human beings are continuously bombarded by electromagnetic energy, including waves from radio transmitters, infrared rays from heat lamps, and ultraviolet rays from the sun and quartz lamps, without receiving any visual sensation as a result of being in contact with these sources. It is only a portion of this *electromagnetic spectrum* that determines the visible world. The wavelengths of some of the waves of the electromagnetic spectrum are extremely short; for example, cosmic rays are only about 4 trillionths of a centimeter in length. Other wavelengths, such as those of radio waves, may be as long as 2 to 3 miles (3–5 km). The rays of wavelengths to which the eye responds lie in about the middle of this spectrum, namely, from 400 to 800 nm. Figure 3.4, an illustration of the electromagnetic spectrum, indicates the range of wavelengths for various parts of the spectrum.

Speed of light

Light travels at a speed of 186,000 miles per second (300,000 km/s). It is many times faster than sound, as is evident by the fact that we see a lightning flash much sooner than we hear the thunder that follows. Each

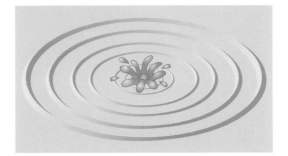

Figure 3.1 Light travels in a wave motion, as demonstrated by ripples in a still pond when a stone is thrown.

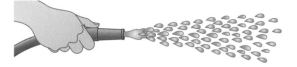

Figure 3.2 One theory is that light behaves as water droplets shooting out of a hose.

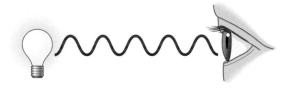

Figure 3.3 Light travels not in a straight line but in a wave motion.

wavelength is the distance from the crest of one wave to that of the next, whereas the *frequency* is the number of wavelengths passing a given point in 1 second. The product of these two quantities is equal to the *speed* of the electromagnetic radiation (*velocity* is the speed in a particular direction).

The speed of light in air is greater than that in other transparent media. For example, the speed of light in ordinary glass is only about two-thirds of the speed in air. However, we designate the wavelength of light in terms of its speed in air.

How do we measure intensity of a light source?

Light intensity is traditionally measured in terms of *footcandles*, a standard dating from preelectricity times. The light from a single candle falling on a surface at a distance of 1 foot illuminates the surface with an intensity of 1 candle per square foot. This is the premetric unit of measurement of light. If we hold a candle near a book in order to read, we soon find that as we move the candle away from the book, there is a distance at which the illumination is insufficient to permit us to read. The illumination of light on a surface is inversely proportional to its distance from the light source (Figure 3.5). The luminance of an object depends on the light reflected, and the equivalent visual sensation is one of brightness. An illumination of 10 footcandles is sufficient for ordinary indoor tasks; 30 footcandles is adequate for sewing and reading, although we often choose a reading lamp that will give us as much as 50 footcandles (Table 3.1).

Because the original standard candle cannot be easily reproduced, it has been replaced by a group of carbon filament lamps operated at a carefully prescribed voltage and maintained in the vaults of the U.S. Bureau of Standards. In modern usage, the amount of illumination, or illuminance, is referred to in terms of lumens (the International System

1,000,000 th of a millimicron   Kilometer

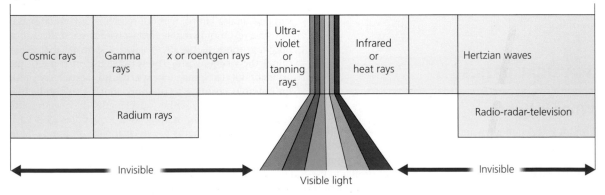

Figure 3.4 Electromagnetic spectrum.

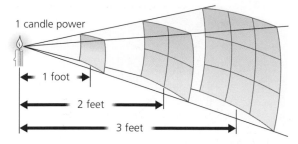

Figure 3.5 Illumination is inversely proportional to the distance of the surface from the light source.
(Modified from Adler FH: Physiology of the eye. 4th ed. St Louis: Mosby, 1965.)

Table 3.1 Recommended minimum footcandles	
Venues and tasks	**Minimum footcandle level**
Auditoriums	15
Waiting rooms	15
Building corridors and stairways	20
Libraries	70
Art galleries	30
Reading rooms	30
Study desks	70
Store interiors	30
School chalkboards	150
Kitchen work surfaces	50
Prolonged sewing	100

of Units [SI], commonly known as the metric system) per foot rather than candles per foot.

Color

The dispersion of white light into its many component colors was first demonstrated by Sir Isaac Newton, who allowed a narrow beam of light to pass obliquely through a prism and then intercepted the transmitted light, which appeared as colored bands or as a spectrum on a screen. The colors he found were spread into definite bands that the normal eye identified as red, orange, yellow, green, blue, and violet. The sequence of hues was always found to be in the same order. Newton called these bands of color the *spectrum* and he called the spreading effect caused by the prism *dispersion*. He was the first to show that white light is really a mixture of all colors. We enjoy everyday examples of this phenomenon of light breaking up into its constituent colors. Rainbows, for example, are produced by the dispersion of light into its spectral parts by droplets of rain or mist in the air.

Each wavelength range has a particular color hue. Red, having the longest wavelength, is deviated least by a water droplet or a prism and therefore appears at one end of the spectrum. Violet, which has the shortest wavelength, appears at the other end of the spectrum (Figure 3.6).

Rays of light and the spectrum

A single *ray of light* is the path of a single corpuscle of light traveling through a tiny aperture through two successive screens.

A *pencil of light* is a group of rays that diverges from its point source. It might pass through the aperture of one screen but would not make it through the aperture of the other.

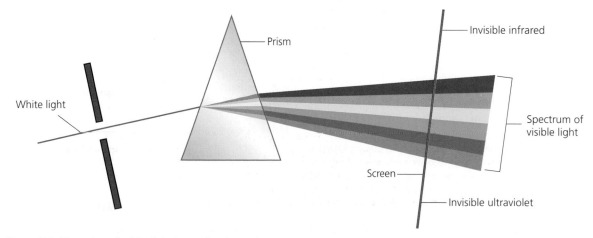

Figure 3.6 Dispersion of white light into colors by a prism.

A *beam of light* is a group of pencils of light. A relatively large aperture is required to admit a beam.

Each filament in an electric bulb has a number of beams and pencils of light. These beams diverge and overlap one another. At close range, they strike an object and create overlapping shadows that are poorly defined. The further the light source, the more parallel are the beams of light. That is why shadows framed from the sun are sharper and more finely etched than those coming from an artificial light source.

Where rays of white light pass through cut glass, they frequently are broken down into lights of varying wavelengths. The longest wavelength is red, followed by orange, yellow, green, blue, and violet.

Red	650–750 nm
Orange	592–650 nm
Yellow	560–592 nm
Green	500–560 nm
Blue	446–500 nm
Violet	400–446 nm

The fragmentation of white light yields the visible spectrum. There are other wavelengths not visible to the eye, including ultraviolet, infrared, x-ray, radio, and electromagnetic.

White light is not regularly broken up unless it travels into and through a different medium such as water droplets or glass. It is important to realize that the various wavelengths travel forward or outward at the same speed. Only their vertical vibrations differ in frequency. Thus the speed of violet light in air is the same as yellow, red, or green – that is, 186,000 miles per second.

When white light enters the eye, all these light waves are moving at the same speed but with a different vibration. These waves fuse, giving the sensation of white even though they travel through the eye, which has a different index of refraction than air.

Bending of light

Most people will have observed that a straight pole placed in a clear pond no longer looks straight but appears to be bent at the surface of the water. Fish under the surface of the water appear to someone fishing to be at a different place from where they actually are (Figure 3.7). This phenomenon is due to *refraction* of light.

If light travels in a straight line, how does one explain this apparent bending of light? Snell discovered the law behind this everyday phenomenon: it was explained by assuming (and this assumption was later proved correct by experiment) that light travels at different speeds in different media. We have stated that light travels in a vacuum at 186,000 miles per second. However, as it travels through other media, such as water or glass, it travels at a slower

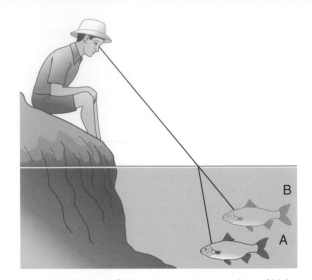

Figure 3.7 Bending of light when entering a medium of higher index of refraction. The real fish is at A, although the boy sees it at B.

velocity. The rate at which light travels through water is 140,000 miles per second (about 225,800 km/s).

Other media, such as glass and the chambers of the eye, also retard the velocity and alter the direction of light. The ratio of the speed of light in a vacuum to that in a given medium is called the *index of refraction* of that medium. This index, which is a comparison of the speed of light through a particular medium to its speed through air, can be expressed as follows:

$$\text{Index of refraction} = \frac{\text{Speed of light in air}}{\text{Speed of light in substance}}$$

For water this index is:

$$\frac{186\,000}{140\,000} = 1.33$$

Thus the index of refraction of a substance determines the speed of light through it. The index of refraction of the common optical media can be expressed as follows:

Air = 1.00
Water = 1.33
Aqueous humor = 1.336
Cornea = 1.37
Lens cortex = 1.38
Lens nucleus = 1.40
Crown glass = 1.49
PMMA (polymethylmethacrylate) plastic = 1.52
Flint glass = 1.65

How light can alter its direction

If rays of light pass from the air through another medium, such as a plate of glass, and pass perpendicularly to the

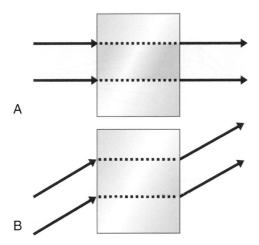

Figure 3.8 (A) Light passing perpendicularly through a plate of glass remains unchanged in direction. (B) Light passing obliquely through a plate of glass is displaced laterally but continues in the same direction.

glass, they will be slowed down somewhat but will emerge along the same line on which they entered the medium (Figure 3.8A). If, however, these rays pass obliquely at any angle to the plate of glass, they will be bent a little at the surface. The oblique rays closest to the glass will enter the glass first, and these rays will be slowed down first on their pathway through the slower medium (Figure 3.8B).

This is similar to the slowing-down effect when a line of soldiers marches at an angle toward a deep sandbar (Figure 3.9). The soldiers who first enter the sandbar will be slowed down first, whereas those at the extreme end will continue at their original speed until they reach the sandbar. This will result in a bend in the straight-line formation. This same effect occurs when a beam of light strikes a glass surface at an oblique angle.

GEOMETRIC OPTICS

Terminology

- **Divergence.** Rays of light from any luminous point of light will spread out or diverge (Figure 3.10A).
- **Convergence.** When a bundle of rays is brought together, the rays are said to converge (Figure 3.10B).
- **Parallel rays.** Light rays are assumed to be parallel if they emanate from a distant light source, such as the sun (Figure 3.10C).

A ray of light entering a medium is called the *incident ray* and the same ray emerging from the medium is called the *emergent ray*. The angle that the incident ray makes with the perpendicular surface of the medium is called the *angle of incidence*. The angle the ray makes within the medium by its change of direction is called the *angle of refraction* (Figure 3.11).

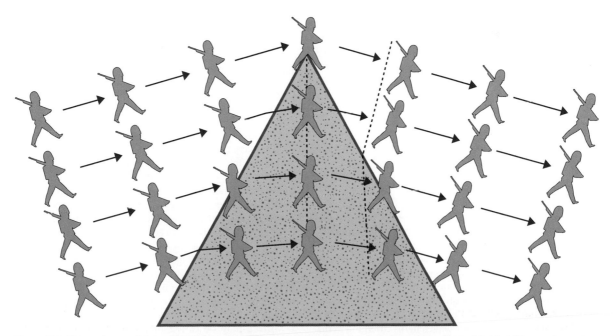

Figure 3.9 The pathway of the soldiers' march is changed by a sandbar. This is similar to the effect of light striking a glass prism.

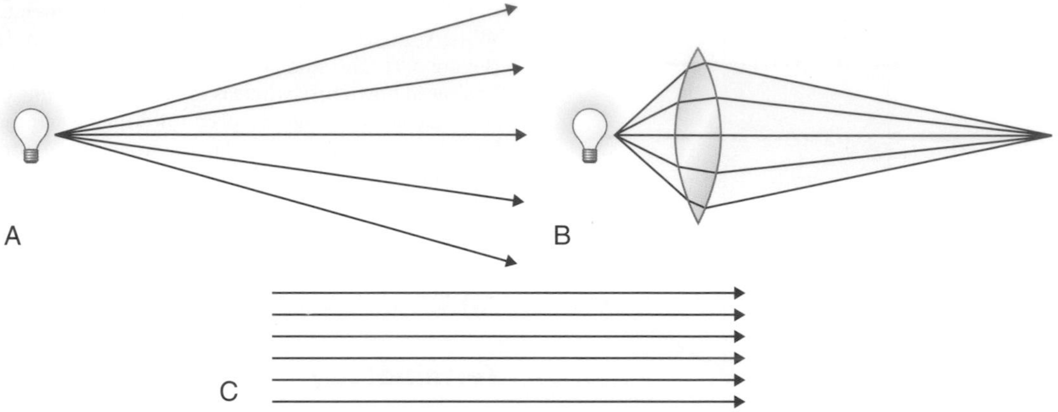

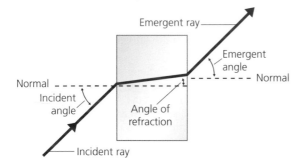

Figure 3.10 (A) Divergence. (B) Convergence. (C) Parallel rays.

Figure 3.11 Incident and emergent rays of light through glass.

The relationship between these two angles and the index of refraction of the medium through which the ray of light passes is the basis of *Snell's law*, a fundamental law in optics that governs the refraction of light by a transparent substance. Snell's law states:

$$\frac{\text{Sine of angle of incidence }(i)}{\text{Sine of angle of refraction }(h)} = \text{Index of refraction}$$

It is on this constant relationship of the incident angle, angle of refraction, and index of refraction of the medium that all lens design depends.

Dispersion

If a spectrum of light travels through a glass with parallel sides, then the deflection of light is such that the emerging rays are parallel to the direction of the original incident rays. The white light may enter a new medium such as glass, be broken up into its spectral components, and then fuse on the way out into a white bundle of rays.

If a ray of light goes through a glass whose sides are not parallel, the white light will be broken up into its spectral components with the various wavelengths emerging in different directions. This effect, called *dispersion*, results in

colored fringes found around anything viewed through prisms or unevenly cut glass. The dispersion value of different types of glass varies, depending on its index of refraction (Figure 3.12).

Color

White light is made up of beautiful colors. This easily can be seen when a narrow beam of white light is passed through clear plastic, which bends the white light at different angles. Sir Isaac Newton, a famous English scientist, made this discovery in 1666. When mist disperses white light it gives rise to the rainbow. Red, green, and blue are the primary colors. In dim light, more sensitive cells in the rods of the retina take over, which explains why we see mainly black and white as it gets darker.

Mirrors and reflection

One way of changing the direction of light is to allow light to rebound from a surface and thus be thrown in another direction. This rebounding of light is called *reflection* and certain laws govern its behavior. Any reflecting surface, such as glass, water, or metal, can reflect light. Because glass and water transmit light primarily, their reflection is secondary. Many other examples of reflecting surfaces are found in nature, such as a still pond or lake (Figure 3.13).

Mirrors illustrate this phenomenon best. They are primarily silver-coated glass, which allows a minimum transmission of light while reflecting the greater portion of the light. Mirrors obey a law that *the angle of incidence equals the angle of reflection* (Figure 3.14). An analogous situation occurs when a billiard ball strikes the rubber cushion of a billiard table. The angle at which the ball strikes the edge of the table is equal to the angle of the caroming ball (Figure 3.15).

Mirrors may be *curved* or *planar*. Curved mirrors are of two types: *concave* or *convex*. *Concave mirrors* reflect

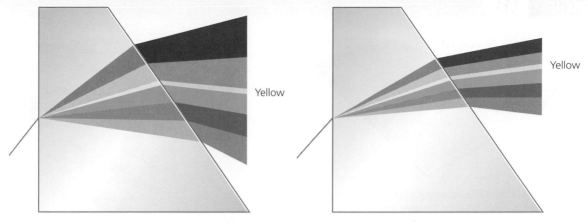

Index 1.60
Dispersion high

Index 1.50
Dispersion low

Figure 3.12 Dispersion factor of light through oblique glass with different indexes of refraction.

Figure 3.13 Reflection. A still lake acts as a mirror.

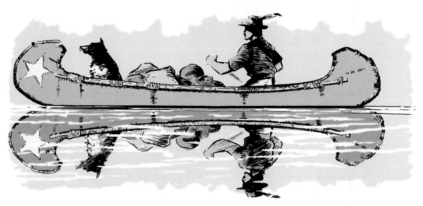

Figure 3.14 Reflection from a plane mirror.

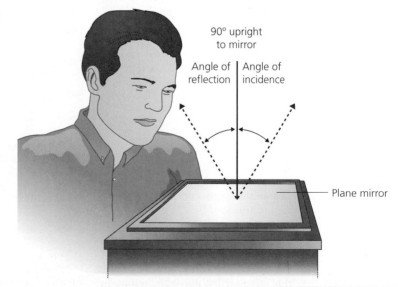

90° upright to mirror

Angle of reflection | Angle of incidence

Plane mirror

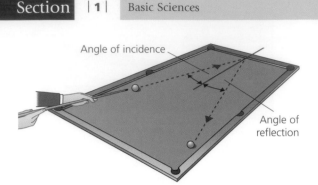

Figure 3.15 Billiard table. Movement of a billiard ball against the cushion of the table observes the same laws as the reflection of light from mirrors.

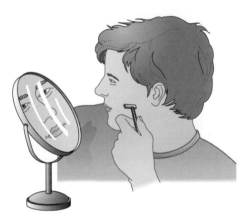

Figure 3.16 Concave shaving mirror. The image is magnified.

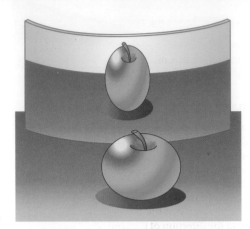

A

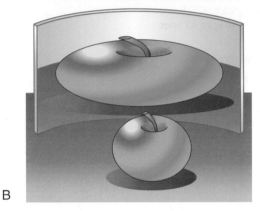

B

Figure 3.17 (A) Reflection from a convex mirror; the image is minified. (B) Reflection from a concave mirror; the reflection is magnified.

light in front of them, so that if an object is placed before the focal point of a mirror, its image is magnified. This property is used to great advantage in the production of mirrors for shaving (Figure 3.16). *Convex mirrors* reflect light away from their principal axes, so that if objects are placed before them the images will appear behind the mirrors in smaller size (Figure 3.17). One application of this second type of mirror is used in retail stores, in which store managers can observe large areas through small mirrors (Figure 3.18).

Lenses

Spectacle lenses were invented in about the 13th century and telescopes in the 17th century. In the past 100 years binoculars, cameras, projectors, periscopes, spectroscopes, and many other optical instruments have been developed with refinements of lens design; all have depended on the knowledge human beings have gained concerning the properties of lenses. Lenses were originally made of glass but are now also made of plastic. The main feature of curved lenses is their ability to bend rays of light.

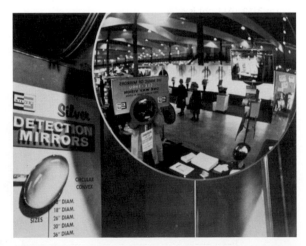

Figure 3.18 Convex mirrors used to prevent shoplifting. The minified image of the store allows easy scrutiny of a large area.

How do lenses bend rays of light?

The basic principle of all lenses may be considered best by a discussion of prisms. One may consider a lens as being made up of prisms.

What is a prism?

A *prism* is a triangular piece of glass or plastic with an *apex* and a *base*. Rays of light, entering from air and going through a prism, bend toward the base of the prism. This phenomenon is related to the oblique surface of the prism and its medium (Figure 3.19A).

The magnitude of the prismatic effect depends on the size of the angle at the apex of the prism. Light always is bent in the direction of the base of a prism. When one looks through a prism, however, the object of regard appears displaced toward its apex (Figure 3.19B).

How are prisms measured?

Prisms used in ophthalmology are calibrated in diopters. By definition, *1 prism diopter* (D) is that prism which appears to displace an object 1 cm at a distance of 1 meter from the eye (Figure 3.20). At 0.5 m, if the object is displaced 1 cm, then the dioptric power of the prism is 2.00 diopters. At 2 m, if the object is displaced 1 cm, then the dioptric power is 0.50 diopter. This is expressed by the formula:

$$P = C/D$$

where:

$P =$ Prism power
$C =$ Displacement of object in centimeters
$D =$ Distance from prism in meters

The use of prisms

Prisms are used in ophthalmology in the following devices and procedures:

1. Ophthalmic instruments such as gonioscopes and ophthalmoscopes
2. Measurements of muscle balance of the eye in cases of strabismus. A prism can alter the direction of light so that the projection of the deviating eye is

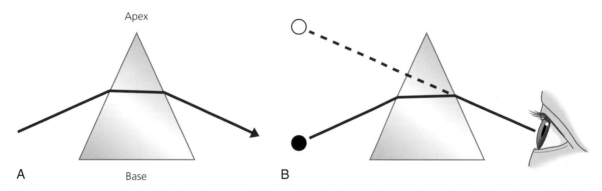

Figure 3.19 (A) Light is deviated by the prism toward its base. (B) The observer views an object through the prism and the object appears to be displaced toward its apex.

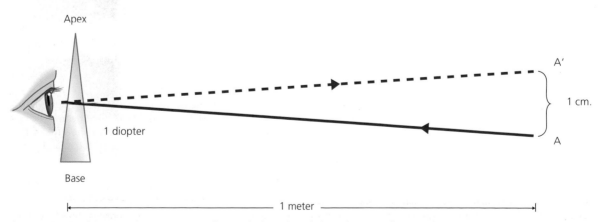

Figure 3.20 An object at point A appears to be at A' when viewed through a 1.00 diopter prism at 1 meter.

the same as its fellow eye, and, in effect, it corrects the sensory alignment of the eye without disturbing the motor alignment

3. Spectacles to correct muscle imbalance, especially those of a vertical nature
4. Eye exercises for muscular imbalance, such as convergence insufficiency

Prisms may be used as reflectors or mirrors. A ray of light usually travels through a piece of glass but there is a *critical angle* in which light is reflected rather than refracted. Any light rays striking a glass surface at an angle smaller than the critical angle will be refracted through the glass. When light hits the glass at an angle greater than the critical angle, the rays of light will be reflected as though the glass were a silvered mirror.

Convex lenses

A *convex lens* is a piece of glass in which one or both surfaces of the lens are curved outward. If two prisms are placed base to base (Figure 3.21A) and the middle corners of the prism are smoothed off, a convex lens is created (Figure 3.21B).

Alteration in the radius, or curvature, of the lens alters its point of convergence or focal point. A more curved lens will bend rays of light to a shorter focus than will a less curved lens. Lenses are considered as positive lenses, or *plus lenses*, if they converge rays of light to a focus behind the lens (Figure 3.22).

Concave lenses

A *concave lens* is a piece of glass in which one or both surfaces of the lens are curved inward. If two prisms are placed apex to apex (Figure 3.23A) and the straight surfaces of the prisms are then curved, a concave lens is created (Figure 3.23B).

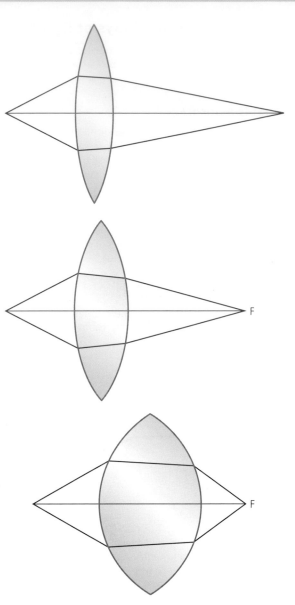

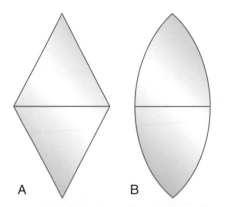

Figure 3.21 (A) Two prisms placed base to base. (B) A convex lens derived from (A) by smoothing off the middle corners.

Figure 3.22 Convex lenses. As the curvature of the lens increases, the focal point moves closer to the lens. Also the more curved the lens, the greater is its power.

With a concave lens, the emergent rays of light diverge after refraction and thus cannot be focused behind the lens. If, however, we extend the direction of the rays of light backward, we can draw an imaginary focus in front of the lens. Thus this lens is called a negative lens or *minus lens* (Figure 3.24).

Up to this point the lenses under discussion have all been spheres. The convex lenses are *converging lenses* and the concave lenses are *diverging lenses*. Converging means bringing together and diverging means spreading apart and that is

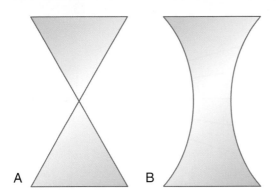

Figure 3.23 (A) Two prisms placed apex to apex. (B) A concave lens derived from (A).

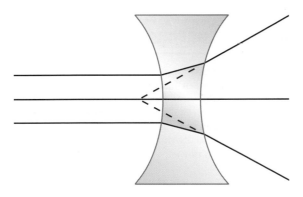

Figure 3.24 Concave lens demonstrating an imaginary or virtual point of focus in front of the lens.

what these lenses do to rays of light. Variations of the spherical lens occur when the curvatures of the anterior and the posterior surfaces are not the same (Figure 3.25).

Focal length

In any lens the ray penetrating through the center of the lens is undeviated, but all the rays on either side will

converge to or from a point. This central ray, or *axial ray*, travels along a line called the *principal axis* of the lens. The rays on either side, or *paraxial rays*, converge to a point on this principal axis, which is called the *focal point;* the distance of this point from the center of the lens is called the *focal length* (Figure 3.26).

A lens must be considered in terms of its focal length. The power of a lens is equal to the reciprocal of its focal distance measured in meters. The power is expressed in units called *diopters*.

The formula for conversion of focal length into diopters of lens power is:

$$D = 1/f$$

where:

$D =$ Power of lens in diopters
$f =$ Focal length in meters

For example:

Lens with focal length of 1 m $= 1/1 = 1.00$ D
Lens with focal length of 2 m $= 1/2 = 0.50$ D
Lens with focal length of 4 m $= 1/4 = 0.25$ D
Lens with focal length of 1/4 m $= 1/0.25 = 4.00$ D
Lens with focal length of 14 $= 1/0.25 = 4.00$ D

To clearly capture the image from a convex lens, a screen must be placed at its exact focal point. An example of this is shown in Figure 3.27.

In a convex lens the focal point always is behind the lens and therefore convex lenses are considered positive (Figure 3.28). With concave lenses, however, the focal point always is in front of the lens, erect and virtual. Concave lenses are designated as minus lenses.

Until now we have considered point sources and point focal points. With regard to an object such as a tree, each point on the tree will have its own focal point in terms of a plus lens system (Figure 3.29). The image behind a convex lens is always real, behind the lens, and inverted. (A real image is one that can be captured by a screen or photographic film.)

When an object is placed before a positive lens, a sharp image is formed at its focal point.

To determine the focal length and the power of the lens, one must know the distance of the object from the lens and

Figure 3.25 Lens forms. (A) Biconvex; (B) planoconvex; (C) convex meniscus; (D) biconcave; (E) planoconcave; (F) concave meniscus.

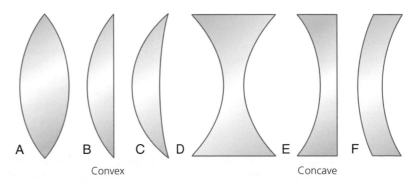

Convex   Concave

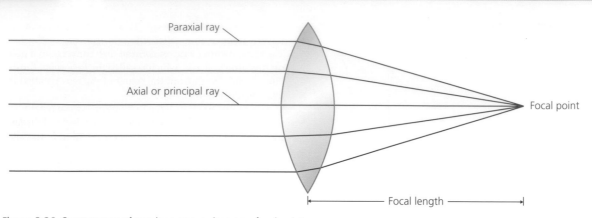

Figure 3.26 Convergence of rays by a convex lens to a focal point.

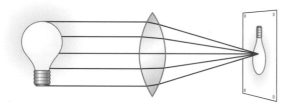

Figure 3.27 A real inverted image of the light bulb is seen when the screen is placed at the focal point of the convex lens.

the distance of the image from the lens. The following formula is used:

$$1/u = 1/f = 1/v$$

where:

u = Distance of object from lens
f = Focal length of lens
v = Distance of image from lens

If any two of these factors are known, then the third can easily be derived. A simpler method to determine the focal length of a lens is to use the formula:

$$U + D = V$$

where:

U = Distance in centimeters that object is in front of lens
D = Dioptric power of the lens
V = Distance in centimeters that object is behind the lens

Once one determines the D, or dioptric value of the lens, one can use the formula $D = 1/f$ and if one uses "cm," one can divide the formula $D = 100/f$(cm) to determine the focal distance in centimeters.

SPHERICAL ABERRATION

Because the periphery of a lens has a different curvature from its center, rays of light striking the lens at its edge do not come to the same focal point as when they strike the lens at its center (Figure 3.30). To eliminate problems caused by this aberration, grinding techniques have been developed. Spherical aberration becomes a problem only with lenses of high power.

CHROMATIC ABERRATION

The edges of spherical lenses act as a prism. However, on passing through a prism, light is broken down into its spectral components. Therefore, color fringes can appear when light passes through a lens. This is particularly noticeable when dealing with lenses of high power. Chromatic aberration can be largely corrected by changes in the shape and index of refraction of the lens. Flint glass has a greater tendency to produce chromatic aberration than does crown glass. This aberration can be corrected by combining two lenses having different indexes of refraction.

If chromatic aberration is excessive, the image formed by the optical system will be fuzzy with colored fringes. There are ways to reduce this color distortion.

1. A light source that has light of only one wavelength (lasers) or a narrow band of wavelengths (sodium vapor lamps) may be used.
2. A filter may be used to take out all but a few wavelengths. Good camera lenses reduce chromatic aberration with appropriate filters.
3. A doublet lens works if one lens has a low index of refraction (crown glass) and the other a high index of refraction (flint glass). This combination is called an *anachromatic lens*. The two lenses of equal dispersion

Figure 3.28 Focal distance varies with the power of the lens. (A) Plus, or convex, lens: the point focus is behind the lens. (B) Minus, or concave, lens: the point focus is in front of the lens.

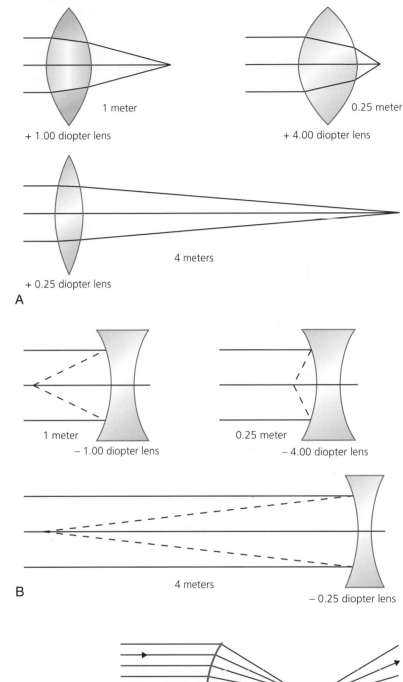

1 meter

+ 1.00 diopter lens

0.25 meter

+ 4.00 diopter lens

4 meters

+ 0.25 diopter lens

A

1 meter

− 1.00 diopter lens

0.25 meter

− 4.00 diopter lens

4 meters

− 0.25 diopter lens

B

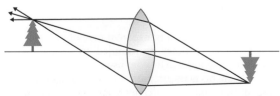

Figure 3.29 Image of a tree through a convex lens is behind the lens, real and inverted.

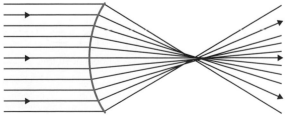

Figure 3.30 Spherical aberration. The rays of light on refraction by the lens converge to a meeting area rather than a single focal point.

value nullify each other, and the chromatic aberration that results is below that of a single lens.

CYLINDERS

A sphere has the same power in all meridians, whereas the cylinder has two principal meridians; one is called the *power* meridian (which has the power of the lens) and the other is called the *axis* (which is only a reference of the cylinder; it has no power).

Cylinders have the shape of a slice of a pipe or bicycle tire in that they are curved sharply in one direction but not at all in the other direction.

The curvature of a lens in one direction conveys the power of that lens and is called the *meridian* of the lens. The image of a cylinder, however, lies 90 degrees away from the meridian of power. This position is the plane of the *axis* of the lens. Therefore, we have two terms: a meridian, which denotes the power of a cylindric lens, and the axis, which denotes the image of the lens, this image being always 90 degrees away from the meridian. Cylindric lenses, as in the trial case, always are denoted by the axis; for example, +1.00 axis 90 has 1.00 diopter of power at 180 degrees but it will form an image at 90 degrees.

Spherocylinders are a combination of a sphere and a cylinder. Such a lens system has two radii of curvature, each with its own focal point and image. For example, in Figure 3.31 the rays of light from meridian x–x focus at X, whereas the rays from y–y focus at Y.

The area between the two focal points of a spherocylindric combination assumes a conoid shape, which is called *Sturm's conoid*. This optical effect is illustrated in Figure 3.31. At A, a section of the bundle of converging rays will be in the form of a horizontal ellipse but at C it will be in the form of a vertical ellipse. At B, the bundle forms a circle called the *circle of least confusion*. The circle of least confusion represents the dioptric average of the spherocylinder. In

refraction, the conoid of Sturm is "collapsed" so that both the vertical and horizontal foci are placed on the retina. In a situation in which one focus is already on the retina, a simple cylinder will move the other focus back or forward to the retina.

A spherocylindric lens really comprises two lenses, each of different power in the two principal meridians, which are 90 degrees apart. The dioptric powers of these two components should be considered separately. For example, +7.00 D sph − 1.50 cyl × 90 means that the spherical power is +7.00, the cylinder is −1.50 diopters and its axis is 90 degrees. The power of that cylinder is at a right axis to the cylinder. Thus the power in the horizontal meridian is +5.50 D.

TRANSPOSITION

Transposition is the process of changing the prescription from a plus cylinder to a minus cylinder, or from a minus cylinder to a plus cylinder, without changing its refractive value. The rules of transposition are based on the principle that when two cylinders of equal power and like sign are crossed at right angles, they produce the effect of a spherical lens of the same power as one of the cylinders.

The rule for transposition of all compound lenses is as follows: *Add the cylinder power to the sphere power algebraically, change the sign of the cylinder, and change the axis of the cylinder by 90 degrees.* The following are examples of typical transpositions:

- Transpose the following prescription to a minus cylinder: +2.00 + 1.00 × 90. Adding +2.00 and +1.00 algebraically, we obtain +3.00 as the new spherical power. Changing the sign of the cylinder to minus and the axis by 90 degrees, we find +3.00 − 1.00 × 180.
- Transpose the following prescription to a plus cylinder: +1.00 − 3.00 × 70. Adding +1.00 and −3.00 algebraically, we obtain −2.00 as the spherical power. Changing the sign of the cylinder to plus and the axis by 90 degrees, we find −2.00 + 3.00 × 160.

PRACTICAL ASPECTS OF OPTICS

Fiberoptics

A *fiberoptic bundle* has a transparent core of material with a high refractive index surrounded by a material of lower refractive index. The core usually is plastic or glass. The rim can be glass or even air. Most fibers are tiny, being only 0.003 to 0.005 inch (0.008 − 0.013 cm) in diameter.

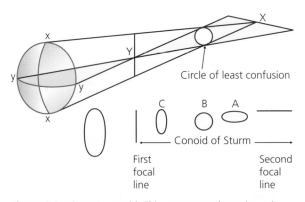
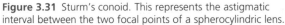

Figure 3.31 Sturm's conoid. This represents the astigmatic interval between the two focal points of a spherocylindric lens.

Light moves along these plastic cores because of total internal reflection. The optical effect is created by the differences in indexes of refraction. Total internal reflection occurs when light moves from a material with a higher index to one with a lower index. Light leaves the pipes at the end of tubing, where it is intense and concentrated. Most of the bundles are parallel to one another, the result being a coherent fiberoptic bundle or image conduit. Coherent fibers are used in computer output terminals as well as in many electrooptical devices.

Gonioscopy

The principle of internal reflection is a problem to an observer who has to examine the eye. Parts of the eye are not visible because light cannot get out of the eye. For instance, the angle structures of the anterior chamber are not visible because of total internal reflection.

Light has to get through the cornea for the examiner to see the angle structures. At the cornea – air interface, however, an abrupt change from a high to a low index of refraction occurs, which causes total internal reflection exactly like that of the fiberoptic tube.

If a contact lens is applied to the cornea, then light can pass through the cornea into the contact lens, which has a refractive index higher than the refractive index of corneal tissue. Once the light is past the cornea, it can travel to the eyepiece and be seen either through a mirror, as noted in the Goldmann lens (Figure 3.32), or through simple

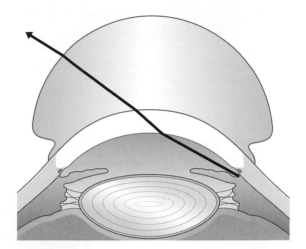

Figure 3.33 The Koeppe lens, which gives a direct view of the angle of the anterior chamber.

refraction, as noted in the discussion of the Koeppe lens (Figure 3.33).

Telescopes

There are two types of telescopes: the astronomical or inverting and the galilean or noninverting.

Astronomical telescope

Both the objective and the eyepiece are of positive power. The primary focus of the eye lens coincides with the secondary focus of the objective lens. They are separated by the distance equal to the sum of their focal lengths. A real image is formed in the focal plane of the objective. The image is inverted and its size is determined by the power of these lenses. The eye lens acts as a simple magnifier and forms a vertical image at infinity.

This telescope, as the name implies, is used in astronomy. Because the stars are so far away, the fact that the image is inverted is not of practical concern.

Galilean telescope

The galilean telescope uses a negative eye lens and positive objective. Again, the two lenses are situated so that their focal points coincide. The focus of the negative lens, however, is on the other side of the lens, so that the two are separated by the difference of the absolute values of their focal length.

The image from this telescope is not inverted because of the negative eyepiece. The erect image has allowed industry to use these basic optical principles to manufacture surgical loupes. These consist of *a galilean telescope* combined with an "add" on the front to allow for close work.

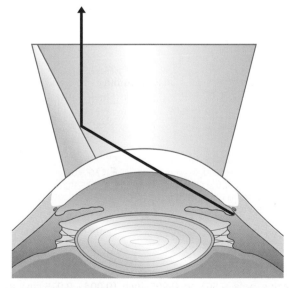

Figure 3.32 The Goldmann lens, which gives an indirect view of the angle of the anterior chamber.

OPTICAL ILLUSIONS

Optics takes us into the fascinating field of optical illusion. In this area geometric optics is affected by our perceptual senses and our interpretation of what we see. The saying "seeing is believing" is not always true because we are influenced greatly by background effect, as well as the effect of certain lines on each other and their interpretation by the brain. Figure 3.34 shows examples of some of the illusions that can be created.

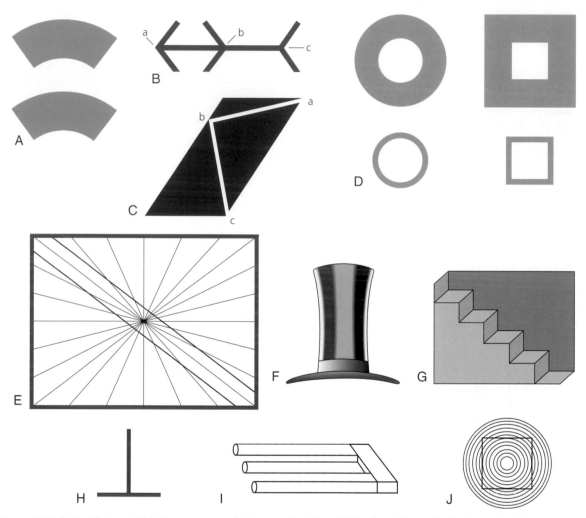

Figure 3.34 Optical illusions. (A) Both arcs are exactly the same size. (B and C) The line ab is exactly the same as bc. (D) Upper circle and square are crowded by the large black borders and appear smaller. Both upper and lower inner circles and squares are the same size. (E) The red oblique lines are straight but they appear curved. (F) The height of the crown appears greater than the width of the brim. Both are the same size. (G) This may appear as a staircase or as overhanging masonry. (H) The height appears greater than the base. (I) Are there three prongs? (J) The red square is a true square and not distorted in any way.

Questions for review and thought

1. How does light travel?
2. What is the cause of the dispersion of white light produced by a prism?
3. Draw a diagram of the electromagnetic spectrum.
4. List the sequence of color hues in the spectrum.
5. What is the law of mirrors?
6. Which type of mirror magnifies: concave or convex?
7. What is a prism?
8. Draw the focal points of a concave lens and of a convex lens, respectively.
9. What is a cylinder?
10. What is Sturm's conoid?
11. What aberrations are there with high minus spectacles (greater than 5.00 diopters)?
12. What are aspheric lenses?
13. How do you find the optical center of a lens?
14. Name some common defects found in glass.
15. What is a galilean telescope?
16. When you are looking through a prism, does the image jump to the apex or the base?

Q   Self-evaluation questions

True–false statements

Directions: Indicate whether the statement is true **(T)** or false **(F)**.

1. A light entering a prism is deflected toward the apex of the prism. **T** or **F**
2. Chromatic aberration occurs when white light enters a new index of refraction and emerges broken into its spectral components. **T** or **F**
3. The speed of red light is considerably slower than the speed of white light. **T** or **F**

Missing words

Directions: Write in the missing word in the following sentences.

4. Placido's disc uses the front surface of the cornea as a _____.
5. A fiberoptic bundle works by _____ reflection, in which the light strikes the wall of the bundle at an angle greater than the critical angle.
6. Yellow lenses act as _____ filters.

Choice-completion questions

Directions: Select the one best answer in each case.

7. If the mechanical center of a lens is changed by edging, what happens to the optical center?
   a. It remains where it was on the lens.
   b. It is displaced toward the edge most shortened.
   c. It is displaced according to Prentice's rule.
   d. It shifts laterally but never vertically.
   e. None of the above.
8. Aberrations of a lens include:
   a. spherical aberration.
   b. astigmatism of oblique pencils.
   c. chromatic aberration.
   d. pincushion and barrel distortion.
   e. all of the above.
9. Convex mirrors make the size of the image:
   a. smaller.
   b. larger.
   c. larger if the object is placed within the focal point of the lens.
   d. smaller if the object is placed within the focal point of the lens.
   e. none of the above.

A   Answers, notes, and explanations

1. **False.** A prism is a wedge-shaped piece of glass that bends light toward its base because of a change in the direction of light waves. It creates this alteration of direction because of the change in the index of refraction between light traveling in air and light traveling in glass. When light emerges from the prism, it undergoes another change in direction toward the base.

   Although the light is deflected toward the base of the prism, the observer sees it toward the apex. By bringing together images separated in space by a heterotropia of the eyes, prisms are used diagnostically to assess the type and magnitude of a strabismus and to treat diplopia.

2. **True.** Chromatic aberration is seen naturally in rainbows. White light penetrates a suspended droplet of water and is

A Continued

broken up into its spectral components. Clinically, chromatic aberration is seen in patients who have corneal edema. The most common occurrences are in persons with severe or acute glaucoma or those wearing ill-fitting contact lenses. The liberated edema fluid breaks up the intact bundle of white light, and patients complain of seeing halos around lights. Frequently a mucous blob on the cornea will do the same thing, so that not all chromatic aberration occurrences indicate pathologic conditions. Some lenses have a higher chromatic aberration than others. For instance, lenses of flint optical glass have a greater tendency to chromic aberration than lenses of barium optical glass. Flint glass has a greater tendency to chromatic aberration than does barium.

3. **False.** All the colors, whether they are reds, blues, greens, or oranges, have exactly the same speed of light, which is 186,000 miles per second. A wavelength is the distance from the top of one wave to the top of the next, whereas the frequency is the number of waves passing in 1 second. Red light may have a longer wavelength than blue but this indicates only its vertical vibration. All colors, white included, travel at the same speed.

The speed of light depends on frequency × wavelength. When the wavelength is shorter, its frequency is increased so that the speed of white versus colored light remains the same.

4. **Mirror.** Placido's disc uses the cornea as a mirror. The disc is used to detect keratoconus. The cone-shaped deformity of the cornea is reflected in the distortion of the annular rings, which appear irregular and oblong on the cornea. Placido's disc is used in a clinical photographic system to give accurate topographic analysis of the central and peripheral sections of the cornea for contact lens fitting. The distance between the rings can be translated into radii of corneal curvature. Reflection from the cornea as a mirror is the basic principle of all keratometers. The image from the keratometer is reflected and brought into focus. A doubling device is used to keep the images aligned. The amount of focusing required to yield sharp corneal images gives the K readings.

5. **Internal.** If light strikes any optical surface at an angle greater than the critical angle, the light, instead of passing through that surface, will be totally reflected.

This principle is well established. Some ophthalmoscopes are based on total reflection by virtue of light striking a prism. In fiberoptic bundles the light is inside the bundle and cannot escape because the angle of incident light exceeds the critical angle and the outer coat of the light has a low refractive index. The light emerging from this fiberoptic bundle is compressed, intense, and very high in illumination. It is a pure light because none of it escapes or is broken down to its spectral components.

Fiberoptic illumination has become an integral part of the illuminating systems used in ophthalmic microsurgery. The commercial uses of the fiberoptic system are numerous and include everything from Christmas tree decorations to illuminating systems for space travel.

6. **Haze.** Yellow lenses are basically haze filters. Skiers and hunters use yellow lenses to reduce haze and improve definition. They are not useful in night driving because they reduce the light entering the retina when lack of contrast is already a problem.

7. **a. It remains where it was on the lens.** Obviously, the center of the lens remains where it is, regardless of how the lens is edged. However, high fashion dictates the shape of the frame and with radical lens designs the optical centers can be shifted in the frame itself and in relation to the eye.

Large frames that contain strong prescriptions, that is, −5.00 diopters or more, frequently slide down the nose with reading. The effect of gravity drops the lens, and the vertex distance of the lens to the eye is changed. With plus lenses it increases the prescription; with minus lenses it does the reverse. Also, unwanted base-up prism is added with plus lenses, with the opposite, or base-down, occurring with minus lenses.

The optical center and the mechanical center do not coincide. The optical center of a lens is that place of the lens that does not contain unwanted prism. It is the point detected on the lensmeter where the rays of light come into focus. The optical center should be in line with the eye. The mechanical center is the geographic center, and in a perfectly round lens it coincides with the optical center. The optical center, not the mechanical center, concerns us.

If the optical center is shifted in the frame, then unwanted prism will occur. If the optical center is shifted outward and the lens is a plus lens, then base-out prism will be added.

The optical centers of the lenses always should be marked and compared with the interpupillary measurements – the distance from the center of one pupil to the other.

8. **e. All of the above.**

Spherical aberration: The image from a spherical lens is never a single point because the central and paraxial rays form more concentrated images than those rays that pass through the periphery of the lens.

The degree of spherical aberration depends on:

1. the aperture of the system; it is reduced by closing down the size of the aperture.

2. the precise form of the lenses used; the error can be reduced, making the curvature of the anterior surface greater than the curvature of the posterior surface.

3. the curvature of the lens; the fault can be diminished by making the peripheral curves less sloped; these are called *aplanatic surfaces*.

A   Continued

Astigmatism of oblique pencils: If light rays strike a lens at an angle instead of perpendicular to it, the image will be distorted in a form similar to that produced by a cylindric lens. Some light rays will strike the lens early and some later. The extra distance has to be traveled by the later rays to strike the lens. Moreover, a flatter section of the lens will be encountered by these rays. The resultant image will be astigmatic, sharp in one direction and fuzzy in the other. If the light rays strike a lens perpendicularly, this type of lens distortion does not occur.

Chromatic aberration: This is discussed in answer 2.

Pincushion and barrel distortion: Distortion occurs when the magnification of the peripheral parts of the lens is different from that of the central area. Pincushion distortion occurs when the peripheral magnification is greater than that of the central magnification. Barrel distortion occurs when the peripheral magnification is less than that of the central magnification.

9. **a. Smaller.** Concave mirrors magnify the image of the object only if it is placed *within* the focal point of the mirror. Cosmetic mirrors always are concave, and the face has to be placed close to the mirror to have its image enlarged and in focus.

   Convex mirrors reduce image size. They are commonly used as survey mirrors in retail stores where large areas of the store can be seen with the aid of a convex mirror.

Pharmacology

Pharmacology deals with the basic properties of drugs, their actions, their fate in the human body, and their known side effects. This chapter deals primarily with some of the drugs that act on the eye, either directly by local application or indirectly by systemic absorption.

GENERAL PRINCIPLES

Locally applied medication

Ophthalmic preparations placed directly in the eye are available in solution, suspension, or ointment forms. Solutions usually are instilled in the conjunctival sac and do not interfere with vision. The main disadvantage is that their duration of contact with the eye is short and therefore they require frequent instillation. Polymers often are added to solutions to enhance contact time. Although ointments remain in contact with the eye for prolonged periods, their tendency to reduce vision by creating a greasy film over the surface of the cornea limits their daily usefulness. Ointments frequently are used for bedtime therapy because of their prolonged contact time; in addition, they are less readily washed out with tears. They also are valuable for use in children who are crying (Table 4.1).

Preparations used in the eye have certain basic requirements regarding tolerance, tonicity, sterility, stability, and penetration.

Tolerance

Eye medications should cause minimal irritation or stinging of the eye. Tolerance of the medication by the eye depends on the solution's having an ideal acid–base balance. The acid–base balance is denoted in terms of its pH.

Solutions that have a pH greater than 7 are *alkaline,* whereas agents with a pH less than 7 are *acid* (for example, boric acid solution has a pH of 4.7). Most ophthalmic solutions have a pH that varies from 3.5 to 10.5. Any solution with a pH within this range causes minimal irritation to the eye (Figure 4.1).

Tonicity

The *tonicity* of a solution refers to the concentration of the chemical in that solution. Normal saline solution, or a 0.9% sodium chloride equivalent, has a tonicity approximately that of tears and is therefore well tolerated by the eye. Solutions with a high concentration of a chemical, however, are hypertonic and thus can be quite irritating. However, solutions low in concentration of a chemical (hypotonic solutions), such as water, are equally objectionable in producing irritation of the eye. Ideally, the closer the concentration of the drug to normal tears (0.9% sodium

Table 4.1 Comparison of characteristics of ophthalmic solutions and ophthalmic ointments

Characteristics	Solutions	Ointments
Instillation	Easier	More difficult
Contact time	Shorter	Longer (slower movement through nasolacrimal drainage)
Irritation on instillation	Frequent	Rare
Discharge retention	No	Yes
Skin allergic reactions	Few	More frequent
Blurred vision	No	Yes (film spreads over eye)
Local symptoms (burning, stinging)	More frequent	Less frequent
Readily contaminated (requires preservatives)	Yes	No
Stability a problem with storage	Yes	Less likely

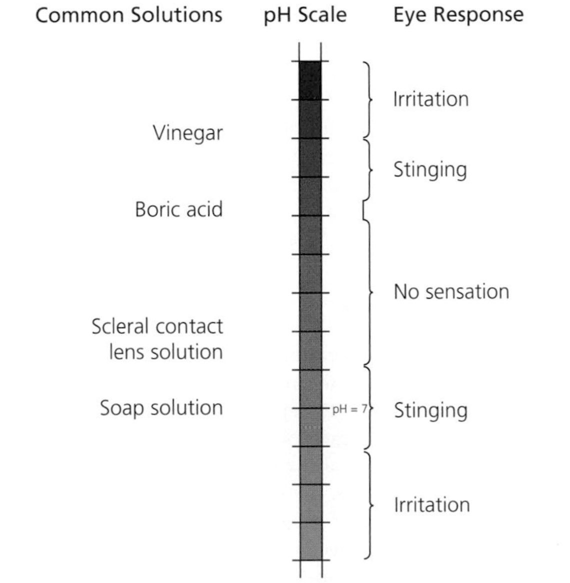

Figure 4.1 The eye responds by stinging and irritation when the pH varies from 7.
(Illustration courtesy of J. Krezanowski.)

chloride equivalent), the less irritating the drug will be. In some cases in which a high concentration of a locally applied drug is required, this ideal may not be achievable.

Sterility

Solutions must be free from bacterial contamination. This can be achieved either by autoclaving or by passing the solution through bacterial filters. Today most solutions are manufactured in a sterile manner by drug companies. To ensure sterility for long periods, preservatives are usually added. A good preservative should be well tolerated by the eye, nonallergenic, and inhibit the growth of bacteria and fungi. About 95% of all commercially available ophthalmic products are preserved with (1) benzalkonium chloride, (2) chlorobutanol, or (3) organic mercurials, chiefly thimerosal and phenylmercuric acetate. For eye surgery, however, the preservative drugs are usually eliminated to make the product less irritating to the open tissues. The solutions for eye surgery are available in sterile individual-dose units. For contact lens solutions, these preservatives often are too toxic to the cornea, and less irritating preservatives are incorporated.

Once a sealed bottle is opened, it is no longer considered sterile. Organisms may enter an open bottle with ease. The most notorious organism found in ophthalmic solutions, including antibiotic drops, is *Pseudomonas aeruginosa*, which can destroy an eye in 48 hours. This organism's predilection for fluorescein solution has led to the development of dry fluorescein-impregnated paper, because this organism cannot survive in a dry environment.

Stability

Solutions must be reasonably stable and not deteriorate or lose their effectiveness. Drugs such as phenylephrine hydrochloride (Neo-Synephrine) and epinephrine oxidize in the presence of air and bright light and consequently are often packaged in dark or opaque bottles. Some drugs require a special base to provide stability. Eye ointments are prepared in either a petrolatum base or a water-soluble base because these bases have proved to be stable. Drugs such as oxytetracycline (Terramycin), which are relatively unstable for any length of time in solution form, have a long shelf life in ointment form and are generally prepared this way.

Penetration

Eyedrops penetrate the eye directly through the cornea and into the anterior chamber of the eye. They do not, however, penetrate far behind the crystalline lens and therefore cannot reach the back, or posterior portion, of the eye. The cornea acts as a barrier to many drops by virtue of the lipid content of its epithelium, which functions as a barrier to all medications not soluble in fat. Eyedrops also must have water-soluble properties to penetrate the remaining portion of the cornea. Thus agents that penetrate the eye well are those that have both fat- and water-soluble properties.

Drugs penetrate the cornea better if they are instilled directly over its surface. When corneal penetration is of utmost importance, the patient should be asked to look down and the drop should be placed above so that it will flow over the cornea.

Alternative routes of medication

Subconjunctival injections

Injections may be administered under the conjunctiva. The subconjunctival medication gains access to the eye by absorption into the bloodstream by the episcleral and conjunctival vessels. *Subconjunctival injections* are used primarily in the treatment of intraocular infection.

Continuous-release delivery

Discs impregnated with drugs permit continuous delivery of medication 24 hours a day for a full 7 days. A small membrane, sandwiching medication, is inserted into the lower conjunctiva by the patient and it gradually releases its medication. Pilocarpine can be incorporated in the Ocusert and over a period of 7 to 8 days it is steadily released at a rate of 40 µg per hour. Lacrisert provides a continuous release of hydroxypropyl cellulose for lubrication in patients with dry eyes.

Retrobulbar injections

Drugs may be administered by injecting medication through the skin of the lower lid, the point of the needle emerging behind the eyeball. *Retrobulbar injections* of a local anesthetic are often used to paralyze the extraocular and eyelid muscles and anesthetize the eye before commencement of intraocular surgery.

Intracameral injection

An injection may be given into the anterior chamber at the start of cataract surgery to enhance patient comfort under topical anesthesia. The injection of 0.5 mL of preservative-free 1% lidocaine (Xylocaine) has resulted in a dramatic improvement in patient comfort, with a decrease in light sensitivity. This advance has led to essentially painless cataract surgery without the use of retrobulbar or peribulbar injections. Vancomycin and other antibiotics may be used.

Systemic medication

The term *systemic* drugs refers to those drugs that are taken orally or by injection subcutaneously (under the skin), intramuscularly (in the muscle), or intravenously (into the vein). These routes of administration are usually chosen because of some disease in the posterior part of the eye or orbit that cannot be reached by locally applied medication. In particular, conditions such as cellulitis, uveitis, and acute allergic reactions often require systemic medication.

COMPLICATIONS OF LOCALLY ADMINISTERED DRUGS

Allergic reactions

Many ophthalmic preparations can cause contact allergic reactions involving primarily the skin of the lids and the conjunctiva. Because hypersensitivity develops as a result of the patient's exposure to the agent, allergic reactions usually follow repeated application of the medication. Thus a delay in time occurs between the reaction to the use of a particular drug and the development of a state of hypersensitivity. This delay in time can be weeks, months, or years and is referred to as the *induction period*.

Once the hypersensitivity state is established, further instillation of the agent serves only to aggravate the allergic response. In the skin, allergic reactions may consist of edema, redness, vesiculation, scaling, and oozing, depending on the patient's sensitivity. In the conjunctiva the most common reaction is either marked chemosis or swelling or low-grade congestion and redness of the conjunctival tissues. Differentiation should be made between an allergic response and an ocular irritation caused by the drug. Some patients with allergies complain of itchiness. In many cases, however, differentiation between the two can be made only by a smear of the discharge of the conjunctiva that reveals the typical cell of an allergic response: the eosinophil.

One of the most common ophthalmic preparations to cause allergic reactions of the skin of the eyelid is atropine. Of the antibiotics, neomycin is most likely to create a hypersensitivity state and induce an allergic response (Figure 4.2).

Toxic reactions

Some drugs can produce irreversible damage within the eye or cause systemic disturbances within the human body. Echothiophate iodide (Phospholine Iodide), used in glaucoma, can cause cataracts, iris cysts, and retinal detachments. If this drug is absorbed systemically in sufficient quantities, it may cause nausea, vomiting, diarrhea, bladder cramps, and cardiac irregularities. One can reduce systemic absorption of eye medication by applying gentle finger pressure to the inner corner of the eyelids, over the lacrimal sac, for 1 minute when instilling drops. This will prevent drops from passing through the nasolacrimal duct to the back of the throat, where they are absorbed.

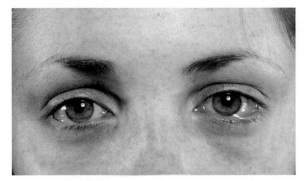

Figure 4.2 Allergic conjunctivitis with swelling of the bulbar conjunctiva.
(Reproduced from Spalton D, Hitchings R, Hunter P: Atlas of clinical ophthalmology. 3rd ed. St Louis: Mosby, 2004, with permission.)

Discoloration of the eye

Pigmentation of the conjunctiva may occur after the prolonged use of epinephrine, silver nitrate, or silver–protein compound (Argyrol). Epinephrine (Adrenalin) causes black spots in the lower conjunctival sac. Silver–protein produces a slate-silver discoloration of the conjunctiva.

Undesirable side effects

Some undesirable side effects may occur. For example, topically applied steroids can:

- Raise the intraocular pressure and cause glaucoma
- Potentiate the growth of viruses, which in herpes simplex infection can cause widespread corneal damage
- Potentiate the growth of bacteria
- Cause delay in wound healing

Pigmentary changes in the macula with loss of vision may occur in patients using chloroquine (antimalarial also used in treating rheumatoid arthritis and systemic lupus erythematosus), phenothiazines (antipsychotic) or indometacin (a nonsteroidal antiinflammatory drug [NSAID]). Oral contraceptive agents may cause migraine-like syndromes, as well as retinal vascular occlusions. Cataracts can occur after the use of antiglaucoma medication such as echothiophate iodide.

Idiosyncrasy

An idiosyncrasy is a constitutional peculiarity in which an individual reacts in a bizarre fashion to a drug. For example, an unexpected reaction to cocaine may occur and the person may develop tremors, motor excitability, or convulsions and may even collapse.

Loss of effect by inactivation

Some ophthalmic solutions may lose their potency if not stored properly. For example, if exposed to light and heat, epinephrine turns brown and loses its effect. Patients receiving epinephrine derivatives should be warned of this contingency and told to keep their eyedrops in a cool, dark place, such as the refrigerator. Prostaglandins are heat sanative.

Spread of infection

In some offices, hospitals, or clinics, where a single bottle is used for a group of patients, the dropper easily can become contaminated. Consequently, infection may spread from patient to patient. This hazard can be eliminated by using small sterile disposable bottles of medication or by limiting the use of the eyedrops or ointment to one individual. When eyedrops are used, care must be exercised that the tip of the eyedropper does not touch the lashes or the eye, so that contamination of the dropper and the eye solution is avoided (Figure 4.3). Some regulatory commissions recommend that bottles of ocular medications be discarded after being opened for 28 days.

PRESCRIPTION WRITING

In some US states the pharmacy boards require that all prescriptions be written as printed or typed (but not as cursive) on special approved prescription paper that protects against altering. Other regulatory regulations may require that prescriptions be electronically written/transmitted. Ophthalmic assistants should be knowledgeable on their state's requirements.

Physicians use many symbols for writing prescriptions. These symbols provide a direct communication from the physician to the pharmacist. The use of Latin symbols today is an anachronism, yet several Latin symbols are retained because of tradition and for brevity (Table 4.2). The following is the format for prescription writing; the setup is shown in Figure 4.4.

1. The patient's name, address, and date of prescription
2. The name of the drug and the percentage of concentration or the dosage of each unit (the drug usually is written out in full to avoid any confusion)
3. The amount of the drug to be supplied, headed by the symbol M or Mitte, which signifies the quantity
4. Sig or S, from the Latin *signa*, "to mark," or in English, "label," which indicates to the pharmacist what directions to label on the medicine
5. The signature of the physician with notation "substitution permitted" or "dispense as written"

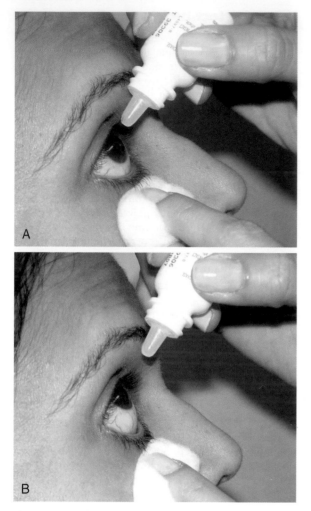

Figure 4.3 Instillation of eyedrops. (A) Incorrect method. Note contamination of tip of bottle by lashes. (B) Correct method. Note tip of bottle is held free of globe and lashes.

6. Possibly some notation at the bottom of the prescription, for example, "may be repeated 2 times," "refill prn for 1 year," or "no refill."

AUTONOMIC DRUGS

The body contains an involuntary nervous system, which is not under our direct control. This system acts to protect the body, provide nutrition and elimination, and carry on daily regulatory activity. The autonomic nervous system is affected by our emotional behavior. The typical "fear" reaction causes our pupils to dilate, our skin to sweat, and even our hair to stand on end.

Table 4.2 Abbreviations and symbols used in prescription writing

Abbreviation or symbol	Meaning
RX	take thou
g	gram
h	hour (*hora*)
q	every
hs	bedtime (*hora somni*)
qs	quantity sufficient
od	right eye (*oculus dexter*)
os	left eye (*oculus sinister*)
ou	both eyes (*oculi uterque*)
mg	milligram
<	less than
>	more than
aa	equal parts (*ana*)
Sol	solution
Ung	ointment
ʒ	dram
oz	ounce
tsp	teaspoon
gt, gtt	drop, drops (*gutta, guttae*)
M	mix (*misce*)
bid	twice a day (*bis in die*)
tid	three times a day (*ter in die*)
qid	four times a day (*quater in die*)
q4h	every 4 hours
ac	before meals (*ante cibum*)
pc	after meals (*post cibum*)
non rep	do not repeat (*non repetatur*)
ad lib	as much as wanted (*ad libitum*)
ss	half (*semis*)
aq	water
prn	as the situation demands (*pro re nata*)

Dr John Doe

170 Bloor Street West
Cleveland, Ohio

Name:	Miss J. White
Address:	227 Sankta Ave.

℞ Date: Jan. 4 Year

Inscription:	Diamox tab. 250 mg
Subscription:	M: 100
Signa:	Sig.: Tab. t.i.d.
Signature:	John Doe, M.D.

Substitution Permitted / Dispense as written

Repeat x2

Figure 4.4 Example of a prescription form.

The *autonomic nervous system* is subdivided into the *sympathetic* and *parasympathetic* nervous systems. Drugs that mimic the action of these two opposing types of involuntary nervous systems are said to be *sympathomimetic* and *parasympathomimetic*, respectively. Sympathomimetic drugs such as epinephrine and phenylephrine act directly on the end organ; they are sometimes called *adrenergic agents*. Parasympathomimetic drugs either act on the end organ in a manner similar to that of acetylcholine or interfere with the action of the enzyme *cholinesterase*, which destroys the acetylcholine normally produced in the tissues. Pilocarpine acts directly on the end organ, whereas eserine, dipivefrin (DP), and echothiophate iodide represent inhibitors of cholinesterase. Some drugs act on the end organ to block the action of the parasympathetic system; they are called *parasympatholytic (cholinergic blocking) agents*. Atropine, homatropine, and cyclopentolate are representative of this group.

Autonomic drugs that affect the eyes are divided into mydriatic, cycloplegic, and miotic agents, which comprise most of the commonly used eye medications.

Mydriatic and cycloplegic agents

Mydriatic drops act on the iris musculature and serve to dilate the pupils. *Cycloplegic* drops act not only on the iris by dilating the pupil but also on the ciliary body, paralyzing the fine focusing muscles so that the eye is no longer able to accommodate for near vision (Figure 4.5). Cycloplegic drops are essential in the refraction of children's eyes and for iritis therapy. Mydriatic agents are primarily used to dilate the pupil for intraocular examinations.

Mydriatic agents

Mydriatic agents with little or no cycloplegic effect are phenylephrine, hydroxyamphetamine, eucatropine hydrochloride, epinephrine, and cocaine.

Phenylephrine hydrochloride (Neo-Synephrine) is available in strengths of 2.5% and 10%. The latter exerts a rapid dilating effect in about 15 minutes and wears off in 1 to 2 hours. Adverse responses with 10% topical phenylephrine have occurred within 20 minutes of the last application of this drug. Some of these patients were treated with application of a cotton pledget of the drug, some by subconjunctival injection, and others by irrigation of the lacrimal sac. A number of deaths have resulted from myocardial infarction and some patients have required cardiac and pulmonary resuscitation for treatment of cardiac arrest. Another group of patients had a marked rise in blood pressure, tachycardia (fast heartbeat), or reflex bradycardia (slowing of the heart). The local ocular reaction reported was massive subconjunctival hemorrhage.

This drug should be used very cautiously or not at all in patients with heart disease, hypertension, aneurysm, or advanced atherosclerosis. Only the 2.5% solution should be used in older adults and in infants. Phenylephrine hydrochloride dilating drops are not recommended for use in low-birthweight infants. The 10% solution should not be used for irrigation. When the drug is used, a cotton pledget should be held over the lacrimal sac for 1 to 2 minutes. Patients who are taking antidepressants or monoamine oxidase (MAO) inhibitors should be treated with caution. These patients may exhibit a significant increase in heart rate.

Phenylephrine is used most commonly as an adjunct to the parasympatholytic drugs (for example, tropicamide [Mydriacyl] and cyclopentolate [Cyclogyl]) to dilate the pupil for ophthalmoscopy. Despite these serious complications with 10% phenylephrine, no serious adverse effects have been reported with the ophthalmic use of 2.5%, though dizziness, fast, irregular or pounding heartbeats, increased blood pressure, and trembling have been reported.

Epinephrine (Adrenalin) exerts a mild mydriatic effect.

Cocaine is primarily a strong anesthetic agent but also exerts a mild mydriatic effect. It can be used to establish the diagnosis of Horner syndrome. It allows one to determine whether a small pupil is part of this syndrome or whether it is due to other causes such as a congenital asymmetry of pupil size (physiologic anisocoria).

The drugs that act as pure mydriatic agents exert their effect by stimulating the dilator muscle of the iris.

Cycloplegic agents

Cycloplegic agents act by paralyzing the sphincter muscle of the iris, and thereby producing iris dilation, and by paralyzing the ciliary muscle, which inactivates accommodation.

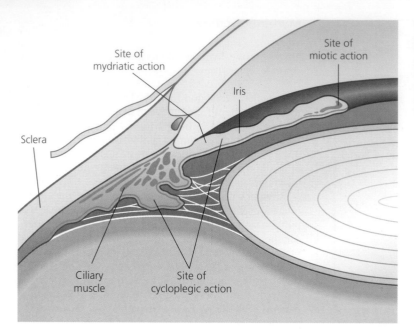

Figure 4.5 Sites of action of mydriatic, cycloplegic, and miotic agents. Mydriatic drugs act on the dilator muscle of the iris. Cycloplegic drugs act by inhibiting the sphincter muscle of the iris and by paralyzing the ciliary muscle. Miotic drugs act by stimulating the sphincter muscle of the iris, causing the pupil to constrict.

Examples of cycloplegic agents are atropine, homatropine, scopolamine, cyclopentolate, and tropicamide.

Atropine (Isopto Atropine, Atropine-Care, generic), available as 0.5% and 1% solutions and ointment, is one of the most powerful cycloplegic and mydriatic agents. After atropine has been instilled in an adult eye, it requires 10 to 14 days for accommodation to return and the pupil to return to its normal size. With children the local effects on the eye are similar but systemic complications are more common. The side effects of systemic absorption in children consist of rapid pulse, fever, flushing, and mouth dryness. Systemic absorption of atropine can be reduced by applying pressure over the lacrimal sac. Atropine may cause allergic manifestations in the form of an eczematoid rash around the eye and conjunctival injection. Parents should be instructed in the method of giving the drops and in observing for signs of local or systemic toxicity. Adverse reactions should be reported immediately to the ophthalmologist's office so that proper steps can be taken.

Homatropine (Isopto Homatropine, generic) is a weaker cycloplegic than atropine and is available in strengths of 2% and 5%. Its effect wears off faster than atropine and accommodation returns in 1 to 3 days.

Scopolamine (Isopto Hyoscine) is midway between atropine and homatropine in duration of action. Scopolamine produces fewer allergic responses than atropine and thus is used as a substitute for it.

Cyclopentolate (Cyclogyl, Cylate, AK-Pentolate, generic) is available in strengths of 0.5%, 1%, and 2%. It has a rapid onset of effect (30 minutes) and a duration of action of 6 to 24 hours, which makes it an ideal agent for office use.

Occasionally children can show signs of systemic toxicity not unlike that seen with atropine.

Tropicamide (Mydriacyl, Tropicacyl, generic), 0.5% and 1%, exerts its effects in 20 to 40 minutes and wears off in 4 to 6 hours. It is a relatively weak agent for paralyzing accommodation and is used primarily for its dilating ability when ophthalmoscopic examination is required.

Cycloplegics are used in the treatment of iritis to relieve ciliary muscle spasm and produce pupillary dilation. The latter is important in preventing the iris from binding down to the lens to form posterior synechiae. These agents are commonly used to inactivate the ciliary muscle for the purpose of objective refraction (Table 4.3). The eyes of darkly pigmented persons dilate with difficulty and hence require stronger concentrations and repeated instillations to obtain an adequate effect. Drugs such as atropine and homatropine are not used routinely in adult eye refraction because of the prolonged delay in accommodation and pupillary function.

Miotics

Miotics act by stimulating the sphincter muscle of the iris, which in turn causes constriction of the pupil (see Figure 4.5). These agents are used in:

- The treatment of open-angle glaucoma because they improve the outflow of aqueous humor from the anterior chamber of the eye
- Angle-closure glaucoma because they withdraw the congestion of iris tissue from the angle structures

Table 4.3 Routines for common cycloplegic agents

Drug	Strength	Frequency
Atropine	Younger than 2 yr, 0.5% Older than 2 yr, 1%	Under 5 yr, three times daily for 3 days before examination
Homatropine	2%, 5%	One drop every 15 min for four applications 1 hour before examination
Cyclopentolate	0.5%, 1%, 2%	One drop every 5 min for two applications 30 min before examination
Tropicamide	0.5%, 1%	One drop every 5 min for two applications 20 min before examination

- The management of convergent strabismus by reducing accommodative effort (used in place of glasses, especially for children younger than 2 years)
- The treatment of accommodative insufficiency, in which they may play a small role

Direct-acting miotics

Pilocarpine hydrochloride (Isopto Carpine, Pilopine-HS Gel, generic) may range in strength from 0.25% to 6% and have a duration of action of 4 to 6 hours. Pilocarpine is a stable, inexpensive, and reliable drug. The local side effects may consist of:

- Ciliary spasm, which may produce a headache, especially in young patients
- Decreased vision in patients with cataracts inasmuch as the pupil is made smaller, which allows less light to enter the eye
- Allergic or toxic reactions that involve the lids and conjunctiva

Systemic side effects are uncommon. Pilocarpine is most commonly used in the chronic care management of open-angle glaucoma and acute care treatment of angle-closure glaucoma.

Carbachol (Isopto Carbachol) is available in strengths of 1.5% and 3% and has a slightly longer duration of action than does pilocarpine. It is absorbed poorly through the cornea and is usually prescribed for patients who are allergic to pilocarpine or for those whose condition cannot be adequately controlled by pilocarpine.

Cholinesterase inhibitors

Cholinesterase inhibitors are drugs that inactivate an enzyme in the body called *cholinesterase*. As a result,

another chemical, called *acetylcholine*, which is normally inactivated by cholinesterase, is freely permitted to exert its effects. The effect of acetylcholine is similar to that of the direct-acting miotics.

Physostigmine is found in strengths from 0.25% to 0.5%. It is used more frequently in the ointment form because drops are unstable and irritating to the eye. It is a fairly powerful miotic and is frequently combined with pilocarpine in resistant cases of glaucoma. There is a high incidence of allergy to physostigmine. Combinations of miotics are generally not recommended. However, the combination of pilocarpine and physostigmine medication is sometimes advocated because these two drugs are able to reinforce each other. Physostigmine is not commercially available in the United States.

Echothiophate iodide (Phospholine Iodide), 0.03% to 0.25%, is a powerful and long-acting agent. It has been shown to produce cataracts and iris cysts with prolonged usage. It should be kept refrigerated because it deteriorates at room temperature.

Side effects

The long-acting anticholinesterase agents are the most likely to produce side effects both locally (in the eye) and systemically. *Local effects* include:

- Ocular discomfort and pain resulting from ciliary body spasm (most apparent during the initial phase of treatment, usually subsiding as treatment continues)
- Induced myopia with blurred vision for distance
- Cataracts
- Retinal detachment
- Iris cysts

Systemic effects include:

- Headaches
- Sweating and salivation
- Nausea, vomiting, and diarrhea
- Lethargy and fatigue
- Cardiac arrest and fall in blood pressure

DRUGS THAT LOWER INTRAOCULAR PRESSURE

With the introduction of *timolol maleate* (Timoptic, generic) in 1978 new programs of research toward pharmaceutical agents that do not affect the pupil or accommodation began. Timolol is a nonselective beta-adrenergic receptor blocker that acts to decrease the formation of aqueous humor. The drug is available in 0.25% and 0.5% strengths, and dosage ranges from 1 drop daily to 1 drop twice daily with or without other antiglaucoma medication.

Adverse reactions are generally uncommon, but if they are present and significant they may lead one to discontinue the medication. Ocular side effects include corneal anesthesia, a punctate keratopathy, and an allergic blepharoconjunctivitis. Systemic reactions consist of bronchospasm in those with underlying pulmonary disease, bradycardia, hypotension, central nervous system disturbances (for example, confusion and hallucinations), and gastrointestinal disturbances (for example, nausea and diarrhea). Timolol should be used with caution in patients with known contraindications to systemic use of beta-adrenergic receptor blocking agents, such as patients with obstructive pulmonary disease (for example, asthma and emphysema) and cardiovascular disease (for example, congestive heart failure, bradycardia, heart block, and hypotension).

Because of its excellent therapeutic response, its low frequency of application, and its generally uncommon adverse reactions, timolol has gained widespread use in the ophthalmic community. Levobunolol (Betagan, generic) is equivalent to timolol. Carteolol (generic) is also available and has fewer adverse effects on lipids.

In an attempt to decrease the systemic side effects so that it can be used in patients with asthma and emphysema, betaxolol (Betoptic S, generic), a selective beta-blocker, was developed. Although fewer pulmonary effects are seen with this drug, they have not been totally eliminated. In addition, the fall in intraocular pressure is not as great with betaxolol as with timolol, a nonselective beta-blocker.

A sympathomimetic agent, *dipivefrin hydrochloride* (Propine, generic), is available in a 0.1% concentration for application of 1 drop twice daily. The drug has a 17 times greater penetration through the cornea than epinephrine alone; therefore, the amount necessary to achieve a similar therapeutic response is significantly less. This reduces the systemic side effects, which may include an elevation in blood pressure, tachycardia, and headache. Ocular side effects may consist of an allergic blepharoconjunctivitis, a punctate keratopathy, and cystoid macular edema. The latter condition is seen in aphakic patients and has been reported to occur in up to 30%. The macular edema is reversible when the medication is discontinued.

Other drugs used to lower intraocular pressures include apraclonidine hydrochloride (Iopidine), which is available in 1% strength for postlaser intraocular pressure spikes and 0.5% for long-term use. Topical dorzolamide 2% (Trusopt) is a major advance in decreasing aqueous inflow. Its side effects are few. A newer group of prostaglandins is available and effective in one-time daily doses. Latanoprost 0.005% (Xalatan) increases uveoscleral flow, but at the risk of changing iris color. Others that have followed in this group include travoprost (Travatan, Travatan-Z) and bimatoprost (Lumigan). They are available in 2.5 mL, 5 mL, and 7.5 mL sizes. By using once daily there is less toxicity to the cornea. Cosopt is a combination of dorzolamide

hydrochloride and timolol maleate. Combination drugs that are on the market include Combigan (brimonidine tartrate 0.2% and timolol maleate) and Simbrinza (brinzolamide 1.0% and brimonidine tartrate 0.2%).

The drug armamentarium against glaucoma has been greatly aided by the use of drugs, taken orally or intravenously, that lower the intraocular pressure. Those commonly used are the carbonic anhydrase inhibitors, glycerol, urea, and mannitol.

The *carbonic anhydrase inhibitors* block the formation of aqueous humor and thereby lower the intraocular pressure. Examples include acetazolamide (Diamox, generic), 125-mg, 250-mg tablets, and 500-g timed-release capsules; dichlorphenamide (Diclofenamide Daranide), 50-mg tablets; and methazolamide (Neptazane, generic), 25- to 50-mg tablets. Side effects of these drugs are:

- Numbness and tingling of the hands, feet, and tongue
- Drowsiness and fatigue
- Kidney stones
- Gastrointestinal upsets (nausea and vomiting)
- Mild skin eruptions
- Blood disturbances

Glycerin is a thick, viscous liquid in a 50% solution given in an oral dosage of 1 to 1.5 g/kg of body weight and is used to lower the intraocular pressure in acute narrow-angle glaucoma and before intraocular surgery. Because of its overly sweet taste, it is mixed with orange juice or lemon juice to make it more palatable. It can cause nausea, vomiting, or headaches.

Mannitol (Osmitrol) is administered intravenously in 5% to 20% solution, with a total dosage of 0.5 to 2 g/kg of body weight given over a period of 30 to 45 minutes. It is used interchangeably with urea. Along with urea and glycerol, mannitol has a large molecular structure that draws fluid out of the eye and other tissues into the vascular tree of the body.

ANESTHETICS

Topical anesthetics

Topical anesthetics in drop or ointment form are applied directly to the eye to abolish corneal sensation. Surface anesthesia of the cornea permits the application of instruments such as the tonometer for the measurement of intraocular pressure. Topical anesthetics are also used to perform surgery on the eye, remove foreign bodies, and facilitate examination with lenses such as the goniolens. Cocaine, the prototype of the group, is a naturally occurring drug. The remainder of topical anesthetics are synthetic. Cocaine is rarely used as an anesthetic because it causes damage to the corneal epithelium and produces pupillary dilation. However, it is considered useful when removal of the corneal epithelium is desired, as in epithelial debridement for dendritic keratitis. Commonly used topical anesthetics are proparacaine hydrochloride (Proxymetacaine, Alcaine, Paracaine, Ophthaine, Ophthetic, generic) 0.5%; tetracaine hydrochloride (Altacaine, Pontocaine, Tetcaine, generic) 0.5%; cocaine 1% to 4%; benoxinate hydrochloride. The suffix "-caine" appended to the name of the drug usually indicates that the drug is an anesthetic.

An inflamed eye is much more difficult to anesthetize because the blood vessels carry away the anesthetic. For mild anesthesia, such as tonometry, 1 or 2 drops are sufficient, but to remove a foreign body deeply embedded in the cornea, more drops may be required at 1-minute intervals.

To avoid a self-inflicted corneal abrasion it is important that the patient be cautioned against rubbing the eye for a short period after topical anesthesia.

Side effects

Local anesthetics are capable of producing contact allergy. Some anesthetics, such as butacaine, have fallen into disfavor because of a frequent tendency to produce allergic reactions. Side effects do occur, though they are minimal with proparacaine and tetracaine, but cocaine has significant side effects, including:

- Irregularities in the corneal epithelium
- Restlessness and delirium
- Irregular respiration, chills, and fever
- Convulsions
- Cardiovascular disorders

Toxic reactions to cocaine result from central nervous system stimulation and may require the rapid administration of a short-acting sedative to counteract them.

Injectable anesthetics

Local anesthetics by injection are used in ophthalmology to produce:

- Anesthesia of the globe
- Anesthesia of the eyelid
- Paralysis of the muscles that move the eye and the eyelid
- Paralysis of the facial muscles

Commonly used agents are procaine hydrochloride (Novocain) 1% to 4%, lidocaine hydrochloride (Xylocaine) 1% to 2%, and prilocaine hydrochloride (Citanest) 1% to 2%. These agents may be combined with epinephrine, which constricts the blood vessels. The purpose of producing vasoconstriction is to reduce the vascularity of tissues and minimize bleeding. These agents also reduce the amount of local anesthetic absorbed by the blood vessels, thereby prolonging the duration of anesthesia. In addition, local anesthetics may be combined with hyaluronidase, which spreads the anesthetic throughout the tissues, thereby producing more prompt and widespread anesthesia.

Side effects

Injectable anesthetic agents may cause:

- Depression of blood pressure
- Depression of respiration
- Stimulation of the central nervous system, leading to nervousness, dizzy spells, nausea, and convulsions
- Depression of the central nervous system, leading to respiratory or circulatory collapse

Management of toxic side effects

The ophthalmic assistant should be prepared to render assistance in the event of a reaction to a local anesthetic.

Fainting

The following action should be taken when a patient faints. Check the airway and breathing. If indicated, call 911 and begin rescue breathing and cardiopulmonary resuscitation (CPR) (see Chapter 49). Loosen tight clothing around their neck. Raise the person's feet, about 12 inches, above the level of the heart. If the person has vomited turn the head to the side to prevent choking. Keep the person lying down for a minimum of 10 to 15 minutes in a cool and quiet area. If this is not possible, sit the person forward with the head between the knees.

Central nervous system stimulation

If tremors or convulsions occur, the ophthalmic assistant should attempt to restrain the patient to avoid self-injury. Again, encumbrances around the neck should be loosened. The ophthalmologist may wish to give the patient diazepam (Valium) to control the reaction, so this should be available and ready to use.

Respiratory emergency

A patient who has difficulty in breathing should be watched carefully. If respiration ceases, artificial resuscitation may become necessary. Today, mouth-to-mouth resuscitation is the treatment of choice. Human immunodeficiency virus (HIV) precautions should be adhered to.

Allergic reaction

Severe allergic reactions or idiosyncrasies to drugs may occur that require immediate specific therapy. This is particularly important to the ophthalmologist in view of the increasing number of surgical procedures and fluorescein angiographic examinations being performed in the physician's office. Any patient developing generalized itching, skin rash, difficulty in breathing, or a rapid and weak pulse after administration of a drug should be considered as having an allergic reaction.

Once an acute allergic reaction is suspected, the following prompt treatment is indicated:

- Epinephrine injected subcutaneously or intramuscularly
- Oxygen
- Corticosteroids injected intravenously
- Tracheostomy for laryngeal edema not responding to the aforementioned methods

The ophthalmic assistant should know where to immediately procure and have available for the ophthalmologist:

- Oxygen
- Epinephrine
- Diazepam
- Intravenous cortisone
- Spirits of ammonia or smelling salts
- Syringes with needles

ANTIALLERGIC AND ANTIINFLAMMATORY AGENTS

Corticosteroids

Corticosteroids are hormones that either are derived from the adrenal gland or are synthetically produced. Cortisone was the first hormone to be isolated. Other steroid preparations are modifications of cortisone, developed to improve and minimize the side effects. For diseases of the eye, steroids are used primarily because they reduce the inflammatory and exudative reaction of diseased tissues. In this regard they are invaluable because they reduce swelling, redness, cellular reaction, and, the final stage of tissue repair, scarring.

Steroids may be given topically or systemically (Table 4.4). Topical steroids are generally used for disorders involving the anterior segment of the eye. Systemic steroids are used for diseases of the posterior segment of the eye and for acute allergic reactions of the eyelids (Table 4.5).

Temporal arteritis

Although steroids are useful in a large variety of ocular conditions, they must be administered with good indication, by the proper route (Table 4.6) and under the supervision of a physician. These precautions are necessary because of the sinister complications of these agents both in the eye and in the body (Table 4.7).

Table 4.4 Topical steroid preparations

Drug	Concentration (%)
Cortisone acetate suspension	0.5
Cortisone acetate ointment	1.5
Hydrocortisone acetate suspension	0.5, 2.5
Hydrocortisone acetate ointment	1.5
Prednisolone acetate	0.12, 1
Prednisolone phosphate	0.125, 1
Dexamethasone phosphate	0.1
Dexamethasone ointment	0.5
Betamethasone solution	0.5

Table 4.5 Systemic steroids commonly used and their equivalent dose

Drug	Dose (mg)
Cortisone acetate	25
Hydrocortisone	20
Prednisone	5
Prednisolone	5
Triamcinolone	4
Methylprednisolone	4
Paramethasone	2
Dexamethasone	0.75
Betamethasone	0.5

If a patient is receiving steroids, the ophthalmic assistant should inquire into his or her medical background. Patients with conditions of diabetes, hypertension, tuberculosis, and peptic ulcers, if given steroids systemically, often will have an exacerbation of their disease.

Steroid therapy is used in the following eye diseases:

- Contact dermatitis of the eyelids and conjunctiva
- Blepharitis
- Phlyctenular conjunctivitis and keratitis
- Ocular pemphigus
- Vernal conjunctivitis
- Acne rosacea keratitis
- Interstitial keratitis
- Sclerosing keratitis
- Chemical burns of the cornea and conjunctiva
- Marginal corneal ulcers

Table 4.6 Common routes of steroid administration for ocular inflammation

Condition	Route
Conjunctivitis	Topical
Blepharitis	Topical
Episcleritis	Topical
Keratitis	Topical
Scleritis	Topical and systemic
Anterior uveitis	Topical and subconjunctival
Posterior uveitis	Systemic and subconjunctival
Endophthalmitis	Systemic and subconjunctival
Optic neuritis	Systemic
Temporal arteritis	Systemic
Sympathetic ophthalmia	Systemic and topical

- Iritis
- Iridocyclitis
- Most forms of posterior uveitis
- Sympathetic ophthalmia
- Herpes zoster ophthalmicus
- Scleritis and episcleritis
- Pseudotumor of the orbit
- Temporal arteritis
- Optic neuritis

Nonsteroidal antiinflammatory drugs

Topical ophthalmic preparations of *nonsteroidal antiinflammatory drugs (NSAIDs)* have been demonstrated to possess a variety of properties of potential benefit to ocular patients. These include analgesic properties, antiinflammatory properties, the ability to prevent intraoperative miosis during cataract surgery, and efficacy in the treatment and prevention of cystoid macular edema. An important pharmacotherapeutic action is the blockage of prostaglandin synthesis.

NSAIDs have been shown to be effective in decreasing ocular symptoms of allergy. The medication can be used as a substitute for topical steroids. Although not as potent as steroids in the relief of allergic symptoms, NSAIDs have a significantly reduced complication rate. Studies have shown that ketorolac (Acular) and diclofenac sodium (Voltaren) are effective in the treatment of ocular pain associated with refractive surgery such as radial keratotomy, photorefractive keratectomy, or automated lamellar keratoplasty and laser-assisted in situ keratomileusis (LASIK). The substantial pain relief significantly decreases the need for oral analgesics and greatly improves patient quality of life in the days immediately following surgery. NSAIDs may cause burning and stinging on instillation. Hypersensitivity reactions are uncommon, especially with preservative-free NSAIDs.

Mast cell stabilizers

Mast cells play an important role in allergic reactions by liberating a variety of chemical mediators such as histamine.

Table 4.7 Side effects of steroids

Ocular effects		Systemic effects
From local application	**From prolonged systemic use**	
Glaucoma	Decreased resistance to infection	Water and salt retention
Proliferation of bacteria	Delayed wound healing	Mental disturbance
Overgrowth of fungi	Papilledema	Hypertension
Proliferation of viruses, especially herpes simplex	Edema of face and eyelids	Sweating
Decreased wound healing	Cataracts	Generalized weakness
Cataracts	Glaucoma	Wasting of skeletal muscles Demineralization of bones Thrombophlebitis Delayed wound healing Bleeding problems Menstrual irregularities Acne Decreased resistance to infection Growth retardation in children

The mediators are responsible for reducing the symptoms and signs of allergy, such as itching, redness, and swelling. *Mast cell stabilizers* prevent the degranulation of mast cells and hence decrease the clinical features. They are most effective clinically when given as a prophylactic treatment before the degranulation of mast cells. Available mast cell stabilizers include cromolyn sodium (Crolom, generic), lodoxamide tromethamine (Alomide), and olopatadine hydrochloride (Patanol). Lodoxamide also inhibits the attraction of eosinophils.

Antihistamines

Antihistamines are effective in relieving the clinical features of acute allergy. They act by blocking histamine receptors. Medications in this class include levocabastine (Livostin) and olopatadine (Patanol).

Antihistamines have a dual role not only in blocking histamine receptors but also preventing release of cytokines and eosinophils that are involved in an allergic response. Cromolyn sodium is an example.

Antiinfective preparations

Antiinfective agents have a wide range of activity against Gram-positive and Gram-negative organisms. They are active against superficial infections such as conjunctivitis, keratitis, corneal ulcers, blepharoconjunctivitis, meibomitis, and dacryocystitis.

There are three large families of antiinfective preparations: antibiotics, antiviral agents, and antifungal agents.

Antibiotics

Antibiotics are chemical substances that can inhibit growth of bacteria and other microorganisms. Some antibiotics act by inhibiting bacterial growth and are called *bacteriostatic agents,* whereas others act by directly killing bacteria and are therefore called *bactericidal agents.* Antibiotics can be differentiated into families. The most prominent are the *aminoglycoside antibiotics* (examples include tobramycin and gentamicin) and the *fluoroquinolone antibiotics* (such as besifloxacin, ofloxacin, and ciprofloxacin).

Bactericidal agents commonly in use are penicillin, streptomycin, polymyxin B, bacitracin, neomycin, vancomycin, ampicillin, tobramycin, gentamicin, ofloxacin (Ocuflox), and ciprofloxacin. Bacteriostatic agents in common use include tetracycline, erythromycin, sulfonamides, and amphotericin B.

Ideally an antibiotic should be selected when the organism responsible for the infection is identified and its sensitivity to antibiotics established. However, it is impractical to withhold therapy until cultures are made and sensitivity is determined. Early treatment is as important as selecting the right drug for the offending agent. Therefore, most ophthalmologists use broad-spectrum antibiotics to treat infections around the eyes until cultures and smears have been made and sensitivity has been determined.

Many patients are seen in an eye doctor's office with an unresolved bacterial infection of the eye because of indiscriminate use of antibiotics. Often the infective component clears but a hypersensitivity develops to the very medication the patient is industriously pouring into the eye. The more medication put into the eye, the worse the situation becomes. Hypersensitivity reactions from antibiotics most commonly occur with the use of compounds that contain neomycin, but they also result from the use of sulfa derivatives.

Another complication in the treatment of bacterial infection of the eye results from *inadequate dosage* and *infrequency of administration* of antibiotics. Antibiotics are given only occasionally by the systemic route for the treatment of ocular infections because greater concentrations of the drug can be achieved topically or subconjunctivally. With topical administration, drops are preferred to ointments because drops do not retain the discharge or interfere with vision. Many infections, however, persist because antibiotic drops are not given frequently enough.

The newest generation of antibiotics is the *quinolones.* The classification has been difficult and depends on their broader spectrum of activity and the reduction in microbial resistance. Two new fourth-generation quinolones at the writing of this text are moxifloxacin (Vigamox) and gatifloxacin (Zymar). These are added to the previous third-generation quinolones levofloxacin (Quixin) and second-generation ciprofloxacin (Ciloxan) and ofloxacin (Ocuflox). All of the quinolones have a common basic cortelone core. More fluoroquinolones are coming on the market to help patients. These are aimed at increasing the bacterial coverage and reducing bacterial resistance (Table 4.8).

Topical antibiotics chosen for ocular infections are those with a wide spectrum of activity and those that are seldom used systemically. The advantage of these broad-spectrum antibiotics is that they provide complete coverage and

Table 4.8 Ocular fluoroquinolones

Generation	Drug	Concentration (%)
4th	Moxifloxacin (Vigamox)	0.5
4th	Gatifloxacin (Zymar)	0.3
3rd	Levofloxacin (Quixin)	0.5
2nd	Ciprofloxacin (Ciloxan)	0.3
2nd	Ofloxacin (Ocuflox)	0.3

minimize the dangers of hypersensitivity reactions. Antibiotics such as fluoroquinolones, bacitracin, and polymyxin B are frequently used because they affect both Gram-positive and Gram-negative bacteria.

Recent studies have shown that the frequent topical application of fluoroquinolone antibiotics is effective in the treatment of corneal ulcers. In the past, specifically made "fortified antibiotics" were the mainstay of corneal ulcer therapy. These drugs had to be formulated by a pharmacist, which frequently delayed the initial treatment. The fluoroquinolone antibiotics are available in over-the-counter preparations ready for treatment.

Frequent application of ciprofloxacin (Ciloxan, generic) in an eye with an epithelial defect, such as a corneal ulcer, has occasionally been associated with precipitates. These will gradually clear when the drug is discontinued.

Continuous indiscriminate use of antibiotic drops may lead to the development of resistant strains of bacteria. Also, other strains of bacteria may proliferate if they do not fall within the sensitivity spectrum of the drops used.

Systemic antibiotics become necessary when the internal or deeper structures of the eye or adjacent tissue are invaded by bacteria. Conditions such as endophthalmitis, orbital cellulitis, or chorioretinitis may require judicious use of systemic antibiotics. Such antibiotics, however, can cause serious side effects (Table 4.9). Chloramphenicol (Chloromycetin) in oral forms was formally withdrawn from the US market per the US Food and Drug Administration in July 2012 due to the risk of serious and life-threatening injuries such as bone morrow depression, aplastic anemia, and even death. Myasthenia-like syndromes, with induced weakness resembling myasthenia gravis, may occur with streptomycin, neomycin, kanamycin, polymyxin, bacitracin, and colistin. Skin

rashes may occur because of allergic reactions to the penicillin group of antibiotics and, on rare occasions, severe serum sickness, angioneurotic edema, and even death may result.

Sulfonamides have a wide spectrum of activity and are effective against some of the larger virus-like agents as well as bacteria. Hypersensitivity reactions to sulfa drugs may be severe, and patients should be questioned about any history of allergy to this drug before its use.

The most commonly used topical sulfonamides are acetyl sulfisoxazole (Gantrisin solution 4% and Gantrisin ointment) and sulfacetamide sodium (Sodium Sulamyd 10%, 30%; Bleph 10; Isopto Cetamide 15%; generic).

Antivirals

The antiviral agents as a group initially had been slow in developing. This is partly because the virus invades the cell structure; antivirals must therefore kill the virus without killing the cell and causing damage. By the time the virus has invaded, there is a time delay before signs or symptoms appear. Antiviral pharmaceuticals are used to treat virus-caused ophthalmic conditions such as herpes simples and herpes zoster.

Historic ophthalmic antivirals are:

- Idoxuridine [IDU] (Herplex, Stoxil) – Topical
- Vidarabine (Vira-A) – Topical

Some current ophthalmic antivirals are:

- Trifluridine [TFT] (Viroptic and generic) – Topical
- Acyclovir (Zovirax and generic) – Oral and intravenous
- Famciclovir – Oral
- Ganciclovir – Topical, intravenous

Ideally, an antiviral should have properties that can work on viruses without causing damage to human cells, is cost effective, and is readily available. As we learn more about virus behavior this may come about.

The first antiviral agent, 5-iodo-2-deoxyuridine, though no longer available in the United States, had been invaluable in the treatment of herpes simplex infections of the cornea. This drug, like the other antivirals, interferes with deoxyribonucleic acid (DNA) synthesis of the virus to produce a virus that cannot function as an infective agent. This drug frequently is referred to as idoxuridine (IDU), or its manufacturing trade names of Herplex or Stoxil may be used.

IDU is used topically for the treatment of herpes simplex and vaccinia keratitis. It is of greatest benefit against the epithelial forms of herpes simplex infections. No serious side effects or contraindications are known in the use of IDU as an ophthalmic solution. This drug is given by instilling 1 drop in the affected eye every hour during the day and every 2 hours during the night until the lesion has cleared. It should be stored in a cool place.

Vidarabine (Vira-A) 3% is an antiviral ophthalmic ointment, specifically for herpes simplex. It is useful for early cases of herpes simplex of the cornea and can be used in cases of herpes resistant to IDU. It does not appear to have any effect on other viruses.

Table 4.9 Some adverse effects of systemically administered antimicrobial drugs

Drug	Possible toxic effect
Ampicillin	Anaphylactic reactions
Clindamycin	Pseudomembranous colitis
Erythromycin	Stomatitis; gastrointestinal disturbance
Gentamicin	Hearing defect; kidney damage
Meticillin	Allergic reactions; rarely bone marrow depression and renal damage
Nafcillin	Similar to those of meticillin
Oxacillin	Similar to those of meticillin
Sulfisoxazole	Allergic reactions; bone marrow depression
Sulfacetamide	Similar to those of sulfisoxazole

Trifluorothymidine (TFT) or trifluridine (Viroptic), is an antiviral agent used in the treatment of herpes simplex keratitis. It is available as a 1% solution, and the usual dosing schedule is a frequency of every 2 hours when the patient is awake. TFT has been shown to effectively heal 97% of ulcers and to be highly effective in treating diseases resistant to IDU and adenosine arabinoside (Ara-A) or vidarabine. The drug's penetration of the cornea and anterior chamber has been shown to be superior to that of other antivirals.

Acyclovir (Zovirax) is a newer antiviral agent that is administered in oral form. The drug can be metabolized only in cells that have been infected by the herpes virus, and therefore uninfected human cells will not be affected by the drug. Acyclovir has been shown to be effective in shortening the course of disease in herpes zoster (shingles) and in severe cases of herpes simplex.

Other current antiviral agents for systemic or intravitreal administration include cidofovir – intravenous, foscarnet – intravenous, valacyclovir – oral, and valganciclovir – oral.

Antifungal agents

Fungal infections of the eye are uncommon, but when they do occur they can be devastating, especially when treatment is delayed. Antifungal agents generally act by binding to the fungal cell wall. This leads to changes in permeability that result in death of the organism. The most commonly used antifungal agents include the following three.

- Natamycin (Natacyn), or pimaricin, is available in a 5% suspension. Because this drug penetrates tissues very poorly, it is useful only when applied topically
- Amphotericin B (Fungizone) also can be administered topically, subconjunctivally, intravitreally, or intravenously. The drug is highly irritating when used topically and may be toxic to the kidneys when administered intravenously. Use of this drug should be reserved for severe infections or resistant organisms
- Ketoconazole (Nizoral) is available for oral administration. Unlike amphotericin, however, it is generally well tolerated. Significant adverse reactions include liver toxicity.

Antiparasitic agents

Acanthamoeba, a ubiquitous parasite found in soil and water, is capable of causing severe keratitis. The infection is most common as a complication of contact lens wear. Agents that have provided some success in the treatment of this parasite include dibrompropamidine 0.15%, polyhexamethylene biguanide (PHMB) 0.02%, chlorhexidine, and neomycin. Corticosteroids are contraindicated.

Decongestants

Decongestants are solutions that shrink the size of the conjunctival blood vessels and in doing so eliminate excess eye redness. These solutions are used to provide symptomatic relief of eye irritation and watering caused by hay fever, smog, and smoke and to relieve eye fatigue resulting from driving, excessive reading, and close work.

Some common decongestants are phenylephrine (Zincfrin solution, Prefrin, Neo-Synephrine), tetrahydrozoline (Visine), and naphazoline (Vasocon, Privine). A common result of use of these drugs is rebound hypersensitivity with recurring redness.

Decongestants are often called vasoconstrictors (such as phenylephrine) and may be contraindicated in infants and adults with narrow angles. They may bring on an attack of narrow-angle glaucoma. Also, a 10% dose may cause an increase in blood pressure or ventricular arrhythmia and even death.

Antiallergic agents

A number of pharmaceutical agents are specifically used during the allergy season (Table 4.10). Some are combinations of the previously mentioned decongestants and histamine blockers.

Table 4.10 Pharmaceuticals used in the treatment of seasonal allergic conjunctivitis

Drug category	Trade name	Generic name
Antihistamine	Optivar	Azelastine
Mast cell stabilizer	Crolom	Cromolyn
Antihistamine	Emadine	Emedastine
Antihistamine/mast cell stabilizer	Elestat	Epinastine
NSAID	Acular	Ketorolac
Antihistamine/mast cell stabilizer	Zaditor	Ketotifen
Antihistamine	Livostin	Levocabastine
Mast cell stabilizer	Alomide	Lodoxamide
Antihistamine/decongestant	Vasocon-A	Naphazoline/antazoline
Antihistamine/decongestant	Naphcon-A, Visine-A	Naphazoline/pheniramine
Antihistamine/mast cell stabilizer	Alocril	Nedocromil
Antihistamine/mast cell stabilizer	Patanol	Olopatadine
Mast cell stabilizer	Alamast	Pemirolast

NSAID, Nonsteroidal antiinflammatory drug.

CONTACT LENS SOLUTIONS

With the proliferation of contact lens solutions, three important factors should be considered in choosing a system: safety, efficacy, and cost. Most contact lens solutions contain more than 95% water. The solution formation depends on the addition of preservatives, wetting agents, buffers, surfactants, cleaners, and disinfectants.

Contact lens requirements call for disinfection but not sterilization; although the incidence of eye infection from contact lenses is low relative to millions of wearers, the hazard is always present. Sterilization is the complete destruction of all forms of microbial activity. Disinfection is the destruction of all vegetative bacterial cells, but does not include spores. Common contact lens solution preservatives include organomercurials (for example, thimerosal, chlorhexidine, and ethylenediaminetetraacetic acid [EDTA]).

Contact lens solutions can cause toxicity or hypersensitivity reactions manifested as conjunctival redness, punctate keratopathy, or corneal infiltrates. Therapy consists of recognizing the potential cause of these symptoms and switching contact lens solutions.

STAINS

Fluorescein is an ocular stain used to show defects or abrasions in the corneal epithelium. The pooling of fluorescein on small corneal defects is best seen by means of ultraviolet or cobalt blue light for illumination. The danger with this agent in solution form is contamination with *Pseudomonas aeruginosa (Bacillus pyocyaneus)*, which appears to flourish in fluorescein. Sterile dry fluorostrips are available commercially to prevent this complication. High-molecule fluorescein has been used with soft contact lenses. The high molecule of fluorescein does not penetrate the pore structure of the soft lens and consequently does not ruin the contact lens during examination.

Rose bengal is a red dye that has an affinity for degenerating epithelium. Similar to fluorescein, it will stain areas in which the epithelium has been sloughed off. The dye also stains cells that are damaged or unprotected by native mucoproteins. Unlike fluorescein, however, intact nonviable epithelial cells of the conjunctiva or cornea will stain brightly with rose bengal. The stain is helpful in making the diagnosis *of keratoconjunctivitis sicca* or other conditions associated with dryness of the conjunctiva and cornea. Paper strips are moistened with several drops of sterile balanced salt solution.

Other vital stains include *lissamine green*, which is generally available as sterile impregnated paper strips. The technique is simple. Apply a drop of sterile saline or artificial tear to the tip of the paper. Ask the patient to look up and insert the paper gently to the inferior conjunctiva.

Lissamine is used to stain dead and degenerating epithelial cells. Toxicity has not been reported in a 1% concentration. It acts similarly to rose bengal but is less irritating. It may be used to detect early dry eyes, which show stain of the nasal conjunctiva. It also may be used to detect a poor tight contact lens fit.

SIDE EFFECTS OF SYSTEMIC MEDICATION

Many oral medications can cause adverse effects on the cornea. Chloroquine, hydroxychloroquine, and amiodarone can cause a vortex keratopathy. Chloroquine can cause a bull's-eye maculopathy. Tamoxifen, canthaxanthin, and nitrofurantoin can cause maculopathies. Steroids may cause high intraocular pressures, cataracts, ptosis, and viral infections. Aspirin may cause retinal hemorrhages.

Questions for review and thought

1. What is meant by pH? What effect does it have on the patient's acceptance of a drug?
2. How can sterility of a drug be achieved?
3. What is the role of preservatives, and which are the commonly used preservatives?
4. What are the common routes of giving medication to obtain an effect on the eye?
5. What is meant by allergy?
6. How can contamination of eyedrops and spread of infection from eyedrops in the office or hospital be eliminated?
7. What information would be contained in a typical prescription for phenylephrine eyedrops, for acetazolamide tablets, and for atropine ointment?
8. What is the action of cycloplegic drugs? How does it differ from that of mydriatic drugs?

Continued

9. List some mydriatic and cycloplegic agents.
10. Name some clinical uses for miotic agents.
11. Name some systemic drugs that lower intraocular pressure.
12. Name some side effects of cortisone therapy.
13. Without referring to the text, list as many clinical uses for cortisone medication to the eyes as you can.
14. Define the major ocular drug categories and identify the categories of commonly used drugs.
15. What is the principal action of decongestants? Why do they "whiten" the eye?
16. Corticosteroids act to suppress inflammation. Name some topical steroid drops.
17. What topical drugs are most prone to create ocular allergies?
18. What are the side effects of giving atropine ointment to children?
19. Which ocular drugs require refrigeration?
20. What are the side effects of pilocarpine?
21. What are some of the side effects of acetazolamide?

Q Self-evaluation questions

True–false statements

Directions: Indicate whether the statement is true (**T**) or false (**F**).

1. Eyedrops penetrate the eye directly through the cornea and anterior chamber of the eye. **T** or **F**
2. Topical medication applied directly to the eye may be absorbed into the body system and produce side effects. **T** or **F**
3. Cycloplegic agents paralyze the sphincter muscle of the iris but do not interfere with the ciliary muscle. **T** or **F**

Missing words

Directions: Write in the missing word(s) in the following sentences.

4. Echothiophate iodide (Phospholine Iodide), which is used in glaucoma, belongs to the class of _____ inhibitors, which inactivate the enzyme in the body called _____.

5. The pupil dilates poorly with cycloplegics in those patients with darkly pigmented irises and in those persons with any of the following medical conditions: _____, _____, _____.

6. Another name for epinephrine is _____.

Choice-completion questions

Directions: Select the one best answer in each case.

7. The tonicity of an ophthalmic solution refers to the:
   a. concentration of the chemical in the solution.
   b. acid–base balance as noted by the pH.
   c. sterility as noted by the level of contamination.
   d. stability of the solution.
   e. solubility of fats.

8. In which of the following are steroids not administered systemically?
   a. Blepharitis
   b. Uveitis
   c. Endophthalmitis
   d. Optic neuritis
   e. Cranial or temporal arteritis

9. Which of the following agents is capable of controlling the herpes simplex organism?
   a. Chloramphenicol
   b. Gentamicin (Garamycin)
   c. Trifluridine (Viroptic)
   d. Homatropine
   e. Fluorescein

A Answers, notes, and explanations

1. **True.** Eye medication in drop form penetrates directly through the cornea by first passing through the epithelium, which acts as a barrier to most medications that are insoluble in fat. The drops must then have water-soluble properties to penetrate the remaining portion of the cornea. Thus agents that penetrate the eye well are those that have both fat- and water-soluble properties. Consequently, manufacturers have designed bases for solutions that will permit the penetration of these drops through the cornea into the anterior chamber of the eye. Eyedrops do not, however, penetrate far behind the crystalline lens of the eye and therefore do not reach the posterior portion of the globe.

2. **True.** A small quantity of drops may be absorbed through the conjunctival vessels but a large portion may pass through the nasolacrimal duct system and be absorbed by

A   Continued

the nasal mucosa directly into the bloodstream. The flush that is often produced when atropine is used in small children is a direct result of the systemic absorption of this drug. Pressure over the lacrimal sac with a cotton ball during the instillation of eyedrops will often prevent the passage of the drops into the nasolacrimal system and thus prevent systemic absorption of eye medication.

3. **False.** Cycloplegic agents such as homatropine, atropine, and cyclopentolate paralyze the sphincter muscle of the iris, which dilates the pupil and the ciliary muscle, which inactivates accommodation. Thus after using a cycloplegic agent, the patient is not only unable to accommodate for near distance and reading but also has a widely dilated pupil that can produce photophobia (light sensitivity) for periods ranging from 1 hour to several days, depending on the medication used.

4. **Cholinesterase.** Cholinesterase inhibitors are a group of drugs that inactivate cholinesterase in the body. As a result, acetylcholine is permitted to exert its effects freely and act directly as a miotic on the iris. It has been utilized in the management of open-angle glaucoma.

5. **Diabetes, syphilis, or posterior synechiae.** These conditions cause increased vascularity and structural changes in the iris, which impair dilation of the pupil with cycloplegic agents. This effect, however, does not occur in the early stages of diabetes but only in the long-standing cases of diabetes associated with retinopathy.

6. **Adrenalin.** Adrenalin or epinephrine is a sympathomimetic drug that exerts its effect by acting directly on the end organ. In the eye it may exert its effect by dilating the pupil, constricting the blood vessels and lowering intraocular pressure. If used over a prolonged time in the eye, it is capable of producing a brownish cast in the lacrimal sac.

7. **a. Concentration of the chemical in the solution.** The tonicity of an ophthalmic solution refers to the concentration of the chemical in that solution and its relationship to that of the tears. If the tonicity of the solution is relatively close to that of tears, the ophthalmic drops will be well tolerated by the eye. If, however, there is a high concentration of salts in the solution so that it is 'hypertonic,' then the drops will be irritating. Similarly, drops that are low in salt concentration or 'hypotonic,' such as water, also will produce irritation of the eye.

8. **a. Blepharitis.** Systemic administration of steroids is not without hazard and its use is confined to those conditions in which the benefits of steroid therapy cannot be achieved by a local topical route. By systemic administration, the adverse effects may result in water and salt retention, swelling in and about the face and eyelids, mental derangements, hypertension, gastric disturbances, accentuation of diabetes, increased blood glucose level, delayed wound healing, and a number of other medical problems.

9. **c. Trifluridine** (Viroptic). Trifluridine has been effective in inhibiting the herpes simplex virus by interfering with the early steps of DNA synthesis. It can be used in cases resistant to IDU or vidarabine.

Microbiology

*Michael A. Ward**

Microbiology is the branch of science that deals with microscopic, unicellular, and cell-cluster organisms. The major microbial categories that may be associated with eye infections are *bacteria, viruses, fungi,* and *parasites.* A basic understanding of microbiology is helpful for the ophthalmic assistant, who may be required to take smears, stain the appropriate slide, and assist in taking a culture.

In everyday life we are constantly in touch with microbes. We wash our hands to lower the number of microbes on our outer skin. We disinfect wounds for the same reason. We cover our sneezes and wash our fruit to prevent getting or spreading infectious diseases. We add chlorine to our water supply to inhibit the growth of *pathogenic* (disease-causing) bacteria. We do many things to control the growth of bacteria, but most bacteria are helpful in our daily lives. In fact, we could not live without the help of certain bacteria that exist in and on our bodies.

For example, bacteria in our gut are necessary for absorption of certain vitamins. Some bacteria actually educate our immune system and help to protect us against pathogenic microbial invaders. Certain species of bacteria are normal inhabitants of specific geographic areas of the body and their numbers are controlled by the local environment's moisture, temperature, and available nutrients. However, when such bacteria (say from the gut) get into the wrong place (like the eye) they have the potential to cause disease.

The eye is subject to the same types of infections that may occur in other parts of the body. Microorganisms are everywhere in our environment, and fortunately the eye is very resistant to infection. Our intact epithelial skin surface resists most microbial invaders. Any break in the skin of the outer eye can act as a portal of entry for microbes, at which point if a significant concentration of microbes, an *inoculum,* is present it may overcome our ocular defenses and cause an infection. Ocular trauma, surgery, radiation, severe surface dryness from exposure or inadequate blinking, lid abnormalities, and corneal degenerative changes may create surface disruptions that leave the eye more susceptible to infection. Persons with normal ocular surface structures may still be susceptible to diseases if their ability to defend against infectious agents is compromised. A compromised immune system can be present in patients with diabetes, acquired immunodeficiency syndrome (AIDS), and those taking immunosuppressive agents such as oral steroids.

A variety of organisms can cause ocular disease of the eye (Box 5.1). These infectious agents have a predilection for certain sites of the eye and usually vary in their severity in causing ocular disease. By far the most common infections result from bacterial and viral organisms. Bacteria are larger than viruses and easily may be seen under magnification by a light microscope. Bacteria range in size from

---

*Images in this chapter are courtesy of Michael A. Ward, unless otherwise stated.

feature is whether the organism stains blue (Gram positive) or red (Gram negative) with a special stain referred to as *Gram stain*. The organism's color after Gram staining is referred to as its Gram character. A bacterium's Gram character tells us about its cell wall make-up and therefore which antibiotics may be useful.

The *coccus* is a round bacterium that arranges itself in a variety of patterns, each with its own characteristics. Certain strains of *Staphylococcus* spp., *Streptococcus* spp., and *Neisseria* spp. are sometimes referred to as pyogenic or pus-producing bacteria. *Staphylococcus* spp. are Gram-positive organisms that may appear in grape-like clusters or, more commonly, singly or in pairs. Staphylococci frequently are present on the skin and may give rise to boils and styes. Not all staphylococci are pathogenic (disease causing); *Staphylococcus epidermidis* is a normal floral organism that lives on our skin and seldom causes disease. *Staphylococcus aureus*, however, is the species most commonly associated with skin infections. A particular type known as methicillin-resistant *Staphylococcus aureus* (MRSA) is a bacterium responsible for several difficult-to-treat infections in humans. It is increasingly reported as a pathogen in skin and other tissue infections. Hospital-acquired MRSA infections are on the decline, but community-based MRSA infections are on the rise.

Streptococci are bullet-shaped Gram-positive cocci that are usually arranged in pairs and short chains. Of the streptococcal organisms, the most common agent to affect the eye is *Streptococcus pneumoniae* (also known as *Pneumococcus*, *Diplococcus*). When causing disease, this organism possesses a polysaccharide (slime) capsule. The encapsulated form of this organism protects it from our body's defenses. Although *Pneumococcus* is a common cause of lobar pneumonia, it also can be the cause of conjunctivitis, a corneal ulcer, or an infection inside the eye referred to as *endophthalmitis*.

The bacterial genus *Neisseria* is a Gram-negative cocci. The species *Neisseria gonorrhoeae*, also known as the gonococcus, and *Neisseria meningitidis*, also known as the meningococcus, are diplococci (paired) and have a characteristic kidney-bean shape. They are the causative agents of gonorrhea and meningitis, respectively. These organisms are very invasive and rapid in their destruction.

0.2 to 5 μm and viruses from 0.005 to 0.1 μm. Viruses cannot be seen with a light microscope but can be indirectly viewed with electron microscopes.

BACTERIA

Bacteria can be categorized in different ways (Figure 5.1). They are commonly classified by morphology (shape), Gram character (dyed color), and ability to live in and use oxygen. Morphologically there are three basic shapes: the round *cocci*, the rod-shaped *bacilli*, and the helix-shaped *spirochetes* (Figure 5.2). Although the shape can be used to classify the organism, another important differentiating

Figure 5.1 Bacteria.

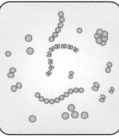
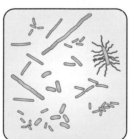
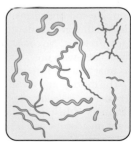
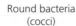

Round bacteria (cocci)   Rod-shaped bacteria (bacilli)   Spiral bacteria (spirilla)

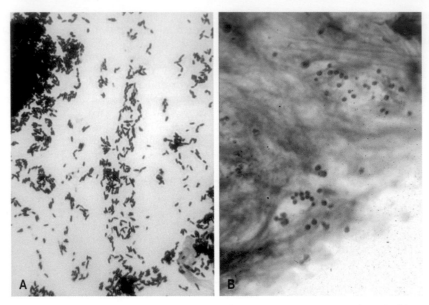

Figure 5.2 Gram stain showing Gram-positive rods on the left (A) and Gram-positive cocci on the right (B). *(Courtesy of Hans E. Grossniklaus, MD.)*

Another group of bacteria are the bacilli. All the members of this group are rod shaped, the rods being long or short, plump or slender, curved or straight, smooth or beaded. Commonly affecting the eye are the Gram-negative rods, *Haemophilus* spp., *Serratia* spp., and *Pseudomonas*. Historically the organism *Pseudomonas aeruginosa* has been considered the most devastating Gram-negative bacillus because of its very rapid and destructive potential. *Pseudomonas* is an opportunistic pathogen. It cannot usually penetrate our intact skin and it causes disease only when given an opportunity such as a corneal abrasion. It is the most common cause of corneal ulcers in patients wearing contact lenses. Unless treatment is initiated early, the organism can cause significant visual loss.

Gram-positive bacilli that affect the eye include *Corynebacterium* spp., *Bacillus* spp., and *Mycobacterium* spp. Corynebacteria are anaerobic rods that are part of our normal flora and live just beneath the outer skin layer. *Bacillus* spp. are soil organisms that seldom cause disease but are devastating in their destruction when involved in intraocular infections. Mycobacterial keratitis is rare but is often associated with previous ocular surgery. It is very difficult to treat and often results in poor visual outcomes.

The third group, the spiral-shaped organisms as found in *Treponema pallidum*, comprises small organisms whose diameter is below the range of resolution of the routine light microscope and which are rarely associated with ocular disease.

The positive identification of bacterial organisms by microscopic shape and staining reaction alone is not usually possible, and culture characteristics are often necessary. The ophthalmologist, however, may frequently make a presumptive diagnosis in association with the clinical picture, but the microscopic picture always remains an important aid.

VIRUSES

Viruses are very different from bacteria. They are made of the genetic material ribonucleic acid (RNA) or deoxyribonucleic acid (DNA), never both, plus a bit of protein. They are obligate intracellular parasites that cannot live on their own. Viruses are very small organisms (5–300 nm) that are not visible through a light microscope. Viruses multiply by injecting their genetic material into suitable host cells. Once inside, they commandeer the reproductive machinery of the host cell and reprogram it to make more viruses.

Our bodies acquire immunity to most viruses during the course of a viral infection so we can fight off a repeat infection by the same strain of virus in the future. However, our bodies are not capable of immunity to all viruses, notably herpes simplex and human immunodeficiency virus (HIV). The herpes simplex virus lives dormant in the nerve ganglia and when activated travels along the nerve root to invade the corneal epithelium and may give rise to a dendritic (branching) or geographic corneal ulcer. The virus can be identified by scraping the advancing edge of the corneal ulcer and inoculating the specimen into a cell culture system.

In most cases, however, the clinical diagnosis of herpes simplex virus is readily apparent and a scraping is unnecessary.

A common disease known as epidemic keratoconjunctivitis (EKC) is caused by an *adenovirus*. Adenoviruses are highly contagious and may affect the upper respiratory tract, the conjunctiva, and the cornea, causing fever, lymph gland enlargement, conjunctivitis, and keratitis. Varicella zoster virus causes chickenpox in children and is responsible for causing a vesicular eruption on the skin referred to as *shingles* in adults. It resides in the trigeminal nerve ganglion (CN-V) and is therefore restricted to only one side of the face, stopping at the midline. Some patients may develop ocular involvement that most commonly manifests as keratitis or iritis.

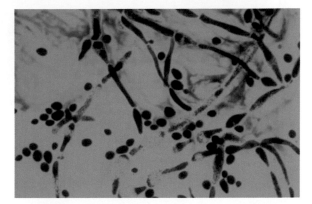

Figure 5.4 *Candida albicans.* Note both yeast and hyphae.

FUNGI

Fungal ocular infections are much less common than bacterial and viral infections. Molds and mildew are fungi. Athlete's foot and ringworm are two common skin diseases caused by fungi. Fungi are larger than bacteria and grow either as a mass of branching interlacing filaments (Figure 5.3) or as rounded yeast forms. They are typically found in soil and moist environments.

Ocular fungal infections are more likely to occur in the outer eye, cornea, and occasionally in the lacrimal sac. Ocular mycoses (fungal infections) are typically associated with trauma involving plant matter. A typical history is one in which a patient's cornea is scratched by a twig or leaf, and several days later the eye becomes red and inflamed. The most common fungal infection of the eye is caused by *Candida albicans* (Figure 5.4), which is a common yeast that also grows on moist skin and on mucous membranes as normal flora, but may overgrow and cause disease. Other fungi that may cause eye infections are the branching fungi *Aspergillus* spp. and *Fusarium* spp., both being more common in warm and moist climates. The largest outbreak of fungal keratitis ever recorded occurred in 2006; it was caused by a *Fusarium* sp. and was associated with a newly introduced contact lens multipurpose lens care product.

OTHER MICROBES

Chlamydial organisms are technically classified as bacteria but deserve a classification of their own. They are intracellular parasites that are larger than viruses but smaller than most bacteria. Chlamydia is the most widespread sexually transmitted bacterial disease in the United States. In North America the most common chlamydial eye disease is adult inclusion keratoconjunctivitis, which is usually spread from an infected sexual partner. Chlamydia may be transferred to infants while passing through the birth canal and result in an eye infection called ophthalmia neonatorum (eye disease of the newborn). Outside of North America, such as North Africa, the Middle East, and South Asia, another chlamydial disease, trachoma, remains epidemic and a serious cause of ocular morbidity. Diagnosis of inclusion keratoconjunctivitis can be made by obtaining a scraping of the conjunctiva and looking for inclusion bodies (microscopic foreign particles) in the cytoplasm of the epithelial cells. In infant chlamydial disease the probability of finding inclusion bodies is higher than in adults. A culture or specialized immunofluorescent test also can be used to confirm the diagnosis.

Protozoa are small single-celled parasites that eat bacteria and infrequently may cause ocular infections. *Acanthamoeba* and *Microsporidia* are two protozoa capable of affecting the eye. *Acanthamoeba* can cause significant ocular morbidity. The organism is ubiquitous; it can be found in fresh water, soil, swimming pools, and hot tubs. It is

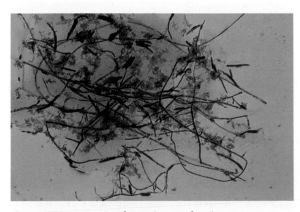

Figure 5.3 Gram stain of *Fusarium* sp. fungi.

Table 5.1 Cytology in eye scrapings

Finding	Possible diagnosis
Polymorphonuclear cells	Bacterial
Mononuclear cells	Viral
Eosinophils	Allergy
Inclusion bodies	Chlamydia
Giant cells	Herpesvirus

capable of causing keratitis, which can progress despite the best available medication. Unhygienic contact lens use is the major risk factor for acquiring this infection; it feeds on bacteria in the contact lens case. This risk is increased when wearers use homemade saline, rinse lenses with tap water, or swim while wearing contact lenses. Corneal transplantation may be required to restore vision but unfortunately there is approximately a 30% recurrence rate of the parasite in the graft. Microsporidia are small simple single-celled parasites that may infect compromised hosts. They are most commonly found in HIV-positive individuals and occasionally in other compromised hosts, such as those on prolonged steroid use. They are too small to be seen by simple light microscopy but may be detected by immunoassay or electron microscopy.

Bacteria, viruses, fungi, chlamydia, and parasites are among the causes of infectious inflammations of various parts of the human body, including the eye. Various terms are used to denote the specific site of inflammation, as noted in Table 5.1. Each part of the eye is susceptible to attack by a large variety of organisms that have in common a predisposition to attack these specific areas.

CLINICAL INDICATIONS FOR SMEARS AND CULTURES

Smears are obtained and cultures are grown to identify causative organisms of an ocular infection. A smear is a sample of discharge or tissue cells obtained by scraping. Gram and Giemsa stains are commonly used; Gram stain is used to examine for bacteria and Giemsa stain is used for cytology. Although many ocular infections occur in which a clinical diagnosis can be made and smears and cultures are unnecessary, in a number of specific conditions, laboratory studies are desirable:

- Acute purulent conjunctivitis or chronic conjunctivitis (Figure 5.5)
- Conjunctivitis in the newborn infant

- Corneal ulcers that possibly have a bacterial, fungal, or parasitic cause (Figures 5.6 and 5.7)

Less commonly, infections of the lids, tear passages (Figure 5.8), intraocular structures (endophthalmitis), or wounds (for example, after surgery or trauma) may result, which require smears and cultures by a variety of specialized techniques.

Cytology is the study of cell types; conjunctival cytology is useful in differentiating types of ocular inflammations. The *conjunctiva* is a clear, loose, vascular tissue that reacts to infection by becoming irritated with inflammatory cells and edematous fluid. Microbial organisms may be difficult to find in smears but the type of inflammatory cells that predominate may give a clue as to the type of infection (Table 5.2). The presence of polymorphonuclear leukocytes (PMNs) is most characteristic of bacterial infections, lymphocytes of viral infections, and eosinophils of allergic

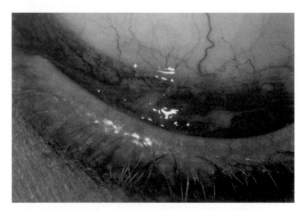

Figure 5.5 Adult *Chlamydia* inclusion conjunctivitis. Note conjunctival follicles and discharge.

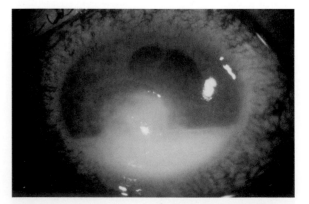

Figure 5.6 *Streptococcus pneumoniae* corneal ulcer with hypopyon.

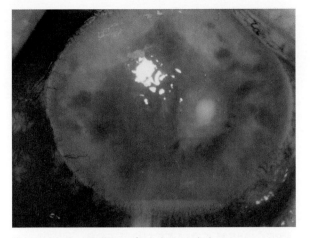

Figure 5.7 *Aspergillus* sp. fungal corneal ulcer.

Table 5.2 Inflammation of the eye

Part affected	Condition
Lids	Blepharitis
Cornea	Keratitis
Conjunctiva	Conjunctivitis
Tear sac	Dacryocystitis
Uveal tract	Uveitis
Iris	Iritis
Ciliary body	Cyclitis
Iris and ciliary body	Iridocyclitis
Choroid	Choroiditis
Retina	Retinitis
Optic nerve	Optic neuritis
Inner ocular coats	Endophthalmitis
All ocular coats	Panophthalmitis
Orbital tissue surrounding eye	Orbital cellulitis

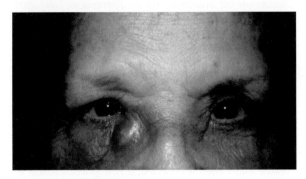

Figure 5.8 Dacryocystitis.

conditions. Smears are of particular importance in conjunctivitis of the newborn infant. Gram- and Giemsa-stained smears can help to differentiate among the likely causes of chlamydia, gonorrhea, or herpesvirus.

The cornea is one of the few tissues in the body without blood vessels; it commonly reacts to infection by ulcerative necrosis. Smears are an important aid to early diagnosis, particularly in bacterial and fungal corneal ulcers. Results of the smears are usually available within minutes to hours and allow the ophthalmologist to choose antimicrobial agents that are generally effective against bacterial or fungal organisms. Culture results usually are available within 1 to 3 days, which allows a modification of the initial antibiotic therapy so as to achieve the best possible clinical response. The etiologic agents of bacterial ulcers vary somewhat with regard to geographic location and patient population. *Pseudomonas* tends to be the most common cause in the southern United States and *Staphylococcus* the most common in Canada and the northern United States.

TAKING SMEARS

For rapid diagnosis, smears obtained from infective material are most valuable. A smear is a sample of discharge or infected tissue that is placed on a glass slide. To obtain a good sample of a superficial tissue, a gentle scraping with a platinum spatula may be done. The actual sampling of infected tissues should be performed by the ophthalmologist or under his or her direct supervision. All corneal lesions must be sampled by the ophthalmologist because this type of operative procedure has certain hazards. The material for culture and smear is taken from the advancing edge of the corneal lesion with a platinum spatula, scalpel blade, or swab. The ophthalmic assistant, however, may easily obtain the sample of conjunctival discharge found in the lower fornix in cases of conjunctivitis. The exudate is collected with a small sterile swab or platinum spatula, either from the lower cul-de-sac or from the inner canthus (Figure 5.9). It is spread as thinly and evenly as possible on the surface of a clean glass slide. The slide then can be stained for bacterial or cytologic differentiation and identification. When a culture is taken, it is important to avoid contamination of the applicator by the lashes and lid margin.

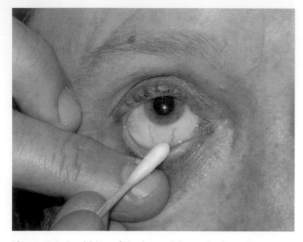

Figure 5.9 Swabbing of the lower lid margin for culture.

MAKING A STAIN

The routine stains of smears that may be performed by the ophthalmic assistant in the office are Gram stain for bacteria and fungi and the Giemsa and Diff-Quik (Baxter Diagnostics) stains for determining tissue cell type or the presence of inclusion bodies. Inclusion bodies often are characteristic of certain types of infection. Gram stain is useful in determining the type of bacteria or fungi responsible for the infection, whereas the Giemsa and Diff-Quik stains are useful in determining the inflammatory cellular response to a particular agent.

The ophthalmic assistant should learn about Gram, Giemsa, and Diff-Quik stains. Diff-Quik is used in place of Giemsa as a rapid stain used for cytology. Giemsa stains are time-consuming and are seldom used today.

Gram stain for bacterial identification

1. Fix smear by gentle heating
2. Cover with crystal or gentian violet solution for 40 to 60 seconds
3. Rinse with water
4. Cover with Gram's iodine for 1 minute; pour off solution
5. Decolorize with 95% ethyl alcohol or acetone for 5 to 10 seconds
6. Rinse with water
7. Cover with Safranin counterstain for 40 to 60 seconds
8. Wash with water, blot, and dry

Gram-positive organisms stain dark blue/purple and Gram-negative organisms stain red/pink.

Diff-Quik stain for cytologic identification

1. Dip slides in Diff-Quik fixative for 10 seconds (10 dips).
2. Dip slides in Diff-Quik solution 1 for 10 seconds (10 dips).
3. Dip slides in Diff-Quik solution 2 for 12 seconds (12 dips).
4. Rinse slides with distilled or deionized water and let them dry.
5. Dip in xylene.
6. Mount.

SPECIMEN COLLECTION FOR CULTURE

Cultures are an important aid in diagnosis of infections. Cotton, synthetic, or calcium alginate tipped swabs are used to collect specimens from the eyelids, conjunctiva, or cornea for culture. The physician may want to inoculate the specimen directly onto culture media in the office or send the specimen swab to the laboratory for plating on the appropriate growth media. Specimen collection swabs with transport media (culturettes) are commercially available to keep organisms viable while in transit. The swab may be moistened in the transport media or other sterile fluid before specimen collection and then immediately placed into the transport liquid and taken to the microbiology laboratory.

Once a specimen is collected, it is important that it be immediately inoculated onto the proper culture medium and incubated at the proper temperature for best results. In the bacteriology laboratory the swabs are routinely plated on nutrient-rich culture media (Figure 5.10).

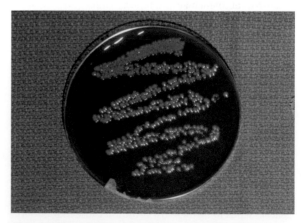

Figure 5.10 Bacterial colonies of *Serratia marcescens* on a chocolate agar plate.

Specific culture media are used to grow particular organisms. The most common types of nutrient-rich culture media include blood agar, chocolate agar, thioglycolate broth, and Sabouraud-dextrose agar. Blood agar is a medium enriched with 5% sheep's blood. It will grow most aerobic bacteria and can differentiate bacterial colonies that produce hemolysin, an exotoxin that lyses red blood cells. Some pathologic species of streptococci (e.g., the responsible organism for strep throat) produce hemolysin on blood agar, lysing the red blood cells and thereby creating a clear zone around the colony. This allows the physician to confirm or rule out the presence of pathologic streptococci by looking at the culture plate. Chocolate agar is a very rich growth medium and is used to grow fastidious organisms such as *Haemophilus* and *Neisseria* spp. There is no chocolate in chocolate agar; it is a nutrient agar with 10% sheep or horse blood that has been heated to release nutrients from the blood cells, which gives it a chocolate-brown appearance. Any organism that can grow on blood agar can grow on chocolate agar. Thioglycolate broth is a liquid growth medium that is used to grow anaerobic bacteria. The broth chemically removes oxygen to maintain an anaerobic environment. It is important that the specimen be completely submerged into the thioglycolate broth to protect it from oxygen. Sabouraud-dextrose agar is used to grow yeast and fungi while suppressing bacterial growth. Bacteria can usually be identified within 24 hours. Viruses and chlamydia are not grown on these culture media.

Chlamydia and fungi require specific cell cultures for growth and identification, which may take 1 to 3 weeks for results. These specimens are collected and placed in viral/chlamydial transport media, placed on ice (4°C), and transported to the microbiology laboratory for culture.

When the physician orders a specimen to be sent for "culture and sensitivity," the request is to isolate and grow the bacteria and then test the organisms for sensitivity to a standard battery of antibiotics. Discs soaked in various antibiotic solutions are placed on the culture medium along with the bacteria to test which antibiotic will inhibit the growth of susceptible bacteria. If the bacterium is sensitive to a particular drug, an area of "no growth" will be visible around the disc.

OTHER AIDS TO IDENTIFY ORGANISMS

Biopsies have some value in the diagnosis of ocular infections. A biopsy is the removal of a piece of tissue, which is

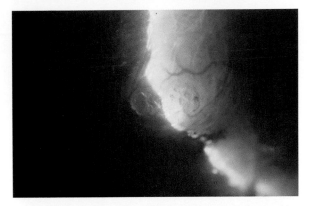

Figure 5.11 Eyelid lesion (molluscum contagiosum) caused by a virus.

then either fixed in preservative (e.g., formalin) and sent to the pathology laboratory or placed unfixed in a sterile jar and sent to the bacteriology laboratory for culture. An example of a condition that is readily diagnosed by a biopsy is the molluscum nodule on the lid margins, which is caused by a large virus (Figure 5.11).

Skin tests are another diagnostic aid that may be performed in the office or hospital clinic. Various infections such as tuberculosis, toxoplasmosis, and some fungi produce a skin reaction if the patient has been infected.

SUMMARY

Many known causes of eye disease may be attributed to infectious agents such as bacteria, viruses, chlamydia, fungi, and parasites. Other unknown causes of diseases may also someday be ascribed to these organisms as improved techniques in isolating and identifying microbes develop. Unfortunately only the exterior portions of the eye are readily available for routine sampling for identification of organisms. However, the ophthalmologist may sample the aqueous and/or vitreous fluids for culture by aspirating through a syringe and needle.

Questions for review and thought

1. Name some common sources of bacteria, viruses, and fungi in your everyday environment.
2. Name some common viral conditions affecting the body.
3. What is the most destructive bacterium affecting the outer portion of the eye?
4. What is the most common viral condition affecting the cornea?
5. Choroiditis refers to inflammation of the choroid; retinitis refers to inflammation of the retina. If all the coats of the eye are inflamed, what is the appropriate term?
6. Outline a procedure to follow in obtaining a smear and staining it to identify bacteria.
7. Explain how a culture specimen is obtained.
8. Organisms may affect the interior of the eye, making it impossible to obtain smears and cultures. Discuss the value of skin tests.
9. What tests can be used to detect infection in the body?
10. What organisms are regarded as normal inhabitants of the eye?
11. Describe conditions that enhance bacterial growth. Give clinical examples.
12. Describe conditions that enhance viral growth. Give clinical examples.
13. What is the best culture medium for bacterial growth?
14. What is the difference among infection, inflammation, and irritation?
15. What is meant by a bacteriostatic drug? Give an example. What is a bactericidal drug? Give an example.
16. What virulent bacterial organisms can survive only in a fluid environment?

Q Self-evaluation questions

True–false statements

Directions: Indicate whether the statement is true (T) or false (F).
1. A dendritic ulcer of the cornea is classically caused by the herpes simplex virus. T or F
2. The organisms that infect the eye can always be immediately and positively identified by microscopic shape and staining reaction. T or F
3. Viruses can be identified by means of light microscopic examination. T or F

Missing words

Directions: Write in the missing word in the following sentences.
4. The _____ and _____ stains are useful in determining the cellular response to a particular agent.
5. Inflammation of the inner ocular coats is called _____.
6. The basic medium used to culture bacteria in ophthalmology is _____.

Choice-completion questions

Directions: Select the one best answer in each case.
7. Conjunctivitis caused by this infectious agent often produces enlargement of the preauricular lymph node.
   a. *Staphylococcus*
   b. *Pneumococcus*
   c. *Haemophilus*
   d. Adenovirus
   e. *Streptococcus*
8. Which of the following is most likely to be responsible for the transmission of epidemic adenovirus keratoconjunctivitis?
   a. Finger-to-eye transmission
   b. Applanation tonometry
   c. Fluorescein solutions
   d. Kissing
   e. All of the above
9. A 30-year-old male laborer has a densely infiltrated corneal ulcer 10 days after an abrasion to the central cornea. A hypopyon is present. Which is the most appropriate immediate procedure?
   a. Give him an antibiotic drop and tell him to return in 3 days if it has not improved.
   b. Presume that the patient has a fungal keratitis and start him on therapy with an antifungal agent.
   c. Make a smear and obtain specimens for culture, then start the appropriate therapy once the laboratory has informed you of the result.
   d. Make a smear and take specimens for culture, start antibiotics appropriate for Gram-negative and Gram-positive organisms, and admit him to the hospital.
   e. Because a hypopyon is present, assume the patient has an endophthalmitis and will need to be treated with the full endophthalmitis regimen.

A Answers, notes, and explanations

1. **True.** The herpes simplex virus is one of the most common viruses affecting the eye. The virus invades the corneal epithelium and gives rise to a dendritic ulcer, which usually affects the central portion of the cornea. The ulcer is almost always unilateral and may affect any age group. A history of cold sores on the face can be elicited in approximately 55% of cases. The infection often recurs in the same eye, and the lesion may be precipitated by the following triggering factors: fever, menstruation, cold, emotion, and overexposure to sunlight. Herpesvirus can be cultivated on the chorioallantoic membrane of a developing chick embryo. The virus also has a typical cytopathic effect on HeLa cell cultures.

2. **False.** It is not usually possible to positively identify an organism by means of microscopic shape and staining characteristics, and often it is necessary to obtain a smear and culture the bacteria. A presumptive diagnosis, however, may be made by considering the clinical picture along with the microscopic shape and staining reaction.

3. **False.** Viruses are the smallest organisms that invade the body. Most cannot be seen by present-day forms of light microscopy, and special techniques such as electron microscopy are necessary for diagnosis.

4. **Wright** and **Giemsa.** The routine stains used to determine cell structure and the presence of inclusion bodies are Wright and Giemsa stains. These allow the cellular response to a particular agent to be determined. Classically, in acute bacterial conjunctivitis the predominant cells would be polymorphs; in viral conjunctivitis, lymphocytes; and in allergic conjunctivitis, eosinophils. The detection of inclusion bodies is of importance in the diagnosis of inclusion conjunctivitis. Gram stain is used mainly for the detection of bacteria.

5. **Endophthalmitis.** Endophthalmitis is a rare condition that usually manifests as a decrease in vision, pain, conjunctival redness, and vitreous haze. In most cases the infection follows a penetrating eye injury or surgery for glaucoma or cataract. In rare instances it is the result of a blood-borne infection. If all three coats of the eye, as well as the vitreous, are involved by the inflammatory process, the condition is called a *panophthalmitis.* It is very difficult to determine clinically whether the patient has an endophthalmitis or a panophthalmitis.

6. **Blood agar.** Cultures are used to determine which infective agent is responsible for a lesion and the sensitivity of the organisms to various drugs. Blood agar is the basic medium used in ophthalmology. Other media used are as follows:

a. Chocolate agar: gonococci, *Haemophilus influenzae*
b. Blood agar enriched with vitamin K: *Actinomyces israelii*
c. Löwenstein-Jensen: *Mycobacterium tuberculosis*
d. Sabouraud-dextrose agar: fungi

Culture specimens from both eyes should be obtained, even though only one eye is involved. When the specimen is obtained, contamination of the applicator by the lashes and lid margins should be avoided.

7. **d. Adenovirus.** Viral conjunctivitis is characterized by generalized injection of the conjunctiva, minimal discharge, and profuse tearing. The preauricular lymph node is commonly enlarged in adenovirus infections, and occasionally the patient may have an associated sore throat and fever. Bacterial conjunctivitis is associated with a profuse discharge, which may cause the lids to adhere, and the patient may have difficulty in opening the eyes on awakening. In addition, a history of a sandy, scraping feeling often is obtained. The conjunctiva is diffusely injected and it is rare for the preauricular lymph node to be enlarged. Answers *a, b, c,* and *e* are all common bacterial causes of conjunctivitis.

In summary, the following table aids in differentiating viruses from bacteria.

	Viral	Bacterial
Tearing	++	−
Discharge	−	++++
Injection	++	+++
Preauricular node	+++	−
Sore throat and fever	+++	+

8. **a. Finger-to-eye transmission.** This question emphasizes the fact that medical personnel who touch lids, conjunctiva, and other ocular tissues must wash their hands between patients when patients with ocular infections are examined. The physician's office is the source of many epidemics of adenovirus infection. In many epidemics the spread has been traced to finger-to-eye transmissions; many patients with the infection have not had applanation tonometry.

9. **d.** This patient in all probability has a bacterial corneal ulcer and requires urgent treatment with antibiotics that will be effective against both Gram-positive and Gram-negative bacteria. Once the organism has been cultured, the antibiotic can be modified appropriately. The presence of the hypopyon does not necessarily imply an endophthalmitis. In all probability, it is a "sterile" reaction to the infected corneal ulcer.

Chapter | 6 |

Office efficiency and public relations

A well-run office is important not only for the efficiency of the staff but also because it keeps patients essentially happy. The roles of the secretary, bookkeeper, receptionist, and even the filing clerk in a busy office are important. Familiarity with the overall practice is necessary: not only the handling of patients but also the back-up services required such as completing insurance forms, reports, collecting, billing, and accounting.

HOW TO MAKE PATIENTS HAPPY

Making patients happy is not just good practice; it may even prevent lawsuits. Patients are ambassadors of goodwill for the practice. The secret to making patients happy lies in developing good communication skills. These communication skills start with an attitude of empathy and caring and letting patients know directly and indirectly that they are important. This attitude is reflected not only by what the physician says and does but also by what the office staff say and do and how psychologically comfortable the patient is made to feel in the office environment. There are a number of ways in which the office staff can show their caring.

1. Do not keep patients waiting for long periods. One of the key factors affecting patients' overall rating of a practitioner is the time spent waiting in the reception area. Waiting time is a major cause of patient dissatisfaction, which increases dramatically when waiting time exceeds 30 minutes. Office schedules cannot always be controlled, especially if emergencies occur. For those physicians who are chronically behind schedule, the staff should take a close look at how appointments are made and try to prevent snarl-ups in the schedule. If delays are unavoidable, patients should be told why they are waiting and how long

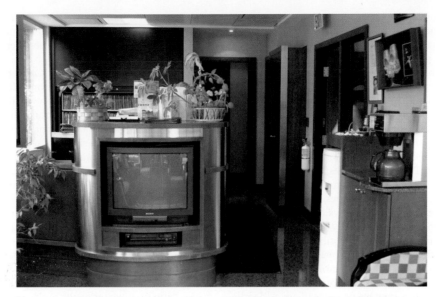

Figure 6.1 The waiting room should be pleasant and well decorated to make the patient comfortable.

the wait may be; this helps minimize the aggravation. In addition, interesting materials should be available to help patients pass the time. These include topical and current magazines or video educational material with television sets in the waiting room (Figure 6.1).

2. Make patients feel important. The first contact the patient has with a physician's office should be courteous, respectful, and personalized (Figure 6.2). This can include little gestures of kindness, such as the nurse asking after a recent baby, the receptionist asking for a preferred appointment time, or the physician inquiring after an ailing family member or recalling some details of an earlier conversation.

It is also appropriate for physicians to stand up and shake a patient's hand when first greeting a patient and to touch patients in a neutral manner (on the arm, shoulder, or hand) during the course of a consultation. These gestures convey empathy, friendliness, and concern. It is critical to convey information in a tone that is neither patronizing nor too technical so that the patient understands the basic problem and what is going to be done to help correct it.

The physician should make eye contact with the patient being examined. Older adults often find it offensive if the physician directs advice to the younger person who may be accompanying them. Patients are often reluctant to ask questions, and it is better to err on the side of too much information rather than give insufficient information. Finally, physicians should not make patients feel they are too busy to listen to their problems, because patients may not only go elsewhere but also be thoroughly dissatisfied and litigious.

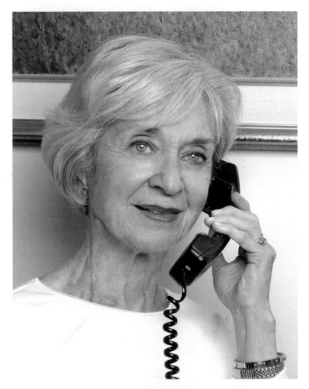

Figure 6.2 An ophthalmic assistant should be warm and courteous and make the patient feel at ease.

3. Create space for comfort. Surprisingly small details, such as how the furniture is arranged, can make a difference in overall patient response. In an eye practice a desk intervening between a patient and the

ophthalmologist often serves as a barrier to communication. It is much better to have a direct, closer interaction with the patient. Both intimacy and empathy are given a head start by placing the chairs near each other to eliminate any broad expanse of space between physician and patient.

4. Respect a patient's right to privacy. Any discussions of fees with the physician or receptionist should be conducted privately so that details of these conversations are not overheard by a room full of strangers. Confidentiality is important.

5. Look the part. People do not respond well to individuals with long hair or those dressed in blue jeans, sports shirts, athletic shoes, and sports socks. To earn patient respect, the physician and staff members should be dressed in conservative attire, the men wearing shirts and possibly ties and the women wearing suits, dresses, blazers, or dress pants. A consistency in color among the staff or laboratory coats may serve the purpose of professionalism. Nametags of the staff are a friendly gesture.

6. In the examining room, pay attention to detail. Unclean examining rooms make patients uneasy, especially when evidence from previous examinations is clearly visible. Cleanliness is an important image for patients, so provide hand sterilizers, for example (Figure 6.3). Interruptions during an examination can be particularly annoying. A loud intercom system undermines privacy and is unprofessional except for emergencies. Small conveniences, such as a coat rack in the waiting room, along with soothing decor, plants,

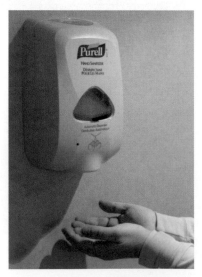

Figure 6.3 A hand sanitizer for staff and patients is useful to show that the office cares.

and art prints, all help to create the impression of a pleasant, welcoming environment and a caring physician. Redecorating every so often may be a good plan.

7. Master communication skills. Conversation is an important factor in making or breaking the physician–patient relationship. Here are a few tips:
   - Be up-front. Give information right at the beginning of the visit and not at the end. One can talk while examining with a slit lamp, retinoscope, and so on. Friendly conversation is appreciated
   - Be creative. Use everyday language to explain what is wrong and how you are planning to correct it
   - Be personal. Ask questions about patients' families, social life, and work situations so that they feel they have not been forgotten from one visit to the next. Make notes on charts about patients' interests and concerns for recall at future visits
   - Be caring. Put a hand on the patient's shoulder or arm to convey empathy but do not overdo this with members of the opposite sex
   - Be prepared. If you have something that needs to be shared with a patient's family, ask them to come in from the waiting room and share the information with them
   - Solicit patient feedback. Confirm that what you have told the patient has been understood by asking the patient to relay the information back to you. This is particularly important for educating patients about care systems for contact lenses. Too often patients leave the office unable to manage their contact lens care systems. Written information will ensure that the message gets across. Handouts are very important and are even more effective if they are personalized
   - Be human. Patients want human beings looking after them. It is perfectly acceptable to tell patients that you also feel bad when the news you have for them is bad.

8. Be fair in all matters of finance. Charge fairly for your professional services but do not overcharge. Be fair in providing refunds to patients who prove to be unsuited for contact lens wear. Always look at the situation from the standpoint of the patient. Maintain goodwill at all costs.

9. Never ever put anything on the records that would be damaging if the records appeared in a court room, for example, the patient is crazy.

New patients and returning patients

Normally in an eye practice, there is a 10% to 20% annual increase in new patients. This is important for growth of a practice and for interest. One should record on a month-to-month basis this ratio compared with old patients returning. If the trend of new patients is downward, one has to look at internal marketing. Is everyone being asked for a referral? Is the telephone answered by a recording? Is the telephone voice bright, cheerful, and welcoming? One may even consider more external marketing and promotional items. Is a definite percentage of revenues allocated to this?

The telephone

The telephone is usually the first contact the patient makes with the office. These calls must be handled in a manner that will reassure the caller, provide confidence in the office, and at the same time protect the doctor from unnecessary interruptions. The receptionist who answers the phone must have the wisdom of Solomon to permit access to the services on the basis of priority. The staff should answer the phone personally most of the day.

Use of answering machines should be kept to a minimum. Having to respond to a "Press 1, Press 2" command is a turn-off to many.

Basically two symptoms require immediate attention: pain and loss of vision. Pain can mean anything from acute glaucoma to a corneal abrasion. Whatever the cause, it requires attention. Loss of vision is more difficult to assess. Sudden loss of vision can be a result of a central retinal artery occlusion and should be seen immediately. Other symptoms to be given top priority include transient loss of vision in one eye (carotid artery disease) or flashes of light (retinal detachment).

The telephone should be operated efficiently. Current systems include call forwarding, digital punch systems, conference call systems, and music or information that comes on when the patient is placed on hold. Telephone equipment provides for on-hold messages. This is an ideal opportunity to improve public relations and add some form of promotion for your practice, for example, an on-hold message such as, "We appreciate that your time is valuable. We will be with you as soon as possible. Thank you for holding." This is an important service for busy lines. An adequate number of telephone lines is needed so that the patient does not spend an excessive amount of time listening to busy signals. The use of physician lines, "hotlines," and outgoing unlisted lines is valuable for a busy office.

Frequently called numbers need not be dialed if memory call-through systems are used. Video display units make dealing with a caller easier. For example, if the caller has a swollen red eye, that patient will be seen immediately even if there is a language or articulation problem that prevents understanding the patient's complaints.

When the telephone rings, it should be answered at once. The receptionist should not permit the line to ring and ring while completing bookkeeping or other duties. The patient becomes more impatient and difficult to handle with each ring. It is an act of courtesy to permit the caller to hang up the phone first when the conversation is finished. Otherwise, it might seem as if the receptionist is trying to get rid of the patient.

Patience, finesse, and tact are needed to handle many patients on the telephone. The ophthalmic assistant should try to wear a smile at all times. Although callers cannot see the person to whom they are speaking, they can readily sense an attitude over the telephone. The ophthalmic assistant will be called on to help, advise, and sympathize with many patients. Calls should be screened carefully so that the ophthalmologist may answer nonurgent calls at a convenient hour. Sometimes the physician will want the ophthalmic assistant to take calls from patients reporting on their condition or requiring information, or the physician may want to receive all calls from patients personally.

It is important that all telephone messages be recorded on a pad. Memory should never be trusted; a busy schedule often makes memory very short. It is a good idea to use a telephone message pad with a duplicate or carbon copy. If the physician wishes a call returned, the assistant has a copy of the name and number. It also is a handy record of incoming messages and telephone numbers.

Memory joggers

Some individuals remember names well; others remember numbers. Some forget appointments and social dates quickly. There are activities that minimize forgetfulness and can make one more efficient. The old concept of "write it down" applies to all of us.

1. Make notes of everything that you think you may forget. These can be made on small pieces of paper, a BlackBerry, iPhone, or iPad, but should be transcribed into an active memory list some time later.
2. Keep a daily calendar that is all in one place for writing down appointments, entertainment events, and other personal events. Begin early not to trust to memory.
3. Try to learn at least one new thing daily. If it is an eye disorder or new disease, then write it down and look it up later when time permits.
4. Repeat information to yourself a couple of times. As the day progresses repeat the information once again.
5. Attend local seminars and record vocabulary you find unfamiliar to look it up later.

Risk management

The telephone is an important vehicle for interviews and assessment of the patient's problems. Many patients will telephone with emergency problems. Remember that the caller may be confused, distraught, rude, or even unable to give a clear account of what is occurring. Skillful management by the telephone receptionist may be sight saving and perhaps even lifesaving. Therefore, the staff member should be courteous, compassionate, efficient, and informative in telephone conversations.

The Board of Directors of the American Academy of Ophthalmology has offered the following guidelines to reduce litigation risks:

- Always confer with the doctor if you have questions relating to the call.
- Take down the caller's number and promise to call back if in doubt about the correct answer to a question.
- Avoid giving general medical advice or discussing diagnoses.
- Answer questions in a friendly but noncommittal manner and refer to the ophthalmologist for definitive answers.
- Do not forget to return the call as soon as possible because often the patient is extremely anxious.
- Try to determine the following:
  - The caller's name, address, and telephone number
  - The essence of the problem
  - When the symptoms first occurred and their duration.

The following list includes typical emergencies that require immediate attention:

1. Chemical contact with the eyes and face. Alkali burns are extremely urgent matters. Patients should have emergency care at the scene of the accident by copious washing before they are brought to the ophthalmologist's office. An acceptable measure would be to fill a basin or bucket with tap water and immerse the patient's head into the water with the eyelids open under water
2. Severe eye, head or face injury, particularly a perforating eye injury
3. Acute or partial loss of vision
4. Recent onset of pain in or around the eye
5. Postoperative pain, infection, or increased redness or decreased vision
6. Recent bulging of an eye
7. Recent onset of flashing lights, floaters, curtains, or veils across the vision
8. Recent onset of double vision
9. Recent change of pupillary size
10. Recent onset of droopy eyelid
11. Foreign bodies in the eye
12. Urgent consultations requested by other physicians.

If the patient has an emergency problem and the physician is unavailable, it is best to advise the patient to see another physician or obtain emergency room care immediately. One outstanding admonition that hangs over the head of every physician is that of "abandonment." One cannot abandon patients, particularly those in the immediate postoperative period. This carries sensitive legal implications.

It is important not to release any information regarding a patient without a legally valid written authorization. A caller who identifies him- or herself as a close relative desiring information should be asked to speak to the physician in the patient's presence.

Remember that all recommendations by the American Academy of Ophthalmology are only examples of important considerations. They should be supplemented by instructions from the ophthalmologist and experienced staff members.

Returning telephone calls

Patients' telephone messages should be responded to on the same day and within a reasonable period of time if possible, otherwise the office staff may have to deal with aggravated patients. Waiting until the end of the day to return patients' telephone calls can be a burdensome task; staff members are fatigued and it may be difficult to reach the patients. In addition, while waiting for their call to be returned, patients have had an opportunity to think about their problems more and become anxious.

Patients appreciate a quick response. Further, the patient who knows that the call is being made between patient appointments may be less likely to waste time with casual questions. If it appears that the call will take a long time, the staff member can arrange to call the patient back at a later time or encourage the patient to make an appointment to come in to the office.

Telephone manners

A telephone call is usually the first contact a patient has with the ophthalmologist's office. The following rules ensure a good impression:

1. Personality is revealed by voice and language. How you speak and what you say are the two most important factors in handling telephone calls. The voice should be clear, courteous, friendly, alive, and precise. Pronunciation should be clear, with lips placed about half an inch from the mouthpiece. Cultivate an attractive, well-modulated voice with pleasing inflections. You should try to make your voice attractive, just as you would try to make your appearance attractive. The impression that is created for the person calling depends on the inflection and tone of your voice. The impression you make—good, poor, or indifferent—reflects on the ophthalmologist and the office. You are the ophthalmologist's representative.
2. Use well-selected, appropriate words and phrases (Box 6.1). Express yourself with a business-like

Box 6.1 **Telephone techniques**

Do not say	Say
When do you want to come in?	Would you prefer a morning or afternoon appointment?
The doctor is booked up until____.	The doctor is scheduled at that time. He can see you at_____.
The doctor is running late.	The doctor was interrupted in his schedule today.
I call to remind you that_____.	I called to confirm or verify_____.
Cancellation.	Change in schedule.
Checkup.	Examination.
Are you an old patient of Doctor__?	Are you a former or established patient of Doctor_____?
You misunderstood.	There was a misunderstanding.
Are you a patient here?	When did we see you last?
Are you on welfare or Medicare?	What type of health insurance coverage do you have?
What is your problem?	Can you tell me what your problem is so we can schedule you properly?

7. Be calm and steady and avoid excitement or abruptness even when the lines become busy. Keep your remarks short. The longer you talk, the more irritable the person on the line or on hold becomes.

8. It has been said that people prefer to talk to those who speak at roughly the same speed as they do, that is, a fast-speaking caller is happier being dealt with by a fast-speaking person. They seem to bond. Therefore, match the speed of your voice as well as the tone to the caller.

9. Try not to abandon the telephone at lunch to an answering service. Rotate the incoming calls among staff members. An answering service should be used sparingly because personnel are not skilled in handling patient questions nor do they have access to the appointment book for schedules.

10. Never repeat personal information you may hear, no matter how unimportant it may seem to you.

11. If answering services are used after hours, train them well in what to say in response to a few basic questions that might be asked. Typed script responses can be helpful.

12. Do not hesitate to ask for the repetition of words or names if you are in doubt. Many names sound very much alike but are quite different. Foreign names given by persons with an accent should be repeated or spelled slowly until they are understood. To ensure accuracy, repeat numbers, amounts, addresses, and other important items.

13. Have paper and pencil ready for messages and obtain accurate and complete information, including correct name, address, and telephone number in duplicate.

14. Keep a list of frequently called telephone numbers.

15. Sit properly. Poor posture produces fatigue early in the day, and fatigue becomes reflected in your voice.

16. Do not photocopy a medical chart and give it to a patient unless authorized by the ophthalmologist. There may be a lawsuit pending.

17. Avoid discussion of fees unless so instructed.

18. Avoid any discrimination. Everyone has the right to receive equal treatment to services regardless of race, ancestry, color, place of origin, citizenship, creed, sex, sexual orientation, age, marital status, or disability. This discrimination may be an act, decision, or communication that imposes a burden on them or denies them a right or benefit that others may enjoy.

19. Ophthalmologists may restrict their practice to a subspecialty but should make recommendations or suggestions for ongoing care to a colleague. The referral should be made in a timely manner. The ophthalmic assistant may aid in this referral.

conciseness in a courteous manner. Use the terms "please," "thank you," "I am sorry," and other expressions of appreciation and regret with a tone of sincerity, which will be quite obvious to the listener. Do not try to cut the person off with constant interjections. Above all, be understanding.

3. Ask who wishes to speak to the doctor. The doctor may not wish to speak to a brother-in-law or a stockbroker but may be receptive to calls from an industrial nurse.

4. Tell patients that the doctor can best answer a call after hours. There is more time and less disruption of normal service. Make sure the doctor receives all patient calls. It is good public relations to ensure that those calls are returned by the doctor on the same day.

5. The office should have enough lines so that busy signals are kept to a minimum. Use a *private line* for any outgoing calls and keep these to an absolute minimum. Avoid personal calls.

6. Avoid putting people on hold unless absolutely necessary. If you must put someone on hold, explain the situation and ask if the person would like to hold or would prefer that you return the call in a few minutes. If the choice is to hold, *thank the person for being patient* as soon as you return to the line. Remember, courtesy is very important.

Office personnel should always remember when answering the telephone that they are important representatives of the doctor and can assist immensely in the building of a

---

Box 6.2 Pet peeves of callers

1. Receive a recording too many times
2. Doesn't introduce oneself. Doesn't use their name. Treats them like a number
3. Put them on hold before they have had a chance to speak
4. Keep them on hold too long without returning to the telephone
5. Transfer them to people who can't help them: "the runaround"
6. Promise to call them back and never do
7. Accidentally disconnect them, particularly a long-distance call, without getting their name or telephone number

---

Box 6.3 Establishing rapport with patients

Sentences of goodwill

"Thank you for holding, Mrs. Brown."

"How may I help you?"

"It's very important that you come in right away."

"I'd like to verify some information to ensure that your medical record is current."

"Could you please repeat the appointment information to me, Mrs. Jones, so I can make sure I communicated clearly?"

Responding to angry patients

"I understand how you feel.'

"Hello, Mrs. Jones. This is Tammy Smith, Dr. Brown's assistant."

"That's understandable, Mrs. Jones."

"I'll be happy to see that the doctor calls you by 5:00 p.m. How can we reach you?"

---

reputation. They must be master psychologists tuned in to the emotional ills and pressures of the public. In many cases a voice is the only contact that the telephone patient has with the office. Therefore, the office must be represented with courtesy, dignity, and a spirit of service, with personnel giving clear and complete answers promptly.

Kim Fox, in her book *Telephone Power*, suggests the seven pet peeves of callers. She also outlines ways of establishing rapport with patients (Boxes 6.2 and 6.3).

SCHEDULING APPOINTMENTS

It is difficult in an ophthalmology office to be on time. Because many patients require dilating eyedrops, it means everyone must wait at least 30 minutes. Therefore, waiting

patients are always present. If emergencies or difficult cases are added, then the normal waiting time can be extended to 1 hour. Waiting is tedious. No one likes to sit beside a total stranger for prolonged periods. Patients become irritated and their tempers grow short. The irritability spreads and affects the entire staff. A hostile patient does not foster good doctor–patient relations.

If waiting is a fact of the office environment, the best way to prevent a potentially disruptive situation is to explain on the patient's arrival that a wait of 30 to 45 minutes may be required to allow for eyedrops and a preliminary examination before the patient sees the ophthalmologist. It does not change the reality of waiting but at least the person knows what to expect and, more important, the reason for the delay. If it is a reasonable explanation, most patients will understand and accept the distress of sitting around. Occasionally a patient will be unreasonable and short-tempered but one cannot satisfy everybody. The assistant should always forewarn patients about the necessity of waiting for the doctor and explain why. Available coffee, tea, or soft drinks along with a TV monitor help goodwill.

The waiting game can produce bitterness on both sides. For the physician, the patient who does not show up for an appointment, or shows up late, has kept the clinician waiting. Some physicians charge for missed appointments. A valid case can be made for doing so, because time is the major commodity for the professional. Many patients feel the same way. Who is to say that a physician's time is more important than anyone else's? Some patients have billed their physicians for lost time spent uselessly in a waiting room. Of course, these views represent the extremes of the doctor–patient dispute.

It is difficult to control the size of an eye practice and simultaneously retain patient goodwill. A well-trained ophthalmic assistant can be the solution, in whole or in part, to the doctor's dilemma. The ophthalmic assistant responsible for telephone appointments acts in the role of doorman to the practice. The assistant is, after all, the first contact the patient has with the office. He or she can attract or discourage new patients or drive away old ones.

The ophthalmic assistant may not be primarily responsible for the scheduling of appointments but should act in a supervisory capacity to see that the physician's appointment schedule is not overcrowded. Any appointment system must be formulated to suit the particular working habits and peculiarities of the physician involved. Appointments must be generously spaced and an adequate amount of time allocated for any special procedures that are to be performed. An efficient appointment system makes allowance for the fact that many patients will require eyedrops. Special consultations for problem cases will require additional time apportioned to the patient's visit. Emergencies often arise during the course of the day and blocks of time may be set aside to permit the efficient, smooth handling of these emergencies with minimal disruption of the existing schedule.

No one should rely on memory in recording an appointment. All appointments must be marked in the appointment book, preferably in pencil so that they can be erased in case of cancellation. A more efficient way to handle appointments is a computerized scheduling system. This allows instant recall if someone calls in about a future appointment. This is now the most common way, but it depends on a staff person who is computer literate.

In making an appointment it is important to spell the name of the patient correctly. The telephone numbers, both home and business, should be obtained in case it is necessary to contact the patient to alter the time of the appointment. The appointment time should be repeated to the patient at least once, so that there is no misunderstanding about the date and time. Whenever possible, patients should be given the first available appointment time suitable for their needs. Tactful questioning of the patient should reveal who referred the patient, whether it was a physician, an optical house, an optometrist, or another patient. It is a matter of good public relations to note this person in the appointment book, as a reminder when the patient arrives.

More time should be allowed for first visits because the doctor will require and usually will wish to spend more time examining new patients. When special tests or procedures are anticipated, such as visual fields or minor surgery, they should be noted and suitable time permitted. The appointment book should be marked in advance whenever the physician is attending meetings or conferences so that double bookings do not occur, to avoid cancellations and rescheduling.

It is false economy to book patient appointments too close together and not leave adequate time for individual staff, department, and all-staff meetings, or to fail to put major policies and group decisions in writing. Hallmarks of the most successful practices include:

- Doctor breakfast or lunch meetings to communicate as colleagues
- Roundtable sessions to solve specific problems at a set time
- General staff meetings
- Suggestion boxes strategically placed
- An annual retreat
- A written procedure and policy manual
- Weekly staff bulletins
- Email communication to staff

BOOKING THE ARRIVING PATIENT

When a patient arrives at the office, certain documentation procedures must be performed to obtain the vital information necessary for the complete charting of the patient. The area of introduction of the patient to the staff should be pleasant. Files should be readily available.

If the receptionist has a good memory, greeting the patient by name on arrival is good public relations. If not, tact in obtaining vital information is important. Many patients will be reticent about giving their age, particularly in front of other patients. Insurance numbers and statistics on financial affairs must be tactfully handled. If a verbal request for information does not provide sufficient confidentiality, a blank information card on a clipboard can be given to patients to complete while they are seated and then returned to the receptionist. This is preferable to asking for confidential information in front of others.

All patients should be given a warm welcome, just as if they were being received into a home. They should feel wanted and comfortable no matter how busy the office situation at the time. Each person should be treated as an individual. Some personal detail that may have been noted previously should be inquired after if the receptionist knows the patient.

Records of patients seen previously will be obtained from the files. If the patient has never been seen before, a new record is opened and all the vital information recorded. The name and address must be printed carefully and clearly on each record card in a standard, readily identified area of the card.

Once the day begins with the scheduled appointments, it is important that there be minimal delay in the processing of each patient. Before the patient is seen by the ophthalmologist, politeness, kind words, and a cheerful "hello" will go a long way in promoting goodwill for the ophthalmologist and the office. The office assistant should always speak to the patients and assure them that they will be seen shortly by the doctor.

In ophthalmology, because eyedrops are usually instilled and the patient must wait a given length of time, a proper flow of patients into different rooms should be planned. The placing of patients into designated rooms by the ophthalmic assistant will ensure proper attention by the ophthalmologist with minimal delay. Patients with sore or painful eyes should be seated in the waiting room in such a position as to avoid facing glaring lights.

THE RECEPTION ROOM

Once in the office, the patient should not have to wait more than 15 minutes before being shown into an examination room. Those 15 minutes in the reception room should be comfortable and pleasant.

A wide variety of current reading material will occupy patients as they wait. Chairs should be spaced so that each patient has elbow room and does not feel cramped up to another person. As a courtesy to patients who find cigarette smoke irritating, you might post a sign that reads "Smoking not permitted in this health care facility."

Many offices have educational brochures available that explain common eye ailments. The reception room is a perfect place to circulate patient information brochures or past newsletters and to dispense information about the practice. Brochures might contain information on office hours, insurance, emergencies, and new medical developments for eye conditions.

The decor of the reception room should create a bright, cheerful atmosphere. Artwork, photographs, plants, and fresh-cut flowers will assist. Depending on the doctor's wishes, the assistant may choose to have coffee, juice, or water available to patients on request. A TV monitor with low or no sound may be of help

Avoid personal conversations with other staff members or on the phone with friends because these often can be overheard by patients. Staff must be professional at all times.

RUNNING LATE

No matter how carefully an appointment system is planned, delays and waiting periods will occur in a busy ophthalmic practice. Unlike other specialists, who can control to a certain extent the number of return visits, ophthalmologists, because of the number of emergencies encountered coupled with demands from referring physicians, have difficulty in adhering to a fixed schedule. Ironically, the qualities that make them run late are the qualities that make them available to patients. When an emergency patient calls, an ophthalmologist says, "Yes, come in and I will take care of you." When a patient talks about ailments (or problems that may be causing the illness), a good doctor will not shove the patient out the door just to stick to a schedule. When confronted with a complicated eye problem requiring extensive testing, a competent ophthalmologist, no matter how busy, will take the time to arrive at the diagnosis that sometimes may be not only sight saving but also lifesaving.

When the doctor is running late, if the waiting patients begin complaining, the ophthalmic assistant should give them a little insight into these facts.

SCRIBES

Scribes are a major time saver for an ophthalmologist in the recording of information. They can increase the productivity of the office and reduce patient waiting time.

Some ophthalmic assistants train to be a scribe for the examining ophthalmologist. They must be familiar with ophthalmic vocabulary as well as vocabulary shortcuts, symbols, and testing equipment. They should have legible handwriting. Ophthalmic scribes can save time in an office not only by recording the examination details but also by prewriting prescriptions for drugs and spectacles for the

licensed doctor's signature. They also assist when reemphasizing instructions while the doctor sees the next patient. Ophthalmic assistants' knowledge will increase by virtue of the fact they will eventually see and hear about every ophthalmic disease, disorder, and treatment.

Another advantage of a scribe to an eye practice is that it often improves handwriting in charting because of the knowledge gained. Forms are often delegated to the scribe to fill in then return to patients immediately, rather than by mail.

The ophthalmologist should verify that clinical notes and forms are completed accurately.

Scribes' signatures should be placed for medical legal purposes, and on electronic records, scribes should have their own password. Some scribes may be licensed in their state to write prescriptions.

MAKING FUTURE APPOINTMENTS

If a repeat appointment is required within the next 2 to 3 weeks because of iritis, conjunctivitis, glaucoma, or postoperative care, this appointment should be made at a designated time that does not overcrowd an already crowded appointment book. Usually these repeat visits are short so they can be scheduled before other regular appointments or integrated into the appointment system by a reserved block of time at the end of the appointment system.

It also is important for working patients that repeat appointment times be given early in the day. A minimal amount of delay is expected in the appointment system at that time because unexpected emergencies tend to occur as the day progresses.

FINANCING

There are a number of financing companies that provide excellent resources to finance expensive procedures for the uninsured or underinsured surgical patient. These companies also provide handouts, newsletters, emails, and support staff to inform patients of the availability of financing for surgery.

RECALL CARDS

Recall cards probably are the single most important vehicle an office has to maintain a regular, steady flow of patients. Many patients need to see an ophthalmologist only every 3, 6, or 12 months. Keeping a record of when they are due for their next examination is a method of ensuring that they receive continuing eye care, particularly for glaucoma or postoperative patients. It is difficult to provide the quality of eye care necessary if people forget or neglect to check their eyes. A recall card is a friendly reminder inviting them to call the office to schedule an appointment at their earliest convenience.

The best way to establish a recall card system is to set up a tickler file and keep it near the last person to speak with the patients before they depart from the office. At that time the physician's notes can be read and a recall postcard addressed with the month of suggested return on it. It is then filed in the tickler file according to month. At the beginning of each month the recall cards that are in the file for the following month should be sent out. Some offices like to follow up the recall card with a personal telephone call. Future appointments may be made as far ahead as 1 to 2 years in an appointment book or computer. It is important to remind these patients by card or by telephone at least 1 to 2 weeks before the appointment. Rescheduling may be required if the date selected is no longer convenient for the patient.

AUTOMATED VOICE MACHINES

There are several companies offering telephone assistance for offices to optimize patient communication. We are familiar with the TeleVox system, which provides caller ID on all incoming calls, prompts the caller to transfer to specific departments—such as to schedule appointments—and provides extensions to speak to live personnel. The system messages can be customized and changed to suit the priorities of the office.

The system can also be used for appointment reminders for scheduled patients, at an appropriate time 2 to 3 days ahead of their appointment. This can be achieved by simply entering the database of upcoming patients and can essentially reduce the "no show" rate by 35%. This also provides an opportunity to fill the appointment holes with transfers, emergencies, referrals, and so on, and helps raise the overall efficiency of the office.

The recall message can be produced in several languages, a nice touch for some, which may help to reach out to patients who have never returned.

FILING

Filing is an important aspect of everyone's everyday practice. If a file is lost or misfiled, a great deal of valuable information may be lost, including measurements that may be impossible to obtain again. The doctor may have to spend considerable time trying to recover information. Anyone may remove files from the filing system, but only one person should be delegated the responsibility of refiling. When a file is misplaced, everyone may be called on to aid in the search for the file. Often the file may have been removed for reports, letters, surgery, and so on.

Most ophthalmic offices have a central filing system, with files placed in alphabetic order. These systems may be further subdivided by an active drawer, which includes files of patients who are under active treatment and who will be returning within the next 4 weeks. Some hospitals and offices file their charts under a numeric system. This is more efficient and minimizes lost files, but it requires additional work. Each chart is numbered in order of being opened and it is filed accordingly. Cross-references are made of all names, in alphabetic order, and even double cross-referenced so that any special foster names or married names are indexed. In an alphabetic system of filing, the controversial order of names such as those beginning with Mac and Mc and names such as DeForest are filed according to an agreed-on procedure, which must be known to all. In addition, common names such as Brown, Smith, and Lee should be arranged in the order of the initial of the patient's first name. The numeric filing system eliminates these challenges and minimizes the number of misfiled records.

It has been our practice to separate the financial from the clinical records for each patient seen. With the advent of Medicare, we have found it expedient to change our patient processing routine so that the financial records, including billing and posting, are prepared at the time of the patient's office visit. The first statement and an account for submission to the insurance company can be given to the patient at this time.

Laboratory and x-ray reports, along with letters from other physicians, must be appended to the patient's chart and brought to the attention of the eye doctor. It is unacceptable to simply file such letters with the chart until the next patient visit without them being seen by the eye doctor.

Missed appointments and cancellations should be noted on the patient's chart and brought to the doctor's attention. Sometimes important litigation hinges on this type of information.

Files should be purged at least annually to allow more space. Outside storage is an option if space is limited. Files of known deceased patients and very old files should be purged regularly and sent to a shredding service or shredded onsite if available. One should establish a year date for the last visit (e.g., 7 years, 10 years) before deleting a file. The practitioner's office should have a policy for length of retention of medical records that follows state or provincial laws and advice of the practice's malpractice insurance company.

ELECTRONIC MEDICAL AND HEALTH RECORDS

Electronic medical records (EMRs) and electronic health records (EHRs) are a computerized medical records system created in organizations that deliver health care such as hospitals, integrated delivery networks, clinics, ambulatory surgical centers, and health care provider offices. These records make up a health care information system that allows for storage, retrieval, and modification of the health care record.

The terms electronic medical records and electronic health records are often used interchangeably, though technically EMRs represent a duplicate of a paper-based charting, whereas EHRs are electronic records with the ability for electronic exchange of patient data from practice setting to practice setting. These electronic records can contain a wide range of patient data including patient demographics, medical history, medications, allergies, immunizations, vital signs, physical examination findings, laboratory tests, radiologic images, photos, prescriptions, and billing and insurance information.

EHRs are being heavily promoted by federal and state governments, insurance companies, and large medical institutions as a system to help physicians and office staff better care for patients before, during, and after health care encounters. Because of these promotions EHRs are being incorporated into many health care provider offices. They are ways to improve efficiency, promote quality improvement, overcome poor penmanship that contributes to medical errors, and offer standardization of forms, terminology, and abbreviations. They allow for data input for collection of epidemiology and clinical data. Barriers to adoption of electronic records include start-up costs, system maintenance costs, and training costs. Patient privacy issues are of concern with electronic records because of their portability and potential access by unscrupulous users and unauthorized individuals.

PRESCRIPTION PADS

Each prescription for a medication should be signed by the prescribing doctor. Blank prescription pads should be kept in a drawer so a patient (or staff member) is not tempted to steal a pad and self-prescribe a narcotic or other medication.

OFFICE EQUIPMENT

Equipment is an important factor in office efficiency. The ophthalmologist or office manager must constantly be on the watch for new business machines that may improve office efficiency. These include calculators, postage meters, copiers, and fax machines. One also must watch for new ideas in billing procedures and form procedures that will be helpful. Floor and wall coverings that reduce noise should be used. Seats should be arranged to relieve back strain. Stamping and sealing envelopes by machine greatly facilitate the speed of these procedures. The telephone

system should be reviewed with the telephone company to ensure that one has the most efficient system available and that proper lines of communication are established between rooms, through either the telephone or an intercom system.

The personal computer, which is now standard in the ophthalmic office, is discussed in detail in Chapter 49.

Ophthalmic equipment is very precise and must be kept in perfect working order. Basic principles to consider include the following:

1. Keep the machines (slit lamp, keratometer) covered when not in use.
2. Regularly check the accuracy of such devices as the Radiuscope, keratometer, and lensometer.
3. Learn to maintain the instruments, from changing a bulb in the projector to attaching a topogometer.
4. Make sure regular maintenance is performed for such instruments as the automatic refractor, keratometer, pneumotonometer, and corneal topography machines.

PERSONAL QUALITIES FOR IMPROVED OFFICE EFFICIENCY

Avoiding interruptions

Before leaving the office at night, create a to-do list for the next day and prioritize the order. Organize a special me or personal hour (preferably early in the morning) and turn all phones and distractions off. Tell your coworkers you want "peace and quiet" to do a special project. You will probably complete this in half the time! Do not become distracted by other folders or emails on your computer; if you have a door, close it. If you work in a cubicle, put up a "do not disturb" sign, and if appropriate devote at least 1 to 2 hours a day to uninterrupted work. Tell other assistants what you are doing and they will probably do the same.

The attitudes of each of us are based on our likes and dislikes and are expressed in our words, our actions, and our behavior. Some of these attitudes become habits, some of which are helpful and some harmful to ourselves, the people we work with, and the patients we greet. The ophthalmic assistant should analyze these attitudes and try to eliminate those that are inappropriate.

An attractive personality depends on an expression of physical, mental, social, and moral qualities. Physical qualities give first impressions to people we meet. Our appearance, voice, manner, energy, and bearing portray a first impression to the patient. Social qualities are developed through our everyday contacts with people. To make a favorable impression one must be considerate of others, cooperative, and courteous and show tact, cheerfulness, and kindness. In addition, patience and sympathy must be part of one's personality. These attributes create a pleasant and stimulating atmosphere in the office.

Mental qualities include intelligence, a keen observation, a retentive memory, and an ability to concentrate and apply oneself. The ophthalmic assistant must be orderly, accurate, and careful in conduct, show an ability to intelligently and quickly answer the many questions that patients ask, and above all show a good sense of humor.

Moral qualities, the foundations of character underlying everything else, include honesty, sincerity, loyalty, and trustworthiness. The ophthalmic assistant should have the courage and determination to do the right thing, regardless of the consequences. These qualities provide an important guideline to the daily behavior of the ophthalmic assistant who works with the public. An assistant can review the effectiveness evaluation to see how he or she rates (Box 6.4). Self-evaluation can be important.

IMPROVING THE PATIENT EXPERIENCE THROUGH SERVICE RECOVERY

It has been said that "a happy patient will tell one other person of their great experience. An unhappy patient will tell five." This adage is no longer accurate. With the widespread use of Twitter, Facebook, and sites such as YouTube, an unhappy person can now connect with literally millions of others with very little effort and in a very short time. This highlights the need to ensure the best possible patient experience, especially if some type of service issue occurs.

There are two types of service issues: expected and unexpected. The expected is handled by proactive methods and established triggers that start the service recovery process. These mishaps include the usual examples of the doctor being late and emergencies arising in the clinic. Communicate early with patients about problems or delays, and offer sincere apologies. A tool kit with gift cards for coffee or a

---

Box 6.4 Rating effectiveness as an ophthalmic assistant

Dependability

Trustworthiness in carrying out instructions and assignments
Excellent
Above average
Average
Below average
Unsatisfactory

Productivity

Achievement of satisfactory quantity of work
Excellent
Above average
Average
Below average
Unsatisfactory

Adaptability

Reception of new ideas and methods; adjustments to changes in work
Excellent
Above average
Average
Below average
Unsatisfactory

Cooperation

Tact: willingness to assist; agreeable compliance
Excellent
Above average

Average
Below average
Unsatisfactory

Accuracy

Exactness, professional skill
Excellent
Above average
Average
Below average
Unsatisfactory

Initiative

Performance in analyzing problems, accepting responsibilities, planning necessary action, and following through
Excellent
Above average
Average
Below average
Unsatisfactory

Individuality

Personal appearance, neatness, behavior on job
Excellent
Above average
Average
Below average
Unsatisfactory

nearby restaurant, taxi vouchers, and other goodies also can be useful.

The unexpected mishaps are a bit more complicated, such as patients arriving on the wrong day or making unreasonable requests. First, one needs to know how to recognize these situations through tell-tale signs; patient body language, tone of voice, anger, or silence. Then one must be prepared to listen, ask questions, and listen again.

Respond with HEART, which stands for*:

Hear. "Please tell me what has happened. I'd like to know how I might help you today." Hear what the patient has to say by truly listening. The biggest gift you can give another is your full attention. Try not to formulate a response while the patient is speaking; just work to understand his or her point of view.

Empathize. "I know what you mean. It can be difficult. I understand what you might be feeling." People want to have their feelings validated. Expressing understanding goes a long way toward helping defuse a tense situation.

Apologize. "I'm sorry that this happened. Please accept our apologies for this delay. I know that your time is valuable." Give a simple apology without blame. Be sincere.

Respond. "How would you like it resolved? We'll be addressing this by..." Make sure to follow up with the patient. Set a timeline for any responses or additional actions, and be sure to stick to it. Give the patient your contact information so that you can be contacted if further questions arise.

Thank. "Thank you for bringing this to my attention. I appreciate you letting me know about this." No one wants to be considered a problem, and these occasions should be looked at as opportunities for improvements. Without someone pointing out issues, larger problems can occur in the future.

What can be expected from patients? Three possibilities are:

Those who have had a great experience: no problem, they're happy

Those who have had a bad experience and no one responds to it: they're unhappy

Those who have had a bad experience that is resolved: these patients are the happiest of all

This isn't meant to be a case for making patients unhappy, but a case for the power of service recovery. Complaints are a gift and the schoolbook from which we can learn. Handling complaints skillfully can actually lead to staff satisfaction. It feels good to resolve a conflict, and the payoff of a happy patient is priceless. Responding with HEART will pay great dividends to patients, staff, and the practice.

---

*Contributed by Melissa Jones, MEd, COE, OCS.

SECRETARIAL DUTIES

The ophthalmic assistant may be required to compose or type letters to insurance companies, physicians, or suppliers. Although the dictator of the letters is responsible for clarity, thought, and completeness, the typist must be given credit for proper setup and form of the letter. Margins must be clearly laid out, paragraphs introduced properly, and punctuation correctly placed. The visual setup of the letter is as important as the wording: both contribute to the impression the receiver will form about the office.

As time goes on, many types of form will become routine and standardized. Even letters will have a standard form of setting up introductory paragraphs and conclusions. The best way of doing things becomes standard. No matter what it may be, there is a best way of doing it, whether it is folding and sealing a letter, putting on a stamp, setting up a letter, or filing a carbon copy. Once these standards are discovered and established, the wasteful and useless movements are eliminated.

HANDLING THE OPHTHALMOLOGIST'S SCHEDULE

Eye doctors are usually busy people; consequently considerable demands are made on their time in the office, in the hospital, and in extra activities. They may be required to fulfill teaching roles and speaking engagements and become involved in community work. From time to time these additional involvements will be made known to the ophthalmic assistant. When they interfere with existing schedules, the assistant should try to ensure that the office and the hospital are organized to accommodate these changes.

The assistant must ensure the appointment book is not overcrowded so that the physician is not constantly delayed in attending meetings or giving lectures. There are times when the ophthalmologist will have to cancel appointments for an emergency, a court case, or an illness. If the physician will be unable to be at the office for an appointment and knows beforehand, the patient should be notified by telephone or letter. Sometimes the appointment may require cancellation by fax. This will be more costly but it is necessary to prevent putting the patient to the inconvenience of coming to the office. The catch word is "rescheduling" and not canceling.

HANDLING SALES REPRESENTATIVES

Sales representatives from the various drug and optical firms attempt to bring the latest information on new products and changes in products to the physician. Some come only occasionally to the ophthalmologist and some come frequently. No matter how busy, the doctor usually prefers to see these salespeople. A few minutes spent with a sales representative may make the ophthalmologist knowledgeable on a valuable new therapeutic tool. Sometimes, however, the physician may be too busy to see a salesperson and may wish the ophthalmic assistant to obtain all the pertinent information and to summarize the contents of the individual reports or to obtain summaries and abstracts of these. Practical experience can teach the assistant how to make a good abstract and then present it to the ophthalmologist at a more leisurely moment or at the end of the day.

The ophthalmic assistant will soon become familiar with the various representatives from the pharmaceutical and optical firms who visit the ophthalmologist. All physicians are interested in receiving firsthand information about their products. One must, however, discriminate between these sales representatives and magazine salespeople, peddlers, and the like. Sales representatives always present cards, are never abusive, and never attempt to get into the doctor's office under false pretenses. Accordingly, they should be greeted graciously. When seeing the representatives, the assistant should explain how busy the doctor is at the given time and how much of the practitioner's time they may have. The doctor is then in a position to close the interview when he or she chooses. If it is inconvenient for the clinician to see a sales representative at the time of his or her call, the caller is entitled to an explanation and should be asked to return at a more convenient time when the physician will be able to see him or her.

In addition to these individuals, there may be many callers who take up the doctor's time unnecessarily. The ophthalmic assistant may be very useful in graciously handling these callers, talking to them, and diverting them. For example, insurance salespeople and those who sell stocks and bonds can be diverted from office hours to a more convenient time, if the doctor wishes to see them. If the caller does not wish to state the nature of business and the ophthalmic assistant knows that the doctor does not wish to be disturbed by such visitors, the caller should be asked to write a letter to the clinician about the matter.

HANDLING MAIL

The doctor should receive mail in an orderly fashion. Personal correspondence is kept together, as is correspondence relating to patients, such as x-ray and laboratory reports and consultation letters. Drug company correspondence is compiled and kept separate from advertisements and medical journals. Such organization expedites the doctor's review of the mail. The accounts should be given to the personnel primarily responsible for them. Before the doctor is presented with an insurance form to complete, the patient's record should be obtained and a certain amount of the form completed by the secretary or ophthalmic assistant.

MEDICAL ETHICS

Physicians are bound by a code of rules and customs to which they are expected to adhere. The background for this code is the Hippocratic Oath, named after Hippocrates, a Greek physician of the fifth century BC who is called "The Father of Medicine." Hippocrates gave sound and shrewd descriptions of many diseases and thus raised the ethical standards of medical practice. The Hippocratic Oath is a beautiful and inspiring statement that was demanded of the young physician about to enter the practice of medicine (Box 6.5). It placed medicine on a scientific foundation, freeing it from superstition, philosophy, and religious rites.

Box 6.5 Oath of Hippocrates

I swear by Apollo the Physician, by Aesculapius, by Hygeia, by Panacea, and by all the gods and goddesses, calling them to witness that according to my ability and judgment I will in every particular keep this, my Oath and Covenant: To regard him who teaches this art equally with my parents, to share my substance with him and, if he be in need, to relieve his necessities; to regard his offspring equally with my brethren; and to teach them this art if they shall wish to learn it, without fee or stipulation; to impart a knowledge of the art by precept, by lecture, and by every other mode of instruction to my sons, to the sons of my teacher, and to pupils who are bound by stipulation and oath, according to the Law of Medicine, but to no other.

I will follow that regimen which, according to my ability and judgment, shall be for the welfare of the sick, and I will refrain from that which shall be baneful and injurious. If any shall ask of me a drug to produce death, I will not give it, nor will I suggest such counsel. In like manner I will not give a woman a destructive pessary.

With Purity and Holiness will I watch closely my life and my art. I will not cut a person who is suffering from a stone, but will give way to those who are practitioners in this work. Into whatever houses I shall enter, I will go to aid the sick, abstaining from every voluntary act of injustice and corruption, and from lasciviousness with women or men, with freemen and slaves.

Whatever in the life of men I shall see or hear, in my practice or without my practice, which should not be made public, this will I hold in silence, believing that such things should not be spoken.

While I keep this, my Oath, inviolate and unbroken, may it be granted to me to enjoy life and my art, forever honored by all men; but should I by transgression violate it, be mine the reverse.

Today the Hippocratic Oath serves as a foundation on which the highest standards of medicine are practiced.

The principles of medical ethics have been developed over the course of centuries as medicine has evolved. Many of these writings may seem old-fashioned now because they are no longer needed, but others have never varied. Although the Hippocratic Oath concerns itself only with the relationship between the physician and the patient, modern medical ethics also govern the relationship of the physician to the community and to fellow physicians. Even though the overall knowledge and technology of modern medical science are vastly superior to those of ancient times, the universal theme of "self-discovery"' has not changed since the days of Hippocrates. The ophthalmic assistant should be acquainted with the fundamental rules of medical ethics, because his or her actions will reflect on the ophthalmologist.

One of the principles of medical ethics is strict secrecy, which must be observed regarding all matters pertaining to the patient. It is not ethical to criticize the work of another physician to a patient. If a physician has inadvertently expressed some opinion to the ophthalmic assistant in private, the assistant may, out of loyalty to the ophthalmologist, wish to show superiority to the patient by voicing criticism of the other physician's treatment. This is strictly against medical ethics.

A physician must be careful to avoid exaggerated publicity or connection with any incident that has news value, especially of a sensational kind. When newspaper reporters call at the office for information or a statement by the physician, they should be transferred directly to the ophthalmologist, who is fully cognizant of responsibilities both to the public and to fellow medical colleagues. Discretion in this area belongs solely to the doctor.

Each physician has occasion to refer patients to outside agencies for some form of service or for the purchase of optical or medical supplies. Patients often ask for the name of an individual or organization from whom they may obtain these services. Their confidence in the opinion of their ophthalmologist is an important consideration in deciding whom to consult and where to go. The names, addresses, and telephone numbers of those physicians or optical firms in whom the ophthalmologist has a measure of confidence and to whom he or she might refer patients must therefore be known to the ophthalmic assistant and must be kept in such a way that the list can be consulted readily. A list should be kept available of agencies such as the local institute for the blind, diagnostic laboratories, and organizations that deal with the perceptually handicapped child.

IN THE PHYSICIAN'S ABSENCE

The ophthalmic assistant can be of immense help to a physician who presents papers at meetings of medical societies, writes articles or books, or undertakes research work. Physicians who communicate findings to the scientific world usually do extensive writing. The assistant can be of invaluable aid in assembling research or reference material and in editing manuscripts. The time when the physician is away from the office for meetings or holidays can be put to good use in this area. The ophthalmic assistant with a leaning toward writing may prefer this phase of work to all others and be instrumental in obtaining reference materials, in searching the Internet, cumulative indexes and libraries for material on the pertinent subject, and in assembling these for the attention of the ophthalmologist. This work, whether it is for a lecture, article, or book, will provide insight into many new facets of ophthalmology.

AIDS IN PUBLIC RELATIONS

1. At one time or another, every ophthalmic assistant will be confronted with an office full of patients waiting at their appointed times while the ophthalmologist has been delayed. The assistant should attempt to reappoint patients who do not have an urgent problem and those who cannot afford to wait. If reappointments or delays are required, the patient is entitled to an explanation of this inconvenience. Because the physician's day is usually devoted to providing service to others, such explanations can be freely candid. Most patients appreciate the demands constantly made on the physician's time and are usually quite fair in thoughtfully considering these delays. For those patients who prefer to wait in the office, refreshments should be offered if the facilities are available.

2. The waiting room should be kept clean and neat at all times. Magazines without covers should be removed and broken toys removed or repaired.

3. The ophthalmic assistant should always be neat, fresh, and well groomed. Extreme styles of clothing should be avoided; make-up should never be excessive. Colognes/perfumes should be avoided as some patients may be sensitive/allergic. Uniforms may be worn. Nametags are desirable.

4. As much as possible have the same member of staff deal with the same patient. Maintain eye contact and a pleasant expression. Smile! Separate work duties from home and personal duties.

5. Patients should be called from the waiting room with a soft and friendly voice that rings with hospitality. If a patient has poor vision, the tone of voice should remain unchanged. Many people approach the partially sighted as though they had lost their other sensory functions and tend to speak in a loud voice or even shout.

6. However, not all patients are blessed with good hearing. The ophthalmic assistant may be required to

speak in louder tones in communicating with the hard-of-hearing patient.

7. The ophthalmic assistant should attempt to have patients remove overshoes, overcoats, and scarves before entering the ophthalmologist's inner office. Coat racks should be available. This invariably saves time and allows patients to be more comfortable for the examination.

8. Children may be led by the hand to the examining room (Figure 6.4). A small toy or gift may establish better rapport with the child.

9. Personalizing a practice can be done in many ways. Look around the office. Is everyone wearing a name badge? Do the nurses, assistants, and technicians have cards with their name and title on them so patients can call directly and ask them questions? When the physician enters the examining room, does the technician introduce the patient to the ophthalmologist? Are visual aids available (Figure 6.5)? Hearing aids can be helpful for the hard of hearing (Figure 6.6).

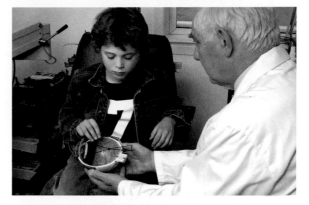

Figure 6.5 Visual aids to demonstrate problems.

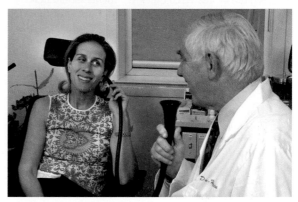

Figure 6.6 A hearing trumpet can be used for the hard of hearing.

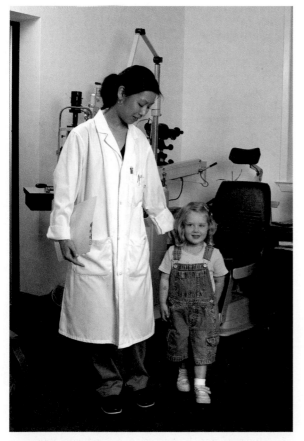

Figure 6.4 Handling the young child.

10. Because of the increasing number of senior citizens who come to ophthalmology offices, some doctors are beginning to offer some form of transportation within a certain radius. This is a great service to seniors who might not drive or to surgery patients who are temporarily unable to drive. A limousine or van that seats six to eight people can be used to pick patients up and return them to their homes. When patients call to make an appointment, the assistant can tell them that on Tuesday and Thursday mornings, for example, a transportation service is available to those living within a 5-mile radius of the physician's office and are having surgery. Would they like to take advantage of such a service? Scheduling transportation requests ahead of time will allow the driver to plan an effective route for picking up patients. The driver should be a patient, courteous person with an excellent driving record and a personality that will make the passengers feel comfortable and safe. Advertising a service such as free transportation is bound to increase telephone requests by new patients for further information

about your office and its services. At a time when more and more new patients are "shopping" for physicians, a service such as free transportation will draw attention.

11. No matter how minor or short a surgical procedure or hospitalization is according to medical standards, it is of major importance to the patient and should be acknowledged as such by the office personnel. Following up surgical procedures with a call from someone in the office or sending a gift such as a plant to a recuperating patient is an extremely courteous and personal gesture. Often a personal note from the physician will boost the patient's morale beyond anyone's expectations. Surgical patients always should be given priority scheduling for follow-up appointments, and any questions they may call in with should be answered quickly. Patients should never feel that the physician or office personnel are ignoring them now that the surgery is over! Developing a special protocol for handling surgery patients will, in the long run, boost the physician's practice. Patients love to talk about their surgeries; let what they say about your office be positive and flattering.

12. Keep records of where new patients are coming from. Have a tracking form that you keep next to the appointment book. When new patients call for an appointment, ask them who referred them to the office. If they are responding to an advertisement and your office runs more than one advertisement, ask them *specifically* which ad they read. Enter the information on the tracking form. At the end of the month review the number of new patients and where they came from.

13. Listening to patients correlates well with a willingness to recommend a practice. Thank-you cards should be sent to current patients who referred new patients to the office. A sample message is shown in Box 6.6. Handwritten signatures are best!

Each of these points contributes to the overall feeling of personalization that is desired in a medical practice. Patient handling is as much a part of medicine as diagnosis and treatment.

Box 6.6 **Sample thank-you card for patient referrals**

Dear _____,
    Thank you for referring _____ to our office. We appreciate your confidence in us. We look forward to continuing to serve you and will always make time available for you, your family, and friends.
    Sincerely,

PATIENT SURVEYS

Ultimately the patient is the one to determine just how pleasant, efficient, and effective an office operation is. An office might set a plan into action thinking that the patients will love it and the fact may be that none of the patients have even been aware of its existence!

Feedback from patients can be very valuable, but office personnel must ask for it. Few patients, unless they are angry about something, will voluntarily mention that they had to wait slightly longer than usual the past two or three visits, or that the reading material in your reception room is outdated and sloppily tossed about.

Patient information surveys are forms you can devise that contain 10 to 15 questions about how patients experience the office, from the time they call to make an appointment to the time they pay for their service and depart. Questions should be worded positively and be followed by definite choices.

For 1 month, as each patient leaves the office, he or she is handed a survey form together with a stamped return envelope. Office personnel explain to the patients that if they would be so kind as to complete this survey and return it at their earliest convenience this would provide assistance in maintaining an office that can best serve their needs. Most people will be more than happy to respond. A suggestion is that they do not sign the survey form so that it will remain anonymous and be truly reflective of their opinion. When a substantial number of surveys have been returned, someone in the office tallies the results, which can be discussed at the next office meeting.

PUBLICITY

The major goal of publicity is to stimulate an interest in and public awareness of the physician or the organization. A good public relations program can accomplish many objectives, for example:

- Create an intense interest for a timely event, for example, anniversary of the practice.
- Be part of an ongoing promotion.
- Promote the physician's image.
- Generate goodwill for the office and physician.
- Highlight any awards for the doctor or practice.

Public relations offers several advantages over other types of promotional tools. Marketing consultants such as Robert Shropshire and Mike Malley can often help a practice in identifying the best features of a practice. Items that are taken as routine for a practice may have an enormous interest for the general public and can be emphasized. Consultants can help phase in new aspects of the practice by professional writing and can advise on proper professional presentations. They also can negotiate best pricing in media advertising. Consultants also are knowledgeable in putting the best foot forward for the practice.

Cost

Advertising and publicity make use of the media to reach the public, but public relations tends to be less expensive. Both result in publicity. Unlike advertising, publicity coverage is inexpensive. In most cases the only expense for public relations is for paper, postage, mail announcements, and, for large users, a public relations firm.

Size of the audience

Public relations can tell the story to thousands of potential patients, possibly millions with the use of mass media. Although the benefit of targeting potentially interested people may be significant, publicity directed toward the general public results in fast and effective communication.

Credibility

Public relations lends an air of credibility that is missing in advertising. If one is interviewed on the 6 o'clock news or quoted in the daily paper, the public tends to perceive the interviewee as an expert. Media attention is usually perceived by listeners and viewers as an endorsement of a product, service, or cause.

Effect

Public relations is persuasive. It can shape public opinion, mold personal images, and even reverse negative attitudes.

Versatility

Public relations can be used to place one in a spotlight at almost any time or any place one chooses. By taking advantage of carefully selected media opportunities, one can expand into new areas of practice.

Longevity

Public relations offers longevity and provides a permanent record. A person who has been mentioned in the media can show the clipping to potential clients, quote it in advertising, or use it as a means to gain more publicity.

ADVERTISING

Advertising is seen as a device to ensure that physicians are competitive and that their fees are dictated by the market. Medical advertising should be factual (one cannot claim to be the best cataract surgeon in a given state without being able to prove it) and informative, listing hours of work, the physician's specialty, and practice restrictions. Above all, the advertisement should be in good taste and have regard for not annoying competing ophthalmologists in the area. The foes of advertising are upset over the loss of dignity that results from using a commercial vehicle to promote a medical reputation. Good advertising can yield results in months that formerly took years to develop on the basis of word-of-mouth recommendation.

SUMMARY

Office efficiency depends on adaptation to patient needs, as well as skill in combining an effective program for telephone responses, handling of patients in the office, filing and recording data, and providing good public relations through publicity and patient management. The goodwill that evolves from this combined approach to office efficiency will have a long-lasting effect in ensuring return visits of patients who are pleased with the services provided.

Questions for review and thought

1. Discuss the appointment system in your office (or make up an appointment system), in particular how you would work emergency appointments into the system.
2. What are some personal qualities of an ophthalmic assistant that greatly enhance his or her ability to get along with people?
3. How may you use your time best when the ophthalmologist is away at meetings or on holidays?
4. How do you handle the small, frightened child? The patient who is almost blind? The patient who is deaf?
5. Mrs. Johnson arrives in intense pain from overwearing her contact lenses. How do you handle this situation?
6. A very important person arrives in the office and, in spite of a number of people waiting ahead of him, he insists on being taken next. How do you handle this situation?
7. The waiting room is crowded. An angry patient says the doctor is running a factory and begins to be abusive. How do you handle such a person?
8. You are applying for a job as an ophthalmic assistant. The doctor questions your value to him or her. What would you say to indicate that you could improve his or her efficiency?
9. Write several on-hold messages for callers who are waiting anxiously for the telephone receptionist to return to the line.

Q Self-evaluation questions

Office problems to solve

Office efficiency is promoted through the work of intelligent, responsible people using the faculties of cooperation, creativity, industry, interest, and sensitivity. Problems that may arise in the office often do not have a cut-and-dried solution. Each situation is unique and requires individual attention. The following problems and brief discussions on how to handle them touch on some areas of difficulty that might be encountered. We have included some of our ideas, but there are a multitude of others that we encourage you to explore.

Problem 1. A patient calls and demands an immediate appointment because he is having a problem with his eyes. He sounds quite hysterical to you and the symptoms do not seem to indicate an emergency. What do you do?

Problem 2. The doctor is away for 2 weeks. Shortly after his or her departure, an important letter arrives in the mail and requests a speedy acknowledgment or reply. What should you do?

Problem 3. The doctor has asked you to reschedule some appointments because of a change in his or her surgical schedule. You have been unable to reach a patient by phone and the appointment is a week away. How should this be handled?

Problem 4. A patient arrives for an appointment and you are unable to locate her chart. How do you handle this situation?

Problem 5. The doctor is running late in his or her appointments. How would you handle the delay with newly arriving patients?

Problem 6. A sales representative arrives and insists on seeing the doctor even though the waiting room is crowded. How do you handle this situation?

Problem 7. What information should you obtain from patients or referring physicians' offices when they call to make an appointment?

Problem 8. It is sometimes difficult to see our own surroundings objectively. It is an interesting and informative exercise to imagine that you are a patient coming into the ophthalmologist's office for the first time. What is your initial reaction to this office? Is it clean, bright, and pleasant or stuffy and forbidding? Was your initial contact with the receptionist pleasant? Did you feel relaxed and comfortable with his or her manner, or did he or she seem harassed, overworked, or hostile? Did you find the waiting room to be well lit, with an interesting assortment of neatly displayed magazines, inviting you to enjoy your wait? Or did you find yourself peering at a tattered 3-month-old periodical in an overheated, overcrowded waiting room?

Problem 9. It has been the assumption throughout these questions that you are an employed ophthalmic assistant. Perhaps you are not. Perhaps you are embarking on a search for employment in this field. You will, then, have to prepare a résumé of your skills, experience, and training. You also will have to be prepared for an interview (or several interviews) with ophthalmologists. Consider the initial impression you want to make on them and the qualities and abilities you want to convey. Do you present yourself as a dependable, cooperative person who can meet challenges and accept responsibilities? Is your appearance neat and professional? You want to go into an interview feeling good, looking good, and emanating confidence in your ability to do the job and your eagerness for the opportunity to do so. How do you plan on doing this?

A Answers, notes, and explanations

Answer 1. There are a few ways to handle this situation. You could tell the patient that you are fully booked and that he can try to reach another physician who might be able to see him on a more immediate basis. You are, however, risking feelings of ill will by turning away this patient. You could inform the patient that he can be placed on a cancellation list and will be notified when an opening becomes available. This means you have taken the responsibility of diagnosing this problem as not urgent. Can a telephone conversation with an upset and frightened patient tell you this?

A third alternative is not to take it upon yourself to diagnose the patient's condition. Take down all the symptoms he is experiencing, get his phone number, pull his chart, and give the message to the doctor. The physician knows his or her patients, as well as possible serious potential problems, and should make the final decision as to what should be done.

Answer 2. The letter should not be left to vegetate for 2 weeks. If the matter is very pressing, contact the doctor. However, even important correspondence may not be extremely urgent. A courteous and considerate way to handle this would be to send the correspondent a brief note explaining that the doctor is away until a certain date and the letter will be answered promptly on his or her return.

Answer 3. You can make a note to call the patient the following day; the person may be out just for the day. This means that you must not forget to place this call on the next day. However, chances are that the patient has given you only a home number and cannot be reached there during the day. Therefore, if you are relying on this single mode of communication, you will have an irate patient to handle 1 week hence if the person arrives for the appointment.

A Continued

It is probably best to send a note as soon as you find it difficult to reach the patient by phone. Rather than leave it another day and waste precious time, post a note advising of the canceled appointment and provide an alternative date. This is easy and convenient and saves patient anxiety and the feeling of having been overlooked.

Answer 4. You could ask her to sit in the waiting room while you look for the chart. However, if you cannot find it within a reasonable time, you are delaying the patient. If you put her name on a blank chart, you would leave the doctor with an embarrassing problem.

It is best to explain to the patient that you are unable to locate her chart at the moment (this should be said after you have thoroughly searched the various areas where it might be). You should tell her that it will take a bit of time to check the files and make up a duplicate chart for today to keep her from waiting. Reassure her that her chart will be located.

Answer 5. It is easiest, but most unwise, to avoid the situation and hope that no one will complain about the delay. This is inconsiderate to the patient who may have another appointment to keep, who must get back to work, or who simply does not appreciate being kept waiting a disproportionate length of time.

One can directly inform an incoming patient that the doctor is running late (because of emergencies, a delay at the hospital, or whatever the case may be) and, unfortunately, there will be a longer than usual wait. Because the patient is being inconvenienced, offer a choice of waiting or rescheduling the appointment.

Answer 6. Some doctors will see sales representatives when they drop by; others prefer to have the ophthalmic assistant make an appointment for these brief visits or have the representative come at the end of the day.

If the practice is busy, as the crowded waiting room would indicate, it is best to form a consistent policy with sales representatives. The pharmaceutical representative will quickly learn when and how the ophthalmologist is available.

If a representative insists on seeing the doctor, present the doctor with his or her card and let the doctor decide what to do. You will find, however, that most sales representatives who come to your office will be courteous and cooperative. It is up to the ophthalmic assistant to set a mutually accommodating manner for visits to be made with maximum efficiency and minimal time lost.

Answer 7. You will need the patient's full name and phone numbers, home and business. Ask if the patient has been to the office previously; if not, you should record the person's mailing address. This is needed if you have to change the appointment and the patient cannot be reached by phone.

It is also helpful to know the basic nature of the problem or the reason for the appointment; that is, a postoperative check, a complete eye examination for a driver's license, a minor surgical procedure, an ocular injury, a contact lens problem, and so on. This information will help you in the scheduling of time for the appointment and in your preparedness for the patient.

When scheduling a consultation appointment, you will need the referring physician's name and, preferably, the nature of the patient's problem. If the patient has undergone any tests related to this particular problem, request that copies be forwarded to you before the appointment date.

Answer 8. Try to go through this mental experiment. Chances are you might see some things you had never before realized existed and that are in need of change or improvement.

Answer 9. This is a personal evaluation and an exercise well worth doing as a method of providing yourself with a self-assessment, as well as learning to put your best foot forward.

Chapter | 7 |

History taking

A history is the story of a patient's medical disorder. By means of the history the physician attempts to reconstruct the stages of disease as it has progressed. To elicit a history, the physician must ask questions about the patient's symptoms. Thus a history is really a series of specific questions linked in an orderly sequence. When a specific problem is identified in the response, specific questions are directed to elicit more detail. This chapter deals with a method of asking questions so that the patient's chronicle will be orderly, concise, and complete.

Two types of patients are seen in an ophthalmologist's office: the patient who desires a routine ocular examination combined with a refraction and the patient with symptoms of an ocular disorder. Unfortunately it is often impossible to distinguish between the two on the basis of a history. Each patient, then, must be questioned as though one expects to find some ocular disease.

Language problems frequently cause concern for both the ophthalmic assistant and the patient. Appendix 10 gives some commonly asked questions in foreign languages. The help of a translator and particularly a family member is valuable.

ORGANIZATION OF A HISTORY

The history should be subdivided to maintain organization. Many charts have the organization stenciled or printed on them. Regardless of the charting method used, an ophthalmic history should include the following:

- Chief complaint
- History of present illness
- History of past health
- Significant medical illnesses
- Previous eye disorders
- Previous surgery, both ophthalmic and general
- Medications currently used and their duration of use
- Allergies
- Inhalants
- Contactants
- Ingestants
- Medications
- Family history of ocular disorders
- Myopia
- Strabismus
- Glaucoma
- Blindness
- Occupation
- Type of work
- Industrial hazards

Although many complaints are strictly ocular in nature, others are a manifestation of poor general health or emotional problems. Occasionally patients may be taking medication that they do not realize affects the eye and will not reveal this aspect of their history unless specifically asked. For example, a patient with a duodenal ulcer may be given propantheline bromide (probanthene), an atropine-like drug that inactivates the ciliary muscle. Such a patient would consult the ophthalmologist because of difficulty seeing at near.

HISTORY PROCEDURE

In pursuing a history, the ophthalmic assistant should attempt to be precise and pertinent. With some patients an inquiry into previous health can result in a saga of each and every contact they have had with a physician. The patient, who may not know what is important and what is irrelevant, must be guided by questions. Frequently patients will state that they enjoy excellent health but when asked what medications they are taking, will respond that they are taking pills for hypertension, injections for diabetes, and iron for anemia. The patient does not connect a general systemic disorder with an ocular problem, yet all the diseases mentioned have serious consequences within the eye itself.

The ophthalmic assistant should be aware of his or her position to receive privileged information. The covenant that binds the patient and physician and allows private information to be transferred from one to the other also applies to the ophthalmic assistant, who works as an extension of the physician. Patients can be frank in discussing their ailments only when they feel confident that complaints are being aired for analysis, not for public consumption. Information garnered during a history should not be revealed to one's family, friends, or even fellow workers. A seemingly slight betrayal, such as revealing the patient's age, may have disastrous consequences and place the office in an awkward position.

The ophthalmic assistant should not refrain from asking a particular question because it appears to be too private or embarrassing. If the history is conducted in a frank and professional manner and the questions are posed with tact and good taste, the patient will reveal even the most private matters, just as he or she would remove a shirt for a chest examination. Above all, patients must have confidence in the professional ethics of the persons who treat them.

Some patients will not reveal the full pertinent history to the ophthalmic assistant. Normally this is not a vote of no confidence if the assistant's demeanor and manner of questioning are professional, but rather a failure of the patient to understand completely the importance of history taking. The occasional patient will refuse to speak to anyone except the physician about any eye problems. This is the patient's privilege. These patients should be treated with the same degree of tact and professionalism as the others.

Tactfully one should inquire about previous ophthalmologist or optometrists visited and their investigations and diagnosis. If reluctance to reveal this information is encountered, one should not pursue.

The assistant should not attempt to interpret or expand a statement made by the patient, because sorting out the information will waste the eye doctor's valuable time, thus negating the intention of the ophthalmic assistant.

The organization of questions is a prerequisite to completeness and to a program for efficiency. A routine should be established so that each patient is asked the same basic questions, preferably in the same manner. Of course, the dialog will differ as the complaints of the patients differ but the sameness of the structural questionnaire will give a certain firmness to the ophthalmic assistant's approach and provide an excellent source of data for review or research.

A routine that may be followed in careful history taking is described in the following sections. As with all routines, it provides guidelines and should not rigidly be followed.

GENERAL INFORMATION

Included under general information are the essential facts that should appear at the beginning of every chart (Figure 7.1). These include the patient's name, address, date of birth, and work and home telephone numbers. It also is helpful to note the source of referral. If a patient has been referred by a medical doctor, a letter to that physician is necessary. The patient's family physician, even though not the source of referral, should be noted on the chart. At times the ophthalmologist may detect, through the ocular examination, signs of a general medical condition, such as hypertension or diabetes, and will want to write to the family physician of these findings despite the fact that a referral was not solicited. For billing purposes the type of insurance plan and policy number should be recorded. Ophthalmic assistants should try to become acquainted with the various insurance plans used in their particular locale. In some instances the wording on a bill may be the sole difference between whether or not the patient receives reimbursement. Certainly, limitations to any particular insurance plan should be explained to the patient. Finally, inquiry should be made into the patient's place and type of employment.

CHIEF COMPLAINT

The chief complaint constitutes the headlines of any ophthalmic history. In a sentence or two the ophthalmic assistant should write down the main reason for which the patient has come to the ophthalmologist for advice and help. In this context the prime question should be direct, simple, and forthright: "How do your eyes trouble you?"

Name:	Norman Deer
Address:	39 Roxborough Road
Telephone:	923-4117
Referred by:	Dr Peters
Family doctor:	Dr Peters
Employed by:	Westinghouse
Occupation:	Clerk
Type of insurance:	Blue Cross
Insurance No.	464-347-213
Age:	50 – Birth date 4/6/1949

Chief complaint:	Difficulty with fine print
History of present illness:	Past 6 months difficulty in reading stock reports. Distance vision fine. No other eye complaints.
Past health:	Diabetes 12-year duration
Medications:	Metformin 500 mg BID
Allergies:	Penicillin, sulfa
Family history:	Glaucoma in mother

Figure 7.1 Typical history.

Many times the patient responds, "That's what I'm here to find out!" The patient may reply concisely or give a long, rambling account of various symptoms. If the patient cannot provide focused answers on the main issue after repeated questioning, the ophthalmic assistant should record what he or she regards as the most serious problem among the patient's symptoms. Commonly described chief complaints are *pain, loss of vision, eye fatigue,* and *blurred vision for near.* One must then proceed to pin down the specifics of the complaint such as date of onset, cause, and duration.

HISTORY OF PRESENT ILLNESS

After the chief complaint is recorded, the patient should be questioned in greater detail about the main symptoms. When did the problem begin and under what conditions?

In other words, what was the patient doing when something was first noted to be amiss? Was the onset slow or rapid in development and did it affect one or both eyes? Once the onset of the patient's symptoms has been recorded, their development and progress should be noted. What did the patient do after they began? Did the person consult a doctor, a friend, or a pharmacist? Did he or she take any medications internally or place any in the eye? Did the symptoms appear to become worse or abate? Was the problem relieved by taking any medication or stopping a particular activity? In other words, what aggravated it and what made it better? The patient should be asked how long a particular symptom has been present and whether it tends to recur.

The pertinent points regarding the most common ophthalmic complaints are reviewed in Table 7.1 to aid the ophthalmic assistant in evaluating symptoms and possible causes

Loss of vision

Very few patients actually will state that they have lost vision, unless, of course, they have become blind because of some unfortunate tragedy. Most patients complain of blurred vision and state this problem in terms of a limitation of function. Blurred vision may assume many forms.

Blurred vision secondary to an error of refraction

Hazy, foggy, or blurred vision, if it occurs at a particular distance, usually indicates a refraction error. The myope cannot see in the distance and the hyperope may have difficulty at near. It is the patient with astigmatism who has difficulty seeing both in the distance and at close range. Even with astigmatism, however, poor visual acuity is not evenly distributed, inasmuch as this type of patient will generally see better at close range because of the magnification afforded by proximity. Most patients with refractive errors have a specific visual disability limited to specific activities.

Blurred vision for close work

A patient whose vision is blurred for close work usually is a presbyope and may complain of an inability to read the stock market report or a number in the telephone book.

Blurred vision for distance work

In this instance the patient is not apt to be a young adult for whom a fresh diagnosis of myopia is about to be made. The patient who is in school most often will complain of

Table 7.1 Ocular symptoms and their possible causes

Symptom	Possible causes	Symptom	Possible causes
Symptoms indicating urgency		Blurred vision in the elderly	Macular degeneration Cataracts Ischemic optic neuropathy
Pain in the eye	Chemical burn Flash burn to cornea Keratitis Glaucoma Iritis Temporal arteritis Retrobulbar neuritis	Persistent tearing in one eye	Dacryocystitis Blocked tear duct Entropion, ectropion Trichiasis Chalazion Bell's palsy
Sudden loss of vision	Macular degeneration Retinal artery occlusion Retinal detachment Retinal vein occlusion Retrobulbar neuritis	Enlarging nodule on lid	Basal cell carcinoma
		Foreign body sensation	Corneal foreign body Corneal abrasion Herpes simplex keratitis
Transient loss of vision	Carotid artery disease Migraine Papilledema Severe hypertension	**Significant symptoms that should be seen as soon as possible**	
Diplopia	Myasthenia gravis Thyroid disorders Diabetes Third nerve palsy from any cause	Gritty feeling	Dry eye syndrome from any cause Conjunctivitis Ocular irritation: dust, wind, ultraviolet lights
Ptosis	Third nerve palsy Diabetes Myasthenia gravis	Headaches	Often tension Hypertension Brain tumor Migraine, cluster headaches, etc.
Flashes of light	Retinal detachment	Blurred distance vision in adult	Diabetes Cataract Macular edema
Trauma	Blow-out fracture of orbit Hyphema		
Symptoms requiring prompt attention		Spots before eye	Retinal tear Vitreous detachment
Discharge and matting of lids in morning	Conjunctivitis	Pain behind eye	Sinus disease Thyroid disorders Orbital tumor (rare) Aneurysm of the carotid artery (rare)
Red eye	Any external disease of eye		
Swelling of lids	Bilateral blepharoconjunctivitis Acute allergies Thyroid disease	Eruption on skin	Atopic allergy Seborrhea Herpes zoster Drug reaction
Halos around lights	Angle-closure glaucoma Cataracts		

inability to see the blackboard. The patient who drives an automobile will state that road signs appear to be quite fuzzy, especially at dusk. Occasionally a patient will recognize this problem by noting that the television set appears fuzzy only to him or her. With regard to television, mothers often become very alarmed when their children sit close to a television screen. This is not usually a symptom of myopia because children like sitting close to the screen for two reasons. First, they enjoy the magnification because big things are easier to view and, second, the closer they are to the screen, the greater is their sense of involvement with the story being told.

Blurred vision secondary to organic disease

The patient with organic disease has difficulty seeing things at all times regardless of the activity. The patient who has a cataract or macular degeneration will be limited in both distance (driving) and at near (reading). The patient with a cataract sees as though looking through a frosted glass window and the patient with macular disease finds things missing when looking straight ahead and so must look at them askew.

Loss of central vision

With loss of central vision patients discover that they are unable to see clearly straight ahead but that they have retained peripheral vision (Figure 7.2). When looking at a face, they may state that the face appears gray or indistinct, whereas the background around the face appears to be clearer. Such a patient commonly sees better in dim illumination. The visual acuity in the affected eye usually is poor. This symptom, if sudden in onset, usually means a disorder of the macula or the optic nerve.

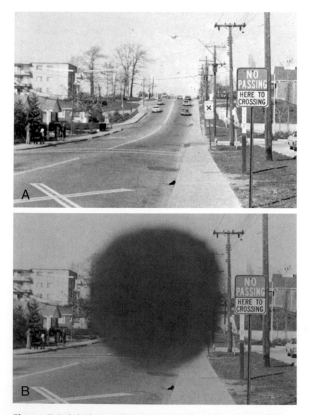

Figure 7.2 (A) The road as it appears to a person with normal central and peripheral fields of vision. (B) Loss of central field. The central field of vision is indistinct, whereas the peripheral field of vision remains clear.

Distorted vision

Distortion of vision is most commonly a sign of macular edema. The patient with this symptom usually complains that objects appear minified and slightly fuzzy and that their contours are curved rather than straight. Visual distortions also are common in patients, such as high myopes, who wear very thick lenses.

Night blindness

The patient with night blindness finds difficulty in seeing things in the early evening, and this difficulty becomes much worse as night falls. Such a patient behaves as though blind in movie theaters, dark rooms, and so forth, yet can see clearly straight ahead in daylight. Eventually the patient suffers visual field restrictions, which make driving and, later, ordinary ambulation difficult even during the day (Figure 7.3). This symptom may be a manifestation of retinitis pigmentosa or vitamin A deficiency.

Transient gray-outs or blur-outs of vision lasting several seconds in one or both eyes

Although this symptom appears to be inconsequential, it often is of great importance. This obscureness of vision may be a symptom of papilledema (swelling of the disk as a result of increased intracranial pressure), carotid insufficiency, or arteriosclerosis.

Inability to see to the right or to the left

This symptom follows a profound field loss in which the patient loses half the field of vision. Such a patient, when reading the visual acuity chart, sees letters on half the chart only and sees them clearly to the 20/20 line of the unaffected side. Usually the patient has difficulty in any visual tasks, such as driving, reading, or even ordinary ambulation (Figure 7.4). When this occurs on the same side in both eyes, one has to be suspicious of brain involvement of the opposite side.

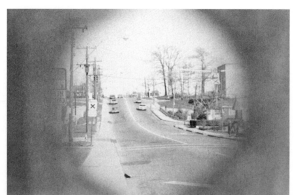

Figure 7.3 Restricted peripheral visual field. The central field is clear.

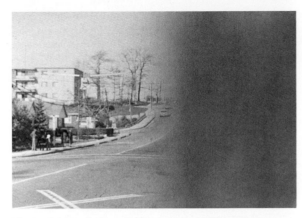

Figure 7.4 Restriction of vision in the right visual field.

Ascending veil

The patient may see a dark shadow ascending like a fog arising in the lower field of vision. This symptom is frequently an ominous indicator of a retinal detachment occurring in the superior retina (Figure 7.5).

Headaches

Headaches are a challenge for all medical personnel. Commonly the patient with a headache has been referred by the family physician, who, unable to find an organic cause for the complaint, has sent the patient to an ophthalmologist for further assessment. Unfortunately, most headaches are not caused by a refractive error or a correctable disorder within the eye, and the ophthalmologist must often report to the family physician that there appears to be no ocular cause for the patient's headaches. Although the symptom of headache is difficult to evaluate, it must be treated with respect because this complaint may indicate many sinister conditions, such as severe hypertension or brain tumor. Of importance in the assessment of any headaches are the following:

1. *Family history of headaches.* In many of the vascular headaches, such as migraine, a positive family history is frequently obtained.
2. *Onset and duration.*
3. *Severity.*
4. *Associated symptoms.* In this regard the ophthalmic assistant is really searching for other findings associated with the headache. For example, the patient with a migraine headache sometimes sees an aura before the onset of the headache. This aura usually consists of flashing lines in zigzag formation, extending from the central area to the periphery and lasting approximately 20 minutes. Other important associated symptoms that should be noted are nausea, vomiting, blackouts of vision, fainting spells, weakness of an arm or leg, numbness of the fingertips, and difficulties with coordination.
5. *Relationship of the headache to visual activity.* Do the headaches follow prolonged periods of close work, or do they appear when the patient rises in the morning? Obviously, headaches caused by errors of refraction will not appear at night, during sleep, or on awaking.
6. *Character of the headache and its location.* A notation should be made of the nature of the patient's headache, whether it is vice-like, throbbing, or dull, as well as its location, that is, in or above the eyes or in the temple regions.

Asthenopia

Asthenopia is a wastebasket term denoting a number of sensations that accompany uncorrected refractive error and problems in ocular motility. Included in this ocular wastebasket of symptoms are the complaints of:

- General eyestrain
- Eye fatigue after reading
- Pulling sensations
- Inability to focus
- Heaviness of the lids after reading
- Sensitivity to sunlight or fluorescent light
- Tendency to fall asleep after reading one or two pages
- Burning, itching, and watering of the eyes with reading

In addition to refractive errors, these symptoms may be a result of chronic conjunctivitis, allergy, lack of tears, an emotional disorder, or fatigue. The patient with asthenopic complaints is apt to be vague and elusive in describing symptoms. Because the disability tends to be

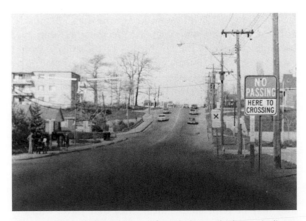

Figure 7.5 Ascending dark veil from below, which may indicate a retinal detachment from above.

minor, lapses of memory are frequent and the patient often is reduced to repeating that "the eyes just don't feel right."

Red eye

The most common cause of a red eye is acute conjunctivitis. The salient features of conjunctivitis are discharge, pain, and blurred vision.

Discharge

The discharge of conjunctivitis can vary from being profuse and watery to being rather scant or purulent. During the day, of course, the discharge tends to drain and is wiped away with handkerchiefs and tissues, but during the night it tends to accumulate and dry. Thus the patient with conjunctivitis complains that the lids are stuck together in the morning, the lashes being matted together in the dry discharge.

Pain

Normally there is no pain with simple conjunctivitis unless the cornea is involved. A secondary keratitis is a common accompaniment of conjunctivitis, especially if the offending organism is *Staphylococcus aureus.* The patient usually complains of a sandy or scratchy feeling or of the sensation of a foreign body in the eyes.

Blurred vision

Because the clarity of the optical media is not affected by conjunctivitis, visual loss is not a prominent complaint in this condition. Because of the discharge over the surface of the cornea, however, the vision in the affected eye may be hazy. Occasionally such a patient even complains of seeing halos around lights.

In cases of conjunctivitis it is helpful to gain information regarding the source of the infection. Inquiry should be made into the presence of a similar disorder appearing in relatives or friends. Detection of the source of the infection may be very important, especially in crowded institutions such as childcare facilities, schools, camps, dorms, or military barracks, where infection can travel through an entire group. It also is important to ask the patient if treatment has been started either by the family physician or by the patient.

Other causes

The red eye also is a manifestation of *acute iritis* and *acute narrow-angle glaucoma,* although the incidence of these two conditions is far less than that of *acute conjunctivitis.* The diagnosis of *acute glaucoma* can virtually be made over the telephone. The onset of this condition is sudden and dramatic, with the entire triad of pain, loss of vision, and congestion of the globe occurring within a matter of 30 minutes. The pain of acute glaucoma, unlike that of conjunctivitis, is intense, and the patient may have associated nausea and vomiting. Also, the visual loss is profound and frequently the vision is reduced to hand movements or counting fingers. The only real distinguishing feature between acute glaucoma and acute iritis, in terms of symptoms, is the difference in the onset of the two conditions. Iritis takes hours or days rather than minutes before it becomes fully developed.

The differential diagnosis of the common causes of an inflamed eye is outlined in Table 7.2.

Double vision or diplopia

The patient with true diplopia reports seeing two objects instead of one. This symptom occurs when there is an acquired loss of alignment of the eyes, so that each eye does not project to the same place in space. Loss of ocular alignment is a common finding in children with strabismus. Children with strabismus, however, do not see double because they are capable of suppressing the vision in one eye to avoid the confusion of double images. Adults are not as adaptable as children and are disabled by double vision (Figure 7.6). They have faulty spatial orientation and projection and complain of dizziness, inability to walk straight, and inability to reach accurately toward an object in space. If the diplopia results from the loss of alignment of the eyes, then covering one eye will always eliminate the second image.

Occasionally the patient may have monocular diplopia. With monocular diplopia the double vision persists when one eye is closed. It is important to make this distinction in the history. Binocular double vision always is caused by the development of a weak or paralyzed extraocular muscle. The loss of alignment results from the fact that an opponent muscle carries the eye over to one side, being unopposed by the palsied muscle. For example, if the right lateral rectus muscle (6th nerve) becomes paralyzed, the left medial rectus muscle would carry the eye inward toward the nose (esotropia) (Figure 7.7).

Monocular diplopia is quite uncommon and may be caused by an extra pupil or cataracts, or it may appear in the recovery phase after strabismus repair.

Floating spots and light flashes

Virtually everyone has seen, at some time or another, small spots before the eyes. They may appear singly or in clusters; they may be punctate or linear; they may travel with the movements of the eye or against them. These floaters are most apparent when the illumination is high and when

Table 7.2 Differential diagnosis of common causes of the inflamed eye[a]

	Acute conjunctivitis	Acute iritis[b]	Acute glaucoma[c]	Corneal trauma or infection
Incidence	Extremely common	Common	Uncommon	Common
Discharge	Moderate to copious	None	None	Watery or purulent
Vision	No effect on vision	Often blurred	Markedly blurred	Usually blurred
Pain	Mild	Moderate	Severe	Moderate to severe
Conjunctival infection	Diffuse; more toward fornices	Mainly circumcorneal	Mainly circumcorneal	Mainly circumcorneal
Cornea	Clear	Usually clear	Steamy	Change in clarity related to cause
Pupil size	Normal	Small	Moderately dilated and fixed	Normal or small
Pupillary light response	Normal	Poor	None	Normal
Intraocular pressure	Normal	Usually normal but may be elevated	Markedly elevated	Normal
Smear	Causative organisms	No organisms	No organisms	Organisms found only in corneal infection

From Chang DF. Ophthalmologic examination. In: Riordan-Eva P, Cunningham ET, Jr, editors. Vaughan & Asbury's general ophthalmology. 18th ed. McGraw-Hill Medical, 2011.
[a]Other less common causes of red eyes are noted in the text.
[b]Acute anterior uveitis.
[c]Angle-closure glaucoma.

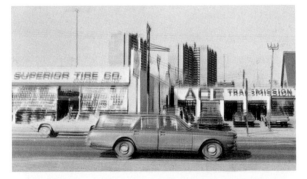

Figure 7.6 Double vision. The images are just slightly displaced vertically.

one is gazing at a clear surface. The most common situations in which they are seen include looking up at a clear summer sky, gazing against a blank white wall, and reading.

These floaters usually are caused by the formation of small particles in the vitreous body and are generally innocuous. However, floaters may, on occasion, be indicative of a more serious derangement within the eye. They may be caused by cells in the vitreous from an active iridocyclitis, or they may be secondary to a retinal tear, hemorrhage, or a detachment.

Tearing

Tearing as an isolated event occurs most commonly as a result of a blockage of the nasolacrimal duct. In infants it results from failure of the duct to become completely canalized. Although tearing is most often a sign of a blocked nasolacrimal duct, it also can be caused by congenital glaucoma, foreign bodies in the cornea, or inturned lashes. Every child with tearing should be assessed carefully.

In adults tearing is a less specific symptom. It may occur as a result of entropion, chronic conjunctivitis, allergy, or obstruction of the nasolacrimal duct. In taking the history of a patient whose primary complaint is tearing, one must note the duration of tearing, whether it appears to come from one eye or both, and associated findings such as redness of the eye or discharge.

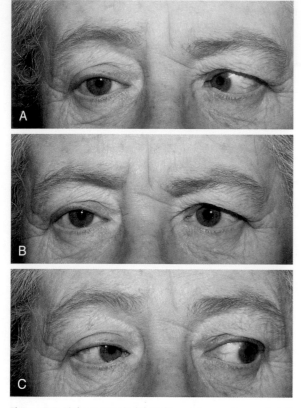

Figure 7.7 Right esotropia (A) Right eye does not move to left (B) Right eye moves only partially out to left (C) Right eye turns left normally.
(Reproduced from Spalton D, Hitchings R, Hunter P: Atlas of clinical ophthalmology. 3rd ed. St Louis: Mosby 2004, with permission.)

PAST HEALTH, MEDICATIONS, AND ALLERGIES

Patients should be asked about their general health at present and its status in the past. In particular, diabetes, hypertension, cardiac disorders, and arthritis should be mentioned. Many systemic disorders have ocular manifestations. If a positive history is obtained, the ophthalmologist can direct the examination with greater purpose.

Equally important is obtaining a history of any medications the patient may be taking. Often the patient will not know the name of the medication but will refer, for example, to a green tablet and a yellow tablet, as though the color of the pill or tablet were its identifying mark. When possible, the ophthalmic assistant should call the patient's pharmacy to identify the exact name of the medication the patient is taking. If this is not feasible, the patient should

be asked the purpose of the medication. Usually most patients are aware of the general function of medications and will state that the pill is for reducing swelling in the legs or relieving high blood pressure.

Inquiry also should be made into the presence or absence of allergies. In general, five types of allergic responses should be inquired about:

1. Allergy to drugs (taken internally or applied topically)
2. Allergy to inhalants (dust, pollens, and so forth)
3. Allergy to contactants (cosmetics, woolens, and so forth)
4. Allergy to ingestants (food allergies)
5. Allergy to injectants (tetanus antiserum)

FAMILY HISTORY

It is helpful if inquiry is made into the familial history of the more common ocular defects. In particular, the presence or absence of such familial diseases as myopia, strabismus, and glaucoma should be asked about. A negative family history does not rule out a genetic familial propensity. Many patients really do not know the ocular status of their relatives, whereas others, being very family proud, are reluctant to confess to any weaknesses in the lineage.

Common familial disorders

- Migraine
- Retinitis pigmentosa
- Retinoblastoma
- Color blindness
- Nystagmus
- Albinism
- Sickle cell anemia
- Choroideremia
- Keratoconus
- von Recklinghausen's disease (elephant man's disease; neurofibromatosis)
- Marfan's syndrome
- Diabetes
- Hereditary macular degeneration (Stargardt's disease)

TIPS IN HISTORY TAKING

The ophthalmic assistant should follow a systematic order in taking an adequate history:

1. Identify the chief reason why the patient has sought an eye examination.
2. Identify any secondary problems the patient has that are referable to the eye.
3. Identify any systemic or general illness the patient presently has and any medication being taken.

4. List past ocular disorders or operations.
5. Determine whether the patient is wearing contacts or spectacles and, if so, how old they are and when the last eye examination occurred.
6. Be succinct but also go into detail about any specific ocular problem that arises. General questions regarding any abnormality may be important, such as time and duration, family involvement, and so on.
7. Record any previous therapy and the response.

SCRIBES*

Scribes are a new subspecialty interest among ophthalmic assistants. They sit and work side by side with their employing ophthalmologist and are in the room with the patient and doctor while the patient history and examination are being performed. They are the official recorder of what transpires. He or she should sign the records as noted on page 104. Sometimes records end up in the hands of lawyers, and legible writing or typing and correct information are a must.

Scribes are a valuable asset because the specific details in recording are often overlooked by the doctor, who is busy responding to the patient's questions or giving specific instructions. Scribes can record details on the go. In addition the patient may forget some aspect of the instructions, and the ophthalmic assistant can explain or repeat them. The scribe may become the best known contact for the patient to call back a few days later.

Scribes have become vital to many ophthalmologists. Although scribes were often used before the implementation of electronic health records (EHRs), the use of scribes in ophthalmology in recent years has exploded. Trained scribes, or medical assistants or technicians acting as scribes, allow the physician to see patients more efficiently, with the added bonus that paper charts are often more legible!

"Let me introduce my scribe _____, who will type or write while I review your chart and complete your examination. Then we will discuss our plan." This sentence is a quick and elegant way for the physician to convey to the patient who the "extra" person in the examination room is and that person's role in the patient's care. A scribe allows face-to-face interaction between the provider and the patient that is lacking when the physician must turn his or her back on the patient to write or type.

It is crucial for scribes entering data in the EHR to be computer savvy—the best scribes type more than 70 words per minute—and familiar with medical and ophthalmic terminology and abbreviations. Like all medical personnel, scribes must abide by the Health Insurance Portability

and Accountability Act (HIPAA) privacy rules, and as an unlicensed individual, cannot practice independently. The scribe is present during the patient encounter and records the actions and words of the physician as they occur. Scribes may not interject their own observations or impressions into the medical record, but with time and training, often anticipate and respond to the physician's needs in the clinic.

Physicians and other licensed providers may rely on the review of systems (ROS) and past, family, and social history (PFSH) obtained and recorded by the scribe; however, this task is often assigned to the certified ophthalmic medical technician. The technician who does the workup for a patient cannot also be the scribe for that patient, because it is not clear in the electronic audit trail when that person was functioning as a technician or as a scribe. Technicians, scribes, and physicians must use their own log-ins in EHRs, which can sometimes slow down the examination; however, there are electronic swiping devices that may be used to quickly change personnel log-ins. It is crucial that scribes do not document findings under the provider's log-in.

Scribes serve as a physician extender in EHRs or on paper. Some examples of other duties commonly performed by a scribe include:

- Input of examination into EHR while the physician dictates
- Edit note per physician request
- Pend medications, tests, orders (for provider to sign)
- Retrieve printouts of refractions, medications, and orders
- Input return visits or follow-up appointments as needed
- Instill eyedrops under the physician's or other licensed provider's order
- Upload test and imaging results
- Fill out surgical consent forms and witness consent signature
- Hold eyelids, and retrieve instruments and drops for physician
- Direct patients to "in-process" waiting, photography, laboratory results, or check-out areas

Scribes typically DO NOT:

- Assist with procedures
- Triage
- Draw up medications
- Schedule patients

When a scribe enters information on a paper medical record and correction is needed, the provider must add and sign an addendum to the scribe's note, rather than cross out or alter what the scribe has written or typed. On electronic records the physician may override the scribe's documentation. The provider must sign an attestation that he or she has reviewed and supervised the scribed chart, whether paper or EHR, and attest to its accuracy and completion. The scribe's attestation may be as simple as "Scribed for Dr. ____ by _____ date/time," and must be legible!

---

*Contributed by Carol J. Pollack-Rundle, BS, COMT.

In March 2015, the Joint Commission on Allied Health Personnel in Ophthalmology (JCAHPO) announced the release of a new Ophthalmic Scribe Certification (OSC). The certification examination is designed to test the knowledge of ophthalmic scribes and ophthalmic medical personnel who create and maintain patient medical records under the supervision of an ophthalmologist. These records include the documentation of a comprehensive patient history, physical examination, medications, laboratory results, and other pertinent patient information.

In addition to recognizing JCAHPO's certification of ophthalmic assistants, technicians and medical technologists, the Centers for Medicare & Medicaid Services (CMS) includes certified ophthalmic scribes to enter electronic medication, laboratory, or radiology orders into electronic health record systems. The examination content covers history taking, ophthalmic patient services and education, ophthalmic terminology, medical ethics and legal issues, and medical notes/records.

A scribe's responsibilities are ultimately controlled by the regulatory requirements and policies established by their health care setting, and the level of risk an employer is willing to accept. As the use of scribes becomes even more prevalent, the potential for expanded legal guidance and direction grows. Practices should monitor federal, state, and regulatory changes to ensure their practices consistently meet compliance with standards.

SUMMARY

The role of the ophthalmic assistant in obtaining a history will, of course, vary with the attitudes and opinions of the supervising eye doctor. Some eye doctors prefer to expand on a skeleton history, whereas others prefer to do the entire questioning themselves. Whatever duties are assigned to

the ophthalmic assistant should be performed as efficiently and expeditiously as possible. Events of a history should be chronicled in breadth rather than in depth. A few short sentences under each heading usually are sufficient to cover an office history. It would be neither appropriate nor efficient for the ophthalmic assistant to spend an hour documenting the patient's complaints. The patient should be left as fresh as possible for examination by the eye doctor.

The analysis of the importance of symptoms is a difficult task because a symptom is merely an expression of disordered function. It depends not only on the patient's condition but also the person's ability to define the trouble with lucidity. Exaggerations, distortions of complaints, irrelevancies, vagaries, and lapses of memory tend to lead the examiner astray. A good historian should not interpret for the patient. If a given history is not precise, a vague statement of the patient's actual complaints should be recorded. The interpretation of the history is the domain of the physician, who will assess all the findings from the history, physical examination, and pertinent laboratory investigations to arrive at a final diagnosis.

The ophthalmic assistant, in obtaining a history, should try to combine the qualities of a good police officer and a kindergarten teacher. The patient's interrogation should be directed toward obtaining the facts. The spirit of that interrogation should be calm, sympathetic, and patient. If possible, the ophthalmic assistant should try to make some notation on the chart of a personal nature, such as the patient's interests and hobbies, occupation, recent accomplishments, or recent tragedies. Such notations are helpful to the eye doctor in establishing rapport with the patient and setting the mood for the interview. Of course, on revisits it is gratifying to the patient to be recognized as a human being rather than as an eye problem. Office personnel should not forget to ask patients about their gardening, their recent vacation, or the progress of their golf. It is all part of a good history.

Questions for review and thought

1. A patient complains of sudden loss of vision in one eye. Outline a series of questions that will bring out the essential features of the problem.
2. Double vision may indicate a paralysis of one or more muscles of the eye. What factors are important in identifying the seriousness of the condition? What muscles might be affected?
3. List the factors that will strengthen the professional components of the ophthalmic assistant's behavior.
4. List the various factors necessary to complete a proper insurance claim in your area.
5. A patient complains of seeing small floating objects in his vision. Outline a series of questions that will bring out the highlights of the history.

6. What is eyestrain?
7. For what conditions is the family history important?
8. Outline a useful sequence to follow in obtaining a good history.
9. What common systemic illnesses have an effect on the eye?
10. What medications should be recorded that affect the eye?
11. What color coding is used on miotics and mydriatic eye medications?
12. List and describe the essential elements of a complete problem-oriented medical case history.

Self-evaluation questions

True–false statements

Directions: Indicate whether the statement is true **(T)** or false **(F)**.

1. History taking is a confidential experience between the patient and the technician who is involved in the questioning. **T** or **F**
2. The most significant question to be asked is, "What medications are you taking?" **T** or **F**
3. The patient should be allowed to speak freely of all his or her problems while the technician is taking a history. **T** or **F**

Missing words

Directions: Write in the missing word(s) in the following sentences.

4. The most common cause of blurred vision is a
   _____.
5. Patients who are unable to see in movie theaters or in the evening are said to have _____.
6. An ascending veil in the lower portion of one's vision is an indicator of a possible _____.

Choice-completion questions

Directions: Select the one best answer in each case.

7. Which of the following is not normally considered in the differential diagnosis of an inflamed, red eye?
   a. Acute conjunctivitis
   b. Acute iritis
   c. Acute glaucoma
   d. Keratitis
   e. Dacryocystitis
8. Which of the following is not part of a history?
   a. Chief complaint
   b. History of past health
   c. Family history of eye disease
   d. Visual assessment
   e. Medication currently used

A   **Answers, notes, and explanations**

1. **True.** The confidentiality of the patient's symptoms is most important. Although some patients may not care who hears their symptoms, many others are disturbed by discussing their problems in public. In addition, some teenagers, indigents, public figures, or highly nervous people require individualized attention to their problems and frequently are offended when their problems become known to others. It may be of no consequence to ask the age of a teenager, but asking the age of a woman who has recently gone through menopause when other people are within earshot may evoke a large measure of hostility. Questions such as those that relate to medications taken may be important to the ophthalmologist, but must be asked privately of the patient.

2. **False.** The most significant question is, "What is your chief complaint?" It is essential to select efficiently the key problem for which the patient has sought help from an ophthalmologist. Once the essential problem or problems have been identified, then the nature of surrounding involvements can be more effectively detailed. The recording of the history becomes important because if it is clearly itemized, the ophthalmologist can minimize time spent in finding the essential facts and avoid the confusion of a mass of disorganized information. Complaints should be reduced to succinct and compressed expressions related to the character and date of onset.

3. **False.** Allowing patients to ramble in a disconnected way serves no purpose except to allow them to get things "off their chest." The most effective way to take a history is for the examiner to guide the direction of the interview so as to bring out the salient features and to jog the memory of the patient for details pertaining to the relevant complaint. In addition, the interviewer must detail other areas in the interview that the patient normally would not have considered. In this way, one can arrive at an accurate and significant history that will have a meaningful and reliable effect in determining the diagnosis.

4. **Refractive error.** In an ophthalmologist's office the most common thing people complain about is some blurring of vision for either distance or near. For most people who seek eye attention, it usually is the myopia that leads to the visit, whether the person has been referred by school or the department of motor vehicles or has just noticed a tendency to squint. In older adults it is the presbyope who requires glasses for reading and seeks attention for blurred vision at near. Although numerous organic diseases affect loss of vision, these are in the minority in an ophthalmologist's practice; however, they always have to be considered when the eye cannot be refracted to a normal visual acuity or when the history suggests more detailed organic loss.

5. **Night blindness.** A number of tests have been developed to determine the levels of light sensitivity and dark adaptation. The term *mesopic acuity* refers to vision under

A | Continued

reduced illumination. A number of disease processes affect dark adaptation and produce night blindness. Such conditions as retinitis pigmentosa initially affect the rods that are abundant in the periphery of the eye and are responsible for mesopic vision by gradually obliterating them so that the patient is unable to navigate in the evening, in movie theaters, and in dimly lit rooms. Other diseases affecting vision under reduced illumination include retinal and choroidal arteriosclerosis, retinal abiotrophies, choroideremia, Oguchi's disease, and hypovitaminosis. The test equipment for dark adaptation and mesopic vision is usually complex and expensive compared with equipment for visual field studies or color discrimination, and consequently it is often unavailable in most practitioners' offices.

6. **Retinal detachment.** When the retina separates from its underlying base, the sensory component is lost and a field of vision that is proportionate to the detached retina becomes diminished. To the patient this manifests as a loss in one or another portion in his or her field of gaze. It may go unnoticed until it begins to affect the macular area of the eye. The patient then responds by complaining of an ascending veil.

7. **e. Dacryocystitis.** This is an inflammation of the lacrimal sac or tear sac that results in a swelling over the tear sac portion. It occasionally spills bacteria into the conjunctival sac, resulting in a secondary conjunctivitis. It is frequently a painful condition that requires antibiotics, hot compresses, and occasionally surgical intervention for resolution to occur.

8. **d. Visual assessment.** Visual assessment is part of the patient's physical examination and is part of the objective measurements. The history is related to the person's complaints and past and present health, along with medications and family history. Any objective measurements are part of the physical examination. The diagnosis of any condition depends on both the history and the physical examination.

Chapter | 8 |

Preliminary examination

Preliminary examination saves the doctor time in assessment of the patient. A preliminary examination of the eyes trains and alerts the ophthalmic assistant to the numerous variations and abnormalities that occur around the eye and the eyelid. It provides a fascinating change from routine duties and challenges the assistant to sharpen diagnostic acumen and develop an interest in the many major and minor diseases and disorders of the eye.

VISION ASSESSMENT

Vision should be assessed both with and without glasses on a standardized chart, and each eye should be tested independently. It has been found that the normal eye can easily distinguish two points separated by an angle of 1 minute to the eye. By convention, most visual acuity charts are constructed so that the sections of a letter subtend 1 minute of arc. Each letter is printed on squares made up of five parts in each direction so that the whole letter to be identified subtends a 5-minute angle to the eye (Figure 8.1).

Visual acuity (VA) is determined by the smallest object that can be clearly seen and distinguished at a distance. The commonly used Snellen charts consist of letters carefully designed to subtend a 5-minute angle to the eye at certain specified distances (Figure 8.2). Generally speaking, 20 feet (6 m) has been considered a practical distance for assessing vision for distance, and the charts have been calibrated with this in mind (Figure 8.3). At 20 feet the distant rays of light from an object are practically parallel and very little effort of accommodation is required. In rooms that are shorter than 20 feet, mirrors may be used to achieve the required distance. Also charts may be proportionately reduced in size to compensate for a room with a shorter working distance.

The results of vision testing are expressed as a fraction. The numerator denotes the distance the patient is from the chart letters and the denominator denotes the distance from the chart at which a normal person can see the chart letters. For example, if a person reads the 20/20 line at 20 feet, visual acuity is 20/20 (VA = 20/20). If the person reads the 20/60 line at 20 feet, visual acuity is 20/60 (VA = 20/60). This actually means that the person can see at 20 feet a letter that a normal person can see at 60 feet (18 m).

Generally, in the Western Hemisphere visual acuity charts are designated in feet, whereas in Europe the metric system is used (Table 8.1).

A quiet area should be selected for testing visual acuity. The chart should be fastened at eye level on a light, uncluttered wall that has no windows nearby to avoid glare. The recommended illumination on the wall chart is 10 to 30 footcandles, but many offices use projected types of vision charts or retroilluminated charts (see Figure 8.3). The general illumination in the room should not be less than one-fifth the amount of illumination on the chart.

In assessing vision the examiner places an occluder over one of the patient's eyes without exerting any pressure on the eye. The patient is then asked to read the chart. The smallest line of letters identified is noted. Adjacent to the line is a notation such as 20/20 or 20/40. The line read clearly is recorded as 20/20 or whatever the case may be. If one or two letters are missed in the line, this may be recorded. For example, if the patient sees the 20/20 line but misses one letter, visual acuity should be recorded as 20/20 − 1.

The patient who is unable to read the largest letter is asked to walk toward the chart; the distance at which he or she begins to read the large letter is recorded as the numerator. For example, 4/200 indicates that the patient was 4 feet from the 20/200 letter. If it is impossible for the patient to distinguish the large letter, the examiner holds his or her fingers before the patient's eye in good light and the vision is recorded as the farthest distance at which the fingers can be counted. For example, if the patient can accurately count the number of fingers the examiner is holding up 3 feet (1 m) away, this is recorded as counting fingers at 3 feet. If the patient cannot distinguish fingers, the examiner should wave a hand in front of the eye.

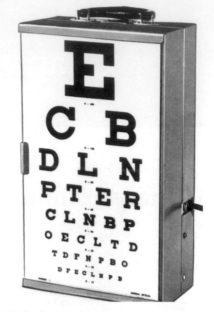

Figure 8.3 Snellen visual acuity chart.

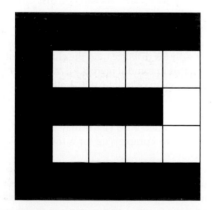

Figure 8.1 The letter E. Each section of the letter subtends 1 minute of arc. Whole letter subtends 5 minutes of arc.

Table 8.1 Conversion table of visual acuity	
Meters	**Feet**
6/6	20/20
6/7	20/25
6/9	20/30
6/12	20/40
6/18	20/60
6/24	20/80
6/30	20/100
6/60	20/200
6/90	20/300
6/120	20/400

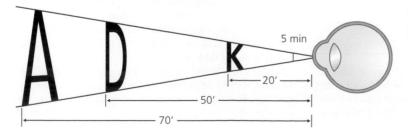

Figure 8.2 Each letter on visual acuity chart subtends a 5-minute angle to eye independent of distance.

If the patient perceives hand movements, the vision is recorded as HM, or hand movements. If the patient cannot even detect hand movements, the room is darkened, a test light is shone into the eye from the four quadrants, and the patient is asked to point in the direction of the light. If the patient can accurately point to light, vision is recorded as light projection. If the patient cannot distinguish the position but is able to just detect the light, the visual acuity is recorded as light perception. If the patient is unable to detect light at all, the vision is recorded as absent light perception.

Illiterate patients and preschool children may be tested by charts made up of numbers, pictures (Figures 8.4 and 8.5), E's (Figure 8.6), or Landolt's broken rings. In the commonly used E test, the child points in the direction of the E either with a finger (Figure 8.7) or with a handheld cutout E. The modern cutout E's are made of plastic. With Landolt's broken-ring test the child merely identifies where the break in the ring occurs (Figure 8.8).

The New York Association for the Blind has modified the readily identifiable pictures of the Schering chart into flash cards that can be held 5 or 10 feet (1.5 or 3 m) from the young child. This distance is more practical for the child and test results can be readily converted to the 20/20 system. The revised Sheridan-Gardiner test for young or intellectually disabled children is a test in which the child is shown a number of letters at either 20 feet (6 m) or 10 feet (3 m), is given a corresponding key chart, and is asked to hold the chart and identify the corresponding letter. The

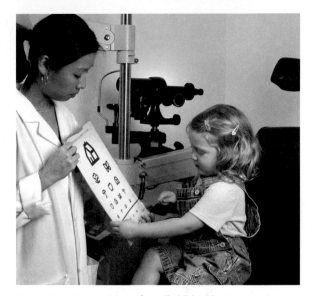

Figure 8.5 Testing vision of small child with pictures.

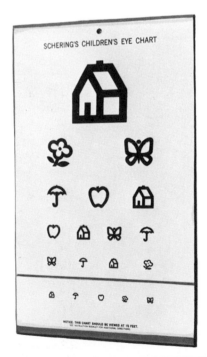

Figure 8.4 Picture visual acuity chart.

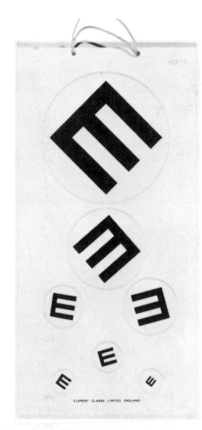

Figure 8.6 E chart with rotating E's.

THE 'E' GAME

1. First ask the child to point three fingers in the same direction that you point your fingers:

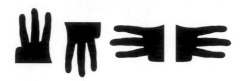

2. Then tell him to consider the E as a table with the arms of the E representing the "legs of the table".

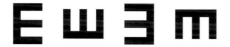

3. Show the E in different positions and ask the child to point his three fingers in the direction of the "legs of the table".

4. Vary direction in which the fingers point. Be sure the child understands the game before testing.

Figure 8.7 Three-finger E test.

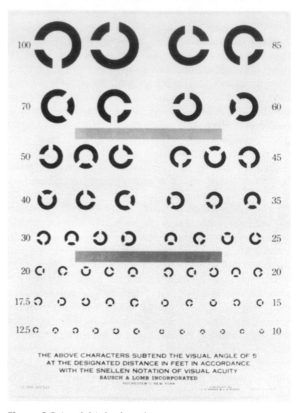

Figure 8.8 Landolt's broken-ring test.

letters in the distance are shown in sequence at the proper distance and the child identifies them by pointing to the key chart.

For near vision the examiner holds the near vision card at normal reading distance, and the child indicates on the key card the letters that he or she can identify.

A miniature toy set may be used to test the young child. The child is asked to match a toy with one held or projected 10 feet (3 m) away. Young children may also be tested by their ability to see and pick up marbles of varying sizes on the floor.

It is often difficult to accurately measure visual acuity of young patients, especially preschoolers. Henry F. Allen, MD, has designed a set of four plastic cards to be used as a preschool vision test (Figure 8.9). The test is a valid index of visual acuity recorded in terms of a 30-foot (9 m) denominator. It is intended for preschool children, and results have been reliable for children ages 2 and over. It is also useful for intellectually disabled older children and for illiterate adults. It can be used for mass screening or for individual testing. No pretraining of younger children is necessary, as is frequently the case with the E game.

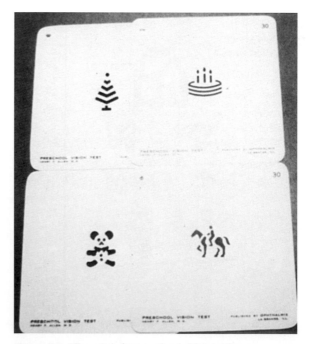

Figure 8.9 Allen cards for preschool vision testing.

The pictures are shown at close range to the seated child with both eyes open and the child is asked to give a name to each picture. The pictures most eagerly received are most likely to be useful. One eye is then occluded and the examiner presents the pictures, in sequence, while backing away from the child. The greatest distance at which three of the pictures are accurately recognized by each eye is then recorded as the numerator of a 30-foot denominator. For example:

- OD = 15 feet (4.5 m): vision = 15/30
- OS = 10 feet (3 m): vision = 10/30

Comparison of the visual acuity of the child's two eyes is more important than absolute values obtained. Normal children between the ages of 2 and 3 can usually identify the pictures at 12 to 15 feet (3.5–4.5 m). Children between ages 3 and 4 can usually identify them at 15 to 20 feet (4.5–6 m). Adults with good visual acuity can recognize them at distances greater than 30 feet (9 m) in good light. A difference of 5 feet (1.5 m) between a child's two eyes is probable cause for referral.

If the child is shy in the presence of the examiner, it has been found that giving the cards to the mother often produces adequate responses.

For infants younger than 2 years of age, a gross estimation of visual acuity can be obtained by simply flashing a light into each eye consecutively. If the child is able to fixate on the light centrally and steadily, vision may be assumed to be grossly normal. If the child's fixation is eccentric but steady, the child's vision is probably below normal. If the fixation pattern is unsteady and eccentric, vision is probably extremely poor and the eye defective. An infant should be able to follow a light by the age of 3 months and reach for toys by the age of 4 to 6 months.

When visual acuity is tested, the following points should be noted:

1. Whenever there is doubt about the child's motivation, intelligence, or attention, the E game should be used because it is unnecessary for the child to make a judgment concerning a visual symbol.
2. A false idea of visual acuity will be obtained if an isolated letter is presented to the patient rather than a line of letters. This is particularly true in persons with amblyopia ex anopsia, who may have 20/40 or 20/50 vision when tested with isolated letters and only 20/200 vision when asked to identify letters in a series.
3. There can be differences in recognition of letters in the same line. The letter L is considered the easiest letter in the alphabet to identify and B the most difficult. The letters T, C, F and E are progressively more difficult.
4. Vision should always be tested with and without the patient's glasses so that a comparison between the two can be made.

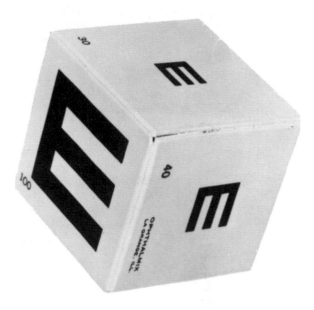

Figure 8.10 E cube used for practicing E game at home.

5. In children, visual acuity testing should not be prolonged and fatiguing. Children are easily distracted and may fail to respond to conventional visual acuity tests because of loss of interest or short attention span.
6. The child who cannot comprehend the organization of the E game should receive practice at home. Parents can be given a small E printed on a card or an E cube (Figure 8.10) or they can cut out the letter E from a piece of cardboard. It is best if a game is made of visual acuity testing. The E can be regarded as a table and the child asked to point a finger in the direction of the legs of the table.
7. In all visual acuity measurements the assistant should note any consistent pattern in the letters missed by the patient. For example, failure to see the nasal or temporal half of the chart may indicate a serious field defect, with loss of vision of half the visual field of each eye.
8. If both eyes are tested together, it is usually found that each eye reinforces the other, so that binocular vision tends to be slightly better than the vision of each eye tested separately.
9. A false visual acuity will be obtained if the patient partially closes an eye or squints. This causes a decreased pupillary aperture and thus allows only central rays to enter the eye, giving much better vision than the patient would normally have. It is important for the patient to keep the eyes wide open.
10. The patient should be observed during testing to prevent peeking around the occluder.

Illiterate patients often say they cannot see rather than admit ignorance. It is important to obtain their confidence and coax them to read a number or illiterate E chart.

11. One of the earliest video acuity testers was developed at Baylor College of Medicine and marketed by Codman-Mentor. It used a keyboard microboard processor, which transmitted finger input to high-contrast television monitors. These monitors displayed perfectly spaced letters or tumbling E's. There were two screens, one for the examiner to watch and control and one for the patient to look at. The apparatus was faster for vision assessment than standard projection charts, and there were zoom capabilities to increase or decrease the size of the letters.

12. Newer and more sophisticated computerized vision testing apparatuses are available from manufacturers such as Haag-Streit, M&S Technologies, Reichert Technologies, Topcon Medical Systems, Stereo Optical Company, and Woodlyn. Features of these devices include high-resolution LCD displays, three-dimensional (3D) capabilities, wireless remotes, randomized and customized optotypes including Early Treatment Diabetic Retinopathy Study (ETDRS) ability and a wide range of test charts, calibration for variable room lengths, pediatric special videos, and fixation targets as well as patient education videos.

Early treatment diabetic retinopathy study chart

The ETDRS chart was developed in 1982 and then revised in 2000 by the National Eye Institute for use in the Early Treatment Diabetic Retinopathy Study. The chart (Figure 8.11) comprises a set of letters originally created by Louise Sloan, using the design of the LogMAR visual acuity chart that consists of letters (optotypes) arranged in standardized typeface, spacing, and size. It differs from the Snellen chart in that there is an equal number of letters per row, the rows and letters are equally spaced on a log scale, and the individual rows are balanced for letter recognition difficulty. Experts believe that the chart provides a more accurate and reproducible measurement of visual acuity than Snellen chart testing. The ETDRS chart has the same number of letters on each line (five), but the size of the letters on a line decreases based on a geometric progression. The ETDRS chart has become the preferred or required chart used in most clinical trials. The standard test is performed at a distance of 4 meters.

Use of pinhole

The pinhole disc, if placed before the eye, eliminates peripheral rays of light, improves contrast, and generally

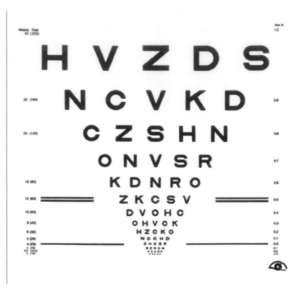

Figure 8.11 Early Treatment Diabetic Retinopathy Study (ETDRS) visual acuity chart.
(From www.nei.nih.gov by National Eye Institute, National Institutes of Health. https://nei.nih.gov/photo/visual-acuity-testing.)

improves vision to almost within normal limits if the patient has a refractive error. The pinhole disc thus serves to differentiate visual loss caused by refractive errors from poor vision resulting from disease of the eye. In the latter condition vision is not improved when a pinhole disc is placed before the eye (Figure 8.12).

Dynamic visual acuity

Visual acuity measured in an office setting is artificial. The eyes are steady, the body is still, and the target is immobile. In real life, as we walk down a street, the eyes are in motion, the body is displaced both forward and vertically, and the object of regard is rarely still. We look at things in action. This type of acuity is sometimes called kinetic vision or dynamic visual acuity.

Kinetic vision, or moving vision, cannot be measured but it is known that acceleration reduces acuity. The faster one travels, the worse one's vision becomes. Body displacement spoils good vision. Try reading on a truck with poor shock absorbers. Fast eye movement is also a detriment to seeing clearly. It is impossible to follow a tennis serve traveling at more than 100 miles (160 km) per hour.

Contrast sensitivity

Another aspect of vision that has proven of interest is contrast gradient visual acuity. This is a measure of the acuity when hampered by poor contrast. A person can have

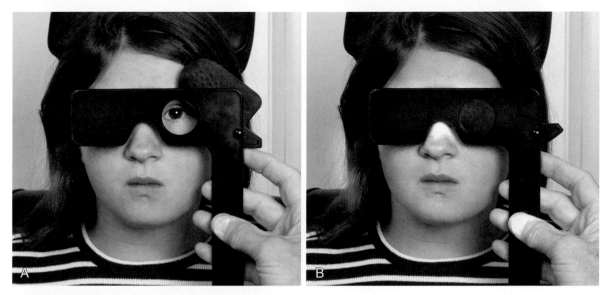

Figure 8.12 Assessment of pinhole vision. (A) Left eye open. (B) Pinhole inserted.

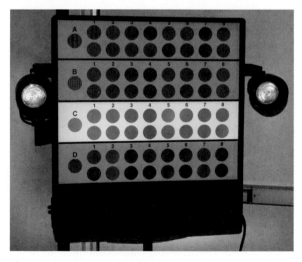

Figure 8.13 Contrast sensitivity test.

20/20 Snellen acuity and complain of poor vision. Snellen acuity measures only an individual's ability to see small, high-contrast images. The visual contrast test can assess the entire spectrum of images and contrast. An individual with cataracts or night blindness may see well in daytime but see poorly at night or on cloudy days when there is little contrast. Vision in the real world can be evaluated more realistically (Figure 8.13).

Contrast sensitivity testing measures vision that resembles real-life situations more closely than the Snellen chart. Contrast sensitivity could probably be detected with photographs of real-life situations with different variations in their contrast; however, this is not practical and reproducible. Consequently, contrast sensitivity charts or machines are used. The contrast sensitivity chart presents a pattern of stripes of varying contrast, size, and orientation. The patient is asked to describe the orientation of the stripes. If the patient answers correctly several times, it is assumed that he or she is able to see these objects at that particular size and contrast. Many sizes and contrasts are presented to determine whether the patient has normal or decreased contrast sensitivity.

Contrast sensitivity tests may be presented as a wall chart with grids of varying size and contrast and a recording pad and instruction for analyzing the results. A smaller chart for near vision testing is also available. The Pelli-Robson chart (Figure 8.14) determines the contrast required to read large letters of a fixed size. In this chart the contrast varies but the letter size remains the same. In the Regan contrast sensitivity chart low-contrast letters of different sizes are shown to the patient. In the Ginsburg Functional Acuity Contrast Test chart, sine-wave gratings tests special frequency (sizes), and levels of contrast are used to plot a contrast sensitivity curve.

In some practices patients are evaluated for contrast sensitivity before and after fitting contact lenses. If the fit is incorrect or the lens is not properly designed, the contrast sensitivity may decrease. This may be even truer with bifocal contact lenses. In addition, lenses often spoil with protein accumulation. Protein deposition reduces their contrast sensitivity while providing good Snellen acuity. In addition, contrast sensitivity testing can help to determine improvement in macular degeneration after use of nutritional supplements and to evaluate treatment response in patients with glaucoma.

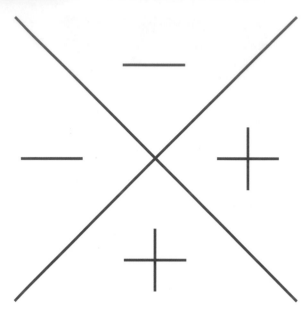

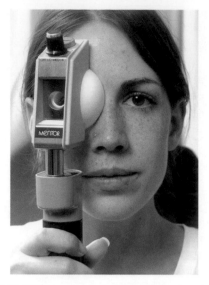

Figure 8.15 Brightness acuity tester (BAT) developed by Jack Holladay to test visual effect of bright sunshine on patient with cataracts.

Figure 8.14 Pelli-Robson contrast sensitivity chart. *(From Bowling B. Kanski's clinical ophthalmology. 8th ed. Philadelphia: Elsevier; 2016.)*

The use of contrast sensitivity tests has become important in refractive surgery. The use of lasers and radial keratotomy to alter the shape of a normal eye so that there is a reduction in myopia must be accompanied by an evaluation. Contrast sensitivity is an important hallmark of the final visual acuity in a person and is much more reliable than Snellen acuity.

Glare testing

Visual acuity may degrade considerably in the presence of bright light. This is particularly true if there are opacities in the media, such as a posterior polar cataract. A number of glare test devices are available on the market (true visual acuity [TVA], brightness acuity tester [BAT], Eye Con) that create a dazzle effect and identify the person whose vision is reduced by glare. The BAT (Figure 8.15), developed by Jack Holladay, delivers three controlled degrees of light when the eye is viewing a Snellen target. Vision with opacities in the ocular media, cornea, lens, posterior capsule, and vitreous, when under the effect of bright light, degrades considerably and provides a true visual acuity in ambient lighting.

In glare testing the patient looks into the machine or at some Snellen letters arranged on a wall chart. The examiner then turns on lights that shine directly into the patient's eyes. The lights have been calibrated to imitate the brightness of headlights coming toward the patient at night, both high and low beams. With the lights on, the patient is instructed to read the letters on the chart. The acuity is measured after glare testing is recorded. With high-beam light, this usually falls off considerably if lens opacities are present.

The Miller-Nadler glare tester is commonly used to test for visual discrimination during bright daylight conditions. It consists of a tabletop viewing screen and a slide projector with 17 slides of varying sizes of land, dot, sea, and rings. The slides are projected onto the viewing screen. With each successive slide, the background is made progressively darker, thus decreasing contrast. The projector screen acts as a glare around the edge of the slide and shines into the patient's eyes. The ability or inability of a patient to detect breaks in rings of smaller size and lower contrast correlates with loss of functional vision outdoors in bright sunlight.

Macular photostress test

This is a sensitive test for detecting macular dysfunction such as cystoid macular edema, central serous retinopathy, and senile macular degeneration. Under conditions of bright light such as produced by the BAT (see Figure 8.15), these disorders are slow to recover vision. Normal recovery to bright light is 0 to 30 seconds but it becomes prolonged to more than 1 minute in patients with maculopathies.

Potential acuity

Potential acuity meter

It is often difficult to see behind a dense cataract, or even an early cataract, to give a good estimate of the potential visual acuity of any particular eye. The cataract often partially obscures the fundus so that evidence of optic atrophy, retinal detachment, and macular disease cannot be determined. Although B-scans can sometimes determine retinal detachments, the subtle retinal defects such as macular edema, macular degeneration, and other vitreoretinal defects are often difficult to determine.

The Guyton-Minkowski potential acuity meter (PAM) is a small apparatus that attaches to a slit lamp. The patient looks into a small aperture in the machine and sees the Snellen acuity chart. The examiner can control the position of the acuity meter, shine it through the pupil, and direct it through particular sections of the patient's crystalline lens. Even patients with mild to moderate cataracts are not totally dense to this light and there are small breaks between opacities. The examiner shines the light through one of these small breaks; the patient can see it unobstructed by the cataract and can then read down the Snellen chart. This has important prognostic significance for determining what the acuity will be following cataract surgery. It lets the physician know that the retina and media are intact and gives an estimate of potential visual acuity.

Interferometer

The interferometer is an apparatus similar to the PAM. Instead of a Snellen chart that is imaged on the retina through breaks in the cataract, the interferometer shines red laser light or white achromatic light directly through the opaque portion of the cataract. The light is not blocked by lens opacity and passes through unchanged. Laser light in a pattern of stripes, either red or white depending on the type of machine, is separated by black stripes of equal size. The width of the stripes can be changed. The patient is asked to name the orientation of each grid as the width is changed, to estimate acuity. As the stripes become smaller, it becomes more difficult to detect which way they are pointing. If the patient can name the orientation of several grids with very thin stripes, it is assumed that the retina can resolve images at that visual level and should approximate good postoperative acuity.

Retinometer

The Heine (Heine Optotechnik GmbH & Co., Germany) Lambda 100 Retinometer (interferometer) operates on the principle of the Maxwellian view: a microaperture is illuminated by a halogen bulb through a red filter and imaged by an optical system into the patient's pupil. The optical system consists of two lenses between which optical grids with variable spacing can be positioned in the parallel beam that passes through them. The resulting diffraction forms a circular test pattern with equally spaced red and black lines on the retina. The distance between the lines corresponds to that of the Snellen E (Visus $1 = 33$ lines/degree of visual angle). The orientation of the lines can be selected by means of a prism in 45-degree steps. Because the beam in the pupillary plane is very narrow (a few tenths of a millimeter), a tiny "window" in the opacity of the lens is enough to allow the light to pass through for a successful examination.

The PAM, the interferometer, and the retinometer give only an estimate of the potential acuity. A patient's acuity may be much better or worse than what was expected.

Near vision testing

Near vision charts are designed to be read at 14 to 16 inches. In patients with accommodative loss, as in patients with early presbyopia, a corrective lens is required to record the near vision. The near vision is recorded as the smallest type that can be comfortably read at the distance at which the card is held. Test cards are available in a wide variety of forms, such as printed paragraphs, printed words, music, numbers, pictures, and E's (Figure 8.16).

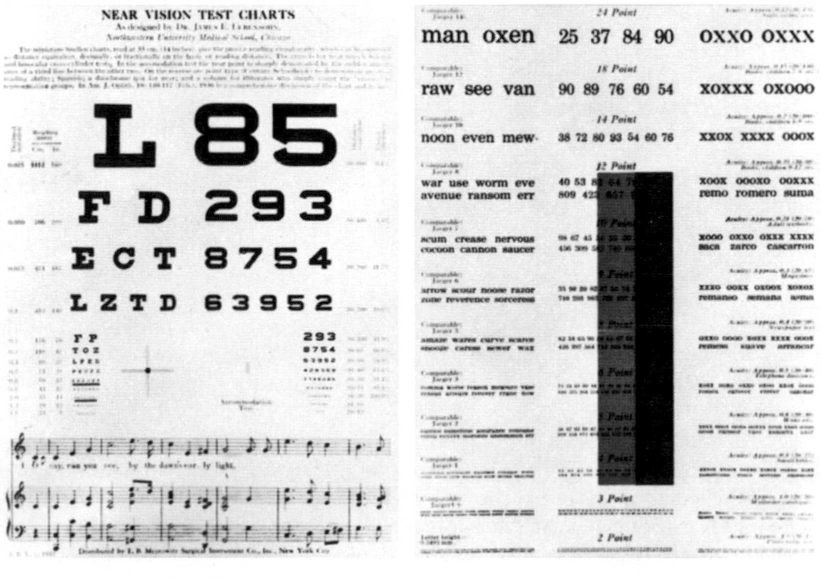

Figure 8.16 Lebensohn reading chart.

Near vision for normal individuals may be recorded as 14/14, J2, or N5. The term 14/14 has the same meaning as the Snellen fraction in that the patient is able to read, at 14 inches (35 cm), small print that is easily seen by a normal individual. The term J2 refers to the Jaeger system. In the latter part of the 19th century Jaeger designed a system of readable print and arbitrarily assigned numbers, beginning J1, to the various sizes. The term *N5* refers to the printers' point system; the print ranges in size from N5 to N48.

Near vision in children does not always correspond to the vision taken in the distance. Children can usually read despite significant refractive errors because they can hold reading material close to their eyes and thereby obtain magnification by the powerful range of accommodation.

MEASUREMENT OF GLASSES

Before the refractive status of a patient is evaluated, it is important to know the previous prescription. The ophthalmic assistant should be very familiar with the technique of neutralizing lenses and arrive at the prescription of the glasses the patient is wearing.

The lensmeter is an instrument designed to measure the prescription of an optical lens (Figures 8.17 and 8.18). (Lensometer is the trade name of the American Optical Company. All other manufacturers refer to lens-measuring equipment as lensmeter, Vertometer, Vortexometer, or Focimeter.) Lenses are made up of either spheres or cylinders or a combination of both. By using a target area on the

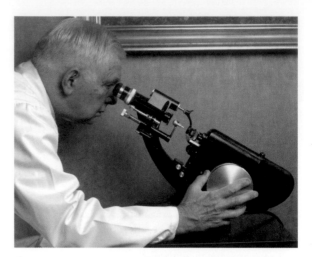

Figure 8.18 Measurement of spectacles with a lensmeter.

lensmeter, one can determine the exact prescription of any lens. All targets have some means of identifying two meridians that are at right angles to each other.

Many types of lensmeters are available. Each manufacturer publishes a manual showing how their instrument is used because the instruments vary in approach. Some work in minus cylinders with plus spheres. Some manual instructions are in plus cylinders for all readings; others are in minus. Therefore, the user may be confused when confronted with an unfamiliar instrument.

Although the instruments vary, the eyepiece on all lensmeters (except the projection type) must be adjusted to compensate for the user's refractive error, if any exists, or all readings will be inaccurate. The examiner should perform the following procedure:

1. Turn the power-focusing wheel until the target is not visible.
2. Turn the eyepiece fully counterclockwise.
3. Look through the eyepiece and turn it slowly clockwise until the grid or reticule just comes into focus. The correct position is the place where it first comes into focus. If in doubt, repeat.
4. Bring the target into sharp focus. The reading should be zero. If it is not, repeat. If zero cannot be obtained, set the power wheel to zero, turn the eyepiece counterclockwise to blur the reticule, then clockwise until the target and reticule just come into clear focus. Note the number on the scale around the eyepiece for quick, future adjustment.

If the examiner wears distance glasses while making this adjustment of the eyepiece, they should be worn every time the lensmeter is used. If the examiner prefers to use the instrument when not wearing glasses, then the eyepiece adjustment should be made without them. It is important to be consistent.

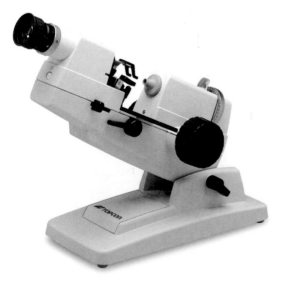

Figure 8.17 Topcon lensmeter.
(Courtesy of Topcon Europe Medical B.V; www.topcon-medical.eu.)

Lensmeters fall into two categories: those using the American crossed-line-type target (Figure 8.19) and those using the European dot-type target (Figure 8.20). Both types are accurate, providing the correct technique is used. The target type therefore is a matter of individual choice and of the operator's familiarity with a specific type.

The American crossed-line-type target consists of solid straight lines at right angles to one another. A single line runs in one direction and three parallel lines run in the opposite direction (Figure 8.21). The whole target can be

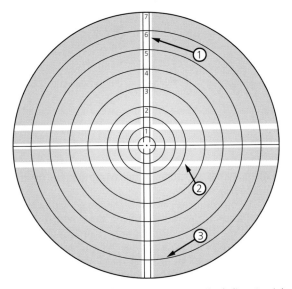

Figure 8.19 American lensmeter target. 1, Single line; 2, triple lines; 3, rings to measure prism in lens.

rotated 360 degrees for determining cylinder axis. At the beginning, it is easiest to measure a lens with this type of lensmeter by following five simple rules:

1. Place the spectacles on the base so that both left and right lenses are resting on the holder. This prevents rotation of the lens and inaccurate axis reading.

2. Focus the single line. Rotate the lines by using the axis wheel so that the single line gives readings closest to zero for both the plus and the minus spheres. This is then marked down as the sphere component.

3. Focus the triple line and record the difference from the single line to the triple line. This is the cylinder portion. For example, if the single line is at +1.00 and the triple line is at +3.00, the prescription will be +1.00 + 2.00.

4. Rotate the axis wheel so the target is on axis when the triple lines are continual. Mark down this axis; this is the axis of the cylinder (for example, +1.00 + 2.00, axis 90). If the single line and the triple line are in focus at the same time, the lens is a sphere.

5. In determining the reading addition in a bifocal lens, move the lens up to the reading segment and then focus again on the triple lines. The difference from the recording of the last triple line to the new triple line in focus is the reading addition. This is always recorded as plus.

If the examiner initially focuses the single line so that it is closest to zero, both the cylinder and the sphere will have the same sign (plus or minus).

In some cases the examiner may wish to record all prescriptions in terms of plus cylinders. In doing so, it is necessary to first bring the single and then the triple lines in focus. By rotating the axis wheel, the examiner can arrange that the triple lines come into focus when more plus is

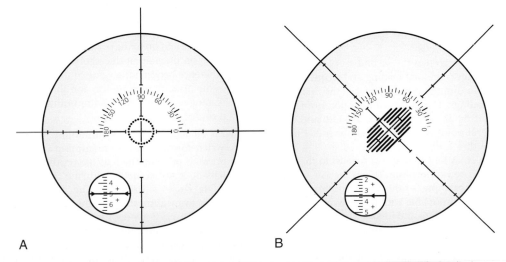

Figure 8.20 European lensmeter test target. (A) Test target with spherical lens. (B) Test target with spherocylinders.

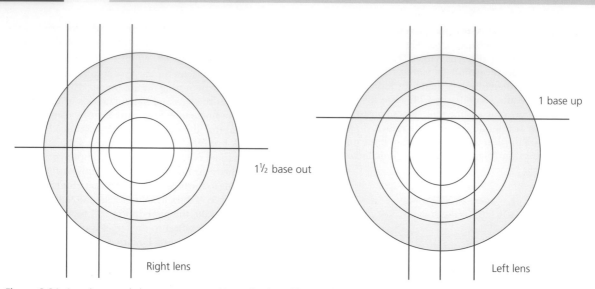

Figure 8.21 American-made lensmeter target. Neutralization of lens with prism incorporated. Note that displacement of target by prism is always recorded in terms of base of prism.

introduced, thereby ending up with cylinders recorded as plus.

The European dot-type target consists of a circle of dots (or variation thereof) that does not rotate. Instead, a protractor grid rotates in the field of view to determine the cylinder axis. The power of a spherical lens is determined by bringing the dots into sharp focus and then reading the power (see Figure 8.20).

The power of a toric or cylindric lens is determined as follows.

1. If a lens contains a cylinder, the target will appear as a system of focal lines. These lines focus in two positions, one perpendicular to the other. First, focus the target so that one of these lines is in focus. The reading closest to zero is marked down as the spherical component (for example, +1.00).

2. Focus the target so that the second set of lines is now perpendicular to the first reading and record the difference in dioptric powers between the first and second readings. This is the cylinder portion. For example, if the first focal point is at +1.00 and the second focal point is at +3.00, then the prescription will be +1.00+2.00.

3. Adjust the cross line so that it is parallel to the focal lines on this second reading. This is the axis of the cylinder (for example, +1.00+2.00, axis 90).

    NOTE: It is impossible with a very weak cylinder to identify a cylindric lens and its axis when the dots are in focus. (When the user is unfamiliar with this instrument, the most common error is that the axis is off by 90 degrees.) There will be no difficulty with stronger cylinders because the dots will smear into distinct lines and aligning the axis grid offers no problems.

The technique for neutralizing a lens with a weak cylinder is as follows. First, rock the power-focusing wheel on either side of the target's focus point and note how the individual dots "bloom" or go out of focus. If the blooming is spherical, you have a spherical lens. If the blooming is oval, you have a cylindric lens. While rocking the focusing wheel, rotate the target protractor or reticule to line it up with the direction (axis) of the oval blooming or smearing of the circular dots. After establishing the cylindric axis, determine the spherical and cylindric power.

4. In determining the additions in a reading bifocal lens, move the lens up to the reading segment and then focus again on the lines at the second focal point. The difference between the value of the second focal point in the distance prescription and that found in the reading segment is the reading addition. This is always recorded as plus.

With all lensmeters it is important (1) to center the lens well before reading the prescription and (2) to measure the prism, if present. The lens has a prism if the center of the lens does not coincide with the center of the target. There are circles surrounding the central target of the lensmeter to measure the amount of prism. The distance between each circle represents 1 prism diopter. It is easy to see at a glance how far the optical center of the lens is displaced in prism diopters from the center of the target. Figure 8.21 illustrates a prism in a lens with the American type of target.

Universal method of using any lensmeter

Many projection instruments make reading of the lens prescription easier. The following method works with any lensmeter, standard or projection type, using any type of target:

1. Place the lens to be measured (in frame or otherwise) in the lensmeter on the table, convex side toward you, with the lens surface firmly against the instrument and with no tilt. Tilting a lens will introduce an error that may result in an inaccurate axis and cylinder power. This is a common error made by the inexperienced user in measuring the bifocal segment. Finding the addition of a fused-glass bifocal requires a special technique, which is covered in detail later.
2. Center the target, then set the power to zero. Move the power wheel from zero to a point well beyond the focus of the target and then back toward zero to the point where the first target meridian or dots come into focus. Take the reading. This is the spherical power.
3. Continue rotating the power wheel in the same direction (do not reverse direction) to bring the second meridian into focus. The algebraic difference is the cylindric power. The sign of the cylinder is opposite that of the sphere. Note the axis of the second meridian. This may be correct or exactly 90 degrees off.
4. Make this check. If the target line or smeared dots are nearly horizontal, the axis is going to be near zero or 180 degrees. If the target line or smeared dots are nearly vertical, the true reading will be near 90 degrees.

This procedure is the same with all makes of lensmeters, and the user actually has a check on a possible cylinder axis error. The user may be in doubt, however, when the axis is near 45 or 135 degrees, in which case another pair of glasses should be tried (or a cylinder from a trial case) to identify which line on the target, or the grid, gives the true axis.

This universal method gives plus cylinder results with minus spheres and minus cylinder results with plus spheres.

Once the user has mastered the instrument, he or she will have no difficulty in modifying the method to work only in plus or only in minus cylinders if this is wished, rather than transposing mathematically from one to the other.

Prism, with the base in any direction, is measured by concentric circles and the displacement of the target. The circles may be in 0.50 or 1.00 prism diopter steps. In addition, some lensmeters have a Risley rotary-type prism as an integral part of the instrument; its secondary use is to center the target for accurate axis reading in a prismatic lens.

Addition

To find the addition of a bifocal lens less than 3.00 diopters, the difference in power between the distance and the reading portions must be found. First, the distance power should be found in the conventional manner, holding the lens being tested in the instrument with the rear surface (usually concave) away from the eye. Second, the reading power should be found, holding the lens in the same position, rear surface away from the eye. If the bifocal is less than 3.00 diopters, the previously mentioned method will produce a correct reading to within 0.06 of a diopter, which is an insignificant error.

For all bifocals greater than 3.00 diopters, the following is the only procedure that gives accurate results:

1. Check the distance portion in the manner indicated previously. This step is identical in checking all lenses and gives an accurate result as to the power of the distance portion.
2. The bifocal must now be reversed in the instrument. Hold its front (usually convex) surface away from the eye and check the distance portion at a spot about the same distance above the center as the point at which you will check the reading power is below the center. In the case of aspheric surfaces, measure the distance through its optical center.
3. Note the finding made through the distance portion. Now check the power through the reading, again with the convex surface away from the eye. Subtract the power of the distance portion found from the reading power to determine the addition.
4. When making all readings, the lens must be firmly against the lensmeter stop, its surface at right angles to the axis of the lensmeter. In some lensmeters it is advisable for the operator to hold the lens in position with his or her fingers and not rely on the lens holder.

Automatic lensmeters

Space-age technology has once again simplified the operator portion of arriving at spectacle measurements. Although costly, this technology will save time and improve accuracy in a busy office. A lens analyzer measures in a single operation the sphere, cylinder, axis, and prism of a lens (see Figure 8.22). The values are digitally displayed and can be recorded, if desired, on a paper tape by the built-in printer. This instrument eliminates the focusing and target alignment tasks, which require a fair amount of skill with a conventional lensmeter. It also does the mathematic tasks of computing cylinder power and of computing the add value of the bifocal segment. The lens analyzer has the unique ability to position spectacle lenses at a given interpupillary distance and then to use prism information collected to compute the net prismatic effect of the spectacle pair. These measurements are made very rapidly. The instrument uses a white light source and a ray trace-type system to make its measurements. It can also measure the amount of ultraviolet lens transmission to let one know exactly how much protection the wearer has.

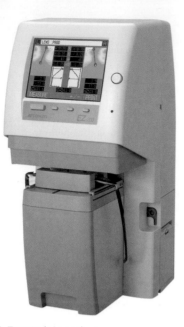

Figure 8.22 Topcon lens analyzer.

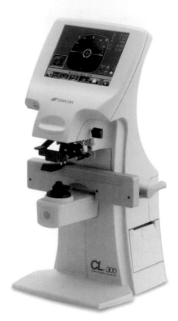

Figure 8.23 Automated lensmeter from Topcon.

The minicomputer in the lens analyzer is used to operate a hard copy printer, to make add computations when bifocals are measured, to change the display cylinder convention, to change round-off modes, and to make special tests for errors and improper measurements, in addition to its primary mode of calculating and displaying the basic lens values. When a spectacle pair is measured, the printed copy records the lens values for both lenses labeled "left" and "right" with sphere, cylinder axis, and prism shown, plus the net prism for the pair. This automatic lensmeter operates on a standard electric power source. The newer Lensometer has a communication link with the phoropter for more rapid refraction.

Rodenstock Instruments manufactures a series of lensmeters in their AL Series. These instruments are fully automated with touch screens and built-in printers. Depending on the instrument in the series, they offer simultaneous measurements of lens power and ultraviolet (UV) transmission, automated detection and measurements of progressive lenses, prismatic lens measurements, pupillary distance (PD) measurements, refractive index calculations, precise lens marking, and a contact lens mode.

The Autolensmeter, manufactured by Acuity Systems, similarly is a microprocessor computer that provides ophthalmic and contact lens reading with accuracy. Pressing one button provides a sphere/cylinder and shows both on a display panel and on printed tape. Pressing another button causes horizontal and vertical prisms to be displayed. The "add" button automatically computes the additional power on multifocal lenses. The Autolensmeter also simplifies the measurement of progressive power lenses.

Topcon makes a lensmeter that is fast and reliable. It also detects if a bifocal is present in a progressive add. There is a color screen that simplifies readings. The instrument provides a printout and it can be integrated into a computer (Figure 8.23).

1. All optical parts of the lensmeter, as well as the spectacle lens, should be kept clean with a soft cloth and lens-cleaning solution.

2. In unusual situations, the spherical power may extend beyond the range of the lensmeter scale. If this occurs it may be necessary to insert neutralizing or opposite-power lenses in the lensmeter to bring the target into focus. The final figures are approximate only.

3. Prisms may be detected by counting the number of rings from the center crossmark that the optical center of the lens is displaced. The direction of the base of the prism can be read directly. For example, if the optical center of the lens is displaced two rings temporally from the center of the crossmarks, then the amount of prism present in the lens would be 2.00 prism diopters, base out.

4. If the center of the lens cannot be detected in the field of the target, loose prisms may be required to bring the optical center of the lens to fall within the area of the target. Some lensmeters incorporate the variable-adjusting Risley-type prisms (see Chapter 9) for this purpose.

ACCOMMODATION

Accommodation is a mechanism by which the eye internally adjusts to changes in the proximity of an object before the eye to maintain a clear image on the retina. This change in the total power of the eye is affected by alterations in the radius of curvature and the thickness of the eye's lens. Increasing the radius of curvature of the anterior face of the lens and increasing its thickness add power to the eye as an optical instrument.

Measurement of amplitude of accommodation

Proximity method

Small print, such as J3 type, is held at a comfortable arm's length and gradually brought closer. The distance at which the patient reports blurring of the letters is measured in centimeters and expressed in diopters. To convert the centimeter measurement into diopters, this measurement should be divided into 100. For example, if the patient detects blurring of the print at 20 cm, the range of available accommodation would be from infinity to 20 cm and the power of accommodation would be 100/20 or 5.00 diopters. It is important that each eye be tested individually and that the patient wear full-distance correction for the test. If the patient is too presbyopic to comfortably hold reading material, an auxiliary lens, such as +2.50, is added to the patient's correction. The amplitude of accommodation is then measured and +2.50 subtracted from the total findings.

Triple line test

In this test two small vertical lines, as found on the Lebensohn chart, are brought toward the patient. The near point is reached when the patient sees three lines instead of two.

Effect of age

The ability of the eye to make these changes in focusing adjustments is greatest in childhood, when the crystalline lens is softest and most malleable. The range of accommodation declines rather precipitously with age as the lens becomes harder. A 10-year-old child has 14.00 diopters of accommodation and a near point of 7 cm, whereas a 40-year-old adult has only 4.50 diopters of accommodation and a near point that has receded to 22 cm (Table 8.2). This means that a 45-year-old man cannot see fine print closer than 22 cm without the assistance of reading glasses.

Table 8.2 Accommodation and near point of the emmetropic eye

Age	Near point in centimeters	Available accommodation in diopters
10	7	14.00
20	9	11.00
30	12	8.00
40	22	4.50
45	28	3.50
50	40	2.50
55	55	1.75
60	100	1.00
65	133	0.75
70	400	0.25
75	Infinity	0

CONVERGENCE

Convergence is an act by which the eyes are turned toward each other to view an object in the midline plane situated close at hand. It is measured by having the patient look at a small target such as a pin, letter, or toy (Figure 8.24). The near point of convergence is that point at which fusion can no longer be maintained and one eye deviates outward. The patient may report seeing double at the moment one eye begins to drift outward. The near point of convergence (NPC) is measured in centimeters.

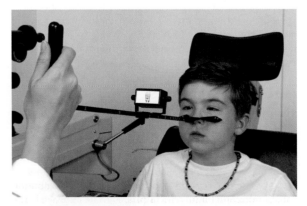

Figure 8.24 Measuring the near point of convergence.

The following points should be kept in mind when measuring convergence:

1. It is a voluntary act that requires the cooperation of the patient and the ability to respond to the test with alertness. If the patient is tired or debilitated at the time of testing, the near point may be unusually remote. If the patient is a distractible, uninterested child, again the near point cannot be adequately measured. For these reasons, the near point of convergence is not regarded as a reliable and completely reproducible test in terms of value.

2. This test requires normal fusion; it cannot be performed if one eye is amblyopic.

COLOR VISION

Defects in color vision may be congenital or acquired. Congenital color defects occur in about 8% to 10% of males and in only 0.4% of females. This defect is transmitted through the female and appears predominantly in the male. Acquired color blindness may occur after diseases of the optic nerve or central retina.

Congenital color blindness may be partial or complete. In the completely color-blind patient, visual acuity is reduced and the patient usually has nystagmus. All colors appear as various shades of gray. Fortunately, this form of color blindness is rare. The partial form is a hereditary disorder transmitted through the female, who usually is unaffected. In the majority of patients, the color deficiency is in the red–green area of the spectrum. With the deficiency in red, this color appears less bright than for the normal individual and thus mixtures of colors containing red are often confused with other colors. Deficient color vision of the red–green variety may pose problems for sailors, drivers, pilots, and textile designers. Absence of blue color is very uncommon.

Tests for color blindness are multiple and varied and consist of matching colored balls or yarns, the red–green lantern test and the most popular test, isochromatic plates.

In clinical practice it is sufficient to test with one of the pseudoisochromatic plates. More scientific approaches to color vision testing (such as the Nagel anomaloscope) are available but are not generally useful for routine clinical practice.

Ishihara test plates

The Ishihara book consists of a series of pseudoisochromatic plates that determine total color blindness and red–green blindness. These plates are viewed by the observer under good illumination. They consist of dotted numbers of one color against a background of another color (Figure 8.25). If color vision is normal, the dots stand out and the patient can read the appropriate number. A person with normal sight may see one number, whereas the

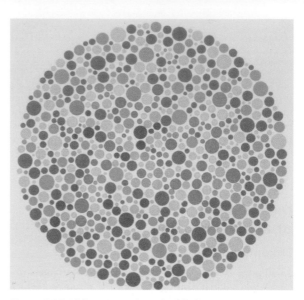

Figure 8.25 Ishihara's test for color blindness.

color-blind person viewing the same plate would interpret the dots as forming a completely different number. For patients unable to read numbers, plates are present in the album with colored winding lines that may be traced.

Hardy-Rand-Rittler plates

This test is no longer manufactured but may still be found in ophthalmic offices. This series of pseudoisochromatic plates includes plates for yellow–blue color blindness as well as red–green color deficiency (Figure 8.26). The background is a neutral gray on which a series of colored circles, crosses, and triangles are superimposed. These geometric designs are present in higher and lower saturations of color to detect the degree of color vision deficiency. Under proper illumination, the observer is required to detect the geometric designs present on each plate. With this color vision test, not only can a graded diagnosis be made (mild, medium, or severe) but also the yellow–blue defects may be differentiated as well as the red and green.

Although it is possible to memorize the numbers on the round Ishihara plates, this is impossible with the Hardy-Rand-Rittler (H-R-R) test because the patient must identify not only what symbols are seen on each plate but also how many and in what quadrant. To ensure against malingering, the plates may be presented right side up, sideways, and upside down. As a result, the malingering patient will have no clues to guide him or her.

Colormaster

Colormaster is a sophisticated, completely automatic and programmable computerized form of presenting color

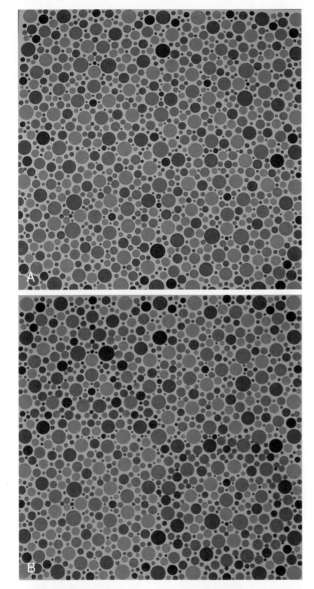

Figure 8.26 (A) and (B) American Optical Hardy-Rand-Rittler test for color blindness.

sequences of constant hue, saturation, and brightness to an individual. This computer has both clinical and research importance because of its repeatability and reliability.

DEPTH PERCEPTION

Depth perception is the highest quality of binocular vision because it provides the individual with judgment concerning depth, based on the coordinate use of the two eyes together. A prerequisite for depth perception is good vision in each eye, overlapping visual fields, and normal alignment of the eyes in all positions of gaze. The four main tests available are the fly test, the Wirt stereo test, the Worth four-dot test, and the biopter test.

Fly test

The patient is provided with polaroid lenses and asked to touch the wings of a fly. If the patient has depth perception, the wings will appear to stand out before the picture (Figure 8.27). This patient will have gross stereopsis of approximately 3600 seconds of arc (when tested at 40 cm).

Wirt stereo test

Animals in three lines are shown to young school-aged children or even to preschoolers who seem able to grasp the idea of the test (see Figure 8.27). If all three lines of animals are correctly selected, the patient has stereopsis of approximately 100 seconds of arc.

The raised rings in nine frames are shown to older children, adults, or even younger children, if possible, depending on the child's alertness. If all nine groups are correctly selected, it may be assumed that the patient has normal stereopsis of approximately 40 seconds of arc. In this portion of the test, two groups must be missed in succession for the examiner to stop the test. For example, if the patient correctly selects groups 1 through 6 and misses groups 4, 7, and 8, number 6 is counted as the patient's maximum amount of stereopsis.

Worth four-dot test

In the original Worth four-dot test, one white disc, one red disc, and two green discs are presented to the patient, who is wearing spectacles with a red-free green lens before one eye and a green-free red lens before the other eye, thus allowing both the patient's eyes to see the white disc. However, the eye covered with the red lens will see, in addition to the white disc, only the red disc. The eye covered with the green lens will see, in addition to the white disc, only the two green discs. The patient is then asked to report the number of discs seen. If four discs are seen, both eyes are functioning. If three discs are seen, then the eye behind the green lens is seeing (the two green and one white) and the eye behind the red lens is suppressing. If two discs are seen, then the eye behind the red lens is seeing and the one behind the green lens is suppressing. If five discs are seen, then another problem is indicated (the eyes are not fusing and muscular imbalance is suspected) (Figure 8.28).

Variations on this test include the Project-O-Chart slide, wall-mounted internally illuminated tests or the flashlight form (Figure 8.29). The symbols shown may be four discs set in a diamond pattern or a disc, a cross, a triangle, and a square. For children, a picture presentation in colors of a clown, a seal, and a ball may be used. In all these tests red and green spectacles are worn.

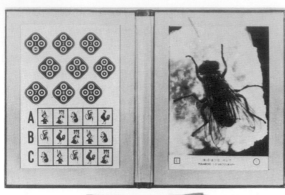

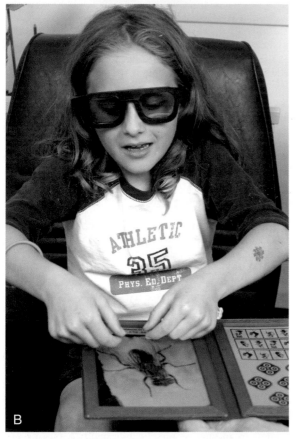

Figure 8.27 (A) and (B) Wirt and fly tests for depth perception.

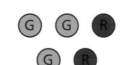

A. Left eye suppression   B. Right eye suppression

C. Esotropia: no suppression   D. Exotropia: no suppression

E. Normal 4-dot response:
no suppression

Figure 8.28 Worth four-dot test. (A) and (B) The suppressing eye. (C) and (D) Muscle imbalance and no fusion. (E) Normal four-dot response. *R,* Red lens before right eye; *G,* green lens before left eye.

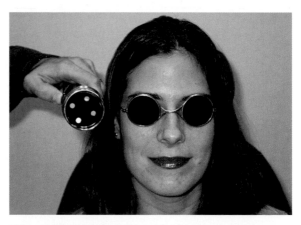

Figure 8.29 Worth four-dot test to detect suppression. *(From Kaiser PK, Friedman N, Pineda II, R. The Massachusetts Eye and Ear Infirmary illustrated manual of ophthalmology. 4th ed. Philadelphia: Elsevier/Saunders; 2014.)*

Biopter test

This instrument has the fundamentals of a home stereoscopic viewer in which slightly different images are presented to each eye (Figure 8.30). The sensation of depth is appreciated by the slightly disparate images.

EXTERNAL EXAMINATION

Although the ophthalmic assistant cannot expect to substitute for the trained eye of the ophthalmologist in recognizing abnormalities of the eye and the eyelid, an awareness of

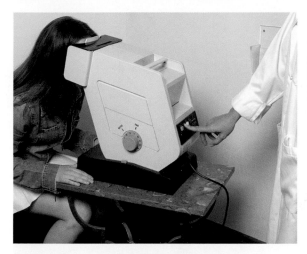

Figure 8.30 Biopter test for depth perception.

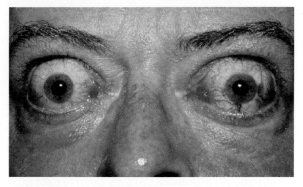

Figure 8.31 Proptosis of both eyes with lid retraction as a result of hyperthyroidism.
(Reproduced from Spalton D, Hitchings R, Hunter P. Atlas of clinical ophthalmology. 3rd ed. St Louis: Mosby; 2004, with permission.)

abnormal external features, with documentation of such on the record, will aid the ophthalmologist in the recording of these abnormalities, as well as alerting him or her to problems that are incidental to the main complaint of the patient. This exercise also helps instill an awareness of and interest in unusual eye problems, whether they are abnormal or pathologic.

The ophthalmic assistant should begin the external examination of the eye by systematically noting the symmetry of the orbits, the eyelashes, the lid margins, the conjunctiva, the lacrimal apparatus, the sclera, the cornea, the iris, the anterior chamber, the pupil, and the lens.

Symmetry of orbits

In proptosis (exophthalmos), in which one eye protrudes, the upper lid is often retracted and there is exposed sclera above and below the cornea (Figure 8.31). Another method of determining the presence of proptosis is to stand behind the patient, draw the upper lids upward, and note which eye appears to bulge more. The ophthalmologist may record the degree of proptosis with an instrument called an exophthalmometer (see Figures 10.35 and 10.36).

Eyelashes

Cilia, or eyelashes, are hairs on the margins of the lids. They are located in two rows, totaling about 100 to 150 cilia on the upper lid and half that number on the lower lid. The bases of these cilia are surrounded by sebaceous glands (glands of Zeiss). Infections of these glands result in a common stye. The average life of a cilium is from 3 to 5 months, after which it falls out and a new one grows in to take its place. If the cilium is pulled out, the new one replacing it reaches full size in about 2 months. If the

cilia are cut short, as is sometimes done preceding surgery on the eye, regrowth is rapid and lashes may appear normal in a few weeks. Some glaucoma medications (e.g., latanoprost [Xalatan], travoprost [Travatan Z], and bimatoprost [Lumigan RC]) may cause the lashes to become darker and longer.

Lid margins

The lid margins should be observed for any redness, scaling, or discharge, indicative of blepharitis. The position of the lid margin also should be noted. It should be tight against the globe and not sag outward (ectropion) or inward (entropion). The punctum on the medial aspect of the lower eyelid should not be visible without depressing the lower eyelid. The more common affections of the lid margin are styes, chalazions, and growths.

Conjunctiva

The bulbar conjunctiva is readily visible. The caruncle is seen as a fleshy mound of tissue at the inner canthus. The palpebral conjunctiva of the lower eyelid is seen by depressing the lower lid while the patient looks toward the ceiling. The palpebral conjunctiva lining the upper eyelid can be seen only by everting the upper lid. Eversion of the upper eyelid is carried out by grasping the lashes of the lid between the thumb and index finger and turning the eyelid over a cotton-tipped applicator or other blunt instrument such as a thin plastic or metal rod. It is important that the patient be asked to look downward to relax the levator muscle. With eversion of the upper eyelid the tarsal conjunctiva is visible and the meibomian glands running vertically from the lid margin are easily seen. The conjunctiva should be inspected for follicles, discharge, color, and growths such as pterygium and pinguecula.

Lacrimal apparatus

The tear film that covers the surface of the eye is composed of the following three layers:

1. A superficial oily layer derived from the meibomian glands and the sebaceous gland of Zeiss. It prevents evaporation of the underlying tear layer.
2. The tear film, which is the middle layer, is secreted by the lacrimal gland and the accessory glands of Krause and Wolfring.
3. The deepest layer is the mucoid layer and is secreted by the goblet cells of the conjunctiva.

The tears are normally carried from lateral to nasal sides along the lid margin. When they reach the opening of the lower lid, the punctum, they drain into the nasolacrimal duct and finally into the nose. Blinking spreads the tear film over the eye but also moves the tears toward the punctum with each blink. Tears contain albumin, globulin fractions, and an antibacterial enzyme called lysozyme. Tear antibodies make up the gamma globulin protein fraction. Tear production may decrease 30% or more in a person older than 50 years.

The presence of tearing in the absence of any other signs of inflammation should be noted. Distension and chronic inflammation of the lacrimal sac may cause a small, smooth elevation in the lacrimal fossa between the inner canthus and the nose. Pressure inward on this area causes the contents of the lacrimal sac to be expressed by way of the puncta onto the conjunctiva. It should be noted whether the contents from the lacrimal sac are tears, mucus, or purulent material.

Deficiency of tears is best measured by Schirmer's test (Figures 8.32 and 8.33). In this test a standardized filter paper, 3 by 20 mm, is inserted in the unanesthetized lower fornix of each eye at the junction of the middle and nasal third of the lower eyelid margin. With the eyes gently closed, these strips become moistened by the tears. The amount of paper moistened can be measured with a millimeter ruler and recorded. Some strips have a methylene blue bar that indicates the amount of tear flow.

Normally the lacrimal gland, under the irritation of a piece of filter paper, should produce sufficient tears to wet at least 10 mm of the paper in 5 minutes. This may be slightly less in older adults. Any tear production less than 10 mm indicates a dryness of the eye and that the condition of xerosis may be present. Carefully performed Schirmer's tests often reveal lower secretions of tears, which could cause minor ocular complaints such as dryness, burning, or a sandy or gritty feeling. This test also may be helpful for contact lens wearers to determine whether there are sufficient tears for comfortably wearing contact lenses.

A variation of the test is Schirmer's test number two, which is accomplished by placing an anesthetic drop into

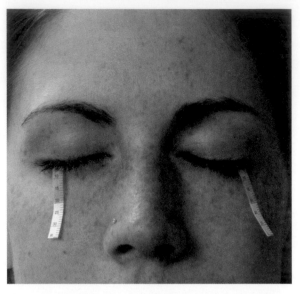

Figure 8.32 Schirmer's test to detect tear deficiency. A filter paper strip is permitted to remain in contact with the eye for 5 minutes. Wetting effect is measured.

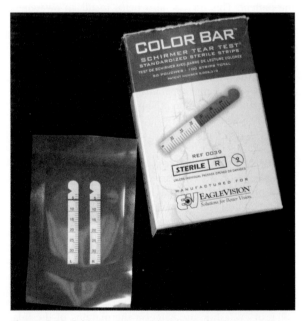

Figure 8.33 Schirmer paper with color evaluation on strip.

the conjunctival sac before the Schirmer paper is inserted. The purpose of the topical anesthetic is to eliminate the reflex tearing caused by the paper itself.

The TearScope (Eagle Vision and Keeler) is an interesting instrument for analyzing the tear film in vivo. It is useful for assessing dry eye symptoms and in contact lens work when one wants to know whether the tear film is stable or whether punctal plugs are required. This instrument can be held in the hands or attached to a slit lamp. It measures the break-up time of tears and tear film with fluorescein-stained tears.

Sclera

The normal sclera is visible beneath the conjunctiva as a white, opaque, fibrous structure. Blue discoloration of the sclera may be normal in a very young child because of the sclera's thinness and the underlying prominence of the dark choroid. Blue discoloration in an adult invariably indicates a pathologic condition; it may signify a tumor, a thinness of the sclera with a protrusion of the underlying uvea (staphyloma), or a nevus. In older adults the sclera may appear yellowish because of the presence of fat and other degenerative substances.

Cornea

The cornea is the first and most powerful lens of the eye's optical system. The radius of curvature of the average cornea that can be measured with the keratometer in the central region is 7.8 mm. The refractive index of the cornea is 1.376, which gives the cornea a power of 48.8 diopters. The concave posterior surface that faces the aqueous has a power of 25.8 diopters, which gives the entire cornea a power of 43.00 diopters or about 70% of the total refractive power of the eye.

The reaction of the cornea to disease is unique. Being avascular, it cannot easily fend off infection. The surface layer of the cornea, the epithelium, is easily disrupted but it fully regenerates when injured. Injury to the epithelium occurs with flash burns, contact lens injuries, abrasions, and superficial corneal foreign bodies. Most infections and injuries usually involve only the corneal epithelium. Bowman's layer shows little resistance to pathologic conditions. It is easily destroyed and never regenerates. Descemet's membrane is quite strong and highly resistant. The endothelial cells may die, and they never regenerate. Neighboring endothelial cells enlarge and fill in the gap of dead cells. Thus the total endothelial cell count in any given area, when viewed by specular microscopy, may drop considerably. If the cornea becomes swollen, it loses its shape and transparency so that loss of vision is common. Total corneal swelling occurs with acute glaucoma, and the cornea may develop a ground-glass appearance.

The normal cornea should be smooth, shiny, and free of irregularities. In children the corneal diameter should not exceed 11 mm. Corneal enlargement 12 mm or greater is strongly indicative of congenital glaucoma. In older adults a white ring is frequently present near the corneal

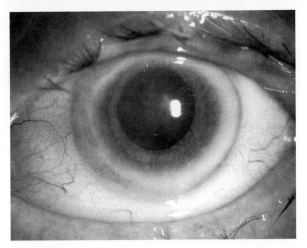

Figure 8.34 Arcus senilis caused by deposition of cholesterol and lipids in the peripheral cornea. A common aging process. *(Reproduced from Spalton D, Hitchings R, Hunter P. Atlas of clinical ophthalmology. 3rd ed. St Louis: Mosby; 2004, with permission.)*

periphery. This creamy white ring is a result of the deposition of fat and is called the arcus senilis (Figure 8.34).

The cornea is normally free of blood vessels. The presence of blood vessels indicates a pathologic condition and disease. Blood vessels in the cornea are best seen with a slit-lamp microscope but can be appreciated with strong focal illumination and the magnification of an ophthalmic loupe. Corneal edema often can be seen with the naked eye because of its characteristic ground-glass appearance. Corneal opacities may be detected by oblique illumination with a small flashlight.

Corneal sensation should be tested with a small wisp of cotton directly applied to the cornea. In this test the patient is instructed to look up. Normally a blink response should occur if the corneal sensation is intact. It is important that the patient not see the cotton approaching the eye because the visually evoked response of seeing a foreign object approach the eye causes a blink. Because of the wide range in individual response, comparison of the corneal reflexes of the two eyes is most useful. Loss of corneal sensitivity follows herpes simplex virus and brain disease involving the fifth nerve.

Use of fluorescein, rose bengal, and lissamine green stains

Fluorescein is an ocular stain used to show defects and abrasions in the corneal epithelium. The pooling of fluorescein on small corneal defects is best seen by means of ultraviolet or cobalt blue light for illumination. This causes the fluorescein to fluoresce. There is a danger with fluorescein in solution form. It becomes easily contaminated with

Pseudomonas aeruginosa, which appears to flourish in fluorescein. Sterile dry fluorostrips in which fluorescein has been impregnated are available to prevent this complication. The fluorescein strip should be moistened with a drop of saline and applied to the lower fornix. This will cause liquid fluorescein to replace the tear film. The ulcer or denuded epithelium will be visible as a brilliant green.

Rose bengal is a red dye that has an affinity for degenerated epithelium. Similar to fluorescein, it will stain areas in which the epithelium has been sloughed off. However, unlike fluorescein, intact, nonviable epithelial cells of the conjunctiva or cornea stain brightly with rose bengal. The stain is helpful in diagnosing keratoconjunctivitis sicca or other conditions associated with dryness of the conjunctiva. If the dye stains devitalized epithelium of the nasal bulbar conjunctiva, a diagnosis of keratitis sicca may be made. The technique is to apply at least 10 mL of sterile balanced salt to the test rose bengal strip.

If available, lissamine green can be used as an alternative to rose bengal. It is less irritating.

Iris

The iris normally is clear to inspection. The irides of both eyes are generally the same color. The color depends on the amount of pigment in the stroma and posterior layer of the iris. A heavily pigmented iris appears brown, whereas a lightly pigmented one appears blue. Interestingly enough, there is no blue pigment in the iris. In the blue iris, the light passes through the nonpigmented stroma and strikes the pigmented epithelial cells on the back of the iris so that light of longer wavelength (red) is absorbed and that of shorter wavelength (blue) is reflected.

A difference in the color between the two irides (heterochromia) may be indicative of a congenital abnormality, iris tumor, retained intraocular foreign body (siderosis), or old iritis.

If a light is brought to bear on the iris at close range against the sclera (transillumination), the light may seem to glow in a patchy way in areas where there has been marked pigment loss. This can occur with some forms of glaucoma (pigmentary), after iritis, or with albinism. Freckles on the iris should be noted because iris freckles are frequently associated with intraocular malignant melanomas. Near the root of the iris lies the dilator muscle. When dilation occurs, at a maximum, the pupil may be 9 mm or greater in diameter. When maximally contracted, it may be only 1 mm.

The iris is normally well supported by the underlying lens. Tremulousness of the iris (iridodonesis) usually means the presence of a dislocated lens. Tremulousness of the iris, or undulating movements of the iris structure, is best seen by having the patient look quickly from one point of fixation to another. Near the aperture is a sphincter muscle that constricts the pupil. In the center of the iris,

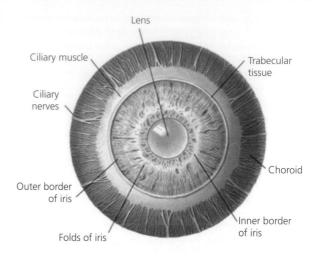

Figure 8.35 Frontal drawing of the eye showing the iris and pupil (lens).
[From Head and Neck Imaging. Mafee, Mahmood F.; Som, Peter M. Published January 1, 2011. © 2011. (Modified from Sobotta Atlas of Human Anatomy © Elsevier GmbH, Urban & Fischer, Munich.)]

running radially around the pupil and forming a circular web, are the blood vessels of the iris. If the lens is absent (aphakia), the iris loses its support, flattens, and deepens the anterior chamber. It may become tremulous.

A defect in the iris is called a coloboma. A coloboma, which indicates absence of some portion of the iris, may be the result of previous surgery or a congenital abnormality.

Muddiness of the iris is a term used to express the general loss of clarity of the pattern of the iris. It is caused by inflammatory exudates in the anterior chamber or on its surface. Normally the textured surface of the iris and the white markings of the iris vessels are easily visible (Figure 8.35).

Anterior chamber

By shining a small penlight from the side, one can make an estimation of the depth of the anterior chamber. If the anterior chamber is shallow, it should be so recorded because the patient may be prone to narrow-angle glaucoma.

Penlight examination for estimating the depth of the anterior chamber

It is important to evaluate the anterior chamber depth in all patients but especially before dilating their pupils.

The depth of the anterior chamber can be estimated by holding a penlight temporal to the eye near the limbus and parallel to the iris plane. Shine the light across the front

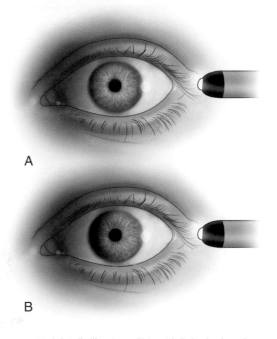

Figure 8.36 (A) Fully illuminated iris with little shadow denotes a deep anterior chamber. (B) Partially illuminated iris with a wide shadow denotes a shallow anterior chamber.

of the iris and toward the nose of each of the patient's eyes. Observe the degree of shadow formation on the iris between the nasal pupillary border and the nasal limbus. A completely illuminated nasal iris with possibly a small rim of shadow just inside the nasal limbus denotes a deep chamber (Figure 8.36A). A wide shadow on the nasal portion of the iris (Figure 8.36B) denotes a shallow chamber. The shadow projected onto the nasal iris denotes that the angle is narrow because the iris is bowed forward and blocks the path of light. Though the oblique penlight test lacks the sensitivity or specificity of a Van Herrick test (a test that uses a slit lamp to create an optic section beam at approximately a 60-degree angle at the limbal cornea that is then compared with the width of the corneal section and the width of the shadow adjacent to it) or gonioscopy, it can be used as a useful tool in detecting a shallow anterior chamber without the use of a slit lamp. An appropriate referral by the ophthalmic assistant to the ophthalmologist can help prevent an acute angle-closure glaucoma precipitated by pupillary dilatation.

Pupil

The ophthalmic assistant can test pupillary function with no special instrument except a small light. The following points should be noted in the examination of pupillary function.

Pupillary reflexes

For assessment of the direct light reflex, the patient should be seated in a dimly illuminated room, with the light evenly distributed throughout the room. A small light is brought from the side and shone directly into the pupil (Figure 8.37). The normal direct light response causes constriction of the pupil on that side.

For assessment of the consensual light reflex, light is directed into one eye while the second eye is observed. An intact consensual response to light causes constriction of the pupil of the unilluminated eye.

Normally when an object is viewed close at hand, three associated reactions occur: (1) convergence of the eyes toward the object, (2) accommodation, and (3) pupillary constriction. These three reactions to near should not be considered a true reflex because one may occur without the other. For example, the pupil may be dilated with a mydriatic agent and the patient may still be able to converge his or her eyes.

The swinging flashlight test compares the direct and consensual reflexes in the same eye. The examiner projects the light on the patient's eye and allows the pupil to go through the phases of initial constriction to a minimum size and subsequent escape to an intermediate size. At this point the examiner quickly swings the light to the other eye, which begins at the intermediate size and goes through the phases of initial constriction to a minimum size and subsequent escape to an intermediate size. Again, as soon as that pupil redilates to the intermediate size, the light is swung to the first eye and a mental note made of the intermediate (starting) size and briskness of the response to light. These characteristics should be exactly the same in both eyes as the light is alternately swung to each eye.

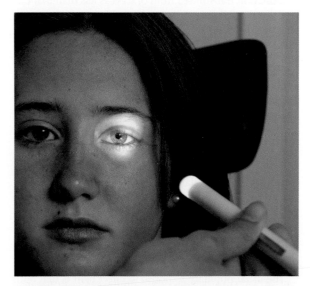

Figure 8.37 Testing pupillary light reflex.

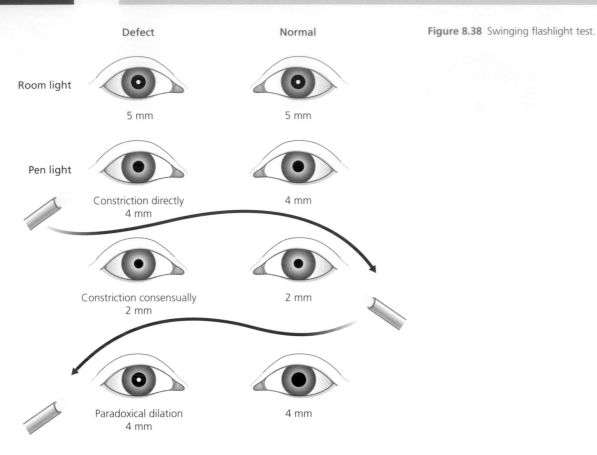

Figure 8.38 Swinging flashlight test.

During the swinging flashlight test, if the amount of light information transmitted from one eye is less than that carried by the fellow eye, immediate dilation of the pupil, instead of the normal initial constriction, may be noted when the light is swung from the good eye to the defective eye. This characterizes an afferent pupillary defect or the Marcus Gunn pupil (Figure 8.38).

Relative afferent pupillary defect test

When a patient complains of decreased vision in one eye with a normal-looking macula, retina, and nerve, it is important to recognize the presence of disease and identify which part of the ocular system is responsible for the vision loss. If the initial ocular examination appears normal, testing for a relative afferent pupillary defect (RAPD) is a way to implicate or rule out optic nerve disease. Even in the presence of significant macular disease, this test will be negative. If the patient has a positive RAPD, then one can diagnose optic nerve disease.

The usual pupillary response to direct light is that both pupils contract equally if there is no abnormality of the pupil's iris, muscle, or stroma. When moving a light rapidly from one eye to the other, both pupils should maintain their degree of contraction. If one is slow in moving the light so that neither eye is dazzled, then the initial response from the first eye is lost and even in a normal status both pupils will partially dilate. In the case of an RAPD the pupillary response is different. When one shines a light in the good eye, both pupils constrict. Then when one shines the light in the other eye, an optic nerve that is injured will transmit light but to a lesser and slower degree. As a result, when the light is moved from the good to the bad eye, the central nervous system interprets this as a decrease of light being presented. The central nervous system's response is to dilate both pupils to let more light in. This dilation response occurs in both eyes, despite only one eye being affected.

Some ophthalmologists and neurologists perform an additional test for prognosis using neutral density filters. The filters are increased in front of the normal eye until the RAPD is equalized and abolished. Others do not find this test to be clinically useful.

The takeaway of a positive RAPD test is that it is a sign of optic nerve disease.

Size

The size of the pupil varies with age, the color of the iris, and the refractive error. The pupil tends to be largest in blue-eyed young children who are myopic. Conversely, the pupil tends to be smaller in infants and older adults. The pupils should normally be equal in size. Failure of a large, dilated pupil to constrict to light is most commonly caused by a cycloplegic drug such as atropine. Such a pupil is 7 to 8 mm in diameter, spherical, and immobile when light is shone into the eye. Dilation of a pupil to 5 to 6 mm can result from paralysis of the third cranial nerve. The pupil may also be large, immobile, and unresponsive to the direct application of light because of severe afflictions of the retina and optic nerve that result in blindness. However, such a pupil can be distinguished from the dilated pupil because of paralysis of the third nerve by testing the consensual reaction to light. If the lesion is a result of a third nerve palsy, the size of the pupil in the affected eye remains unchanged when the light is directed into the fellow eye. If the pupillary dilation is a result of disease of the retina or optic nerve, the consensual light reflex produced by shining light into the sound eye will produce a constriction of the pupil in the affected eye.

The pupil may also be dilated and fixed to direct light stimulation and consensual light stimulation after an episode of acute narrow-angle glaucoma. However, this pupil is characteristically oval.

Bilateral constriction of the pupils (miosis) is most commonly caused by glaucoma medication, such as pilocarpine. Small, pinpoint pupils are characteristically found in morphine addicts. Unilateral constriction of the pupil occurs with iritis, interruption of the sympathetic pathways of the eye, and irritative lesions of the cornea.

Psychic influences such as surprise, fear, and pain markedly dilate the pupil. Dim light also dilates the pupil, whereas bright light constricts it. At times the pupil is constantly contracting and dilating; this is called *hippus*.

During sleep the pupil is constricted. This is such a constant finding that it serves as an aid in differentiating true from simulated sleep.

Any irritation of the cornea or conjunctiva such as an abrasion results in constriction of the pupil.

Shape

The pupil is normally round and regular. Irregularities in the shape of the pupil may result from congenital abnormalities, inflammation of the iris, trauma to the eye, and surgical intervention (Figure 8.39). Trauma may cause tears of the iris in the form of a wedge-shaped defect, either at the pupillary margin or at its base (iridodialysis). A corneal laceration with prolapse of the iris may result in the drawing up of a segment of the iris to the site of the laceration (adherent leukoma). In severe iritis, the iris may be bound down to the lens by adhesions (posterior synechiae), and irregular changes may occur in the shape of the pupil.

Equality of size

The pupils should be equal in size and react equally to direct light stimulation, consensual light stimulation, and near objects. In the light of an ordinary room, the diameter of the normal adult pupil is between 3 and 5 mm. If the two pupils are unequal in size, the condition is called anisocoria. Anisocoria may be harmless but it is never physiologic. Inequality of size may be caused by a tonic pupil (Adie's syndrome). In this condition, which can be mistaken for a partial third nerve palsy, the pupil responds to light stimulation very slowly. Adie's syndrome is diagnosed by instilling a low dose (0.125%) of pilocarpine,

Figure 8.39 Variations in pupillary size and shape. (A) Dilated or mydriatic pupil. (B) Constricted or miotic pupil. (C) Full or sector iridectomy. (D) Peripheral iridectomy. (E) Congenital coloboma of iris. (F) Iridodialysis. (G) Posterior synechiae.

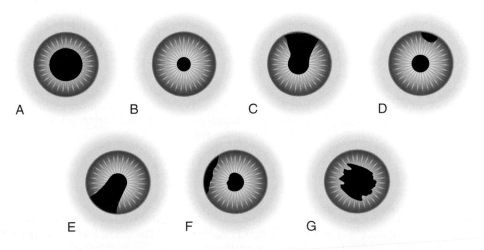

which can result in the constriction of the tonic pupil caused by cholinergic denervation hypersensitivity, whereas a normal pupil will not constrict with such a low dose of pilocarpine.

Disorders of pupillary function may involve many of the previously mentioned factors together. For example, Argyll Robertson pupils, one of the classic signs of late syphilis, are small, irregularly shaped, and nonreactive to either direct or consensual light stimulation but reactive to near stimulation.

Differential diagnosis of a dilated pupil

A dilated pupil may be caused by third nerve palsy, trauma, Adie's pupil, or acute glaucoma, or it may be drug induced.

Third nerve palsy

If the dilated pupil is fixed, the cause may be third nerve palsy. This condition may be associated with ptosis and a motility disturbance, characterized by the eye being deviated out and down. The pupil responds to constricting drops, such as pilocarpine. This is a neurosurgical emergency, and the possibility of an intracranial mass lesion must be ruled out.

Trauma

Damage to the iris sphincter may result from a blunt or penetrating injury. Iris transillumination defects may be visible with the ophthalmoscope or slit lamp and the pupil may have an irregular shape.

Adie's pupil

In Adie's pupil, the pupil responds better to near stimulation than to light. The condition is thought to be related to aberrant innervation of the iris by axons that normally stimulate the ciliary body. Absent knee jerks are usually associated.

Acute glaucoma

The patient may complain of pain and/or nausea and vomiting. The eye is red, vision is diminished, intraocular pressure is elevated and the pupil is middilated and poorly reactive.

Drug-induced dilation

Iatrogenic or self-contamination may occur with a variety of dilating drops, such as cyclopentolate hydrochloride (Cyclogyl), tropicamide (Mydriacyl), homatropine, scopolamine, and atropine. The pupil is fixed and dilated and, unlike in third nerve palsy, does not respond to constricting drops.

Differential diagnosis of a constricted pupil

A constricted pupil occurs in Horner's syndrome or iritis and may be drug induced.

Horner's syndrome

Other signs of Horner's syndrome include mild ptosis of the upper lid and retraction of the lower lid. The difference in pupillary size is more notable in dim light because adrenergic innervation to the iris dilator muscle is diminished.

Iritis

Slit-lamp examination shows keratitic precipitates and cells in the anterior chamber and a prominent ciliary flush. The intraocular inflammation stimulates pupillary constriction.

Drug-induced constriction

Iatrogenic or self-induced pupillary constriction may be caused by a variety of drugs, including pilocarpine, carbachol, and echothiophate iodide (Phospholine Iodide).

Lens

The entire lens is normally not visible without the aid of a slit-lamp microscope. However, an advanced cataract may be seen with the naked eye, because it causes a gray, opaque appearance in the pupillary aperture.

Blinking

Most people blink 15 times per minute. The duration of a blink is approximately 0.3 to 0.4 second. The average period between blinks is about 2.8 seconds in men and just under 4 seconds in women. Spontaneous blinking does not produce a discontinuity of vision in spite of the fact that vision is interrupted during the blink. Continual squeezing of the eyelids together is called blepharospasm. It occurs as a result of inflammatory diseases of the anterior segment, Parkinson's disease, and stress.

EXAMINATION OF THE OCULAR MUSCLES

The six extraocular muscles in each eye are innervated by a total of three nerves. The action of specific muscles can vary, depending on the position of the eye when it is innervated. Table 8.3 shows the general relationships that apply.

The examiner should determine the range of ocular movements in all gaze positions (Figure 8.40). Limited movement in any gaze position can be documented as 21, minimal; 22, moderate; 23, severe; or 24, total. For example, a patient with right sixth nerve palsy can be recorded (Figure 8.40B). Figure 8.40C shows a record of a blow-out fracture to the right orbit with entrapment of the inferior rectus muscle and limitation of upward gaze.

Table 8.3 Extraocular muscle innervation

Innervation	Muscle	Primary action
Third nerve	Superior rectus	Up and out
	Medial rectus	In
	Inferior rectus	Down and out
	Inferior oblique	Up and out
Fourth nerve	Superior oblique	Down and in
Sixth nerve	Lateral rectus	Out

The corneal light reflex test is a simple practical evaluation of muscle imbalance for patients who cannot cooperate sufficiently for prism cover testing or who have poor fixation. The Hirschberg method is the most popular and is based on the premise that 1 mm of corneal light reflection corresponds to 7 degrees or 15 prism diopters of ocular deviation of the visual axis (Figure 8.41). This is a "guestimate" method that may be quantitated and refined by the use of prisms, as in the Krimsky method.

The alternate cover test is perhaps the most widely used for detecting and measuring strabismus, tropia, or phoria. It is reliable and easy to perform and it requires no special equipment. The test is conventionally used at both distance and near, with and without glasses, with the eyes being examined in the primary position. To ensure fixation in very young children, the fixation object should be an interesting and detailed article, such as a brightly colored toy. Once the examiner is sure that the child is looking at the fixation object, an occluder is interposed in front of one eye. If the left eye is occluded, the following possibilities may ensue:

1. The right eye, which is deviating, may move horizontally (esotropia is a move inward; exotropia is a move outward) or vertically (hypertropia is a move up; hypotropia is a move down), indicating that the child has a manifest strabismus (Figure 8.42).

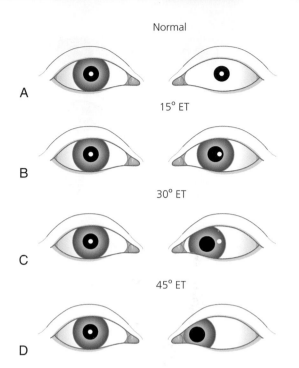

Figure 8.41 Hirschberg's method of estimating deviation by light reflex.

2. The right eye may wander slightly, indicating that the fixation of the eye is defective or absent, as may occur with gross amblyopia.
3. There may be no movement of the right eye, indicating that this eye is straight.

The procedure is then repeated, this time covering the right eye without allowing the patient to become binocular during testing. Manifest strabismus is revealed by observation of any movement of the uncovered eye to take up fixation when the occluder is placed before the other eye.

Occasionally a child may be referred who appears to have an ocular deviation but there is no detectable strabismus. This condition is called pseudostrabismus. In most instances

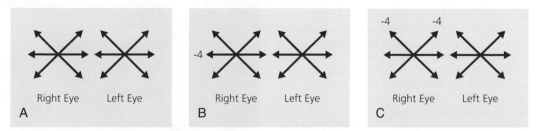

Figure 8.40 (A) Method for examining and recording ocular motility. (B) Record of sixth nerve palsy of right eye. (C) Record of right orbital blow-out fracture and limited upgaze.
(From Stein HA, Slatt BJ, Stein RM. A primer in ophthalmology: a textbook for students. St Louis: Mosby; 1992.)

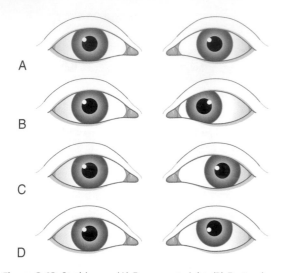

Figure 8.42 Strabismus. (A) Eyes are straight. (B) Esotropia. (C) Exotropia. (D) Hypertropia of left eye.
(From Stein HA, Slatt BJ, Stein RM. A primer in ophthalmology: a textbook for students. St Louis: Mosby; 1992.)

the appearance is caused by the presence of prominent epicanthal folds that extend from the upper lid, cover the inner canthal region, and blend into the medial aspects of the lower lid. This is a false impression of a turn, more noticeable when the child turns the eye to either side. A full discussion of ocular muscle deviations is offered in Chapter 43.

INSTILLATION OF EYEDROPS AND OINTMENT

Frequently the assistant is requested to instill various types of liquid medications into the patient's eyes. There are wrong ways and right ways to do this.

All drops, with the exception of topical anesthetics, are placed into the inferior cul-de-sac with the patient looking up. With the dropper bottle in the right hand, the left forefinger is used to depress the lower lid, making a small pocket of the cul-de-sac. With the patient's eyes in the elevated position, the dropper bottle is brought over to and close to, but not touching, the cul-de-sac. One drop is placed in the pocket so formed. More than 1 drop is a waste of solution because the total capacity of the cul-de-sac is ⅙ of a drop.

Topical anesthetic drops, such as those used when intraocular tension is being measured or before the ophthalmologist removes sutures from the eye, are placed in the eye with the patient looking down and with the solution directed to the 12 o'clock position of the sclera near the limbus. With the dropper bottle in the right hand, the upper lid is elevated with the left thumb. While the patient looks down, the right hand with the dropper bottle is placed close to, but not touching, the lashes and the solution is expressed at the 12 o'clock position of the sclera.

There are two reasons for the different manner of instilling medications into a patient's eye. First, solutions placed in the lower cul-de-sac with the patient looking up are those medications designed to either dilate the pupils or place a particular medication in contact with the eye for a period of time. Second, when solutions are dropped into the eye, the patient will blink; when the patient's eyelids close, the cornea goes up underneath the upper lid (Bell's phenomenon). If a topical anesthetic has been placed in the lower cul-de-sac, as the patient blinks and the cornea travels upward, the maximum amount of topical anesthesia is going to be obtained on the inferior portion of the sclera. However, because the eye is being anesthetized for measurement of intraocular tension, the cornea must be anesthetized. When the patient looks downward as the topical anesthetic is placed in the eye at the 12 o'clock position, the blinking causes the cornea to travel upward and thus to come into contact with the topical anesthetic just applied, thereby rendering a more complete and well-distributed area of corneal anesthesia.

When ointments are required, a small amount (about ¼ inch, or 6.4 mm) is instilled into the lower cul-de-sac as the patient looks up (Figure 8.43).

When *not* to dilate before asking the eye doctor

1. The depth of the anterior chamber is very important. If the depth is shallow because of a narrow angle, there is a risk of precipitating angle-closure glaucoma. Do not dilate.

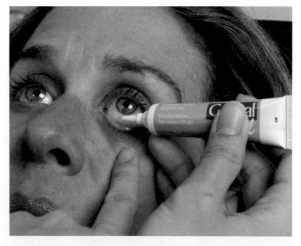

Figure 8.43 Instillation of ophthalmic ointment.

2. Before cataract extraction with implantation of an iris-supported intraocular lens. Do not dilate. These implants were popular in the early 1990s, but are no longer used. The dilation of the iris in these patients could result in a dislocated intraocular lens.

3. If the patient is undergoing neurologic observation and pupillary signs are being followed, dilation may alter the diagnosis and confuse the attending physician. Do not dilate until the neurologist or neurosurgeon thinks it is safe to do so.

OPHTHALMOSCOPY

The ophthalmoscope, invented by von Helmholtz in 1851, permitted analysis of the interior of the eye during life. For the first time, this allowed recognition of changes in the eye grounds, providing valuable information in the diagnosis of disease of the general system, as well as of the eye itself.

There are two types of ophthalmoscopes: direct and indirect. The indirect ophthalmoscope permits binocular vision with depth perception (stereoscopic vision). It also permits a wider field of view of a given area. The image is inverted in this type of ophthalmoscope. The indirect ophthalmoscope may be used in the operating room without contamination and permits indentation of the sclera and a better view of the periphery of the fundus. It provides more intense illumination and frees the hands for operative manipulation.

However, the direct ophthalmoscope is the one most popular for all practitioners (Figure 8.44). This permits a greater magnification (×15). It is easier to use with small or undilated pupils and is mechanically easier to use. This ophthalmoscope contains a number of spherical lenses that help the practitioner to focus. However, there are no cylindric lenses, so that if the individual has an astigmatic error of refraction, it cannot be compensated for. The direct ophthalmoscope enables the examiner to use the power of the subject's eyes as a magnifying system to see the retina as an erect picture.

Ophthalmoscopy is best performed in a dimly lit room to facilitate pupillary dilation. However, for better inspection of the fundus, the pupil should be dilated with a mydriatic agent such as phenylephrine 2.5% (Table 8.4). This does not inhibit accommodation. With heavily pigmented irides, a stronger mydriatic agent is required. Drops such as cyclopentolate (Cyclogyl 1%) or tropicamide (Mydriacyl 1%) should be instilled. These drops do affect accommodation. When inserting a mydriatic cycloplegic drop, one should be sure that the chamber angles are deep. If not, angle-closure glaucoma may be induced.

The examiner stands directly in front of the patient and examines the patient's right eye with the examiner's own right eye and the left eye in a similar fashion. This permits the examiner to be closer to the patient. Both of the

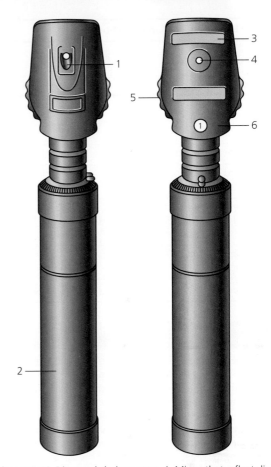

Figure 8.44 Direct ophthalmoscope. 1, Mirror that reflects light into patient's eye with viewing hole (4) above, through which examiner looks. It is in this viewing hole that positive or negative lenses can be superimposed to adjust focus. 2, Handle where battery power is supplied. On top of handle base is rheostat for light adjustment. 3, Headrest bar, which goes against examiner's forehead. 4, Viewing hole. 5, Focusing wheel. While holding ophthalmoscope, examiner can use index finger to move wheel to adjust lenses in hole at (4). 6, As dial wheel (5) is moved, power of lens is indicated in this small window. *(From Coles W. Ophthalmology: a diagnostic text. Baltimore: Williams & Wilkins; 1989.)*

examiner's eyes are kept open. The patient is asked to look at the opposite wall over the shoulder of the examiner. The cornea, anterior chamber, and lens structures are first carefully examined at a distance, usually about 15 inches between the patient and the examiner. The examiner gradually approaches the eye of the patient, carefully noting the cornea, anterior chamber, and lens structures, until a red reflex appears. This red reflex is a combination of the reflex from the choroidal vasculature and the pigment epithelium (Box 8.1).

Table 8.4 Drops used in refraction

Drug	Onset of maximum cycloplegia	Duration of activity	Comment
Atropine sulfate 0.5%, 1%	45–120 min	7–14 days, especially in a blue-eyed child	Not used routinely except for the assessment of accommodative strabismus in children
Scopolamine hydrobromide 0.25%	30–60 min	4–7 days	Used in atropine-allergic patients
Homatropine hydrobromide 2%, 5%	30–60 min	3 days	Requires half hour to an hour to take effect and lasts 3 days; not used routinely
Cyclopentolate hydrochloride 0.5%, 1%, 2% (Cyclogyl)	30–60 min	6–24 h	Active in 30–60 min; two sets of drops given 5 min apart; a good rapid-acting cycloplegic drop for office use
Tropicamide 0.5%, 1% (Mydriacyl)	20–40 min	4–6 h	A good drug for office use with an effect similar to Cyclogyl

Modified from Stein HA, Slatt BJ, Stein RM. A primer in ophthalmology: a textbook for students. St Louis: Mosby; 1992.

Box 8.1 **Tips on ophthalmoscopy**

1. If the examiner has any significant astigmatic error, he or she should wear corrective glasses.
2. A smaller light spot should be used for astigmatic eyes to minimize distortions from toric corneas.
3. The cornea and anterior structures of the eye should be examined from a distance of 1 foot (30 cm) through the sight aperture of the ophthalmoscope. The examiner then moves to within 1 inch (2.5 cm) of the eye to observe the retina.
4. The patient should be asked to gaze on all quadrants to observe the peripheral retina. Each arteriole is followed out to the periphery.
5. To avoid coming too close to the patient's eye, the examiner may put his or her middle finger forward and rest it against the patient's cheek. This provides a proprioceptive method of determining how close the examiner is to the patient.

For purposes of orientation, the optic disc is first identified. The disc is an oval structure that represents the site of entrance of the optic nerve. The color and shape are noted. It is usually light pink and may have a central yellowish white depression called the physiologic cup, created by a separation of the nerve fibers. The depression may be large and occupy up to half of the disc. At the base of the cup are grayish spots representing the opening of the lamina cribrosa, the connective tissue layer through which the fibers of the optic nerve pass. The cup size is noted and the margins of the disc are observed. The margins of the disc are sharp and distinct, except for the margins of the upper and lower poles, which may be slightly fuzzy.

The blood vessels are then examined. From the disc the retinal arterioles and veins emerge and bifurcate, then extend toward the four quadrants of the retina. The central retinal vein, which is usually found lateral to the central retinal artery, is larger and darker red. The examiner observes for venous pulsation, which, if present, suggests there is no papilledema because this disappears early. These veins branch into retinal vesicles and arterioles; the retinoles are darker. Retinoles and arterioles cross over and under each other, but an arteriole never crosses over an arteriole, nor does a retinole ever cross a retinole.

Approximately 2 disc diameters away from the optic disc and slightly below (about 1 mm) its center is the macula, about 5.5 mm in diameter. The macula is a small avascular area that appears darker red than the surrounding fundus. At the center of the macula is a glistening oval reflex called the fovea. At its center is the foveola, which has no rods but a high density of cones. This area is a vascular capillary-free zone. This saves the foveola from vessels that obscure visual acuity. Underlying choriocapillaries supply this capillary-free zone.

Cilioretinal arteries arising from the ciliary circulation are seen in about 20% of patients and account for the blood supply to the macular region in these individuals. This is an important fact when occlusion of the central retinal artery occurs, in which the cilioretinal artery provides continual nourishment to the macular region and maintains central acuity. In young people, a second reflex, which appears as a glimmering halo, may surround the entire macular region.

Each quadrant of the fundus is examined in turn. For the examiner to see as much of the peripheral retina as possible, the patient should be asked to look in the direction of the quadrant under study. The examiner follows out the arterioles in that particular quadrant to the extreme limit. The color of the fundus is usually an even red hue but it varies with the general pigmentation of the underlying choroid and the general pigmentation of the individual. The background is bright orange-red in people of fair complexion, whereas it is deeper brick-red in darker individuals. Some details of the choroidal vessels may be seen in fair individuals and in the periphery.

Most ophthalmoscopes have two or more beam lights of different sizes. The smaller beam light is particularly useful for viewing the fundus through small pupils, such as those found in narrow-angle glaucoma patients under treatment with pilocarpine. It eliminates some of the glare around the pupil from reflex scattering from the iris. Cobalt blue filters may be present as an aperture disc in the ophthalmoscope. These are used for fluorescein studies of the fundus as well as examination of the cornea with fluorescein strip papers. Ophthalmoscopes sometimes contain a target so the patient can fixate on the center of the grid for viewing the macular area.

VISUAL FIELDS

Visual field testing is important in a thorough workup of a patient to screen any possible interference in the nerve pathways from the eye to the brain. It is discussed more fully in Chapter 19.

SUMMARY

The use of abbreviations (Table 8.5) is generally to be condemned in public institutions, where the abbreviated word may not be understood by all. However, in private offices it may be helpful and save time. The best record and the one that is the easiest to understand is a small sketch of the pathologic condition seen on inspection (Figure 8.45).

Table 8.5 Commonly used abbreviations

Symbol	Meaning
VA	Visual acuity
od	Oculus dexter (right eye)
os	Oculus sinister (left eye)
VOD	Vision right eye
VOS	Vision left eye
ou	Oculi uterque (both eyes)
RE	Right eye
LE	Left eye
EOM	Extraocular muscles
NPC	Near point of convergence
NPA	Near point of accommodation
℞	Prescription for eyeglasses or drugs
Δ	Prism diopter
D	Diopter
T	Tension

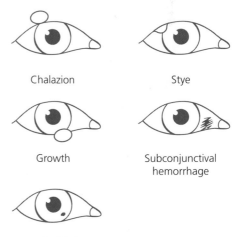

Chalazion   Stye

Growth   Subconjunctival hemorrhage

Embedded foreign body

Figure 8.45 Diagrammatic recording of external abnormalities.

Questions for review and thought

1. Discuss what is meant by 20/20 vision; 20/40 vision.
2. Describe a routine to be followed for checking distance vision; for checking near vision.
3. How do you check the vision of an illiterate patient?
4. Describe vision testing in children.
5. If a patient cannot identify the large E on the chart, how can you assess lesser degrees of vision?
6. Describe your method of determining the prescription of a pair of glasses.
7. How do you measure the add on a cataract bifocal?
8. Describe how prisms can be measured on the lensmeter that you use.
9. Describe a method of measuring the near point of accommodation. What is the importance of this test?
10. Describe a method of measuring the near point of convergence. What is the importance of this test?
11. What are some methods for testing color vision?
12. Describe some rough tests for depth perception. What factors impair depth perception?
13. Outline a routine for examination of external features of the eyelids and eye.
14. How are the pupillary light reflexes tested?
15. What are Schirmer's test number one and number two? How is each performed?
16. Outline a method of transposing plus cylinders to a minus prescription, using the formula $+1.00 + 2.00 \times 90$.
17. Where does the lid margin normally lie on the cornea when the eye is open? How can you tell if it is drooped or retracted?
18. Outline a method of appraising vision in a man with dense cataracts and less than 20/200 vision.
19. What is the normal blink rate? What does increased blink rate usually mean?

Q Self-evaluation questions

True–false statements

Directions: Indicate whether the statement is true **(T)** or false **(F).**

1. In visual acuity recordings, 6/12 is equal to 20/60 vision. **T** or **F**
2. In occlusion nystagmus, the vision is improved when the one eye is occluded. **T** or **F**
3. Shining a light in the eye not being examined is a valid way of doing a pinhole assessment of vision. **T** or **F**

Missing words

Directions: Write in the missing word in the following sentences:

4. When neutralizing lenses, the displacement of the target by the prism is always recorded in terms of the _____ of the prism.
5. A 10-year-old boy has 14.00 diopters of accommodation. A 45-year-old man has _____ of accommodation left.
6. Defects in color vision are present predominantly in _____.

Choice-completion questions

Directions: Select the one best answer in each case.

7. The following tests are suitable for color vision testing.
   a. The Worth four-dot test
   b. The Ishihara test plates
   c. The fly test
   d. All of the above
   e. None of the above
8. Depth perception requires:
   a. good vision in each eye.
   b. overlapping visual fields.
   c. normal alignment of the eyes.
   d. all of the above.
   e. none of the above.
9. Proptosis is a sign of:
   a. thyroid disease.
   b. adult glaucoma.
   c. ptosis.
   d. hypertension.
   e. all of the above.

A Answers, notes, and explanations

1. **False.** 6/6 vision in meters is equivalent to 20/20 vision; 6/12 vision in meters is equivalent to 20/40 vision. In Canada and the United States, visual acuity charts are designated in feet, whereas in Europe the metric system is used.

2. **False.** Occlusion nystagmus is a congenital condition in which nystagmus and esotropia may be induced by covering one eye and decreasing vision. The decrease in light sensation is enough to cause the other eye to oscillate. Such children, when given routine vision tests, score poorly because the examiner fails to look for this condition. In these children, the eye that should be occluded can be fogged with a +10.00 diopter lens to allow proper vision in the other eye.

3. **True.** A pinhole disc before the pupil improves vision to normal limits if the loss of vision is a result of a refractive error. The pinhole test separates refractive visual loss from pathologic visual loss. With disease, a pinhole over the pupil makes vision worse. Shining a light in the other eye causes both pupils to constrict and is a simple way of achieving the pinhole test.

4. **Base.** If the lens has a prism, the center of the lens does not coincide with the center of the target. The displacement measured in circles of expanding radii is a measure of the power of the prism and is recorded as base in, out, up, or down. The distance between each circle represents 1.00 prism diopter. With the new automatic devices, prism power is digitally recorded and the results are instant.

5. **3.50 diopters.** The decline in accommodation is most striking between ages 30 and 40 when it drops from 8.00 to 4.50 diopters. It is caused by atrophy of ciliary muscle and loss of elasticity of the lens of the eye. Unfortunately there is no way to halt the process; thus it is inevitable that everyone eventually needs reading glasses, except near-sighted people, who merely take their glasses off.

6. **Boys.** Congenital color defects, red–green being the most common, are transmitted by the female and appear predominantly in the male. In fact, 8% to 10% of males are color deficient. Total color blindness is another matter; it is rare and very disabling and causes blindness and nystagmus in children.

7. **b. The Ishihara test plates.** Ishihara test plates are those most commonly used for the detection of color deficiency. Other devices such as the Nagel anomaloscope are superior in detection of possible defects and in quantifying them. The Ishihara plates, however, are inexpensive to purchase so they can be used by every industrial or school nurse. They are simple to use, no expertise is required, and the results are reproducible. It is basically a color vision screener and not an analyzer.

8. **d. All of the above.** Most authorities believe that depth perception cannot be acquired. If there is a congenital strabismus and the eyes are straightened at age 3 years, that child will not have depth perception. Having poor depth perception may not be of practical importance because there are so many monocular clues to judge distance. Pilots need it in the rare instances that they have to make a visual landing. Athletes, like baseball or tennis players, are also handicapped without depth perception.

9. **a. Thyroid disease.** Protrusion of the eyes is usually measured with the exophthalmometer. When it occurs in one eye, it frequently indicates a retrobulbar mass, a hemangioma being most common. But when it occurs in both eyes, it means thyroid disease until proved otherwise. Deposits of fat, hyaluronic acid-like material, and inflammatory cells cause the typical bulging of the eyes.

Chapter 9

Visual function and impairment

Bernard R. Blais, Harold A. Stein

INTRODUCTION

There are many ways of looking at anything depending on perspective.

Artists all recognize this. Famous ones have unique perspective. Some have altered color value in the cones of their retina, for example, yellow-blue blind.

One alters one's perspective when placed in large or small lecture rooms. Magicians can create visual illusions and fool us into seeing things that are not there or making things disappear before our eyes. Houdini made an elephant disappear on stage in front of a large audience.

ASPECTS OF VISION LOSS

Vision loss can be observed from many different points of view. The most commonly used set of aspects is the International Classification of Impairments, Disabilities, and Handicaps promoted by the World Health Organization (WHO), and the International Classification of Diseases. The aspects and ranges of vision loss are also the subject of a recent standard of the International Council of Ophthalmology.

TYPES OF VISION

The basic structure of the eye is shown in Figures 1.1 and 1.2. The retina contains receptor cells, rods, and cones, which, when stimulated by light, send signals to the brain (as described in Chapter 1). These signals are subsequently interpreted as vision.

Most of the receptors are rods, which are found predominantly in the periphery of the retina, whereas the cones are located mostly in the center and near periphery. There are approximately 17 rods for every cone.

According to the duplicity theory of vision, the rods are responsible for vision under very dim levels of illumination (scotopic vision) and the cones function at higher illumination levels (photopic vision).

This dual-receptor system allows the human eye to maintain sensitivity over an impressively large range of ambient light levels. Between the limits of maximal photopic vision and minimal scotopic vision, the eye can adapt rather effectively to changes in brightness of as much as 1 billion times. The sensitivity of the eye automatically adjusts to changes in lumination.

Although the human eye can function over a vast range of brightness, the retina is sensitive to damage by light, such as from lasers, bright flashlights (more than 600 lumens), or unprotected sun gazing or bright computer screens. This potential for light injury exists because the optics of the eye can concentrate light energy on the retina by a factor of 100,000 times.

Both rods and cones function over a wide range of light intensity levels and at the intermediate levels of illumination. They function simultaneously. The transition zone between photopic and scotopic vision where the level of illumination is equivalent to twilight or dusk is called mesopic vision.

Photopic, mesopic, and scotopic vision

Photopic vision

- Cone photoreceptors/color vision
- Resolves fine detail 20/20 or better: high acuity
- Functions only in good illumination

Mesopic vision

- Both rods and cones function over a wide range of light at simultaneous levels.
- Intermediate levels of chromatic function simultaneously.
- Twilight or dusk occurs in a mixed rod/cone mode.
- Ambient illumination should be from dim to dark.
- No surface (including reflective surfaces) within the subject fields should exact the chart luminance.

Scotopic vision

- Uses rod photoreceptors
- Occurs in very low light levels
- Exhibits poorer quality vision
- Is limited by resolution (usually 20/200 or less) for acuity
- Provides ability to discriminate only shades of black and white (confirmed by noting that at dusk different colors of the flowers in a garden become virtually indistinguishable)
- Provides enhanced sensitivity and low detection threshold under marked reduced illumination

Absent color vision

The luminance shows typical situations in which the eye would be in each operating mode. The ambient light level created by the sun level is almost independent of position until the sun falls to 5 to 10 degrees above the horizon. The eye's contrast sensitivity is roughly constant when the sun is much above the horizon. Once the sun is over the horizon, twilight begins and the change from photopic to mesopic and eventually to scotopic vision begins. Pure scotopic operation occurs only when there is no significant light source. Even good moonlight can prevent full scotopic operation.

Adaptation—the response to changing levels of stimulation, which for photoreceptors means light—also differs for rods and cones. Because the cones have three separate "channels," the overall sensitivity is lower and the rods are much more sensitive than cones at lower levels of light. Because of the nature of human visual response, these levels are typically measured in terms of luminance (candela per unit area), but on a logarithmic scale. This means that differences of 1.33:1 or 1:0.75 are the smallest discernible steps, despite the seemingly large changes in the associated luminance values.

LUMINANCE VERSUS ILLUMINATION

Luminance is a photometric measure of the luminous intensity per unit area of light traveling in a given direction. It describes the amount of light that passes through or is emitted from a particular area, and falls within a given solid angle. According to the International System of Units (SI), luminance is candela per square meter (cd/m^2).

Luminance is often used to characterize emission or reflection from flat, diffuse surfaces. The luminance indicates how much luminous power will be perceived by an eye looking at the surface from a particular angle of view. Luminance is thus an indicator of how bright the surface will appear. In this case the solid angle of interest is the solid angle subtended by the eye's pupil. Luminance is used in the video industry to characterize the brightness of displays. A typical computer display emits between 50 and 300 cd/m^2. The sun has a luminance of about 1.6×10^9 cd/m^2 at noon.

Luminance is invariant in geometric optics. This means that for an ideal optical system, the luminance at the output is the same as the input luminance. For real, passive, optical systems, the output luminance is *at most* equal to the input. As an example, if you form a demagnified image with a lens, the luminous power is concentrated into a smaller area, meaning that the illuminance is higher at the image. The light at the image plane, however, fills a larger solid angle so the luminance comes out to be the same assuming there is no loss at the lens. The image can never be "brighter" than the source.

MEASUREMENT AND ASSESSMENT OF VISUAL LOSS

When considering visual functioning, we can perceive many different aspects of vision loss, depending on our point of view and the interventions, such as surgery and rehabilitation.

In considering how various causes may result in structural changes, such as scarring, atrophy, or loss, the focus is on the tissue. However, structural changes do not reveal how well the eye functions as a whole. For that we must widen our view from the tissue to the organ, and a clinician is needed to measure aspects of organ function, such as visual acuity, visual field, and contrast sensitivity.

Yet knowing how the eye functions does not disclose how a person functions. Our perspective thus has to expand even more to encompass the individual level and consider tasks such as reading, mobility, and face recognition. For this perspective, various vision rehabilitation professionals are needed to work with a patient. Beyond this scope, the person has to be viewed in a societal context and assessed for how all of these changes have an effect on the person's participation in society, such as causing job loss or reducing quality of life. The goal of all of these interventions is to ensure the patient is satisfied with the resulting condition.

ASPECTS OF VISUAL IMPAIRMENT

When organ functions are reduced, we speak of impairments. The most common *ocular visual impairments* are a result of ocular disorders. More recently, increased attention is being given to cerebral disorders, which may cause *cerebral vision impairment*. In infants and children the cause may be perinatal cerebral ischemia, in adults it may be traumatic brain injury, and in older adults it may be a stroke. Cerebral visual impairments may cause abnormal visual functioning, which can be captured under the term *visual dysfunction*.

VISUAL FUNCTIONS

Ophthalmology has unique tools that can measure *visual function* with great precision. Those with the greatest effect on general functioning are (1) *visual acuity* and (2) *visual field*, followed by (3) *contrast sensitivity*. Many other functions such as color vision, stereopsis, light and dark adaptation, and psychophysical and electrophysiologic tests (e.g., electroretinography, visual-evoked potentials) can assess visual function but they are poor predictors of functional consequence. Because loss of visual acuity has many different causes, it is a good screening test, but adds little to the differential diagnosis. Yet whatever its cause it can help in predicting the effect on activities of daily living (ADL).

Measurement and assessment of functional aspects

The different functional aspects are measured and assessed in very different ways. Visual functions measure how the eye functions by varying one parameter at a time in a simplified, artificial environment. For example, the visibility of test objects depends on their size, contrast, and illumination. If we vary the size while keeping contrast and illumination constant, we create a *contrast sensitivity* test, like the CV-1200. If we vary the illumination while keeping size and contrast constant, we perform a *dark adaptation* test. Each test provides a threshold value for the measured stimulus parameter. The threshold criterion is generally defined as the response level that is 50% greater than guessing. Threshold measurements are chosen not because threshold performance is the most relevant performance level for ADL, but because they enable more precise psychophysical calculations.

For visual functions we measure the variable stimulus needed for a fixed response; for functional vision we measure the variable performance for a fixed task, either objectively (timing, error rate) or subjectively (questionnaires).

Finally, we must consider the societal context, or quality of life. For subjective judgments such as making and keeping friendships, social skills, and self-confidence, measurement is more difficult. The ultimate goal is satisfaction, which describes the subjective balance between individual achievements and individual expectations

Parameters of ocular function

1. Macula function
2. Provides binocular vision
3. Visual acuity (VA) better than 20/200
4. Central vision less than 10 degrees
5. Stereopsis
6. Color vision

Analysis

Basic visual functions and essential ADL are:

1. Acuity testing for:
   - Monocular (each eye) and binocular (both eyes) vision
   - Both distance and near visual acuity
   - With and without correction (the person's eyeglasses or contact lenses, intraocular lenses)
2. Stereopsis findings as a baseline; note subsequent changes, if any
3. Color perception, of the three visual hues
4. Visual fields to determine visual acuity from the fovea to the ciliary body
5. Muscle balance (distance and near), also called binocular balance. The examination should be for vertical and horizontal phorias
   - General limits of normal functional balance are set for far and near vision when performing the tests.

Ocular (visual screening)

Step-by-step procedures must be completed for all screened personnel. These steps are based on procedures instituted in the Purdue studies for WWII workers: 150,000 employees tested.

Verified by the US Army in 2010 for usefulness for all active duty and civil service employees.

Peripheral

1. VA worse than 20/200
2. Peripheral visual fields more than 10 degrees
3. Scotopic vision—night vision—exclusion area of macula/fovea control

Preventive medicine guidelines, CPT codebook's evaluation/management guidelines, requirements

1. Ocular history, which includes a general overview of the individual's visual history
2. Complete visual (ocular) screening examination
   a. Visual acuity quantitative bilateral tests are measured for far, at infinity (at minimum and especially in pediatrics), for near, and for intermediate distances (based on job description); contrast sensitivity is done periodically; all examinations are performed with and without corrective devices (i.e., glasses, contact lenses).
   b. Color vision
   c. Gross visual fields
   d. Heterophoria/heterotropia (horizontal and vertical) and depth perception
   e. Intraocular tension (e.g., puff tonometers) by separate glaucoma screening

WHY PERFORM VISUAL SCREENING

Visual function and visual tasks can analyze anatomic and structural changes caused by disease or injury. Also included here is a discussion of the relationship of these functional changes to the visual requirements of ADL or specific occupational requirements.

The precision and accuracy with which the eye can contrast that of the most sophisticated camera. It has unique focusing capabilities, and its ability to work with the brain allows people to undergo special training (e.g., finding specific details or characteristics in a product such as a flaw in a factory-made part). The eye also can differentiate and distinguish between subtle shades of color and images under conditions of high and low contrast.

Aspects of vision loss and function

Vision loss can be observed from many different perspectives in addition to those of the patient, whether it is the treating physician, a family member, or a caregiver. Each aspect is different but they all revolve around the same clinical case and reveal something about the patient.

Functional vision

Functions describe how the eyes and the visual system function. Functional vision describes how the person functions. When organ functions are reduced, they are referred to as impairments. The most common *ocular visual impairments* are caused by ocular disorders. More recently, increased attention is being given to cerebral disorders, which may cause *cerebral visual impairment*. Cerebral vision impairments may cause abnormal visual functioning, which can be considered under the term *visual dysfunction*.

Another scenario involves screening patients with an identifiable defect during an evaluation required by federal law for entrance into a work position, such as the evaluation that a pilot might undergo. In particular, the Americans with Disabilities Act (ADA) of 1990 requires that an individual be evaluated to determine whether that person is qualified to fulfill the essential tasks of the position, with or without accommodation, without significant increase in risk to self or others.

Binocular vision

Binocular vision (seeing with two eyes) is normal and confers three benefits: it makes hard-to-see objects easier to detect, it enlarges the total field of view, and it improves a person's capacity to distinguish small differences in depth.

The most distinctive benefit of using two eyes derives from the fact that because they are horizontally separated, they do not have exactly the same view of the visual world. The small differences between the images in the two eyes are systematically related to the arrangement of objects in depth, providing information from which the visual system is able to distinguish small differences in the distances at which objects lie. This capability, known as *stereopsis*, is most beneficial for making fine depth judgments, especially when objects are nearby (i.e., within arm's reach).

For all three of these capabilities (enhanced acuity, field of view, and stereopsis) the brain must properly combine information from the two eyes.

If the vision in the two eyes differs substantially, the brain may be able to combine the information in a unified view *(binocular single vision)* or may be unable to use the differences between the images to distinguish small differences in the depth. Binocular vision can be disturbed even though each eye alone is functioning normally. Abnormalities in the brain, or improperly coordinated movements of the eyes, or misalignment of them, can disrupt normal binocular vision. When the brain is unable to combine information of the two eyes, a person may experience double vision *(diplopia)* or *binocular rivalry*, a sometimes haphazard switching of the eyes from one eye to the other. Failure to combine information from the two eyes can lead to a reduced ability to use small differences in depth. Moreover, under some circumstances, vision of the two eyes might conflict, making vision poorer than if one eye alone were used.

Binocular vision (simultaneous images with two eyes) is normal and confers three benefits: (1) it makes hard-to-see objects easier to detect, (2) it enlarges the total field of view, and (3) it makes a more effective depth perception.

Monocular vision is one-eyed vision. A person with monocular vision usually has one of the following:

- Suppression
- Amblyopia
- Tropia
- Disease
- Trauma

Visual acuity quantitative bilateral tests are measured for far (or at infinity), for near, and for intermediate distances (based on job description); all examinations are performed with and without corrective devices (i.e., glasses, contact lenses).

A visual acuity test may be an evaluation for those especially who have had cataract implant operations or refractive surgery or are older.

Contrast sensitivity

Contrast sensitivity (CS) determines the lowest contrast level that can be detected by a person for a given size target. Normally a range of target sizes is used. Unlike visual acuity, CS measures two variables, size and contrast; acuity measures only size.

Figure 9.1A demonstrates normal contrast, whereas Figure 9.1B demonstrates a loss of contrast in which the image is hardly visible. CS measures the degree to which the visual system can discriminate between adjacent areas of light and dark. Unlike measures of static focal acuity such as the Snellen test, measurement of CS does not yield a single figure, describing performance. It does, however, detect functional vision loss often caused by early eye disease. Moreover, it can produce a more sensitive and comprehensive measurement of visual capability and performance than is provided by Snellen visual acuity alone.

The causes of CS loss are many, and the consequences are substantial. It is important to enhance contrast in the environment for people to avoid falls on steps or curbs and to function in situations such as driving in fog or rain.

The human visual system is discretely sensitive to visual information of different sizes. Measuring the angular size rather than the actual size of the element in the optic array is preferred because the visual size (the image projected on the retina) varies with the object's actual size and distance to the subject. In this way, size and distance are compressed into a single figure.

The three designated channels (mechanisms) within the visual system correspond roughly to low, medium, and high spatial frequencies (number of cycles per degree of visual angle). Low spatial frequencies provide general position, medium spatial frequencies provide general position and general shape, and high spatial frequencies provide edges and fine details.

TESTING

Early tests used repeating bars called sinusoidal gratings. The most common test now is the Pelli-Robson test, which uses letters with sharp edges that are more like actual objects. The gratings, however, are used for test purposes because it is possible to control both contrast and spatial frequency and because more common scenes require a complex apparatus to produce.

The result of a test on CS on the Commercial Drivers Report is called a contrast sensitivity modulation transfer function (MTF). The test generally measures CS (the inverse of the threshold contrast at which an observer can just discriminate the grating) over a range of spatial frequencies. The differential sensitivity across this range yields the modulation transfer function.

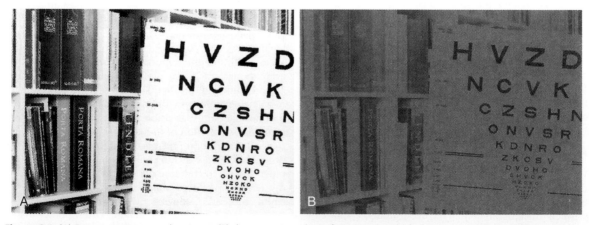

Figure 9.1 (A) Demonstrates normal contrast; (B) demonstrates a loss of contrast in which the image is hardly visible.

EVERYDAY VISUAL EXPERIENCE

Standard tests of visual acuity, for example Snellen optotypes, generally measure resolution of fine detail at high contrast (black on white). However, in everyday visual experience, most objects are seen against a diffuse background or with other objects at moderate or intermediate levels of contrast. The visual scene is typically made up of large and small objects with coarse outlines, intermingled with fine detail and producing a mixture of stimuli that include gradual transitions between areas of light and dark, as well as abrupt transitions and sharp edges.

Clinically measured visual acuity, therefore, cannot assess a person's capacity to distinguish and identify a wide variety of different images. Selective loss of intermediate and low spatial frequencies may produce disturbing visual symptoms in subjects with nominally normal visual acuity, as measured with standard high-contrast sharp-edged optotypes.

The MCC uses reading rather than letter acuity, which can capture a larger retinal area than letter recognition. It presents both high-contrast and low-contrast targets on the same side of the same card, ensuring that both are read at the same distance and under the same illumination. It also makes visible the difference between the high-contrast and low-threshold contrast without additional calculations (Figure 9.2).

Stereo depth perception: far

The ability to judge relative distances when all clues except binocular triangulation are eliminated is referred to as stereo depth perception. The test for this ability requires simultaneous use of both eyes. In cases in which the subjects have little or no vision in one eye, the test should be eliminated.

Occasionally an individual with good acuity scores fails to fuse the right and left eye patterns. The experience is a doubling or overlapping of images. The examiner begins by asking the subject who is wearing polarized lenses to look at sign number one and indicate if the ring at the bottom seems to float out closer to the eyes than the other three rings. If the answer is yes, then the subject is asked to look at sign number two and indicate which ring floats out, proceeding to signs three, four, and so on (Figure 9.3).

Scoring with stereo test

The examiner's use of patience is extremely important here because the test often requires of the subjects a few extra moments per sign. Subjects should be encouraged to keep trying. It may be necessary to occlude one eye and then remove the occlusion to give subjects an opportunity to readjust their focus. The test is continued until, as in previous tests, subjects give two consecutive wrong answers. The score is the last number answered correctly before those consecutive misses.

Color perception

Color perception should be tested monocular with the use of the six reproduced Ishihara pseudoisochromatic plates, which measure the ability to see red and green hues (Figure 9.4). This test detects the presence of a color deficiency but does not classify it as to type. A total of eight numbers can be seen by color-normal individuals in the six circles. Individuals with low visual acuity (20/50 or less) may fail this test.

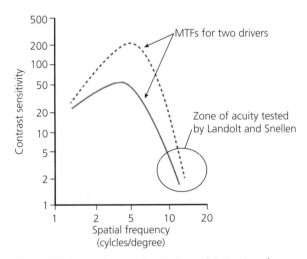

Figure 9.2 Contrast sensitivity. *MTFs*, modulation transfer functions.

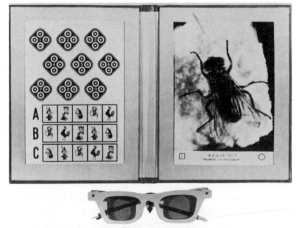

Figure 9.3 Wirt and fly tests for depth perception.

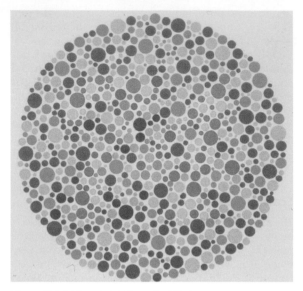

Figure 9.4 Ishihara's test for color blindness.

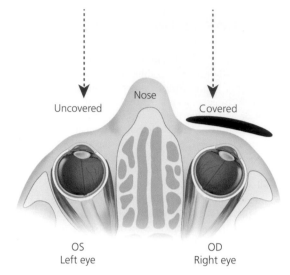

Figure 9.5 Heterophoria.

Recent advances in psychophysical understanding of color vision defects has led to the use of the American Optical Test to include the alternate color perception tests using the Hardy-Rand-Rittler (HRR) test symbols the industrial use of color shading in the functional use and safety requirement (e.g., patient may have need for up to 88 different color shades). These symbols consist of the triangle, letter X, and circle depicted in various colors, and they are used to detect the presence of color deficiencies along protan, deutan, and tritan color confusion lines. The HRR plates do not classify as to type of defect. That is determined with follow-up testing using the HRR pseudoisochromatic plate book.

Individuals with low visual acuity (20/50 or less) in both eyes may fail color vision testing. The cause of failure in some cases may be low visual acuity rather than faulty color perception. Individuals with low acuity should be identified in the visual acuity section of the vision test series.

Phorias

Heterophoria

Heterophoria is a condition in which both eyes are directed in the same direction except when one eye is covered. The eyes are parallel when both are open but when one eye is covered, the covered eye moves away from the other eye. When an occluder is removed from the eye, the eye then straightens. This is also known as a phoria (Figure 9.5).

Phorias describe the relative directions of the eyes during binocular fixation on a given object in the absence of an adequate fusion stimulus. With normal binocular vision and with both eyes open, subjects will see a single target in space. Because the phoria indicates a latent deviation of the eyes, dissociation is required to determine the amount and direction of the deviation. The examiner evaluates the subjects' vision under dissociation with the use of a prism to determine whether their lines of sight are parallel or if they diverge or converge.

For an examiner to reveal phoria, the cover–uncover test can be used. Cover one eye of the subject with a card and have the subject look at your fingertip. Move the finger around to break the normal reflex that holds a covered eye in the correct vergence position. Then hold your finger steady and uncover the eye. It may be seen to flick quickly from its correct position. If the uncovered eye moves from outward in, the person has exophoria. If the eye moves from inward out, the person has esophoria. If no movement is detected, the person has orthophoria (Figure 9.6). It is quite normal for most people to have some amount of exophoria or esophoria.

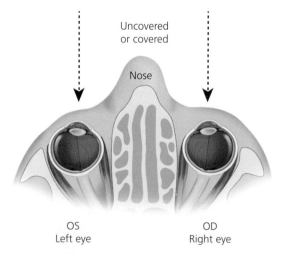

Figure 9.6 Orthophoria.

Heterophoria can be lateral (horizontal) or vertical. A lateral heterophoria can be either an exophoria or eso-phoria. *Exo* means "turning outward," away from the nose, whereas *eso* means "turning inward," toward the nose. In an exophoria, if the right eye is covered, it will drift outward under the cover. As soon as the right eye is uncovered, it will move back in and fixate on the target again. The same actions occur for esophoria, although the drift is inward.

Lateral phoria

Vertical phoria

The test for vertical phoria measures, in 0.5 prism diopter steps, the relative posture of the eyes in the vertical plane when all stimuli to binocular fixation are eliminated.

INTERVENTIONS FOR REHABILITATION

The four aspects of vision loss are not independent but form a loose chain of cause and effect. Rehabilitation, therefore, involves manipulating each of these links to achieve the least possible handicap or the greatest possible participation.

Rehabilitation involves a team of different professionals, and the effects of their interventions must be measured with different yardsticks. Thus it is important that all evaluators not only understand their own responsibilities and the differences in various approaches, but also have a basic familiarity with corresponding issues of the other team members as well.

Understanding ophthalmic equipment

Today, more than ever, the ophthalmologist's clinical acumen is enhanced by the many instruments available that facilitate the determination of refractive errors of the eye, the detection of muscular imbalance, and the magnification and visualization of the interior structures of the eye. This chapter deals with ophthalmic instruments, their purpose and mode of use, and their advantages and limitations.

EQUIPMENT USED FOR REFRACTION

Determining the refractive error of an eye permits the ophthalmologist to prescribe lenses that enable the patient to obtain the best possible visual acuity.

Projector and projector slides

The projector provides a means of projecting, on a silver screen, test letters and characters that can be used in assessing visual acuity.

It consists of a housing for a bulb, an opening for introduction of different target slides, and a lens system that can be focused onto a silver screen. The housing for the bulb is made readily accessible for interchange of bulbs when bulbs darken or burn out. Rheostats may be introduced into the power circuits to lengthen the life of the bulb. The lens system and slides should be kept clean and dust free.

Projectors provide a means of illuminating (1) a horizontal row of test letters or characters, (2) a vertical row of test letters or characters, and (3) a single-test letter or character, and may allow the introduction of red–green to illuminate the letters.

The use of red and green letters is the basis of the duochrome test and a means of fine-tuning the refraction. In this test, half the panel is illuminated in red and half the panel in green. Under the duochrome principle, green is normally focused in front of the retina, whereas red, having a longer wavelength, is focused behind the retina for the emmetrope. Therefore, a patient seeing the letters on the green panel more clearly than those on the red panel is hyperopic, requiring more plus to bring the red wavelengths onto the retina. The patient seeing the letters more clearly on the red panel is myopic, requiring more minus to bring the green onto the retina. The emmetrope sees both equally blurred. The duochrome test thus provides a means to arrive at the final correcting lens for the refractive error present.

Available projector slides have a large variety of test targets and specialized tests for refraction. Commonly available slides include:

- Snellen test letters
- Landolt (split circle) rings
- Numbers
- E's
- An astigmatic clock
- A picture chart
- A Worth four-dot test

Projectors may be controlled by remote control units. The use of remote control units is especially important if projectors are installed in inaccessible places or areas that are awkward for the examiner to control.

Trial case and lenses

The trial case is a tray of lenses and accessories used to determine the refractive error of an eye. These lenses are individually marked in the strengths of the dioptric power of each lens, as well as in the direction of axis of the cylindric lenses. The trial case consists of:

- A pair of plus spheres ranging from +0.12 to +20.00 diopters
- A pair of minus spheres ranging from −0.12 to −20.00 diopters
- A pair of plus cylinders ranging from +0.12 to +8.00 diopters
- A pair of minus cylinders ranging from −0.12 to −8.00 diopters
- Accessory lenses
- Trial frame

These lenses are designed to fit a standard trial frame. Each lens is encircled by a metal rim for protection. Handles are provided with spheres for ease of handling and are optional with cylinders. The choice is governed by the type of trial frames used. Cylinders with handles are used with the trial frames illustrated in Figure 10.1, but not with simple types having no revolving cylinder lens carriers. Handles would interfere with the free rotation of the cylinder in the latter type. The cylinder is marked with reference to its axis and not the meridian. Thus the position on the cylinder, as marked on the lens, is the axis of zero power and indicates the position of the image on the retina.

Accessory lenses available in a trial case are:

- An occluder lens
- A pinhole disc
- A stenopeic slit
- A Maddox rod lens

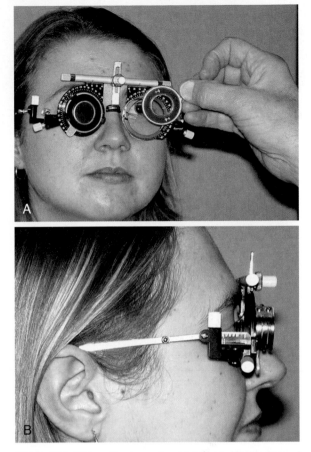

Figure 10.1 (A) Inserting lenses in a trial frame. (B) Side view of trial frame.

- Prisms ranging from 0.50 to 6.00 prism diopters
- A red glass filter lens

Use of trial lenses

Trial lenses are not used routinely because they have been eclipsed by the *refractor* or *phoropter* (see following text), which offers the ophthalmologist the speed of exchange of lenses in a completely enclosed housing. The trial lens, however, has a place in determining the refractive error of children who are intimidated by the massive bulk of the refractor, or whose narrowly set eyes cannot be positioned properly behind the openings in the refractor (Figure 10.2). Bifocals are prescribed by use of the trial frame with lenses because the patient can best judge a comfortable working and reading distance with the head bent and the eyes lowered in a natural reading position. Trial lenses are also used in refraction of aphakic and high-myopic eyes because it is expedient that the correcting lenses and the spectacles that the patient receives approximate each other with reference to their

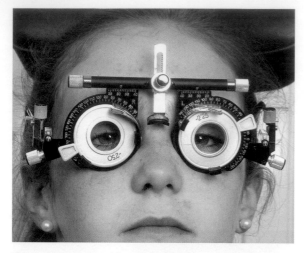

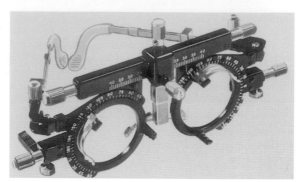

Figure 10.3 Trial frame.

Figure 10.2 Testing vision with trial frames and lenses.

distance from the eye itself. Trial lenses must be used when low visual aids in the form of high-plus prescription lenses are used.

The trial frame is essentially a frame capable of holding a group of three or four trial lenses for each eye. It has adjustable earpieces and an adjustable bridge that alters the interpupillary distance. Some trial frames have an adjustment for tilting the frames toward the reading position. In high-minus and high-plus prescriptions, the proximity of the lens in the frame to the eye (vertex distance) must be measured. This aids the optician in duplicating the prescription. The calibration scale incorporated on the outer side of the frame can be used for this purpose, but is not really an accurate method of making this measurement. Modern trial frames have a thumbscrew mechanism on the side of the trial frame to rotate the front lens carrier, which is used to house the cylinder. This enables the cylinder to be rotated to the proper axis.

The front surface of the trial frame is marked off in degrees from 0 to 180 (Figure 10.3). By convention, frames are labeled in a counterclockwise direction beginning on the right-hand side of the horizontal meridian.

Refractor or phoropter

The refractor consists of the entire trial set of lenses mounted on a circular wheel so that each lens can be brought before the aperture of the viewing system by merely turning a dial (Figures 10.4 and 10.5). In addition to the conventional spheres and cylinders, accessories are available including a polarizing lens, a pinhole, a Maddox rod, and a working lens for retinoscopy. There are many types of refractors on the market, varying in the number of accessories available and the mode of housing these accessories. Fundamentally, these refractors are of the same design and purpose.

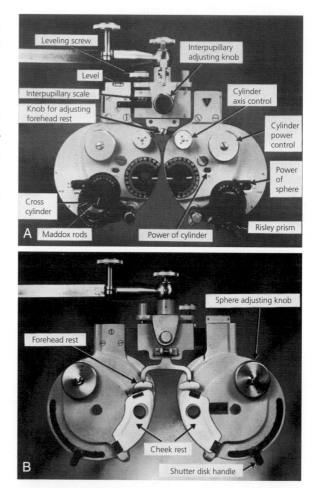

Figure 10.4 Greens' refractor (older type). (A) Front view. (B) Back view.
(Courtesy of Bausch & Lomb Co., Rochester, NY.)

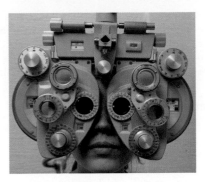

Figure 10.5 Improved Greens' phoropter II.

We shall discuss the Bausch & Lomb Phoropter II (manufactured by Reichert) because it is a typical example of the devices available. (The terms *phoropter* and *refractor* are often used interchangeably.)

Body

The body consists of two disc-like casings that house the lenses. The entire instrument is mounted on a pole or a hydraulic stand. A forehead rest ensures that the patient is correctly positioned and that the eyes are as close to the lens system as possible. The knobs at either end on top of the phoropter adjust the interpupillary distance for the individual patient. If the patient has a head tilt or a vertical muscle imbalance, the phoropter may have to be tilted so that one aperture is higher than the other. Leveling adjustment knobs are adjacent to the interpupillary distance knobs.

Lenses

For each eye there are large circular discs that contain spheres and cylinders. These lenses may be presented individually or in combination. A large dial on the back surface of the phoropter introduces spheres in units of 3.00 diopters (some older models may be 4.00 diopters). A *side wheel* can be rotated to introduce spheres in small jumps of a quarter of a sphere. The total spherical power is read on the front casing. Plus spheres are recorded in white and minus spheres in red. The range of spherical lenses is from +20.00 to −28.00 diopters.

Phoropters are available in either plus or minus cylinders, but never both. Cylinders are introduced by the top knob on the front surface of the phoropter in units of 0.25 to 2.50. If higher cylinders are required, auxiliary cylinders of 2.50 can be flipped in front of the lens system, extending the range to 5.00. Additional loose auxiliary cylinders may be added to extend the range to 7.50 diopters. Astigmatism may be corrected to 0.12 diopter by introducing an auxiliary cylinder of 0.12 diopter. All cylinders have an axis that is controlled by a small knob,

about which the accessories rotate. Markings on the front surface are in degrees, from 0 to 180, with individual axis markings in 5-degree intervals.

Aperture control handle

A small handle on the side of each eye of the phoropter controls the aperture. By moving the handle up or down, one may introduce the following:

1. An occluder to block out one eye
2. A pinhole disc
3. A +0.12 sphere, which can raise the total spherical power of the combination of lenses by 0.12 diopter
4. A retinoscopy lens, which may be custom ordered according to the distance at which retinoscopy is performed (the usual retinoscopy lens ranges from +1.00 to +2.00 spheres and is introduced by the control handle for retinoscopy and removed for subjective testing)
5. Prisms, 6.00 diopters base-up before the right eye and 10.00 diopters base-in before the left eye
6. Maddox rods, vertical and horizontal

From time to time, the complete phoropter should be returned for cleaning of lenses.

Auxiliary lenses

Auxiliary lenses include cylinders of 0.12 and 5.00 diopters for each eye (the phoropter has lenses available in either plus or minus cylinders, but not both), and cross cylinders of 0.25, 0.37, and 0.50 for each eye.

Accessory equipment

Accessory equipment includes Risley's prisms to measure muscle imbalance, a cross-cylinder holder, and a reading-card holder. The *cross-cylinder holder* is geared to follow the cylinder axis control. The cross cylinder is inserted in a double ring of metal, the outer ring being fixed, whereas the inner ring, which holds the cross cylinder, is capable of being flipped or turned to reverse its position. The *reading-card holder*, attached to the front of the phoropter, permits the holding of a reading card at a variable distance from the phoropter. The reading-card holder is a rod, calibrated in inches, centimeters, and diopters, and it is capable of presenting four test cards to the patient.

Aids in care of refractor/phoropter

1. If the lenses are dirty, they should be cleaned with a lint-free swab slightly moistened with either alcohol or ether. Ammonia or ammonia-containing cleansers should not be used. Lenses may be dried with a tissue.
2. Do not put fingers, pens, or pencils in the front aperture to see if a lens is in place because the marks left are extremely difficult to remove. The rear apertures are often protected by a cover glass.

3. The instrument should not be lubricated because the design of the instrument is such that no interior oiling is necessary. It may be helpful at times to oil the bearings on which the cross cylinder and the Maddox rod ride.
4. Cleaning material should not be used on the numbers and workings that indicate lens power. These should be cleaned with a dry, soft cloth.
5. The forehead and cheek rests are removable and should be cleaned periodically with cotton moistened in 70% alcohol solution.
6. The instrument should be covered with a plastic cover when not in use.

Retinoscope

The retinoscope is the most valuable instrument in determining the refractive error of an eye (Figures 10.6 and 10.7). It is useful in determining the total objective refractive error of an eye and may be the only means of assessing

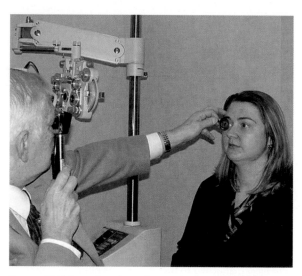

Figure 10.6 Procedure for retinoscopic examination.

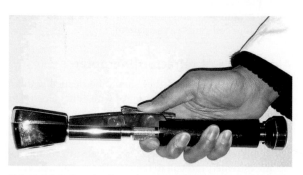

Figure 10.7 Copeland streak retinoscope.

refractive error in infants and small children. It is also useful for the objective estimation of the refractive error in people who cannot read, are learning disabled, are debilitated and uncooperative, and have speech loss. There are two basic types: the spot retinoscope and the streak retinoscope.

Spot retinoscope

The spot retinoscope is designed so that the refractionist can look down the center of a slightly diverging beam of light through the pupil of the patient's eye. The modern retinoscope has a light source in the handle of the instrument, shining upward, which strikes a mirror set at 45 degrees. The beam is therefore turned through 90 degrees.

The mirror may be semisilvered or may have a hole through its center through which the refractionist can look. Therefore, an area of the patient's retina is illuminated and the refractionist sees this as a red-reflected glow. This is termed a *reflex*.

In the eye with no refractive error, the rays of light come to a focus on a point on the retina and the refractionist sees the whole pupillary area lit with a red glow. This is analogous to an automobile's headlight, in which the whole 6-inch (15 cm) circular diameter of the headlight appears to be illuminated, whereas the source of this illumination is a small filament in the bulb, about 5 mm long, positioned correctly at the point of focus of the optical system of the headlight. Moving the retinoscope away from the pupil extinguishes the red reflex.

If the patient is myopic, the rays of light from the retinoscope will come to a focus in front of the retina, cross at this point, and illuminate a relatively larger area of the retina behind the focal point. If the light source is moved across the pupil, the rays of light from the retinoscope, pivoting on the focal point, will move the illuminated area on the fundus in a direction opposite to that of the retinoscope. This apparent shift of the illuminated area is termed an *against motion*. The refractionist therefore adds minus lenses before the patient's eyes to move the focal point back onto the retina. When he or she has the correct combination of lenses, the movement of the light across the pupil causes no movement of the reflex, it merely turns on and off.

If the patient is hyperopic, the ray of light from the retinoscope, when going through the eye, would focus at a point behind the retina (if the retina does not block the rays of light). Lateral movement of the retinoscope across the pupil causes the area illuminated on the retina (pivoting about the focal point) to move in the same direction as the retinoscope, indicating that the eye is hyperopic or far-sighted. This shift is termed *with motion*. The refractionist then adds plus lenses to bring the focusing point up to the retina until the *on and off* light reflex appears without any apparent movement.

In summary, if a retinoscope beam produces *with motion* of the red reflex, the patient's eye is hyperopic or far-sighted and needs plus lenses to correct the condition. If the retinoscope beam produces *against motion,* the patient is myopic or near-sighted and needs minus lenses to correct the refractive error.

If the eye is astigmatic, it will exhibit two powers on axes at 90 degrees to one another. The retinoscope is then used to correct the power on one axis and then on the other. A cylindric prescription can be obtained in this manner with use of spheres alone, but generally cylinders are added, as well as the spheres, until the *on and off reflex* is observed on all axes.

All the aforementioned theory depends on the patient's relaxed accommodation (that is, the patient's looking at some object 20 feet [6 m] away) and on parallel rays of light entering the eye and coming to a focus on the retina. The light source of the retinoscope, held about 18 inches (0.5 meter) from the patient during retinoscopy, produces diverging, not parallel, rays of light from the retinoscope. Therefore a +2.00 diopter lens (in the refractor, known as the retinoscopy lens) is put in the trial frame so that the divergent rays from the retinoscope are in fact parallel when they enter the pupil. The power of this lens depends on the working distance of the refractionist; for example, if he or she works at 0.5 meter (18 inches), this would be a +2.00 diopter lens.

Some refractionists prefer a working distance that requires a +1.50 diopter retinoscopy lens.

The final prescription, taken from the lenses in the trial frame or on the phoropter, is reduced by the working distance power to determine the distance prescription of the patient.

Streak retinoscope (see Figure 10.7)

The same principles that apply to the spot retinoscope also apply to the streak retinoscope. In the streak retinoscope the light source is a straight-line filament of the bulb. There is a condensing lens between the mirror and the bulb so that the filament itself may be focused onto the patient's eye as a straight line. By means of a movable sleeve that envelops the whole retinoscope, the bulb may be rotated and moved up and down to adjust its focus. Because the light source is a streak of light rather than a cone, if the eye is not emmetropic the area of the retina illuminated becomes a straight line rather than a spot. If astigmatism is present, it is very easy to determine its axis because the streak, playing externally across the patient's face and trial frame with its axis graduation, will not be at the same angle as the streak seen on the retina. The retinoscope streak is rotated until it parallels the streak on the retina and the axis is thereby established. (See Chapter 11 and Figure 11.13.)

From this point the procedure is basically the same as with a spot retinoscope and lenses are added until the reflexes on both axes exhibit no with or against motion when the streak is passed across the pupil.

Accessories used in refraction

Cross cylinder

The cross cylinder consists of a plus and a minus cylinder set at right angles to each other, with a handle set midway between the two axes (Figure 10.8). The axis of the plus cylinder is marked in white and the axis of the minus cylinder marked in red. Cross cylinders are available in dioptric strengths of 0.12, 0.25, 0.50, and 1.00.

The cross cylinder is a refining instrument that determines the exact axis of the astigmatic error and the exact power of the cylinder. The method of use is described in Chapter 11.

Pinhole disc

The pinhole disc is a small disc with a small central opening that eliminates peripheral rays of light, permitting only the central rays to pass through. The pinhole disc permits the examiner to differentiate poor vision caused by refractive errors from poor vision resulting from disease of the eye. Generally, vision that can be improved with a pinhole disc usually can be improved by spectacle lenses.

A multiple pinhole disc serves the same purpose as the pinhole disc, but is an easier device to use because the patient does not have to search for a solitary tiny central hole (Figure 10.9). The patient is asked to view a small line of print with one eye occluded and with the pinhole disc placed before the other eye. If looking through the pinhole disc improves the patient's visual acuity above the uncorrected vision, the findings are recorded as *vision with PH* (pinhole). Corrective lenses often improve vision to the level obtained with the pinhole disc.

Distometer

The distometer is a caliper used to measure the vertex distance (Figure 10.10). The vertex distance is the distance from the cornea of the patient's eye to the back surface of

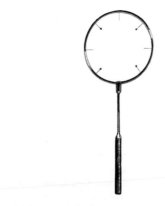

Figure 10.8 Cross cylinder.

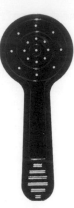

Figure 10.9 Multiple pinhole disc.

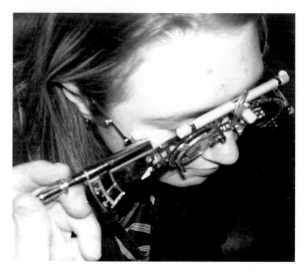

Figure 10.10 Measuring vertex distance with a distometer.

the lens inserted in the trial frame, refractor, or glasses. The distometer consists of a scale in millimeters, an indicator, a movable arm, and a fixed arm.

To use the distometer the examiner places the fixed arm of the caliper on the closed lid of the eye and the other arm against the back surface of the lens. The separation between the posterior surface of the lens and the eyelid is recorded on the millimeter scale. One millimeter is incorporated in the calibration of the distometer to allow for the thickness of the eyelid to arrive at the correct vertex distance. It is important to measure the vertex distance on all high-plus or high-minus lenses; the power of the lens in the trial frame or refractor may change when the lens is moved to a new location in the spectacle frames.

For example, if a +12.00 diopter lens in the trial frame is 10 mm from the cornea but the correcting lens in the spectacle frame is 13 mm from the cornea, a +11.50 lens will be required at this position to give the patient the same visual acuity. The vertex measurement by the distometer permits the dispensing optician to calculate the effective power of a lens required in the final prescription when there is disparity between the distance of the position of the trial frame lens to the cornea and the final spectacles. To calculate the change in the power of a lens, one may refer to small disc or vertex conversion tables (see Appendix 12).

In such a case, if the optician has adjusted the prescription to compensate for this closer vertex distance fitting (an ideal for comfortable vision), the lensmeter reading of the patient's glasses will not correspond with the prescription on the patient's records, either in sphere or in cylinder. The only part of the prescription that will remain the same is the axis.

Halberg and Janelli clips

The Halberg or Janelli trial clip (Figure 10.11) eliminates the need for measuring the vertex distance. The clip is designed to accommodate two trial case rings (or, in the case of the Janelli, three case rings), a sphere, and a cylinder. The trial clips are placed on the patient's glasses; by over-refracting, one can arrive at the prescription with proper effective power for that particular frame. This is extremely important in the high-minus or high-plus prescriptions.

The clips also are useful for small children wearing glasses, when it is not possible to use a conventional trial frame or refractor.

Of major importance in preliminary assessment of refractive errors is the autorefractor. Some have subjective components, some have vision assessment capability,

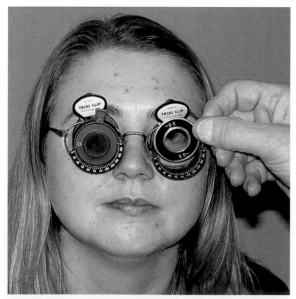

Figure 10.11 Halberg trial clip used to refract over spectacles.

and others have keratometer assessments. (See the section on autorefractors in Chapter 11.)

EQUIPMENT USED TO DETECT MUSCLE IMBALANCE

Maddox rod

The Maddox rod is a group of either red or colorless parallel glass rods that together act as a cylinder (Figure 10.12). The purpose of the Maddox rod is to dissociate the eyes and prevent them from fusing. The Maddox rod accomplishes this by changing the size, shape, and color of a point of light to a line, or streak, of light so that fusion is impossible. The relaxed fusion-free position of the eyes can then be measured easily.

The Maddox rod lens is useful in detecting (1) the presence and amount of a heterophoria, which is the fusion-free position of the eyes, and (2) the presence and amount of a heterotropia, which is a manifest deviation of the eyes not held in check by fusion.

The grouped, red cylindric rods of the Maddox lens convert a white point source of light into a red line running perpendicular to the axes of the Maddox rod. To detect vertical heterophoria, the examiner holds the Maddox rod before one eye with the rods in a vertical position before the eye. The eye behind the Maddox lens perceives a point source of light as a horizontal red line. If the patient, with both eyes open, sees the red line passing directly through the white point source of light (which is viewed by the other eye), a vertical muscle imbalance is not present. With the Maddox rod lens before the right eye, if the patient sees the red line lower than the point source of light, then the patient has a *right hypertropia* or a *right hyperphoria* (Figure 10.13). If the red line is above the point source of light, a *right hypotropia* or a *right hypophoria* is present. By convention, vertical deviations of the eye are always

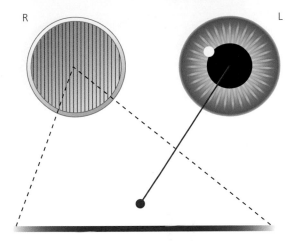

Figure 10.13 Right hyperphoria or right hypertropia. With the Maddox rod held vertically before the right eye, the horizontal red line appears below the point source of light.

designated in terms of the higher eye, so that in the latter example a right hypotropia would be designated as a *left hypertropia* (Figure 10.14). The Maddox rod test should be carried out both at near (16 inches [40 cm]) and distance (20 feet [6 m]).

If the Maddox rod is rotated so that the rods are placed horizontally before the eye, the patient will perceive the red line in the vertical direction. If the Maddox rod is held before the right eye of the patient and the line appears on the right side of the light, then *esophoria* or *esotropia* is present (Figure 10.15). If the line appears on the left side of the light, then *exophoria* or *exotropia* is said to exist (Figure 10.16).

The Maddox rod may also be used to detect torsion *cyclophoria* and *cyclotropia*. Torsion is the result of those ocular muscular anomalies that cause the eyes to rotate in a

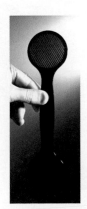

Figure 10.12 Handheld Maddox rod combined with occluder.

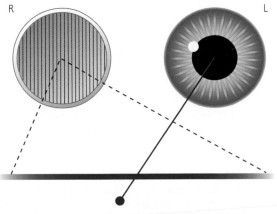

Figure 10.14 Left hyperphoria or left hypertropia. With the Maddox rod held vertically before the right eye, the horizontal line appears above the point source of light.

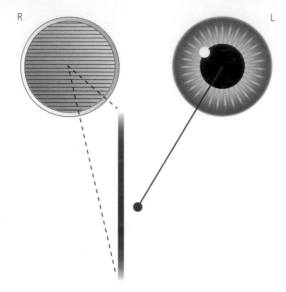

Figure 10.15 Esophoria or esotropia. With the Maddox rod held horizontally before the right eye, the vertical red line appears on the right side of the point source of light.

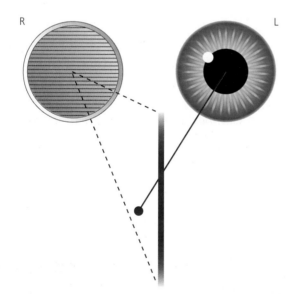

Figure 10.16 Exophoria or extropia. With the Maddox rod held horizontally before the right eye, the vertical red line appears on the left side of the point source of light.

clockwise or counterclockwise fashion. To detect torsion, a red Maddox lens is placed before one eye and a white Maddox lens before the other eye, with the rods of both lenses held in the same direction. If the patient sees that the red line and white line are not parallel, then torsion is present, as well as cyclophoria or cyclotropia.

A prism is needed to measure a phoria or a tropia with a Maddox rod. For example, if the patient has a right hypertropia and reports seeing the red line below the point source of light, base-down prisms are placed before the Maddox rod in increasing strengths until the patient states that the red line runs through the light. The amount of prism required to center the red line on the small light is then a measure of the vertical muscle imbalance in prism diopters.

Prisms

A prism is a triangular, or wedge-shaped, piece of plastic or glass that has the property of displacing a bundle of light toward the base of the prism (Figure 10.17). If the prism is placed before an eye, an object viewed in front of the prism will appear to be displaced toward its apex.

Prisms are used in measuring the presence and the amount of any tropias or phorias. The tests most commonly used to measure ocular muscle imbalance with prisms are the Krimsky test, the Maddox rod prism test (discussed previously), and the prism cover test.

In the *Krimsky test* the observer notes the position of the corneal reflexes when a small light is shone into the eyes. The examiner notes where this reflex is centered in the fixating eye. Prisms are then placed before the deviating eye until the position of the reflex in the pupil of the deviating eye is located in the same position as that of the fixating eye. For example, if the patient's right eye is turned in, the light reflex may be found overlying the temporal margin of the pupil and base-out prisms would be required to displace this reflex to a more central position.

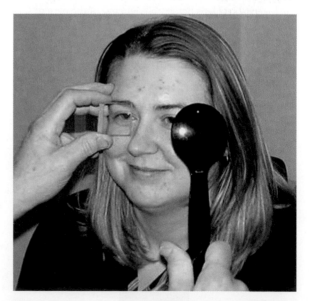

Figure 10.17 Prism cover test. Handheld prisms are introduced to neutralize a deviation.

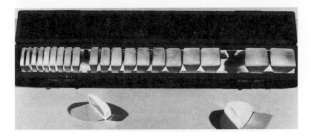

Figure 10.18 Loose or individual prisms set.

The basis of the *prism cover test* is to displace the image of the deviating eye by the use of prisms so that it falls on the macula of that eye. Thus each eye projects to the same point in space, and covering one eye does not require any movement of the other eye to take up fixation. The amount of prism diopters required to achieve this endpoint is a measure of the deviation (see Figure 10.17). The mechanics of this test are discussed in Chapter 43.

Types of prisms available are the loose prism, horizontal and vertical prism bars, and Risley's rotary prism.

The *loose* or *individual prism* is made of plastic or glass. These prisms are supplied in low powers in standard trial lens sets and in a full range of powers in individual prism boxes (Figure 10.18).

Horizontal and vertical prism bars (Figure 10.19) are fused prisms amalgamated into a single bar of gradually increasing strengths. These prisms may be set in a horizontal direction (base in or out) or in a vertical direction (base up or down). The prism bar is principally used to measure the amplitude or power of fusion. It is sometimes used in the cover–uncover test for measuring strabismus in children because it permits rapid examination in a patient whose patience and attention may be limited.

Risley's rotary prism (Figure 10.20) consists of two counterrotating prisms mounted in rings, one in front of the other. These rings are easily rotated in opposite directions by a small thumbscrew. When the two bases are rotated so that they lie behind one another, their effective power is additive. When the apex of one prism is rotated so that it lies behind the base of the other, the effective power is zero. Thus Risley's rotating prism provides a rapid and simple increase in prism power strength so that a deviation may be rapidly adjusted and measured without the delay in introducing individual prisms before the eye.

INSTRUMENTS USED TO DETERMINE POWER OF LENSES

Several instruments are available to assist the ophthalmologist and the ophthalmic assistant in accurately determining the strength of the lenses the patient has been wearing.

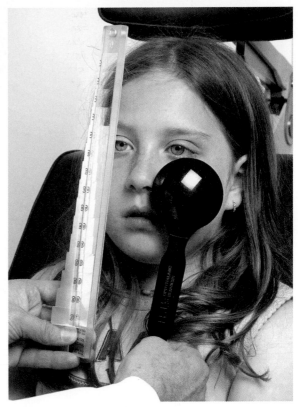

Figure 10.19 Prism bars used to measure the amplitude or power of fusion.

Lensmeter

The lensmeter (sometimes called Lensometer or Vertometer) is used to determine (1) the dioptric vertex power of a lens, (2) the axis, (3) the optical center of a lens, and (4) the presence of a prism and the direction of its base. It consists of an illuminated target, a holder for the glasses to be measured, an adjustable eyepiece, and an optical system designed to focus on an image in the anterior focal plane of the lens to be measured.

To use the lensmeter, see the detailed instructions in Chapter 8.

Geneva lens measure

The Geneva lens measure measures the radius of curvature of the lens surface and records it in diopters. The instrument consists of a dial with a revolving hand and three pins projecting from the instrument. The approximate dioptric power of the lens can be determined by placing the surface of the lens against the pins and then rotating the lens by 90 degrees. If the reading on the scale remains constant, no cylinder is present on that side. The algebraic sum of the

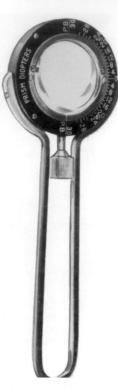

Figure 10.20 Risley's rotary prism.

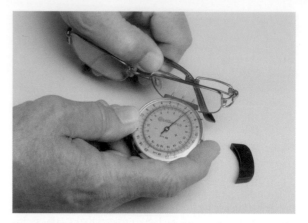

Figure 10.21 Using a lens clock to measure the curvature of a lens surface to determine the dioptric power of the lens

readings from the front and back surface of the lens represents the dioptric power of the lens (for example −2.00 sphere on one side and +6.00 sphere on the other side is equivalent to a +4.00-sphere lens). If the reading is not uniform over the entire surface of the lens, the difference between the lower and higher readings represents the amount of cylinder present. The disadvantage of the Geneva lens measure is that the gauges are calibrated for crown glass only and are subject to considerable error in determining the axis of the cylinder. The gauge gives incorrect measurements for hard resin (plastic) lenses, for aspheric surfaces, and for invisible progressive bifocals.

The use of the Geneva lens measure is that occasionally when glasses are made the base curve may have changed considerably so that the patient may develop headaches and eyestrain. The gauge can help in identifying this cause (Figure 10.21)

INSTRUMENTS USED TO EXAMINE THE INTERIOR OF THE EYE

Ophthalmologists enjoy the unique privilege of being able to examine, by direct visualization, the interior of a vital organ. They can study the retina, which is a modification of nervous tissue, the head of the optic nerve (optic disc), and the state of the retinal blood vessels, which to a large degree mirror the state of other blood vessels of the body not visible to inspection. Because many systemic and neurologic diseases first manifest by alterations within the eye, the use of the ophthalmoscope and other such devices has assisted in bringing ophthalmologists into closer contact with their medical colleagues in related fields.

Direct ophthalmoscope

The ophthalmoscope was invented more than 100 years ago by Hermann von Helmholtz. Von Helmholtz's work was based on the observations of Ernest Brücke, a well-known Viennese physiologist, who 4 years earlier had reported noticing a red light in the pupil of a young man standing in the auditorium of the university as the chandelier light reflected from the student's eye in a direction corresponding to that of his own visual axis. With the popularization of the ophthalmoscope, a wealth of blinding diseases could be understood, and investigation of their cause and treatment began.

The ophthalmoscope consists fundamentally of a light source, a viewing device, and a reflecting device to channel light into the patient's eye. The reflecting device can be a mirror or a reflecting prism. If the patient and examiner are both emmetropic, then light from the patient's retina will be in focus for the examiner. If, however, either the patient or the examiner is hyperopic or myopic, the spherical lenses must be used to overcome their refractive error. Because the ophthalmoscope contains no cylindric lenses, astigmatic errors of refraction cannot be compensated for. Thus if a patient has a large amount of astigmatism, a crystal-clear view of the fundus cannot be obtained. The direct ophthalmoscope enables the examiner to use the power of the subject's eye as a magnifying system to see the retina. Although the field of vision is somewhat restricted compared with that seen with the indirect ophthalmoscope, the magnification is greater, being approximately ×15 for the former and ×5 for the latter (Figure 10.22).

To facilitate pupillary dilation, ophthalmoscopy is best performed in a darkened room. For a better inspection of the fundus, however, the pupils should be dilated with a weak mydriatic agent, such as 2.5% phenylephrine. With heavily pigmented irides, a stronger mydriatic agent, such as 10% phenylephrine, should be used but with *caution*. Because there have been deaths recorded from the application of a single drop, 10% phenylephrine should *not* be routinely used. It should *never* be used with patients who have hypertension or cardiovascular disease. If it is imperative to dilate the pupils of these patients, then cyclopentolate (Cyclogyl) or tropicamide (Mydriacyl) should be used. Pupillary dilation with drops usually is performed in all new patients and in those with extremely small pupils.

The examiner stands directly in front of the patient and examines the patient's right eye with his or her own right

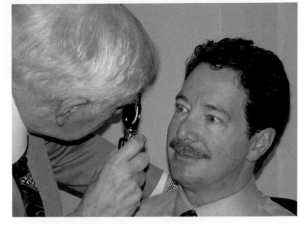

Figure 10.23 Use of the direct ophthalmoscope to detect pathology in anterior segment and fundus of eye.

eye and the left eye in similar fashion (Figure 10.23). The first structure in the fundus noted, for purposes of orientation, is the optic disc. The disc is an oval structure and represents the site of entrance of the optic nerve (Figure 10.24). It is usually pink and may have a central white depression, called the *physiologic cup*. The margins of the disc are sharp and distinct except for the margins of the upper and lower poles, which may be slightly fuzzy. From the disc the retinal arterioles and veins emerge and bifurcate; they extend toward the four quadrants of the retina. The retinal vein, which usually is found lateral to the retinal artery, is larger and darker red.

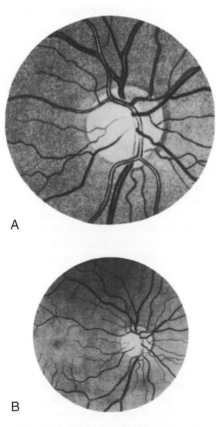

Figure 10.22 (A) Fundus as viewed with the small aperture of the direct ophthalmoscope. Note the magnification obtained but the restrictions in the fields seen. (B) Fundus as viewed with the indirect ophthalmoscope. Note the larger field of view, reduced magnification, and inverted image.

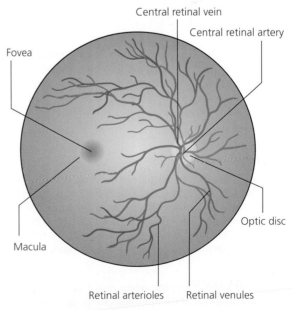

Figure 10.24 Fundus of eye.

Approximately two disc diameters away from the optic disc and slightly below its center is the *macula*. The macula is a small avascular area that appears deeper red than the surrounding fundus. In heavily pigmented individuals the macula may have a darker hue than the adjacent fundus. In the center of the macula is a glistening oval reflex called the *fovea*. In young people a second reflex, which appears as a glimmering halo, may surround the entire macular region. Each quadrant of the fundus is examined in turn. To see as much of the peripheral retina as possible, the examiner should ask the patient to look in the direction of the quadrant under study. The color of the fundus is usually an even red hue, but it varies with the general pigmentation of the eye, as well as the individual's pigmentation.

Because the disc of the ophthalmoscope lens permits very close observation of an object, the ophthalmoscope usually examines the lens, the iris, the cornea, and the external eye.

Special devices on the ophthalmoscope

Red-free light

Although a true red-free state cannot be obtained with the yellow-green filters found in many ophthalmoscopes, the filters do serve a purpose. Viewing the fundus with a relatively red-free filter makes the retinal blood vessels appear black and retinal nerve fibers more prominent. The macula stands out against the greenish-gray background of the fundus as a golden-yellow oval patch. The use of red-free light for examining the fundus is particularly valuable for detecting minute superficial hemorrhages, holes in the retina, and early degenerations of the macula.

Red light

Red filters diminish the contrast between the retinal blood vessels and the retina. However, melanin pigment, which absorbs red rays, contrasts strongly with the surrounding red fundus. Red light illumination is therefore of value in differentiating hemorrhage from pigmented tumors that contain melanin.

Polarized light

Incorporation of two polarizing filters into the optical system, which polarizes the light leaving the ophthalmoscope, minimizes irritating reflections from the patient's cornea. The only problem with the general use of polarized light is that the intensity of the illumination has to be greatly increased to compensate for the filtering effect of the two polarizing filters.

Slit illumination

In the construction of the ophthalmoscope the insertion of a slit or a diaphragm in the course of the illuminating system simply reduces the illumination. For focal high-intensity illumination, better results are attained when the slit is directed from a slit-lamp microscope and the fundus is viewed with a contact or Hruby lens. The use of a slit lamp is valuable in estimating the level of various areas of the retina.

Aperture discs

Most ophthalmoscopes have two or more aperture discs of different sizes. The smaller apertures are particularly useful for viewing the fundus through a small pupil, such as that found in glaucoma patients under treatment.

Cobalt-blue filters

These are used for fluorescein studies of the fundus.

Many types of ophthalmoscopes are available. Electric-power ophthalmoscopes offer the advantage of illumination that is more controlled and of higher intensity.

Indirect ophthalmoscope

The indirect ophthalmoscope was invented by Dr. C.J.T. Rooter only 1 year after von Helmholtz's invention of the direct ophthalmoscope. The indirect ophthalmoscope permits the examiner to see more of the retina in one glance than the direct ophthalmoscope allows. Because of its construction, the instrument also accommodates a larger and brighter light source, which permits the examiner to penetrate moderate cataracts and to see retinal detail. Usually, however, the pupil must be dilated to use this device.

For indirect ophthalmoscopy, the patient's eyes must be fully dilated with a mydriatic agent. The examiner holds a convex lens in front of the patient's eye and through a viewing device attached to the headband of the indirect ophthalmoscope, the examiner sees a real, inverted image at the focal point of the handheld lens (Figures 10.25 and 10.26). The size of this aerial image varies with the dioptric strength of the lens used. Most commonly used is a +20.00 diopter lens.

The fundus camera is simply an enclosed indirect ophthalmoscope with a camera back.

Relative merits of direct and indirect ophthalmoscopes

The *direct ophthalmoscope* permits a greater magnification ($\times 15$), is easier to use with small or undilated pupils, and is mechanically easier to use. The *indirect binocular ophthalmoscope* permits binocular vision and depth perception, permits a wider field of view of a given area, is easier to use in the operating room without contamination, permits indentation of the sclera and thus a better view of the periphery of the fundus, provides more intense illumination, and frees the hand for operative manipulation.

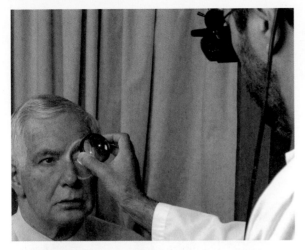

Figure 10.25 Examination with indirect ophthalmoscope.

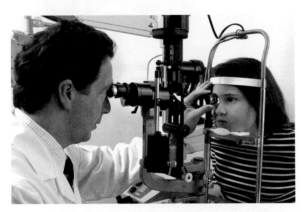

Figure 10.26 Examination of the fundus with lens.

Transilluminator

Transillumination is used when the media are too cloudy to permit inspection of the fundus and the examiner suspects the presence of an intraocular tumor. The transilluminator (also called a muscle light or a Finhoff light) consists of a handle and a small, narrow tip that contains a heat-free or insulated high-intensity light source. The beam of the transilluminator is passed over accessible areas of the sclera and in normal cases a bright red glow comes from the pupil if there are good transmissions from any point where the light is applied. If the light passes over the site of a solid tumor, the brilliance of the glow in the pupillary space will be diminished and an outline of the tumor revealed. The transilluminator is also useful for providing a bright source of illumination for the inspection of the external eye, the lids, and the iris reflex.

INSTRUMENTS USED TO STUDY THE ANTERIOR SEGMENT OF THE EYE

Slit-lamp microscope

Use of slit lamp

This instrument is used to illuminate and examine under magnification the anterior segment of the eye. The slit-lamp microscope enables the observer to view binocularly the conjunctiva, sclera, cornea, iris, anterior chamber, lens, and anterior portion of the vitreous, and it permits the detection of disease in these areas. The slit lamp is the heart of an ophthalmologic examination. The watch glass on a watch appears relatively clear when viewed from the front, yet when a penlight is directed obliquely at the edge of the watch glass, it brings out scratches and smears that are not easily seen in normal lighting. Similarly, the front surface of the eye and the interior of the eye can be seen more clearly when light is placed obliquely and there is backscattering of the light. Allvar Gullstrand of Stockholm, who won the Nobel Prize in 1911 for his studies on the optics of the eye, realized that a very special system was needed to see structural details in these so-called transparent tissues. Thus the first Gullstrand slit-lamp microscope was developed.

Attachments to the slit-lamp microscope permit examination of the angle structures, ciliary body, and fundus. The attachment of an applanation tonometer permits measurement of the intraocular pressure. Photographic attachments enable photography of the anterior segment of the eye. The slit-lamp microscope is of special importance in conditions such as dendritic keratitis, corneal foreign body, and early lens changes, which are better diagnosed and treated by having a well-illuminated and highly magnified view of the area.

Design of slit lamp

Slit-lamp microscopes have an illumination system combined with a microscope set on an instrument table fitted with a head- and chin rest.

The *illuminating system* is controlled by a transformer with adjustable ranges of voltage to provide intense illumination when required. Good illumination is about 5 million lux units. Controls are placed on the illuminating arm to (1) narrow the beam of light to a narrow slit, (2) vary the length of the slit to a small pinpoint of light, (3) introduce color filters to provide a green and a deep cobalt blue to the beam of light, (4) rotate the slit, and (5) adjust the angle between the slit beam and the microscope's line of sight. A Kodak Wratten yellow filter no. 15 may be advantageous when used in conjunction with a cobalt-blue filter to enhance contrast visibility of fluorescein staining of the eye.

The newer slit lamps are designed so that the illuminated slit remains sharply in focus with the microscope at all times. The illuminating system may be shifted to illuminate the eye from any angle and may be altered so that the beam falls to the side of the area to be viewed.

The *instrument table* and *headrest* permit adjustment to make the patient more comfortable. A fixation light is usually attached to the headrest to enable the patient to maintain fixation.

The microscope is attached to a movable stage operated by controls to permit focusing. In the new models there is a joystick type of control. The microscope, along with the illuminating system, is adjustable in both the side-to-side direction and the up-and-down position. The microscope itself is composed of an *eyepiece* (with extra eyepieces for higher magnification) and an *objective*. The eyepiece is individually adjustable to enable the examiner to neutralize his or her own error of refraction. Without interrupting the examination, the examiner can increase the magnification power of the objective from ×6 to ×40. Some microscopes have a smaller range of magnification. Some have zoom optics. It has been found that a magnification of ×15 is very good for routine use. Additional magnification may be achieved by changing the eyepiece to that of a higher power.

Types of slit lamps

Several models of slit lamps are available. Each has special features that make it valuable. Available slit lamps include Haag-Streit (Figure 10.27), American Optical, Bausch & Lomb Thorpe, Carl Zeiss Nikon (Figure 10.28), and Topcon.

Technique of slit-lamp examination
(Figure 10.29)

Both the patient and the examiner are seated. The patient places the chin on the chin rest and the forehead against the headrest. The chin rest and the microscope are adjusted so that the beam of light falls on the cornea. The fixation light is adjusted in front of the eye not being examined to position the patient's other eye for the examination. The light is adjusted to a narrow beam and directed from the side onto the cornea. The microscope is set for the low power and the eye is examined. A single-level control on the microscope permits movement and focusing in depth on the cornea and the anterior structures of the eye. Methods of illumination with the slit lamp include direct and indirect illumination, sclerotic scatter, retroillumination, and diffuse illumination. Although the beam of the slit can vary in length and width, the longer and wider beam is used to examine lids, cornea, conjunctiva, and sclera. The fine beam and short beam are used to examine fine details and produce a Tyndall effect when directed at the aqueous and vitreous. When these contain protein they flare, and even white and red cells can be observed with the magnification of the microscope.

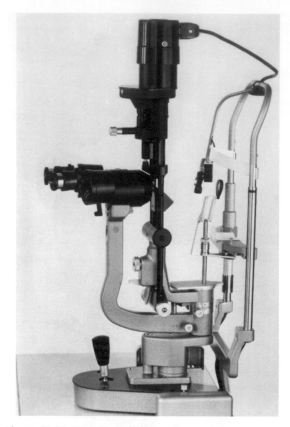

Figure 10.27 Haag-Streit slit-lamp microscope. *(Courtesy of Haag-Streit.)*

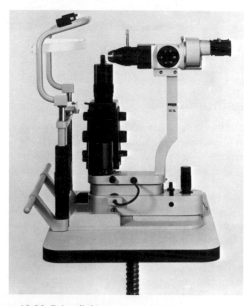

Figure 10.28 Zeiss slit lamp. *(Courtesy of Carl Zeiss Ltd.)*

A slit-beam cross-section of a normal cornea

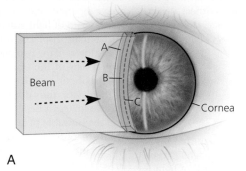

A

Corneal diseases and defects

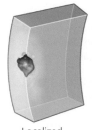
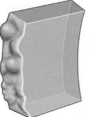
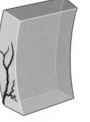
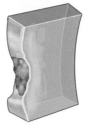

B

| Localized edema | Bullous keratopathy | Corneal vascularization | Corneal scarring | Corneal ulcer | Keratoma |

Corneal epithelial defects

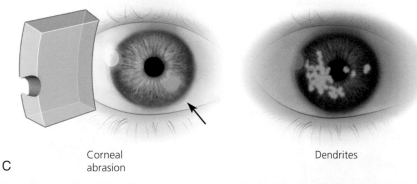

C

Corneal abrasion   Dendrites

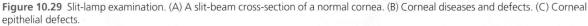

Figure 10.29 Slit-lamp examination. (A) A slit-beam cross-section of a normal cornea. (B) Corneal diseases and defects. (C) Corneal epithelial defects.
(Redrawn from Leitman, Gartner, Henkind: Manual for eye exams. 4th ed. Oradell, NJ: Medical Economics Co Book Division; 1978.)

The slit lamp provides increased magnification of the cornea and conjunctiva, including the palpebral conjunctiva. One can visualize under magnification the effect of deposits or scratches on a contact lens surface placed on the cornea.

Focusing with the microscope is performed by the central joystick. The interpupillary distance must be adjusted for binocularity. The patient must be positioned comfortably at the proper eye level. One should maneuver the beam to the correct position and define the slit width to the optimum width. About 1 to 2 mm is best. Start with a low magnification and build up to a higher magnification.

Check the lid margins and punctum first. Then look at the bulbar conjunctiva to assess hyperemia. View the superior and inferior conjunctiva and the everted lid for papules or follicles. Then sweep the beam across the cornea under high magnification and look for corneal defects including opacification, edema and striae, folds, and microcysts. Check the depth of the anterior chamber and the iris for variants from normal.

Slit-lamp attachments

Hruby lens (Figure 10.30)

The Hruby lens is a −55.00 diopter lens constructed to permit the examination of the vitreous body and the fundus of the eye under slit-lamp illumination and magnification. The lens is placed before the eye and the pencil of light is directed through the center of the Hruby lens toward the posterior portion of the eye. The microscope is then focused on the fundus.

Fundus contact lens

This is a handheld contact lens inserted onto the anesthetized eye. Before the lens is placed in the eye, a drop or two of methylcellulose is placed on the concave side of the lens. The contact lens permits the examination of the fundus of the eye. In comparison with the Hruby lens, the contact lens eliminates the air interface between the lens and the eye and thereby eliminates anomalies of corneal curvature and corneal irregularities.

Pachymeter

Some slit lamps (such as the Haag-Streit model 900) have attachments to measure accurately the thickness of the cornea and the thickness of the anterior chamber. The optical pachymeter is available in two different models: one for measuring the thickness of the cornea and one for estimating the depth of the anterior chamber.

This measuring device consists of two plano glass plates—one above the other edge to edge—that are placed above the right ocular of the slit lamp and divide the projected beam of light entering the slit lamp equally about a horizontally displaced midway line.

The lower of the two plates is fixed perpendicularly to the optical axis of the objective, but the upper plate can be rotated about a vertical axis by turning the scale segment of the device, thus doubling the image. The separation of the two images is dependent on the angle between the fixed and the movable plates.

When observed through the split-image eyepieces, one of the two images in the upper field and one in the lower field, not being needed for the measurement, are displaced prismatically. Thus the measuring points lying in the optical split image can be brought exactly into coincidence.

For measuring corneal thickness, the endothelium and the epithelium are used as measuring points. For measuring the depth of the anterior chamber, the epithelium and the anterior surface of the crystalline lens are the measuring points.

In addition to the optical pachymeter, the ultrasonic pachymeter has gained more widespread use for the measurement of corneal thickness. Its ease of use and ready portability make it much simpler to use. Ultrasonic waves are passed through the cornea to provide a digital readout of the corneal thickness. The head of the pachymeter is either of the solid type or fluid filled. The probe is applied directly to the anesthetized cornea. The readouts are given in micrometers of the thickness of the cornea. Some pachymeters are also able to measure the thickness of the epithelium (Figure 10.31). This instrument has application in keratoconus detection and for patient selection for refractive surgery. Handheld pachymeters are also available.

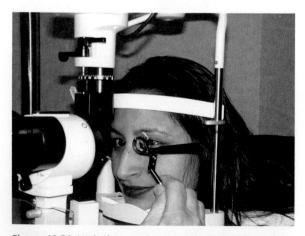

Figure 10.30 Hruby lens used to examine the fundus under magnification.

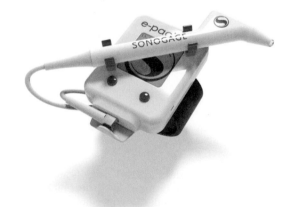

Figure 10.31 Ultrasound pachymeter that measures corneal thickness and epithelial thickness.
(Courtesy of Sonogage Inc., Cleveland, OH.)

INSTRUMENTS USED TO EXAMINE THE ANGLE STRUCTURES OF THE EYE

Goniolens

The goniolens is used to examine the ciliary body, the periphery of the retina, and the angle structures. Normally these areas are inaccessible for direct examination. The use of the goniolens is the only method for detecting angle-closure glaucoma, to determine whether the angle is open or closed. The lens is of value in locating preferential surgical sites of drainage in glaucoma and for evaluating the cause of failure after glaucoma surgery. There are two basic types of goniolenses: those using mirrors in their construction to enable the observer to see into the angle and those using the prismatic effect of a very-high-plus lens to accomplish the same purpose. The mirror-type goniolens deflects a beam of light into the opposite angle of the anterior chamber (Figure 10.32). The image of this illuminated angle is reflected along the same course and is visible through the objective lenses of the viewing microscope.

All the goniolenses available are of the contact lens type. The lens is placed on the anesthetized cornea, with a thin layer of fluid separating the lens from the cornea. Usually this is goniogel, but a tear gel works well.

Available contact goniolenses include the following:

1. The *children's goniolens*, which is small to conform to the small cornea
2. The *single-sided goniolens*, which requires rotation to view the complete periphery of the angle of the anterior segment
3. The *four-sided goniolens*, with all four mirrors inclined at the same angle, permitting the examiner to view the complete circumference of the angle without rotation of the goniolens

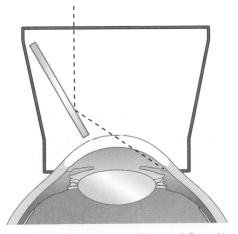

Figure 10.32 Goniolens. A beam of light is deflected into opposite angle of the anterior chamber.

4. The *Goldmann three-mirror contact lens*, with each mirror inclined at a different angle, thus permitting a view of the periphery of the retina and a view of the ciliary body, as well as the angle structures of the anterior chamber
5. The *Koeppe contact goniolens*, which is applied to the cornea, with saline solution or methylcellulose interposed, and which is used with the patient in a reclining position and the examiner viewing the angle structures through a handheld gonioscope
6. The *operating goniolens*, which is similar to other contact goniolenses except that one side is partially removed to permit access of a goniotomy knife for surgery on the angle structures

The first four lenses mentioned are used in conjunction with a slit-lamp microscope.

Posner diagnostic and surgical gonioprism

Although the principle of the Posner diagnostic and surgical gonioprism is certainly not new, the device is a good modification over existing instruments. This lens is used for viewing the anterior chamber and consists of a highly polished, truncated, silver-surfaced pyramid, with a plain anterior viewing surface over four mirrors, all inclined at 64 degrees, forming the sides of a pyramidal lens. The lens is used with a 45-degree angle so that the entire 360 degrees of the anterior chambers can be observed by locating the lens 11 degrees in either direction, making a small adjustment in the slit-lamp beam. It is an ideal lens for use in children or in patients with a small palpebral fissure.

A modification of this lens is the lighted surgical gonioprism, which was designed by Jerald L. Tennant. This lens is illuminated by a lighted halogen fiberoptic system that aids in viewing the alignment of feet of the anterior chamber that support an intraocular lens. It was designed primarily for viewing anterior chamber lens implants, particularly at the conclusion of the implantation procedure. The gonioprism is placed on the cornea at the position of the feet of the intraocular lens and is examined in relationship to the angle.

Gonioscope

The gonioscope is essentially a handheld microscope combined with an illuminating system used in conjunction with the goniolens for gonioscopy of the angle structures. The gonioscope may be balanced on counterweights over ceiling pulleys for ease of handling. In using the gonioscope, the examiner places a contact goniolens on the patient's cornea while the patient is in the recumbent position and then examines the complete angle structure through the magnification of the handheld gonioscope (Figure 10.33).

165

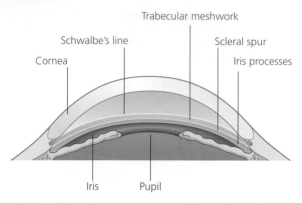

Trabecular meshwork

Schwalbe's line

Scleral spur

Cornea

Iris processes

Iris

Pupil

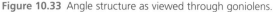

Figure 10.33 Angle structure as viewed through goniolens.

INSTRUMENTS USED TO ASSESS THE CORNEA

Keratometer

It is necessary to obtain the exact radius of curvature of the cornea. This can be accomplished with the ophthalmometer (keratometer), which is used in fitting contact lenses. Keratometry is the measurement of the central anterior curvature of the cornea. It is valuable in eye examinations, particularly for detecting and measuring corneal astigmatism. The keratometer consists essentially of a target that is imaged by the cornea and telescoped to observe this image. The measurement of the target image reveals the corneal curvature in diopters with the variation in curvature (astigmatism). The keratometer is invaluable in cases of irregular astigmatism, asymmetric astigmatism, oblique astigmatism, conical cornea (keratoconus), and nystagmus. The Bausch & Lomb keratometer is the standard on which other keratometers are based (Figure 10.34 and see Chapter 14).

Figure 10.34 Measuring correct curvature with the Bausch & Lomb keratometer.

A lightweight, handheld autokeratometer was developed by Alcon Systems. A rechargeable battery located in the handle provides several hours of use. Its accuracy appears comparable with that of traditional keratometers. It is of clinical value in hospitals, permitting early postoperative measurements after cataract and corneal transplantation. Because of its easy portability, its use in the clinical setting can minimize the number of keratometers required for a well-equipped office.

This keratometer, which is fully automatic and computerized, allows the operator to measure the vertical and horizontal base-curve values of the cornea and the angle of maximum difference between the two base curves and to calculate astigmatism. These measurements, which can be taken while the patient stands, sits, or reclines, are stored automatically in terms of the right and left eyes and are displayed in either diopters or millimeters. An automated line-up system ensures that the keratometer is in line during measurements.

To take a measurement, one presses on either the right- or left-eye button. When a ring of green lights illuminates, the pupil is centered in the ring and a red blinking light is centered over the pupil. The patient is asked to fixate on the central blinking red light and the keratometer is stabilized by the examiner's free hand on the patient's forehead. The keratometer lights are then aligned until eight green lights are located in an "X" formation around the red fixation light. The holding button is then released. The green lights turn off and there is a long chirp. This records the measurement of that eye. The procedure is then repeated on the fellow eye.

The Humphrey autokeratometer shows both the shape and the vault of the cornea. It uses infrared rays and measures an area 2.6 mm centrally. The Canon automatic keratometer K1 uses a xenon light and does the keratometer measurement in 0.1 second.

Specular microscope

The specular microscope is covered in Chapter 41.

INSTRUMENTS USED TO DETERMINE TEAR FLOW

Dacryocystography/lacrimal scan

Dacryocystography (DCG) and lacrimal scan are imaging techniques that are occasionally used to evaluate the lacrimal outflow system in patients who report persistent tearing. DCG is the best anatomic test for determining the actual site of obstruction in the lacrimal outflow system. With the patient lying down, a drop of topical anesthetic is placed in the palpebral aperture. Both lower puncta are simultaneously intubated and injected with low-viscosity oil. Serial radiographs are taken during injection.

The lacrimal scan is the most physiologic test to date. It simulates passage of the tears through the lacrimal excretory passages without the use of invasive instruments. The test does not, however, give the same detail as the DCG in determining the actual obstruction site. The lacrimal scan determines whether the tearing is caused by the inability of the lids to promote tear flow into the lacrimal passages or by an obstruction of the outflow system. A drop of technetium sulfur colloid is placed on the marginal tear strip of each lower lid while the patient is sitting upright. No anesthetic is necessary because the drop is nonirritating and has the same pH and osmolarity as tears. Pictures are taken by a specialized gamma camera that uses less than 2% of the radioactivity of routine x-ray studies. The photographs are taken every 10 seconds for the first minute and then every minute for 20 minutes, after which time the patient's eyes are wiped and a final picture is taken.

INSTRUMENTS USED TO MEASURE INTRAOCULAR PRESSURE (TONOMETER)

The tonometer, which is designed to measure the intraocular pressure, is used in the most important single test in the detection of glaucoma. There are two instruments in common use: the applanation tonometer and the indentation tonometer (e.g., the Schiøtz tonometer). These two types are compared and a number of instruments using these principles are discussed in Chapter 25.

SPECIAL INSTRUMENTS

Exophthalmometer

The exophthalmometer is an instrument designed to measure the forward protrusion of the eye. This instrument provides a method of evaluating and recording the progression and regression of the prominence of an eye caused by disorders such as thyroid disease and tumors of the orbit. Instruments commonly in use are the Luedde and the Hertel exophthalmometers.

Luedde exophthalmometer

The Luedde exophthalmometer is simply a transparent ruler calibrated in millimeters. One end is notched to fit easily into the bony prominence of the lateral orbital margin. The observer, standing at the side of the patient whose gaze is directed forward, sights the apex of the cornea through the transparent plastic rule and then records the forward protrusion of one eye at a time in millimeters.

Hertel exophthalmometer

This instrument consists of a horizontal calibrated bar with movable carriers at each side. Each carrier consists of mirrors inclined at 45 degrees to reflect both the scale reading and the apex of the cornea of profile. Notches on the side carriers are placed on the bony lateral orbital margins of the patient. The patient is then asked to fixate on a point on the examiner's forehead. The apex of the cornea of each eye is superimposed on the millimeter scale reading by the inclined mirrors. The examiner records the measurement of each eye, alternately viewing with the right and left eye. The distance along the horizontal bar also is recorded as the base figure so that the carriers will be set at the same base for comparison at subsequent readings. This instrument provides a reliable comparison of the forward protrusion of each eye in relation to the bony orbit (Figures 10.35 and 10.36).

Placido's disc

Placido's disc is a flat disc on which have been painted alternating black and white rings that encircle a small central round aperture (Figure 10.37). The disc is used in evaluating the regularity of the anterior curvature of the cornea. Its relative simplicity makes it a useful instrument for detecting early stages of keratoconus.

In an examination using Placido's disc, the patient is placed with a strong light behind one shoulder; the examiner observes the cornea through the central hole of the disc. The reflections of the rings on the cornea are free of distortions if the cornea is normally curved. If the cornea has an irregular curvature, considerable distortion of the concentric rings will occur. An electric Placido's disc, or keratoscope, has been designed for controlled illumination and convenience.

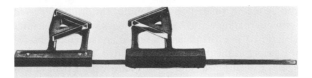

Figure 10.35 Hertel exophthalmometer.
(Courtesy of Bernell.)

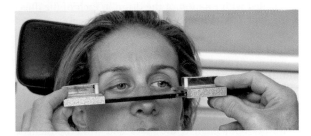

Figure 10.36 Hertel exophthalmometer used to measure protrusion of the eye.

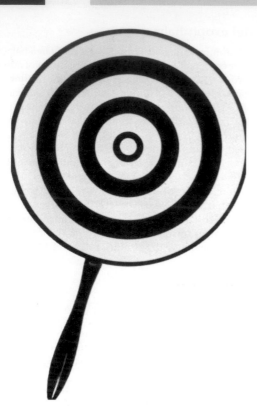

Figure 10.37 Placido's disc, used to identify corneal irregularities.

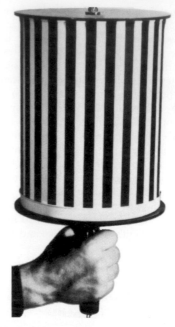

Figure 10.38 Optokinetic drum.

Optokinetic drum

The optokinetic drum consists of a handle and a drum that can be readily rotated on the handle. The drum is covered with alternating vertical white and dark stripes or pictures (Figure 10.38). The patient is seated and asked to observe the stripes as the drum is slowly rotated. The drum is held 1 foot (30 cm) away and rotated slowly from right to left, then from left to right, and finally upward and downward. The quick, jerky refixation movements the patient has to make in viewing the revolving stripes produce a jerk nystagmus of the patient's eyes. Normally this jerk nystagmus can be elicited with rotation of the drum in each of the directions tested. A failure to elicit a jerk-nystagmus type of response in one direction often indicates severe and serious neurologic disease.

A simplified optokinetic tape, designed by Dr. J. Lawton Smith, is a useful alternative to the larger drum. Its chief virtue is that it can be carried in the pocket. It consists of a series of 2-inch (5 cm) red squares sewed onto a 4-inch (20 cm) tape approximately 3 feet (1 meter) in length. A further refinement is the black and white optokinetic tape, which retracts into a carpenter's type of measuring tape cartridge.

Ophthalmodynamometer

The ophthalmodynamometer is an instrument designed to measure the pressure in the ophthalmic artery and its parent vessel, the internal carotid artery (Figure 10.39). It is used primarily to diagnose conditions resulting in a lower pressure in these main arteries. In particular, it is used in the diagnostic workup of cases of carotid insufficiency, carotid thrombosis, and carotid stenosis.

For this test it is best if two examiners are present. One examiner applies the instrument to the globe, increasing the force applied in small increments, while the other visualizes the state of the retinal vessels (Figure 10.40).

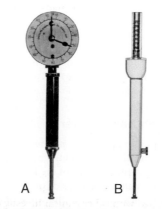

Figure 10.39 Bailliart ophthalmodynamometer. (A) Dial type. (B) Plunger type.

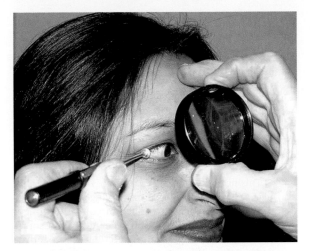

Figure 10.40 Measurement of ophthalmic artery pressure using an ophthalmodynamometer.

Visualization can be achieved by use of either the direct or the indirect ophthalmoscope.

The patient should be seated comfortably and the pupils dilated with a mydriatic agent. Local anesthetic drops are instilled into the eye before application of the ophthalmodynamometer. The assistant places the instrument over the bulbar conjunctiva in the horizontal meridian of the eyeball, temporal to the limbus, and gradually increases the force to the eye as the examiner regards the retinal vessels on the surface of the disc. Once the intraocular pressure has been raised sufficiently to cause a pulsation of the central retinal artery, a reading is taken. This is the diastolic pressure recorded in grams. As the compression of the globe is continued, the central retinal artery finally ceases to pulsate, collapses, and appears completely blanched. At this point another reading is taken; this reading represents the systolic pressure in grams.

For best results three readings of both the systolic and the diastolic pressure for each eye are made, with the patient in both the upright and the reclining positions. The recordings of pressure in grams can be converted using tables to millimeters of mercury.

Most ophthalmologists, before performing ophthalmodynamometry, also record the intraocular tension in each eye and the blood pressure in each arm.

A pressure difference of 20 between the two eyes is considered significant. Because one-third of patients with a diagnosis of a stroke are found to have disease of the carotid arteries, this test has proved most valuable. It is a simple, nontraumatic method of detecting cerebrovascular disease. However, because both false-positive and false-negative results do occur with this test, the results always must be correlated with other clinical investigations.

The Dynopter was introduced by the American Optical Company to overcome some of the defects inherent in applying scleral pressure to the globe to cause collapse of the central retinal artery. The Dynopter is used with the slit lamp in a manner similar to that for the applanation tonometer. No ophthalmoscope is required. The eye must be anesthetized because the pressure is applied to the cornea rather than to the sclera, as is done with the older types of instruments. After the eye is anesthetized, the slit beam is used to view the optic disc through the microscope while a contact lens exerts increasing pressure on the cornea. The graded pressure dial is turned until the first pulsation of the central retinal artery is obtained. This is the diastolic pressure. The observer then turns the dial until sufficient pressure is exerted to stop all blood flow. This is the systolic pressure. Readings are then taken and recorded. This method provides a greater degree of accuracy and repeatability than others. It is not possible, however, to obtain measurements on the recumbent patient.

Doppler test

The Doppler test has virtually replaced the ophthalmodynamometer as a test of carotid flow. The test measures the flow of the internal and external carotid arteries directly. It is less subject than the ophthalmodynamometer to instrumental and operator errors. If the internal carotid artery of the neck is narrowed by atheromatous plaques, then the flow pattern distal to the obstruction site will be reduced and irregular. The turbulence of flow may be so great that the sound may be audible with a stethoscope placed directly over the internal carotid artery. This sound is called a *bruit*. With transducers in the instrument, however, the precise measurement of flow can provide more accurate information regarding carotid artery patency. This test is used for people with central retinal artery occlusions, transient ischemic attacks, and cerebrovascular accidents.

Automatic refractors

Sophisticated automatic refractors that, in effect, perform retinoscopy and in most cases are designed to be operated by the ophthalmic assistant have come onto the market. These instruments do not produce a refraction from which a pair of glasses should be made. The present ones do no more than an automatic retinoscopic or objective refraction. It is essential that the results obtained with these machines be refined by a subjective refraction. In a busy office, however, they save a great deal of time. See Chapter 11 for a more detailed description of autorefractors.

COMPUTERIZED CORNEAL TOPOGRAPHIC ANALYSIS

There has been increased research and growing interest in the field of corneal topography, that is, measurement of the curvature of the anterior corneal surface. With the capabilities of modern computers and software technology, it has become feasible and practical to precisely analyze the radius of curvature (millimeters) and corresponding refractive power (diopters) at thousands of points across the corneal surface.

Computerized corneal topography is a logical advance from the basic principles of keratometry and photokeratoscopy developed during the 20th century. Photokeratoscopy provides the user with only qualitative information about the curvature of the cornea and changes that accompany surgery, contact lens wear, and progressive corneal abnormalities. The keratometer yields quantitative data, but only at four points. These points are located at approximately the 3-mm optic zone along two perpendicular meridians. One pair of points is aligned along the steepest axis of the corneal surface, with the second pair 90 degrees away. Each pair of points is averaged across its respective meridian to yield two K values, which approximate the cornea's central refractive power. The keratometer has fundamental limitations in that it is able only to measure points along the annulus of the 3-mm optic zone and it assumes orthogonal symmetry of the flat and steep axis of the cornea.

Topography provides a color-coded representation of the cornea's shape and monitors corneal curvature changes from the apex to the periphery.

See Chapter 40 for more details.

Visual field equipment, tangent screens, and perimeters

See Chapters 19 and 20 for a discussion of visual fields.

DIAGNOSTIC ULTRASOUND: A-SCAN AND B-SCAN

Ultrasound was first used in World War II; the sound waves were used to locate submarines under water. In a variety of ophthalmic disorders, diagnostic ultrasound provides information that cannot be obtained in any other way. This is especially true in eyes with opaque media that preclude ophthalmoscopic examination. Intraocular use is stressed because space does not permit a detailed description of the somewhat more difficult field of orbital diagnosis.

Two common types of ultrasound waves are used. The A-wave is a single-beam, linear wave that is directed in a probing manner to detect interference along its pathway. It travels like a beam of light in a straight direction. A B-scan consists of a series of these impulses sent out by a moving transducer that are amalgamated into a two-dimensional image. This not only minimizes possible missed areas but also gives a clearer picture of the underlying pathologic condition. The B-waves are used to detect tumors of the orbit or eye that cannot be identified by any other means. The sound waves, like light waves, pass through certain tissues and are reflected by others. When the sound wave meets firm tissue, such as is found in a tumor mass, the waves are reflected off its surface. The rebounding waves are received by a transducer, which turns the sound energy into electrical impulses that are amplified and displayed on an oscilloscope in a visible pattern called an *ultrasonogram* or *echogram* (Figure 10.41). Homogeneous tissue, such as normal lens vitreous or aqueous humor, does not reflect ultrasound and produces no echoes. A cataractous lens produces intralenticular echoes. In some centers, ultrasound is used to aid the surgeon in locating a foreign body in the eye.

B-scan ultrasonography also has been effective in diagnosing many ocular tumors, especially choroidal malignant melanomas. Drs. K. Ossoinig and Fred Blodi reported a 95% accuracy using a standard B-scan echogram in a large series of choroidal malignant melanomas.

B-scans differ from A-scans in that they are more complex. An A-scan is a linear echo, and the reflection of this linear ultrasound can indicate the position of the cornea, the lens, and the retina. The B-scan is similar, but it extends above and below the horizontal to sweep the contents of

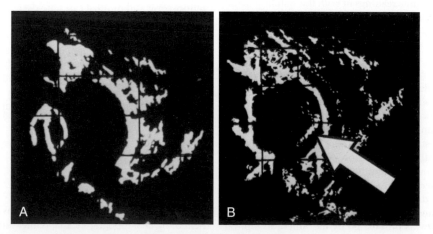

Figure 10.41 B-echogram. (A) Normal. (B) Showing retinal detachment *(arrow)*.

the globe. Both A- and B-scanners are available from several manufacturers as portable devices.

C-scan techniques also are available and are used in diagnosing orbital disease. The C-scan uses a transducer to cover a small aperture. It images soft tissue within the span of a corollary plane that is recorded on polaroid positive–negative film. The corollary plane scans across the axis of the optic nerve. C-scan techniques are used primarily for optic nerve lesions, especially tumors.

A detailed discussion on diagnostic ultrasound can be found in Chapter 42.

RADIOACTIVE PHOSPHORUS

One test to detect whether an ocular or retroocular tumor is benign or malignant is determination of the radioactive uptake of the tissues. It is known that cancerous tissues proliferate rapidly. Certain highly malignant tumors (especially malignant melanomas) take up and retain certain radioactive elements, particularly radioactive phosphorus (^{32}P), to a greater extent than do normal tissues. In this test the ^{32}P is injected intravenously and the radioactivity is assessed on the surface of the eye by a Geiger counter 24 and 48 hours after the injection. The major difficulty in this test is that the counter has to be directly over the tumor. With tumors at the back of the eye it is difficult to place the tip of the counter accurately. In addition to this mechanical difficulty, some tumors simply do not give a high count. Other tumors such as retinoblastoma, the most common eye tumor in children, rarely show any alteration in the radioactive uptake of ^{32}P.

A positive ^{32}P test result, then, is of value in providing corroboration for the presence of an actively growing malignant tumor; however, a negative result is of little value because it does not indicate the absence of a tumor.

ELECTRORETINOGRAPHY AND ELECTROOCULOGRAPHY

Electroretinography (ERG) responses are described as photopic (light adapted) or scotopic (dark adapted). Although the rods outnumber the cones 13 to 1 in the normal human retina, the cones account for 20% to 25% of the ERG response amplitude. The response of the dark-adapted eye to white light breaks down to an early corneal negative A-wave; a corneal positive B-wave; a slower, usually positive C-wave; and, in some mammals, a small D-wave. The resting potential of the normal retinal axis is measured by a silver disc electrode mounted in a scleral contact lens.

An electrical potential exists between the cornea and the retina of the human eye. This potential can be altered by changes in the intensity of light entering the eye, the wavelength of that light, and the state of adaptation of the eye, that is, whether it is light adapted or dark adapted. In some disease states the resting potential is altered and the ability of the electrical potential to be changed by these other factors is abnormal.

There are basically two types of retinal receptors: the rods that serve vision in dim light and the cones that mediate daylight vision and color vision. The electroretinogram reveals disease of either the rod population or the cone population, or both.

For this test, electrodes incorporated into a contact glass are placed directly onto the eye. Eye movements disrupt the values of the test, so the patient must be old enough to fixate on a target, which keeps the eyes still. Because they are unable to cooperate, very young children do not make good subjects for this test.

Total loss of electrical activity can be recorded in siderosis bulbi (caused by retained iron foreign bodies in the eye), in stages of retinitis pigmentosa, and in severe vitamin A deficiency. Selective degeneration of the rods, as manifested by night blindness, also can be detected by this method because the electrical reaction during dark adaptation is faulty. Selective involvement of the cone, as seen in congenital total color blindness, also is revealed by the inability of the eye to electrically respond during conditions of light adaptation.

Electrooculography (EOG) measures the standing potential between the electrically positive cornea and the electrically negative back of the eye. It indicates the activity of the RPE and photoreceptors cells. Diffuse or widespread retinal pigment epithelium (RPE) disease is required to significantly affect the EOG response. The EOG is always abnormal when the ERG is abnormal and therefore provides useful information only when the ERG is normal. One of the current diagnostic uses for the EOG is in Best's vitelliform macular dystrophy.

ERG and EOG are generally preformed in university centers. Expert technical knowledge is required to perform these tests and to interpret their results.

LASERS

The laser (covered more completely in Chapter 34) is a device that amplifies light waves. The name itself is taken from the beginning letters of *l*ight *a*mplification by *s*timulated *e*mission of *r*adiation. Intense beams of light have many practical implications, but in the eye their virtue is that the laser beam may be directed through the pupil to the retinal structures for repairing retinal holes and tears and destroying blood vessels.

The ruby laser emits a beam that creates a heat reaction in the pigment epithelium of the retina, binding the epithelium of the retina to the underlying choroid; it also aids the sealing of retinal holes in a retinal detachment when the retina is adjacent to the choroid. The blue-green light of the argon laser is superior to the red light of the ruby laser in treating certain blood vessel diseases of the eye because it is absorbed by the red blood pigment, which resists the red light of the ruby laser. The argon treatment is a feature in diabetic retinopathy and other retinal conditions such as Eales' disease, in which vessels grow abnormally and bleed easily; sickle cell anemia, which produces sludging of blood in peripheral eye vessels; and several congenital vascular conditions that cause blindness.

It has been well established that argon or neodymium-yttrium aluminum garnet (YAG) laser treatment is a good alternative to the invasive surgery of a peripheral iridectomy in producing a hole in the iris. The former is painless and causes minimal inflammation, which is normally handled by application of steroid drops for about a week. It is most useful in treating angle-closure glaucoma or aphakic pupillary block glaucoma, or in opening an incomplete surgical iridectomy. The Abraham iridectomy lens, a modified Goldmann type of fundus lens, may be valuable in delivering a more intense laser beam to the iris. Blue eyes are more difficult to penetrate than brown eyes because of the lack of the heat-absorbing pigment in blue irides. Laser trabeculoplasty involves using the laser for shrinkage of the trabecular meshwork.

The excimer laser has been developed for two specific uses. First, it enhances vision so that combined myopia and astigmatism, or hyperopia and astigmatism, can be eliminated or refractive errors can be significantly reduced. Second, it has significant use in removing corneal scars and corneal dystrophies, stopping recurrent corneal erosions and smoothing out corneal surfaces after surgery for conditions such as pterygium. The current influence of the excimer laser on refractive errors is more thoroughly discussed in Chapter 36.

SUMMARY

The ophthalmic assistant should become knowledgeable about the workings of each instrument in the office. It is important to keep the instruments clean and all lenses free of dust and grease by using a lint-free cloth. The ophthalmic assistant should be able to change bulbs in every instrument inasmuch as the use of the instrument depends on a functioning bulb and an intact power supply. An active inventory of the replacement bulbs in the office should be kept so that bulbs always are available. Another area of expertise that should be developed is calibration of the tonometers. In addition, the ophthalmic assistant should know the purposes of each piece of equipment and what information can be derived from its use. For a more comprehensive look at new imaging equipment see Section 4 (Ocular imaging).

Questions for review and thought

1. What is the purpose of the red-green test on the projection equipment? Explain the test.
2. Discuss the power and range of the various types of lenses and auxiliary lenses on the lens tray that you have in the office.
3. How can you tell the power of a prism in the standard lens tray?
4. How can you differentiate a cylindrical lens from a spherical lens in the lens tray?
5. What is the purpose of the pinhole disc?
6. What is meant by a retinoscopy lens in a standard refractor? What is its power? Why?
7. What is the difference between phoria and tropia? What instrument is used in detecting these conditions and how?
8. Explain the principle of either the spot or the streak retinoscope.
9. What is meant by vertex distance? How is it measured in a trial frame? In a spectacle? In a refractor?
10. What are the prisms used for?
11. What is the prism cover test?
12. Discuss the relative merits of direct and indirect ophthalmoscopy.
13. What is the purpose of a goniolens?
14. Draw the endpoints of the two half circles from the applanation tonometer as seen when a true reading of the intraocular pressure is to be obtained.
15. What is the value of the ophthalmodynamometer? What does it measure?
16. How can you determine whether a lens is concave or convex without using instruments?
17. What is the exophthalmometer? Describe how either the Luedde or the Hertel exophthalmometer is used.
18. How is ultrasound of value in ophthalmology?
19. Outline the value of automated refractors in clinical ophthalmology.
20. Compare the advantages of automated refractors versus retinoscopy and subjective refraction.
21. Outline the disadvantages of automated refractors versus retinoscopy and conventional subjective refraction.
22. Discuss inherent errors that can occur in the use of an automated refractor.
23. What is instrument myopia?
24. What are the drawbacks to introducing an automated refractor in practice?

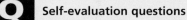

Q Self-evaluation questions

True–false statements

Directions: Indicate whether the statement is true **(T)** or false **(F).**

1. In the duochrome test, a near-sighted person sees the letters more clearly on the red panel. **T** or **F**
2. Trial frames and lenses are better than the phoropter in determining the refractive status of the aphakic person or a person with high plus or minus lenses. **T** or **F**
3. The Maddox rod is used to dissociate the eyes and prevent them from fusing. **T** or **F**
4. Manual objective refractors require significant operator skill and time. **T** or **F**
5. Automated objective refractors require significant operator skill and time. **T** or **F**
6. Some automated refractors provide for subjective refinement. **T** or **F**

Missing words

Directions: Write in the missing word(s) in the following sentences:

7. The radius of curvature of any lens can be measured simply by using a _____.
8. Phenylephrine is an excellent mydriatic for dilating pupils. The safest or most commonly used concentration of this drug is _____.
9. The optic disc is best examined with _____.
10. Objective refractors may be used to replace _____.
11. Automated objective refractors still require _____ testing.
12. When an assistant using an automated refractor requires the patient to provide responses to questions, this is considered a _____ refraction step.

Choice-completion questions

Directions: Select the one best answer in each case.

13. If the media are opaque, which of the following tests can be used to determine whether an intraocular tumor is present?
    a. Transillumination
    b. Ultrasound A- or B-scan
    c. ^{32}P
    d. All of the above
    e. None of the above
14. The Hruby lens is:
    a. a −55.00 diopter lens.
    b. a jeweler's loupe.
    c. a lens for detecting the intraocular pressure.
    d. a lens for viewing Schlemm's canal.
    e. none of the above.
15. The results of an automated refractor are least affected by:
    a. large pupils.
    b. cataract.
    c. small pupils.
    d. irregular astigmatism.
    e. corneal scarring.
16. To incorporate an automated refractor in a practice, one usually does not need to:
    a. designate a staff person to be responsible for testing.
    b. provide more housing space.
    c. increase the capital cost.
    d. have a maintenance service agreement.
    e. have a large-volume practice.
17. An accurate automated refraction result usually is found in:
    a. a patient with moderate cataract.
    b. improper alignment of the patient's eyes.
    c. high astigmatism (greater than 7.00 diopters).
    d. macular degeneration.
    e. irregular corneal surface.

A Answers, notes, and explanations

1. **True.** Green normally is focused in front of the retina because of its short wavelength. Therefore, a near-sighted person whose entire image is focused in front of the retina would see letters on the red side of the chart more clearly. Red has a longer wavelength and is seen more clearly by the larger eye of the myopic person. The person whose near-sightedness has been overcorrected, however, will see the green letters more clearly. The duochrome test is useful in determining the type and end point of the refractive error.

2. **True.** It is useful that the correcting lenses and spectacle lens that the aphakic patient and all patients with high plus or minus lenses finally wears are similar with respect to the distance of the lens from the eye and its tilt. With four-drop lenses, trial aphakic spectacles are provided so that the margin of error is minimized. Even without minimal effective diameter (MED) lenses or four-drop lenses, trial frames are still the best way of arriving at the aphakic person's, or those with high-plus or high-minus lenses, final prescription inasmuch as the measurement for vertex distance is more reliable. The Halberg clip is an excellent method for determining the true spectacle correction.

3. **True.** This is done by changing the shape and color of the image of one eye. The rod converts a point of light to a linear rod by virtue of cylindric rods that run across it. The red line always runs perpendicular to the axes of the Maddox rod.

4. **True.** To operate manual objective refractions, a person needs skill and time for the alignment and adjustment steps.

5. **False.** Automated objective refractors require little skill by the ophthalmic medical assistant. Skill is required when the patient is not aligned properly or moves during the testing procedure.

6. **True.** Some automated refractors have a subjective component in which the assistant will question the patient as to changes in vision. The instrument can add or subtract both sphere and cylinder to refine the prescription. This is considered a subjective refinement.

7. **Geneva lens measure.** The disadvantage of this instrument is that the gauges are calibrated for crown glass only. Moreover, the axis of the cylinder is not precisely determined.

8. **2.5%.** Recently deaths have been reported with the use of 10% phenylephrine; this concentration should *not* be used for routine dilation. The weaker solution should be used routinely. Phenylephrine should *not* be given to patients with hypertension or active cardiovascular disease. When it is given, care should be taken to occlude the punctum so that minimal drainage into the nose and minimal systemic absorption occur.

9. **The direct ophthalmoscope.** The direct ophthalmoscope permits greater magnification so that the fine details of cupping of the disc are easily observed with this instrument. The indirect ophthalmoscope offers a wider field of vision, but it is not as good for examining disc detail such as mild cupping, slight pallor, pits or holes, and the growth of delicate new blood vessels off its surface.

10. **Retinoscopy.** The automated refractors can give a beginning prescription for refinement on a subjective basis. This simulates retinoscopy and becomes a starting point for refraction.

11. **Subjective.** Subjective testing is most important after using an automated objective refractor. The refractor provides only the starting point; one must still obtain individual responses to the given refractive finding.

12. **Subjective.** The word *subjective* means that the patient, who is the subject, has input into the final results.

13. **d. All of the above.** Probably the most widely used test for an intraocular mass when the media are too cloudy to permit direct examination is the B-scan ultrasound. It is precise, easy to perform, and painless. Permanent records can be obtained. The location and type of a retrolental mass often can be detected with this method.

14. **a. A −55.00 diopter lens.** The Hruby lens is a −5.00 diopter lens for viewing the fundus. It is not as good as a fundus contact lens, but it has the advantage that the retina can be examined without placing an instrument on the eye.

15. **a. Large pupils.** Large pupils do not affect the result of the automated refractor. In fact, the opposite is true. Small pupils may yield no information, often because of misalignment.

16. **e. Have a large-volume practice.** Automated refractors can be valuable in any type of practice, whether it is small volume or large volume. They can provide a reference point similar to retinoscopy. The cost effectiveness may have to be questioned if the practice is relatively small, however.

17. **d. Macular degeneration.** Macular degeneration is a dysfunction of the eye's cones. The actual refractive error is not altered, although the vision is markedly reduced centrally. Consequently, the automated refractor usually provides reliable results as far as the refractive finding is concerned.

Chapter | 11 |

Refractive errors and how to correct them

Almost all patients who enter an ophthalmologist's office require a determination of the refractive status of their eyes, for either diagnosis or treatment. Only by correcting the patient's refractive error can the ophthalmologist distinguish between visual loss caused by organic disease and that caused by a refractive error. Any visual loss not amenable to correction by lenses is regarded as a pathologic condition. Unexplained visual loss not corrected by glasses must always be investigated.

Many patients, regardless of their problem, be it fatigue with driving or headache, expect to receive a pair of glasses to remedy their complaints. Some patients are methodic about having their glasses changed every year or every 2 years; they believe that glasses, like tires, will wear out in time. Others think that glasses have a therapeutic effect on the eyes, maintaining them in good performance and preserving their integrity. Vision, especially in younger individuals and the presbyopic patient, may deteriorate with time, necessitating a change in correction but the health of the eye is not affected, for better or worse, regardless of changes made in the glasses. There is some evidence, however, that in the young, plus correction may prevent the normal loss of hyperopia and minus correction may exacerbate the development of myopia.

Glasses function to improve visual performance, to relieve the symptoms of refractive errors and muscular imbalance of the eyes, and to prevent suppression of one eye in children younger than 5 years, when the refractive difference between the two eyes is great. This chapter deals with the signs and symptoms of refractive errors and the therapy available for their treatment.

EMMETROPIA

The emmetropic eye is a normal eye in which all the rays of light from a distantly fixated object are imaged sharply on the retina without the necessity of any accommodative effort. This is a relatively uncommon condition (Figure 11.1).

AMETROPIA

There are three basic abnormalities in the refractive state of the eye: hyperopia or hypermetropia, myopia, and astigmatism.

Hyperopia

The hyperopic or far-sighted eye is one that is deficient in refractive power so that rays of light from a distant object

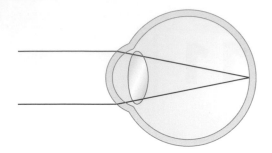

Figure 11.1 Emmetropic eye. Parallel rays of light come to a focus on the retina.

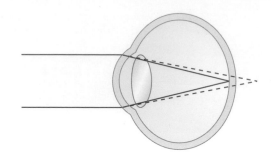

Figure 11.3 Manifest hyperopia. Accommodation by the lens of the eye brings parallel rays of light to focus on the retina.

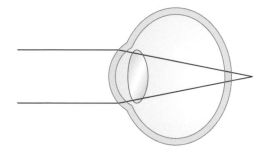

Figure 11.2 Hyperopic eye. Parallel rays of light come to a focus behind the retina in the unaccommodative eye.

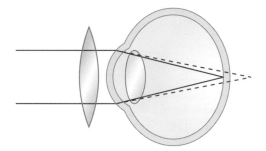

Figure 11.4 Absolute hyperopia. A convex lens is required to bring rays of light to focus on the retina.

come to a focus at a point *behind* the retina with respect to the unaccommodated eye (Figure 11.2). Consequently, the image that falls on the retina is blurred and can be brought into focus only by accommodation or by placing a plus, or convex, lens in front of the eye. The convex lens supplies the converging power that the eye is lacking.

Cause

In most cases of hyperopia, the chief cause is a shortening of the anteroposterior axis of the eye. Such an eye is smaller than the normal, or emmetropic, eye. At birth almost all human eyes are hyperopic or shorter than normal, to the extent of 2.00 or 3.00 diopters. With growth, the eye lengthens and approaches the normal length of an adult eye. Each millimeter of shortening of the eye is represented by 3.00 diopters of refractive change. This shortening of the globe results in *axial hyperopia*.

Another cause of hyperopia is found when the front surface of the eye (the cornea or lens) has less curvature than normal so that the image formed is focused at a point behind the normally placed retina. This is called *curvature hyperopia*.

From a practical standpoint, the cause of the hyperopia is not of great importance. What is significant is whether the accommodative system of the eye can supply an additional plus power to correct the hyperopic error. Young people are usually not handicapped by hyperopia because of their excellent range of accommodation.

Types

Hyperopia may be latent, manifest, or absolute. A *latent hyperopia* is the portion of the hyperopic error that is completely corrected by the eye's own accommodation. The compensation is so complete that any attempt to place a plus lens in front of such an eye will merely blur the vision. *Manifest hyperopia (facultative hyperopia)* is the element of the refractive error that can be corrected either by convex lenses or by the patient's own accommodation. In both latent and manifest hyperopia *the patient has normal visual acuity* (Figure 11.3). *Absolute hyperopia* is the portion of the refractive error that is not compensated for by accommodation (Figure 11.4).

To understand the three types, consider the following case. A 32-year-old man is found to have a visual acuity of 20/50. A +1.00 lens is given, which improves his vision to 20/20. This means that the patient has 1.00 diopter of absolute hyperopia. It is found, however, that the patient can still see 20/20 if an additional 1.50 diopters are placed before the absolute correction. Thus the patient is found to have 1.50 diopters of manifest hyperopia. A cycloplegic examination is performed and it is found that the patient requires 3.50 diopters of plus lenses to enable him to see 20/20. Of the 3.50 diopters, 1.00 diopter we know has been accounted for in the form of *absolute hyperopia*, 1.50 diopters were present as *manifest hyperopia*, and 1.00 diopter remains in the form of *latent hyperopia*. Such a patient requires 1.00 diopter, will accept up to 2.50 diopters, but cannot be given the full hyperopic correction of 3.50 diopters.

Role of cycloplegia

Cycloplegic drops paralyze accommodation and thereby prevent the accommodative effort required to compensate for hyperopia. Therefore, under cycloplegic examination all of the hyperopia is uncovered. Full correction of hyperopic errors, however, can never be based on cycloplegic findings because correction of the latent factor will only blur distance vision. The findings may be unreliable, however, in the management of accommodating esotropia. Cycloplegic examination indicates the magnitude of the refractive error. Noncycloplegic examination reveals the acceptability of a particular correction.

Symptoms

In the young the condition may cause no symptoms, because a healthy youngster has an ample reserve of accommodation and, if hyperopic, accommodates for distant and near objects without being conscious of the act. Thus a 5-year-old may have 4.00 diopters of hyperopia and not require any spectacle correction whatsoever. It is usually in older adults that the symptoms of hyperopia become apparent, as educational demands and the time allotted for close work increase and accommodative reserves decrease (Figure 11.5).

The symptoms of eyestrain are many and varied. They include headaches, burning of the eyes, and a pulling sensation of the eyes. These symptoms are generally related to the constant excessive accommodation that is required for close work. In older patients no symptoms may appear until the power of accommodation has diminished to the extent that the near point is beyond the range of comfortable reading distance, so that close work has to be held

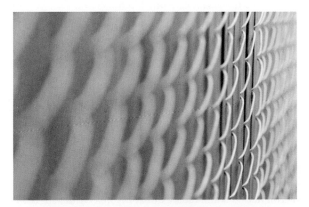

Figure 11.5 Hyperopic vision. Note that the fence in the foreground is fuzzy, whereas the distance is clear.

farther away than usual to be seen clearly. The greater the degree of hyperopia, the sooner this symptom arises; therefore, presbyopia commences at an earlier age than usual in the uncorrected hyperopic eye.

Treatment

The treatment of hyperopia is based on the patient's symptoms, occupation, and ability to compensate for close work. In the very young the treatment of hyperopia is usually unnecessary. The only exception to this rule occurs with *accommodative strabismus*. In this condition part or all of the strabismus may be corrected by the use of convex lenses, which decrease the need for accommodation and thus for the associated excessive convergence.

In older adults hyperopia always is corrected to improve near vision. Some believe the facultative component is never fully corrected unless the patient complains of fatigue and headaches. Whereas a 5-year-old may be oblivious to 4.00 to 5.00 diopters of hyperopia, a young college student may be very distressed by the presence of even 1.00 diopter of hyperopia. Such a patient needs to wear glasses only when the demands on accommodation are the greatest, that is, for performing close work. Some doctors, however, believe that the facultative component should be fully corrected.

In a middle-aged person, reading glasses become a necessity. The decline in accommodative power becomes so great that the patient is totally unable to see at a comfortable reading distance without convex lenses. Moreover, the power of the lenses exceeds the absolute and facultative demands of the hyperopia so that the patient can see comfortably with reading glasses for close work but the vision is totally blurred when these lenses are used for distance vision.

Older adults, particularly those between 55 and 65 years, find it difficult to accommodate even 1.00 diopter. This type of hyperopic patient usually needs convex lenses for both distance vision and close work.

Myopia

Myopia, or near-sightedness, is that condition in which parallel rays of light come to focus at a point just in front of the retina with respect to the unaccommodated eye (Figure 11.6). The myopic eye has basically too much plus power for its size. The myope has a fixed far point in space. For example, a person with 1.00-diopter myopia can see an object clearly if it is 3 feet (1 m) from the eye (Figure 11.7).

Types

In *axial myopia* the eyeball is too long for the normal refractive power of the lens and the cornea. Parallel rays of light are brought to a converging point usually somewhere in the

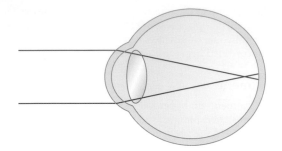

Figure 11.6 Myopic eye. Parallel rays of light are brought to a focus in front of the retina.

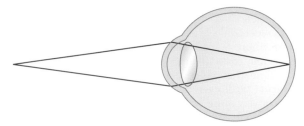

Figure 11.7 The myope can see clearly to a fixed far point in front of the eye.

vitreous in front of the retina. This type of eye is larger than normal.

In *curvature myopia* the eye is of normal size but the curvatures of the cornea and lens are increased.

Index myopia is a result of a change in the index of refraction of the lens. This is witnessed in two pathologic states: diabetes and cataract. In diabetes the lens loses water because of the high level of blood sugar in the anterior chamber, and therefore its index of refraction increases. In the cataract patient, the lens becomes increasingly hard because of the constant lamination of lens fibers being pushed to the center of the lens. The hard inner core increases the index of refraction of the entire lens structure, thereby increasing the converging power.

Cause

Almost everything has been blamed as a cause of myopia: diet, obesity, allergy, lighting conditions, vitamin deficiencies, and even wearing glasses too much or too little. Controversy and heated debate have raged about whether excessive close work or reading is a primary cause of myopia.

Much research and clinical investigation have been carried out in trying to understand the development of myopia. The results, however, have been inconclusive.

In the great majority of cases the near-sighted eye is longer than the normal eye. Just as some people are tall and some are short, so some people are far-sighted and some

are near-sighted. The near-sighted eye has grown longer than normal.

Most authorities agree that some myopia is familial, passed from one generation to another as a dominant trait. In fact, it is uncommon to find a myope who does not have one parent or siblings with a similar condition.

In the past the causes of myopia were a subject of heated debate and its treatment was often based on speculative theories. One school of thought held that myopia was a result of an excessive accommodative effort. In this regard children often were given bifocals to prevent them from using their own accommodation to see objects at near. Often limitations were placed on them at school and the child was allowed to use the eyes for homework only for a period not exceeding 1 hour. A variation of this line of thinking led to the undercorrection of myopia. Because these children could never see adequately at a distance, they would not use their accommodation. It was believed that not making an effort at accommodation would prevent the progress of the myopia.

Another group believed that myopia was caused not by excessive accommodation but by a lack of it. The contention was that a myope has to make less of an accommodative effort at near than an emmetrope or a hyperope. Therefore, to increase the circulation to the ciliary muscle and improve the health of the eye, this group advocated overcorrecting the myopia so that the individual would have to accommodate more than necessary.

Another prevalent speculation was that myopia was a result of a vitamin deficiency, especially during the growing years. To cope with this deficiency, calcium and vitamin D were prescribed during the active growth period, especially during adolescence, when myopia was thought to increase the most.

One group believed that myopia was related to deficient lighting conditions while children were reading. With this in mind, many parents became alarmed if they discovered their children reading in bed during the twilight hours and using only the available natural light.

Refractive surgery has become popular as a way of treating myopia (see Chapter 32). With the higher degrees of myopia, removal of the lens (lensectomy) has been advocated as a way of countering myopic effects. Some of these patients were treated by replacing the lenses of their eyes with artificial lenses. Other operations for the relief of high myopia included shortening the eyeball or flattening a central portion of the cornea.

The overwork theory of accommodation excess in myopia has been resurrected. It has been shown that some groups of students seem to have a higher incidence of progression of their myopia than do individuals who leave school at an early age and who do not do any close work. Furthermore, some doctors treat myopia by placing atropine or homatropine drops into myopic eyes to relax the ciliary muscle.

Progress

Myopia is rare at birth. It usually manifests after the fourth year of life. Its progression is relatively constant until the time of puberty. At that time the myopia may change alarmingly and progress rapidly, requiring changes of glasses every 6 months. Normally the myopia becomes arrested when full maturity is reached. Therefore, the ages between 20 and 40 years are relatively quiet and the myope's correction may remain virtually unchanged during this period except for a condition called progressive myopia.

Symptoms

The most outstanding symptom of myopia is inability to see objects clearly at a distance. Near vision is always good (Figure 11.8). Myopic children often regard this as the natural order of life: objects in the distance are fuzzy, whereas those at close range are clear. In many cases the myope is not detected until the school runs a visual screening program. Older children often learn of their condition when they discover that classmates sitting beside them can see the blackboard with ease, whereas they see it only with difficulty.

The antics of the near-sighted movie cartoon character Mr. Magoo are well known. The humorous episodes in which Magoo mistakes a gorilla for his wife make us laugh, but they also make us aware of the danger and menace that a near-sighted person can be to society. Just imagine what a hazard Magoo would be on today's highways!

Many myopic children have a tendency to squeeze their lids around their eyes to create the effect of a pinhole camera. This is one expedient the myope uses to obtain better vision in the distance. The constant squeezing of the lids, however, may lead to headaches and general eyestrain. Squinting is not a substitute for spectacles.

Progressive myopia

Occasionally myopia develops in early childhood and reaches alarming degrees. Children younger than the age of 10 who have myopia of −6.00 diopters or more often develop secondary visual complications because of the elongation of the eyeball and a thinning of the sclera (Figure 11.9). These complications, such as seeing spots before the eyes because of vitreous degeneration, may be relatively harmless. Others, such as retinal degeneration and detachment and macular hemorrhage, may be more serious. Invariably, all myopia more than 10.00 diopters in magnitude is axial, that is, associated with an elongated eyeball. Because of these complications, the myope in particular should be examined yearly, not only for alteration of the spectacle correction but also for a thorough retinal examination.

Treatment

Most doctors feel myopia should be fully corrected at all times so that the person can enjoy comfortable and clear distance vision (Figure 11.10). Some doctors, however, believe that myopia should be undercorrected and that the myope should read without glasses. They believe this prevents a further increase in myopia. The full correction, however, enables the myope to establish a normal relationship between accommodation and convergence. Myopic children require no special inducements to wear their glasses. These children, on receiving their glasses, soon learn to enjoy the sharp, clean edges of clear vision and will reach for their glasses the first thing on arising in the morning.

Moreover, myopes are among the most conscientious regarding reappointments. Although they do not initially recognize their own visual defect, once they receive glasses they become acutely aware of the progress of their myopia and changes in the clarity of things.

People with myopia of high magnitude, such as 4.00 diopters or greater, are slightly handicapped by the fact that their image size is smaller. A high myopic lens placed at a distance

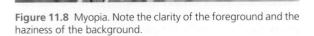

Figure 11.8 Myopia. Note the clarity of the foreground and the haziness of the background.

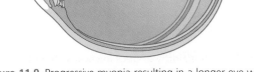

Figure 11.9 Progressive myopia resulting in a longer eye with thinning of the sclera.

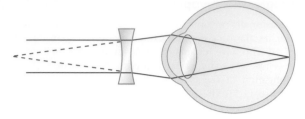

Figure 11.10 Myopic eye. A concave lens brings parallel rays of light to a focus on the retina.

from the eye has a minifying effect. This effect may be offset by the use of contact lenses. Not only is the image size more normal with contact lenses, but also the aberrations of the thick lens are eliminated and the field is enlarged. The use of contact lenses in high myopia, that is, −10.00 diopters or greater, is especially recommended because in these ranges secondary disadvantages of spectacle correction are great.

Astigmatism

Astigmatism is the condition in which rays of light are not refracted equally in all directions, so that a point focus on the retina is not attained.

Types

Regular astigmatism

Regular astigmatism is a refractive condition that is amenable to correction by cylinders. The axes of the principal meridians of the astigmatism are at right angles to each other. If the axis of the astigmatism deviates from either horizontal or vertical meridians, generally the deviation is symmetric in the two eyes.

Regular astigmatism may be subdivided into the following groups:

In *simple astigmatism* one of the focal lines always falls on the retina; that is, one meridian is emmetropic. The other meridian may have its focus behind the retina or in front of it. The condition then is referred to either as *simple hyperopic astigmatism* or as *simple myopic astigmatism,* respectively (Figure 11.11A–B).

In *compound astigmatism* the rays of light are refracted so that both focal points lie either in front of the retina or behind it. The former is referred to as *compound myopic astigmatism* and the latter as *compound hyperopic astigmatism* (Figure 11.11C–D).

In *mixed astigmatism* one focal point lies behind the retina, whereas the other focal point lies in front of it (Figure 11.11E).

Irregular astigmatism

If the cornea has been damaged by trauma, inflammation, scar tissue, or developmental anomalies so that a geometric

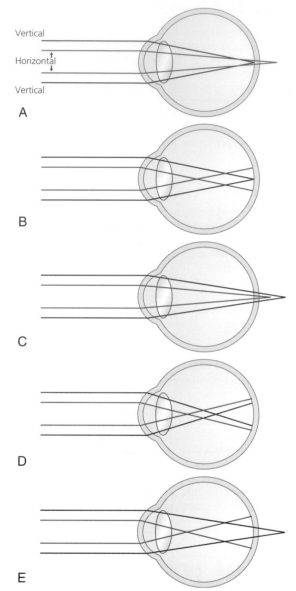

Figure 11.11 (A) Simple hyperopic astigmatism. The vertical bundle of rays is focused on the retina; the horizontal rays are focused behind the retina. (B) Simple myopic astigmatism. The vertical bundle of rays is focused on the retina; the horizontal rays are focused in front of the retina. (C) Compound hyperopic astigmatism. Both focal points fall behind the retina. (D) Compound myopic astigmatism. Both focal points lie in front of the retina. (E) Mixed astigmatism. The vertical rays come to a focus behind the retina; the horizontal rays focus in front of the retina.

form is not adhered to, the resultant condition is called *irregular astigmatism.* In view of the irregularity of the corneal surface and the lack of any geometric form, this condition usually cannot be completely corrected by cylinders.

Cause

In most instances astigmatism results because the radius of curvature of the cornea is not equal in all directions. Although at birth the cornea usually is a perfect sphere, by the age of 4 years it loses its spherical qualities. The horizontal axis (vertical radius) of the cornea becomes more steeply inclined so that rays of light are refracted more acutely than those rays being refracted along the vertical axis of the cornea. This type of astigmatism is commonly referred to as *with-the-rule astigmatism*. The astigmatism in which the vertical axis (horizontal radius) of the cornea is stronger than the horizontal one is referred to as *against-the-rule astigmatism*. In the formative years astigmatism may alter in small increments, but its axis usually remains relatively unchanged.

Although astigmatism most commonly results from a cornea that is not spherical, in some instances the astigmatism may be the result of an unequal bending of light by the crystalline lens, the so-called *lenticular astigmatism*.

Problems of astigmatic individuals

Because neither the horizontal nor the vertical axis forms a point focus, the person with an astigmatic condition usually chooses the more normal, or emmetropic, axis for seeing. If the two axes are equally in focus, then the vertical focal line is, as a rule, preferentially chosen. The object being viewed will appear somewhat indistinct.

Consider an individual with an astigmatic problem in which the vertical axis is focused on the retina and the object of regard is a cross. Each point of the cross that is imaged on the retina is elongated in a vertical direction. The horizontal line therefore appears as a series of short vertical lines that elongate into a broad, blurred band; in the vertical line, the vertical strokes are superimposed and cover each other so that the whole line appears sharply defined and black, with only the uppermost and lowermost of the vertical lines having a vertical, brush-like appearance (Figure 11.12).

Obviously the most common complaint of the patient with astigmatism is inability to see at both distance and near, whereas the hyperopic person normally can see efficiently at a distance and the myope sees quite adequately at near.

As with other refractive errors, the astigmatic patient uses many compensatory movements to improve vision. There may be a tendency to half close the lids to make a horizontal slit between the lids and cut off the rays in one meridian. Reading matter may be held very close to the eyes to obtain a large, even though blurred, retinal image.

REFRACTOMETRY AND REFRACTION

Refractometry is defined as the measurement of refractive error and it should not be confused with the term *refraction*. Refraction is defined as the sum of steps performed in

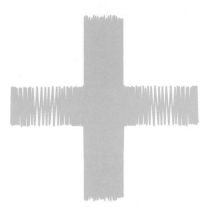

Figure 11.12 Distortions of points of light are in a vertical direction. The horizontal band is fuzzy except at the end; the vertical band is sharp except at the end.

arriving at a decision as to what lens or lenses (if any) will most benefit the patient. These steps include, in addition to refractometry, measurement of visual acuity, measurement of accommodative ability, and the exercise of clinical judgment. Refraction, often referred to as an art, is generally considered to require a license for its practice and constitutes a major activity of ophthalmology and optometry.

Refractometry, however, is strictly limited to clinical application of optical principles. This measurement function can be performed at the highest level of precision by technicians and, in some cases, even by sophisticated instruments and computers.

The exercise of clinical judgment included in the foregoing definition of refraction refers to a consideration of such factors as the patient's occupational requirements, muscle balance, impairment of vision by other than refractive error (such as cataract, macular degeneration, or suppression amblyopia), the extent and type of refractive error present, and even the emotional "set" of the patient with respect to wearing glasses. (For some patients, even though there may be a significant error, the maximum benefit is achieved by prescribing no lenses at all.) Refractometry may be classified in several different ways: preliminary versus refining, objective versus subjective, and cylinder versus sphere. These classifications are integrated in Table 11.1.

Methods of refractometry

For convenience, refractometric methods are considered here under two headings: objective and subjective. Objective methods provide the advantage of permitting measurements to be made without requiring the patient to give answers; adequate measurements can be made in patients who are unable or unwilling to answer questions but who cooperate to the extent of fixating a distant target. The disadvantages of objective methods are that they require a moderate-sized or dilated pupil and they cannot be relied

Table 11.1 Classifications of refractometry

	Sphere	Cylinder
Preliminary		
Objective (retinoscope and objective separators)	Approximate	Approximate
Subjective (dials and cylinders)	—	—
Refining		
Subjective (cross cylinder)	—	Precise
Subjective (duochrome)	Precise	Precise

on to provide data that are sufficiently accurate to provide the basis of a prescription. The advantages of subjective methods are that they can be performed even when the pupil is very small and they provide data that are much more precise and reliable; their use, however, is limited by the amount of patient judgment and participation required.

Steps for refractometry

At the beginning of any refraction, a decision must be made about whether to use drops and, if so, what drops to use (Table 11.2).

Cycloplegic drops

Most refractionists use cycloplegic drops on anyone up to the age of 20 years. The drops impair the power of accommodation by inhibiting the ciliary muscle. They also dilate the pupil. Thus the drops have two basic functions:

1. They arrest accommodation or focusing, which in a young person with a powerful accommodative ability may not be achieved any other way.
2. They dilate the pupil to make a retinal examination more complete by exposing a greater part of the peripheral retina.

The drawback to drops is that adult patients who drive to the examination have to return home with blurred vision, photophobia, and fear.

Systemic absorption of the drugs in Table 11.2 can cause a toxic reaction. For instance, atropine can cause a fast pulse, a fever, and a skin rash. To minimize the systemic absorption of these drops, pressure should be exerted with a cotton ball or tissue held over the tear sac for a minute after the drop is instilled in the eye.

The next step in the process of refraction is to check the old glasses for power and optical centration. Frequently the refractionist uses this information as a basis for refining the prescription or for the overrefraction.

Lensmeter

A *lensmeter* records the optical center of the lens, its power, and the axis of the correcting cylinder, including its power.

Table 11.2 Drops used in refraction

Drug	Onset of maximum cycloplegia	Duration of activity	Comment
Atropine sulfate 0.5%, 1%	45–120 min	7–14 days, especially in a blue-eyed child	Not used routinely except for the assessment of accommodative strabismus in children
Scopolamine hydrobromide 0.25%	30–60 min	4–7 days	Used in atropine-allergic patients
Homatropine hydrobromide 2%, 5%	30–60 min	3 days	Requires half an hour to an hour to take effect and lasts 3 days; not used routinely
Cyclopentolate hydrochloride 0.5%, 1%, 2% (Cyclogyl)	30–60 min	6–24 h	Active in 30–60 min; two sets of drops given 5 min apart; a good rapid-acting cycloplegic drop for office use
Tropicamide 0.5%, 1% (Mydriacyl)	20–40 min	4–6 h	A good drug for office use with an effect similar to Cyclogyl
Phenylephrine hydrochloride 2.5%	30–60 min (no cycloplegia)	30 min–2 h	Little effect on accommodation; 2.5% most commonly used because of potential systemic effects. Avoid 10%

Modified from Stein HA, Slatt BJ, Stein RM. A primer in ophthalmology. St Louis: Mosby; 1992.

The newer lensmeters are fully automated and digitalized. These basic mechanical lensmeters are accurate but require some technical expertise. Details are presented in Chapter 8.

Notation of the axis of the cylinder must be precise inasmuch as a patient will not tolerate a large deviation from his or her old prescription, especially in high degrees of astigmatism.

RETINOSCOPY

The retinoscope is the most useful instrument in the refractionist's armamentarium. Retinoscopy is the chief objective method of determining the refractive error of an eye (see Figure 10.6). It is the only way to assess the refractive error in children, people who are illiterate, people who speak a different language from the examiner's, and people who are too confused, suffer from dementia, or are ill to add a precise subjective component to the total refraction.

The retinoscope has a viewing system and an illuminating system. The viewing system consists of a small aperture at the head of the retinoscope that enables the examiner to see. The illuminating system shines diverging rays of light into the patient's eye. This light enters the patient's eye and is reflected back again as a reflex in the patient's pupil. This reflex appears as a red-orange glow with a slight shadow around it. The vergence of the rays of light that leave the patient's eye depends on the refractive error of that patient. In a myope the rays leave converging, in a hyperope the rays leave diverging, and in an emmetrope the rays leave parallel.

The degree of divergence of the rays that leave the illuminating system of the retinoscope depends on the distance of the retinoscope from the patient's eye. Most ophthalmologists use a working lens in the phoropter or trial frame to account for this distance. The working lens conventionally is held at 66 cm, being a +1.50 diopter lens, or at 50 cm, being a +2.00 diopter lens. If the patient is far-sighted, the examiner will see, in the patient's eye, a reflex that moves *with* the movement of the retinoscope. In this instance plus lenses are added until there is no movement at all; in other words, until the refractive error has been neutralized. The working lens is then removed or subtracted and what is left in the trial frame is a measure of the hyperopia. Usually +1.50 or +2.00 diopters are subtracted to allow for the working distance of 66 or 50 cm, depending on the arm length.

If the patient is a myope, the movement of the examiner's retinoscope will create a movement of the reflex that is opposite to the movement of the retinoscope. In this instance the examiner places concave lenses or minus lenses in front of the patient's eye until the "against" motion is converted to a nonmoving reflex.

The reflex seen in the patient's pupil becomes much brighter and moves much faster as the refractive error becomes reduced. In other words, small refractive errors have a bright and fast reflex, whereas large ones have a dull and slow reflex. The reflex fills the entire pupillary space when the refractive error has been eliminated.

The following list provides aids to retinoscopy:

1. The patient should be looking at a distant object of regard at least 20 feet (6 m) away.
2. The patient's left eye should be examined with the examiner's left eye and vice versa.
3. Plus cylinders should be used in astigmatic cases because it is easier to see "with" motion.
4. Small differences in astigmatism are difficult to see, yet most astigmatism is 1.00 diopter or less. The power of the correcting cylinder should be moved forward and backward as a check for accuracy.
5. The eye not being measured should be fogged or occluded. The patient should not be told to close one eye during retinoscopy.
6. Irregular reflexes will appear in the following cases:
   a. Keratoconus
   b. Corneal scarring
   c. Cataracts
   d. Dirty soft contact lenses
   e. Warped corneas from poorly fitting hard contact lenses
   f. Lens subluxation
   g. Postsurgical corneas.

Streak retinoscope

There are two main types of retinoscopes: the spot retinoscope and the streak retinoscope. The Copeland streak retinoscope has been the most popular. Other streak retinoscopes are the Nikon, the Welsh-Allyn, the Keeler, and the Reichert. The last three retinoscopes work by holding the bar on the handle down, whereas the Copeland and the Nikon work by holding the bar up.

Many ophthalmologists use the streak retinoscope (Figure 11.13). The streak reflex illuminated in the pupil can be aligned easily with an astigmatic error. Moreover, it can be rotated to any desired meridian. With the streak retinoscope, the point of neutrality sometimes is evidenced by a cleavage in the streak (scissors reflex) so that half the streak moves in one direction and the other half moves in the opposite direction.

The light source for the streak retinoscope has a linear filament. From this source a divergent collection of light rays strikes the person's pupil. The alignment of the rays from the linear filament is made possible by the adjustable sleeve on the instrument, which provides rotation of the bulb.

Streak retinoscopy is largely plus cylinder retinoscopy, that is, corrected with plus cylinders. A mirror in the instrument bends the path of light at right angles to the vertical orientation of the handle so that light can move across the space between examiner and patient. When the sleeve is up, a planomirror effect is created. The sleeve-down position

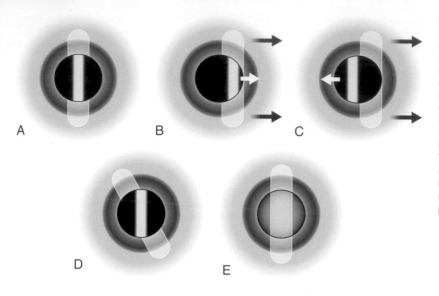

Figure 11.13 Reflexes produced by the streak retinoscope. (A) Normal. (B) "With" movement. The reflex moves in the same direction as the retinoscope, indicating a hyperopic eye. (C) "Against" movement. The reflex moves in the direction opposite to that of the retinoscope, indicating a myopic eye. (D) Streak is not uniform in size, speed, or brightness over the entire aperture. The band is more prominent in one meridian, indicating astigmatism. (E) Neutralization point. There is no movement of the reflex and the pupil is filled with a red glow.

produces a concave mirror effect. Thus with sleeve up, the most traditional position, diverging rays are emitted (planomirror effect), whereas in the sleeve-down position converging rays are formed (concave mirror effect).

A retinal reflex is found in the pupil when light from the retinoscope is shone into the patient's eye. The movement of this fundus reflex will yield information as to the presence of myopia, hyperopia, or astigmatism. The instrument must be moved to elicit the reflex in the pupil. The movement is perpendicular to the axis of the streak. When the streak is vertical, the movement of the instrument is sideways.

It is important to remember that the light in the patient's pupil is reflected from the retina so that a total picture of the refraction is obtained.

The working distance must be taken into account in retinoscopy. Most refractions use a 22-inch (66 cm) distance, which, translated into diopters, is an added plus lens of +1.50 diopters. If the person is emmetropic, with this lens no movement will be present in the light reflex of the patient's pupil. The neutralization point can be as much as 0.50 diopter of accuracy. If the patient is hyperopic or far-sighted, the reflex will become a "with" movement (the reflex moves in the same direction with the movement of the retinoscope). If the eye is myopic, there will be an "against" motion from the neutral state (Figure 11.14).

With a far-sighted eye, plus lenses are added until neutralization occurs. The added plus spheres are then a measure of the total hyperopic refractive error. The same approach occurs with myopia, except that concave lenses are used.

Many practitioners prefer to use the "with" motion because it is easier to see compared with an "against" motion. This can be done by overcorrecting myopic eyes or by reversing the position of the sleeve.

Neutrality of the objective refraction can be determined by the following:

1. **The brightness of the reflex:** the closer one comes to neutralizing the refractive error, the brighter the reflex.
2. **The speed of the light movement:** when the light movement is dull and slow, it means the refractive error is still considerable.
3. **The size of the reflex:** the reflex fills the entire pupil when the neutrality is reached.

A large pupil makes it easier to recognize the motion of the reflex. For this reason, pupillary dilation is helpful in most cases.

With astigmatism, the speed, brilliance, and size of the reflex will be considerably different in one meridian compared with the other principal meridian. Each band of light is neutralized separately and the difference in diopters measures the degree of astigmatism. In all computations, one must reduce the value of the working lens by +1.50 or +2.00 diopters.

AUTOREFRACTORS*

Several refracting instruments have been introduced over the past few years. These include manual objective refractors, automatic infrared retinoscopes, and sophisticated subjective refractors that can modify the results to obtain the optimum visual acuity. Some are quick and easy to use; some take longer and require more operator skill.

*The authors thank David L. Guyton, MD, for his contribution to this section.

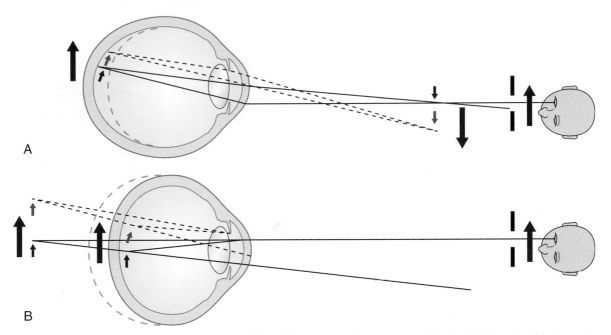

Figure 11.14 Movement of images on retinoscopy. (A) Myopia: real upside-down image creating "against" motion. (B) Hyperopia: virtual upright image creating "with" motion.

All of these automated refractors are designed to be managed by the ophthalmic assistant without the need for extensive knowledge of refractometry techniques. Some have subjective components that can refine the readings, some have the capability to assess the patient's vision, and others provide keratometer readings of the cornea.

Historical development

Automated refractors date back more than 100 years, but only recently have some of them become successful. There have been three major problems in obtaining the necessary accuracy. First, many automated refractors have used only small portions of the patient's pupil to make the measurement. Because of the optical irregularity present in many eyes, the refraction obtained through small portions of the pupil may not be valid for the entire pupil. Such optical irregularities are easily visible during retinoscopy, and the automated refractors have no better way to deal with these than does retinoscopic examination. Second, maintaining proper alignment of the automated refractor with the patient's eye was difficult with many of the early instruments. To lessen this problem, automatic tracking capability has been added to some of the newest automated refractors. Third, and most important, most automated refractors have been placed in box-shaped instruments that cause the awareness of near. Patients tend to accommodate when looking into these boxes, even though the visual targets within the boxes may be imaged optically at infinity.

Accurate refraction is impossible in the presence of accommodation, and this so-called instrument myopia has been a continuing problem for automated refractors. Various fogging techniques or "free-space" techniques are used to try to overcome the problem of instrument myopia.

Objective refractors

These instruments focus on the ability to determine the corrected refraction that will give the optimum vision. The objective refractor requires minimal cooperation on the part of the patient except to hold still and look straight ahead. The subjective refractors, on the other hand, require responses from the patient, particularly in the final refinement step of the refractive measurement.

Manual objective refractors

In the 1930s several instruments known as *objective optometers* appeared in Europe. The operator focused or aligned a target pattern on the patient's retina to determine the refraction. These manual objective refractors still are used in many parts of the world in preference to retinoscopy. They are less expensive than the other automated refractors, but require more time and more operator skill. Patient cooperation is essential and instrument accommodation is common when cycloplegia is not used. The objective optometers use only small portions of the eye's optics for the measurement and alignment is critical, limiting the accuracy of the findings. One of these refractors, the Top-con, uses infrared light for the alignment and measurement process so that the patient is not dazzled by the bright white-light target pattern used in other models.

Automatic objective refractors

Automatic objective refractors first became available in the 1970s, using infrared light to refract the eye automatically either by retinoscopy or by similar principles. The first instruments in this group were the Safir Ophthalmetron, the 6600 Auto-Refractor, and the Dioptron, now all discontinued. The infrared light refractors give good results in healthy eyes with medium to large pupils, but accuracy decreases in the presence of immature cataracts, corneal haze, or pupils less than 3 mm in diameter.

Operation of autorefractors is extremely simple and the measurement time is rapid, requiring only 1 second or less for most of the instruments. The refractive results obtained, however, must be regarded as only preliminary. Accuracy is good enough to identify 'no change' refractions and to monitor postoperative refractions until stable, but the results are not reliable enough to serve as the basis for prescribing glasses or contact lenses. Refinement by subjective techniques is recommended before prescribing.

Combination objective/subjective refractors (Figures 11.15 and 11.16)

Subjective capabilities have been added to several automatic objective refractors. For example, visual acuity can be measured through these instruments both before and after the refraction. Also, sphere, cylinder, and axis can be adjusted manually according to the patient's responses

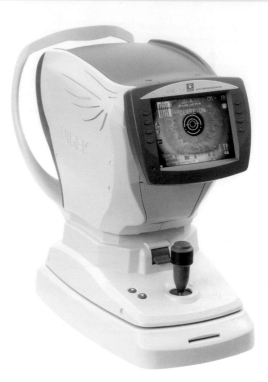

Figure 11.16 Nidek ARK-1 s Auto Refractor and Keratometer. *(Courtesy of Marco Ophthalmic, Jacksonville, FL, www.marco.com.)*

to various targets presented. Cross-cylinder testing is incorporated into most of these instruments, with successive views of the two cross-cylinder choices. The objective portion of the refraction with these instruments is the same as with the other automatic objective refractors.

The subjective capabilities of each of the combination refractors may be used, if desired, for refinement of the refraction. Considerable operator skill and knowledge of refracting techniques are necessary for optimal subjective refinement with these instruments and there is still the problem of instrument myopia in patients up to the age of 40.

Automated subjective refractors

Two automated refractors with purely subjective capabilities were on the market for about 10 years. The first to appear was the Humphrey Vision Analyzer in the mid-1970s. The Vision Analyzer used a novel optical system to refract the eyes in "free space," using a concave mirror 10 feet (3 m) from the patient. Even the method of refraction was novel, using smeared-out astigmatic line targets in two independent meridians 45 degrees apart to arrive at the final cylinder and axis. The Vision Analyzer required an entire room, however, and was somewhat complicated

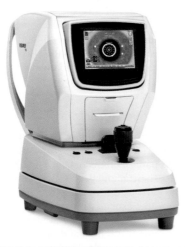

Figure 11.15 Zeiss VISUREF 100 Auto Refractor and Keratometer. *(Courtesy of Zeiss, UK, www.zeiss.co.uk.)*

to administer. It provided both binocular and near testing capabilities, unique among the automated refractors.

Because hyperopic patients often accommodated to the plane of the mirror of the Vision Analyzer, overrefraction capabilities were added, creating the Humphrey Overrefraction System. The eyes were refracted while the patient wore glasses, and the results were trigonometrically added to the power of the glasses.

Remote-controlled refractors

Several refractors or phoropters have been motorized in recent years and equipped with remote-controlled keyboards. These are designed to be operated by the skilled refractionist because the techniques of refraction are not automated and still require full knowledge of refractive procedures. These remote-controlled refractors are expensive. Their major advantages are to impress the patient and to ease the practitioner's back strain. Retinoscopy can be performed in the usual manner through these instruments, and accuracy is comparable to that obtained with conventional manual refractors.

Accuracy of measurement

The automatic objective refractors still create problems of irregular refraction in the patient's eye, maintenance of alignment of the instrument with the eye, and instrument myopia. Although accuracy is within 0.25 diopter of the subjective refinement in more than 80% of cases, it is not always obvious which measurements are incorrect, necessitating subjective refinement of most refractions. With a visual acuity check built into some of the objective instruments, valid information can be obtained at least to identify "no change" refractions and to monitor the stability of the refraction after surgery.

The automated subjective refractors were highly accurate but required more operator skill. They also were not free from the problem of instrument myopia, and repeat measurement under cycloplegia was sometimes necessary in younger patients. The patients had to be 8 or 9 years old to respond reliably to the subjective refractors, whereas with the objective instruments, refraction sometimes can be effected in patients as young as 3 or 4 years.

To date, neither a purely objective nor a purely subjective instrument has fully replaced conventional refracting techniques; that is, it is precisely the combination of an objective starting point and subjective refinement that yields the most reliable results throughout the widest range of patients. It is not surprising that automated refractors are evolving into combination objective and subjective instruments, but the subjective portion still requires knowledge of refracting techniques and at least a moderate amount of experience for optimal results. It is likely that more sophisticated methods for subjective refinement will be developed within the next few years, decreasing operator dependence of the present instruments.

Errors with automated refractors

Some of the errors that occur with automatic refractors include the following:

- The individual patient can accommodate to the instrument.
- Reflection over the patient's current glasses can occur.
- Some autorefractors do not provide vision as an endpoint; consequently, if there is an error in the printout, the examiner does not know if the measurement is reliable.
- Peripheral light from the room can affect the reading; thus a dimmed room is required.

In our experience, autorefractors act as an automatic retinoscope and do not provide good subjective refraction. The examiner should place the findings in a phoropter or trial lens case and test the patient subjectively. Autorefractors, however, do provide a reliable starting point in a refraction procedure and for an inexperienced retinoscopist the autorefractor may be even more reliable than a retinoscope. Many of the newer autorefractors also rely subjectively on the machine and add, which is a large advantage.

Where are we going with automated refraction?

As autorefractors become more accurate than conventional techniques, there is no question that the concept of autorefraction is here to stay. The combination objective and subjective instruments with full subjective refinement capability appear to be the final common pathway for both the objective and subjective types. In spite of the impressive capabilities of the newest instruments, their incorporation into an office practice must be carefully planned. Scheduling of patient appointments and proper sequencing of examinations must be arranged to prevent the automated refractor from obstructing the flow of patients. Operators must be trained properly and substitute operators must be available. Service and maintenance for the instruments must be arranged and be available quickly when needed. Instrument operators must learn to recognize when either the patient or the instrument is having problems and to "flag" such cases for special consideration or repeat refraction by conventional techniques. Practitioners must learn when to trust the instruments and when not to and must provide feedback to the ophthalmic assistant if any learning is to occur. It is precisely the absence of such feedback that has limited the usefulness of automated refractors in many practices.

Patients generally are impressed with the automated instruments, and most do not seem annoyed that less time may be spent with the practitioner. Most practitioners initially expect too much from the automated refractors but eventually come to regard them as a valuable second opinion unbiased by knowledge of the patient's old prescription. The time will come, however, when the instruments are made less operator dependent, simpler, and more reliable. Then the practitioner will need only to exercise the art of prescribing rather than to take time with the tedium of manual refraction and retinoscopy.

Of clinical importance is the new tendency to integrate keratometric measurements and corneal topography with the autorefractor for a more detailed analysis of the refracting components of the eye. The wavelight or orbscan that is used by the refractive surgeon gives reasonably accurate refraction endpoints.

SUBJECTIVE REFINING OF REFRACTION

Once a preliminary estimate of the refractive error has been made by retinoscopy, the information is placed in a phoropter or trial frame. The patient's clinical responses to changes of spherical and astigmatic lenses are then noted while progressively smaller and smaller visual acuity letters are presented to the patient for evaluation. Special procedures often are used in the refining of the final refractive error. These procedures include tests for astigmatism and the duochrome test.

Astigmatism tests

Two methods are primarily used for determining the axis and the power of the correct cylinder: the astigmatic dial or clock and the cross cylinder.

Astigmatic clock

The astigmatic clock has black lines intersecting at a common point, with the ends separated by 30- or 10-degree intervals (Figure 11.17). The patient is seated at the normal refracting distance from the chart (20 feet [6 m]) and asked to select the blackest line on the chart. The blackest line corresponds, of course, to the axis of the rays of light that are most in focus. Therefore, the correcting cylinder is placed 90 degrees away from the blackest line; either positive or negative cylinders may be used. Positive cylinders bring the most hyperopic focal point forward and collapse the astigmatic interval so that the focal point is either on the retina or in front of it. Minus correcting cylinders reduce the astigmatic interval and push the point of focus either on the retina or behind it.

When the astigmatic dial is being used, it is usually wisest to use minus cylinders and reduce the astigmatic component by eliminating the myopic focal point.

The astigmatic component is resolved when the two principal axes on the clock are equally distinct and all lenses are equally in focus. Before asking the patient which

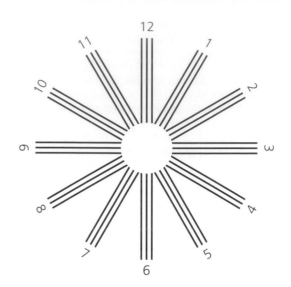

Figure 11.17 Astigmatic clock.

line on the clock is the darkest, the examiner should blur the patient's vision to about 20/50 on the myopic side. This is done because a myopic state tends to inhibit accommodation. After the patient has selected the blackest line on the multiple dial chart, his or her attention is directed to a second chart that has only two lines that can be maneuvered to any position. The lines are set according to the most in-focus and out-of-focus axis. Then minus cylinders are placed before the eyes, with the axis 90 degrees from the blackest line, increasing their strength approximately 0.25 diopter at a time, until the blackness and distinctness of the two lines are the same. To ensure that the eyes are maintained on the myopic side or in a fogged state, it is advisable to add 0.25 diopter of plus sphere for each 0.50 diopter of minus cylinder that is used. Once all the lines appear dark and equally distinct, the myopic error can be reduced by use of minus spheres.

In using the astigmatic clock with the spokes set 30 degrees apart, the examiner should ask the patient, in terms of hours on the clock, which line appears blackest. The smaller number of the clock hours is then multiplied by 30 degrees to determine the correcting axis. For example, if the 2 to 8 line is the blackest, then 2 times 30 is 60 and 60 degrees is the axis of the correcting cylinder.

If two lines appear equally black—that is, 1 to 7 and 2 to 8—then a mean between the two is taken and the axis of the correcting cylinder is determined that way. In the latter case it would be 1.5 times 30 and 45 degrees would be the axis of the correcting cylinder.

Cross cylinder

A cross cylinder is a lens consisting of two cylinders of equal power but of opposite designation, one being plus and the other minus, their axes set 90 degrees apart. In most cross cylinders the red marks indicate the minus axis and the white the plus axis. The entire lens is mounted in a ring, with a handle placed halfway between the plus and the minus axes (see Figure 10.8).

A cross cylinder is used to determine the axis of the correcting cylinder and to check on this axis and the power of the correcting cylinder.

The cross cylinder produces a mixed astigmatism of equal amount but opposite power in the two principal axes of the cylinder. To determine the *true axis of the correcting cylinder*, the patient wears full correction in the trial frame or the refractor, as determined by either a subjective astigmatic dial test or retinoscopy. The patient is then instructed to fixate on a line of letters that he or she can comfortably read. The handle of the cross cylinder or the axis of the lens of the phoropter is placed in alignment with the axis of the correcting cylinder already in the trial frame. The cross cylinder is then flipped from position 1 to position 2 and the patient is asked to comment on the clarity of the two positions of the cross cylinder. If the letters appear equally blurred at positions 1 and 2, then the axis of the correcting cylinder in the patient's trial frame or phoropter is assumed to be correct. If one position is clearer than the other, the correcting cylinder is shifted in that direction. If the refractionist is using minus cylinders, the cylindric correction is shifted in the direction of the red dot that indicates the minus power of the cross cylinder. The opposite is true if the refractionist uses plus cylinders. A cross cylinder is most successfully used when it is held in a stationary frame, such as the refractor. This ensures proper alignment of the handle of the cross cylinders when the cross cylinder is changed.

Once the axis of the correcting cylinder has been determined, then the *power of the correcting cylinder* is investigated. This is accomplished by placing the handle 45 degrees away from the axis of the correcting cylinder in the trial frame or refractor. In this position the plus or minus cylinder of the cross cylinder is parallel with that of the correcting cylinder. Again the patient is asked to observe whether there is any difference in the clarity between positions 1 and 2. If there is a difference in the clarity, cylinders are added or subtracted, depending on whether plus or minus cylinders are used, until the clarity of the letters becomes the same, regardless of which side of the cross cylinder is flipped.

A prism in the cross-cylinder technique is incorporated in the Topcon refractor and is available as an accessory for other refractors. This device doubles the image so the patient is able to view two test charts simultaneously with one eye and to determine the clarity of the charts with the two positions of the cross cylinder. Additional cylinder or axis shift can be altered until the ultimate endpoint is reached when both lines are equally distinct.

It is immaterial whether one uses a cross cylinder or an astigmatic dial chart for the correction of astigmatism.

The results are equally valid with both techniques. The efficiency by which one obtains a good refraction depends more on the skill of the refractionist than on the technique used.

Irregular astigmatism

In irregular astigmatism the refraction in different meridians is irregular. Usually when irregular astigmatism is found, there is an associated pathologic condition of the cornea. Two of the most common causes of irregular astigmatism are corneal scarring from any cause and the developmental condition called *keratoconus.*

The diagnosis of irregular corneal astigmatism is best facilitated by using Placido's disc. This is a large, flat disc painted with concentric black and white circles (see Figure 10.37). It is held in front of the eye, and the reflexes are observed through a hole in the center of the disc. The distortion of the circles on the cornea is usually readily visible.

The treatment of irregular astigmatism by conventional cylinders is virtually impossible. The best method of treating either corneal scarring or keratoconus is usually with a contact lens. If the treatment of irregular astigmatism by contact lenses is unsuccessful, often a corneal transplant becomes necessary.

Spherical equivalent

Occasionally in refraction, especially if the patient is an adult who has never worn glasses and requires a large astigmatic correction, the refractionist uses the spherical equivalent. Essentially the cylinder is reduced, and half of that reduction is added algebraically to the sphere. For example, assume that the patient's correction is a +3.00 sphere combined with a +6.00 diopter cylinder, axis 180. Let us say in this instance that the refractionist decides that this cylindric correction would be too great for the patient to accept at once, and the decision is to reduce the cylinder by 1.50 diopters. Then the refractionist would add +0.75, or half the reduction, to the sphere. The resulting prescription would then read +3.75 sphere combined with +4.50 cylinder at axis 180. If one wishes only to determine the spherical equivalent expressed as spherical, the following examples apply: $-2.00 + 1.00$ at axis $180 = -1.50$ sphere and $+2.00 + 1.00$ at axis $180 = +2.50$ sphere.

Duochrome tests

Duochrome tests are based on the fact that light of longer wavelengths (red) is refracted by optical systems less than light of shorter wavelengths (blue or green). In the *red–green duochrome test* the projector screen is illuminated through a filter that is red on one side and green on the other. Another form of duochrome test requires the patient to look at a point source of light through a cobalt-blue glass filter. This type of glass is peculiar in that it transmits light in two "bands" of wavelengths that are widely separated: one in the red and the other in the blue.

On one hand, if the red–green test is used and the patient has insufficiently corrected myopia, then the letters on the red side will stand out blacker, clearer, and sharper. They require more minus for the green to be as distinct as the red. On the other hand, if the same myopia is overcorrected and made artificially hyperopic, then the letters against the green background appear blacker, clearer, and sharper. The sphere is adjusted until letters on both sides are of equal quality. In the latter case, they require plus levels for the red to be equally distinct. Similarly, with use of the *cobalt-blue test*, the person with undercorrected myopia perceives a blue circle with a red center, whereas the person with overcorrected myopia perceives a red circle with a blue center. The red–green test is more commonly used than the cobalt-blue test.

Duochrome tests are useful only in refining spherical power, contributing nothing to the determination of cylinder power or axis. Therefore, the most appropriate use of a duochrome test is as an endpoint determination in refraction.

ANISOMETROPIA

Anisometropia is a condition in which there is a difference in the refractive error of the two eyes. If the difference in the refractive error of the two eyes is slight, binocular vision is easily attained. Each 0.25 diopter difference between the refraction of the two eyes causes 0.5% difference in size between the two retinal images, and a difference of 5% is probably the limit that can be tolerated. Moreover, inasmuch as accommodation is a bilateral act in that it occurs equally in both eyes, there is no internal adjustment that one eye can make to compensate for this difference in refractive error. Because of difference in image size, fusion of images of unequal size becomes impossible. Normally a 1.50 diopter difference in the refractive errors between the two eyes is quite easily managed with the retention of binocular vision. In large errors, in which the difference amounts to 1.50 to 3.00 diopters, fusion can take place for large and gross objects. With greater differences, some adjustment in binocular vision occurs. For example, the child may learn to alternate his or her vision, that is, to use one eye for distance and one eye for near. This is especially apt to occur when one eye is far-sighted and the other near-sighted.

If the refractive error is negligible in one eye and great in the other eye, the individual tends to suppress the image in the eye with greater refractive error. This is especially true if the eye involved has a large astigmatic error, so that vision for both distance and near is foggy. The constant habit of suppression leads to loss of vision or *amblyopia from disuse*.

This condition is preventable because useful vision can be retained if the error in the defective eye is corrected early enough in life and the use of the eye is encouraged at the time by suitable patching or other exercises.

ANISEIKONIA

Another problem caused by unequal refractive errors is the development of *aniseikonia*. In this condition the differences in the size of the retinal image affect the patient's spatial judgments. This is not a common complaint and it is most readily found in people who use spatial judgments at all times in their daily work. People such as carpenters, interior designers, engineers, and artists are most prone to speak of disorders in spatial perception. These patients complain of visual discomfort, fatigue, headaches, distortion of objects, slanting of tables, dipping of surfaces, and so forth. Diagnosis of this condition is made with the patient's history and simple screening tests; for example, the patient reports a rectangular card as trapezoidal. Measurement of aniseikonia can be performed with a special instrument called a *space eikonometer*.

Treatment

When anisometropia occurs in children, especially those younger than 12 years, every attempt should be made to induce them to wear the full correction. For adults, especially when the difference is only between 2.00 and 4.00 diopters, the full correction again should be given, and they should be encouraged to bear with this correction despite symptoms. Often after 3 to 4 weeks of wear, the symptoms of eyestrain disappear and adults become comfortable with their lenses. In older patients the visual discomfort often becomes intolerable, so that it is frequently advisable to undercorrect the eye with the higher refractive error.

Anisometropia and aniseikonia are treated more successfully today with contact lenses, particularly in the young child who has not yet developed amblyopia. Prisms correct the secondary muscular imbalance; iseikonic glasses also are used to treat this problem.

APHAKIA

Aphakia is a condition in which the crystalline lens is absent from the eye. This may be caused by removal of a cataractous lens, or by displacement of the lens from the pupillary space by trauma.

Today implant surgery is performed in most countries, but there are still a dwindling number of patients who have cataract surgery in earlier years without benefit of an implant.

Correction of aphakia is perhaps the most difficult task for the refractionist. The intraocular lens (IOL) today represents the most suitable form of visual rehabilitation after cataract surgery. When indicated, a contact lens may be used. With a contact lens the magnification is only 7%, compared with 33% for an aphakic spectacle lens. The visual adjustments and distortions with a contact lens are considerably reduced compared with those with spectacles. However, the tendency is toward implants in all new cataract procedures. This is called *pseudophakia*. Fortunately, *accommodating IOLs* permit the aphake to read.

Perhaps one of the most disturbing aspects of aphakic vision is the *jack-in-the-box phenomenon*. In this situation the aphakic person finds an object through the edge of the spectacles and looks toward it, only to see that it is gone. *Aphakic vision, even though it results in 20/20 vision, requires a complete visual reorientation*. Spatial relationships, distances, and spatial judgments are all altered with this new type of vision.

An aphakic eye can never work together with a normal eye. This is because an aphakic eye essentially is a very far-sighted eye and the anisometropia induced is too great to overcome. Unless one uses a contact lens on the operated eye, it will not coordinate with the unoperated eye.

1. The optical centers must be exact because even a slight error causes a prismatic displacement with a thicker aspheric correction.
2. The distance of the trial lens from the eye and the eventual spectacle glass also must correspond. The distance of the eye from the trial lens (vertex distance) can be measured with a distometer. If this notation is put down on the prescription card, the opticians can make the suitable adjustment in power.
3. The periphery of the lens must be ground off. This type of lens is referred to as a lenticular aphakac lens. The lenticular aphakac lens serves to reduce the weight of the glass and abolish the extreme aberrations occurring from the periphery of a normal aphakic spectacle. Newer forms of aspheric spectacles are less curved in the periphery with use of an aspheric front surface instead of a lenticular design.
4. The frames must fit comfortably on the nose and be set straight. Fortunately, the era of aphakia is over because every cataract removal operation is replaced by an intraocular lens.

WHEN TO REFRACT AFTER CATARACT SURGERY

Historically it was taught that at least 6 weeks were required after a cataract operation before aphakic lenses could be prescribed. The final prescription was then given when, after a recheck 1 week later, the prescription was still the same. With small-incision cataract surgery, the time has been compressed considerably. Some surgeons use the keratometer as a guide and perform refraction when the K readings are stable between two visits.

There has been a marked change in cataract surgery. The phacoemulsification and femtosecond laser method has become accepted and is in widespread use. This method requires only a 1- to 3-mm incision. These patients are mobile almost as soon as the procedure is finished and they can undergo refraction early. Almost all patients today receive lens implants, and the refraction must be performed over the implant. Often glare of the implant can be a problem to the retinoscopist. The surgeon must make the decision as to the timing of a preliminary refraction.

Refractive points specific to the aphakic and pseudophakic person

The aphakic (no lens implant) and pseudophakic person may not have a healthy eye, and the vision may not be refined to 20/20 or 6/6. The eye may have suffered surgical trauma, such as cystoid edema of the macula, or may have macular degeneration. Cataract patients generally are older adults and may have degenerative ocular manifestations such as glaucoma or optic atrophy. A multiple pinhole may be used to start refraction to assess the potential of the eye.

The use of retinoscopy may be awkward in many ways. The patient who has no accommodation and has hazy vision cannot fixate accurately. The eye may move because of lack of fixation or lack of attention and concentration. If the patient does not hold the eyes steady, erratic and confusing scissor movements of the retinoscopy reflex may occur. Also, the axis and the amount of astigmatism will be difficult to gauge.

We have found keratometry an important reference starting point in pseudophakia, particularly when the retinoscopy shadows are poor.

In pseudophakia, with an intraocular lens, the problems are different. The pupil after an implant procedure may be small, and the retinoscopy shadows are more difficult to assess. If the pupil is small, frequently the surgeon will authorize the use of a mydriatic agent for the refraction. An ophthalmic assistant should not even consider dilating the eyes of a patient with an iris-supported intraocular lens without instructions from the surgeon. Fortunately these lenses are uncommon today. Dilation in older iris-supported implants may be a pivotal step in dislocating the lens. In pseudophakia, retinoscopic examination in the direct visual axis frequently causes disturbing reflections from the intraocular lens surface. These annoying reflections can be avoided by moving side to side until a good reflex is obtained.

Procedure after cataract surgery

After cataract surgery, keratometric reading, which provides the starting point for refraction, can be obtained. Often the glare induced by the intraocular lens implant makes retinoscopic examination difficult. Once the keratometric readings are stable between visits, the final refraction can be considered. The autorefractor, used with dilated pupils, also may provide a good starting point for refraction.

Cataract lens

Aphakic lenses for the person who has had cataract surgery without benefit of an intraocular lens are fast disappearing. Up until the early 1970s almost all patients underwent this procedure and required cataract glasses. Many cases today have been reversed by *secondary implants* or the benefits of contact lenses, thus eliminating the problems induced by aphakic glasses. Despite these advances, some individuals are still wearing these cataract glasses.

The bull's-eye lenticular lens, a bulbous lens mounted on a plano carrier, has given way to the more cosmetically acceptable, highly aspheric lenses. These lenses are lighter and can be dispensed in a fashion frame. The optical effect is outstanding. The field of clear vision is enlarged and the pincushion distortions are reduced to a minimum.

These lenses commonly have up to a 4.00 diopter drop in power at the periphery of the lens. This aspheric effect creates a marked improvement in the patient's cosmetic and functional rehabilitation.

The patient still has a 30% magnification of image size, but other features of lens scotoma, jack-in-the-box phenomenon, distortion, and field limitation, which are present in regular aphakic lenses, are greatly reduced with the highly aspheric lenses. These lenses also are lighter and more comfortable, with less of a tendency to slide down the nose.

Presbyopic intraocular lenses of various designs are rapidly being developed by several companies, and their success rate in offering the presbyopic patient ability to read at distance and near is becoming predictable.

PRESBYOPIA

Everyone becomes presbyopic with age. The accommodative ability decreases because of loss of the strength of the ciliary muscle and hardening of the lens. However, not everyone who is 45 or older needs reading glasses. Myopic patients do not because they can simply take off their glasses to read. Those who are near-sighted in one eye may not be aware of this anomaly and may carry on happily without a reading aid indefinitely. Also the needs of people differ. An architect will require reading glasses long before a waiter will. Some people do not read or sew and have little use for a reading assist at any time. Thus the correction of presbyopia is not just optical. The needs of the individual must be kept in mind. What does the person do? What lighting is available? The brighter it is, the better. How much reading is done and at what distance? Does the person need to look up and down to see distance and near for occupational reasons? Are the person's symptoms genuine, or is stress or anxiety making reading difficult?

Symptoms

The primary feature of presbyopia is an inability to do close work. Initially it manifests as difficulty in seeing the telephone book ("the print is grayer now") or a problem in seeing the menu in dimly lit restaurants. Presbyopic individuals cannot see small print or see without good illumination. They may increase lighting to see clearly. Light adds contrast and constricts the pupil to a pinhole aperture. Some people complain that they have to hold the print farther away, so eventually they are reading with an uncomfortable reach, complaining that their arms have become too short. Other symptoms include fatigue with reading, grittiness of the eyes with prolonged close work, and trouble with threading a needle.

Treatment

Two types of spectacle lenses are available for the treatment of presbyopia: the reading glass and the bifocal (regular, trifocal, or graded). Psychologically, most new presbyopes are much more receptive to the idea of reading glasses. They are referred to as *working glasses, sewing glasses, library glasses*, in other words, by any term that denotes their use rather than the patient's advancing age. Bifocals conjure up a picture of one's grandmother and represent the first step toward declining vigor and old age.

If the patient's distance vision is adequate, reading glasses are usually prescribed first. The patient is, however, warned that the glasses will help only to read at near. They will blur things if they are used for distance work. The patient also is told that with time the reading glasses now prescribed will no longer suffice as accommodation declines. Many patients think that with time the glasses seem to get stronger, rather than thinking that an intrinsic disorder of the eye is becoming more pronounced. Even if the patient requires glasses for distance, it is often best to give the patient a separate pair of reading glasses for close work. Most patients have several friends or relatives who have had difficult times in adjusting to bifocals, and the patients will relate these stories with great relish. For this reason, and for psychologic considerations, the patient is best left to cope with trying to use two pairs of glasses. Once patients have become sufficiently harried trying to use two pairs they will return, asking for bifocals and will adjust to them quite comfortably. The optician can be of great service in helping patients choose the proper bifocal. For individuals who are conscious of their appearance, no-line bifocals are available *(progressive no-line lenses)*.

Some presbyopes complain that their glasses are too strong. When bifocals are prescribed, the near point of accommodation is measured in each eye with the patient's distance spectacles in place. It is customary to give the weakest possible lens that will enable the patient to see at a comfortable working or reading distance. The stronger the lens given for a bifocal addition, the shorter will be the patient's range of focus. This loss of range can be quite disabling for the executive who must see the corner of the desk or for the typist who has to look away at approximately 30 inches (75 cm) to see the typing. Therefore, when lenses are prescribed, it always is advisable to leave some accommodation in reserve. In fact, the rule in prescribing near corrections is to give that correction which will leave half the amplitude of accommodation in reserve.

When strong bifocal additions are required, such as +2.00 to +2.50 or sometimes +3.00, the range of focus is compromised by necessity. For those patients whose occupations demand an intermediate zone—that is, an ability to read at 1 meter—trifocals are used, the trifocal being one-half the strength of the bifocal. Trifocals should not be prescribed with abandon, because to most patients trifocals mean three times as much trouble as "regular" glasses. An individual with a +2.50 correction can see clearly only objects located at about 16 inches (40 cm) away. Anything farther than this distance is fuzzy. Progressive or no-line lenses are another option.

Tests for the correct power

The simplest way to test for the correct power is to allow patients to hold a reading chart at their own preferred reading distance and prescribe the lens that gives the needed clarity. A reading add of less than +1.00 diopter does not offer real assistance, and anything greater than +3.00 diopters makes the focal point too close and the reading distance too narrow to work in.

Why not give all patients a +2.50 add when they are 45 years of age and let them grow into that prescription at 65 years of age? This would be a good idea in cost terms, but a doctor could lose his or her entire practice. The stronger the lens, the greater the weight factor, the aberrations, and the distortions and the closer the work distance.

Visual age considerations are as follows:

- At ages 42 to 45: a +1.00 to +1.25 is appropriate.
- At ages 45 to 50: a +1.50 to +1.75 is a common strength.
- At ages 50 to 65: a +2.00 to +2.50 or even +3.00 is common.

The strength of the add varies with the refractive error, being greater with hyperopic people and the presence of pathologic conditions. Cataracts or macular degeneration may demand the higher magnification gained by closer reading distance, and the strength of the add varies with the individual's needs.

Each eye should be tested individually and a record made as 20/20 or J1 and so on. The reading chart is a simple ready test and is desirable because the patient selects the reading distance. A variable light source helps simulate the patient's own illumination at work or home.

Another method is to test the amplitude of accommodation. This is merely the closest focal point at a given print size. For example, if a person's vision begins to blur at 25 cm, the amplitude of accommodation is 4.00 diopters. The patient is given a lens that leaves half the amplitude of accommodation in reserve. If the patient has to work at 33 cm and requires 3.00 diopters of accommodation, then only a +1.00 diopter add is needed. One-half the amplitude of accommodation is 2.00 diopters. To summarize, the need of accommodation is 3.00; thus the added plus strength of the reading aid is +1.00.

The dynamic cross-cylinder test also is useful. A +0.50 cyl/−0.50 cyl is the one most commonly used. A grid made up of horizontal and vertical lines is the test target. The patient wears the distance correction. If the astigmatism has been properly corrected, the grid lines should be equally clear. The cross cylinder, with minus axis vertical, is added. Plus spheres are added, increasing the power until the vertical lines are clearer. At the same time, spherical power is reduced until the lines are again equally clear. The add is the difference between the total spherical power for near and distance correction.

This test has application for patients in whom the amplitude of accommodation is difficult to measure. It is not a preferred method, however.

Prescription

Patients should be given what they need. A man who works in a factory and walks around with safety glasses requires bifocals. He cannot walk with reading glasses. The same may be said for the musician who must look at the music and see the conductor. This person cannot see in the distance with reading glasses.

Reading glasses should be given in the following circumstances:

1. As a first lens when applicable
2. Whenever one is in doubt about which lens to prescribe
3. For people who spend most of the day reading, writing, or working at a fixed distance

Bifocals should be considered for the following patients:

1. One who requires distance and near vision within moments, for example, a teacher
2. One who already wears distance glasses; two pairs of glasses, one for distance and one for near, are too cumbersome for efficiency
3. One who is disgruntled with reading glasses (no other options are available in a spectacle design and the choice is limited to bifocals or readers)

Do's and don'ts

1. Do not prescribe bifocals for a −1.50 diopter myope. The simplest and cheapest device may be to take off the glasses, which is similar to opening a window; it always is much clearer to look through an open window.
2. Bear in mind that plastic and glass lenses absorb some light transmission.
3. Do not overcorrect the patient's vision. The greatest source of aggravation is with lenses that are too strong.

4. Never prescribe trifocals as an initial lens. A trifocal is used for intermediate range and is half the strength of the bifocal. Usually the bifocal must be a +2.00 diopter in power before a trifocal is valid. The trifocal is +1.00 diopter. This is too complicated and heavy a prescription for a first-time user.

5. Do warn patients of the difficulties and limitations of seamless or no-line bifocals. The no-line or invisible bifocal, often called progressive bifocal, although popular for cosmetic reasons, may induce marked astigmatism when the eyes wander to the sides of the bifocal segment. Some invisible or no-line bifocal lenses have larger clear fields than others, but all contain some limitation of clear, undistorted field in the reading portion. Newer adaptations of these lenses, which go under the trade names of Varilux III (Comfort), Multilux, and Omnifocal, have addressed this problem and have improved the quality of vision, but the fault remains. These lenses are expensive and promise a great deal. Optically they remove image jump and sharp transitions of focal power. Patients should be informed. This problem is covered in more detail in Chapter 13.

6. Do not change the prescription of a bifocal until the fit has been appraised. The top of the segment on flat-top segment bifocals (used to minimize image jump in looking from near to far) should be at the level of the lower lid. If the segment is too high, it will cut into the distance segment. If the segment is too low, it will add plus power to the prescription and the patient will in effect have a stronger spectacle. The fit of a bifocal affects the power, the field of vision, the image size, and the distortion factor. Always look at what the patient is wearing before reordering lenses, especially if the complaint regards a new set of spectacles. The flat-top bifocal is conspicuous. If the patient has strong feelings about the symbolic act of moving into bifocals, then respect this attitude. Some people's jobs depend on looking "young"—for example, entertainers, salespeople, and media people—and these individuals frequently prefer a no-line or progressive bifocal.

7. Always check the reading segment monocularly. Sometimes a difference in the prescription between the two eyes indicates a fault in the distance correction. Most people have equal accommodative reserve, and the bifocal addition should usually be the same. If unequal adds are required, an error in distance correction or some pathologic condition should be suspected.

8. Do not prescribe a bifocal if patients can read with their distance glasses. If patients can read through the distance segment, they often never get used to the bifocal segment. It is an intrusion in the field. Besides, they do not need a reading addition.

9. Look at the reading pattern when deciding between bifocals or reading glasses. Bifocals work well for people who drop their eyes to read, because bifocals do not upset any ingrained visual habits. But for those who lower their heads and always look through the center of the lenses, reading glasses should be considered.

Myths to be dispelled

The following myths need to be dispelled:

Myth 1. *Reading glasses ruin powers of accommodation and contribute to the aging of the eye.* In reality, new bifocal wearers quickly become dependent on and enjoy the reading additions. Further loss of accommodation would have occurred anyway.

Myth 2. *Bifocal wearers, in the main, have a difficult time adjusting to bifocals.* In reality, the vast majority (a clinical guestimate is more than 90%) have no difficulty in adapting to bifocals.

Myth 3. *Bifocals are a hazard when a person walks down stairs.* In reality, myopic persons with vision of this power, without glasses, have no difficulty in descending stairs.

Myth 4. *Bifocals should be worn for racquet sports to see the ball close in.* In reality, they should not be worn. Only distance spectacles are needed. Bifocals are not only unnecessary, they are a hazard to the game itself and create blind spots.

Myth 5. *Presbyopia is a disease and the eyes become weaker with age.* In reality, presbyopia is a normal change in the refractive error associated with the aging process. It is not a disease. The crystalline lens of the eye loses its ability to accommodate because of changes in the lens fibers. Presbyopic individuals see 20/20 for distance and near and merely require different lenses to accommodate their needs. Presbyopic eyes are healthy.

COMPLAINTS: HOW TO ANTICIPATE THEM

Most frames are designed by fashion people in Paris, Italy, or New York and are not particularly practical from an ophthalmic point of view. In the merchandising of lenses, style has become paramount and function downgraded.

A few key points will provide assistance to the patient and prevent much grief at a later date.

1. Jumbo frames are a very poor idea for someone with a large refractive error. People who have worn small frames before and want to move into a high-fashion style should not be encouraged. Large lenses induce large aberrations and increase the weight of the lenses. People will complain of ocular vertigo and blurred vision because of the sliding effect every time they look down.

2. Impact-resistant lenses should always be ordered. In many states and countries this is law, but an ever-present element of neglect or indifference exists and somehow the cheaper lenses occasionally find their way into the market. A lens should be a protection, not a liability. Safety standards for every country are not the same.

3. Bifocals less than +1.25 diopters should not be prescribed. The disadvantages of a new bifocal do not warrant a new device with minimal advantages. Also, people tend to like high magnification when being tested and resent the same prescription in their ordinary lives. The ophthalmologist should not overplus a bifocal. When in doubt the rule is, do not change the glasses.

4. Tints should not be prescribed in lenses for indoor use. A tinted lens reduces contrast and makes reading more difficult. A tint, even though slight, makes driving in dim illumination hazardous. Besides, tints can distort colors. A blue tint can make the person more myopic. When driving at night, it enhances the normal night myopia.

5. When a high prescription has been given, it is important to check that the base curve has not been changed. A change of base curve or a change in the tilt of the lens may induce unwanted aberrations.

6. Glasses for older adults should not be changed unless significant visual gains can be made, at least two lines. Frequently, vision of older adults is undercorrected because of slight hardening or sclerosis of the lens of the eye. These patients often like being a little undercorrected for distance and overcorrected at near.

7. Plastic tends to be softer than glass and scratches more easily. This disadvantage is compensated by the lightness. Plastic lenses also do not shatter, a fact of importance when dealing with a high myope who has lenses that are very thin at the center. Plastic frequently results in a thick lens and may not be desirable as a social lens. This consideration can be dealt with by making the lens one-third thinner with flint glasses, which have a higher index of refraction. These lenses should not be used for children or adults working in industry because they are more brittle.

GLASSES CHECKS AND HOW TO HANDLE THEM: 12 KEY POINTS

When a complaint is received from a patient who is unhappy with new glasses, public relations skills are important. Someone may have made a mistake, so it is best to check the total prescription. Arrogance, dismissal, and clichés like "You will get used to your prescription" will drive the patient to obtain a second opinion and jeopardize the doctor's reputation with that family. The following 12 key points should be checked:

1. Poor centration. It is possible that the lenses are not centered properly. The optical centers of the lenses should be checked and aligned with the eyes.

2. Large frames. The frames may be too large compared with the patient's old glasses. If so, the patient will experience new distortions, particularly from the periphery of the lens. It may be necessary to go back to the old size of frames.

3. Incorrect prescription. The lenses should be checked on the lensmeter. They may not be correct. Not only can the doctor make a mistake, but the optician and laboratory are also capable of the same sin.

4. Vertex problem. The distance the present lenses are set from the eyes should be compared with that of the old spectacles. If the vertex distance is not the same as the old lenses, or has not been corrected in the prescription with refractive errors greater than 4.00 diopters, then the power will be wrong.

5. Frame problems. Do the frames slide up and down the nose with head movement in reading? Parallax may be a factor here.

6. Unwanted prism. Because of faulty centration, prisms may be introduced that cause induced phorias, either vertical or horizontal. This is more common in strong reading glasses.

7. Base curve. Have the new lenses been made up on the same base curve as the old ones? A change may cause difficulty. A Geneva measure may be useful.

8. Stress lines. Are there stress lines in the lenses? Have the lenses been crimped into the frames? Crimping occurs when lenses are inserted in frames under pressure. It downgrades the quality of vision. Perceived through the lenses, crimping can be detected by viewing with a double Polaroid filter (Wilson polarizer) and viewing through the spectacles. If lenses have been crimped in the frames, it will produce distortions in vision (Figure 11.18).

9. Thick lenses. Are the lenses thicker than they need to be for the power involved, resulting in excessive glass to look through centrally?

10. Tilt. Are the lenses tilted adequately for reading or is the patient reading obliquely through the lenses?

11. Correction of nondominant eye. Has the nondominant eye been corrected so that it has far better vision than the dominant eye? This may result in some difficulties. Check for eye dominance.

12. Segment line of bifocal. Is the lens set too high or too low and interfering with some of the visual pathways, particularly during walking or working? Are the segment heights symmetric?

The prescription should be reviewed. The doctor should rerefract and check the sphere cylinder and axis. An axis change of 10 degrees from previous glasses may not be

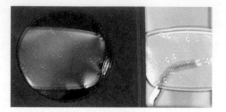

Figure 11.18 The quality of the spectacle lens viewed against a bright background with Polaroid filters can show crimping in frames, producing distortion in glasses that may cause eyestrain or asthenopia.

tolerated even if correct. In higher-cylinder corrections, an axis change of more than 5 degrees may not be tolerated.

If the prescription is wrong, the patient should be told. It is better to admit to an honest mistake and ask the lens company to replace rather than continue a subterfuge.

Cycloplegic drops should not be used for recheck. The prescription may be different with a smaller pupil. Also, the smaller the pupil, the greater the depth of focus, a factor that must be taken into consideration.

SUMMARY

Refraction is an art that requires patience, practice, and contact with many people before excellence is attained. Glasses must fill a particular need, and in the final analysis it is the need and not the refractive error that is paramount. The acme of visual efficiency—20/20 or 20/15 vision—is totally unnecessary in a 5-year-old child but may be vital to a young college student. Experience teaches us how to handle the presbyopic mechanic who must lie on his back and look directly at the undersurface of an automobile; the 65-year-old receptionist-typist who must be able to see across the room, type at 26 inches (66 cm), and read at 16 inches (40 cm); and the old, illiterate person who comes in for a check-up and neither reads, sews, nor does any close work whatsoever. In addition to knowledge of optics and the method of refraction, the refractionist must be congenial and a little talkative, at least enough to be able to assess the patient in terms of profession or work, hobbies, and special interests.

Questions for review and thought

1. Illustrate the convergence of parallel rays in an emmetropic eye, a myopic eye, and a hyperopic eye.
2. With full cycloplegia, one measures 3.00 diopters of hyperopia. Will the patient accept this amount in a pair of glasses? Explain.
3. Why does a young person not require as much hyperopic correction as an older person?
4. What is meant by axial myopia?
5. What are some of the causes that have been suggested for myopia? Which are possible?
6. When does myopia usually stop changing?
7. What is with-the-rule astigmatism?
8. Where is the axis of a minus cylinder in with-the-rule astigmatism? Of a plus cylinder?
9. What is irregular astigmatism? How is it treated?
10. Outline the value of automated refractors in clinical ophthalmology.
11. Outline the disadvantages of automated refractors versus retinoscopy and conventional subjective refraction.
12. Explain how the cross cylinder is used.
13. What is Placido's disc? What is its purpose?
14. Outline some of the problems inherent in the correction of aphakia by spectacles.
15. In a strong plus or minus prescription, of what importance is the distance of the spectacles from the eye? Explain.
16. What is the cause of presbyopia?
17. Discuss the shadows seen on retinoscopic examination of a myope.
18. What is the most common problem in the correction of presbyopia?
19. What is the purpose of a cycloplegic refraction?
20. What is a manifest refraction?
21. What is the greatest difference between the refractive errors of two eyes that are compatible with good fusion?
22. What is meant by eyestrain?
23. Outline methods of dealing with a patient who complains of an inability to wear prescribed glasses.

Self-evaluation questions

True–false statements

Directions: Indicate whether the statement is true **(T)** or false **(F)**.

1. The duochrome test is based on the fact that green is refracted behind the retina. **T** or **F**
2. Myopia is largely a hereditary disorder. **T** or **F**
3. Fogging involves discouraging accommodation by blurring the patient's eyes with plus spheres. **T** or **F**

Missing words

Directions: Write in the missing word in the following sentences:

4. Retinoscopy and the correction of astigmatism are best done with a _____ cylinder.
5. Retinoscopy can yield information on an irregular cornea because of _____ reflexes in the pupil.
6. Vertex distance measurements can be avoided by _____.
7. Automated objective refractors still require _____ testing.

Choice-completion questions

Directions: Select the one best answer in each case.

8. Aphakic spectacles cause which of the following problems?
   a. Magnification by 10%
   b. Barrel distortion
   c. Jack-in-the-box scotoma
   d. Variable vision
   e. Induced astigmatism
9. Presbyopia should first be corrected by:
   a. reading glasses to prevent it from getting worse.
   b. taking off the glasses if the patient is myopic.
   c. vitamin A.
   d. bifocals if the patient does not need a distance correction.
   e. a decrease in illumination.
10. The results of an automated refractor are least affected by:
    a. large pupils.
    b. cataract.
    c. small pupils.
    d. irregular astigmatism.
    e. corneal scarring.

A **Answers, notes, and explanations**

1. **False.** Green is refracted by the optical system of the eye so that a person with normal vision will have green focus in front of the retina and red focus behind the retina. A person who finds the letter on the green side more clearly in focus than that on the red requires plus correction.
2. **True.** Myopia is largely a hereditary disorder, but this is still debatable. Other causes have not been conclusively proved. Other claims of the causes of myopia that are without scientific validity are the following:
   a. Poor illumination
   b. Reading too much, with the eyes too close to the page or without the proper reading posture
   c. Dietary problems, particularly insufficient vitamins
   d. Glasses that have been fully corrected instead of being undercorrected
   e. Wearing glasses (that is, proper correction) too early in life
   f. A disease that makes the eyes "weak"
   g. A lack of proper eye exercises
3. **True.** It is vitally important in the refraction of the eyes of children or young adults to control accommodation so that this element can be eliminated from the tabulation of

a proper prescription. With children, short-acting cycloplegic drops are used. With many adults and in some practices, cycloplegic drops are not routinely used because of practical problems such as a patient with fully dilated pupils trying to drive an automobile on a bright day. Instead of "dropping" the eyes, fogging may be used to eliminate the accommodative component of the refraction. The pupils are not artificially dilated and a visual hazard is not created. The patient can drive home in safety or return to work or school. In addition, no deleterious side effects occur with fogging. It is a natural way to eliminate or reduce accommodation.

4. **Plus.** Plus cylinders are desirable because a "with" movement is easier to view in the pupil than an "against" movement. Because of this optical effect, the chance of making an error of retinoscopy is least when the reflex is neutralized from the plus side.
5. **Distorted or irregular.** The reflexes in the pupillary aperture should be regular and even. A distorted reflex means the corneal surface is irregular. This could be a result of surgery to the anterior segment, early keratoconus, "warping" of the corneal surface by an ill-fitting contact lens, or inflammation such as an old herpes scar.

A Continued

Whatever the cause, a proper refraction cannot be performed because there is no valid method of treating irregular astigmatism with regular lenses.

6. **Overrefraction.** There are two ways of handling vertex problems. One method is to make the calculation with a distometer and make the adjustment from distometer tables. A more accurate method is to overrefract over the patient's present spectacles and use the resultant power in a new prescription for the same frame.

7. **Subjective.** Subjective testing is most important after using an automated objective refractor. The refractor provides only the starting point; one must still obtain individual **responses** to the given refractive finding.

8. **c. Jack-in-the-box scotoma.** Aphakic spectacles do cause an increase in magnification of the image size but it is 30%, not 10%. They also cause distortion but the effect of this **distortion** is a pincushion type, with the sides sloping inward. Variable vision does not really occur with proper lenses. However, many aphakic patients receive a poor fit and the lenses may slide down the nose with reading. This slide is due strictly to the weight of the lens. The newer, lighter lenses control this variability caused by the slide of the frames. Chromatic aberration is a feature of many lenses, not just aphakic ones. Chromatic aberration is the break-up of white light into a spectrum of colors. The jack-in-the-box scotoma does occur with aphakic spectacles, and objects appear to dart suddenly into the peripheral field of the person wearing aphakic spectacles.

9. **b. Taking off the glasses if the patient is myopic.** Presbyopia should be corrected by the simplest device possible. A person who must work and walk around requires bifocals. A presbyope who is in industry requires safety glasses; thus there is no other option but bifocals.

   If the patient is near-sighted, an easy solution is to have that person remove the glasses. It is fast and inexpensive and the optical effect is the best if the vision is between −1.00 and −2.50 diopters.

   Reading glasses do not make presbyopia better or worse. One practical way to postpone presbyopia is simply to direct more light onto the page. An increase in illumination adds contrast, which is an excellent way to obtain greater clarity. It also makes the pupil smaller, thereby producing more of a pinhole effect.

10. **a. Large pupils.** Large pupils do not affect the result of the automated refractor. In fact, the opposite is true. Small pupils may yield no information, often because of misalignment.

Chapter 12

History of spectacles

*Hans-Walter Roth**

ANTIQUITY

No one knows when the earliest vision aids were used. There are no written recordings from early times. No paintings or sculptures showing optical devices or specimens from these times are available; the earliest known representation is in a church mural from the year 1270.

---

*Images in this chapter are courtesy of Hans-Walter Roth, with permission.

The ancients were surely aware of the optical effects of water or glass, for example, the magnifying effect of a drop of water, the enlarged view of a leaf vein seen through a dewdrop, or the visual effect through a spherical transparent jewel of the underlying surface.

Recent findings have shown that the Egyptians and Babylonians knew and used rules of optics. An optically useful lens with a refractive power of approximately +9.00 diopters was unearthed in Nimrod. Two optically polished spheres were found in the tomb of Tutankhamen, currently stored in the National Museum in Cairo.

Several optically excellent quartz spheres representing the eyes of a pharaoh were found among burial gifts. They still can be used as magnifying glasses for reading. Eyes in the statue of the god Horus in the British Museum in London show aspheric corneal surfaces, similar to the corneal curvature of a human eye. Collections of lenses in the museums of Cairo and of Athens indicate that the production of visual aids seems to have developed in parallel with the invention of writing. The rarity of the devices and reports perhaps reflects the limited population requiring such devices (i.e., priests and high public officials).

Earlier writings do not contain references to visual aids. The earliest description of sunglasses was made by Pliny (23–79 BC). He wrote that the Roman emperor Nero used a polished emerald to view the gladiators. He does not mention if the optical surface was spherical, but it is apparent that the light-absorbing nature of the gem made viewing in bright sunlight more pleasant. From the same era one can read complaints by older Roman statesmen that the condition of their eyes made reading of legal texts difficult. It is sure that presbyopia was considered a disease in ancient Rome, but no one documented any treatment with visual aids.

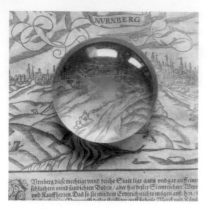

Figure 12.1 Reading stone, manufactured between 1250 and 1300.

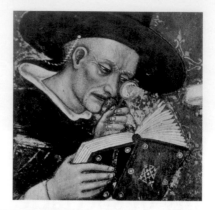

Figure 12.2 Single lens spectacle, Treviso, Italy, 1352.

THE BEGINNING

The earliest mention of a visual aid was the reading stone (Figure 12.1). It was described by the German poet Albrecht in 1270 as a magnifying glass. In the same year Konrad of Wuerzburg wrote about a crystal that enlarged printed letters. The shape and the polished surface reminded him of a large drop of water that when laid on a printed page greatly increased the size of the text. The stone was a polished hemisphere of the semiprecious gemstone beryl, which when laid on a page enlarged the text in all directions. The refractive power was +15.00 to +30.00 diopters, a power too great to correct presbyopia by wearing close to the eye.

EARLY EYEGLASSES

The inventor of spectacles, meaning glasses worn directly on the eyes, is unknown. Ptolemy wrote in about 125 BC concerning the enlarging ability of a spherical glass lens; the Saracen mathematician and astronomer Alhazen published the laws of refraction in 1028. The Oxford Franciscan monk Roger Bacon noted in 1267 that a presbyope could read the smallest printed letters with the aid of appropriately polished lenses.

Classic spectacles that are worn directly over the eyes appeared in more recent times when clear, transparent glass became available at a reasonable price. This first occurred on Murano, a small island near Venice still famous for the production of glass. There was mention of such eyeglasses in the official state documents around 1300. Developments from spectacle manufacturers no longer required that the lens be placed on the text to read; it could now be held in front of the eye. The earliest sample of such a spectacle is a single lens in the Church of Konstanz dating from 1270. The first colored painting showing this type of reading glass, constructed like a magnifier (Figure 12.2), dates from 1352 and is in the church of San Nicolo in Treviso, a small city near Venice. In this church one can also view the first representation of two lenses bound together, called *rivet spectacles*.

RIVET SPECTACLES

The early example in Figure 12.3 shows reading aids as a single lens or a pair of lenses called a *lorgnon*, which developed into modern spectacles. Two such lenses fixed together were designed to be held in front of the eyes to enable binocular reading. The two lenses were attached by a strap riveted to the frame of each lens, which enabled a variable interpupillary distance. This method of fabrication resulted in the name rivet spectacles.

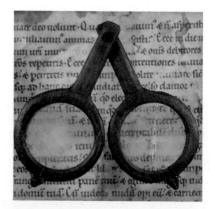

Figure 12.3 Rivet spectacle from about 1390, frame made of wood. Copper wires fix the glasses.

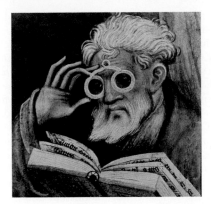

Figure 12.4 Rivet spectacle, from a church painting, 1405, Wildungen, Germany.

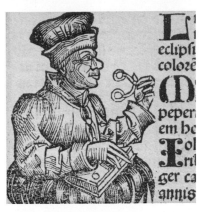

Figure 12.6 First printed example of a rivet spectacle, 1498, edited by Hartmann Schedel, Nuremberg.

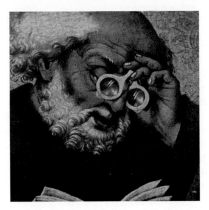

Figure 12.5 Rivet spectacle in a painting from 1466, Rothenburg, Germany.

Representations of this type of spectacle are frequently found in 15th- and 16th-century paintings; they enabled the clergy to read from scripture as is represented in the altar paintings shown in Figures 12.4 and 12.5. The cathedral in Ulm has a stained-glass window dated 1438 showing Peter with a pair of rivet spectacles. The earliest printed representation of a rivet spectacle is in the *World Chronicle* of H. Schedel printed in Nuremberg in 1498. In this illustration noted physicians, researchers, and scientists of that period wore rivet spectacles as signs of their educated background (Figure 12.6).

Samples of rivet spectacles are rare; the oldest were found in the cloister at Wienhausen in Germany. These visual aids had been hidden during a war and forgotten for many centuries. The frames were made of beechwood fixed together with copper rivets. By this simple technique the lenses could be made to fit any interpupillary distance and be centered over each eye.

MANUFACTURE

The increased market resulted in the production of glass reading glasses in Murano either by grinding and polishing or by casting in metal forms. The resultant high cost limited them to those who could afford them. The strength ranged from +2.00 to +3.00 diopters based on the requirements of the reader. This age group was 40 years or older, an age not attained by many in this time.

Glass lens manufacturing did not remain a Venetian monopoly for long. Efforts at duplication and improvements were made in many other countries, but initially Italy remained the only source of the glass. Numerous cities, for example, the free cities of Nuremberg and Augsburg, established firms solely for producing and selling reading lenses (Figure 12.7). These organizations soon established rules and regulations to guarantee quality control and thereby improve the marketability of their products. Competition of cheaper products was a factor; an early

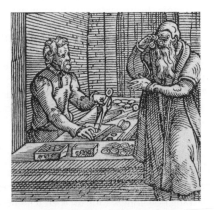

Figure 12.7 Early optic shop, printed 1525.

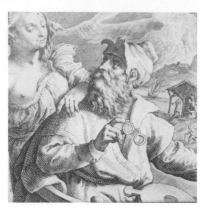

Figure 12.8 Spectacle with leather frame, from about 1560.

conference was held in Nuremberg to codify lens production and define the profession of spectacle manufacturers. To ensure quality control a guild was founded, and in Paris and London the regulations for teaching and awarding of Masters' documents were codified.

Minor improvements were made during the first century of spectacle making: better lens polishing, new methods of stabilizing the positioning of spectacles for reading, and some improvements in lens casting. The 16th and 17th centuries saw the appearance of less expensive spectacles, usually +3.00 diopters intended for presbyopes, framed in leather or iron. Products with horn, copper, or brass frames were made for the clergy or public officials, whereas those framed in gold, silver, or ivory were rarities reserved for the very wealthy.

We know more about the price of spectacles during this era than production details. Although cheap imports from Italy were available, none were reportedly sold through peddlers. Quality spectacles were available only from approved spectacle makers. Lenses framed in horn or leather (Figure 12.8) cost, on the basis of current value and quality, about 5 US dollars. This reflected the cost of currently available cheap glasses produced by mass production techniques.

The use of glasses appears often in paintings of the clergy, merchants, and artists, men whose livelihood required good reading vision. The common folk, for whom reading and writing were not an issue, obviously did not require them. Schools had to be founded in Europe, and printing presses made available before reading glasses became necessary for everybody who could read.

THE FRAME

It is astonishing how long it took for spectacles to be made in the current form. Initially frames were made of wood and later of metal, and a pair was connected with a scissors-like apparatus that could be opened or closed. This rather clumsy mechanism remained unchanged in common use for centuries, although it did not enable the lenses to be set at a fixed distance from the eyes or centered. Rivet glasses had to be held by hand until the 1600s, when someone thought of fixing them in front of the eyes by means of a leather strap or cord wrapped around the head. Others attached the glasses to a man's cap or wig; the variations were boundless. Famous people were shown in numerous paintings and etchings of the period wearing these variations. The Spaniard Benute de Valdes described spectacle wearing in his book dated 1623; the main themes were not only the various configurations but also the grading of lens strengths.

SCISSOR SPECTACLES AND FORK GLASSES

Rivet glasses evolved into scissor spectacles. As the name implies, the frame was scissor shaped, with lenses where the blades would be. Such glasses were useless for reading because the hand holding them blocked the view of the reading matter; this made them better for distance viewing. Most were made of horn and were often embellished with decorations, reflecting the taste of the wearer. Louis XVI of France, who was nearsighted, used costly scissor glasses to view court events.

Napoleon Bonaparte, his brother Jerome, and other noted persons of the Age of Absolutism used scissor glasses to correct refractive problems. They were not in general usage because they covered a large part of the face, especially the mouth.

In 1797 Dudley Adams recommended fixation of the lenses by a forehead band or bar. This not only permitted centration of the lenses along the optic axes of both eyes, but also enabled establishment of the correct interpupillary distance. This new state enabled lenses to be ground for distance vision. Because of the problems associated with the available methods for fixing the position of the lens in relationship to the eyes, many new methods were tried. To improve the comfort of glasses held in place by pressure, small cushions were made that were the precursors of today's nose pads. Another method used horn frames with ridged surfaces, the elasticity of the material enabling them to be held by a relatively small pressure on the bridge of the nose.

Gradually it was realized that there were many people with myopia who needed daily spectacle wear. This necessitated fixed lens positioning in front of the eyes and resulted in production of various models of iron, brass, and precious metals and later, in the United States, frames of buffalo horn. Most lenses were round, but they were available in oval shape in horn frames.

SINGLE LENSES AND MONOCLES

Next to the classic spectacles, the single lens was the most common alternative for many years. The lens could be positioned directly over the eye by hand or other methods. Interestingly, many of these lenses were concave for myopia. In 1585 William Bourne listed such glasses as perspective glasses. About this time, public wearing of spectacles was either frowned upon or forbidden, so single lenses, although difficult to wear, were an alternative. Shortly thereafter, in England, wearing glasses became stylish. Glasses were thought of as jewelry and were worn on a chain around the neck. Because of their ornamental status, they were completed by goldsmiths rather than by opticians.

The common man carried a single lens mounted in a grooved copper wire. Mass-produced versions such as the lorgnon made in Nuremberg (Figure 12.9) were priced for the average person.

Another form of the single lens is the so-called monocle worn by the British King Charles II. This version was held in front of the eye by compression from the musculus orbicularis. The edge of the frame was rounded and often grooved to improve wearing retention (Figure 12.10). Small loops were often attached to the frame to help keep the lens in place. To achieve greater distance between the eye and the lens and to increase comfort, an additional ring, a so-called gallery, was attached to offset the lens frame from the lids.

In 1727 Baron von Stosch appeared in public wearing a monocle. This had an effect on style-conscious people, who immediately adopted this form of eyewear. Scientists warned about the health-related dangers of such wear but this did not halt its use. The monocle increased in popularity for most of the ensuing two centuries, usually among the upper classes and especially military officers.

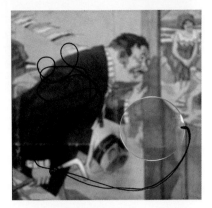

Figure 12.10 Model of a monocle, about 1870.

SPRING SPECTACLE FRAMES

These frames were common in various countries including England into the 18th century. An example was the invention of a variety of elastic metal nose clamps (Figure 12.11). Lenses were framed with metal, wood, horn, or leather. Later the entire apparatus including the metal hoops and nose clamps were made of the same metal, which enabled mass production of less expensive spectacles. These so-called spring frames were the forerunners of the *pince nez* (Figure 12.12). The French physician Joseph Bressy published a patent in 1825 for small, thin steel plates that held the frame on the nose with more or less comfort. Wearing oval lenses became common. Small nosepieces or patches lessened the uncomfortable pressure on the nose. An attached cord prevented the glasses from being dislodged onto the ground or secured them when they were not needed (Figure 12.13).

The variations in form were large. One type used a vertical construction to spread the glasses, another permitted adjustment of the interpupillary distance by moving the

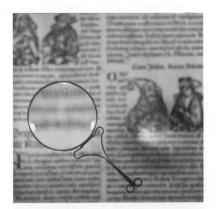

Figure 12.9 Monovision lens in copper frame, Nuremberg, about 1680.

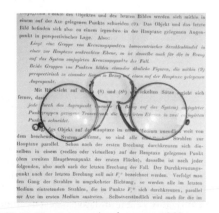

Figure 12.11 Pince nez made of copper, 1860.

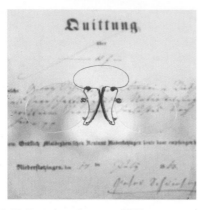

Figure 12.12 Frameless pince nez, 1870.

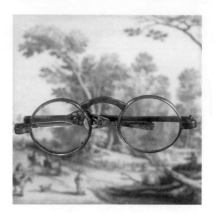

Figure 12.14 Early temple spectacle, brass frame, 1760.

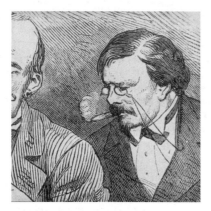

Figure 12.13 Pince nez with cord, 1890.

glasses along a horizontal axis, necessary in the correction of astigmatism with toric lenses.

For more than 100 years, until the time of the First World War, the primary method for visual correction required glasses to be held in place by being clamped to the bridge of the nose. This eyewear became a symbol of position and of intelligence because the main wearers were merchants or teachers. Military officers wore the monocle because other forms of visual aids were officially forbidden when on parade.

TEMPLE PIECES AND CURVED EARPIECES

In 1890 frames with sidebars, called *temple pieces,* were produced, some with curved portions that extended behind the ears. These additions provided a more secure fit on the head. The earpieces were present on the earliest form of temple pieces (Figure 12.14) and gave spectacles the configuration they have today. Extension of the sidebars behind

the ears became common at the start of the 20th century and provided an improved fit.

LORGNETTES

The *lorgnette* (Figure 12.15) evolved from the scissor spectacle; in 1770 George Adam introduced a glass case that could be used to store them. In 1800 the lorgnette was the most frequently used form of glasses and was produced in a multitude of variations. M. Lepage improved the mechanism in 1818 so the connections between the lenses permitted it to be folded. Pressure on a button released the glasses from the case.

The lorgnette was the typical eyewear of the bourgeoisie and was prized by prominent women, who often carried it as jewelry. Finally, by the onset of the last century, this style was converted into spectacles with curved earpieces.

Early glasses were used to correct for presbyopia and had a range of powers between +1.00 and +4.00 diopters. With the awareness of other refractive errors and the knowledge

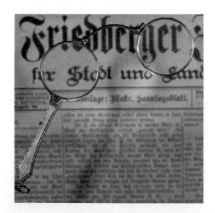

Figure 12.15 Spring glass or lorgnette, brass, about 1850.

that minus lenses could correct myopia, spectacles were developed for distant vision. These improvements brought the need to enable sharp vision at both near and far distance with one pair of glasses. The problem was solved with the invention in 1785 that joined two lenses of different refractive powers, or bifocals. The inventor was the American statesman and scientist Benjamin Franklin. John Hawkins improved the system in 1827 with the development of the trifocal lens.

It is astounding that before 1800 no one was aware that the human cornea has two major refractive zones, one vertical and the other horizontal. The English physicist and physician Thomas Young first reported this, but correction for astigmatism was not possible until 1825 when the Scottish astronomer George Airey created the first astigmatic lens for daily wear. In 1850 the first industrially produced lens containing a cylinder was manufactured by the best-known glass factory of the time, which was located in Rathenow. This commercial availability enabled correction of astigmatism in the general population.

The onset of the 19th century saw the use of biconcave or biconvex lenses. In a series of experiments, the English physician William Wollaston showed how the sharpness of vision can be improved when the refractive capabilities of lenses are better used; for example, in 1804 he reported that acuity can be increased when the concave surface of the lens faces the eye. Johannes Kepler had reported this principle in 1611 with the use of polished meniscal lenses. However, it was not until 1904 that the Danish ophthalmologist Hans Tscherning reported that the refractive benefit could be optimized by the use of so-called periscopic spectacle lenses.

It is amazing that the use of curved earpieces is only 100 years old and that it was not until 1906 that Moritz von Rohr of Zeiss Oberkochen developed the so-called punctal glass to eliminate peripheral visual images.

GOGGLES AND SUNGLASSES

Glasses have uses other than correcting visual anomalies, such as preventing injury from particulate matter or from glare. Pliny reported that Roman nobles viewed through a polished emerald for protection. In the 16th century spectacles were first tinted; this prompted scientific discussions regarding which color provided not only the most wearing comfort but also the greatest protection to the eye. The color of the oldest goggles was either yellow or blue (Figures 12.16 and 12.17), whereas Chinese glasses were tinted gray or yellow.

In 1885 the French ophthalmologist Fieusal was the first to connect glare sensitivity to a range of short-wave light and to recommend light absorption in this short-wave region. In 1912 the Swiss ophthalmologist Vogt reported

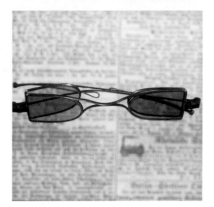

Figure 12.16 Sunglasses, blue tinted, 1750.

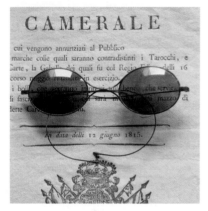

Figure 12.17 Sunglasses without refraction, blue, 1815.

that absorption of infrared radiation led to eye damage. In the following years the glass industry developed absorbing lenses that filtered out dangerous light radiation, permitting only harmless rays to impinge on the eye. Nowadays, more sunglasses than glasses for visual anomalies are worn.

GLASSES IN THE FAR EAST

Glasses are a classic, typical, and essential item in Asian culture. Although it may be assumed that glasses have been part of the culture for many years, there are no accounts in contemporary Chinese literature or encyclopedias indicating this. It is reasoned that Venetian merchants, including Marco Polo, introduced spectacles to the Chinese Empire. It is sure that during the 16th century glasses were imported because there is no record of any local manufacturing. The earliest Chinese-made spectacles had lenses of rock salt or quartz (Figure 12.18)

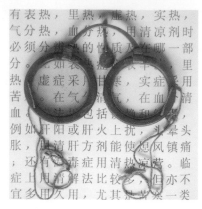

Figure 12.18 Chinese reading glasses, 1690.

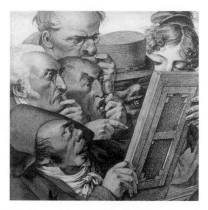

Figure 12.19 The upper class; French color print of 1875.

instead of glass. Also they were made not so much to correct refractive anomalies but to indicate the high social

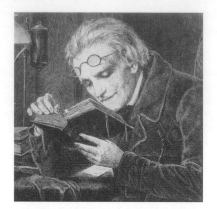

Figure 12.20 Modern spectacle for myopia, 1920.

position of the wearer. The configuration of spectacles copied those manufactured in Europe. In the early 20th century Chinese spectacles were made with curved earpieces.

SUMMARY

The history of spectacles is the history of scientific progress; it is an integral part of our culture (Figures 12.19 and 12.20).

Spectacles have enabled millions of people with visual problems to take part in daily life and to acquire an education. From their beginning as a reading lens made of the gemstone beryl, glasses have improved to include multifocal lenses, contact lenses, and implants into the living eye.

FURTHER READING

Corson R. Fashions in eyeglasses from the 14th century to the present day. London: Peter Owen; 1967.

Court TH, von Rohr M. On the development of spectacles in London from the end of the 17th century. Trans Opt Soc 1929;30:1–12.

Emsley HH, Percival AS. Percival and best form lenses. Man Opt 1963;17:21–3.

Hardy WE. An outline history of British spectacle making from 1629 onwards. Man Opt 1966;151:677–84.

McConnel JW. The history of spectacle lens correction in Germany. Man Opt 1967;20:260–70.

Poulet W. Atlas on the history of spectacles. Bonn/Bad Godesberg, Germany: Wayenborgh; 1978.

Rosen E. Did Roger Bacon invent eyeglasses? Arch Int Hist Soc 1954;7:32–41.

Roth HW. A contribution to the history of contact lenses. Bonn/Bad Godesberg, Germany: Wayenborgh; 1978.

Chapter | 13 |

Facts about glasses*

Melvin I. Freeman, Shoshana (Sue) M. Levine

Virtually every patient who enters an ophthalmologist's or other eye care practitioner's office receives a refraction and most receive a prescription for spectacles. Even if patients plan to use contact lenses as their main corrective device, they should have glasses for backup. Thus the ophthalmic assistant needs some information about the construction and types of spectacle frames and the types of lenses currently used.

Despite an accurate prescription, many patients are unhappy with their glasses because of the design, fit, or prescription. The goal of correcting a refractive error is not only to achieve the best possible vision for each eye, but also to do so with a pair of glasses that match the patient's aesthetics and lifestyle as well. Glasses that make the wearer feel good and look good are more likely to be worn regularly. The purpose of this chapter is to provide a brief résumé of the types of eyeglasses available to the patient, reviewing the advantages and disadvantages of each.

HISTORY

The use of spectacles has its origin in ancient history (Figure 13.1). In the early periods optical glass was of poor quality and was made from scarce pebbles of quartz or semiprecious stones. The first primitive spectacles were balanced precariously on the nose, tied to the ears by means of thread or string or held in the hand as one holds a present-day lorgnette. Their use was confined solely to monks and other learned men of the day. By the 17th century, spectacles were in common use and were elaborately fashioned of gold or silver for members of the aristocracy, whereas tortoiseshell frames were used by members of the upper middle class.

Despite the improvements and refinements in the manufacture and dispensing of frames, the final choice of the right set of spectacles is a personal one, derived not by any scientific formula but by the whims, fancies, and needs of the individual.

Today's fashion industry has influenced frame design tremendously. It is common to see fashionable frames with international designer names (e.g., Prada, Tom Ford, and Salvador Ferragamo). The stigma of wearing glasses has transcended into a fashion statement and has exploded into the sunglass arena. Frame selection has evolved from a simple visual necessity to a method of communicating a personal statement, a fashionable tool for displaying an image one wishes to present.

FRAMES

A frame for every face[†]

As a rule, frames look best when they complement a patient's facial form. Current fashion trends should be taken into account; if the style of the moment is small

---

*Chapter revision edited by Katy Murphy, COA.

[†]Modified from The Vision Council's website *Frame Shapes* (with permission).

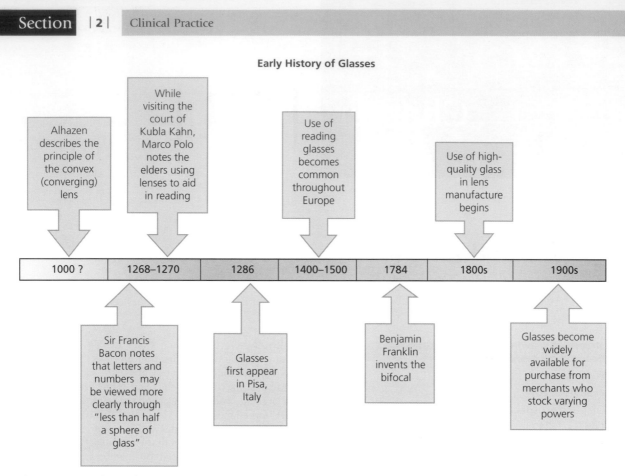

Figure 13.1 Timeline in the history of spectacles

round frames, public demand will lean in that direction. A knowledgeable assistant will be able to tell whether the trendy look suits a particular patient, and if not, what different styles to offer. Here it is best to refer to classic rules for assistance. The first step is to determine which of the seven basic face shapes the patient has: oval, diamond, round, square, base-down triangle, oblong, and inverted triangle (Figure 13.2).

The most flattering eyeglass frames are those that are the right depth and width for the face. Generally, a flattering frame shape is opposite to the face shape. A round face, for example, looks best with a squared, angular frame, not a rounded shape.

The Vision Council's website (www.eyecessorize.com) devotes an entire section to selecting the correct frame shape.

Oval: The chin is slightly narrower than the forehead and the cheekbones are high. There appears to be a natural facial balance. *Best options:* Choose frames that are as wide as or wider than the broadest part of the face. Select frames in proportion to the face size. Most frame shapes are good on an oval face.

Diamond: A small forehead and wide temple area gradually narrow to a small chin. Often, cheekbones are high and dramatic. *Best options:* To widen the forehead and jaw and to minimize the cheekbones and wide temple area, select frames that are top-heavy with sides that are straight or angled outward toward the bottom. Frames should be square, rimless, or shaped with a straight top and curved bottom. Avoid frames with decorative temples that make the middle of the face look wider.

Round: Full face with very few angles that appears equal in height and width. *Best options:* To make the face seem longer and thinner, select oval, slightly curved angular frames that feature high or mid-height temples. Clear bridges and color on the temple area flatter this face.

Square: This face has a broad jawline and forehead, with wide angular cheekbones and chin. *Best options:* To lengthen the face, try subtly curved frames, no wider than the widest part of the face. For a high-style look, experiment with stark, geometric shapes that have color concentrated on the outside corners. Square faces can also wear top-heavy frames, oval shapes with temples in the

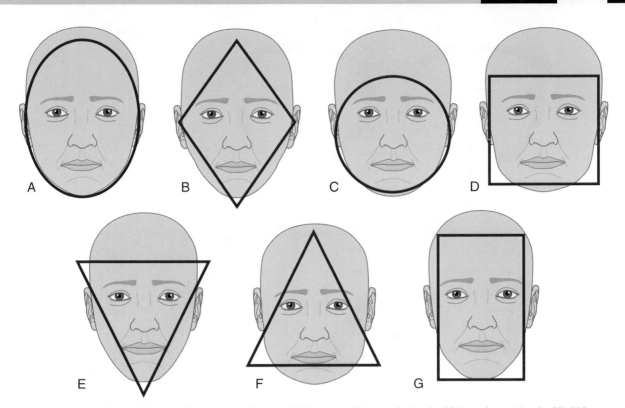

Figure 13.2 Face shapes. (A) Oval. (B) Diamond. (C) Round. (D) Square. (E) Inverted triangle. (F) Base-down triangle. (G) Oblong. *(Modified from photos courtesy of The Vision Council.)*

center, and frames with decorative temples hinged above the eye level.

Inverted triangle: Below a wide forehead, this face shape narrows into high cheekbones and a narrow chin. *Best options:* To add width to the chin and cheeks, select frames that angle outward at the bottom but are no wider than the forehead. Low temples, light colors, and rimless styles balance the face. Frames with rounded tops and square bottoms, aviators, and butterfly shapes are other options.

Base-down triangle: A narrow forehead becomes fuller at the cheeks and chin. *Best options:* Frames should add width to the forehead but soften and narrow the jaw, chin, and cheeks. Flattering frames angle outward at the top corners. They should be as wide as or slightly wider than the broadest part of the jaw. Square, aviator, and metal frames with rimless bottoms are flattering selections, or try top-heavy frames with angled bottoms.

Oblong: This face shape is longer than it is wide and the forehead, cheek, and jawline are comparable in width. *Best options:* To shorten and widen the face, select styles that extend beyond the widest part of the face. Choose frames with decorative temples, strong top bars, and round bottom lines. Round, deep, or square shapes shorten and soften an oblong face.

Although fashion is key to frame design, so too are comfort, durability, and thinness. A wide range of frame materials is available; each has its own characteristics.

Spectacles can be defined as an optical appliance composed of lenses and a frame with sides, called *temples*, extending over the ears. The front, main part of the frame holds the actual lenses in front of the eyes, the pads give support on the nose, and the temples hold the front part in the correct position before the eyes. Frames may be made of metal, rubber, wood, plastic, or a combination of metal and plastic.

Figure 13.3 illustrates the anatomy of frames. Bridge size may be noted as distance between lenses (DBL), which should not be confused with the distance between the (optical) centers (DBC). Temples often are marked with the overall temple length expressed in either inches or millimeters. When two numbers are found on the temple, both overall length and length to the bend are given.

Metal frames

Originally, frames were designed and handmade of silver or solid gold for the aristocracy. These metals have gradually been replaced by other metals, such as gold-filled,

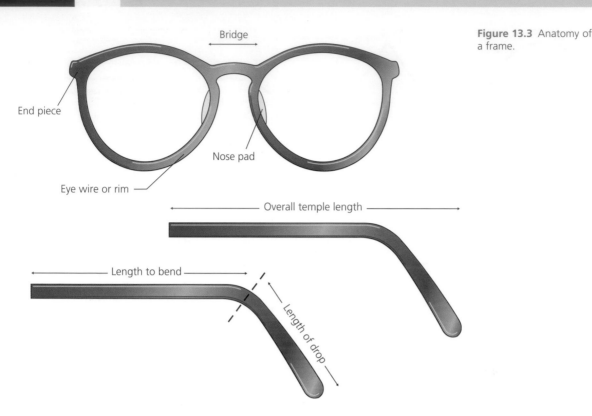

Figure 13.3 Anatomy of a frame.

nickel, aluminum, stainless steel, memory metal such as Flexon, and titanium (Table 13.1).

Plastic and composite frames*

There are two types of plastic frames: those molded to shape from *plastic materials* in an injection-molding machine and higher-quality frames cut to shape from a flat piece of plastic, which is then machined and polished to form the finished frame.

Ophthalmic frames made from different types of plastic and composite materials include the following:

Propionate is a spun cast, easy to manufacture lightweight plastic with translucent colors to rival Optyl. It is easily recognizable and needs only a hot-air blower for adjustments. Propionate holds its shape well but, like all plastic, this feature depends on the manufacturing quality. *SPX* is stronger and more flexible than propionate, enabling the production of very thin plastic frames. If SPX is overheated, it will shrink and not return to its original size. Thus lenses are mounted while the frame is warm or at room temperature.

Cellulose acetate is a common plastic used today that comes in various colors and patterns. It will burn if a flame is held in contact with the material, but is self-extinguishing; when the flame is removed, the plastic will cease to burn. Clear acetate will not change color or yellow with age, and cellulose acetate does not become brittle.

Lucite (Plexiglas, Perspex) is a much tougher plastic and is available in solid colors only (or two-tone or fade-away patterns, produced by laminating two colors). Once the frame is fitted, it retains its shape better than cellulose acetate or nitrate. Lucite does not change color, but manipulation requires much more heat than do other materials.

Nylon (Grilamid, Trogamid) frames are lightweight, hypoallergenic, and relatively unbreakable. They are injection molded and thus of one solid color. Some types are dyed after completion to give the appearance of stock sheet materials also found in cellulose acetate. Nylon requires a high temperature to glaze. Lenses should be cut as close as possible to final size and shape. Because nylon can become dried out, patients should soak the frames in water monthly.

Polycarbonate frames are a good choice for safety and sports use because they have high impact resistance. The frames are clear so they do not block the field of vision. They are not adjustable, but elastic straps and rubber bridge pieces offer flexibility and comfort.

*In part from Stein HA, Freeman MI, Stenson SM. *CLAO residents curriculum manual on refraction, spectacles and dispensing.* Metairie, LA: CLAO Publications, 2001 (with permission).

Table 13.1 Metal frames: characteristics of the most common types in current use

Material	Composition (%)	Features	Adjustment considerations
Nickel/silver	Nickel (18) Copper (64) Zinc (16)	Shock-resistant flexibility Suitable hardness for precision metalwork Some anticorrosion	Cold bend tools Excess heat in soldering will weaken
Monel	Nickel (66) Copper (27) Various (7)	Harder than nickel/silver Very high heat resistance; no weakness from soldering Uses: bridge, temples, sometimes because material is more rigid and stronger	Cold bend tools Monel and nickel/silver solder well together
High-nickel alloy	Nickel (85–90) Chrome (10–13)	10 times more expensive than nickel/silver Extremely hard; used in bridges and endpieces where pressure is high	Cold bend tools Solderable
Stainless steel	Nickel (10) Iron (65) Chromium (19) plus carbon, manganese, phosphorus, sulfur (6)	Extremely flexible Extremely hard Can be made thinner, thus lighter Corrosion immunity	Cold bend tools Cannot be soldered by conventional means
Titanium	A silver-gray element alloyed with other elements	Maximum flexibility of materials used to date Extremely strong; can be made very thin High memory retention Ultralightweight frame material Immune to corrosion High heat resistance	Cannot solder with existing techniques
Aluminum	Alloyed with copper, silicone, iron, bronze, manganese, zinc, chromium	Lightweight frame material Must be made thicker to increase strength Poor corrosion resistance unless colored	Cold bend tools Excessive bending results in weak spots and breakage
Bronze	Zinc (92) Tin (8)	Used only in temples High elasticity while retaining tensile strength Withstands bending	Cold bend tools Adjust at eyepiece
Cobalt		Thin, lightweight, noncorrosive Variety of colors	Difficult to adjust
Memory metals	Titanium and nickel alloy	Flexible and durable Can be twisted and bent without breaking and returns to original shape	Difficult to adjust Design limitations

Polyamide/copolymide is a blend of nylons that is durable, light, and flexible. It holds translucent colors well and is scratch-resistant. Lenses should be edged to exact size and inserted cold into the frame, then the frame can be shrunk by carefully applying heat. Polyamide will shrink if placed in a salt pan.

Optyl is an epoxy resin, weighs 30% less than cellulose-based frames, and is considered hypoallergenic. To insert lenses, edge them slightly oversized and then heat the frame. Do not cool in water. Adjustments should be made by heating and adjusting one part at a time, preferably using a hot-air blower with a narrow opening. The frame will hold its shape until heated again. The temples can be lengthened by heating until soft, then gently stretching.

Thermoplastic polyester elastomer (Hytrel) frames are a polyether–ester block copolymer combining the characteristics of high-performance elastomers and flexible plastic. The frame offers mechanical strength and durability in a flexible component. The material is not affected by a wide range of temperatures and it maintains flexibility and lens retention.

Memory plastic is tough and virtually unbreakable. It is extremely flexible and can be bent or twisted and still maintain its original fit. Its shape is not affected by heat and the color resists scratching, chipping, or wearing off.

Kevlar is made of strong fibers mixed with a hybrid nylon. It is available in limited colors. Lenses should be cut to the exact size, because although Kevlar will not shrink or expand when exposed to heat, it can be softened by heat for lens insertion.

Composite combines Kevlar, polyamide, and ceramic fiber and is used for nonprescription sun lenses as well as prescription lenses. Lenses to be inserted should be cut to exact size with more bevel on the front side. Plastic lenses are recommended and should be inserted cold. Glass lenses require a slight preheating of the frame. The frame should never be heated with lenses inserted, and never to temperatures greater than 160 degrees.

Advantages

The plastic frame is basically rigid and it keeps its adjustment well, once fitted. The colors, patterns, and styles available in plastic are almost limitless. Most frames have fixed plastic pads that rest on the side of the nose. It should be noted, however, that plastic does become brittle with age.

Bridges

There are two basic types of bridges: the *saddle* (Figure 13.4) and the *keyhole* (Figure 13.5). The saddle bridge rests lower

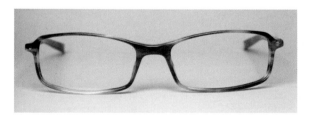

Figure 13.4 Saddle-bridge frame.

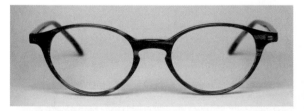

Figure 13.5 Keyhole-bridge frame.

on the nose and creates the illusion of shortening a long nose. A keyhole bridge is more flattering to a round, short nose. Most plastic temples have a metal core for rigidity and strength. Some fronts are braced with metal, buried in the plastic, running across the top of the front from hinge to hinge. These frames are desirable for children and athletes.

Combination frames

A combination frame consists of a metal chassis with a decorative metal or plastic top and two fully adjustable pads (Figure 13.6). Combination frames with movable pads are ideal for patients with high hyperopic or high myopic corrections, inasmuch as the distance of the lens from the eye can be accurately placed, as can the height of the bifocal or trifocal segment. The advantage of movable pads is that they can be moved in the up-and-down adjustment and backward and forward to fit the patient's face. In prescriptions for a heavy lens, these frames should be ordered with jumbo pads (oversized plastic pads), which give a larger weight-bearing surface on the nose and have less tendency to leave marks.

Semirimless frames

Rimless frames look much like combination frames in that there is a decorative top but no apparent metal holding the lens shape. Rimless frames may be of metal or plastic construction. In the case of plastic, there is actually a nylon cord fitted into a groove cut in the edge of the lens that holds the lens to the top. This nylon cord is almost invisible and gives the frame a rimless appearance.

In some metal rimless frames the lenses are held in position by hidden notches in the lenses. The notches are engaged by tabs protruding from the top, but when the frame is viewed from the front the tabs are out of sight behind the top.

Older-model rimless spectacles actually had holes drilled through the lenses and small nuts and bolts placed through these holes to hold the lenses in position (Figure 13.7). This type of rimless frame was easily shattered when dropped and therefore is now practical only when high-index, polycarbonate, or Trivex lenses are used. Modern-day semirimless spectacles have a pressure mount with a post shim to hold the lenses in place.

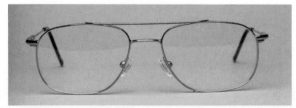

Figure 13.6 Frame with adjustable pads.

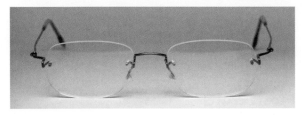

Figure 13.7 Rimless frame.

Frame measurements

Most frame measurements are based on the box system, whereby the lens is enclosed in a rectangle and the distances between opposite sides are taken as the *eye size*. An imaginary line running through the center of the lenses is called the *datum line*. This is a very important line, because all measurements are taken at this point (Figure 13.8).

On the back of a frame are a few figures such as 46 × 22, which represent the lens size (46) and the bridge size (22). All measurements are in millimeters.

The other measurements are for the temples; they vary according to the use for which the glasses are intended and the consequent shape of the temples.

Temples

The temple is the long strut that extends from the lateral aspect of the eyepiece and rests on the ear. The temple length (e.g., 140 mm) is expressed as the overall length from the hinge end to the end that rests behind the ears. Most plastic temples have a metal core for rigidity and strength.

Several varieties of temples are available. The more commonly used types are:

Cable temples (Figure 13.9A). Cable temples sometimes are known as *riding bow* temples or *curl side* temples. The cable temple is either metal or plastic, with the ear portion made of a flexible metal that can be shaped to fit the contour behind the ear. Another type of riding bow temple has a much stiffer metal core covered with plastic. A comfortable fit is possible only when this temple is contoured to the back of the ear. This type of temple is ideal for children and active people, for those who are constantly looking down, or for positions in which the spectacles might otherwise slide off the face.

Straight temples (Figure 13.9B). Straight temples sometimes are called *library* temples. These are ideal for people who constantly take their glasses off and for those in religious orders whose ears are concealed under a habit, making it difficult to put on or take off glasses that have riding bow or other paddle temples.

Paddle temples (Figure 13.9C–E). Paddle temples are sometimes called *skull* temples or *hockey-end* temples. These temples are ideal for general use and are the most common type used today.

Specialty frames

Frame manufacturers produce the majority of frames with standard eye sizes and bridge sizes. This leaves a small portion of the population with unusual facial measurements unable to obtain a correct fit with the commercially produced frames. Fortunately some optical companies will

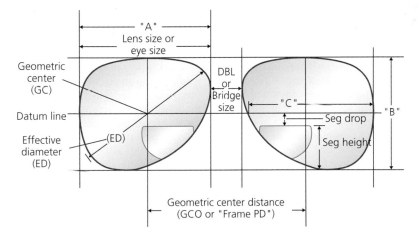

Figure 13.8 In the boxing system, the "A" dimension is the horizontal boxing width. If the frame is properly marked, the eye size will be equal to the "A" dimension of the frame. The "B" dimension is the vertical boxing length. The "C" dimension is the width of the lens along the horizontal midline. This dimension is seldom used today. The "C" dimension should not be confused with the "C-size" of a lens. The C-size of a lens is the distance around the lens, i.e., its circumference. The dispenser uses the C-size to ensure that a lens ordered in isolation (without the frame) will be exactly sized for that frame. *PD,* Pupillary distance; *DBL,* distance between lenses. *(Reproduced with permission from Opticians Association of America: Professional dispensing for opticians. 2nd ed. Philadelphia: Butterworth-Heinemann, 1996.)*

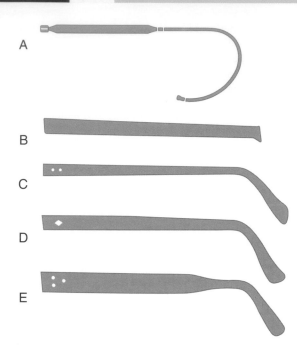

A

B

C

D

E

Figure 13.9 Temples. (A) Cable, riding bow, or curl side temples. (B) Straight or library temples. (C–E) Paddle, skull, or hockey-end.

make frames for this group by hand and will produce frames for special vocational or medical requirements. A few of these are mentioned here.

Frames for individuals with low, flat bridges

Because infants and some people have practically no bridge to their noses, the ordinary plastic frame fits too low on the face and is so close to the eyes that the lenses interfere with the eyelashes. A handmade frame with special nose construction can be made to look like a standard frame yet have the necessary low-set, thickened portion to the bridge so that the spectacles can be properly adjusted in front of the patient's eyes. Before this development, such patients had to be fitted with frames that had adjustable pads to raise the frame and move it away from the face. Today, some manufacturers offer frames which feature a bridge specifically designed to fit this facial shape. These frames are designed with wider pads to move the frame away from the face.

Side shields

There are conditions, such as an anesthetic cornea or a "dry eye," for which it is necessary to enclose the eye between the frame and the face. There are many ways of doing this, but most side-shield constructions are not attractive and usually are bulky, hard, and poor fitting. With the use of a soft,

transparent plastic, a shield can be produced and trimmed with a pair of scissors to exactly fit the individual patient. An added bonus is that it is almost invisible and, being soft and pliable, it does not interfere with the glasses being folded up in the standard manner.

Ptosis crutch

Although the ideal solution in the case of ptosis is an operation, there may be contraindications to surgery. Frames can be fitted with a ptosis crutch, which is a small piece of wire or plastic affixed to the inside of a spectacle frame. This wire can be adjusted to raise the eyelids of the patient so afflicted.

DISPENSING SPECTACLE FRAMES

It is important that spectacles are produced so that the patient, when viewing distance objects, looks through the *optical centers* of both lenses. Consequently it is essential to know the distance between the visual axes through the pupils of the patient, so that the lenses may be correctly mounted in the spectacle frame at the same interpupillary distance. The term *pupillary distance* is abbreviated PD.

Unfortunately the visual axis through the human eye does not pass through the center of the pupil, as one might expect, but varies from patient to patient and is on the nasal side of the pupil. Therefore, any mechanical device that measures from the center of the pupil of one eye to the center of the pupil of the second eye will give a measurement greater than the actual distance between the visual axes of the two eyes.

This error is of little significance if the prescription is a weak one. However, a few millimeters of error will produce a decidedly uncomfortable pair of glasses for those patients requiring unusually strong (greater than ±4.00 diopters) prescriptions: binocular aphakes, myopes, hyperopes, or those with large amounts of astigmatism. Because it is difficult to assess the visual axis or the center of the pupil, the practice is to measure (if both pupils are the same size) from the nasal edge of the pupil on the patient's right eye to the temporal side of the pupil on the patient's left eye (Figures 13.10 and 13.11).

Two PDs are taken, one for distance, where the visual axes are parallel, and one for near, which is the close working distance of the patient.

There is only one accurate method of measuring PD—the *light reflex method*—the result of which gives the distance between the visual axes of the two eyes, rather than the distance between the center of one pupil and the center of the other. The difference between the two methods of measurement may be 2 to 5 mm. There are many optical interpupillary gauges that can give the measurement from pupil to pupil very accurately for distance vision; the PD can then

Figure 13.10 Measurement of pupillary distance. Measurements are made from the nasal edge of one pupil to the temporal edge of the other.

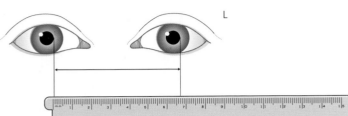

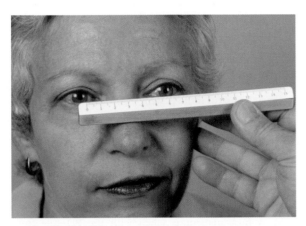

Figure 13.11 Measuring pupillary distance.

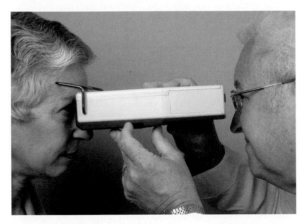

Figure 13.12 Measuring pupillary distance by pupillary gauge.

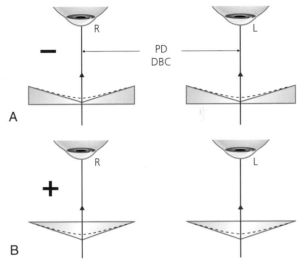

Figure 13.13 (A) Minus or concave lens. Optical center is at its thinnest part. (B) Plus or convex lens. Optical center is at its thickest part. *PD*, Pupillary distance; *DBC*, distance between centers of lenses.

be converted for near vision by means of tables. One gauge on the market today uses the accurate reflex method (Figure 13.12).

Special considerations in measuring PD include the following:

1. If the patient has pupils of different size and the standard method with a PD rule is to be used, the measurements should be made from the nasal side of the limbus of the patient's right eye to the temporal side of the limbus on the other, ignoring the measurements from the pupil.

2. If the patient can see from only one eye, the measurement can be taken for the good eye from the center of the bridge of the nose to the center of the pupil, because an inaccuracy of a few millimeters one way or the other has no significance.

3. If the patient has a squint, the measurement can be taken from the inner canthus of one eye to the outer canthus of the opposite eye, giving a reasonably accurate PD. A better way is to occlude the turning eye and measure from the center of the bridge of the nose to the center of the uncovered eye and then repeat with the other eye covered. The sum of the two measurements is the PD.

The PD is taken so that the optical centers of the lenses will be directly in front of the visual axes through the pupils (Figure 13.13). If the optical centers are not so placed, an unwanted prism is incorporated in the glasses.

The *optical center* can be defined as the thinnest part in the center of any minus lens or the thickest part of the center of a plus lens. Only at the optical center do rays of light go through the lens without bending. To make this clearer, a minus lens can be represented by two prisms, bases out,

215

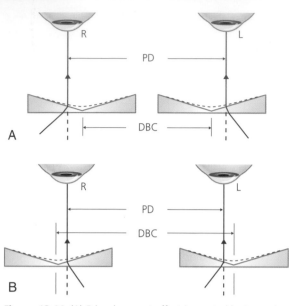

Figure 13.14 (A) Prism base-out effect is created by inward displacement of the optical centers of two concave lenses. (B) Prism base-in effect is created by outward displacement of the optical centers of two concave lenses. *PD*, Pupillary distance; *DBC*, distance between centers of lenses.

and a plus lens, bases in. When these lenses have their centers in line with the visual axes, they are correctly positioned in front of the patient's eyes (Figure 13.14).

If the PD is wrong and the lenses are off-center, the vision is bent by the lenses toward the base of the prism in each case and the object would appear to be displaced laterally. The eyes would have to turn in or out to try to correct this, causing discomfort to the patient. If the lenses are high power, plus or minus, so much prism can be introduced that double vision will result. In the case of a lens of +10.00 diopters, if the PD is out 1 mm then 1.00 diopter of prism that has not been prescribed is introduced into the prescription.

Measuring pupillary distance with a ruler and the reflex method

Most times, the PD is measured with a device called a pupillometer. When checking the PD manually, the following equipment is required:

1. Small PD rule, graduated in millimeters
2. Pinpoint of light, such as a bare bulb of an ophthalmoscope battery handle or a penlight

To take a *distance PD*, the procedure is as follows:

1. Sit approximately 16 to 18 inches from the patient to be examined.
2. Hold the light source immediately under your left eye. Place the PD rule across the bridge of the patient's nose so that it will extend to cover the lower half of both pupils.

3. Make sure the patient looks directly at the light bulb.
4. Place the zero mark of the ruler on the pinpoint reflection of the light on the cornea. Use your left eye for this purpose.
5. Without disturbing the PD ruler and without the patient moving the head, move the light to a position underneath your right eye.
6. Make sure the patient is still looking at the light.
7. Note the measurement on the PD rule of the reflection of the light on the cornea of the patient's left eye. (In doing this you will observe that the pinpoint of light is not in the center of the pupil but at some point nasal of center. The measurement is an accurate one of the distance between the visual axes of the two eyes [incorrectly termed the distance PD for want of a better term].)
8. Note the measurement at the center of the nose (this may be useful if the patient's face is grossly asymmetric).

Obtaining the *PD for near* is done in a similar manner, but the distance between the patient's eyes and the observer's eyes should be adjusted to the appropriate near distance. (It varies from person to person and from occupation to occupation.) The observer proceeds as before. Then the light is placed under one eye and the patient looks at the light. A measurement is taken with the PD rule from the reflection on the cornea of one eye to the reflection on the cornea of the other eye, without moving the light. This will be the "near" PD.

Spectacle frames often have to be chosen for their physical advantages in supporting the lenses that are required. The heavier the lenses, the greater the distribution of weight on the nose. The new technology that has made possible a larger selection of eye fashion may limit the choice of frames for the high myope, high hyperope, and the rare aphake without an intraocular lens.

Spectacle frames, as previously noted, should also provide cosmetic enhancement to the wearer. The design of the frame should take into consideration the contours of the face. In persons with unusually long faces, frames that are noticeably longer horizontally than vertically are very effective in reducing the long appearance of the face. An unusually long nose can be diminished optically by a low-fitting bridge bar. Dark colors accentuate this shortening effect. A small nose can be made to look longer by a slender bridge bar set high up or a keyhole bridge. Frames that are greater in depth at their outer ends than at their middle help to make eyes that are too closely set together appear to be more widely separated; the opposite type of frame helps to mitigate the effect of eyes that are set unusually far apart. Thus an illusion of wide-set eyes can be created by having the frame color fade away at the bridge.

Brightly colored frames complement the natural tones of a light-haired individual, whereas darkly colored frames blend better with a dark complexion. Dark-colored frames draw attention to nose width and should be avoided by people with very narrow or very wide noses.

The actual choice of frames or style is highly personal. A variety of frames are available for both indoor and outdoor sports, for motoring, and for business and social occasions.

The frames should hold both lenses firmly in a direction perpendicular to the visual axes because tilting can introduce optical errors that may be considerable in lenses of high power. Glasses for distance should sit vertically, whereas glasses for reading should be slightly lowered and tilted downward. The frames should be comfortable at all times and cause no irritation of the skin on which they rest, and the lenses should be as close to the eyes as possible without touching the eyelashes.

LENSES

Spectacle lenses are made from plastic, high-index plastic, polycarbonate, Trivex, or glass.

Most single-vision lenses are made up in a curved form rather than the flat form (Figure 13.15).

Optical laboratory statistics for the latter part of 2015 reveal that glass lenses were dispensed for only 3% of patients, polycarbonate lenses for 37% of patients, and plastic lenses for 60% of patients, with high-index plastic lenses accounting for one-third of the plastic lenses dispensed.

Historically, many types of glass were used for optical purposes. The primary glass used for ophthalmic lenses was *crown glass* of 1.523 refractive index. Also used was *flint glass* with a refractive index of 1.62 when a higher refractive index was desired, as in the making of bifocal or achromatic lenses. Flint glass contained lead, which is absent from crown glass. Glass with an index of 1.6 was produced by adding more titanium dioxide to the glass mix. The main advantages of crown glass in optical spectacles were its excellent optical properties and its resistance to scratching.

A higher-index glass was Lantal (1.9) from Carl Zeiss, Germany (Figure 13.16). These lenses were used for individuals with high myopia or hyperopia and were remarkably thin.

Glass lenses, unlike plastic, must be treated to resist breakage. They can be hardened by chemical processes or by heat.

Plastic lenses have about half the weight of glass lenses and are highly impact-resistant. With a center thickness of 3 mm, they can be considered as safety glasses without special hardening techniques. Plastic lenses have a thicker profile than do glass, scratch more easily, and do not protect the eye from ultraviolet light unless properly tinted. High-index plastics (1.50–1.74) are available to further reduce the center thickness to 0.8 mm and therefore the overall edge thickness. High-index plastic is available in photochromic material.

Each manufacturer has an individualized series of base curves for toric meniscus lenses. In theory, to give a "perfect" lens with no distortions, the inside curve should have a radius that coincides with the radius of the rotating eyeball. Thus there would be the same vertex distance between the cornea and the spectacles no matter which way the eye turned behind the spectacles. This would give undistorted vision from edge to edge. However, if glasses were made in this way, the front surface of a high plus lens would be so bulbous and thick and the lens would be of such a small diameter that it would never fill the spectacle frame. It would be cosmetically unacceptable. Therefore, all manufacturers' "corrected" lenses are truly corrected only in the weaker powers. Beyond 5.00 diopters, plus or minus, no lens other than an aspheric lens is a "corrected" one.

A corrected lens is a compromise designed to avoid or minimize the distortions created through the edges of an ophthalmic lens. These distortions include the following:

1. *Chromatic aberration*, in which white light is broken up into its spectral components and observed as color fringes
2. *Spherical aberration*, in which a lens fails to focus a broad beam to a single point

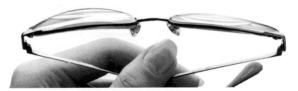

Figure 13.16 Lenses of identical power. Standard index lens on left, high-index lens on right.

Figure 13.15 Types of lenses. Meniscus lenses are designed with a base curve.

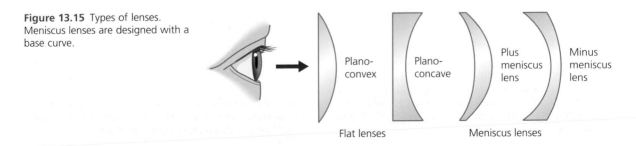

Plano-convex

Plano-concave

Plus meniscus lens

Minus meniscus lens

Flat lenses

Meniscus lenses

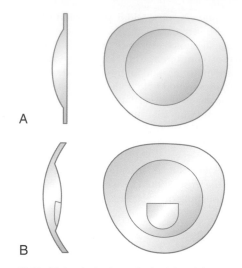

Figure 13.17 Lens distortion. (A) Normal square pattern. (B) Strong concave lenses distort a square to a barrel shape. (C) Strong convex lenses distort a square to a pincushion shape.

3. *Distortion,* which is an aberration that causes objects to appear in other than their true shape. With strong concave lenses, the square is distorted to a barrel shape; with plus or convex lenses, the square is distorted to a pincushion shape (Figure 13.17). Distortion occurs when the eye looks toward the periphery of a lens. It is overcome chiefly by using deeply curved lenses, high base curves, or aspheric lenses

4. *Astigmatism,* which occurs when an oblique ray of light strikes a spherical surface. This type of astigmatism also is reduced to a minimum by deeply curved lenses

Corrected lenses have many designs. There are *meniscus lenses,* which generally are ground on a 6.00-diopter base curve. A *toric lens* is curved like a meniscus lens, but also contains a cylinder that formerly was ground on a convex surface in single-vision glass lenses and on a concave surface in bifocals. In plastic lenses the cylinder is on the concave surface. Most modern cylindric lenses have the cylinder on the concave side and are referred to as *minus cylinder lenses.*

Aphakic lenses

Modern cataract surgery involves inserting an intraocular lens so that the thick aphakic spectacle is no longer required. The new condition is called *pseudophakia,* in which a cataract is removed and an intraocular lens implanted. There are, however, patients in whom a cataract was removed by the intracapsular route without an implant. These patients still wear either contact lenses or aphakic spectacles. The aphakic spectacles have a distortion inherent in their manufacture because of the strong correction. To avoid these distortions, special lens designs have been created to minimize both the distortions and the weight of these lenses. The types most commonly used are (1) lenticular lenses, (2) aspheric lenses, (3) hard-resin (plastic) lenses, and (4) combinations of 1, 2, and 3.

Lenticular lenses

The lenticular lens may be described as a small-diameter, circular, or oval prescription lens (too small to fit a modern frame) mounted on a longer-diameter, thin planocarrier, which is edged to fit the frame (Figure 13.18). The resulting lenticular lens weighs less and is thinner than a full-sized lens of the same power.

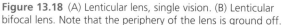

Figure 13.18 (A) Lenticular lens, single vision. (B) Lenticular bifocal lens. Note that the periphery of the lens is ground off.

The main disadvantage of the lenticular lens is that it gives a bull's-eye effect, making it more conspicuous than the full-sized lens. Decentration of a full-sized lens creates a heavy prismatic shape and heavy physical weight.

Aspheric lenses

A standard plus lens suitable for a patient who has had a cataract operation may be optically correct through its center but it gives a progressively stronger effect as the patient's vision moves away from the center to the edge of the lens. This increase in plus power toward the edge, resulting from an increase in vertex distance, causes the pincushion distortions previously mentioned, as well as blurred vision in these areas. Therefore, if a lens is ground with correct power at the center and a drop-off of power toward the edges, distortions and blurring of vision are eliminated or at least minimized. This is the aspheric lens, which is available in plastic (Figure 13.19).

Plastic lenses*

Plastic lenses are made from a very high-quality synthetic resin and have the same qualities as glass but half the weight. They are also highly impact-resistant and are rated as *safety lenses.* They have a cosmetic disadvantage, being thicker than equivalent glass lenses in the higher prescriptions. Plastic lenses are not quite as resistant to scratching as glass, but some manufacturers apply a coating on the plus (outside) surface to make them more scratch-resistant. There are two types of plastic used in lenses: thermosetting or hard resins (CR-39) and thermoplastic resins (polycarbonate).

*From Stein HA, Freeman MI, Stenson SM. *CLAO residents curriculum manual on refraction, spectacles and dispensing.* Metairie, LA: CLAO Publications, 2001 (with permission).

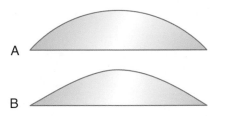

Figure 13.19 (A) Spherical lens, side view. (B) Aspheric lens, side view. Note the flatter curve in the periphery of the lens. This eliminates many of the aberrations of the periphery of the lens and permits a greater field of vision.
(In part from Stein HA, Freeman MI, Stenson SM. CLAO residents curriculum manual on refraction, spectacles and dispensing. Metairie, LA: CLAO Publications, 2001, with permission.)

Plastic hard-resin lenses (CR-39)

The breakability and ungainly weight of glass, especially in higher prescriptions, is the reason that CR-39 is now among the popular lens materials used. The weight of CR-39 is nearly half that of crown glass. This hard resin accounts for a significant number of ophthalmic spectacle lenses dispensed. It has an Abbe number of 58, making it a close second to crown glass in optical quality. The *Abbe number*, an indication of optical quality, is inversely proportional to the *chromatic dispersion* of the specific lens material. In general, the higher the refractive index of a material, the greater is its chromatic dispersion and the lower its Abbe number. The Abbe numbers of ophthalmic lenses vary between 30 and 60.

CR-39 is less expensive than other materials and even without special treatment, blocks 55% of ultraviolet A (UVA) and ultraviolet B (UVB). Its index of refraction is 1.50. It has a density half that of glass (1.32), is highly transparent, demonstrates high impact resistance, and exhibits a very low chromatism.

The chemical name for CR-39 is allyl-diglycol-carbonate. In its basic form CR-39 is a liquid monomer. Polymerization is achieved by treatment with heat and a catalyst. In its polymer form, CR-39 is unmeltable, insoluble, solvent-resistant, and stable. CR-39 can be coated and tinted. It is available in photochromic materials. Its major shortcoming, compared with crown glass, is its tendency to scratch.

More recent developments in thermosetting plastic resins include medium-index (refraction less than 1.56) and high-index (refraction more than 1.56) plastics. These allow for the manufacture of even thinner and lighter lenses than with CR-39. The main disadvantage of high-index plastics, shared with CR-39, is that they are easily scratched, so that protective coatings are necessary. In 2000 a 1.74 index plastic lens was introduced in Japan (Seiko Optical). This aspheric lens has an Abbe value of 33.

Polycarbonate lenses

Polycarbonate is a thermoplastic resin with a carbonated skeleton composed of a succession of carbonate radicals and phenol. It is manufactured in solution. Polycarbonate is a byproduct derived from purified resin chips. Because of its strength, polycarbonate can be used to manufacture lenses with thin centers, producing spectacles that are cosmetically appealing and lighter in weight. Its primary advantages are its impact resistance and its safety. For these reasons, polycarbonate lenses are ideal for use in sports and in safety glasses.

The cost of polycarbonate is slightly higher than CR-39, but polycarbonate lenses come with two built-in add-ons: a scratch-resistant coating and UVA/UVB protection. Polycarbonate blocks all UVA and UVB in the harmful range up to 380 nm. To tint polycarbonate lenses, a scratch-resistant coating impregnated with dye is applied to the back of the lens. AR coatings can be added to improve polycarbonate lens performance.

Similar to other high-index plastic or glass lenses, polycarbonate lenses have a relatively low Abbe number (32). Even so, the resulting chromatic dispersion typically becomes an issue only with strong prescriptions (more than 4.00–5.00 diopters).

Trivex lenses

A newer development in spectacle lens materials is Trivex, manufactured by PPG Industries. Trivex is a triperformance material, exhibiting excellent optics and impact resistance while being thin and lightweight.

This material was initially developed for use in the military, as a type of "visual armor." It is now available for commercial use.

Trivex material is urethane-based, with light cross-linkage. It is prepared by casting and is designed for low shrinkage. It has an Abbe number of 46 and a refractive index of 1.53. It demonstrates good scratch, chemical, and impact resistance.

Lenses made from Trivex material are available in single-vision, progressive, and variable tint designs.

The Optical Laboratories Association (OLA), now the new Optical Laboratory Division of The Vision Council, has advised that polycarbonate or Trivex should be the lens material of choice for children, athletes at their sport, people with an active lifestyle (such as firefighters or police officers), and patients with no or reduced vision in one eye.

Safety lenses*

It hardly seems necessary to remind practitioners, and all health care personnel, that they live in a litigious society. The concept of informed consent is a necessary part of ophthalmic practice. Informed consent includes informing patients about the impact-resistant qualities of spectacle lens materials. Polycarbonate lenses are as much as 60 times

---

*Modified from Stein HA, Freeman MI, Stenson SM. *CLAO residents curriculum manual on refraction, spectacles and dispensing*. Metairie, LA: CLAO Publications, 2001 (with permission).

more impact-resistant than other materials. They can be surfaced as thin as 1 mm center thickness and still pass the US. Food and Drug Administration (FDA) drop-ball tests.

All eye care practitioners have reasons to inform patients about the safety of their lenses beyond the fear of avoiding a lawsuit. Forty-five percent of disabling eye injuries occur at home. This compares with 19% that occur on the job. The American Academy of Ophthalmology reported in 2015 that 125,000 eye injuries occur in the home each year. Therefore, promoting safety lenses as a guard against household hazards, such as oven cleaners and bleach, splattered hot grease, drilling or hammering screws or nails into walls or hard surfaces, curling irons near the face, lawn mowers, and power tools makes good sense. This message becomes even more important for monocular patients.

The first recorded court case in which the choice of optical lens became an issue occurred in 1981 when a Wyoming rancher wearing glass photochromic executive bifocals mounted in a dress frame sustained an injury while roping. Because polycarbonate was so new a product and enjoyed very limited availability and was at the time available only in single vision, the defendant was not granted an award. Subsequently, practitioners have become aware of the importance of optical lens safety considerations and their responsibility to present these considerations to patients. Since 1981, polycarbonate lenses and other protective lens materials have matured and are available in every form of commonly used lens design. The courts have been consistent in ruling that patients should be informed of all lens choices. Not doing so exposes the individual dispensing eyewear to potential damage claims.

When selecting safety or protective eyewear it is important to remember that one should not only choose the appropriate lens material but also select an appropriate frame material to optimize eye and face protection.

No glass lens yet devised is completely shatterproof. However, glass can be treated to resist blows of tremendous force and, should glass safety lenses break, they would crumble into "hailstones" with no sharp splinters to lacerate the eye.

Heat-treated impact-resistant glass lenses

Today the emphasis is on discouraging glass and recommending plastic for patient safety. However, when these lenses are used in industry, they are made of the standard ophthalmic glass; the only prerequisite is that the lens must not be less than 3 mm thick at its thinnest point. For general wear (as in sports or for children) the minimum thickness is 2.2 mm. The lens must be ground, polished, and edged to fit the frame before hardening. The lens is not "case hardened"; that is, the surface is no tougher after treatment than before. It is therefore no more resistant to scratching after treatment than before. Industrial impact-resistant lenses will withstand a blow from a 1-inch steel ball dropped from a height of 50 inches (1.25 m) (Figure 13.20).

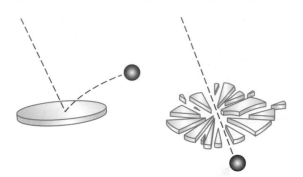

Figure 13.20 Safety lens on the left does not shatter when a steel ball is dropped on its surface.

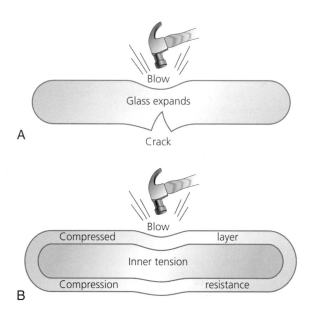

Figure 13.21 Effect of tempering a glass lens to prevent breakage. (A) Untreated lens. (B) Treated lens. A firm outer compressed layer of glass is created by heat. This compressed layer prevents the lens from breaking at a point opposite that of the impact.

The finished lens is heated in an oven almost to its melting or softening point, removed and then rapidly cooled by blasts of cold air on both surfaces simultaneously. The surfaces cool and contract faster than the interior of the lens. Eventually the interior of the lens cools and contracts and pulls the surface of the glass lens into a compression condition (balanced by tension in the interior).

Glass is very strong in compression but pulls apart easily in tension. When one strikes a pane of glass, it does not shatter on the side that is struck. The bending force of the blow exerts itself as a tension (pulling apart) on the side opposite to that struck, and the glass breaks (Figure 13.21).

A blow on the surface of the heat-treated lens (creating the bending force) must be great enough to overcome the compression of the opposite surface and must then put this surface under enough tension to tear the lens apart. Thickness plays a part and the criteria of the American National Standards Institute (ANSI) advise a minimum of 2 mm at the optical center and 1 mm on the edge.

All heat-treated glass lenses may be identified by the fact that they unpolarize polarized light. The *polariscope* is an instrument used to identify an impact-resistant lens. This device consists of two sheets of polarizing filters set with their axes at right angles. Thus no light comes through the combination of the two filters. Inserting the treated lens between the filters upsets the polarized light so that a pattern is now seen through the combination of the filters and the spectacle lens. The shape (Maltese cross) of the pattern seen is no indication of the strength of the lens.

Some glasses on the market are labeled "toughened lenses." These are heat-treated, "hardened" lenses that will withstand blows that would shatter ordinary glass. They are not treated to the point where they would be labeled safety glasses and should not be considered as such.

Another type of safety lens is the *laminated lens,* in which a sheet of plastic is sandwiched between the two pieces of glass. If the lens is shattered, the glass particles adhere to the plastic. These laminated lenses are seldom used today, except for polarized lenses.

Another type of impact-resistant lens is available. A *chemical treatment* is used that results in a lens with impact-resistant qualities far superior to those produced by the heat-treating method. The chemical hardening process consists of placing the finished glass lens in a hot solution of a potassium salt for about 14 hours. In that time the sodium ions in the glass are replaced by potassium ions (which are physically larger than the sodium). During cooling, the potassium ions place the surface into a state of compression which gives an impact-resistant property to the lens.

Unlike the heat-treated lens, this process cannot be detected by polarized light. Failing other indications that the lens has been chemically treated, the drop-ball test is the only way to check such a lens!

Safety lenses are recommended for all children, people engaged in sports, and industrial workers.

Role of protective lenses in sports

Most people's active lifestyles include participation in a sport of some kind. The benefits of sports are many, including stronger community ties and improved personal health. When considering what types of protective equipment will be needed, safety for the eyes should not be overlooked (see Table 21.1).

Role of protective lenses in shooting, hockey, and racquet sports

For individuals who do skeet shooting, there is the risk of being hit by ricochet pellets glancing from targets. Broken pieces from clay targets can careen from the flight path and strike the shooter. Game hunters may risk eye injury directly from tree branches or from pellets deflected off rocks or tree branches and even from the stray shots of other hunters when hunting in heavy grouse or woodcock cover. All shooters should be aware of the danger of blowback that results from a defective shell or gun. Pieces of lead or copper jacketing can sail back to endanger shooters. For shooting range officials and spectators, eye protection is essential.

In the shooting sports, tints may be required. Polycarbonate presently provides the best protection, but lacks the optical clarity in the range of tintability required by shooters. Trivex lenses are an alternative protective lens for sports; they can be tinted. The object of the lens coloration is to develop contrast between the target or game and the background. In trap and skeet shooting, there are four basic colors of clay targets: white, black, yellow, and fluorescent orange. To see these when thrown under different light conditions, one needs colored lenses to bring out the color of the target against the sky. Thus the serious shooter should own more than one pair of glasses to select interchangeable lenses in shooting frames. Shooting lenses should be in light to medium shades so that the pupils will contract more and give a greater depth of focus. Lenses may be coated but can still transmit 99.9% of the light to give the sharpest image possible. In overcast weather conditions, light scattered by water particles in the atmosphere produces a blue coloration. This blue dominance tends to compress the chromatic range and flatten color. The most negative effect on vision is that the blue light is not well focused on the retina but rather in front of it. As the level of blue light increases, visual acuity decreases. Lenses with a light gold or amber color will neutralize the blue effect on overcast days. Skeet shooting or hunting ducks early in the morning or late in the evening requires the use of a high-transmission lens that permits maximum light transfer.

Hockey is another high-risk sport in which there is a likelihood of sustaining eye injuries with permanent loss of vision. Many eye injuries in amateur sports in Canada result in legal blindness. Through efforts of safety committees, manufacturers began developing certified face protectors, which resulted in a marked decrease of eye injuries. All nonprofessional players are now required to wear these protective masks that meet the safety standards.

In racquet sports, serious eye injuries have been increasing over the past few decades. Through the efforts of Doctors Pashby and Easterbrook, eye guards have been developed that withstand the impact of a ball traveling up to 89 miles per hour (144 kilometers per hour). These guards must have full lenses and must not obstruct the player's peripheral view. Attention is focusing on developing shields for badminton players because badminton birds can travel at speeds up to 135 miles per hour (217 kilometers per hour).

By far the most popular protective lenses are polycarbonate lenses and Trivex lenses. As mentioned, these are impact-resistant and outperform plastic, glass-heated, and chemically treated lenses.

Antireflection (no-glare) coating

Artificial office light, computer video display terminals, and handheld phones and electronic devices can cause reflections in untreated glass and create ghost images. This is particularly true with high-index glasses. When light passes through a spectacle lens, some is reflected by the front and the back surface of the lens. Streetlights in the driver's field of view may be duplicated or triplicated. Coat the lens and only one image is seen.

Coating a lens with magnesium fluoride is sometimes referred to as *blooming* a lens. The name comes from the distinctive purplish sheen, similar to the bloom on a ripe plum, seen on the surface of the lens. All camera lenses and optical instrument lenses are bloomed to cut out internal reflections and permit greater light transmission through the glass.

Coating is placed on a finished ophthalmic lens in a vacuum. Magnesium fluoride is heated in a crucible and "fumed" onto both surfaces of the lens. This material is very tough and usually lasts the life of the lens.

The coating, one-quarter of a wavelength of yellow-green light, works by causing the reflection of light off the front and back surfaces of the *coating* to be out of step by exactly one-half wavelength; thus the waves cancel each other out and the reflection is not there. The reflections that *are* seen are from the red and the purple ends of the spectrum, giving the bloomed color in reflection.

Almost all lens coatings are multicoatings. These coatings, which are almost invisible, eliminate the red and the blue ends of the spectrum. The multicoated lenses require special cleaners and antistatic and antifog solutions, as well as a very fine wiping cloth. Hard-resin lenses are commercially available and they too can be coated. Prevencia antireflection (AR) coating is specifically designed to block blue rays from computer screens and handheld devices. New improved Varilux coating adds a 25 E-SPF UV protection.

Sunglasses and tinted lenses

By use of the appropriate chemicals, clear glass lenses may be color-coated in almost any shade or color or even mirrored. If a mask of appropriate shape is placed between the fuming crucible and the lens, a gradient color or gradient mirror coating can be produced. Popular colors available commercially are green, neutral gray, brown, rose, and transparent (one-way) surfaces.

Color coating of ophthalmic lenses gives an even coloring across the whole surface of the lens, whether it is a strong plus or a strong minus lens. The coating, whether it is antireflection, mirror, or color, may be removed chemically in about 10 seconds, should this be necessary.

Almost all sunglasses are clear lenses coated to the chosen color. However, colored-glass lenses are still available that are perfectly satisfactory for plano or weak prescriptions. If the prescription is a high plus, then the color of the glass is darker at the center than at the edges. Conversely, a high minus lens would have a central light spot. Before the advent of the surface coating process, evenly spread color was obtained by laminating a colored plano lens to a clear prescription lens, an expensive process that is no longer necessary.

Colored plastic lenses are clear lenses dyed the appropriate color. Therefore, they have an even color no matter how strong the prescription may be. Gradient tints or even several colors on the same lens can be produced. Plastic lenses can be effective blockers of ultraviolet light, but not of infrared light.

A neutral gray tint has been the most popular color for sunglasses in North America for almost half a century. Because of its neutral absorption of all colors of the visible spectrum, light intensity is reduced without color distortion or imbalance, which is a very important factor when proper color perception is essential, for instance, a pilot having to read various colored dials, gauges, or maps; a telephone lineman distinguishing between color-coded telephone wires; a driver who might have difficulties differentiating colors of traffic signals; a participant or spectator at a sporting event where each team is denoted by the color of their uniforms; or a naturalist watching birds, animals, or flowers. In short, gray lenses should be recommended whenever a patient wants protection from intensive light or glare without loss of color differentiation.

The human eye responds to wavelengths of 380 to 780 nm. Shorter or longer wavelengths do not elicit a visual response but may enter the eyes and cause heating or photobiologic damage. Blocking lenses are valuable. The stratospheric ozone layers help protect the eyes, but holes are appearing in the ozone layer owing to manmade chemicals, especially the fully halogenated methanes (chlorofluorocarbons [CFCs]).

A green lens absorbs most of the ultraviolet and infrared light and transmission peaks roughly at the same point as the luminous curve of the eye. Naturally, violet, blue, orange, or red colors are less distinguishable. Green lenses are recommended for situations with high amounts of reflected light (which contains large amounts of ultraviolet), such as glaciers and open water. They should be recommended for vacations in the tropics and for use during hot weather to protect against (heat) rays. In industry, green lenses of various densities are used for welding and other high light and heat situations. They also have the psychologic effect of "coolness" during hot weather and thus provide comfort to the wearer.

For many years brown tints were very popular in Europe. Brown-tinted lenses are being dispensed more commonly in North America. Brown lenses absorb almost all of the ultraviolet and have a very even progressive curve throughout the visible spectrum. Brown lenses are most useful in moderate to cold climates to protect against ultraviolet radiation and excessive radiation, with the added benefit of creating a "warm" visual environment. Three different tints of brown are available in either glass or plastic lenses.

Except for the cobalt-blue lenses used to judge the temperature in a blast furnace, blue lenses are more a whim of fashion than eye protection.

Yellow-tinted lenses are good absorbers of ultraviolet, violet, and blue. Suppressing this area of the spectrum enhances contrast in the rest of the visible spectrum. A yellow lens is therefore preferred to increase contrast in marginal light conditions, such as hunting at dawn or dusk or driving in foggy conditions, but should not be worn to protect against excessive light.

Other tints, such as pink, purple, and mauve, are deviants of the aforementioned tints and are used mainly as fashion accents.

Cheap sunglasses, usually in injection-molded plastic frames, are sold widely. These are not ground and polished lenses, although they may appear to be. Some lenses are plastic and can be identified as such by "bending" the lens in the frame. Cheap sunglasses are produced from flat, colored-glass sheets of low quality. Circles are cut from the flat sheet and each circle is placed in a metal concave dish having a curve of about 4.00 diopters. The dish is placed in an oven and left until the glass sags, or "drops," to the shape of the dish. The "lens" now has the shape of a ground lens. Lenses made in this manner are called "dropped lenses," and may be identified as such by (1) the shallow curve, (2) the distortions of objects *reflected* on the surface of the lens, and (3) usually some unwanted and unprescribed power. A properly ground and polished lens will show no distortions of reflected light and is usually on a base curve of about 6.00 diopters.

A popular type of sunglass on the market is the polarized sunglass. Such lenses usually are made of plastic but are sometimes found in a laminated form, in which the polarizing filter is sandwiched between two sheets of glass. Polarized sunglasses are available in prescription form.

Apart from the color of the lens, the axis of the polarizing material is placed in the frames so that glare coming off a flat horizontal surface is further darkened. The glasses are good for driving into the sun, because a white, glaring highway will appear dark. People who fish or go boating find that glare off water is reduced considerably when wearing polarized lenses. In rough-surfaced areas, such as grass, they are no improvement over tinted lenses. Brands of polarized lenses include Xperio, KBco, and Drivewear.

The American Academy of Ophthalmology has suggested some guidelines for consumers to follow when purchasing sunglasses (Box 13.1).

Densities

In dispensing tinted lenses, it is important to know the light conditions and environment in which the lenses will be used. Lenses that are too dark will dilate the pupil and visual acuity will be reduced. Should light intensity vary

---

Box 13.1 **Tips on purchasing sunglasses**

1. Ultraviolet (UV) absorption. The most important factor to look for in sunglasses is the indication that they block 100% of UV rays. Check for the manufacturer's label indicating whether the sunglasses are 100% UV absorbent and if they meet the American National Standards Institute (ANSI) guidelines for eyewear.

2. The bigger the lenses, the more coverage and the less damage to the eyes from the sun. Oversized glasses and wraparound-style glasses help decrease UV rays from entering the eyes from the side.

3. The color of the lens and the darkness of the tint are not good indicators of the glasses' ability to filter out UV light. Lens color should cause as little color distortion as possible. Dark gray or dark green tints permit the most normal color vision.

4. The price of a pair of sunglasses is absolutely no indicator of their lenses' ability to absorb UV light.

5. Polarized lenses tend to reduce reflection and glare and are especially effective around water and snow.

6. Photochromic lenses change color in response to sunlight, often preventing the need for two pairs of prescription glasses. Today there is much faster activation and deactivation with new photochromic lenses.

7. Special UV-absorbent coatings are available, which can be applied to everyday glasses. These are often applied to glasses used for skiing, high-altitude flying, and outdoor sports.

8. The US Food and Drug Administration requires that all eyeglass lenses, including sunglasses, be made of impact-resistant glass or plastic. Also the frames must be nonflammable. "Impact-resistant" does not mean that the lenses are shatterproof, but rather that they can withstand moderately sharp impacts.

Modified from American Academy of Ophthalmology EyeSmart: How to choose the best sunglasses. 2015. With permission.

rapidly, such as driving in bright sunlight through shaded areas, vision could be impaired. Therefore, very dark lenses may be recommended only for sailors, people who fish, and hikers. Naturally, for driving long distances through prairies and urban areas, a dark shade is most comfortable.

Providing a medium tint with a gradient mirror gives the patient an opportunity to select the density according to the prevailing light conditions. Naturally, in this respect, the photochromic lenses fill a specific void in the eye protection field. Their ability to adapt to the varying light intensities has made them one of the most sought-after lens materials.

Photochromic (indoor–outdoor) glasses

Photochromic lenses have the chameleon-like ability to change from light to dark and back again. In glass photochromic lenses, silver halide microcrystals impart this changeability and never wear out. The halides darken when exposed to ultraviolet or the blue end of the spectrum. The more popular technology is plastic photochromic lenses. The range of darkening photosensitive plastic lenses has been developed to the point where a pair of glasses can be perfectly clear lenses indoors and a satisfactory sunglass outdoors. Whereas clear plastic lenses transmit 90% to 92% of light indoors (polycarbonate and CR-39, respectively), advanced technology photochromic lenses (in a 1.50 Refractive Index) transmit 89% of light, which makes them indistinguishable from clear lenses indoors. Indoor transmission can also be enhanced with antireflective coatings. The average pair of sunglasses is designed to filter 70% to 85% of visible light and block 100% of UVA and UVB radiation.

The cycling of the modern photochromic lenses happens quickly. Transition lenses darken to a 70% tint within 35 seconds (Figure 13.22). During the reverse process, out of UV radiation for just a few minutes, they return to a 70% clarity. All photochromic lenses are affected by temperature. The range of dark to light is greater in cold weather (winter day) than in hot (summer picnic).

Ultraviolet light boxes are available that allow one to demonstrate the darkening of lenses with ultraviolet light. One can place an opaque tape (or paper) over the lens to see the dramatic effect. Most photochromic lens brands are available in gray or brown. Photochromic lenses are available in a whole host of materials including standard index (1.50), mid-/high index (1.53–1.59), high impact (Trivex and polycarbonate), and super high index (1.60–1.67) and are available in all lens designs from spherical single vision to aspheric single vision, segmented bi- and trifocals, and various no-line multifocals.

Today's modern photochromic lenses are for everyday use and not just for patients with light sensitivity. Like any premium product, photochromic lenses cost more

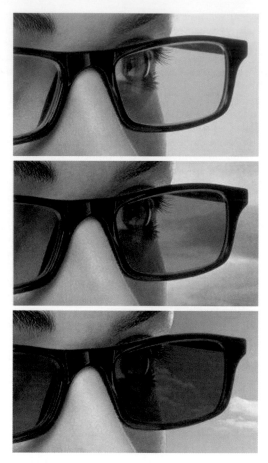

Figure 13.22 Progression of a photochromic tint. *(Courtesy of Transitions Optical, Inc.)*

since they have advanced technology and research and development costs are included in the price. However, they deliver more patient benefits, including convenient protection from glare and UV radiation, and typically have built-in scratch resistance.

Ultraviolet and blue-blocking lenses

Through-and-through tinted lenses that filter out more than 98% of blue and ultraviolet light were developed by Corning Glass Works and Younger Optics. The latter are made in C39 plastic. These lenses, which range in color from amber to red, are called plastic CPF by Corning, and PLS by Younger. They are photochromic in that they darken outdoors and lighten indoors. For the normal individual these lenses provide comfort from glare, reduce haziness, and sharpen vision. The light-colored CPF lenses (CPF 511, CPF 527, and PLS 530) may aid individuals with developing cataracts; the darker red lenses (CPF 550, PLS 540, and PLS 550) may improve functional visual acuity for such conditions as retinitis pigmentosa, albinism, aniridia, and intense photophobia.

The best method of evaluating these lenses is to place a plano-CPF lens over the existing lenses of the patient. Then the examiner turns up the lights of the room and rechecks vision. The patient is asked to go to a bright window and observe the change. If the change is significant, the lenses should be prescribed.

Mirrored sunglasses

A one-way mirror surface can be placed on a clear or colored glass lens to convert it to a sunglass for special purposes.

There are situations in which patients do not wish anyone to see their eyes (perhaps because of permanent or temporary disfigurement). Mirrored sunglasses give this protection and the patient has no trouble seeing through the mirrored lenses. In terms of the patient's vision, the tint can be neutral gray, pink, green, or any other color found in ordinary sunglasses.

Multifocal lenses

Multifocal lenses include all types of bifocals, trifocals, and the so-called invisible bifocals or continuous-vision lenses.

There are two basic types of multifocal lenses: the one-piece, or Ultex, and the fused.

The *one-piece* is so named because the material (glass or plastic) is the same throughout the lens and the power is varied by changing the curvature of the surface on the convex or concave side of the lens. The following types of bifocals and trifocals are of the one-piece construction:

1. All-plastic lenses, with segments on the convex side in almost every case
2. Younger (round-segment) invisible bifocals, with segments on the convex side
3. Progressive no-line design lenses, with no segments but with curvatures on the convex side. Designs from Zeiss and Hoya have curvature changes on both sides (Figure 13.23). The Shamir In Touch design lens has a wider, broader intermediate area, which allows more comfortable reading of handheld phone and electronics screens
4. The Executive, or President, type of bifocals or trifocals in glass or plastic, with segments on the convex side

The *fused* multifocal lens uses glass of two or more indexes of refraction. When the segment with the higher index is countersunk (fused) into the main lens, the surfaces of a fused lens have no change of curvature. The add (that is, the plus dioptric power of the bifocal or trifocal) is governed by two factors: (1) the difference in the indexes of refraction of the various types of glass and (2) the depth of the countersink into which the segment is fused. The following are fused-type glass lenses:

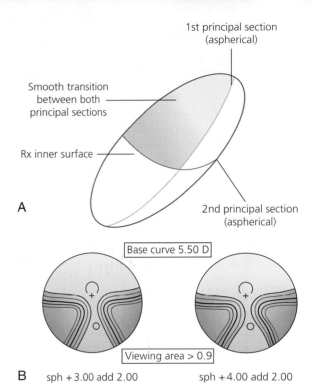

Figure 13.23 (A) Description of atoric prescription surface. (B) Constant visual field size with Hoya IQ lens, at the position of wear.

1. Kryptok or Achromat round-segment bifocals, with segments fused into the convex side
2. Flat-top bifocals and trifocals, with segments fused into the convex side
3. Catraconoid bifocals, with a glass aspheric convex surface and with a flat-top segment buried in the lens (aspheric curvatures are before the reading segments as well as the distance portion; plastic aspheric bifocals have aspheric surfaces for the distance portion of the lens only)

Falling into a category between one-piece and fused lenses are *cement bifocals* (Table 13.2). These comprise two lenses of the same type of glass having the same index of refraction fastened together to form a lens with the characteristics of the one-piece lens. These are rarely seen today but are included here for historical reference. The following explains how a fused bifocal is made:

1. A countersink is placed in a lens blank of appropriate depth and the countersink is finished by polishing (Figure 13.24A).
2. The segment that is merely a small lens of glass with a higher index of refraction than the main lens also is ground and polished to exactly fit the curvature of the countersink (Figure 13.24B).

Table 13.2 Types of bifocals

Type	Advantages	Disadvantages
Cement	Inexpensive (Noted here for historic interest, not widely seen today)	Line of demarcation very visible and collects dirt Poor durability; segment tends to loosen and fall off
Kryptok	Inconspicuous segment Inexpensive	Distinct chromatic aberration when reading segment is more than +1.75 Prism displacement at junction of distance and near segments very noticeable Increases thickness of lens
Ultex	Segment practically invisible No chromatic aberration Light in weight Reading segment on inside of lens and thus protected	More costly Prism displacement
Flat-top	No prism displacement Because of barium segment, chromatic aberration almost eliminated	More costly than Kryptok

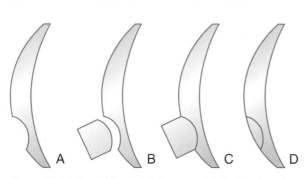

Figure 13.24 Fused bifocal. (A) A countersink is placed on the lens blank. (B) A segment of a higher index of refraction is ground to fit into the countersink. (C) Two lenses are fused together in an oven and cooled slowly. (D) Excess lens material is ground off and polished.

3. The two are fused together in an oven and allowed to cool slowly (annealing), so that no strain is set up inside the lens (Figure 13.24C).
4. The button is then ground off and the whole convex side is finished to a polish. This is the Kryptok or Achromat bifocal with a round segment (Figure 13.24D).

For a flat-top bifocal the process is much the same. The countersink in the main blank is made as previously mentioned. The button, however, is a different shape (Figure 13.25).

A carrier is fused to the top of the flat segment after the contacting surfaces are fined to an optical flat. In fining (the manufacturer's term), a lens curvature is brought from a frosted-glass appearance to a satin finish.

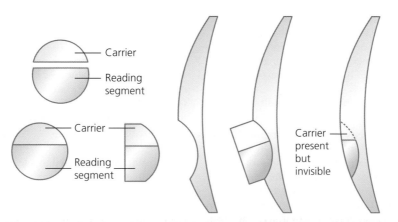

Figure 13.25 Flat-top bifocal. The reading segment is combined with a carrier of similar properties as the main lens. This button is then inserted into the countersink of the main lens, fused and ground off to produce a flat-top bifocal. The carrier is invisible but the segment, being of a different type of glass, can be seen.

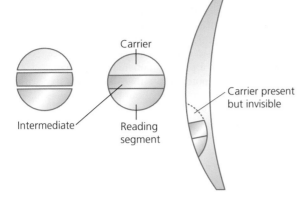

Figure 13.26 Flat-top trifocal. This lens is manufactured similarly to the bifocal, with an intermediate segment interposed between the carrier and the reading segment.

A flat-top trifocal is made in the same manner as a bifocal, but three types of glass form the button (Figure 13.26). The carrier matches the main lens in color and index of refraction, as in the bifocal. The intermediate segment is made of a glass with more bending power (higher index of refraction) than the main lens or carrier, but with less bending power than the reading segment. The intermediate segment is half the dioptric power, in the finished lens, of the reading segment. For example, trifocals with a +3.00 add would have an intermediate segment power of +1.50. Spectacle lenses are made of crown glass with an index of 1.523. Segments are made of barium glass or flint glass (index of refraction from 1.625 to 1.690).

Special flat-top bifocals and trifocals

The Executive bifocal, in plastic, is a modern version of the original Benjamin Franklin bifocal, which has two lenses in one eye wire: the lower half for reading, the upper half for distance (Figure 13.27A).

The modern equivalent is of one-piece construction. The prescription is ground on the concave side and there is a distinct ridge on the convex side where the two powers join. Trifocals are constructed the same way.

Invisible bifocals (progressive-add lenses [PALs])

Multiple invisible or progressive bifocal lenses are on the market. These lenses gradually increase in power as the line of sight travels downward through the lens. An early version of this lens was the Beach bifocal. Other names in this category are Flexsite, Omnifocal, Younger, Truevision, Difinity, and Varilux. Additional entries to the market come from Zeiss, Hoya, Essilor, Nikon, Shamir, and Kodak. The 48% market share of multifocal lenses is divided between PALs at 30.1% and lined bifocals or trifocals comprising 17.9%.

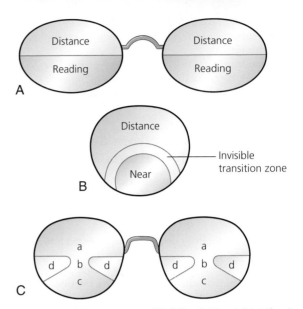

Figure 13.27 (A) Benjamin Franklin bifocal. (B) Invisible bifocal. (C) Multilux or Varilux lens: a, clear distance vision; b, gradual increase in power on axis to coincide with convergence of eyes; c, clear reading area; d, distortion area.

The main difficulty in any lens that gradually increases in power is that vision on either side of a vertical line through the optical center produces unwanted, unprescribed cylindric power, causing great distortion. This is a fault of the Omnifocal and the Beach and, to a lesser degree, of the original Multilux or Varilux lens. The new Varilux lenses are a great improvement over the first generations.

The Flexsite and Younger (Figure 13.27B) bifocals are an attempt to create a one-piece round segment lens, with the segment on the convex side and the dividing line blended on the surface of the lens so that it is invisible. The result is a lens with a correct prescription for reading and for distance vision but with a blurred transition zone between the two. The Younger bifocal is not widely in use, but shown here for historical reference.

The Multilux lens is constructed with a top portion that is a correct distance prescription, which gains in dioptric power toward the periphery; a bottom portion that is a correct near prescription, losing dioptric power toward the periphery of the reading area; and a transitional zone gradually increasing in power from distance to near (the Varilux lens is more widely in use). The chief disadvantage is that there are distortions through this lens in the lower right and lower left quadrants with induced astigmatism (Figure 13.27C). They are successful (as are the Younger bifocals) with some patients who are not bothered by the areas of distorted vision. To help practitioners, the bifocal add is often marked on the lens itself.

Use of Digital or Free form lenses provides a new way to surface lenses that minimizes the amount of distortion caused by light passing through the lens and transfers the optical surface onto a lens, which produces a complex surface with extreme accuracy.

Digital lenses may not neutralize as prescribed due to the alterations that occur during processing of the lens's curves. Although an add may read as +2.37 instead of +2.25, the lens is actually optically correct as prescribed.

Multivision lenses from a patient's point of view (vocational lenses)

Unfortunately there is no one type of bifocal or trifocal that universally meets the visual requirements of all patients. The following are examples of some of the special needs of patients.

1. A presbyopic truck driver may need tinted bifocals, with segments set high enough so that the instrument panel is visible only through the bifocal and with an add of "intermediate" power to give clear vision at 24 inches (60 cm). These glasses, because of the tint, would be unsuitable both for driving at night and for reading because 24 inches is too far for this purpose.
2. A barber needs large segments set much higher than usual because he or she is working at near, with vision almost straight ahead.
3. A bookkeeper or an executive spends most of the working day at a desk, using bifocal segments, and a fraction of the day looking across the office. Thus this person should have "desk bifocals" of the Executive type, with segments set much higher than normal.

All these multivision lenses might be termed *vocational bifocals* and *trifocals*. With the flexibility of current styles and technology, almost any type of segment, shape, size, or positioning—trifocal or bifocal—can be produced economically.

Computer glasses*

Discussing the patient's visual demands in detail helps design just the right lenses for maximum satisfaction. Tens of millions of people spend an hour or more of every working day in front of a computer screen.

Computer lenses are designed for task-specific wear by presbyopes who spend extended time at the computer. Computer lenses offer full-screen vision at intermediate distance, as well as a wide near area to provide transition for looking at the keyboard.

Several computer lenses are available that work well, but as with digital lenses, during neutralization, they may not read as prescribed but will be optically correct.

A computer screen is usually about an arm's length away from the user's eyes. This is different from the near zone for reading and the distance zone, representing an intermediate zone that requires specific add power.

Neither general-wear bifocals nor ordinary progressive lenses work well for many patients older than age 40 who work at computers more than an hour a day. Most desktop computer screens are about 10 to 20 degrees below primary gaze and many are at eye level, making general-wear bifocals ineffective. Computer screens are usually slightly farther away than the effective range for bifocals. As a result, wearers of standard bifocals tilt their head upward and may have to lean forward to see the screen clearly, creating an awkward position.

Progressive addition lenses work better but still not well enough for many presbyopes who work at a computer. These lenses have a narrow range of clear vision for viewing a screen but are not designed for extended gazing at objects in this intermediate range. Progressive addition lens wearers are often left to search for just the right distance to hold their heads from the screen. The viewing area is often restricted.

Patients who use computers only briefly and infrequently can get by with general-wear progressives. Early presbyopes with low adds can sometimes succeed by viewing the screen through the distance portion of their progressive lenses.

The special needs of computer-using presbyopes include a large central area for intermediate viewing and a lower portion for focusing on closer objects. It is important to note the role that the placement of the screen has in making the prescription effective. Usually it is appropriate for a computer monitor to be 24 inches (60 cm) from the eyes at 15 degrees below, rather than the standard 14 inches (35 cm) for reading. Most specialized lenses will work at those levels, and wearers should be advised that reconfiguring their workstations can help improve vision and make the prescription more effective.

Patients wearing progressive addition lenses for general wear are good candidates for the new designs available in response to demand from computer users. One design offers a wide midrange correction at the top of the lens for viewing the computer screen with a wide correction for near work at the bottom. The astigmatic distortion is on either side of the lens and interferes minimally with vision. Another design offers a large central area for intermediate-range viewing, a large near-viewing area at the bottom of the lens, and a small area for distance viewing at the top. The astigmatic distortion is located relatively high in the lens.

For young presbyopes, a single-vision lens dedicated to computer use can be effective. Such lenses are less expensive and provide a large, clear field of vision, and the users still have enough accommodation to see near objects clearly through lenses designed for intermediate distance.

Some patients—usually those already happy with general wear bi- and trifocals—prefer bi- and trifocals specifically prescribed for computer use. For advanced

*From Stein HA, Freeman MI, Stenson SM. *CLAO residents curriculum manual on refraction, spectacles and dispensing*. Metairie, LA: CLAO Publications, 2001 (with permission).

presbyopes, flat-top bifocals designed for computer use can work well. The top of the lens should contain the intermediate prescription for computer use and the bottom area the prescription for near distance. Distance vision will be slightly blurry in this design. For those who work at computers but also need distance vision, bifocals can be prescribed with the upper portion used for distance viewing. For computer users who want some measure of correction at all three distances, a trifocal with larger intermediate segment can be prescribed. For others, there is the variable reading lens, a subcategory of progressive addition lenses. There are computer lenses available such as the Shamir Office lens, a no-line design specifically for intermediate and near. This works well for the monitor and keyboard and allows the wearer to maintain a very comfortable head position for long periods at the computer.

Most popular types of multifocal lenses

The essential factors in a bifocal lens should be that the line of demarcation is inconspicuous, involving no sudden break, that the additional strength of the add does not augment the weight of the lens, and that the segment is large enough to give an adequate field of vision for reading. The line of demarcation, even though inconspicuous, should not interfere with distance vision. Bifocals have an inherent disadvantage in that there is an image jump—an apparent displacement of objects—when one changes the direction of vision from distance to near. Efforts to minimize this image displacement are made by incorporating additional segments with optical centers designed to produce a compensating prismatic effect. There are basically two types of bifocal segments available.

Flat-top segment

The flat-top segment is fused with the optical center lying at the upper portion of the segment; this is of value in treating

low hyperopes and all myopes. It eliminates image jump when looking from near to far. The base-down prism of the main lens is partially neutralized by the base-up prism of the flat-top segment (Figure 13.28A).

Round-top fused segments (Kryptok, Achromat)

The Achromat looks like a Kryptok but is a superior lens because it has less chromatic aberration (color fringing around objects) than does the Kryptok. This lens is used for hyperopic patients. In stronger powers the base-up prism of the main lens is neutralized by the base-down prism of the round segment (Figures 13.28B, 13.29 to 13.31).

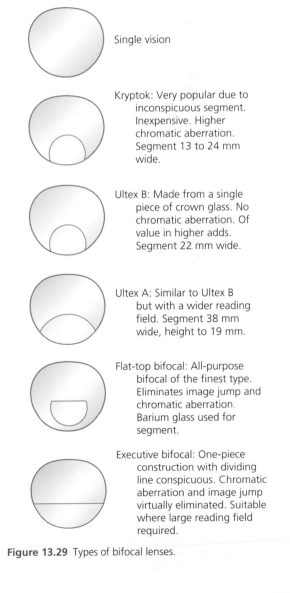

Single vision

Kryptok: Very popular due to inconspicuous segment. Inexpensive. Higher chromatic aberration. Segment 13 to 24 mm wide.

Ultex B: Made from a single piece of crown glass. No chromatic aberration. Of value in higher adds. Segment 22 mm wide.

Ultex A: Similar to Ultex B but with a wider reading field. Segment 38 mm wide, height to 19 mm.

Flat-top bifocal: All-purpose bifocal of the finest type. Eliminates image jump and chromatic aberration. Barium glass used for segment.

Executive bifocal: One-piece construction with dividing line conspicuous. Chromatic aberration and image jump virtually eliminated. Suitable where large reading field required.

Figure 13.29 Types of bifocal lenses.

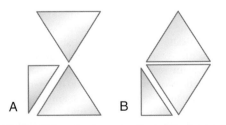

A   B

Figure 13.28 (A) The prism base-up effect of the flat-top bifocal segment counterbalances the base-down effect of the adjoining distance concave lens. (B) The prism base-down effect of the bifocal segment counterbalances the base-up effect of the adjoining distance convex lens.

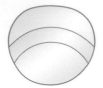

Round-top trifocal: Intermediate segment designed to permit reading in the intermediate zone.

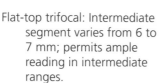

Flat-top trifocal: Intermediate segment varies from 6 to 7 mm; permits ample reading in intermediate ranges.

Executive trifocal: Similar to flat-top trifocal but with a wider field.

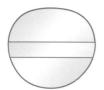

Vocational trifocals: Upper segment may be used to view objects overhead at close range.

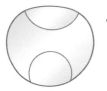

Additional configuration of vocational trifocal

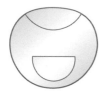

Additional configuration of vocational trifocal

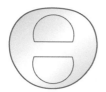

Figure 13.30 Types of trifocal lenses.

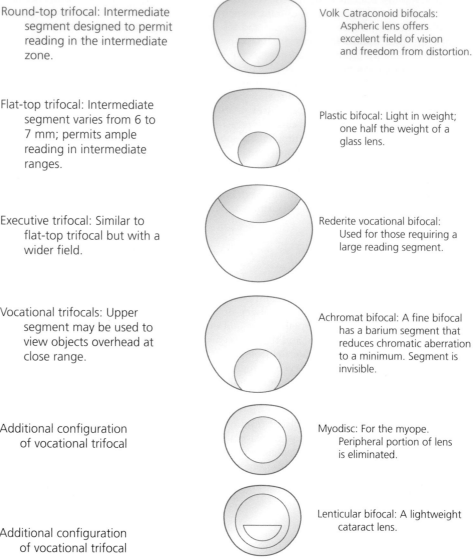

Volk Catraconoid bifocals: Aspheric lens offers excellent field of vision and freedom from distortion.

Plastic bifocal: Light in weight; one half the weight of a glass lens.

Rederite vocational bifocal: Used for those requiring a large reading segment.

Achromat bifocal: A fine bifocal has a barium segment that reduces chromatic aberration to a minimum. Segment is invisible.

Myodisc: For the myope. Peripheral portion of lens is eliminated.

Lenticular bifocal: A lightweight cataract lens.

Figure 13.31 Types of bifocal lenses.

Progressive lenses

Progressive-addition lenses such as the Varilux series are capable of providing a more flexible presbyopic correction. The Varilux I, introduced in 1959, was the first generation of these lenses, which are characterized by distance and near spherical zones that are linked vertically by a progressive corridor and laterally by a continuous surface. Later Varilux lenses were designed to provide not only a progressive surface but also visual comfort. The current market, in keeping pace with the aging baby boomers, has been prolific in the design and manufacture of bifocal progressive lenses. The new progressive lenses with aspheric surfaces dramatically reduce peripheral aberrations, enabling a wider central corridor. The multidesigned progressives are available in reading additions up to +3.50 diopters and astigmatic progressives up to 6.00 diopters. Additional options are available in plastic, glass, and tints. Zeiss, Varilux, and Hoya offer progressive bifocal technology with asphericity in both convex and concave surfaces. This reduces aberrations significantly as spherical and astigmatic powers increase.

Each point on the surface is matched as closely as possible to natural vision. This eliminates unwanted aberration and there is a specific increase in power in the central and peripheral areas. The Varilux 360 lens is a multidesigned progressive-addition lens, with specific changes based on the reading power. A complete range of addition designs goes from 0.75 to 3.5 diopters, which maximizes patient satisfaction at each stage of presbyopia. This lens takes into account not only central vision but also peripheral vision, which is important for patient adaptation and comfort; it also allows easier adaptation than did previous lenses.

The manufacturer suggests that, while a patient looks at one point at eye level, the distance from the center of the pupil to the edge of the frame should be measured. The fitting height varies depending on the choice of lens; it can be as little as 13 mm or as much as 24 mm. One chooses the smallest vertex distance possible between 12 and 14 mm and a pantoscopic tilt between 10 and 15 degrees. The examiner uses the pupillometer to measure PD for far vision; fitting heights are measured from the center of the pupil to the edge of the frame just below. The centering chart is used to check the accuracy of the mounting. The lens is marked for far-vision prism and near-vision power. The fitting cross always should be placed at the center of the pupil (Figure 13.32).

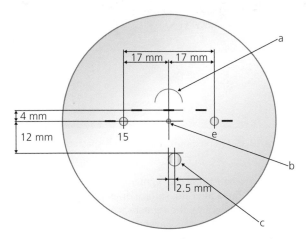

Figure 13.32 Measurements for Varilux II and Varilux Infinity progressive addition lenses. a, Far-vision power; b, prism power; c, near-reading power.

Specific control of asphericity is seen in many of today's progressive lenses. There is a current trend in progressive technology as a growing number of baby boomers are becoming presbyopic.

Handheld devices, such as cellular phones and tablets, have recently been found to emit a harmful blue light. Reacting to concerns about the side effects of this blue light, Essilor, a digital progressive lens maker, is embedding Smart Blue Filter in their products. Other manufacturers are also developing and implementing blue filter blocking lenses to reduce digital eye strain. Further developments in lens technology are expected as we begin to better understand the ocular side effects of the widespread use of digital devices.

Centering of lenses

Glasses should be centered so that the patient looks through the optical center of the lens; otherwise a prismatic effect will be introduced. A prismatic effect of 1.00 prism diopter is produced for every 1 cm of decentering of a 1.00-diopter lens. Thus a 10.00-diopter lens will produce 1.00 prism diopter of deviation for every millimeter that its optical center is displaced. The amount of prismatic deviation can be shown by the formula:

$$P = hd$$

where P = prismatic deviation; h = distance the lens is displaced in centimeters; d = dioptric power of the lens.

Decentering is often intentionally produced. Reading glasses are normally decentered 2.5 mm inward and 6.5 to 8 mm downward inasmuch as the eyes are converged and turned down for reading. Decentering of lenses has been used to correct minor disturbances of ocular muscle imbalance.

Pantoscopic angle

The pantoscopic angle or tilt of the frame is the vertical angle that the frame front makes to the face when the glasses are worn (Figure 13.33). When viewed from the side, it is normal for the lower rims of the frame front to be closer to the cheeks than are the upper rims. The proper pantoscopic angle may range from 4 to 18 degrees. Often

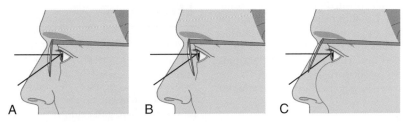

Figure 13.33 Illustrations of vertical angle of spectacle front tilt. (A) No pantoscopic angle (uneven vertex). (B) Proper pantoscopic angle (even vertex). (C) Retroscopic angle required for protruding cheek.
(Courtesy of Jackie Freeman, Bellevue, WA. Reproduced with permission from Stein HA, Freeman, MI, Stenson, SM. CLAO residents curriculum manual on refraction, spectacles and dispensing. Metairie, LA: CLAO Publications, 2001.)

people with extremely protruding eyebrows may exceed this range. This angle permits the eye to focus downward from distance gaze to near gaze and maintain a constant vertex distance. It enables the patient to view reading print directly through the center of the reading addition. This is a very critical aspect of the fitting procedure.

Use of prisms in glasses

A vertical muscle imbalance of more than 1.00 diopter cannot be tolerated by the patient. To compensate for a vertical muscle imbalance, the amount of prism diopter correction needed is determined by the Maddox rod test. Suitable compensating base-up or base-down prisms are incorporated into the lenses. For example, an individual with +2.00 diopters of right hypertropia would require 2.00 diopters of vertical prism to correct the imbalance. This may be given as 1.00 diopter, base down, in front of the right eye and 1.00 diopter, base up, in front of the left eye. Prisms may be used for the treatment of large horizontal phorias and for convergence insufficiency.

If the difference in the refractive error between the two eyes is large, an undesired prismatic effect and a secondary ocular muscular imbalance may be induced when the patient is looking through the bifocal segment. In this situation, a "slab-off"' or a bicentric lens may be required to neutralize the induced prismatic effect. Slab-off is the most common technique used to correct vertical imbalance at near. Slab-offs often are used when the imbalance is greater than 1.5 prism diopters. They are, however, useful only for those with 5.00 prism diopters or less in vertical imbalance on looking downward.

Fresnel lenses and prisms

The Fresnel lens has been used in various ways for many years and has found its way into ophthalmic lenses. It is used in ships' lanterns and in lighthouses as a light-condensing lens but its most modern application is in condensing lenses in projectors and in many of the single-lens, reflex camera viewfinders, where it gives brilliance to the image projected on the ground-glass focusing screen.

A development in ophthalmic prisms is the Fresnel press-on prism (Figure 13.34), which is as thin as a piece of paper and has powers up to 40.00 prism diopters. Like the Fresnel lens, it has visible lines. The thin plastic prism is cut to the shape of a spectacle lens and is pressed onto the lens surface without the use of cement (Figure 13.35). The prism can be easily removed and changed in a few seconds. The advantage of the Fresnel prism is its low weight. It is ideal as a temporary prism over the patient's existing prescription.

Press-on adds

Plastic reading segments are available for instantly turning a lens into a bifocal. After wetting the concave surface of the

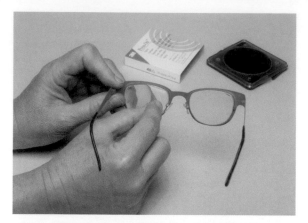

Figure 13.34 Fresnel prism applied to left lens of glasses.

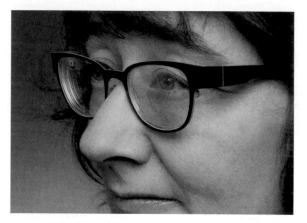

Figure 13.35 Fresnel prism applied to left spectacle lens

glasses, one can press the segments onto the lens, where they will adhere after the surface dries. This is not a long-term solution because the segment will not adhere forever, but it is enormously convenient. They can easily be removed and are a valuable adjunct to sunglasses.

PRODUCTION OF PRESCRIPTION LENSES

On receipt of the prescription from a patient, the dispensing optician notes whether multivision (bifocal or trifocal) or single-vision lenses are specified. If a single-vision lens is required, the optician or the optical laboratory can select from stock an uncut, finished, single-vision lens of the exact power of sphere and cylinder needed. This lens is *laid out* and *edged* (shaped to fit the frame) (Figure 13.36) so that when it is mounted in the frame the axis of the prescription is as specified. Most single-vision prescriptions do not

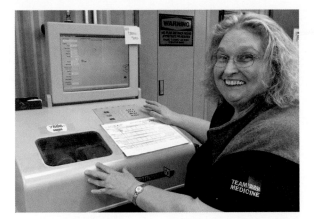

Figure 13.36 Patternless edger in modern optical laboratory.

require surfacing of the lens. Consequently, single-vision glasses can be produced to prescription in a matter of hours if necessary.

The story of bifocals and trifocals is somewhat different. A stock of finished bifocal lenses that can be edged and put into a frame is just not possible (except a limited stock of sphere bifocals). The possible permutations and combinations of sphere powers, cylindric powers, axes, bifocal or trifocal addition powers, bifocal or trifocal segment shapes, and the position of the segment in the finished glasses mean a stock of finished bifocals or trifocals cannot be maintained by even the largest optical companies. These lenses must be custom made. However, lens manufacturers do semifinish multifocal lenses to the point of providing an uncut lens finished on one side with the bifocal or trifocal segment of predetermined power. The patient's prescription as to spherical and cylindric power and axis must be produced on the other side.

In the case of hard-resin lenses and fused-segment bifocals and trifocals, the prescription is placed on the concave surface by diamond-tooled *generators*. The result is a *frosted glass* appearance to the lens. The second step is termed *fining*. A cast-iron lap that exactly fits the prescription generated on the lens is rubbed against the lens under a mixture of fine emery and water. The result of the fining stage is a satin-finished surface. The third and last step again uses a lap, but this time a polishing pad is placed between the glass and the cast-iron lap. A polishing material (such as cerium oxide in water) produces the high polish of the finished lens. From this point the procedure is similar to that for the single-vision lens; that is, the lens is laid out, edged to the shape of the frame, and inserted into the patient's frame.

Because of the necessity of surfacing one side of the bifocal and trifocal lenses and the additional time required for this, multifocal lenses cannot be produced as quickly as can single-vision lenses. They must go to a laboratory capable of doing more than just edging a single-vision stock lens to shape. Very few dispensing opticians have surfacing facilities on their premises. A few have edging machinery but most send their work to optical laboratories. Other companies have injected molding machines or in-house laboratories to convert simple prescriptions in 1 hour. Some offices have "edgers" to convert lenses to fit specific frames.

CARE OF GLASSES

Patients should understand the need for care and cleaning of their glasses. Too often the patient comes to the ophthalmologist wearing a dirty, scratched pair of glasses that has undoubtedly caused blurred vision. The following rules should be observed in the maintenance of spectacles.

1. The frames should be kept clean. The collection of grease and dirt on the frames and the lenses is best removed by washing in soapy lukewarm water. Spectacle lenses should not be cleaned or polished when they are dry, because they may become scratched. Most lenses are coated with scratch-resistant or antireflective coating and should not be cleaned with anything containing alcohol or ammonia; these chemicals can wear away coatings.

2. When not in use, spectacles should be kept in their case. If this is not possible, they should be laid so that they are supported by the folding sidepieces or left standing on their rims.

3. Spectacles should be removed by taking them off with both hands, holding them firmly and close to the hinges. Removing them with one hand causes the frame to bend out of shape or even break.

4. During the winter, lenses frequently mist over and blur vision. Fog-resistant coatings are available, but not recommended because they must be reapplied regularly.

5. In hardened lenses the surface compression layer is only 0.003 or 0.004 inch (0.008 or 0.01 cm) in depth, and a fairly deep scratch could exceed this and thus weaken the safety feature of the lens.

6. Screws in glasses may become loose. Check them when cleaning, and if the lens moves within the frame, have an optician tighten and adjust the frames. Regular visits to the optician for cleaning and adjustment of frames will help keep glasses in the best condition over time.

Questions for review and thought

1. Discuss the manufacture and types of ophthalmic frames.
2. What are the advantages and disadvantages of the different types of ophthalmic frames?
3. How is pupillary distance measured?
4. What is the temple length? What points are measured?
5. What type of glass is used commonly for ophthalmic lenses?
6. What are some of the distortions inherent in lenses?
7. High-power hyperopic lenses usually present a special problem because of their thickness and weight. What type of special lens is available to overcome these problems?
8. Safety glasses are recommended for children, people engaged in sports, and industrial workers. How are they constructed?
9. Sunglasses filter out certain of the color components of white light. Discuss some types of sunglasses that are available.
10. Bifocals are used to provide two focal distances in the same glass. They may be of one-piece or fused construction or even cemented. Draw diagrams to illustrate how fused bifocals are constructed.
11. Special occupations, such as garage mechanics, may require the worker to use a bifocal segment in an uncommon position. Name as many occupations as you can in which the bifocal segment may be required in an unusual position.
12. What are the advantages of the Fresnel prism?
13. Does a large stylish frame size improve or diminish visual acuity in a person with a large refractive error?
14. What lenses would you recommend for night driving?
15. Does a blue lens affect visual acuity?
16. How can thick glasses be made lighter?
17. What types of frames should be avoided because of their flammable potential?
18. What kind of glasses should a welder use?
19. What are the advantages and disadvantages of trifocals?

Q Self-evaluation questions

True–false statements

Directions: Indicate whether the statement is true **(T)** or false **(F).**

1. Cellulose nitrate is the most common plastic used in the fabrication of spectacle frames. **T** or **F**
2. The pupillary distance is the distance from the center of the pupil of one eye to the center of the pupil of the other eye. **T** or **F**
3. The optical center of a lens is the thinnest part of the lens in a myopic correction and the thickest part of a lens in a hyperopic correction. **T** or **F**

Missing words

Directions: Write in the missing word in the following sentences.

4. The primary glass used by opticians is _____ glass.
5. Aphakic lenses tend to distort to a _____ shape.
6. Coating a lens often is referred to as _____ a lens.

Choice-completion questions

Directions: Select the one best answer in each case.

7. The preferred material to be used in children's glasses is:
   a. CR-39.
   b. polycarbonate or Trivex.
   c. high-index glass.
   d. high-index plastic.
   e. none of the above.
8. The invisible bifocal offers:
   a. great vision over the whole lens.
   b. great vision just in a band on either side of the optical center.
   c. great vision nasally where the eyes turn in to read.
   d. best vision in powers greater than +1.50.
   e. none of the above.
9. A Fresnel lens is a press-on lens and:
   a. it can be cut to any shape.
   b. it comes in prisms up to 15.00 diopters as well as in a range of positive and negative lens powers.
   c. it gets dirty easily, peels off, and has to be replaced often.
   d. it causes a drop of vision because the optics are not sharp.
   e. is all of the above.

A   Answers, notes, and explanations

1. **False.** Cellulose nitrate burns fiercely if a flame is brought to it. Today the use of such flammable plastics is not allowed in the make-up of spectacles. A lit cigarette near the frames may ignite them. One of the popular plastics used presently is cellulose acetate, which is desirable because it comes in a variety of colors. It can burn if a flame is held to it but it does not ignite and spread on its own.

   Lucite, a much tougher material, is frequently used. For children, nylon and Optyl frames are popular because they are flexible and virtually indestructible. Flexibility allows the frame to fit any face and prevents snapping, which can occur with the more rigid plastics. Nylon is made up in a limited number of colors but Optyl can be dyed to any color combination.

2. **False.** This distance actually exceeds the true interpupillary distance, which is measured from the visual axis of one eye to the other. The visual axis is a little nasal to the center of the pupil in most instances. Because of the inherent difficulties in measuring visual axis, the PD is normally taken from the nasal edge of the pupil of the patient's right eye to the temporal side of the pupil of the left eye.

   Light reflexes off the pupil can indicate the visual axis of the eye and they are more accurate.

   Two readings should be taken: one for the distance and one for near.

   The PD is an important measurement because many complaints and glass checks stem from a failure of the optician to center the lens to the visual axis of the eye. When this happens, unwanted prism is introduced, and the patient has symptoms.

3. **True.** The optical center of the lens should be marked inasmuch as it does not coincide with the midpoint between the nasal and temporal sides of the frame. Most lensmeters have a marking device to indicate the true optical center of the lens. Some frames are so large and eccentric that the optical centers of the lenses never approximate the visual axes of the eyes. Checking optical centers should be performed on every glass check because centering is the largest source of complaints.

4. **Crown.** Crown glass has been a favorite lens for opticians because it has a lower refractive index and has less of a tendency to color dispersion. However, such lenses are heavy and are particularly cumbersome in higher powers. CR-39, a hard resin plastic lens, accounts for more than 50% of ophthalmic lenses prescribed. The weight of CR-39 is nearly half that of crown glass. Polycarbonate, a thermoplastic resin lens, is used in sport and safety glasses because of its impact resistance.

5. **Pincushion.** A lens that is thick causes distortion because the bending of light at the edge of the lens is not the same as in the middle of the lens. In an aphakic lens, the thickness is in the center of the lens and the lens profile drops off sharply toward the edge. In high myopes, the thickness of the lens is toward the edges, and the distortion created by the thin center moving out to thicken at the periphery causes barrel distortion.

   In aphakic lenses remedies for distortion include: (1) lenticular lenses because they get rid of the lens edge and (2) lenses that are flatter in the periphery because they eliminate the drastic change in power. The four-drop lens does this job well. Basically these lenses fall into the category of aspheric lenses.

6. **Blooming.** The lenses are coated with magnesium fluoride, which is one-quarter of the wavelength of yellow-green light. The coating imparts a purplish sheen to these lenses, similar to bloom on a ripe plum; hence the name.

   The coating is tough and lasts the lifetime of the lens. The purpose of coating the lens is to eliminate annoying light reflections from lights and bulbs.

   A coated lens allows greater light transmission while depressing the amount of internal reflections.

7. **b. Polycarbonate** or **Trivex.** When dispensing eyewear for children, it is important to address the many safety issues relevant to the child, as well as the concerns of the parents. Infants and toddlers are prone to bumping into objects and falling down; older children who play sports, as well as children of any age engaged in normal child's play, will benefit from the added safety of polycarbonate or Trivex lenses in their eyeglasses. It is for this reason more than any other that polycarbonate or Trivex is the material of choice for all pediatric dispensing. With an impact resistance significantly greater than that of CR-39, high refractive index, and lower specific gravity, there is no more suitable material for children. Still, CR-39 remains an option when polycarbonate's slightly higher cost is an issue. Generally speaking, the use of crown glass in children's eyewear is contraindicated.

8. **b. Great vision just in a band on either side of the optical center.** This lens has become very popular because it eliminates the visible presence of bifocals, which to many people means aging. Optically it offers some advantages. It eliminates image jump, as the transition between the distance and near portion is not abrupt. It also confers a continuous increase in power looking down so that a longer band of near focal points is available to the wearer. However, this lens does create lateral astigmatism on either side of the central band of the lens. Many people find the distortion disabling for reading. Some of the newer models of this seamless bifocal are better because the diameter of the clear central zone has been expanded.

9. **e. All of the above.** A Fresnel lens is basically a temporary lens. The advantages of this lens are that it is flexible and lightweight. However, the disadvantages of hazy vision and of lower durability and reliability preclude constant wear.

   It is a good temporary lens for postsurgical cataract cases and for those people with temporary diplopia who require bridge prisms to carry them along until their condition improves.

Chapter | **14** |

Rigid contact lenses: basics

Contact lenses have become a routine part of our armamentarium for visual rehabilitation of the eye. Their use and demand are constantly increasing. More than 20% of the North American population is myopic and many of these people depend on visual correction. Coupled with the increasing use of contact lenses, many myths and fallacies have arisen regarding their indications and contraindications. At the very minimum, the ophthalmic assistant should be able to discuss with the patient the function of a contact lens, its purpose, and its limitations. The ophthalmic assistant can also be of value in some of the technical aspects of contact lens wear, such as method of insertion and removal and, particularly, proper care and storage of the lens itself. This chapter deals with the practical aspects of management of the patient who desires contact lenses, and in particular, rigid contact lenses.

DEVELOPMENT

As early as the 16th century, Leonardo da Vinci conceived and sketched prototypes of modern contact lenses. He experimented by neutralizing his own refractive error by placing his face in a container of water. In the following century René Descartes described and illustrated a glass type of scleral contact lens (Figure 14.1). However, the first practical type of contact lens was produced in 1887. This lens consisted of a glass capsule containing gelatin that was placed in contact with the cornea, with the glass being molded to correspond to the shape of the eye.

In 1932 the first major advance in the design of the contact lens was made. Investigating impressions made from the human eye, Dr. Joseph Dallos found that no two were identical. From this he concluded that it was impossible to fit a contact lens manufactured to a preconceived formula. Dallos then developed a technique of making negative casts of the anterior segment of the living eye. However, his lenses could be tolerated for only limited periods of time because of the excessive weight of the glass and they were difficult to manufacture. In 1938 the first molded scleral contact lens that overlaid the sclera was made from a plastic material called polymethyl methacrylate (PMMA). This lens had many advantages over glass, because it was lighter, shatterproof, and easily moldable.

It was not until 1948 that Kevin Tuohy introduced the first fluidless corneal lens, which was designed to rest on the corneal tear layer. These were large, but later smaller microcorneal lenses were introduced, which made possible a great step forward in the successful wearing of contact lenses.

New crosslinking technology stabilizes thin lens designs for comfort and durability. There are at least 48 different RGP contact lens materials available by 11 different manufacturers. These manufacturers provide their GP material to labs all across the world that produce numerous GP lens designs.

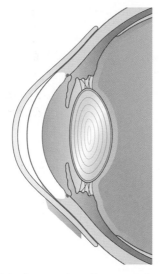

Figure 14.1 Scleral contact lens. The contact lens fits over the cornea and sclera.

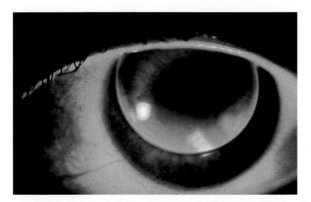

Figure 14.2 The silicone acrylate contact lens is gas permeable. It may be fitted larger than conventional polymethyl methacrylate (PMMA) rigid lenses. Note that the upper eyelid margin is covering the upper portion of the contact lens.

Further developments in rigid lens manufacture came with the introduction of intermediate curves, the practice of refining the edges, and the development of toric lenses. Rigid lens technology made another leap forward with the introduction of silicone and fluorocarbon. When combined with PMMA, these materials make the plastic material gas permeable (Figure 14.2). As a result of these new materials, in most countries today PMMA rigid lenses are rarely used.

The latest advances in rigid gas-permeable (RGP, or GP) technology involve improving the biocompatibility of materials to prevent unwanted deposits from tears. Polysulfone has been used in contact lens polymerization.

OPTICS

The rigid contact lens, for all practical purposes, eliminates the cornea as a major source of refractive error of the eye, because it is the same refractive index (RI) as the fluid in front of it. The fluid interface between the contact lens and the cornea fills out irregularities in the contours of the anterior corneal surface, converting the cornea to a sphere. Thus the fluid may be considered a forward extension of the cornea. If the radius of curvature of the back surface of the contact lens is the same as that of the front surface of the cornea, the refractive power of the contact lens will be the same as that of the cornea. The change in refractive power is produced by altering the curvature of the contact lens, as well as changing the total contact lens power.

HOW THE CORNEAL CONTACT LENS WORKS

A contact lens rests on the cornea just as a small fragment of paper adheres to the wet fingertip by just touching it. The natural moisture on the surface of the cornea is sufficient to create a surface tension and permit the lens to adhere quite strongly.

The back surface of the lens is contoured so that it exactly fits the curvature of the cornea. This curvature can be measured by instruments such as an ophthalmometer (or keratometer), and topographer. It is vital that these measurements be exact because if there is any contact or touch between the cornea and the contact lens, then a scratch, abrasion, or erosion can occur in the superficial layers of the cornea. The contact lens therefore rests on a liquid cushion (tear film) and never on the eye itself. Injury to the cornea is one of the most damaging complications that can result from a poorly fitted contact lens. Not only does it produce a painful red eye that obscures vision, but it also provides a portal of entry for bacteria and other pathogenic organisms to form a corneal ulcer.

The difference between the front surface curvature and the back surface curvature of a contact lens produces the power of the lens.

The edge of an RGP contact lens is thin and polished so that it can gently slide underneath the lid without being dislodged and prevent lid irritation when blinking.

TERMINOLOGY

To appreciate contact lens technology, one should have an understanding of contact lens jargon. The following terminology applies to rigid as well as soft lenses.

The ophthalmometer is an instrument designed to measure the corneal curvature by using the cornea as a front surface mirror. The instrument is most commonly referred to as the keratometer, even though this is actually a trade name of Bausch & Lomb.

In astigmatism with-the-rule the vertical corneal meridian has the steepest curvature, whereas in astigmatism against-the-rule the horizontal meridian has the steepest curvature (Figure 14.3).

In performing keratometry some authors record the flattest meridian first and the steepest meridian next so that a keratometer (K) value of, for example, 44.00 diopters × 46.00 diopters × 85 indicates that the horizontal meridian has a radius of 44.00 diopters and that the vertical meridian has a radius of 46.00 diopters with the axis at 85 degrees. Other authors prefer to always record the horizontal meridian first, regardless of which is the flattest. This value may be expressed in either diopters or millimeters of radius. Table 14.1 gives a comparative value of the K reading in diopters and millimeters. Each 0.05 mm is equivalent to approximately 0.25 diopter, so that a 0.5-mm radius equals approximately 2.50 diopters. Expressed another way, each 1.00 diopter change in the K reading equals approximately a 0.2-mm radius change.

Table 14.1 Diopter to millimeter conversion

Keratometric reading (D)	Radius convex (mm)
47.75	= 7.07
47.50	= 7.11
47.25	= 7.14
47.00	= 7.18
46.75	= 7.22
46.50	= 7.26
46.25	= 7.30
46.00	= 7.34
45.75	= 7.38
45.50	= 7.42
45.25	= 7.46
45.00	= 7.50
44.75	= 7.55
44.50	= 7.58
44.25	= 7.63
44.00	= 7.67
43.75	= 7.72
43.50	= 7.76
43.25	= 7.80
43.00	= 7.85
42.75	= 7.90
42.50	= 7.95
42.25	= 8.00
42.00	= 8.04
41.75	= 8.08
41.50	= 8.13
41.25	= 8.18
41.00	= 8.23
40.75	= 8.28
40.50	= 8.33
40.25	= 8.39
40.00	= 8.44

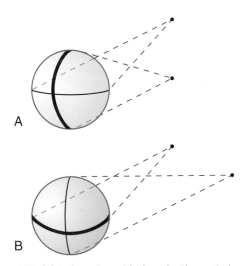

A

B

Figure 14.3 (A) Astigmatism with-the-rule. The vertical corneal meridian has the steepest curvature. (B) Astigmatism against-the-rule. The horizontal meridian has the steepest curvature.
(From Stein HA, Slatt BJ, Stein RM, Freeman MI. Fitting guide for rigid and soft contact lenses: a practical approach. 4th ed. St Louis: Mosby; 2002.)

In contact lens work one usually first considers the flattest K reading. If the back surface of the lens is to be the same radius as K, this is referred to as fitting on K (i.e., if K readings are 44.50/45.00, the base curve of the lens

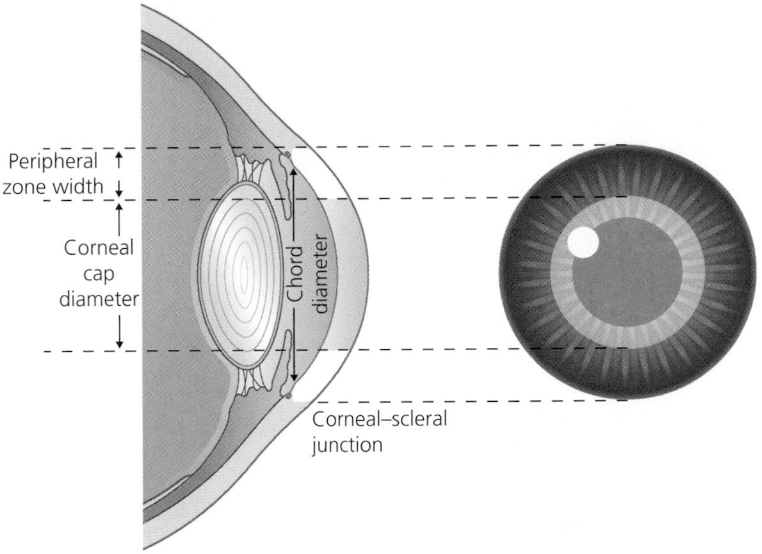

Figure 14.4 Corneal cap, representing the theoretic spherical central zone of the cornea.

(From Stein HA, Slatt BJ, Stein RM, Freeman MI. Fitting guide for rigid and soft contact lenses: a practical approach. 4th ed. St Louis: Mosby; 2002.)

would be 44.50 or 7.58 mm). RGP lenses may be fitted on K, flatter than K, or steeper than K. This may depend on the size of the lens and the corneal astigmatism. Soft contact lenses are generally fitted 3.00 to 5.00 diopters flatter than K.

The corneal cap is the central zone of the cornea. This has a radius of approximately 4 to 6 mm and has a relatively constant spherical radius of curvature (Figure 14.4). The peripheral or paracentral zone of the cornea is the area surrounding the corneal cap and extending to the limbus. It has a much flatter curvature than does the central curve. The rate of flattening does not conform to a mathematic progression, that is, the cornea is not a true ellipse. It is generally described as being aspheric.

Most rigid corneal lenses are either bicurve or tricurve. A bicurve lens has one base curve and one secondary curve (Figure 14.5). A small lens is usually bicurve. An intrapalpebral fit is one that fits within the palpebral fissure limits, and is bicurve. This type of lens is small and steep, with narrow peripheral curves of 0.2 mm and small diameters of 7.5 to 8.8 mm.

A multicurve lens has a base curve and three or more peripheral curves. A tricurve lens usually has a large diameter (Figure 14.6). A contour lens is basically a tricurve lens with a narrow intermediate curve. The blend is the point of transition between the radii of curvature from one curve to another. The sharp junction is removed by making the zone of transition with a curved tool that has a radius value between the values of the two adjacent curves.

An intermediate curve is a curve between the base curve and the peripheral curve.

The total lens diameter or the chord diameter is the measurement from one edge of the lens to the opposite side.

This is a linear measurement and is not related to the circumference of the lens. Most rigid lenses used today have a chord diameter between 8 and 10 mm, whereas the chord diameter of a soft lens usually ranges from 12 to 15 mm. Depending on which end of the scale they fall into, lenses may be referred to as small or large.

The peripheral curve width is the diameter from one edge of a secondary curve to another.

The central thickness of a lens is the separation between the anterior and posterior surfaces at the geometric center of a lens. The higher the minus power, the thinner is the center, whereas the higher the plus power, the thicker is the center.

Tints refer to the coloring available in a lens. They may be blue, brown, gray, or green for rigid lenses. They may be numbered 1 to 3, with number 1 the lightest and number 3 the darkest shade of each color.

A ballasted lens, often referred to as a prism ballast lens, is one that is weighted with a heavier base that orients inferiorly when the lens is worn. A truncated lens is one that is cut off to form a horizontal base. The amputation of the base is usually at the inferior pole of the lens. Truncation is frequently used to add stability to a rigid alternating bifocal lens, or soft toric lens, and to prevent rotation.

Back vertex power refers to the effective power of the lens from the posterior surface. The distance from the back surface of the lens to the focal point is the back focal length; its reciprocal is the back vertex power.

The primary base curve, as well as all other curvatures of a lens, may be expressed in terms of millimeters of radius of curvature. It can also be expressed in diopters: a primary base curve of 43.25 diopters is equal to 7.8 mm. The primary central posterior curve of a lens is designed to conform to the optic zone of the cornea.

239

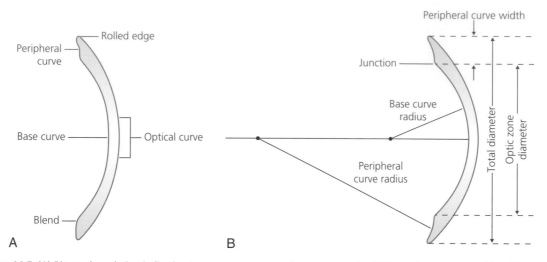

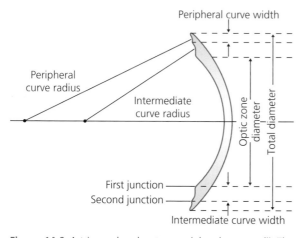

Figure 14.5 (A) Bicurve lens design indicating two curves: a primary base curve and a flatter peripheral curve with rolled edges to permit greater comfort. (B) Same bicurve lens indicating the diameter of the optic zone and the diameter of the peripheral curve. The combination of the two makes up the total diameter of the lens.
(From Stein HA, Slatt BJ, Stein RM, Freeman MI. Fitting guide for rigid and soft contact lenses: a practical approach. 4th ed. St Louis: Mosby; 2002.)

Figure 14.6 A tricurve lens has two peripheral curve radii. The intermediate curve may be very narrow, as found in contour lenses. These lenses have large diameters—9.5 mm or greater—with an optic zone of 6.5 to 7.5 mm, which is just large enough to clear the maximum pupil diameter. The peripheral curves are slightly flatter than the base curves by 0.4 to 0.8 mm, with a width of 1.3 mm. With a standard tricurve lens the intermediate curve is 1 mm flatter than the base curve. The peripheral curve is a standard 12.25-mm radius.
(From Stein HA, Slatt BJ, Stein RM, Freeman MI: Fitting guide for rigid and soft contact lenses: a practical approach, 4th edn. St Louis: Mosby, 2002.)

The optic zone of a lens is the central zone that contains the refractive power and generally corresponds to the central corneal cap of the cornea.

Toroidal or toric lenses (derived from Latin *torus*, "a bulge") are lenses with different radii of curvature in each meridian. The meridians of the shortest and longest radii are called the principal meridians, and they differ by 90 degrees. These lenses are used to correct astigmatism.

A front surface toric lens has an anterior surface that has two different radii of curvature but a central posterior surface that is spherical. Usually a prism ballast is required for orientation.

A back surface toric lens has a posterior surface that has two different radii of curvature and an anterior spherical surface.

In a bitoric lens the anterior and posterior surfaces have two curvatures on the front and back surfaces. The axes of the anterior and posterior toroidal surfaces may coincide or be oblique to one another, but usually they coincide.

The lenticular bowl refers to the diameter of the optical portion of a lens and is used with higher-power lenses.

The posterior apical radius (PAR) refers to the radius of curvature of the back surface of a lens at its apex. This is the area of curvature that will conform to the front surface of the apex of the cornea. Lenses are labeled by the posterior radius at the apex of the lens.

When a base curve of a lens is said to be made steeper, this means that the posterior radius of curvature is decreased (e.g., from 8.4 to 8.1 mm), so that the curvature is now steeper. When the base curve is said to be made flatter, it means that the posterior radius of curvature of the lens is increased (e.g., from 8.1 to 8.4 mm), so that the curvature is now flatter.

The sagittal depth or height of a lens is the distance between a flat surface and the back surface of the central portion of the lens. Thus for two lenses of the same diameter but of different sagittal depths, the lens of the greater sagittal depth produces a greater "vaulting" of the lens and in effect is steeper. This is often referred to as the sagittal vault.

There are two important variables in understanding the mechanism of loosening or tightening a lens. These variables are the diameter and the radius of the lens. If the diameter is kept constant, by changing the radius to a longer radius (e.g., from a 7.8- to an 8.4-mm radius), the sagittal vault or sagittal height of the lens becomes shorter and the lens becomes flatter. The converse is also true (Figures 14.7 and 14.8).

If the central posterior curve (radius) of the lens remains the same but the diameter is made larger (e.g., from 13 to 15 mm with soft lenses or from 8 to 9 mm with rigid lenses), the sagittal vault or sagittal height of the lens is increased and the lens becomes steeper. The converse is also true (Figure 14.9).

For example, if we consider the lens as being part of a similar circle (Figure 14.10) and we take two parts of the circle with different diameters or chords, the portion of the circle with the larger diameter will have a greater sagittal vault.

The wettability of a surface is measured in terms of its contact or wetting angle. In the case of a contact lens this is the angle formed between the tangent to the edge of a drop of water and the surface of a contact lens. The wetting angle, called theta, is expressed as zero if the material is completely wetted by the liquid (Figure 14.11). As the wetting angle becomes greater than zero, the solid surface cannot be completely wetted. As an extreme, if a drop of mercury were to be placed on a glass slide, it would not spread out on the surface but would form a small blob whose angle would be greater than 90 degrees (see Figure 14.11). Some plastics have smaller wetting angles than others; the lower the wetting angle of the plastic, the better the tears will spread evenly over the surface of the contact lens. Wetting solutions reduce this angle and permit better flow of tears and comfort. The lower the wetting angle, the greater is the spread of tears.

Terminology pertaining to oxygen studies has taken on increasing importance in the contact lens literature because of the development of extended-wear lenses and gas-permeable contact lenses.

The oxygen transmission through a given material is a laboratory measurement, often referred to as the DK value, where D is the diffusion coefficient for oxygen movement in lens material and K is the solubility coefficient of oxygen in the material. A coefficient is a measure of a physical or chemical property that is constant for a system under specific conditions. The DK, or permeability, is characteristic of a material obtained in a given condition at a given temperature in the laboratory only. A rule of thumb is that the higher the DK of the material,

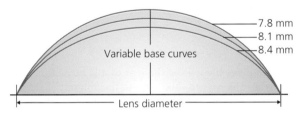

Figure 14.7 If the diameter is held constant, by decreasing the radius of curvature from 8.4 to 7.8 mm the sagittal height or vault of the lens is increased.

(From Stein HA, Slatt BJ, Stein RM, Freeman MI. Fitting guide for rigid and soft contact lenses: a practical approach. 4th ed. St Louis: Mosby; 2002.)

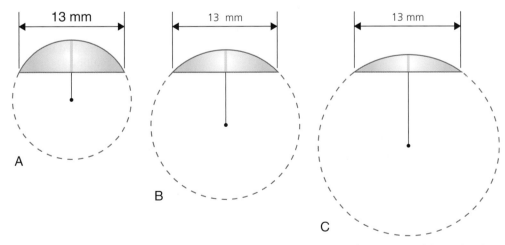

Figure 14.8 (A)–(C) show three circles of increasing length of radius. If the diameter of a given arc of the circle is kept constant, the sagittal height will decrease from (A) to (C).

(From Stein HA, Slatt BJ, Stein RM, Freeman MI. Fitting guide for rigid and soft contact lenses: a practical approach. 4th ed. St Louis: Mosby; 2002.)

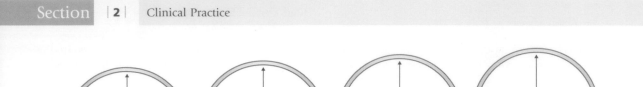

Figure 14.9 When the radius is kept constant and the diameter increased, the sagittal height of the lens is increased and the lens becomes steeper.

(From Stein HA, Slatt BJ, Stein RM, Freeman MI. Fitting guide for rigid and soft contact lenses: a practical approach. 4th ed. St Louis: Mosby; 2002.)

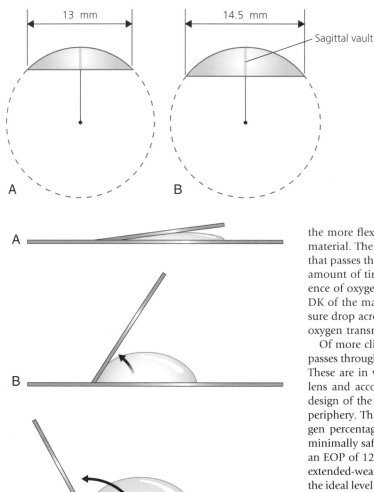

Figure 14.10 If portions of two similar circles are cut off, each with a different diameter, portion (B) with the larger 14.5-mm diameter will have a greater sagittal depth or vault than portion (A) with the smaller 13.0-mm diameter.

(From Stein HA, Slatt BJ, Stein RM, Freeman MI. Fitting guide for rigid and soft contact lenses: a practical approach. 4th ed. St Louis: Mosby; 2002.)

Figure 14.11 Wetting angles. The smaller the wetting angle of contact, the greater the spreading of a liquid over a solid surface. A hard lens is hydrophobic and has a 60-degree angle of contact with water. (A) Low wetting angle. (B) Wetting angle of methyl methacrylate hard lens. (C) Large wetting angle with droplet of mercury.

(From Stein HA, Slatt BJ, Stein RM, Freeman MI. Fitting guide for rigid and soft contact lenses: a practical approach. 4th ed. St Louis: Mosby; 2002.)

the more flexible will be the lens that is made from this material. The oxygen flux refers to the amount of oxygen that passes through a given area of the material in a given amount of time driven by a given partial pressure difference of oxygen across the material. It is a function of the DK of the material, the lens thickness (L), and the pressure drop across the lens (P). DK/L is often referred to as oxygen transmissibility.

Of more clinical importance is how much total oxygen passes through a lens and is permitted to reach the cornea. These are in vivo measurements, which involve the total lens and account for not only the material but also the design of the lens and its thickness in the center and the periphery. This measurement is called the equivalent oxygen percentage (EOP). An EOP of 9% is considered the minimally safe level for daily wear contact lenses, whereas an EOP of 12% is considered the minimally safe level for extended-wear contact lenses. An EOP of 18% is considered the ideal level for extended-wear contact lenses as this is the level for normal physiologic corneal swelling that occurs in the closed eye during sleep.

DESIGNS

Sophisticated corneal contact lens technology has made possible the manufacture of numerous widths, thicknesses, curvatures, and edge designs to aid the modern practitioner.

The contact lens can vary in diameter from 6 to 12 mm. Most people wear lenses with a diameter of 8 to 10 mm. They are generally smaller than soft lenses. The optic zone of the lens varies widely in diameter and may range from 5 to 8 mm, depending on the overall diameter of the lens. Contact lenses are available in monocurve, bicurve, tricurve, multicurve, and aspheric designs.

A secondary, or intermediate, curve is often put on a lens next to the base curve of the optic zone to accommodate the flatter periphery of the cornea. This intermediate curve may be 2.00 to 7.00 diopters flatter than the base curve. A tricurve lens is designed to have secondary curves. The width of these curves is relatively small, such as 0.2 mm. Occasionally, multicurve lenses are designed.

The resurgence of aspheric designs in rigid lenses has aimed to mimic the peripheral flattening of the cornea in a controlled and reproducible manner, thereby eliminating the need for progressively flattening peripheral curves.

The peripheral curve is the outermost curve and is much flatter than the other curves of the lens to conform to the flatter periphery of the cornea. The peripheral and intermediate curves permit a free flow of precorneal fluid under the lens.

To eliminate the sharp edges of the junction lines of these curves, the junctions are blended to give smoothness to the transition of the different curvatures. The blend may be light (the zones are readily identified) or heavy (the zones blend into each other).

Fenestration of hard lenses is valuable only from a historical perspective. Most RGP lens materials cannot be fenestrated because this increases the fragility of the lens. The ability of RGP lenses to transmit gases negates the functional need of fenestration.

Central thickness is an important factor in contact lens comfort. The thinner the lens, the more comfortable but also the less stable is the lens and the more likely it is to warp and break. The thinner the lens, the greater is the oxygen transmission through the plastic.

Edge design of a contact lens is important and is frequently the cause for patient rejection. The edge must be carefully designed, rounded, and polished. If the edge is too thick, it will irritate the eyelid margin. If it is too thin, it will be too sharp (knife edge) and irritate.

Contact lenses can also have cylinder ground into the back surface (back toric lenses), into the front surface (front toric lenses), or into both the front and back surfaces (bitoric lenses). Prism ballast can be incorporated in a contact lens to give weight to the lens and thus prevent rotation. Bifocals of varying design are also available (see Chapter 16)

PATIENT EXAMINATION

Although a careful eye examination is mandatory before a practitioner decides whether a patient is a suitable candidate for contact lenses, certain areas must be delineated in more detail. A complete history of the eye is needed, as well as a history of systemic medications such as oral contraceptives or the possibility of pregnancy. During the inquiry, an assessment should be made not only of the person's reasons for desiring contact lenses but also of personal hygienic habits and the ability to look after the lenses and persevere with the required lens care routines. For obvious reasons, the patient's manual dexterity should be evaluated. Also, the patient's temperament and emotional maturity should be evaluated so that introduction of contact lenses will ensure success rather than frustration and problems for both the practitioner and the patient. In those patients who were dissatisfied with previous contact lenses but wish to try again, one should establish the reason for the previous failure.

More than 95% of patients can wear contact lenses. The following instances preclude their use:

1. Chronic blepharoconjunctivitis from any cause, such as seborrhea or acne rosacea
2. Pterygium formation: with small pterygia, contact lenses can be fitted but larger pterygia may require removal first
3. Seventh nerve palsy (Bell's palsy)
4. Poor hygiene: people who do not keep their hands clean will not keep their lenses clean. Clean fingernails trimmed short are mandatory.
5. Industrial hazards: people who deal with highly volatile acids or bases (alkalis)
6. Severe allergies: most allergic reactions can be suppressed by the use of local antihistamines. However, allergic reactions can reduce wearing time in soft lens wearers and cause papillary conjunctivitis
7. Age: if the need is present, age is no barrier. One-day-old newborn children who have had cataract surgery have been fitted with contact lenses. Older adults, until intraocular lenses became popular, routinely wore aphakic contact lenses
8. Low tear film: avoid serious dry eyes with low tear film.

The TearScope (Eagle Vision and Keeler) analyzes the tear film in vivo to assess its stability and to determine whether there is a dry eye syndrome requiring punctal plugs before contact lens wear. The TearScope measures the break-up time of tears and tear film with fluorescein-stained tears.

A careful slit-lamp microscopic examination of the cornea before the patient begins contact lens wear permits detection of small scars or opacities of the cornea that cannot later be blamed on the contact lens. The eyelids and in particular the undersurface of the upper eyelid should be examined for follicles, papules, and signs of inflammation. The lid margins must be free of blepharitis. Any ghost vessels or signs of new vessel formation on the cornea should be noted and their cause determined.

The patient's eyes should be refracted and the best possible visual acuity recorded. Any muscle imbalance should be measured by prisms, and particular attention should be paid to the phorias.

The corneal diameter can be measured with a handheld ruler, a slit-lamp eyepiece reticle, pupillometer, or a contact lens of known diameter. The most accurate method of measuring a corneal diameter is by applying a contact lens of known diameter or by using a slit-lamp eyepiece reticle. The size of the pupil may be measured by a ruler under room lighting conditions or estimated by a pupillary gauge. The height of the palpebral fissure and the area where the upper eyelid crosses the cornea should be recorded. These factors have an important bearing on the lens design. Lid tension can be estimated by grasping the lid between thumb and forefinger, pulling slightly down and letting go. This will give a rough indication of whether the eyelid is loose or tight. The practitioner should observe the patient to see if the blink rate is reasonably normal. Adequacy of tear production may be measured by the filter paper (Schirmer's) test. Keratometry (described later) is an important basis for the initial lens design required.

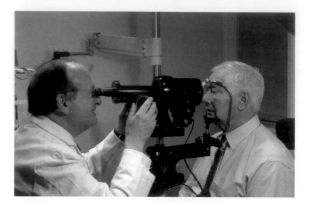

Figure 14.12 Taking a keratometer reading.

FITTING CORNEAL CONTACT LENSES

Measurements

The following measurements are required to fit a contact lens:

- The refractive error of the eye
- The dioptric curvature of the cornea
- The contact lens diameter
- The lens thickness
- The optic zone
- The peripheral curve blending

The refractive error of the eye is determined by conventional methods. Prescription for distance vision is determined in minus cylinders because all contact lenses are manufactured in minus cylinder form. When fitting rigid lenses, the corneal cylinder is disregarded by the fitter because up to 3.00 diopters of the corneal astigmatism can be easily corrected with a rigid spherical lens. The vertex distance of the spectacles should also be recorded, because the dioptric power of a plus lens is increased and that of a minus lens decreased when the spectacle prescription is converted for contact lenses. These changes in the power of the lens are related to the distance from the original spectacle to the cornea and the power of the lens itself.

The dioptric power of the cornea is determined by keratometer readings (Figures 14.12 and 14.13). For keratometer measurements, the patient is seated before the keratometer, with the chin placed on the chin rest. The room should have dim illumination. Two illuminated targets, called mires, are positioned so as to be reflected from the center of the cornea. The observer views the cornea

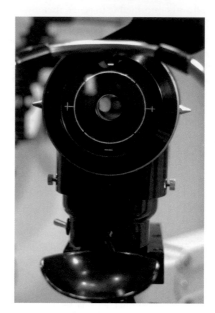

Figure 14.13 Front surface of the Bausch & Lomb keratometer.

through the telescopic system of the keratometer. This light is split by a prism into the images of the vertical and horizontal axis.

The keratometer should be calibrated on a steel ball of known radius at least once every 2 months. Before measurements are taken, the eyepiece must be adjusted to the observer's prescription. The patient should be comfortably seated and the keratometer placed so that the patient must lean slightly forward to place the chin in the chin rest. The patient is then instructed to press his or her head firmly against the forehead rest and to grasp the base of the instrument firmly with both hands to steady the head and to fixate the eyes steadily. The patient is encouraged to open the eyes widely and to blink occasionally. The fitter should be seated with both feet flat on the floor, to be able to operate the instrument without having to strain the neck or slump forward. Once the instrument has been aligned, the mires are positioned so as to be reflected from the center of the cornea. The fitter should constantly keep one hand on the knob that controls the clarity of the mire images and the other hand on the knob that controls the separation of the mire images; otherwise the instrument may be out of focus at the moment the final setting is made.

The Bausch & Lomb keratometer is typical of other keratometers in use (Box 14.1). The illuminated targets, or mires, consist of three illuminated circles, with one circle having a plus sign as an appendage. The central circle has both a plus and a minus sign. At first the central circle appears doubled (Figure 14.14A) until the focusing knob is used to produce a single central circle (Figure 14.14B). The black control cross should always be in the center of the right bottom circle. The next step is to rotate the axis of the keratometer so the plus and minus signs are aligned (Figure 14.14C). Then the horizontal measuring drum is turned so that the plus signs overlap and become single (Figure 14.14D). This is the first *K* reading. The vertical measuring drum is then turned so that the minus signs overlap (Figure 14.14E). This is the *K* reading of the second curvature. In exceptionally flat or steep corneas, readings cannot be taken without accessory lenses to extend the range of the keratometer.

It is common practice to record the horizontal reading first. The difference between the horizontal meridian and the vertical meridian constitutes the corneal astigmatism. As mentioned previously, when the horizontal meridian is flatter than the vertical meridian, the corneal astigmatism is referred to as with-the-rule. If the horizontal meridian is steeper than the vertical meridian, the corneal astigmatism is referred to as against-the-rule. When the corneal astigmatism of the eye differs from the refractive cylinder of the prescription, this difference is referred to as residual astigmatism.

Because the keratometer measures the central zone, or optic cap, of the cornea, which has a diameter of 5 to 7 mm and includes the visual axis of the cornea, this reading should represent the base curve of choice (Figure 14.15). However, the periphery of the contact lens actually rests on the intermediate zone of the cornea, which is somewhat flatter than the optic cap.

Automated keratometers also provide the dioptric *K* value of the central cornea (Figure 14.16). The corneoscope is another instrument that provides a photographic representation of the curvature of the portions of the cornea central to peripheral.

Topographic corneal analysis is the most sophisticated way of analyzing the corneal dioptric values. By a computerized readout with color analysis, a person can determine 6000 keratometry points on the cornea. This provides considerable new information and data on the cornea, which in turn can help determine how much flatter the periphery of the lens should be to the central radius of curvature.

Box 14.1 **Bausch & Lomb keratometer**

I. Adjusting the eyepiece.
   A. Position the occluder.
   B. Turn the eyepiece cap counterclockwise as far as possible; the user should see a blurred cross.
   C. Look through the eyepiece and turn the eye focus. Note the reading on the outer periphery of the eyepiece. Repeat the same set several times to verify the results.

II. Seat the patient comfortably before the instrument and fit the chin securely on the chin rest with the head against the headrest.

III. Level the keratometer to the patient's eye. Set the instrument at 90 and 180 degrees. Put the instrument to one side to align it with the eye. Raise or lower the instrument until the silver pin on the side of the lamp house is lined with the patient's pupil. The patient's head must be positioned vertically and not tilted.

IV. Patient fixation: turn the instrument so that it points directly at the eye to be examined. One should see a tiny bright ring (the mire) in the center of the cornea. The mire should be aligned with the pupil and the patient should see the reflection of his or her own eye.

V. Take the reading: to obtain the proper measurement, Steps A through E should be followed.
   A. Focus the instrument carefully with the focusing knob. The double circle is seen with black crosshairs near the center when out of focus (Figure 14.14A). By turning the knob you should see a single clear circle with a clear cross in the center (Figure 14.14B).
   B. Rotate the instrument to locate the axis plus signs tip to tip. The axis of the cylinder is found when the tips of the two plus signs just touch. Turn the horizontal measuring drum until the plus signs are barely separate and the lines of the plus cylinders appear to be continuous (Figure 14.14C).
   C. Measure the horizontal meridians. Turn the left measuring drum until the plus signs are superimposed (Figure 14.14D).
   D. Measure the vertical meridians. Turn the right measuring drum until the minus signs are superimposed (Figure 14.14E). Actual diopter power of the corneal curvatures can be obtained.
   E. The difference between the two measurements is the amount of corneal astigmatism. Read the axis on the scale and record.

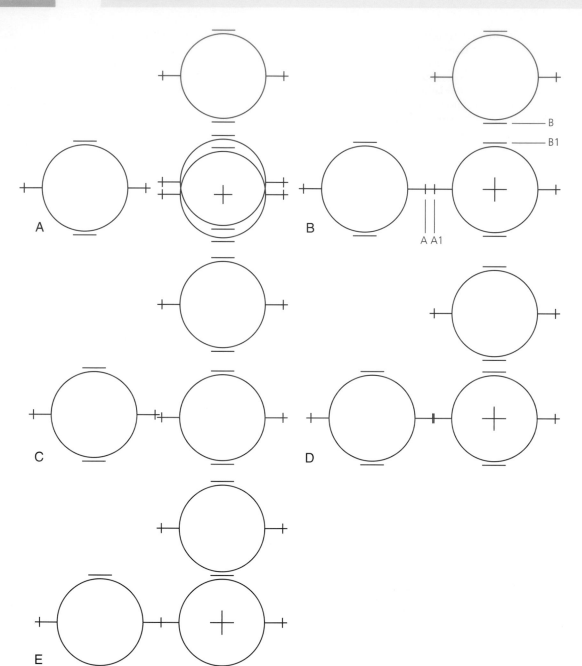

Figure 14.14 (A) Keratometry mires. When first viewed the circles overlap and the + and the − signs are separated. (B) The circles are united by focusing. The +A and A1 are separated. Then the −B and B1 are separated. The central + is focused in the exact center of the central circle. (C) The axis is then aligned. (D) The horizontal plus signs (+A to A1) are united by focusing. (E) The minus signs (−B to B1) are then united. This is the endpoint. Keratometer (K) readings are then read from the rotating focusing knob, and recorded.

Details of this topographic analysis are addressed in Chapter 44.

The size of the rigid contact lens is important. The topographometer is an instrument designed to measure the optic cap or apex of the cornea. In spherical corneas this optic cap is the same in all diameters, but in astigmatic corneas there is a difference in curvature at different meridians. RGP contact lenses are ordered on the basis of the flattest radius

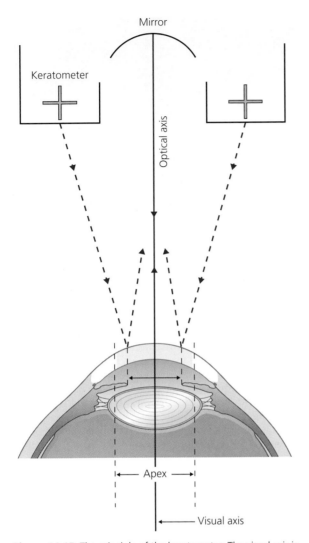

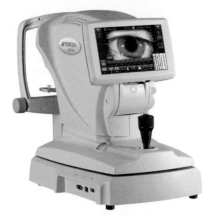

Figure 14.16 Automated Topcon keratometer.
(Courtesy of Topcon Europe Medical BV; www.topcon-medical.eu.)

The optic zone is determined by the difference of the lens diameter and the width of the peripheral curves, which are flatter than the base curve. The peripheral curves are designed to allow tear flow under the lens at the flatter corneal periphery.

Trial lenses

Trial lenses are simply a set of corneal contact lenses of known diameter, power, base curves, and peripheral curves. Most experienced practitioners use a fitting set of corneal contact lenses in conjunction with a keratometer. The use of a fitting set practically eliminates the need for exchanges of lenses. Most experienced fitters agree that the best instrument to evaluate a fit is a contact lens on the eye.

Materials and manufacture

Corneal rigid contact lenses were for many years constructed of PMMA. This material absorbs fluid minimally (less than 2%) compared with the soft lenses, which vary in hydration from 25% to 80%. PMMA has excellent optical qualities, but requires some adaptation because of some discomfort associated with its use and its lack of oxygen permeability. These lenses are fitted smaller than the visible iris diameter, but larger than the pupillary diameter, and are known as corneal lenses.

The PMMA lens is hardly used today and has been superseded by RGP contact lenses. To date, the RGP lenses have been made of (1) cellulose acetate butyrate (CAB) (currently out of use), (2) silicone acrylate, (3) styrene, (4) silicone resin, (5) fluoropolymer, and (6) fluoronated silicone acrylate combinations (fluorosilicone acrylates [FSAs]). These lenses are often referred to as semisoft or flexible rigid contact lenses. These lenses are much more flexible than standard PMMA lenses and have greater

Figure 14.15 The principle of the keratometer. The visual axis is aligned along the optical axis of the instrument so the central front surface of the cornea reflects the mires of the keratometer.
(From Stein HA, Slatt BJ, Stein RM, Freeman MI. Fitting guide for rigid and soft contact lenses: a practical approach. 4th ed. St Louis: Mosby; 2002.)

of the optic cap. Other factors that determine the size of the lens are the width of the palpebral fissure, the prominence of the globe, and the spasticity of the eyelids.

The thickness of a lens is an important factor in comfort. Again, thinner rigid lenses are more comfortable but are less stable and more likely to warp and break. Lenses should be ordered with minimal thickness and be verified by a thickness gauge. In powers greater than −6.00 or +2.50 diopters, a lenticular design is frequently used to reduce the thickness and consequently the weight of the lens. Some ultrathin lenses flex and provide less irritation.

oxygen permeability, which is not found in the standard PMMA lenses. The FSA polymers have advanced in terms of oxygen permeability as well as the wetting angle since their introduction. They have the advantage of being able to correct several diopters of corneal astigmatism and, because of their gas permeability, are able to maintain corneal deturgescence and relieve some of the symptoms of corneal hypoxia. RGP is now being replaced by GP to reflect the high oxygen permeability and other features of these newer materials.

Fitting gas-permeable lenses

The ideal fit for any GP lens is one in which the lens position is high, even when the lens overlaps the superior limbus (Figure 14.17). The upper lid should cover a portion of the lens during the full cycle of each blink. The purpose of the high-riding lens is to tuck the edge of the lens under the lid to avoid lid impact. This "full-sweep" blink also enhances lens surface wetting. The engagement of the upper lid margin with the edge of the lens is a major cause of discomfort. Even a soft hydrogel lens is uncomfortable if it is made small and interpalpebral.

At times, the ideal may not be achieved (Figure 14.18). The position of the upper lid may be too high to cover the upper position of the lens or there may be excessive astigmatism, which, because of the corneal topography, resists the upper motion of the lens. In these cases, the central position may be accepted, provided that the patient accepts this type of fit, or modifications can be made. The lens diameter may be reduced to increase the lid lift or a flatter base curve can be chosen. A central fit on the cornea is adequate, but a low-riding lens is unsatisfactory. When the lens is low, the blink rate is frequently suppressed to a minimum or the blink itself is incomplete. Also, a low lens is frequently a source of lid gap, which causes staining

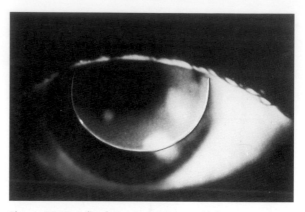

Figure 14.18 A flat-fitting lens riding too high.
(From Stein HA, Slatt BJ, Stein RM, Freeman MI. Fitting guide for rigid and soft contact lenses: a practical approach. 4th ed. St Louis: Mosby; 2002.)

of the cornea at the 3 and 9 o'clock positions. The margin of the upper lid slides over the low lens, and it bridges the nasal and temporal cornea between the edge of the lens and the limbus. Lid gap is especially common with highly myopic refractive corrective lenses because the edges of the lens are prone to be thicker than usual and the trough between the edge of the lens and the margin of the cornea is likely to be deep. Because these lenses are usually of large diameter, the proper edge treatment is essential. A plus edge or configuration for myopic lenses with power greater than −4.00 diopters and a minus edge for lenses +4.00 diopters or greater is usually designed.

Systems for fitting

Inventory fitting

One manufacturer (Syntex Ophthalmics) believes that three diameters of lenses 8.5, 9.0, and 9.5 mm will satisfy almost all requirements for myope patients and lens diameters of 9.5 and 10.0 mm will satisfy most aphakic eyes. If adequate base curves are available, these lenses will simplify fitting.

For myopic patients, the larger 9.5-mm diameter is recommended for levels of high astigmatism and flatter corneas.

Inventory fitting by lenses with preselected diameter simplifies fitting because one has fewer variables to deal with. In addition, one can rely on the quality control in providing lenses and controlled edge designs by one manufacturer.

Lid sensation is directly dependent on the edge finishing. It must not be left thick but thinned out to minimize lid sensation and the uncomfortable fitting of a lens that lies under the upper lid (Figure 14.19). A good reliable laboratory is most important. A soft lens may be more comfortable because of its relatively large diameter and its constant edge position underneath the upper eyelid.

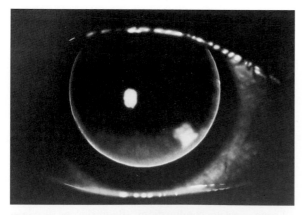

Figure 14.17 Large gas-permeable rigid contact lens with upper edge under upper lid. Normal fit.
(From Stein HA, Slatt BJ, Stein RM, Freeman MI. Fitting guide for rigid and soft contact lenses: a practical approach. 4th ed. St Louis: Mosby; 2002.)

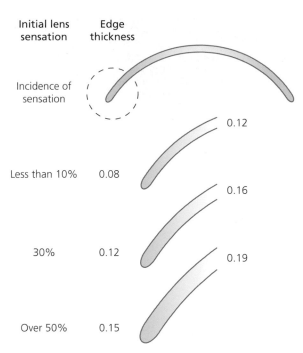

Initial lens sensation	Edge thickness
Incidence of sensation	
Less than 10%	0.08
30%	0.12
Over 50%	0.15

Figure 14.19 Sensation of lens is directly related to edge thickness. Lens edges must be made thin to reduce lens sensation. More than 50% of patients with a lens edge 0.15 mm as noted in the lower lens complain of sensation because of lens–lid impact.

(Courtesy Syntex Ophthalmics Inc., Phoenix, AZ.) (From Stein HA, Slatt BJ, Stein RM, Freeman MI. Fitting guide for rigid and soft contact lenses: a practical approach. 4th ed. St Louis: Mosby; 2002.)

Inventory systems for RGP lenses may see a resurgence because there are a number of good aspheric and spherical stock lenses that fit a broad range of prescriptions and topographies with a relatively small number of lenses (250 or less). Some manufacturers offer a particular design nationally (e.g., Boston Envision). This type of inventory system is good for the moderate to large RGP practice. The important factor in this method is the immediate accessibility to these lenses.

Nomogram fitting

The ideal method of fitting silicone acrylate lenses is from a trial set where the lens is placed on the eye. There are a number of low-volume fitters and occasional fitters who do not wish to maintain a standard fitting trial set, but rather follow a fitting nomogram. We have developed a nomogram that is designed to guide for the best possible starting point in lens selection (Table 14.2). With a nomogram, one may order the lens directly by referring to the nomogram for the initial lens factor. It is essential to have a set of diagnostic RGP lenses in the office. Selection of the initial base curve could be based on the nomogram.

The nomogram takes into account the progressive increase in diameter required for flatter corneas and the decrease in diameter for the steeper corneas. The second factor to take into account is the increased thickness required for the more delicate silicone acrylate lenses to avoid flexure on the cornea. The base curve is selected according to the corneal toricity. If the corneal cylinder is 0.75 diopter or less, select the base curve the same as the flattest *K*. If the corneal cylinder is between 1.00 and 2.00 diopters, add one-quarter of the difference of the two Ks to the flattest *K*, and if the corneal cylinder is more than 2.00 diopters, add one-third of the difference to the flattest *K*.

If the flattest curve of the cornea is 42.0 diopters and the cylinder is less than 0.75 diopter, we would select a lens base curve of 42.0 and diameter of 9.2 mm and provide the laboratory with the details of the peripheral curves.

In developing a nomogram, we analyzed the fit of 987 eyes. We found that 75% could be fitted on a first-fit basis using this nomogram and most of the remainder fitted with fewer than two subsequent lenses.

We also have developed a nomogram for the newer fluoronated silicone acrylate lenses, based on the fitting of 1578 eyes (Table 14.3). This is similar to the silicone acrylate nomogram. According to this nomogram by knowing the *K* reading and the refractive error, one can select the first lens, which will fit 80% of the time.

Special solutions are required for silicone acrylate lenses. Wetting and soaking solutions used at least 15 minutes before insertion condition the lens and improve its wetting angle. They also remove any accumulation of surface deposits.

Special problem solving with gas-permeable silicone acrylate and fluorosilicone acrylate lenses

The goal of the manufacturer when developing a new GP material is to maximize the permeability, stability, and wetting properties of the lens while minimizing depositing. Silicone has the one great feature of being extremely oxygen permeable. It has the downside of being hydrophobic (not-wetting), which can lead to dry eyes, eye scratchiness, and redness. As more and more silicone was added to GP materials to increase DK, manufacturers found that surface wetting decreased and protein depositing increased. Additionally, increased silicone in materials sometimes resulted in lenses that cracked, hazed, and warped. The introduction of fluorine (fluorosilicone acrylates) allowed the silicone content to be reduced (as a result of the oxygen permeability of fluorine), allowing even higher levels of DK materials to be achieved. Research continues and third-generation fluorosilicone acrylate materials have been introduced (e.g., Boston XO2 and FluoroPerm 151) that have significantly increased the permeability of GP lenses into what is sometimes referred to as the "hyper-permeable" range.

Table 14.2 Nomogram for initial lens selection for silicone acrylate lenses

If corneal cylinder <0.75 diopter (D): Select flattest keratometer (K)
  1.00–2.00 D: Add $^1/_4$ of difference of 2 Ks to flattest K
  >2.00 D: Add $^1/_3$ of difference of 2 Ks to flattest K
(All prescriptions greater than +2.00 D should be in lenticular form)

Base curve (D)	Diameter (mm)		Peripheral curves (mm/D)		
	Minus power	Plus power			
40.00 and 40.25	9.6	9.8	0.2/36.00	0.2/31.00	0.2/27.50
40.50 and 40.75	9.5	9.7			
41.00 and 41.25	9.4	9.6	0.2/36.00	0.2/31.00	0.2/27.50
41.50 and 41.75	9.3	9.5			
42.00 and 42.25	9.2	9.4	0.2/32.00	0.2/27.50	
42.50 and 42.75	9.1	9.3			
43.00 and 43.25	9.0	9.2	0.3/33.00	0.2/27.50	
43.50 and 43.75	8.9	9.1			
44.00 and 44.25	8.8	9.0	0.3/34.00	0.2/29.00	
44.50 and 44.75	8.7	8.9			
45.00 and 45.25	8.6	8.8	0.2/36.00	0.2/29.00	
45.50 and 45.75	8.5	8.7			
46.00 and 46.25	8.4	8.6	0.2/36.00	0.2/30.00	
46.50 and 46.75	8.3	8.5			

Table 14.3 Nomogram for fitting fluoronated silicone acrylate lenses

Initial lens selection:
If corneal cylinder ≤0.75 diopter (D): Base curve 0.75 flatter than the flattest keratometer (K)
  1.00–1.75 D: Base curve 0.25 flatter than the flattest K
  >1.75 D: Base curve 0.25 steeper than the flattest K

Base curve (mm/D)	Diameter (mm)	Peripheral curves (mm/D)		
	Plus and minus power			
8.44 and 8.39 mm 40.00 and 40.25 D	9.8	0.3/9.10 mm	0.2/10.50 mm	0.2/11.50 mm
8.33 and 8.28 mm 40.50 and 40.75 D	9.7	0.3/37.00 D	0.2/32.00 D	0.2/29.00 D
8.23 and 8.18 mm 41.00 and 41.25 D	9.6	0.3/9.10 mm	0.2/10.50 mm	0.2/11.50 mm
8.13 and 8.18 mm 41.50 and 41.75 D	9.5	0.3/37.00 D	0.2/32.00 D	0.2/29.00 D
8.04 and 7.99 mm 42.00 and 42.25 D	9.4	0.2/8.90 mm	0.2/10.00 mm	0.2/11.50 mm

Table 14.3 Continued

Base curve (mm/D)	Diameter (mm)	Peripheral curves (mm/D)		
7.94 and 7.89 mm 42.50 and 42.75 D	9.3	0.2/38.00 D	0.2/34.00 D	0.2/29.00 D
7.85 and 7.80 mm 43.00 and 43.25 D	9.2	0.2/8.90 mm	0.2/10.00 mm	0.2/11.50 mm
7.76 and 7.71 mm 43.50 and 43.75 D	9.1	0.2/38.00 D	0.2/34.00 D	0.2/29.00 D
7.67 and 7.63 mm 44.00 and 44.25 D	9.0	0.2/8.70 mm	0.2/9.50 mm	0.2/11.50 mm
7.58 and 7.54 mm 44.50 and 44.75 D	8.9	0.2/38.75 D	0.2/35.50 D	0.2/30.75 D
7.50 and 7.46 mm 45.00 and 45.25 D	8.8	0.2/8.70 mm	0.2/9.50 mm	0.2/11.50 mm
7.42 and 7.38 mm 46.00 and 46.25 D	8.7	0.2/38.75 D	0.2/35.50 D	0.2/30.75 D
7.34 and 7.30 mm 46.00 and 46.25 D	8.6	0.2/8.40 mm	0.2/9.20 mm	0.2/10.50 mm
7.26 and 7.22 mm 46.50 and 46.75 D	8.5	0.2/40.00 D	0.2/36.75 D	0.2/32.00 D

From Stein HA, Slatt BJ, Stein RM. A fitting guide for rigid and soft contact lenses: a practical approach. 3rd ed. St Louis: Mosby; 1990.

Fluorosilicone acrylate materials tend to resist protein deposition but not lipid deposition, and often special cleaning may be required.

Many of the major and disabling complications of PMMA lenses have been eliminated by the use of the new generation of GP lenses. There are still, however, a number of GP lens-related problems that need to be addressed. By understanding these problems and solutions, practitioners are able to direct their attention in achieving happiness and success in lens wear. The Gas Permeable Lens Institute (GPLI) website (www.gpli.info) provides helpful information on GP lenses.

Three o'clock and nine o'clock position staining

There are several causes of 3 and 9 o'clock position staining.

Lid gap

A lid gap occurs mostly with large-diameter rigid lenses. It is particularly prone to occur with GP lenses whose edges have not been properly thinned.

The gap occurs between the margin of the lens and the cornea. The meniscus of tears becomes very thin or absent at this border, creating a lens-induced dry spot. The degree of staining is intense, often associated with episcleritis and formation of dellen. The staining of the cornea is attributable to desiccation of the corneal epithelium and not to corneal hypoxia. It is particularly prone to occur with lenses that ride low, that is, not brought up to a high position with a blink. Poor lid adherence is another cause of a low-riding lens.

The treatment is to make the lens flatter, thinner at the edges, or smaller in diameter.

At times the lens will rise with a blink and then suddenly drop to a low position. Such a lens requires a little alteration; flattening the base curve and blending the peripheral curves frequently solves the problem and permits tear flow.

Poor blinking

The incomplete blinker dehydrates the exposed portion of the eye at the 3 and 9 o'clock positions. Lines of protein accumulation across the lens, caused by dehydration, indicate its presence.

Poor tear film

Some people have an insufficient tear film to support a large-diameter lens. With these people, supplementary tears during the day and a bland ointment at night may be enough to remedy the problem.

Comment

Three and 9 o'clock position staining is more common with large RGP lenses. Despite the intensity of the corneal erosions and episcleritis, patients do not seem to have much pain. Some fitters do not treat the corneal erosion because it may be an asymptomatic condition. This is an error. Breaks in the epithelial integrity should not be tolerated. More often than not, these patients primarily complain of eye redness.

Lens-flexure problems

The softer silicone component that is added to the silicone acrylate mixture combined with the thin-designed lenses permits some flexure with each blink because of the pressure effect of the eyelid on the lens, which may rock on a toric cornea. This phenomenon results in blurring of vision, along with a residual astigmatism that is not corrected by the tear film. The modulus of elasticity measures a material's propensity to deform; as a rule, the higher the modulus, the more it resists deformation. Information on the modulus of a specific GP material may be obtained from the manufacturer.

Against-the-rule corneas create even more lens flexure as the lid sweeps over the lens. Steeper fitting of the lens also creates more opportunity for lens flexures. Smaller lenses may produce even more flexure than the larger-diameter lenses, which have a greater stabilizing force.

The newer fluorocarbon lenses combined with silicone acrylate are even more prone to produce flexure. They are also capable of warping on the cornea and creating a glued-on syndrome. The fluorocarbonated silicone acrylate lens should be fitted at least 0.5 diopter flatter than one would fit the silicone acrylate lens.

These problems of lens flexure are found because the new generation of lenses is being used to correct astigmatism. These problems were apparent with very thin soft hydroxyethylmethacrylate (HEMA) lenses in the early years. Their use for corneal toricity was minimal because one soon learned that the soft HEMA lenses draped entirely over the cornea because they did not have any hard component. These lenses did not significantly correct large measures of corneal astigmatism.

To remedy this problem the practitioner needs to increase the thickness of the lens. This will vary with the degree of corneal cylinder present. As a rule, the thickness should be increased by 20% to 30% for larger lenses and 40% to 60% for smaller lenses, which are more subject to flexure.

The lens should also be fitted high under the upper lid to minimize flexure, which may occur with an interpalpebral lens.

The newest trend in RGP technology is crosslinking of polymers to prevent flexure, especially in thin designs. Thus thinner lenses and more permeable materials can be used with extra comfort.

EVALUATING CONTACT LENSES

Contact lens practitioners should accept only high-quality lenses furnished by the manufacturing laboratory. Lenses arriving from the laboratory should be checked to see whether they have been made to exact specifications. By doing so and by rejecting lenses that fall below standard, the practitioner will keep the laboratory on guard to furnish high-quality material. In addition, adequate evaluation of the lens dimensions will eliminate frustrations in fitting that might be attributed to faulty lens construction. Many unnecessary lens modifications may be prevented if proper lens inspection is performed.

Measuring diameter

The total diameter of a contact lens may be measured by a magnifier that basically consists of a plus lens with a scale. The contact lens is held between thumb and forefinger until one edge is aligned with the zero portion of the scale. The diameter can be read directly from the scale.

An alternative method is to place the contact lens, concave side down, into a ruler with a V-shaped groove (Figure 14.20) until it slides into the lowest area in the groove in which it can no longer move. The measurement is then read directly from the adjacent scale on the plastic bar.

The contact lens may also be measured on a Shadowgraph and its diameter read against the scale of the Shadowgraph (see Figure 14.23).

Contacto Gauge and Radiuscope

Either the Contacto Gauge (Neitz Instrument Co. Ltd, Tokyo, Japan) or the Radiuscope (American Optical Co.,

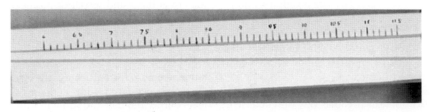

Figure 14.20 V groove to measure hard-lens diameter.

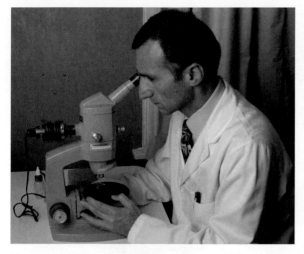

Figure 14.21 Measuring curvature of a contact lens with the Radiuscope.

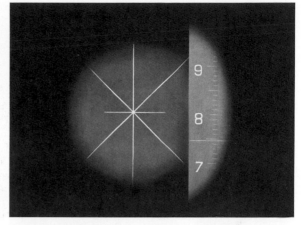

Figure 14.22 Pattern and inside measuring scale in a Radiuscope.
(From Stein HA, Slatt BJ, Stein RM, Freeman MI. Fitting guide for rigid and soft contact lenses: a practical approach. 4th ed. St Louis: Mosby; 2002.)

Buffalo, NY) may be used to measure the base curve of a contact lens (Figure 14.21). This measurement enables the examiner not only to check the accuracy of the lens received from the manufacturing laboratory but also to detect possible warpage of a lens that would be responsible for incorrect fitting.

The following are rules for measuring the concave curve of a contact lens with the Contacto Gauge:

1. Put 1 drop of water in the hollow of the contact lens mount holder. Place the contact lens horizontally in the mount with its concave side upward.
2. Turn on the light. Move the microglide stage to center the contact lens in a position just beneath the objective.
3. While looking through the eyepiece, rotate the coarse adjustment knob clockwise until the spoke-pattern target comes into view. Center the target in the eyepiece by moving the microglide stage. Bring the target into sharpest focus by using the coarse and fine adjusting knobs.
4. Set the dial gauge to zero.
5. Continue to rotate the coarse adjustment knob until the target disappears and the filament comes into view. Continue through the filament until the target reappears (real image). Refine the sharpness of the target by using the coarse and fine adjustment knobs.
6. The radii of curvature readings are now taken from the dial gauge. The short hand in the inner dial is the whole number, for example, 5, 6, or 7 mm. The long hand in the outer dial is the fraction of the whole number expressed in decimal equivalents of hundredths of a millimeter, for example, 0.23, 0.59, or 0.101 (Figure 14.22).

The Radiuscope operates in a similar way. If the convex radius of curvature measurement is desired, the examiner should proceed with either instrument exactly as for the concave measurement, but should place the lens initially in a convex lens mount and float the contact lens with the convex side upward.

Shadowgraph and Contactoscope

The Shadowgraph (Urocon Inc., Hollywood, CA) and Contactoscope (Wesley-Jessen, The Plastic Contact Lens Co., Chicago, IL) (Figure 14.23) use light transmitted through the lens for inspecting contact lenses. The Shadowgraph magnifies a contact lens in cross-section or in front view. Magnification of the contact lens to 20 times its size is accomplished by internal projection on a ground-glass screen. On the screen is a reticule scale graduated in 0.1 mm, which can be used to measure (1) the diameter of the lens, (2) the width of the peripheral curve, (3) the width of any blending area, and (4) the width of the intermediate curve. The blending zone cannot be seen by the naked eye but can be evaluated only under the large magnification created by the Shadowscope. The Shadowscope is also useful in showing scratches on the optical surface of the contact lens, as well as any cracks or nicks in the edge.

The cross-section view of the contact lens shows up the contour of the edge so the edge thickness can be measured, which should be no thicker than 0.12 mm.

To use the Shadowgraph and Contactoscope, the practitioner places the contact lens on a vertically mounted stage to provide a front view of the lens. The image is focused on the screen by a lever under the stage. The lens should be scrutinized for scratches, nicks, and cracks. The screen image can be raised or lowered by a knob on the stage so that the lens can be placed against the measuring scale. The diameter of the lens can then be measured on the scale. The peripheral curve width, the blend width, and the intermediate curve width can then be inspected and measured.

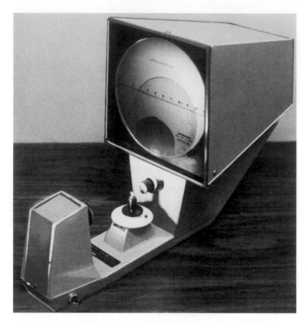

Figure 14.23 Shadowgraph used to magnify and measure a contact lens.

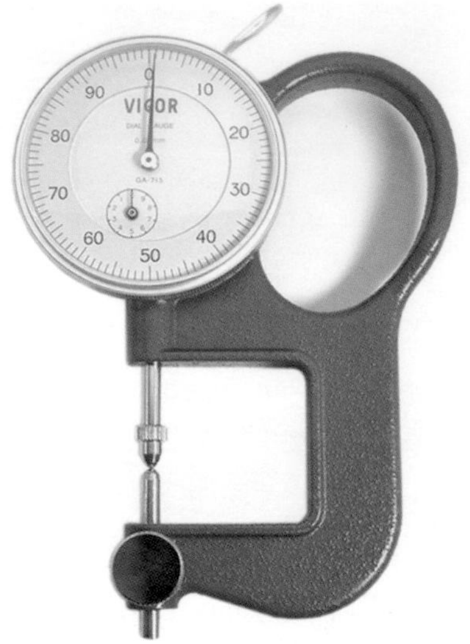

Figure 14.24 Thickness gauge. Before measuring, thickness gauge must be set to zero.
(Courtesy of Vigor Optical, Division of Grobet USA, Carlstadt, NJ.)

To view the lens on the edge, one can either rotate the lens perpendicular to the screen or lay the lens on its convex surface on the stage. The practitioner may need to refocus to get a sharp image of the edge. One can move the stage laterally to project the image of the edge on the reticule scale to measure edge thickness.

Measuring power

The power of a contact lens may be measured on the standard lensmeter. Place the lens concave side down to measure the back vertex power of the contact lens. A small error in the power may arise if the lens is held in place with fingers, particularly with higher-power lenses. To measure the front vertex power, place the lens concave side up on the lensmeter.

Measuring thickness

For measuring thickness, a contact lens is inserted in the thickness gauge, convex side down. The pin of the gauge is allowed to descend slowly until contact is made with the concave surface. The measurement is read from the dial (Figure 14.24).

INSERTION AND REMOVAL TECHNIQUES

It is important that the patient be carefully instructed on how to insert, remove, and care for contact lenses.

Insertion

The hands should always be carefully washed and dried before insertion of the lens. The lens is cleaned and wet before inserting, then balanced, concave side up, on the tip of the index finger. The lens is moistened with contact lens solution or methylcellulose. The right hand should be used for the right lens and the left hand for the left lens, although this may vary with patient preference. The patient looks straight down, chin on chest, keeping both eyes open. The upper lid is then held at the lashes with the fingers of the opposite hand pressing up and against the bony margin of the brow. The lower lid should be held at the lash margin with the fourth finger of the hand that is holding the lens pressing down and against the cheek. The lens finger is then brought straight up to the eye until the lens touches the eye (Figure 14.25). An instant afterward, the lower lid should be released and then slowly the upper lid. It is important to impress on the patient that he or she should not look away at the last moment. The head must always be kept straight and the temptation to turn must be avoided.

In the early stages of learning to insert the lenses, the use of a mirror will help. The patient should learn to insert the lenses without a mirror as soon as possible, because one may not be handy at all times.

Some individuals are more successful in placing a lens on the eye when they do not have to look at the lens coming toward the eye. These individuals should look downward, with the upper lid lifted by the forefinger or middle finger. The lens is then placed on the sclera above the cornea and the upper lid is released. The lens usually centers itself on the eye. As an alternative, one can look up and place the lens on the lower sclera, pushing the lens up with the lower eyelid margin.

Removal

Removal of the lens is much easier. The lens should always be centered and moving freely before removal is attempted. A wetting or lubricating drop placed in the eye before removal can be helpful. The patient should be instructed to look down and to cup the opposite hand under the eye to catch the lens. The forefinger is placed on the outer corner of the eyelid and the lid is pulled aside at the same time the patient blinks (Figure 14.26). The lens will usually pop out.

Another method of removal is the scissors method. In this method the upper lid is held by the forefinger and the lower lid is held by the middle finger of the same hand. The lids are then separated at the lateral margin like when a pair of scissors is opened. The patient is asked to blink at the same time that this maneuver is done.

The two-handed method actually pushes the lids under the lens. One finger of one hand grasps the upper lid and the index finger of the other hand grasps the lower lid. The lids are then pushed toward the contact lens, squeezing it out of the eye.

Centering

Lenses may lodge off-center and thus may appear (1) under the upper lid, (2) under the lower lid, (3) in the outside corner of the eye, or (4) in the inside corner of the eye. The wearer should never panic under these circumstances because a gentle push in the appropriate direction will center the lens easily.

The lens can be centered by feeling for it through the closed eyelid. The patient is instructed to place four fingers on the eyelid and gaze straight ahead. The lens is then massaged toward the center of the eye (Figure 14.27). This can also be done with one finger (Figure 14.28). A lubricating drop is put into the eye before centering.

Do's and don'ts with contact lenses

1. The hands should be washed before handling and inserting contact lenses.
2. It is helpful to wet the finger before balancing a GP lens on it. For soft lenses, a dry finger is preferred.
3. All makeup should be removed. An excellent eye makeup remover is the packet of wipes sold by IMEDS of Montreal (Figure 14.29).
4. The eye should not be rubbed with the lens in place.

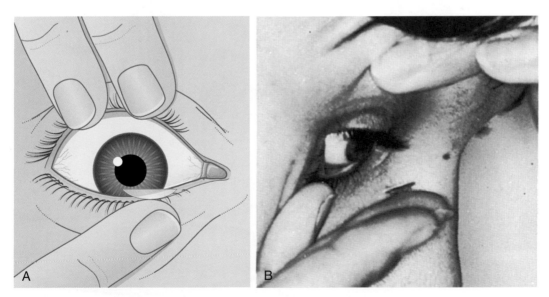

Figure 14.25 Rigid gas-permeable (RGP) contact lens insertion by the patient. (A) The upper lid is retracted by grasping the lid near the margin and pulling it. The left hand is used to elevate the right upper lid. The patient's gaze is directed downward and the lens is carried to the eye by the index finger of the right hand. (B) Incorrect method: the upper lid should be grasped near the lid margin and the lens should rest on the tip of the finger.

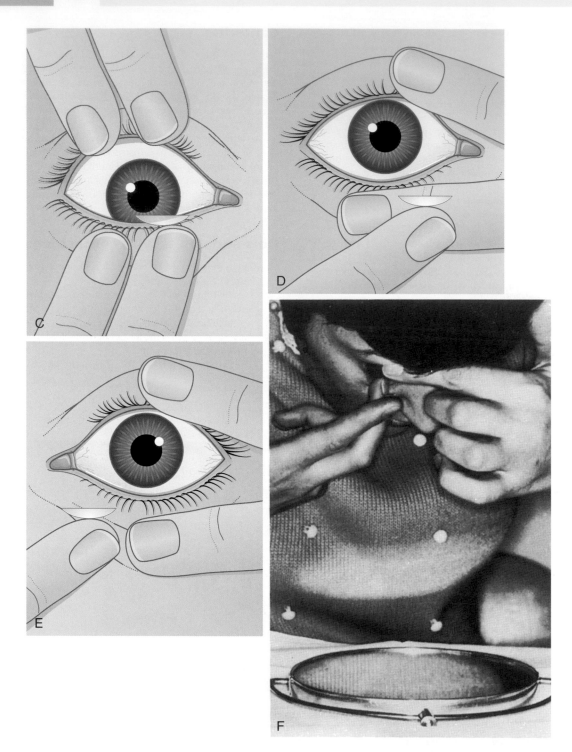

Figure14.25, cont'd (C) For the unsteady or tremulous patient, the middle finger carrying the lens rests on the index finger. (D) The lids are separated by the index finger retracting the upper lid and the middle finger depressing the lower lid. The index finger of the free hand brings the lens to the eye. (E) The lids are separated laterally between the index and middle fingers while the hand opposite the eye carries the lens. (F) Use of a mirror for inserting a lens.

(From Stein HA, Slatt BJ, Stein RM, Freeman MI. Fitting guide for rigid and soft contact lenses: a practical approach. 4th ed. St Louis: Mosby; 2002.)

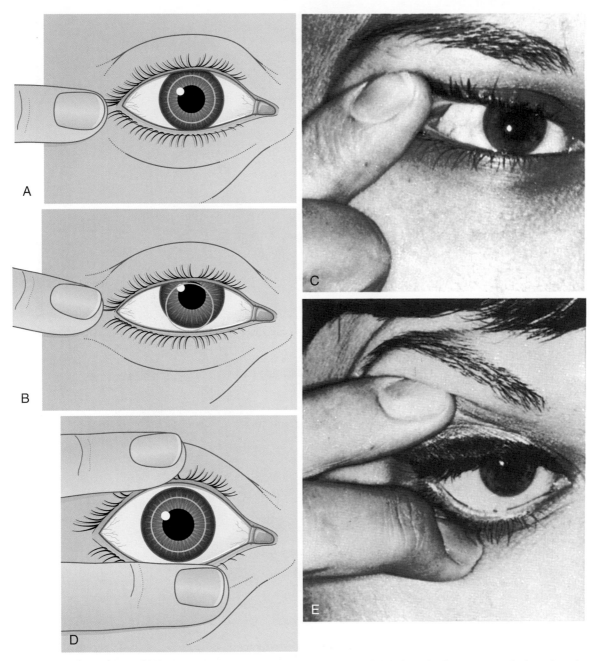

Figure 14.26 Rigid gas-permeable (RGP) contact lens removal by the patient. (A)–(C) The index finger tugs at the lateral canthus in an outward and upward direction. If the lids are held widely open, the edge of the lid margin should engage the lens and dislodge it. (D) and (E) The open-handed scissors method. The lids are opened widely and the index and middle fingers are applied to the upper and lower lids to squeeze the lens off the eye.

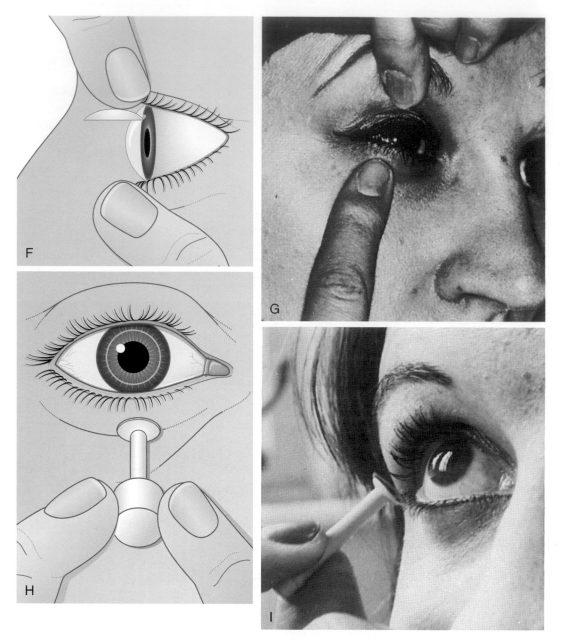

Figure14.26, cont'd (F) and (G) The two-handed scissors method. (H) and (I) The use of a suction cup is best delegated to an assistant to avoid inadvertent application of the cup to the cornea.
(From Stein HA, Slatt BJ, Stein RM, Freeman MI. Fitting guide for rigid and soft contact lenses: a practical approach. 4th ed. St Louis: Mosby; 2002.)

5. After removal, the lenses should be rinsed with saline or rinsing solution to remove secretions.

6. Storage of the lens is in contact lens solution. This permits the lens to be disinfected as well as lubricated on initial wearing. Follow the care instructions carefully for the specific disinfection solution being used to allow for effective disinfection.

7. Lenses should not be rinsed or placed in hot water because they may warp under extreme heat. Tap water use in general should be avoided, especially with soft contact lenses.

8. Beauty aids such as mascara should be used sparingly around the eyes. It is important to insert contact lenses before any cosmetic is applied to the lids. A cosmetic

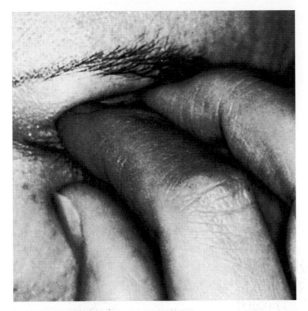

Figure 14.27 Centering the lens by massage.

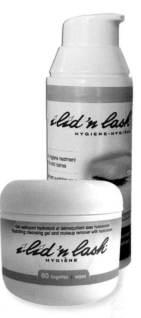

Figure 14.29 Wipes used to remove makeup. The main advantage is that they do not sting or burn.
(Courtesy of IMED Pharma Inc, Dollard-des-Ormeaux, Quebec, Canada.)

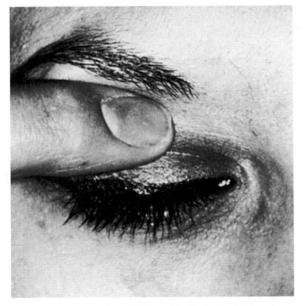

Figure 14.28 Centering the lens with the index finger.

with an oily base should be avoided because any oily agent will gather on the lenses and cause distortion of vision. Similarly, if a facial cleansing agent is used to wipe away a cosmetic, a liquid, nongreasy material is preferable to cold cream or other products with an oily base. Mascara should be used sparingly on the lashes, and only waterproofed brands are advisable. It

should be placed on the very tips of the lashes only. Also, liquid eyeliner is preferred because it does not run or flake as does pencil eyeliner. False eyelashes should be used sparingly or not at all. They are made from human hair, animal hair, or synthetic fibers and are applied with adhesive to either the underside of the lid or the outside lid margin. In many cases the adhesive breaks off and enters the eye, interposing between the cornea and the contact lens and causing irritation and abrasions. Hair spray is also irritating to the corneas. Certainly, anybody wearing contact lenses should use hair spray with caution. The eyes should be closed when hair spray is used and kept closed for several moments until the air clears. Similarly, the eyes should be kept closed when the head is placed under a hot hair dryer because the dryer causes evaporation of tears and a dry eye, which in turn can result in a corneal abrasion.

9. The lens wearer should avoid swimming while wearing contact lenses. The lenses can be washed out of the eye and pathogens present in the water could attach to the lenses.

10. Body-contact sports such as hockey and football should be avoided with RGP lenses in place. Individuals involved in these sports may do best with soft lenses. For activities such as golf, jogging, tennis, or badminton, rigid contact lenses can be worn with confidence.

CARE

Much has been written about the care of contact lenses. Of primary importance are the solutions that are used to minimize the possibility of bacterial contamination and permit relative safety for the eye. It is also important that the lens remain optically clear, free of debris and secretions, so that it will be comfortable when placed in the eye. The number of solutions available is legion, with many having combination features of wetting, cleaning, and soaking. It is thought that the contact lens–tarsal plate interaction is responsible for giant papillary conjunctivitis (GPC), an autoimmune papillitis of the upper tarsal conjunctiva. Wetting solutions minimize GPC.

Superpermeable rigid contact lenses are slightly flexible. The lens wearer should not bend or flex the lenses because they may warp or change shape so as to alter their fit. In addition, they are more fragile and may chip or crack.

The newer rigid lenses should be cleaned after each removal by placing them in the palm of the hand and cleaning the outer as well as the central portions with a suitable cleaner. It is important to use the lens care system prescribed by the eye care doctor and to follow the lens care instructions carefully.

When not being worn, the lenses should be kept hydrated by soaking them in the recommended solution. This will not only disinfect the lenses but also make them more wettable. If the lenses are not going to be used for a long period, periodical change of the solution is recommended; otherwise they should be cleaned and kept dry. The lenses must be cleaned and soaked in conditioning solution before use.

Care of gas-permeable lenses

Giant papillary conjunctivitis occurs with GP lenses but not with the same frequency as with hydrogel lenses. Allergic reactions occur in 1% to 5% of rigid lens wearers and increase to 10% to 20% in soft lens wearers. Soft contact lenses replaced on a frequent replacement regimen, in particular, disposable replacement, can dramatically reduce the occurrence of GPC.

It is important to keep GP lenses clean. Daily nonsensitizing surface-acting cleaners assist in reducing the incidence of papillary conjunctivitis. After the lenses are cleaned, a saline solution, preferably without preservatives, should be used to rinse them. At times, reactions can occur to the saline solutions and the cleaners. It is the preservative thimerosal that is usually the sensitizing agent and, as a result, few care systems today use thimerosal in their formulations. In such cases, nonpreserved saline solution dispensed from an airtight container should be used. Weekly or bimonthly cleaning may be necessary. Soft lens weekly cleaners can be best used for the more thorough cleaning of protein build-up. How does a patient know the lenses are dirty? After cleaning, the lenses should be clear and transparent. If the lens is exposed to a light source, the dirty deposits will become visible instantly.

Wetting solutions

The main function of a wetting solution is to convert the water-repelling surface of a rigid lens into a water-loving, or hydrophilic, surface. Ordinarily the dry plastic, when dipped in water, dries rapidly as the beads of water accumulate in little bubbles on the surface. Once a wetting agent has been used, the water forms a uniform film over the surfaces of the plastic. Thus when a wetting agent is used on a contact lens the tear film spreads easily and evenly on both surfaces of the lens, not only making the lens comfortable by acting as a cushion but also providing excellent refractive properties.

In addition to the wetting property, using a wetting solution helps maintain a clean lens by preventing finger smudges. Once the wetting solution bottle has been opened, sterility cannot be guaranteed and hence most commercial solutions contain a preservative to maintain sterility.

The practice of using saliva as a wetting agent before insertion is to be condemned. Although it does have good wetting characteristics because of a polysaccharide present, the risk of bacterial contamination to the lens is so real as to make the procedure totally unjustified. In addition to other microbes found in saliva, *Pseudomonas aeruginosa* is found in 6.6% of the population. Corneal ulcers resulting from a *Pseudomonas* infection can lead to blindness if not treated quickly and correctly.

Soaking solutions

Soaking solutions are designed to clean the lens of oily and sebaceous secretions that accumulate from the eyelid and conjunctival glands. Soaking the lens overnight in properly designed solutions removes these secretions from the lens. If the lenses are stored dry without adequate cleaning, they will accumulate secretions, which harden on the lens surface to form a film that is difficult to remove except by polishing.

In addition to the function of cleaning, soaking solutions contain germicidal agents that disinfect the contact lens. Although this action is by no means complete, certainly having no sterilizing effect on fungi and viruses, it does render some asepsis to the lens.

Another valuable benefit of soaking a lens overnight is the ability of the plastic to absorb some water. This maintains the lens in a constant curvature, reduces irritation, and maintains good vision.

Cleaning solutions

When a lens is removed from the eye, it is covered with oily secretions, mucus, or crystalline deposits. These materials must be removed before storage. Household detergents are not recommended because they often leave a film on the lens. Patients should clean the lens before storage by applying a few drops of a lens cleaner and rubbing the lens between the thumb and forefinger and then rinsing it well in water. They must avoid such agents as alcohol, acetone, kerosene, or lighter fluid in cleaning plastic lenses. Mechanical (swirl clean) and electrical (sonic clean) cleaning instruments are available for cleaning contact lenses adequately.

Rigid lenses can be polished and cleaned effectively on a modification unit to remove any accumulated film. With some of the newer GP lenses, it is advisable to check with the manufacturer before attempting in-office procedures.

Eyedrops with contacts

Some practitioners recommend eyedrops with high viscosity to reduce lens sensation. Also available are drops that clean and rewet the lenses while the patient is wearing them.

Lens cases are frequently the source of germs that can contaminate contact lenses. It is important that lens cases be kept scrupulously clean. A good routine to follow is to scrub the lens case at least once weekly with a toothbrush and soap. It is important to replace the lens case on a regular basis. Follow your eye doctor's recommendation.

EVALUATING THE FIT

An ideal fit is one in which wear is comfortable, vision is clear and comfortable with minimal spectacle blur, and there are no disturbances of the corneal integrity.

Subjective criteria

Adaptation symptoms

Initially the patient must adapt to the presence of the contact lens, which is basically a foreign body that rides on the surface of the cornea. The adaptive symptoms the patient has in early wear are normal and are distinguished from symptoms caused by poor fit in that they consistently decrease until they disappear as wearing time is increased. The following are some of the symptoms the patient may experience with early contact lens wear:

1. Awareness of the lens. Normally the patient is expected to be aware of the presence of corneal lenses. With time this awareness abates.
2. Photophobia or light sensitivity. Photophobia that persists after the adaptation period is a symptom of corneal irritability. The patient has discomfort and even pain when exposed to normal thresholds of light.

3. Spectacle blur. Foggy vision occurs when the contact lens is removed and glasses are worn. The spectacle blur is caused by edema of the central portion of the cornea, which may be a result of inadequate oxygen transport to the cornea, from either inadequate tear transport to the cornea or a material that has insufficient oxygen permeability characteristics.
4. Reflections. Internal reflections may occur from the contact lens itself or from a lens that decenters.
5. Burning sensation. This symptom of corneal irritability may represent corneal edema, corneal erosion, or excessive eyelid contact.

During the adaptation period, because the patient may have tearing, lid irritation, and excessive sensitivity to light, activities that require good visual acuity should be avoided. Until the adaptation period is complete, the patient should avoid driving a car; working on lathes, grinders, and other high-velocity moving equipment; and doing prolonged close work.

Abnormal symptoms

Symptoms may be caused by poor technique on the part of the patient in the insertion or removal of the lenses. A poor insertion method is a common failing of the novice. Among the hazards of incorrect insertion are the tendencies of the person to flinch, move the eye quickly, thrust the lens against the cornea, or squeeze the lids around the lens.

Symptoms caused by low oxygen (hypoxia) to the cornea tend to become more severe and more constant as the lenses are worn. Lenses that prevent adequate tear and oxygen exchange are referred to as "tight" lenses, but symptoms are essentially caused by starvation of oxygen in the cornea. The symptom of corneal hypoxia is a burning sensation that appears after a comfortable induction period of 2 to 3 hours. Such a lens may not lag with eye movement, will not drop when the lids are pulled away, and shows little or no excursion with blinking. However, if the lens is too "loose," it may frequently slip off the cornea or fall out of the eye.

Poor vision may be a result of a variety of conditions. The power of the lens may be in error, the fit of the lens may be poor, the lens may be warped, or it may have been inserted in the wrong eye.

A distinction should be made between foggy vision that occurs on insertion of the lens and that which arises 2 to 3 hours after contact lens wear. The former is usually caused by incorrect cleansing or mucus under the lens. The latter is usually indicative of corneal edema or corneal hypoxia and is a pathologic finding.

Excessive awareness of a contact lens can be a psychologic problem because it is only an extension of the normal conscious feeling of something foreign on the eye. However, the normal contact lens wearer usually has many periods during the day when he or she is free of this sensation. If the patient should suddenly become aware of the contact lens, this symptom may be indicative of roughened and scratched edges of the lens or the presence of dried secretions on its surface.

A burning sensation is generally attributed to a tight lens, to stagnation of tear fluid between the lens and the cornea, to corneal anoxia, or to damage of the corneal epithelium. In the first three cases the symptom abates on removal of the lens, whereas in the last it does not.

The patient with a foreign body sensation will either harbor a tiny foreign body between the lens and cornea, particularly in dusty areas, or have erosions of the cornea. Any patient who has pathologic symptoms should be told to remove the lenses and be reassessed before wear is resumed.

Abnormal symptoms and signs and the corrections required to eliminate them are discussed further in Chapter 14.

Objective criteria

The fit of a contact lens may be objectively evaluated according to its relationship to the lid margins and its position on the cornea. Ideally, the upper margin of the lens should fit under the upper lid and be free of the lower lid. Blinking action of the lids should raise the lens slightly. The contact lens should be well centered on the cornea and not displaced to either side.

Other objective criteria used to evaluate the fit of a contact lens include (1) fluorescein patterns, (2) alteration of the blink rate, (3) scratches, chips, and roughened edges of the contact lens, and (4) changes in the cornea.

Fluorescein patterns (Figures 14.30 and 14.31)

If the size and movement of the lens in the patient's eye appear satisfactory, the fluorescein test should follow. In this test, fluorescein is placed on the superior margin of the cornea. Fluorescein patterns are best seen with an ultraviolet lamp source for illumination and a slit-lamp microscope or handheld magnifier for inspection (Figure 14.32). The fluorescein dye forms a thin layer between the contact lens and the cornea. The distribution of the dye enables the observer to evaluate the adequacy of the precorneal fluid layer between the contact lens and the cornea.

The patient with a normal corneal contour will have an even and thin layer of dyed tear film centrally surrounded by a slightly deeper ring of fluid peripherally. At the area of marginal touch at the extreme periphery of the lens, the depth of the tear film is minimal. A flat lens, which is a lens with a flatter posterior curvature than the anterior central surface of the cornea, tends to rest on the optic cap of the cornea and touch it (Figure 14.33). At the area of contact there is an absence of the green fluorescein dye (Figure 14.34). A steep lens has a steeper posterior curvature than the cornea and bridges it, making contact at its margin with the peripheral portion of the cornea (Figure 14.35). Peripheral contact tends to cause central pooling of the dye, with a ring of touch marginally (Figure 14.36).

Alteration of the blink rate

Blinking properly is an important factor in the successful wearing of a contact lens. With blinking there is an interchange of tears between the contact lens and the cornea, thereby bringing fresh oxygen and nutrients to the cornea. As tears are produced, they form a small ring around the lid margins. When the lids close, as occurs in blinking, they act like a windshield wiper and sweep the tears over the cornea. When a contact lens is worn, the lids move the lens and a new precorneal tear film is produced, which interchanges with the existing tear film.

A patient whose lenses fit comfortably blinks normally, is free of squinting, and shifts gaze in a normal manner. If excessive blinking develops, it is usually in response to a lens that has excessive movement. Normally the lens makes a small, quick excursion upward with the blink and then gently falls. A loose lens is generally indicative of a flat lens–cornea relationship. A loose lens slides more easily off center and the patient begins to blink excessively trying to recenter the lens.

If the blink rate is reduced and the patient is given to staring, the contact lens may be irritating the eyelid. By opening the eyes wide and controlling the blink rate, the patient avoids the unpleasant contact of the superior margin of the contact lens and the upper lid. The nonblinker may show a reduction in the blink rate from the normal of 12 times a minute, or once every 3 or 4 seconds, to 3 or 4 times a minute.

Changes in the blink rate often occur because of awareness of the contact lens and persist despite a perfect contact lens fit. To avoid this habit, many fitters advocate blinking exercises. The patient is asked to fixate on a distant object and perform voluntary closures of the lid until the lid awareness diminishes in intensity.

Scratches, chips, and roughened edges of the contact lens

Scratches may occur from incorrect handling of the contact lens. If the scratches are central and numerous, they can cause scattering of light and a diminution of visual acuity. Chips and roughened edges may cause erosion of the corneal epithelium by scratching it. Roughened edges may be caused by incorrect cleansing of the lens if the normal secretions and sediment are allowed to collect and dry at the margin of the lens. A contact lens should be examined under magnification to ensure that the lens is free of surface defects and adherent deposits.

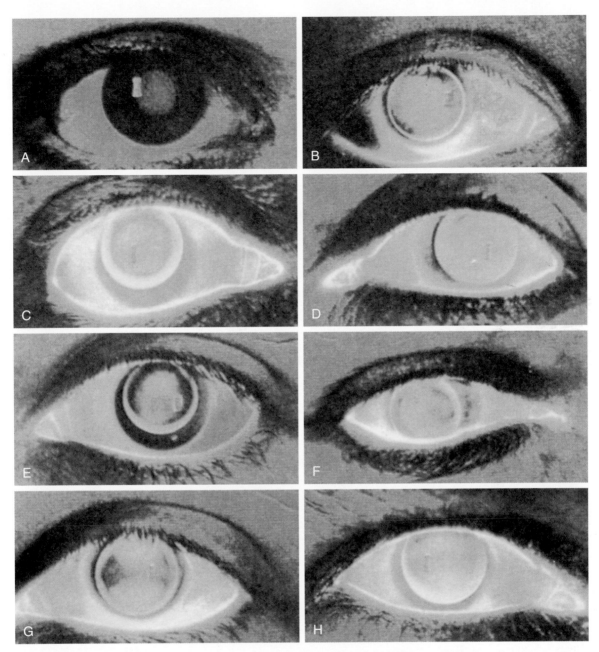

Figure 14.30 Common fluorescein patterns. Corneal lens. (A) Normal fluorescence of the crystalline lens without the instillation of fluorescein. This is a source of confusion to the novice in assessing the fit. (B) Minimal apex-clear fitting in a corectopic patient with the pupil at the limbus at the 12 o'clock position. Note that a more apex-clear lens would show a broader dark band of contact adjacent to the peripheral curve. (C) The apex-clear pattern in the normal eye. Note the fluorescence of the crystalline lens within the pupil. (D) Flat-fitting lens. There is touch at the apex of the lens. (E) Flat-fitting lens. A pool of fluorescein with a curved lower limit is seen above the central touch. (F) Flat-fitting lens. A pool of fluorescein with a curved upper limit is seen below the central touch. (G) Flat astigmatic picture. The other eye of the patient with corectopia is seen in (B). (H) Apex-clear astigmatic pattern in a normal eye.

(A–H reproduced with permission from Duke-Elder S, Abrams D, editors. System of ophthalmology, vol 5: ophthalmic optics and refraction. St Louis: Mosby; 1970.)

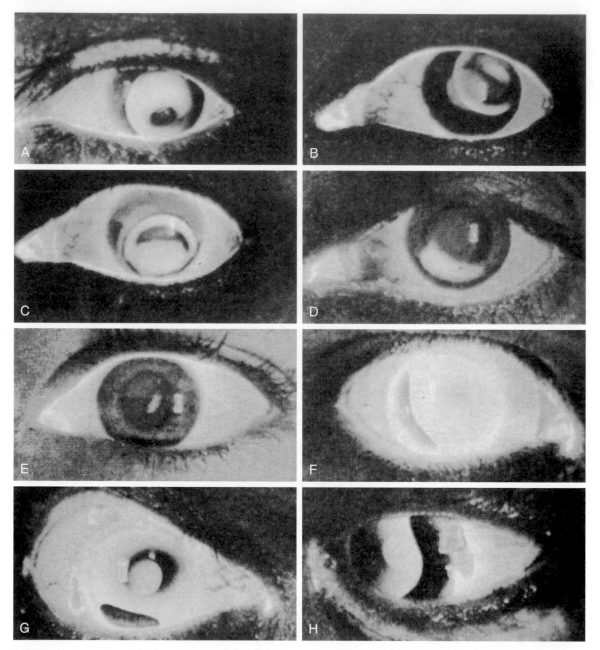

Figure 14.31 Corneal lens. (A) Keratoconus. A hard touch in the area of the cone, lifting off the lens in other areas. (B) Keratoconus, a thin, small lens fitted to the flattest keratometry reading. This lens proved satisfactory. (C) Same case as in (B) with the lens in a lower position, showing a completely different fluorescein pattern. (D) Asymptomatic corneal stain of a superficial punctate type, 6 days after cessation of corneal lens wear. (E) Transient crescentic staining of a granular of punctate type with a corneal lens, differing from that resulting from central corneal edema and not giving rise to any serious complications. Scleral lens. (F) Normal eye, scleral lens. There is a light corneal touch with adequate limbal clearance and a sausage-shaped bubble associated with the fenestration. (G) Central corneal touch. Poor limbal clearance. (H) Nasal corneal touch and enlargement of the bubble on adduction.

(A–H reproduced with permission from Duke-Elder S, Abrams D, editors. System of ophthalmology, vol 5: ophthalmic optics and refraction. St Louis: Mosby; 1970.)

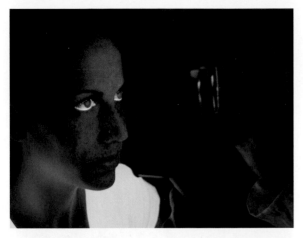
Figure 14.32 Burton lamp used to evaluate fit of contact lens.

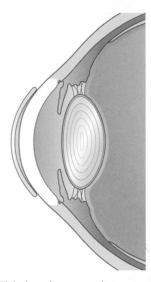
Figure 14.35 Tight lens: base curve is too steep.
(From Stein HA, Slatt BJ, Stein RM, Freeman MI. Fitting guide for rigid and soft contact lenses: a practical approach. 4th ed. St Louis: Mosby; 2002.)

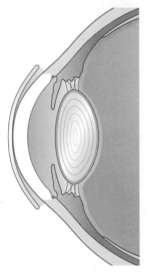
Figure 14.33 Flat contact lens resting on apex of cornea.

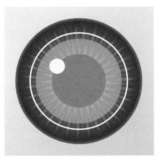
Figure 14.36 Fluorescein pattern of a steep lens. Note absence of dye at the periphery as a result of marginal touch.

Changes in the cornea

Alteration of the surface of the cornea occurs either in the form of diffuse or localized corneal edema or in the form of erosion of the epithelium. Corneal edema results if the contact lens fits so tightly against the cornea that the surface epithelium cannot breathe or become oxygenated. Depriving the cornea of oxygen interferes with its metabolism, which in turn causes the formation of edema. The factors that cause corneal edema are (1) a flat lens, which causes compression of the apex of the cornea; (2) a steep lens, which causes stagnation of tears; (3) a poorly centered lens, which causes pressure in one area; (4) incorrect blinking; and (5) incorrect cleansing of the lens.

Patients complaining of spectacle blur or photophobia that persists beyond the first week or two should be examined for edema. On retroillumination the edema will appear as a smoky area in the center third of the cornea.

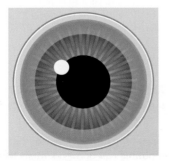
Figure 14.34 Fluorescein pattern of a flat lens. Note absence of dye centrally.

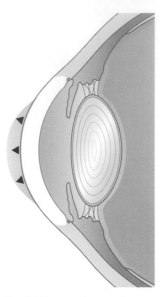

Figure 14.37 The rigid lens produces a discrete type of corneal edema, confined to the corneal cap, which does cause spectacle blur because it produces a radical steepening of the corneal curvature.

(From Stein HA, Slatt BJ, Stein RM, Freeman MI. Fitting guide for rigid and soft contact lenses: a practical approach. 4th ed. St Louis: Mosby; 2002.)

Another method of detecting edema is by keratometry (follow-up *K* readings). Edema often produces *K* readings higher than those originally found (Figure 14.37).

During the adaptation period, edema is almost inevitable. It should not, however, be present after 2 or 3 weeks. If edema persists it will be accompanied by subjective complaints of photophobia, burning smokiness, and spectacle blur. The usual cause of edema is a tight lens resulting from too steep a base curve. However, the peripheral curve may be too shallow or poorly blended, or the lens may be too large.

Erosions of the corneal epithelium may occur because of the incarceration of tiny foreign bodies between cornea and lens. They are visible as slightly depressed spots that tend to take up the fluorescein stain (Figure 14.38). Other causes of corneal erosions, or punctate staining, of the cornea are (1) a chipped or roughened edge, (2) flat peripheral curves, (3) a flat lens, (4) incorrect recentering of a lens, (5) poor insertion and removal techniques, (6) dust or other particles under the lens, and (7) overwearing of lenses.

Corneal edema has become much rarer owing to the development of high-DK GP materials. A patient with corneal edema will complain of blurred vision or veiled vision. In punctate staining the most common symptom is a foreign body sensation of the eyes either during contact lens wear or after the lens has been removed. If a patient continues to wear contact lenses despite signs and symptoms of a punctate keratitis, he or she can easily develop a

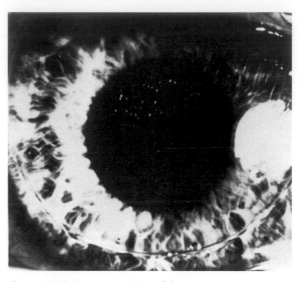

Figure 14.38 Punctate staining of the cornea. *(Courtesy Dr. J. Dixon.)*

corneal scratch or abrasion or, eventually, a corneal ulcer. The occurrence of corneal erosions requires immediate removal of the contact lens and reevaluation of the fit.

ADJUSTMENTS

The most common problems with contact lenses are that they are either too loose or too tight. If the lens is too loose, it may be redesigned to provide greater adherence to the cornea by:

1. Increasing the optic zone diameter
2. Increasing the overall diameter of the lens
3. Decreasing the radius of the optic zone (mm)
4. Decreasing the radius of the intermediate or peripheral curve (mm)

All modifications that produce a tighter-fitting lens require the manufacture of a new lens. A lens can always be adjusted to fit more loosely, but never more tightly. Note that some newer materials do not allow for in-office adjustment.

PROBLEMS ASSOCIATED WITH OVERWEARING CONTACT LENSES

Moderate to severe pain, lid edema, lacrimation, and marked photophobia can occur if contact lenses are worn for too long. These symptoms usually occur if the patient has been too ambitious in the early adaptive period in trying to prolong the wearing time. They may occur as a result of carelessness, as typified by the person who falls asleep while wearing contact lenses. The pain usually occurs 2 to 3 hours after the lenses have been removed and is intense. The patient is usually very agitated and in such distress that examination of the cornea can be made only after local anesthetic drops have been instilled in the eye. The cornea shows diffuse erosions over its apex and stains intensely with fluorescein. This condition usually responds to patching of the eye. Within 24 hours the surface of the cornea is usually clear.

Acute hypoxia of the cornea was a common event with PMMA lenses, but is a rare occurrence with any of the GP lenses. Most of the hazards of insufficient oxygen to the cornea, whether acute or chronic, have been eliminated with GP lenses and, with the newer type of these lenses, extended wear for varying periods is a reality. The oxygenation of the cornea under the closed lid is sufficient to sustain metabolism despite the presence of a contact lens.

USES

The popular thought regarding the use of contact lenses is that they are of value only for cosmetic purposes. It is true that many patients experience a tremendous psychologic emancipation when freed from the burden of heavy, thick, and unsightly glasses, but this is not their primary function. Contact lenses are a wonderful visual aid that can provide vision unobtainable by any other means. They are of particular value to a patient with high myopia. Myopes constitute the largest group of contact lens wearers, probably because of their high degree of motivation.

Contact lenses offer a more normal image size because they are closer to the eye. Just as high-plus cataract spectacles magnify the image on the retina by virtue of lying in front of the eye with an air interspace, high-minus spectacles tend to minify the retinal image. When contact lenses are used for myopia, the retinal image is more normal, enlarging about 10% for a −6.00 diopter lens and much more for a higher-minus lens. Therefore, contact lenses result in a retinal image of more normal size and better visual acuity. They allow an unrestricted field of view because the lenses move with the eyes and the appearance is like that of unaided vision.

Contact lenses also treat irregular astigmatism caused by corneal scarring.

Hyperopic patients form a small portion of those desiring contact lenses, because a far-sighted person needs a comparatively low-powered lens and can usually obtain satisfactory distance vision without glasses.

The patient who has had cataracts removed suffers the same visual disabilities as the high myope and therefore enjoys the same advantages with contact lenses, such as freedom from the weight of heavy glasses, a wider range of field of vision, and a more natural-appearing image. For the aphakic or postcataract patient, spectacles enlarge the image by 33%. With contact lenses, there is a restoration to a more normal image size because the contact lens reduces the magnification to only 7%. In addition, the aphakic individual suffers from many aberrations while looking through the periphery of the spectacle lens. With contact lenses, distortion never occurs because the lens moves with the eye and vision is always obtained through the central portion of the lens.

Nowadays, intraocular lenses are inserted after all cataract removal operations. For patients who had the procedure performed before the advent of intraocular lenses, contact lenses offer restored normal vision. Contacts may make the image size approximately the same size as the image seen by the fellow eye, or at the very least only slightly larger. For patients in whom this is not possible, contact lenses offer a solution to restore normal vision because it makes the image seen approximately the same size as that seen by the fellow eye.

Contact lenses have also been used for children who have undergone surgery for congenital or traumatic cataract.

Keratoconus is a developmental anomaly of the cornea, which is characterized by progressive thinning and an apical bulge of the central portion of the cornea (Figure 14.39). This condition results in irregular myopic astigmatism that cannot be corrected by glasses. Contact lenses flatten the cornea, tend to stabilize the condition, and, by virtue of the fluid interface between the contact lens and the cornea, eliminate irregular astigmatism and permit clear vision.

The cornea may be too thin for repeat laser treatment. Following laser surgery a condition of keractesia may have developed and the only option may be glasses or a contact lens. This condition is an excellent indication for contact lenses. Keractesia is an induced form of thinning of the cornea may be too thin for crosslinking. The only option may be glasses or an RGP contact lens.

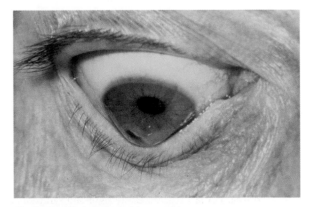

Figure 14.39 An advanced case of keratoconus.

Besides correcting refractive errors, contact lenses may be used to cover unsightly eyes. In these cases the contact lens is colored to disguise disfiguring features of the eye.

Contact lenses also have been useful in treating patients with nystagmus. In these cases vision is improved because the correcting lens moves with the eye. Another use for contact lenses is for a patient with congenital albinism. A small pupillary opening is provided and a collarette of darkly tinted soft lens is produced to protect the patient from excessive glare.

An interesting field of research is under way to investigate the potential of GP lenses for reducing myopia progression (peripheral blur hypothesis). If these studies result in valid scientific evidence, the use of such lenses in young people may become standard practice, in particular in those Asian countries that have a very high rate of myopia.

Many professional people, including actors, politicians, and public speakers, wear contact lenses to improve their appearance before the public. Professional athletes such as hockey players and football players can participate in competitive sports only by being free of the encumbrance and hazard of spectacles. Among athletes, however, soft contact lenses may be the wiser choice because they are less likely to be lost than are rigid lenses.

SUMMARY

One of the major concerns with contact lenses is education of the contact lens patient. Each patient should be instructed about the symptoms that can be expected and tolerated and those that are danger signals and indicate immediate consultation. Also, each patient should be shown the methods of handling the lenses, their insertion and removal, and their storage and hygiene.

Each phase in the adaptation period should be clearly outlined to the patient. The patient must be given an orderly schedule to follow and a routine to perform.

The patient also should be told the function that the contact lens will perform. This function may be optical, therapeutic, or cosmetic. The wearing of contact lenses demands the payment of a price, in attention, care, and finances. The patient should know the benefits and be aware of the hazards.

Questions for review and thought

1. Name factors that contraindicate the wearing of rigid contact lenses.
2. List the advantages and disadvantages of corneal rigid contact lenses.
3. What holds a contact lens in place?
4. What are the characteristics of the plastic used in rigid lens manufacture?
5. Outline a method of evaluating a patient before prescribing contact lenses.
6. The keratometer is an important instrument in evaluating the anterior corneal curvature. Outline a method of performing keratometry.
7. How can you verify the diameter of a contact lens? The radius?
8. Given a patient with $-2.75 + 0.75 \times 90$ and K readings of $43.50 \times 44.50 \times 90$, with normal lid and pupillary opening, how would you compute a possible type of rigid lens for initial trial?
9. What effect would contact lenses have on the visual field of a patient with a -6.00 diopter lens?
10. Describe spectacle blur and its causes.
11. Describe how you would instruct a patient to clean and insert contact lenses.
12. Describe three methods of instructing the patient in lens removal.
13. What is the value of a wetting solution? Name several that are available.
14. What is the value of a lens cleaner? Name several that are available.
15. What are the advantages of using a trial set in contact lens fitting?
16. What is the importance of blinking?
17. What causes corneal edema after wearing of contact lenses?
18. How can a lens be adjusted that is too tight? Too loose?
19. Contact lenses are frequently used for cosmetic or refractive purposes. However, after cataract surgery they aid considerably in overall vision. Why?
20. What is your routine wearing schedule for rigid lenses?
21. What symptoms may be attributed to a loose lens and to a tight lens?
22. List the features of a contact lens that can be modified without making a new lens.

Self-evaluation questions

True–false statements

Directions: Indicate whether the statement is true **(T)** or false **(F)**.

1. The keratometer is an instrument that is used to measure the radius of curvature of the front surface of the cornea. **T** or **F**

2. If the keratometer measurements show a difference in dioptric power from one meridian to the opposite meridian, then irregular astigmatism exists. **T** or **F**

3. With fluorescein staining, if a dark area appears centrally, then the corneal lens is considered too steep. **T** or **F**

Missing words

Directions: Write in the missing word in the following sentences:

4. With-the-rule astigmatism is present when the horizontal meridian is _____ than the vertical meridian.

5. The optic cap is the _____ zone of the cornea.

6. The power of a rigid contact lens may be measured by an instrument called the _____.

Choice-completion questions

Directions: Select the one best answer in each case.

7. Defects in lens material or edge design may be identified by which piece of equipment?
   a. Radiuscope
   b. Shadowgraph
   c. Lensmeter
   d. Keratometer
   e. Profile analyzer

8. A rigid lens that is too loose may result in:
   a. spectacle blur.
   b. burning sensation.
   c. blurring of vision after blinking.
   d. night blindness.
   e. pain after lens removal.

9. Fluorescein patterns may be most helpful in identifying a poorly fitting lens. A lens that shows a large dark central area with an absence of fluorescein is indicative of:
   a. a normal fit.
   b. a steep lens.
   c. a flat lens.
   d. incorrect fenestration of the lens.
   e. none of the above.

A Answers, notes, and explanations

1. **True.** The keratometer measures the front surface of the cornea, which acts as a convex mirror reflecting the mires or images of the keratometer. The keratometer measures only a very limited circular area of the cornea, approximately 2 to 4 mm apart, depending on the manufacturer of the keratometer. The keratometer makes an assumption as to the index of refraction of the cornea.

2. **False.** If the dioptric power from one meridian to the opposite meridian is different, then regular astigmatism is said to exist and the difference in diopters between the two meridians indicates the amount of corneal astigmatism present. When irregular astigmatism exists, the mires are distorted and it is difficult to obtain satisfactory reflecting images from the cornea. Such conditions as keratoconus and scars of the cornea produce irregular astigmatism.

3. **False.** The dark area indicates that there is no fluorescein pattern centrally, which signifies that the lens is touching the central portion of the cornea. This exists when the lens base curve is flatter than the curvature of the cornea so that the central portion of the lens rests on the central portion of the cornea and prevents the dye from entering the center and pooling centrally.

4. **Flatter.** The eye is shaped in some ways like a football whose long axis is positioned horizontally in the palpebral fissures so that the steeper meridian is vertical and the flatter meridian is horizontal. This is known as with-the-rule astigmatism. When this occurs in the opposite direction, it is considered against-the-rule astigmatism.

5. **Central.** The optic cap lies in the central 5 to 7 mm of the cornea, which involves the visual axis of the cornea. This is the area that should be measured with the keratometer in determining the central corneal radius of curvature. This is the area that becomes involved when a rigid contact lens is overworn and edema results, causing fogginess of vision.

6. **Lensmeter.** By holding a rigid contact lens between the thumb and forefinger or letting it rest concave side down, the examiner may measure the back vertex power of a contact lens. The lens should always be placed so that the concavity of the lens lies toward the instrument so that the back power is measured. This is of minor significance in low powers, but in high minus or high plus powers, it may become significant.

7. **b. Shadowgraph.** The Shadowgraph is a type of magnifier and projector that permits the examiner to check the details of the lens material and edge design for chips, roughness,

269

A Continued

or sharpness. Important features such as sharpness or roughness of a rigid lens may be fundamental to the comfortable wearing of rigid contact lenses. It is the edge design, which must ride against and under the eyelid, that tends to produce the lid awareness of a contact lens. The surface quality of the lens as well as defects in material can be identified with the magnification of the Shadowgraph instrument.

8. **c. Blurring of vision after blinking.** A loose lens will often decenter after a person blinks and will ride either to the side or low, resulting in poor vision and fluctuating vision. Burning sensations are a result of hypoxia that develops from stagnation brought on by the accumulation of metabolites centrally from a steep lens that does not permit adequate venting and exchange of tear film. This is a tight lens symptom. Spectacle blur is a result of hypoxia with edema that develops in the central portion of the cornea and is usually a result of either overwear of a contact lens or a tight lens that does not permit adequate tear exchange. Pain following lens removal is also a symptom that there has been corneal hypoxia or complete anoxia brought on by incorrect venting or tear exchange and indicates a tight lens rather than a loose lens.

9. **c. A flat lens.** The absence of fluorescein is indicative that the lens is touching the apex of the cornea so that fluorescein does not intervene between the lens and the cornea. This central touch may cause warpage of the cornea with compression changes on the surface of the cornea. If the lens is too flat, it may rock and usually decenters. Also there may be a flattening of the cornea and an undesirable type of reduction of myopia at the expense of possible permanent structural changes in the cornea. The principle of orthokeratology is to provide very slight changes by central touch so that small degrees of astigmatism can be reduced on a regular basis in this manner. This, however, may result in irregular flattening of the cornea by compression, with resulting induced irregular astigmatism.

Soft contact lenses

There are approximately 90 million contact wearers worldwide. In the United States alone, data indicate that approximately 13% of the population (more than 36 million) use contact lenses for vision correction and it is estimated that the United States represents approximately 40% of the number of wearers worldwide. Most contact lens wearers also own a pair or two of spectacles. Data indicate that in 2015 the number of spectacle units (number of eyeglasses manufactured) worldwide was approximately 3.5 billion.

The soft lenses rival rigid lenses in their quality of vision and surpass them in the realm of comfort and ease of adaptation (Figure 15.1). The two basic types of soft lenses are the hydrogel (hydrophilic) lens, which owes its softness to its ability to absorb and bind water to its structure, and the silicone hydrogel lens, which owes its softness to the intrinsic property of the rubbery material.

HISTORY OF HYDROPHILIC LENSES

In 1960 two young New York lawyers established a company with the unique function of promoting patent exchanges among corporations. Their specialty was combing through the dusty corporate files for idle patents and setting up licensing agreements with other companies interested in putting the dormant ideas to use. In 1965 the men who had established the National Patent Development Corporation suddenly dissolved their patent law business. They had uncovered a patent with so many exciting possibilities that they decided to pick up a license themselves. In effect, they became their own client, eliminating their role as middlemen.

The new material was a plastic that they called hydron. It was developed by Dr. Otto Wichterle, head of the Institute of Macromolecular Chemistry of the Czechoslovakian National Academy of Science and a leading expert on polymer chemistry, and by Dr. Drahoslav Lim. The new material appeared to be like other plastics in that it was a hard

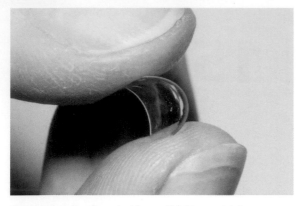

Figure 15.1 A soft contact lens will fold completely.

transparent substance that could be cut, ground, or molded into a variety of shapes. When placed in water or an aqueous solution, however, the tough, rigid plastic became soft and pliable. In this wet form it could be bent between the fingers until the edges met or could be turned easily inside out, yet it would snap back into its original shape quickly. When allowed to dry, the supple waterlogged material became as dry as a cornflake and crushed to a powdery dust if smashed. The substance was subjected to rigorous biologic tests and was found to be inert and fully compatible with human tissue. One of its properties was that although highly elastic when wet, it remained strong and able to hold its shape (Figure 15.2).

The plastic is hydroxyethyl methacrylate (HEMA), a plastic polymer with the remarkable ability to absorb water molecules. Chemically, the polymer consists of a three-dimensional network of HEMA chains crosslinked with ethylene glycol dimethacrylate molecules about once every 200 monomer units. As the water is introduced to the plastic, it swells into a soft mass with surprisingly good

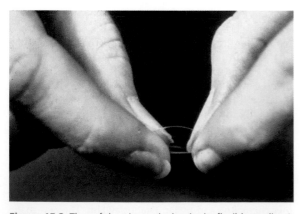

Figure 15.2 The soft lens is sturdy despite its flexible quality. It can be stretched, dried, or crumpled and still retain its integrity.

mechanical strength, complete transparency (97%), and the ability to retain its shape and dimensions.

Five vigorous years of improvements and clinical trials were conducted on the soft lens before the US Food and Drug Administration (FDA) (which considered the lens a drug) approved the lens as a safe prosthetic device of good optical quality. The FDA's caution, after the thalidomide tragedies in which a drug produced severe deformities in the babies of pregnant women, was understandable. Both the public and the practitioner needed protection. In the first phase of research the soft lens was tested with laboratory animals to ensure that it was nontoxic; later it was given to selected practitioners and independent research workers for clinical trials on human beings.

It soon became apparent that the soft lens was an innovation of major importance, with widespread application not only as an instrument for treating diseased corneas, but also as a superior contact lens. In the early stages, however, the therapeutic possibilities of soft lenses overshadowed any other consideration because it appeared that these lenses would replace many conventional treatments of external diseases of the eye.

As the number of contact lens companies throughout the world expanded, a search for newer and better lens plastics and lens designs developed. Many modifications were made as new monomers were discovered and crosslinked to create differing polymers; polyvinyl pyrrolidone (PVP) was added to increase oxygen permeability, and methyl methacrylate (MMA) to create more stiffness to aid in handling ease. Non-HEMA hydrogel polymers were introduced.

Research activity was also directed toward lens designs to correct astigmatism, bifocal corrections, and tinted lenses for cosmetic appearance as well as therapeutic application. Ultrathin and higher-water-content lenses have opened up significant new areas in contact lens development, with increased success rates. In the manufacturing arena the emphasis is on automated computer-driven systems and advanced molding processes.

The most recent developments have been the addition of ultraviolet-screening agents to soft polymers and the amplification of the concept of biomimesis. *Biomimesis* is defined as the ability to create or mimic biologic surfaces. Various approaches have been tried to improve the biocompatibility of materials for use in the human body. The surface properties of foreign materials play a critical role in triggering a biologic response and initiate undesirable and unwanted interactions with proteins and other biomolecules at the material surface. The formation of blood clots on surface materials, dental plaque build-up, and contact lens deposits are examples of the same phenomenon. A synthesized phosphorylcholine added to soft lens material to promote biocompatibility has produced the Proclear lens from CooperVision. Current soft lens research aims to produce a contact lens that replicates the tears in the human eye. Materials with water content as high as 92% are under investigation.

With the proliferation of soft materials, it became necessary to classify lenses in several ways. Classification by water content means that the soft lens contains that percentage of water, for example, low water content (37.5%–45%), medium water content (46%–58%), and high water content (59%–92%). The FDA classifies lenses into four basic groups based on water content and ionicity for the purpose of evaluating disinfecting systems with different lens material groups. With the development of new high-DK materials, a fifth classification group is being considered. The process used to manufacture a soft lens is another method of classification. Lenses may be spin cast, lathe cut, or cast molded; 90% of soft lens production in the world today uses the cast-molded method. Finally, soft contact lenses may be classified by design or function (e.g., daily wear, flexible wear, extended wear, or continuous wear).

Silicone hydrogel lenses with higher oxygen permeabilities are the latest development in soft contact lens material (Boxes 15.1 and 15.2).

ADVANTAGES

The advantages of hydrophilic contact lenses are as follows:

1. Comfort
2. Rapid adaptation
3. Lack of spectacle blur
4. Disposability
5. Minimal lens loss
6. Minimal overwear reaction
7. Lack of glare and photophobia
8. Difficulty in dislodging
9. Protection of entire cornea
10. Attractive alternative for rigid lens dropouts
11. No serious corneal abrasion on insertion

Comfort

These lenses are exceptionally comfortable from the initial period. It is impressive to witness the rapid tolerance of the cornea to the presence of the contact lens. The lack of awareness of a soft lens is due partly to the flaccidity, water content, and thin edges of the lens, which mold to the white of the eye (the sclera). Therefore, there is almost no interference from the upper lids during normal blinking. The lens hugs the eye so closely that the advancing surface of the eyelid just glides over it (Figure 15.3). Its supple quality when wet also contributes to the easy acceptance of the soft lens. Being hydrophilic, or water-loving, it forms a cushioned fluid buffer between itself and the cornea. It also contours itself to the unique shape of the individual cornea. With no hard edges to irritate the eyelid edge and no rigid structure to compress delicate living tissue, there are minimal frictional erosions. Because of its soft qualities,

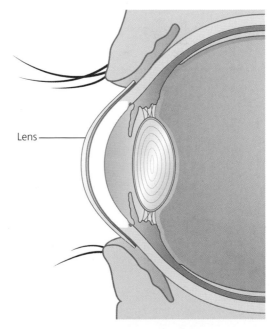

Lens

Figure 15.3 The soft lens fits under the eyelid margins and the advancing lid edge just glides over its surface. This accounts for part of its comfort factor.
(From Stein HA, Slatt BJ, Stein RM, et al. Fitting guide for rigid and soft contact lenses: a practical approach. 4th ed. St Louis: Mosby; 2002.)

a normal tear exchange takes place by diffusion through the lens matrix and under the lens.

A rigid lens has to be fitted according to the precise shape of the cornea. If the fit is poor, or if the laboratory does not make the lens according to exact specifications, a rigid lens will irritate the eye. A soft lens is more flexible on the eye. A wide latitude is possible without corneal injury, and less exacting measurements are required.

Rapid adaptation

Tolerance is extremely high compared with that of the rigid lens. The lenses are frequently comfortable to a new patient within 30 minutes. Wearing schedules can be easily increased to full-time day wear within 10 days.

Lack of spectacle blur

Removal of the lenses permits patients to switch directly to their glasses within 5 to 10 minutes without the spectacle blur that occurs with edema induced by polymethyl methacrylate (PMMA) rigid lenses. Spectacle blur is uncommon because of the diffuse nature of any edema, which spreads evenly over the cornea and does not alter its radius (Figure 15.4).

Disposability

Soft lenses may be replaced on a disposable regimen, for example, replaced daily, weekly, or biweekly, reducing patient discomfort and risk of infection. Soft lenses replaced on a disposable regimen are ideal for occasional or intermittent wear.

Minimal lens loss

With new patients, rigid lenses are sometimes lost in the first 3 months, when handling is still somewhat clumsy. Rigid lenses also dislodge with aggressive sports activities. The technique for removal of a soft lens is such that loss is less frequent than with a rigid lens. The larger size of the soft lens, coupled with the firm adherence of the lens to the cornea with minimal sliding effect, reduces the loss factor considerably. It is rare for a patient to report the loss of a soft lens (Figure 15.5). The lenses do not fall out.

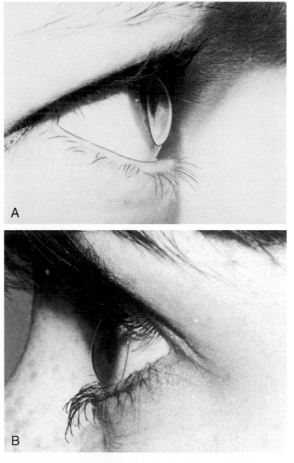

Figure 15.5 Comparison of hard and soft lenses. (A) The hard lens is smaller than the cornea and can be easily dislodged with the edge of the lid. (B) The soft lens is larger than the cornea, hugs the eye tightly, and seldom is displaced even during body contact sports.

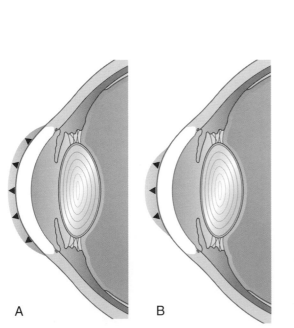

Figure 15.4 (A) The soft lens produces a diffuse area of corneal edema that does not alter the radius of curvature of the cornea and does not cause spectacle blur. (B) A low-DK hard lens produces a discrete type of corneal edema, confined to the corneal cap, which does cause spectacle blur because it produces a radical steepening of the corneal curvature.
(From Stein HA, Slatt BJ, Stein RM, et al. Fitting guide for rigid and soft contact lenses: a practical approach. 4th ed. St Louis: Mosby; 2002.)

Minimal overwear reaction

Every ophthalmologist remembers cases of the overwear syndrome experienced by the old PMMA rigid lens wearer, who appeared at the hospital emergency room in the middle of the night with excruciating pain, having worn these lenses longer than the normal time limit. This problem is virtually eliminated with the soft lens. In older low-DK soft lens material, 2% of patients reported slight corneal edema with halos about lights and a burning sensation of their eyes. At the end of the day no serious disabling disorder has occurred. The edema effect was further reduced by the advent of materials with greater oxygen permeability.

Oxygen is carried to the cornea through the tear film and is replenished through the circulation of tears under the lens and diffusion through the lens. This is the same method by which the cornea receives its oxygen supply under a rigid lens. The evidence of a good tear layer between the soft lens and the cornea has been demonstrated by a French ophthalmologist, Dr. Paul Cochet, who showed spherical particles 1 to 3 μm in diameter passing underneath the lens. When the tear layer has been stained, it has been shown to ripple with the blinking motions of the lids. The respiration of the cornea is provided by tear exchange during blinking.

Lack of glare and photophobia

Glare and light sensitivity are seen almost routinely in the early weeks of rigid lens wear. These symptoms are virtually absent with the soft lens, making it the ideal lens for outdoor athletes such as golfers and tennis players. Also, the generous size of the optic zone means that the pupil is always covered; this minimizes glare.

Difficulty in dislodging

The firm adherence of the soft lens to the eye permits it to be used in body contact sports and reduces embarrassment associated with dislodgment (Figure 15.6).

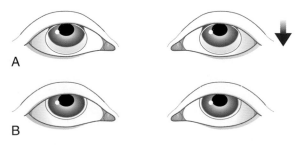

Figure 15.6 (A) With rigid lenses the lenses drop when the tennis player moves his eye up to hit the ball. (B) Soft lenses move with the eye and show only minimal lag; thus they are an ideal sports lens. *(From Stein HA, Slatt BJ, Stein RM, et al. Fitting guide for rigid and soft contact lenses: a practical approach. 4th ed. St Louis: Mosby; 2002.)*

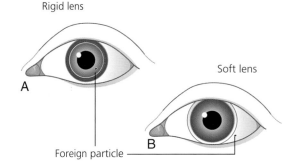

Figure 15.7 The rigid lens permits foreign particles to enter under the lens, whereas the soft lens tends to prevent the entry of foreign bodies under it by its scleral impingement and minimal movement. (A) Foreign body under RGP lens. (B) Soft lens prevents foreign bodies from getting under. *(From Stein HA, Slatt BJ, Stein RM, et al. Fitting guide for rigid and soft contact lenses: a practical approach. 4th ed. St Louis: Mosby; 2002.)*

Protection of entire cornea

Hydrophilic lenses cover the entire cornea. They can be used to reduce corneal exposure for such conditions as facial paralysis and corneal insensitivity (Figure 15.7). In this sense these lenses are used as bandage lenses for entropion, trichiasis, dry eye, and corneal dystrophies.

Attractive alternative for rigid lens drop-outs

A significant percentage of rigid lens patients are unable to persist in wearing their lenses. This intolerance may be the result of dryness as a result of pregnancy, birth control pills, allergies, or a change of environment. Most of these patients readily accept soft lenses and are able to wear them comfortably.

No serious corneal abrasion on insertion

In the rigid lens, incorrect insertion can cause an abrasion of the cornea. This does not occur with the soft lens because of its soft nature.

Cosmetic lenses

Colored and opaque hydrogel lenses to enhance or change eye color have been available since the 1980s.

DISADVANTAGES

The disadvantages of soft contact lenses are as follows:

1. Lack of ability to correct severe astigmatism
2. Variable vision
3. Lack of durability
4. Faulty duplication
5. Deposit formation
6. Modifications impossible
7. Disinfection problems

Lack of ability to correct severe astigmatism

Astigmatism is not easily corrected by conventional soft lenses. The soft lens contours to the eye and corneal astigmatism frequently remain uncorrected. There are, however, a number of special designs of toric soft lenses available to correct astigmatism of dioptric powers up to 4.00 diopters (Figure 15.8).

Variable vision

Despite good fittings, a small percentage of patients become disenchanted because of either poor or variable vision. These problems may result from fitting failures, uncorrected astigmatism, or a dehydration effect from the water-laden lenses. They may also result from deposit formation and lens spoilage.

Lack of durability

Soft lenses are much more fragile than rigid lenses and any rough handling may scratch or tear them. Even with careful handling, they may be sliced by fingernails and may develop nicks at the edges because of the constant pinching and flexing of the lenses during insertion and removal. However, they are much hardier today. The higher the water content or the thinner the lenses, the more fragile they are.

Faulty duplication

Lenses will break or tear and require replacement. Often a duplicate set may be necessary, but duplication of lenses

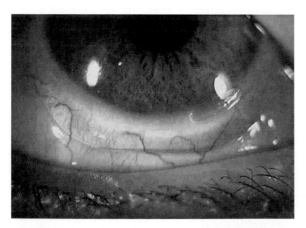

Figure 15.8 Soft toric lens used to correct astigmatism. The flat edge is kept in position by the lower eyelid. (Note: Truncation is rarely used today because of the advent of the newer astigmatic soft contact lens designs.)

(From Efron N. Contact lens practice. 2nd ed. Oxford: Elsevier/ Butterworth-Heinemann; 2010.)

today is of a high standard. Most hydrogel lenses are disposable or frequently replaced and therefore are mass produced.

Deposit formation

Protein, mineral, and lipid deposits may accumulate on the surface of a soft lens more quickly than on a rigid lens (Figure 15.9). Although special cleaning and protein-removing agents are available, strict adherence to their schedules for use is required to eliminate these build-ups

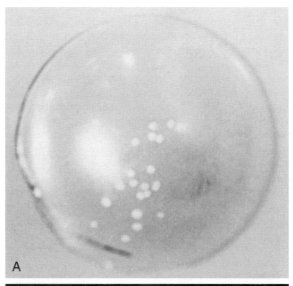

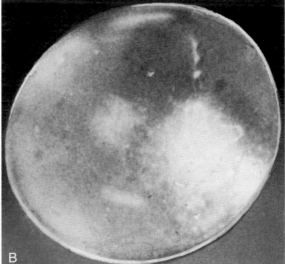

Figure 15.9 (A) Deposits on a soft lens. (B) Protein build-up on a soft lens varies with the duration of wear, the method of sterilization, and the tear composition and concentration of individual patients.

(From Stein HA, Slatt BJ, Stein RM, et al. Fitting guide for rigid and soft contact lenses: a practical approach. 4th ed. St Louis: Mosby; 2002.)

and preserve the life of the lens. New lens developments may minimize deposit adherence.

Modifications impossible

Although a soft lens can be dehydrated to the dry state, it does not form a regular shape in the dry state and accurate modifications are impractical.

Disinfection problems

The routine of disinfecting must be rigidly adhered to, otherwise infection may occur. This applies if the lenses sit in the drawer during illness or vacations, or if there is a temporary "holiday" back to glasses.

Boiling, chemical, and ultraviolet methods of disinfection have their advantages and their drawbacks. In any event, rigid adherence to disinfection procedures is important both for the practitioner who keeps an inventory and for the patient who wears the lenses only occasionally. Fungal growth and bacterial contamination of the lenses may occur because soft lenses can be penetrated more easily by infectious organisms. In addition, protein adhering to the lens surface can harbor bacterial organisms. Another source of infection is the use of stale, dated solutions. Because of the very real possibility of contamination with *Acanthamoeba*, which could result in a serious protozoan infection, tap water and even distilled water is no longer recommended for use in any way with soft contact lenses.

PATIENT EVALUATION

Each patient who visits the office for a contact lens examination requires a complete history and physical examination. History taking should include previous eye disease, recurrence of infection, systemic diseases (e.g., diabetes, neurologic disorders, ocular disorders), current medications, allergies, and general health. In addition, age, occupation, and previous contact lens experience should be recorded. The third factor to consider is the patient's motivation and capability for compliance. A history of allergies might require the patient to use nonpreserved solutions for rinsing.

External examination consists of careful inspection of the cornea, conjunctiva, and fornices. The lids should be everted to detect any underlying pathologic condition and, in particular, note should be made of papillary formation of the conjunctiva. Routine slit-lamp biomicroscopic examination is performed to detect the presence of any corneal disease or scarring. Schirmer's test should be performed to evaluate the adequacy of tear formation. The corneal sensitivity test can be administered (Figure 15.10). The palpebral fissures should be measured; the findings may alter the fitter's judgment about the diameter of the soft lens to be used. Lid

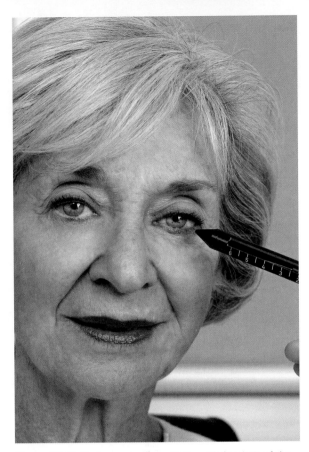

Figure 15.10 Testing corneal sensitivity with fine hair of the Cochet-Bonnet esthesiometer.

tension can be evaluated by grasping the upper lid between thumb and forefinger and holding it upward. A careful refraction should be performed, along with keratometer readings. The pupil and horizontal visible iris diameter should be measured by a ruler, a pupillometer, or a slit-lamp biomicroscope. These measurements also may affect the diameter of the lens selected.

Patient selection

Soft lenses are the lens of choice today. They are ideal for the following individuals:

1. Rigid lens drop-outs because of irritation, a bad experience with overwear, or difficulty in maintaining a rigid daily wearing schedule
2. Intermittent wearers, such as public speakers, athletes, or actors, who want to wear their lenses only occasionally
3. Workers who fear losing a lens at work (soft lenses rarely fall out)

4. Aphakic patients
5. Older adults who are impatient with the prolonged routine in following the rigid lens-wearing schedule
6. Patients with low to moderate astigmatism

The decision to dispense contact lenses to any patient is, of course, a professional judgment and should be made by a professional contact lens fitter.

MANUFACTURE

There are various methods of manufacturing soft lenses:

1. Spin casting
2. Lathe cutting with manual or automated lathes
3. Molding methods

The most common method today of manufacturing soft lenses is a combination of lathe cut and molded. Most steps today are relatively automated, quality control being performed by random sampling.

Spin-cast lenses

The spin-cast process, devised by Bausch & Lomb, produces a highly reproducible lens with a very smooth surface. This means that the lens is so standardized that all replacement lenses are duplicates of the original regardless of where in the world they are purchased. Although this is not difficult for a Coca-Cola bottle, it is a triumph for contact lens assembly.

Bausch & Lomb manufactures its Soflens by means of the spin-cast method. It is derived from a revolving mold that whirls the liquid plastic at high speed. The mold gives the lens its outside curvature. The inside curvature is formed as a result of the speed of rotation, the various surface tensions of the liquid, and the precalculated mathematic relationship between gravitation and rotation. The result is a parabola with an inside curvature that can shorten or lengthen, depending on the speed of rotation. The procedure is basically a kind of pressureless molding.

Because the posterior surface of a spin-cast lens is aspheric, the traditional K readings and the posterior surface's relationship to the base curve do not apply with these lenses. The basic fitting system is based on measurement of the horizontal visible iris diameter and selection of a suitable diameter of lens with proper power. The numeric suffix on the label denotes the lens diameter. A label ending in 4 is a 14.5-mm diameter, a 3 is a 13.5-mm diameter, and the absence of a number is a 12.5-mm diameter.

A combination of the spin-cast and lathing processes has been developed by Bausch & Lomb. This design (e.g., Optima), permits more variables in fitting while combining the high quality of the front surface for crisp optics. Other major soft contact lens manufacturers such as Alcon, CooperVision, and Vistakon have developed their own advanced proprietary manufacturing methods.

Lathe-cut lenses

In the lathe-cut manufacturing process the lens, in the dehydrated state, behaves like a rigid lens. It is cut on a lathe to exact specifications similar to those of a rigid lens. Automated lathes are in fashion and reduce labor. Initially the back surface is ground with a diamond tool and then the front surface is polished and edged. In this method, peripheral curves, blends, and even intermediate curves can be cut for better lens design. Lathed lenses are individually or custom made and a wide variety of parameters can be ground for a better fit. The most important factor in the grinding of the soft lens is that one cannot use the usual polishing compounds that contain water; thus the whole process of grinding and polishing must be performed without any contamination by water.

Lathe-cut lenses are produced for both stock and custom orders, with most using high-tech computer-controlled systems for excellent quality and reproducibility. The most important consideration in cutting soft lenses from a dry button that is later to be hydrated into a hydrogel lens is that the entire process of lathing must be performed under very strict climate control; too much humidity in the laboratory can cause variations in the finished product because the button can absorb moisture from the air. After completion of the grinding process in the hard inflexible state, the lens is placed for several hours in a water bath, where it undergoes swelling and expands to its final state. This swell factor must be taken into account in the grinding of the lens in the hard state.

When the finished lens in a dry state is hydrated for final wet inspection or quality control, the difference or swell factor is 20% to 40%, depending on the polymer material and water content. This factor makes it extremely important for the "dry state" lens to be made to exact specifications. In years past, criticisms of lathe-cut lenses included their inconsistency and that reproducibility could be suspect. Today's lathe-cut lenses, however, compare favorably in quality and reproducibility with those manufactured by any other process.

Molded lenses

The cast-molding process uses precision injection molding of engineered thermoplastic resins to produce lens replica molds. These molds are used in a monomer-casting process to convert crosslinkable lens monomers directly into a finished contact lens form. This process produces an optically finished surface from the mold, thus ensuring accurate reproduction of the lenses.

The FDA receives a constant parade of applications for approval of new lenses. With each lens comes an innovative approach to solving some of today's contact lens problems.

INVENTORY VERSUS DIAGNOSTIC LENSES

Soft lenses may be fitted in one of two ways: from an inventory of lenses, by selecting the lens that gives the best fit and the best visual acuity, or from a trial set of standard diameters and base curves to obtain the proper fit. The fitter can then overrefract to obtain the correct power of the lens and order directly. Alternatively, lenses may be ordered after the fitter makes an educated guess according to K readings, horizontal corneal diameter, and refraction, realizing that a few changes of lenses may be required before the correct lens fit is achieved.

As a result of the large diameter of soft lenses and its effect on sagittal depth, their fit must be much flatter than that of rigid lenses. The average diameter of soft lenses used today is 13.8 to 14.5 mm, requiring that they be fitted 1.0 to 1.5 mm (5.00–7.00 diopters) flatter than K. Because of the large diameter of these soft lenses, they should be fitted appreciably flatter than the flattest K reading of the cornea. Lens diameter and base curve are inversely related. To arrive at essentially the same fit, the base curve of the lens selected should be flattened as the lens diameter is increased; for example, a 12- to 13-mm diameter lens usually is fitted approximately 2.00 to 3.00 diopters flatter than K, whereas a 14- to 15-mm diameter lens has to be fitted approximately 3.00 to 5.00 diopters flatter than K.

Lens selection may be based on one of three methods:

1. Selection of soft lenses based on probable corneoscleral profiles, in which the fitter may select a lens diameter based on the horizontal iris diameter and observe how the lens performs on a given eye
2. Selection of soft lenses with a posterior curvature of radius based on K readings of the cornea, determined by actual measurement of the cornea
3. Selection of soft lenses based on the sagittal value of the lenses, which requires the K reading of the cornea and takes into account not only the posterior radius of the lens curvature but also the diameter of the lens

The fitting criteria are similar for all daily wear soft lenses. Some basic guidelines apply.

1. The hydrophilic lenses are fitted as large as or larger than the diameter of the cornea and range in size from 12 to 15 mm.
2. Small eyes require smaller diameters and consequently steeper base curves, whereas larger eyes are fitted with larger lenses and flatter base curves.
3. Soft standard-thickness lenses generally are fitted flatter than the flattest K reading, usually about 2.00 to 3.00 diopters for the smaller lenses and 3.00 to 5.00 diopters for the larger lenses. The thinner soft lenses (0.06 mm and less) are fitted 4.00 to 7.00 diopters flatter than K because they tend to drape themselves over the corneal surface (Figure 15.11).

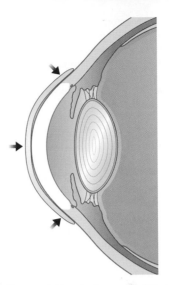

Figure 15.11 Three-point touch. A normally fitting soft lens will rest lightly at the apex and at the periphery of the cornea. *(From Stein HA, Slatt BJ, Stein RM, et al. Fitting guide for rigid and soft contact lenses: a practical approach. 4th ed. St Louis: Mosby; 2002.)*

4. A normal-fitting lens should show a 0.5- to 1-mm lag in the downward direction with each blink and provide good vision before and after blinking.
5. A soft lens that moves excessively (more than 1 mm with each blink) is too flat; a soft lens that moves less than 0.5 mm with each blink is too steep and will limit tear exchange.
6. A soft lens that decenters usually is too flat or too small (Figure 15.12). To correct this problem, a larger-diameter lens or a steeper lens should be selected.

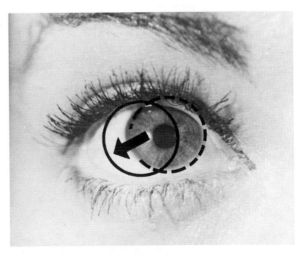

Figure 15.12 Decentration. The soft lens does not center properly; it has decentered outward.

7. The fitter may determine increased steepness or flatness from a table showing the relationship of the diameter to the radius (sagittal values) (Table 15.1). To loosen a lathe-cut lens, smaller diameters in 0.5-mm steps may be fitted or the radius increased in 0.2- to 0.3-mm steps.

8. The lower the water content of the lens, the more durable the lens becomes. The higher the water content, the more fragile is the lens.

9. The thinner the lens, the greater is the oxygen permeability to the cornea. However, a thin lens tears easily and some optical quality may be lost by wrinkling.

10. Hazy vision caused by oxygen deprivation may occur either from wearing a lens that is too tight or from overwearing the lens.

11. Contact lens decentration can be caused by tight eyelids, large corneas, against-the-rule astigmatism, or asymmetric corneal topography.

12. Routine soft lenses do not correct large amounts of corneal astigmatism. In general, astigmatism greater than 1.0 diopter requires correction by toric soft lenses or rigid lenses.

13. With soft lenses, regular fluorescein cannot be used to study tear exchange because it permeates the lens. High-molecule fluorescein can be used, but it is no more effective than evaluating tear exchange by noting the movement of the lens. Fluorescein is helpful in highlighting and assessing corneal pathologic conditions.

14. Heavier lenses usually have to be fitted larger. The lens weight is influenced by its thickness and water content. Polymers of high water content are usually weaker than those of lower water content and require lenses of greater thickness. The increased gravitational pull on a heavier lens has to be offset by use of a larger diameter.

15. The rigidity of a lens is a function of its thickness, its water content, and the unique properties of the polymer from which it is made.

16. When fitting soft lenses, the fitter should aim at fitting the flattest possible lens that will provide good clear vision, center well, and have no effect on the corneal integrity.

Table 15.1 Sagittal relationship of various base curves and diameters			
Diameter	**Radius**	**Diameter**	**Radius**
Flatter		14.0	8.1
12.0	8.7	13.0	7.2
12.0	8.1	14.5	8.4
12.5	8.7	13.5	7.5
12.0	8.4	15.0	8.7
12.5	8.4	14.0	7.8
12.5	8.1	14.5	8.1
12.5	7.8	15.0	8.4
12.0	7.8	15.5	8.7
13.0	8.7	13.5	7.2
13.0	8.4	14.0	7.5
13.5	8.7	14.5	7.8
13.0	8.1	15.0	8.1
13.5	8.4	15.5	8.4
14.0	8.7	14.0	7.2
13.0	7.8	14.5	7.5
13.5	8.1	15.0	7.8
14.0	8.4	15.5	8.1
13.0	7.5	15.0	7.5
14.5	8.7	15.5	7.8
13.5	7.8	Steeper	

LENS INSPECTION

The following routine is important for checking the quality of the lens received. For all soft lenses each factor should be assessed. Because of the manufacturing reproducibility of today's soft contact lenses, lens inspection is typically only done on specialty lenses when there is a concern of an incorrect parameter(s).

Edge and surface inspection

This should be performed with the lens under the microscope. The lens may be held in the hand or placed on a clear glass slide. It may be compared with white paper placed behind it to see whether discoloration has occurred. The lens also can be examined under a hand magnifier.

Diameter

The lens is viewed through a magnifying gauge with a millimeter scale. No pressure must be exerted on the lens to distort the surface.

Base curve

The Soft Lens Analyzer was developed to measure the base curve of hydrogel lenses. In addition, it measures diameter and center thickness and provides close surface and edge inspection on soft lenses as well as rigid lenses. Because hydrogel lenses all contain some percentage of water, accurate measurement is best obtained in the hydrated state. The Soft Lens Analyzer provides a wet cell in which the lens is immersed in saline. The lens is then measured against a series of hemispheric standards with known radii from 7.6 to 9.8 mm in 0.2-mm increments. A beam of light is projected through and around the lens positioned on the standard. This image is projected onto a small built-in screen at ×15. The operator determines the base curve in terms of the lens-bearing relationship to the standard on which it is centered. This system for measuring the base curve of a lens is applicable to all lenses.

Power

This can be determined with a fair degree of accuracy for spin-cast and lathed lenses. The lens is cleaned well and blotted dry with lint-free tissue. It is placed concave side up under a lensmeter. The measurement must be read quickly because this becomes impossible if the lens dries too much. The value of in-office inspection of a soft lens for its power before dispensing it is questionable. Sterility can be compromised and the ability to check lens quality in the practice is poor. Manufacturers use optical, ultrasound, and interferometry to verify the base curve and power of soft lenses.

The evaluation of a good fit depends on the positioning of the lens and its movement on the eye. The basic fitting philosophy is to fit the flattest, thinnest lens that will provide crisp vision before and after the blink, comfortable wear, stable positioning, and minimum metabolic interference.

A well-fitted lathe-cut lens is about 1 to 2 mm larger than the cornea, centers well, and results in a lag of 0.5 to 1 mm or slightly less on upward gaze. If the eye is moved sideways, the lens will lag slightly, but will quickly center and follow eye movements. The eye should be white and the patient able to wear the lenses comfortably all day. The lenses may, however, be too tight or too loose (Figure 15.13).

Tight lens

A tight lens is really a large, or steep, lens and does not appear to have any movement after a blink (Figure 15.14). It is uncomfortable to the wearer and may cause circumcorneal injection and indentation of the sclera adjacent to the limbus. The lens centers well, but vision is frequently blurred or fluctuating (Figure 15.15); after a blink there may be a temporary clearing that lasts a few seconds. Retinoscopy may reveal a dark shadow in the center, which may momentarily clear after a blink. Keratometry will show distortion of the mires, which clear after a blink. All these signs of a tight lens are caused by a lens that is steeper than the central cornea, which results in a gap that separates the lens from the cornea. During a blink the lid smooths the lens across the

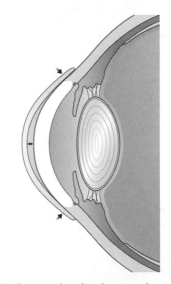

Figure 15.14 Cross-section showing steep lens.
(From Uotila M, Gassett AR. Fitting manual for Bausch & Lomb and Griffin lenses. In: Gassett AR, Kaufman HE, editors. Soft contact lens. St Louis: Mosby; 1972.)

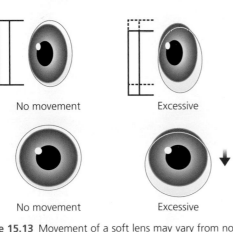

No movement   Excessive

No movement   Excessive

Figure 15.13 Movement of a soft lens may vary from none (tight) to excessive (loose).

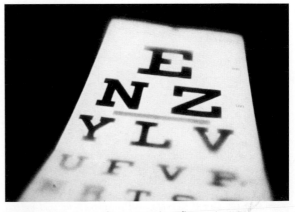

Figure 15.15 A poor fit may produce fluctuating vision.

cornea and there is a temporary central adherence of the lens to the latter. Sometimes a lens that fits well initially gradually tightens (Figure 15.16).

Symptoms and signs of a tight lens are indicated in Box 15.3 and Figure 15.17.

To correct a tight lens syndrome, the fitter must switch to a flatter lens by flattening (decreasing) the base curve or by reducing the diameter of the lens.

> **Box 15.3 Symptoms and signs of a tight lens**
>
> 1. Fluctuating vision that clears immediately after blinking
> 2. Initial comfort that changes to increasing discomfort as the day progresses
> 3. Corneal injection or redness around the circumference of the cornea (see Figure 15.16A and B)
> 4. Corneal indentation; compression of the conjunctiva at the limbus and a dish-like depression that obstructs the normal flow of vessels
> 5. Absent or minimal movement after blinking (see Figure 15.17)
> 6. Keratometry results in which mires that are distorted before a blink clear after it
> 7. Retinoscopic reflex, which is fuzzy at first and clears momentarily

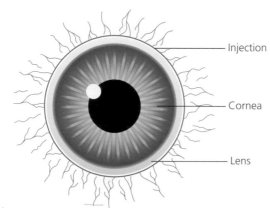

Injection

Cornea

Lens

A

Circumcorneal injection

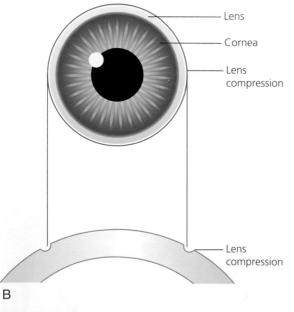

Lens

Cornea

Lens compression

Lens compression

B

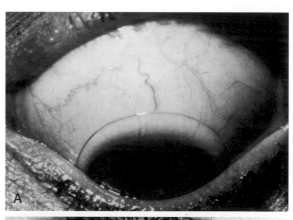

A

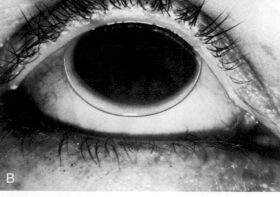

B

Figure 15.16 (A) Circumcorneal injection. Note the considerable vascularity at the limbus. (B) Circumcorneal indentation. The tight lens compresses the peripheral limbal tissues.

(From Stein HA, Slatt BJ, Stein RM, et al. Fitting guide for rigid and soft contact lenses: a practical approach. 4th ed. St Louis: Mosby; 2002.)

Figure 15.17 (A) Slightly tight lens as indicated by minimal movement up on downward gaze. (B) Tight soft lens. Note the lack of lag on upward gaze and indentation in perilimbal area.

(From Stein HA, Slatt BJ, Stein RM, et al. Fitting guide for rigid and soft contact lenses: a practical approach. 4th ed. St Louis: Mosby; 2002.)

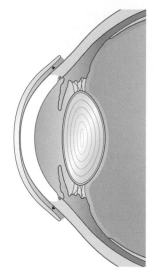

Figure 15.18 Cross-section showing flat lens.

(From Uotila M, Gassett AR. Fitting manual for Bausch & Lomb and Griffin lenses. In: Gassett AR, Kaufman HE, editors. Soft contact lens. St Louis: Mosby; 1972.)

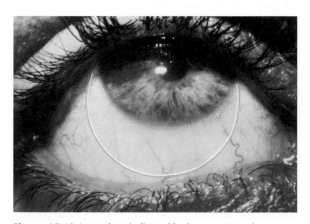

Figure 15.19 Loose lens indicated by lag on upward gaze.

(From Stein HA, Slatt BJ, Stein RM, et al. Fitting guide for rigid and soft contact lenses: a practical approach. 4th ed. St Louis: Mosby; 2002.)

Loose lens

A loose lens is a small, or flat, lens that exhibits excessive movement, lags 2 to 4 mm on downward excursion, and, if extremely loose, may slide off the cornea entirely on lateral gaze (Figure 15.18). A loose lens centers poorly and gives poor, unstable vision. Vision may be good initially, but may decrease two or three lines after each blink, although it may recover rapidly (Figures 15.19 and 15.20). Keratometer readings may show slight distortion of the mires that is increased after each blink. With a loose lens, the edge may roll out and become dehydrated and may fall out of the eye on a blink (Figure 15.21).

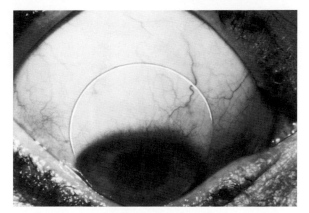

Figure 15.20 Loose lens. On downward gaze the lens rides high. A valuable test to confirm the fitting of a soft lens.

(From Stein HA, Slatt BJ, Stein RM, et al. Fitting guide for rigid and soft contact lenses: a practical approach. 4th ed. St Louis: Mosby; 2002.)

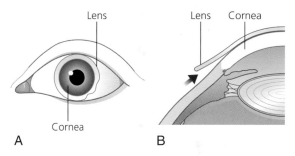

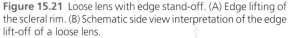

Figure 15.21 Loose lens with edge stand-off. (A) Edge lifting of the scleral rim. (B) Schematic side view interpretation of the edge lift-off of a loose lens.

(From Stein HA, Slatt BJ, Stein RM, et al. Fitting guide for rigid and soft contact lenses: a practical approach. 4th ed. St Louis: Mosby; 2002.)

The signs and symptoms of a loose lens are listed in Box 15.4.

To correct a loose lens, one must switch to a lens that is steeper either by steepening the base curve or by increasing the diameter of the lens.

DISINFECTION

Disinfection of both spin-cast and lathe-cut soft lenses has been tested and found reliable. The major concern is that germs can enter the plastic of the lens and contaminate it. The molecular openings of the hydrogel plastic are so tiny that bacteria and fungus spores cannot invade it. The only ways that bacteria can contaminate an intact lens are by multiplying on its surface or if the surface of the lens is broken. This is more likely to occur if bacteria are present.

1. Variable vision, clear before blink, not clear on blink
2. Excess awareness of lens
3. Poor centering
4. Excess movement (see Figures 15.19 and 15.20)
5. Edge stand-off (see Figure 15.21A)
6. Lens falling out (see Figure 15.21B)
7. Bubble under a lens
8. Keratometry findings that show clear mires that blur after blinking
9. Retinoscopy results that are clear at first and blur after blinking

There are essentially three methods for disinfecting hydrophilic lenses: heat, chemical (including multipurpose solutions and hydrogen peroxide systems), and ultraviolet exposure. Chemical systems are used for lens disinfection by the majority of wearers.

The heat, or thermal, method consists of two steps:

1. The lenses are stored in normal saline solution in the patient's lens case.
2. The lenses are boiled daily in a specially designed automatic shut-off unit. Tests have shown that no actively growing pathogens survive this treatment at a temperature of 82°C (180°F).

Several methods of chemical disinfection are available. These are based on chlorhexidine, quaternary ammonium compound, sorbate, Polyquad, Dymed, and other disinfecting agents as preservatives. Thimerosal was once used but it causes sensitivity.

Boiling routines are a little cumbersome but effective. The only drawback to boiling is that the mucus and protein debris, if not cleaned from the lens beforehand, become coagulated and baked onto the surface of the soft lens. Also, most medium- and high-water lenses cannot be boiled. The lens replacement rate is higher with the thermal method than with the chemical method of disinfection. With chemical disinfection, the germicide rapidly passes into the lens, cleans it, and disinfects it. The lens must be carefully rinsed; if not, it is irritating. Also, some individuals may be sensitive to the chemicals or preservatives in the solution. Thimerosal is a common offender.

The AOSept system, as well as Clear Care system by Alcon, and Peroxi clear adopted by Bausch & Lomb are unique in that they use a saline that contains 3% hydrogen peroxide as a disinfecting solution, combined with a specially treated disc that is in the case at the same time to effect neutralization for a 6-hour period. The Sauflon Company (UK) markets a one-step hydrogen peroxide disinfecting solution that includes a nonionic surfactant cleaner.

Of concern has been the devastating parasite *Acanthamoeba*. It can cause severe keratitis, with pain and ring infiltrates into the cornea. The cyst form is killed primarily by heat, but is resistant to chemical disinfection. Water samples taken in Great Britain from roof cisterns indicated the presence of *Acanthamoeba*. It is recommended that wearers use only commercially available lens care solutions and adhere to the manufacturers' recommended procedures.

CLEANING

Protein is a natural component of human tears. Over time this protein, or mucin, secreted by the glands of the eyelid and found in the tears, tends to stick to the surface of the soft lens and coat it. These deposits are often not noticed until they become thick and vision becomes blurred or the lens becomes slightly irritating. These deposits develop rapidly in some people, whereas others may never have a problem. They can interfere with the action of antibacterial agents in soaking solutions.

Lenses also may become filmed from dirty fingers, hair spray, or smoke. Cleaning is an important part of lens care. Because cleaning can result in the removal of microorganisms, it aids in the disinfection of contact lenses. Theory dictates that the lower the concentration of microorganisms on a lens, the less challenge there will be to the disinfectant, making the disinfection step as effective as possible.

Several prophylactic cleaners for daily care of hydrophilic contact lenses are on the market. They contain various salts at physiologic concentration, preservatives to maintain control of microorganisms, and long-chain nonionic detergents. These surface-acting (surfactant) detergents provide cleaning efficacy. Manufacturers claim that they remove mucoproteins, lipid deposits, and other forms of debris from the contact lens before the lenses are disinfected. These cleaners are not 100% effective, however, and eventually most soft lenses require replacement.

The hands should be washed carefully; special soaps for contact lens wearers are preferred because many commercial soaps contain moisturizers such as lanolin, which may be transferred to the lens surface. The hands are then dried with a clean, lint-free towel before removing the lens. The lens is rubbed on both sides on the palm of the hand with a clean finger, using the lens cleaner, for at least 20 seconds. This lens care step is sometimes referred to as "digital cleaning."

Enzyme cleaners are intended for removal of protein deposits, which accumulate over time and which are resistant to prophylactic cleaning regimens. The enzyme works differently from a detergent: it is capable of breaking down proteinaceous deposits, whereas detergent can remove only loosely deposited matter on the surface. After the lens is cleaned and rinsed with saline solution, it is soaked in the enzyme solution for a minimum of 15 minutes or overnight. Exceptions are the high-water lenses, in which the soaking time may be minimized to prevent enzyme retention by the lens. Then the lens is rubbed and rinsed with freshly prepared saline solution and disinfected before wearing. This procedure should be undertaken at least twice monthly for the soft lenses and even every week if the lenses easily become coated. Current premixed enzyme solutions are added to the nightly disinfecting regime and rinsed off before insertion.

Surfactant cleaning after lens wearing increases the surface clarity and reduces the rate of solution reaction. Dirty lenses are more likely to bind high concentrations of preservative to their surface, thus creating a toxic keratitis or conjunctivitis that results in red eyes. Most patients' lenses are somewhat filmed and dehydrated after a normal day of wear and this makes it more difficult to clean the lenses properly in the evening.

Hydrogen peroxide systems are the most stringent cleaning systems. It is advisable to refer to the manufacturer for details concerning each of the specific products. The standard of hydrogen peroxide systems is ophthalmic-grade hydrogen peroxide 3% to be used after surfactant cleaning. The recommended time for disinfection is a minimum of 20 minutes. Many suggest overnight storage before neutralization of the hydrogen peroxide by means of a catalyst such as sodium pyruvate or catalase. The catalyst can be in the form of a saline storage step, that is, a saline-containing neutralizer into which the lenses are placed after hydrogen peroxide disinfection, or a sodium-catalyst tablet placed directly into the hydrogen peroxide to convert it into saline.

Contact lens care companies have introduced multipurpose, one-step lens-care systems also referred to as MPS. These systems are meant to be "all in one," in which they clean, disinfect, and store the soft contact lenses.

Cleaning routines are part of a preventive maintenance program to ensure longer, more comfortable lens wear as well as longer lens life. The section on disposable lenses discusses at length how regular replacement of soft lenses can be practical and effective. Soft lenses nowadays are replaced daily, every 2 weeks, and monthly so protein build-up is no longer a big problem.

INSERTION AND REMOVAL TECHNIQUES

The insertion and removal of soft contact lenses are different from the techniques used for conventional lenses. The soft lens is inserted on the lower part of the sclera and gently pushed onto the cornea with the lower eyelid. To remove soft contact lenses, it is generally recommended to first slide the lens down with the index finger to the lower sclera and then to pinch off the lens. Before removal the lens should be checked to ensure that there is no adherence to the cornea. A comfort drop (lubricating drop) placed before removal can be an aid.

Older adult patients may have difficulty placing, removing, and handling contact lenses. Normally if this problem cannot be overcome by in-office training, the patient should not receive the lens. In some cases, however, another person might be taught to place, remove, and handle the lenses for the patient. The same is true with children who are being fitted with hydrophilic contact lenses. Insertion devices are available for the soft lens, but they should not be used unless manual attempts have failed.

Insertion by the fitter

The following technique is used for lens insertion by the fitter:

1. Keep nails short at all times.
2. Wash hands and rinse thoroughly to remove all traces of soap. Dry with a lint-free towel. Avoid using oils and creams on your hands before handling the lens.
3. Remove the right lens from the vial or case and place in the eye.
4. Place the lens on the tip of the index finger, concave side up. Have the patient look straight ahead. Retract the lower lid with your middle finger (Figure 15.22).

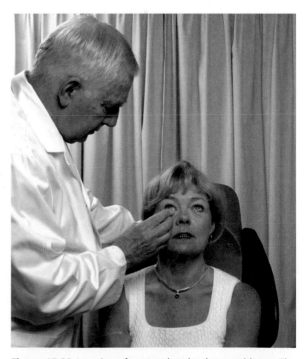

Figure 15.22 Insertion of contact lens by the practitioner. The middle finger retracts the lower lid while the contact lens is gently rolled into the lower conjunctiva.

5. Have the patient look down and slightly nasal. Apply the lens on the sclera. Lift your finger and ask the patient to gaze upward and then look straight. Swirling the lens on the sclera also helps to make it comfortable by introducing tears into the lens and making it isotonic with the tears.

6. Have the patient close the eyes and lightly massage the lid to help center the lens.

7. Repeat the same procedure for the left lens.

Removal by the fitter

The following technique is used for lens removal by the fitter:

1. Wash the hands before removal, as was done for insertion.

2. Be sure the lens is on the cornea and freely moving before attempting removal.

3. Have the patient look up. Place the middle finger on the lower lid and touch the edge of the lens with the forefinger.

4. While the patient is looking up, slide the lens down onto the white of the eye. Bring the thumb over and compress the lens lightly between the thumb and index finger so that the lens folds and comes off easily.

Insertion by the patient

Careful patient instruction in the care and handling of soft contact lenses is frequently left to the ophthalmic assistant. It is important that the patient understand the procedure and care system and comply with it. Failure to comply with instruction is the greatest single cause of difficulties with well-fitted soft contact lenses.

The following technique is used for lens insertion by the patient. For beginners, a large mirror is helpful (Figure 15.23):

1. Keep the nails short and carefully wash and dry the hands.

2. Take the right lens out of the vial either with forceps or by pouring the contents of the vial into the palm of the hand.

3. Rinse the lens with normal saline solution.

4. Place the lens on the tip of the index finger of the dominant hand. With thin lenses, permit the lens to dehydrate for 1 to 2 minutes in air and dry finger.

5. Look at the mirror, retract the lower eyelid with the middle finger, apply the lens on the eyeball.

6. Express any air, remove the index finger, and then slowly release the lower lid.

7. Close the eyes and gently massage the lids to help center the lens (Figure 15.24).

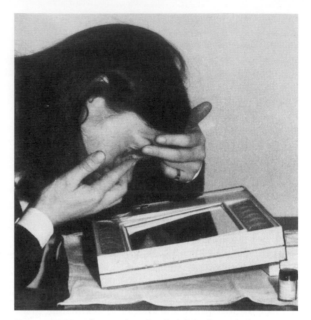

Figure 15.23 A large mirror is a helpful adjunct in inserting a lens.
(From Stein HA, Slatt BJ, Stein RM, et al. Fitting guide for rigid and soft contact lenses: a practical approach. 4th ed. St Louis: Mosby; 2002.)

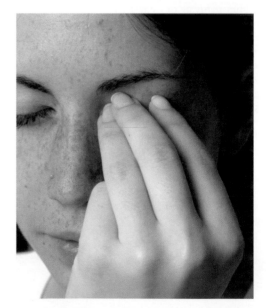

Figure 15.24 Centering the lens through the closed eyelid.

Removal by the patient

The following technique is used for lens removal by the patient:

1. Check vision in each eye separately to be sure the lens is in place on the cornea.

2. Wash hands and rinse thoroughly.
3. Look upward. Retract the lower lid with the middle finger and place the index fingertip on the lower edge of the lens.
4. Slide the lens down to the white of the eye.
5. Compress the lens between the thumb and index finger so that air breaks the suction under the lens. Remove the lens from the eye.
6. Prepare the lens for cleaning and sterilizing according to the recommendations of the manufacturer and the practitioner.
7. An alternative method of removal is to look nasally and slide the lens to the outermost portion of the eye before removal.

TACO TEST

If there is any question of whether the lens is inside out, the "taco test" should be performed (Figure 15.25). In this test the lens is flexed between the forefinger and thumb. If the edges are erect and point inward like a taco, the lens is in the correct position. If the edge appears to fold back in the fingers, the lens is everted and must be reversed. For new ultrathin lenses the taco test may not be valid, however.

PRECAUTIONS FOR WEAR

1. Do not insert lenses if eyes are red or irritated.
2. Do not use tap water, distilled water, or spring water directly in the eye; always use commercially manufactured saline solution.
3. Do not use any solutions with contact lenses other than those specifically recommended.

4. If the lens becomes uncomfortable when first inserted or while wearing, or if vision becomes blurred, foreign material may be present on the inside surface of the lens. The lens should be immediately removed, cleaned, rinsed, and reinserted.
5. Lenses should not be worn in the presence of irritating fumes or vapors.
6. Lenses should not be worn overnight unless specifically advised.
7. If the lens is difficult to remove or difficult to slide down, place a comfort drop (lubricating drop) or two on the eye or a few drops of commercially manufactured normal saline solution. The lens should soon once again move freely and be easily removable.
8. If vision is blurred while wearing the lens, consider the possibility that the lens may be inside out, off center, or not clean, or that the right and left lenses have been switched.
9. If the lens is left exposed to air, it will dry out and become hard and brittle. Should this occur, handle it gently and place it in saline solution and it will again become soft and flexible.
10. If hair spray is used, it should be applied before lens insertion.
11. There are special glasses available for makeup application and removal for the presbyope (Figure 15.26).

WEARING SCHEDULES

Because soft lenses are much more comfortable than rigid lenses, the wearer may be inclined to overwear them beyond corneal tolerance during the first few days. The manufacturers' routine wearing schedules are usually conservative in build-up, but are designed to give maximum protection with minimum risk of corneal edema in the early stages while the eye builds up tolerance to the soft lens.

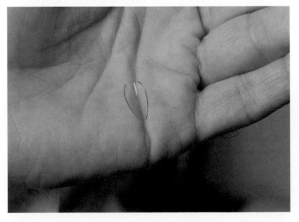

Figure 15.25 Taco test to determine correct side of the lens.

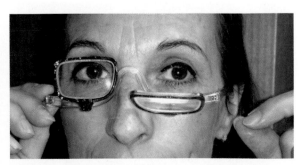

Figure 15.26 Glasses for makeup application and removal.

The difficulty in permitting overnight wear with standard lenses is that blinking does not occur and consequently there is tear stagnation between the soft lens and the cornea, thus not allowing oxygen exchange, with subsequent hypoxia to the cornea. For many people this may result in serious corneal edema in the morning.

Lenses designed for extended wear are discussed in detail later in this chapter.

THIN AND ULTRATHIN LENSES

A major technologic change in soft lens manufacture has been the development of the thin and ultrathin soft lenses, with the central thickness on both measuring less than 0.1 mm and even as little as 0.02 mm. The advantages and disadvantages of these thinner soft lenses are outlined in Box 15.5.

The importance of thin and ultrathin lenses is that they provide exceptional initial comfort. Also, being thin, these lenses allow some diffusion of oxygen and minimize corneal edema formation from hypoxia. Because of their oxygen permeability characteristics, these lenses may be fitted slightly tighter than regular soft lenses and consequently produce more stable vision; thus they are useful for sporting activities. They also appear to reduce the incidence of giant papillary conjunctivitis.

A disadvantage of thin and ultrathin lenses is that they are harder to handle and require more patience on the part of both the fitter and the patient in instruction. Such lenses also have an exaggerated dehydration effect in dry environments. They may damage more easily. In addition, inconsistent vision results from lens dehydration. They may also give a poor quality of vision.

CORRECTION OF ASTIGMATISM

Most failures in soft lens wear occur because the lenses do not adequately correct astigmatism; as a result, vision is poor. The soft lens conforms to the shape of the eye and only about 1.00 to 1.50 diopters of astigmatism can be ignored. This low amount of astigmatism is what is usually found in most lens wearers. However, a number of patients with astigmatism greater than 1.50 diopters can be fitted with soft toric lenses. Many of the toric soft contact lens designs allow for astigmatic correction as low as 0.75 diopter.

Toric lens design

To correct astigmatism, a toric or spherocylindric lens is used (Figure 15.27). The lens must be stabilized so that it does not rotate on the eye. To accomplish this, the cylinder is ground on either the front or the back surface. Current methods available to prevent rotation are:

- Prism ballast lenses
- Truncation
- A combination of prism ballast lenses and truncation
- Double slab-off or thin-zone lenses
- Aspherical back surface
- Posterior toric surface lenses
- Bioflange (thick interior edge)
- Combinations of any of these

Once lens rotation has been stabilized and compensated for, the lens can be constructed with the cylinder incorporated along a given axis, but the lens maintains a fixed axis position. The ability to hold its position is critical to good vision at higher amounts of astigmatism.

Toric lenses have orientation marks on the periphery for positioning purposes. The marks are etched at either 6 o'clock or 3 and 9 o'clock.

Prism ballast

Just as in a rigid lens, a prism can be incorporated into the lens so that the thicker, heavier edge orients to the inferior aspect of the eye (Figure 15.28). A front or back surface toric lens can then be ground in the proper axis to compensate for the astigmatism. These lenses should be fitted

---

Box 15.5 Advantages and disadvantages of thin soft lenses

Advantages	Disadvantages
Initial comfort and adaptation	More easily damaged
Decreased incidence of overwear	More difficult to manufacture; thus quality control may not be as precise
Alternative for highly sensitive people	More difficult to handle
Reduced risk of corneal warpage	Inconsistent vision resulting from possible dehydration
	Tearing easily

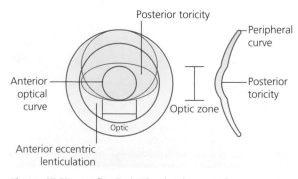

Figure 15.27 Keraflex Toric/Blanchard contact lens.

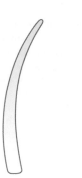

Figure 15.28 Prism ballast to provide weight and stop rotation of a lens.
(From Stein HA, Slatt BJ, Stein RM, et al. Fitting guide for rigid and soft contact lenses: a practical approach. 4th ed. St Louis: Mosby; 2002.)

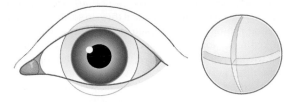

Figure 15.29 Double slab-off soft lens used to correct astigmatism. The lens is made thinner superiorly and inferiorly so that the thinner portions tend to rotate and come to rest under the upper and lower eyelids.
(From Stein HA, Slatt BJ, Stein RM, et al. Fitting guide for rigid and soft contact lenses: a practical approach. 4th ed. St Louis: Mosby; 2002.)

accurately so that they rotate to the final resting position and the cylinder is not misaligned.

These lenses depend entirely on adequate movement and rotation. The eyelids influence the final position of the lens. Tight lids have a considerable influence on rotation of the soft lens and are difficult to fit with an astigmatic soft lens. The position of the lower lid has a stabilizing influence and lenses must be fitted larger for those with wider palpebral fissures.

Truncation

By cutting off a lower segment of the lens, its rotation is stopped by allowing it to lie along the bottom lid for stability. Consequently the lens can have a toric or cylinder portion ground on its anterior surface. Truncation is useful when combined with prism ballast lenses because it eliminates the heavy, thick edge of the prism that lies below. However, few lens designs use truncation as a design parameter for stabilizing lens orientation.

Truncation and prism ballast

Several forms take advantage of both truncation and prism ballast. The lower portion is truncated by 0.75 to 1.5 mm to eliminate the excess weight, the prism ballast. Lid configuration affects the final position of the inferior truncations. The truncated edge must be beveled; otherwise, the lens could cause corneal abrasions. Truncation is no longer commonly used for soft lenses.

Double slab-off

In this method of correcting astigmatism, the superior and inferior portions of the lens are "slabbed off" from the anterior surface, resulting in a lens that is thinner at the top and bottom, but thicker in the exposed portion of the lens (Figure 15.29). The lens rotates so that the thinner portions lie under the upper and lower eyelids. The lids tend to hold the lens in the proper position and a toric front surface can be ground on the lens to correct the astigmatic portion.

Configuration of the eyelid, blinking reflexes, and tension of the eyelids have an effect on the final rotation of the lens. Thus each patient must have a trial fitting with a set of trial lenses, with markings that identify the position of the soft lens at all times. By using a soft lens as a diagnostic lens, the practitioner can incorporate correcting values to arrive at the final lens for incorporation of the cylindric power and axis.

MEDICAL USES

A revolution has occurred in the treatment of corneal diseases by judicious use of soft contact lenses. A large number of patients who could not previously be helped can now use the soft contact lens, which can act as a bandage. It is not a panacea for all diseases but, if well fitted and used wisely with well-selected patients, contact lenses can be of inestimable value to promote healing and epithelial regeneration.

The soft lens acts by delicately covering the cornea and thereby protecting it. Its water-absorbing qualities keep the surface of the cornea moist and well lubricated under the agreeable protective shell. Soft lenses best used as a bandage are those that are extremely thin or those that have a high water content.

Bandage lenses can be used in a variety of medical and surgical situations. These include (1) corneal dystrophies (e.g., bullous keratopathy), (2) corneal erosions (e.g., dry eye, trichiasis, entropion), and (3) after surgery (e.g., corneal graft, and postlaser photorefractive keratotomy [PRK]).

Blisters of cornea (bullous keratopathy)

Bullous keratopathy in its late stages is characterized by blind and excruciatingly painful eyes. In this condition the cornea becomes swollen and the superficial layer of the epithelium is raised into convex mounds. Some of these corneal blisters rupture and, when they do so, there is a raw, burning feeling and often pain in the eyes, along with a marked reduction in visual acuity. The attendant scarring and irregularity of the cornea that follow the rupture of these blisters can, on a cumulative basis, cause permanent loss of vision. This condition is brought on not by lack of oxygen to the epithelium but by damage to the inside layer of the cornea, the endothelium, so that aqueous humor from the anterior chamber can percolate through the cornea.

The introduction of the soft therapeutic contact lens and its popularization by Dr. Herbert E. Kaufman revolutionized the treatment of the disease. A bandage lens is a safe, simple, nonsurgical method of relieving both the pain and the profound visual loss. It can be inserted in the office rather than an operating room. Its application does not require sophisticated surgical expertise and can therefore be performed by virtually every ophthalmologist or ophthalmic technician in any part of the world. Numerous reports in the ophthalmologic literature confirm that these lenses are well tolerated and can be worn continuously for prolonged periods on diseased corneas without adverse effects. In each case the patient is comfortable and may experience improvement in vision as long as the lenses remain in place. For terribly scarred corneas, the only improvement is freedom from pain. Some patients become so frightened of possible reactivation of discomfort that they wear their soft contact lenses 24 hours a day for months without removal.

Fitting of the soft lens for bullous keratopathy is more challenging than fitting for refractive errors. A trial lens may be used. In many cases it may be possible to use an inexpensive soft lens. A properly fitted lens has both central and peripheral contact so that it does not flex in the center with each blink. It may be necessary to fit the lens with minimal or no movement. Extra movement is painful because it erodes tissue under the lens. Because patients with bullous keratopathy wear soft lenses continuously, 24 hours per day, dehydration of the lenses is a concern. Daily lubricating drops are advised. Regular (monthly) replacement gives the best results and keeps the lens comfortable.

For aphakia one can use a planolens to achieve the corneal change; once the cornea improves, however, the refractive power needs to be considered. In some cases it is necessary to use medication, such as hypertonic saline 5%, along with the lens.

Corneal ulcers

An ulcer is a large defect in the tissues and its appearance on the cornea is viewed with alarm. If a corneal ulcer increases in size and grows deep, it can cause perforation of the cornea and a loss of the structures inside the eye, which can herniate through the defect. This usually means loss of the eye. The likelihood of such a contingency is quite real.

Pressure within the eye itself can cause a perforation if there is a weakness of the coats of the eye, such as a thinning of the cornea or sclera. Furthermore, because the cornea is devoid of any blood vessels (a factor that aids in its transparency but prevents the successful mobilization of the body's resources to a damaged site), it is an extremely vulnerable organ. The cases in which soft lenses have been tried have been those in which antibiotics and pressure dressings have failed and the surgeon has had to perform corneal transplantation. The major cause of infection and corneal ulcers is poor hygiene. Dirty hands, nails, and contact lens cases are often most responsible. Contaminated distilled water is also a common cause.

Recurrent corneal erosion

Many people have had a piece of grit fly into the eye and have required professional help to remove it. Once the eye is patched for 24 hours, the cornea repairs itself and the mishap is forgotten, relegated to the domain of unpleasant minor memories. If, however, the eye is injured by anything organic, such as a fingernail, the cornea may heal but break down again weeks or months later.

The entire sequence of the initial accident is relived and the person suffers pain, sensitivity to light, watering eyes, redness of the eye, and marked blurring of vision. The event may seem unreal because there is no antecedent injury the second or third time. Soft lenses may prevent this recurrent breakdown.

Dry eyes

The primary disturbance in keratitis sicca is a result of a gross deficiency of tears, which parches the cornea and causes dryness of its surface so that it develops pits and erosions. Patients with dry eyes complain of a terrible burning sensation that is much worse when indoors. They are constant visitors to drugstores and will buy anything that comes out of a dropper, provided it is wet.

Again, the mechanism by which soft lenses achieve these clinical results is not clear. They do act as a protective bandage and their tendency to retain water probably accounts for their successful lubricant value. In patients affected with this condition, improvement in their general corneal status gives symptomatic relief and improves their vision, in some instances in a spectacular fashion. These lenses are often effective if used in conjunction with artificial tears and local antibiotics that do not contain preservatives. In some cases, however, soft lenses fail to be of help.

Contact lens wearers as well as laser-assisted in situ keratomileusis (LASIK) patients experience dry eye syndrome. In addition, there are many dry eye conditions such as Sjögren's syndrome that can contribute to this dry eye feeling. Anywhere from 15% to 25% of the average population has dry eyes. A Japanese study pointed out that 82% of contact lens wearers had dry eyes. In late stages of dry eyes, the cornea often becomes desiccated and ulcerated and eventually scar formation occurs. Symptoms of dry eyes are listed in Box 15.6.

Medical specialist situations that can lead to dry eyes include:

- Keratoconjunctivitis sicca or Sjögren's syndrome
- Thyroid
- Chemical burns
- Post-LASIK

In the contact lens wearer there is often blurred vision as a result of lens dehydration. The thinner the lens, the more the dehydration occurs. After LASIK, dry eyes can occur in 80% because of the severance of the corneal nerves at the limbus and by the compression of the microkeratome.

The function of the tear film is to hydrate and protect the ocular surface:

- Reduce friction on blinking
- Enhance oxygen to the cornea
- Remove waste and cellular debris
- Protect against infection

A dry eye workup consists of:

- A history
- Schirmer's test
- BUT (break-up time of tears)
- Tear meniscus height
- Rose bengal test for staining of the conjunctiva
- Evidence of lag ophthalmos

The more sophisticated tests such as the lactopheron test and tear osmolarity are rarely used in clinical practice.

The management of dry eyes consists essentially of:

- Copious drops
- Humidifier in bedroom and at work
- Flaxseed or fish oil capsules 1000 mg, two to four times daily
- Swim goggles
- Bedtime patching
- Punctal plugs

Many artificial tears are available for use. If one is using them in any copious amount, the ones that are preservative free are better. Punctal plugs are easily inserted.

There are numerous types available on a temporary or a permanent basis.

Two developments are of interest. Cyclosporine (also, ciclosporin) drops in dilute 0.05% solution (Restasis) correct the inflammatory process that occurs on the conjunctiva and that may give rise to a blockage of the reflux from the conjunctiva to the brain and to the lacrimal gland. Testosterone 3% has also been used in a transdermal patch.

Hormones are said to increase meibomian secretions. Lid hygiene is important and there are surfactant gels that can be applied to reduce the inflammation around the meibomian glands. Of benefit has been the development of a goggle-style sunglass, the Panoptx/7-Eye Orbital Seal, which seals to the skin and protects the eye (Figure 15.30).

Omega-3 fatty acids are a class of essential polyunsaturated fatty acids, the best sources of which are fish oil (from salmon, sardines, and other oily fish) as well as flaxseed, walnut, and canola oils. Eighty-three percent of the population is deficient in omega-3 fatty acids, which have a multitude of other health benefits as well as improving meibomian secretion and retention of tears. The meibomian gland secretions are augmented by the essential fatty acids to produce an oil layer of the tear film and prevent evaporation of tears. We have patients obtain 1000 mg capsules and use 2 to 4 per day.

In addition, there are pilocarpine-type drops such as Salagen that can be taken in pill form to stimulate the lacrimal gland secretions.

Self-medication is a plight of the dry eye patient. Numerous over-the-counter drops, such as vascular astringents, improve the eye's whiteness. At least 20% to 40% of the population use nonadvised medications on their own. The contact lens practitioner should encourage the right choice of tear products. The best are those with minimal toxic preservatives or those that are preservative-free. There are a host of preservative-free tear substitutes that are probably kinder to the cornea. Some come in small individual dispensers for use once or twice during the day. Others are available in 5-mL bottles (e.g., TheraTears and GenTeal).

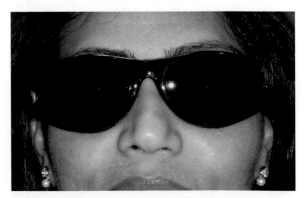

Figure 15.30 Panoptic glasses for dry eye syndrome. Frames cover the periphery of the eyes.

Conclusion

Soft lenses have added a new dimension to the treatment of severe external ocular diseases. They act basically as a protective cover for the cornea, shielding it from irritants and allowing it to rest, much in the same way as a cast permits a broken leg to mend. With the introduction of extremely thin lenses, lenses of high water content, and silicone hydrogel lenses, their potential use has been expanded.

In looking to the future, soft contact lenses may become even more important as current research in the field comes to fruition. Research is under way to determine the use of contact lenses for drug delivery. This field of research is advancing rapidly and there are numerous ocular (and possibly even systemic) drugs that could be administered via this new route. Advantages over drug application via eye drops are many. Another interesting area of research involves development of nanotechnology devices placed into the contact lens to monitor intraocular pressure (IOP) changes continuously. Medical management of glaucoma could then be administered very specifically, possibly using the contact lens itself. It will be interesting to see where this research leads.

EXTENDED-WEAR LENSES

Extended-wear lenses are worn for longer than 16 hours or more (typically overnight). The manufacturing technology has advanced to produce thinner and thinner soft lenses that provide more comfort and more oxygen under the lens. In addition, lenses can be made with a high water content, which also provides more oxygen to the underlying cornea. It has been clearly shown that if the thickness of a soft lens is halved, its oxygen transmission is doubled.

A second factor that has resulted in the availability of extended-wear lenses has been the ability to polymerize soft lens materials and manufacture lenses that absorb more water in their substance. For every 10% increase in water absorption of these materials, there is a corresponding 50% increase in oxygen transmission, so that if water content increases by 20%, the oxygen transmission doubles. Hydrophilic lenses that retain up to 90% water have been developed. Polymer chemists working in this specialized area have developed materials that have satisfactory tensile strength and are durable.

A third thrust has been the development of new fluorosilicone hydrogel materials for soft contact lens manufacture. These silicone-based soft lenses are the newest on the market, with DK values of more than 100. Some of the soft contact lenses manufactured from these new materials have been approved by the FDA for extended wear up to 30 days. As a result, a term has been coined for such long-term extended wear: "continuous wear."

Myopic versus aphakic extended wear

Extended wear for myopia is a completely different problem from extended wear for aphakia. The myopic person is usually younger, with healthier corneas and better tear production, and is usually more capable of learning the insertion, removal, and care techniques for the lenses. In addition, having myopia aids an individual in seeing lenses for insertion, as well as in following care routines. The aphakic person, on the other hand, is usually older, has poor hand coordination, poor tear production and a tendency to form increased lens deposits and is usually less mobile for return visits to the office or clinic. In addition, the aphakic lens is considerably thicker so as to achieve suitable power in the center of the lens, and this impairs some of the oxygen transmission qualities of the lens. The inability of aphakic individuals to accommodate or visualize the lens on their finger makes insertion and removal very difficult.

Problems with conventional extended-wear lenses

Studies suggest that previously available conventional extended-wear soft contact lens did not provide adequate oxygen transmission for continued normal aerobic corneal epithelial metabolism. As a result, in conventional extended-wear soft contact lens patients, one sometimes sees epithelial microcysts and changes in the appearance of the endothelium (morphometric changes). The long-term significance of these effects is unknown, and further research into the effects of extended-wear soft contact lenses is warranted. Any of the following findings is cause for immediate concern:

1. Acute hypoxic episodes
2. Microcysts of the epithelium
3. Giant papillary conjunctivitis (GPC)
4. Neovascularization
5. Striate lines
6. Infiltrative keratitis
7. Superficial punctate keratitis.

Any of the these findings should immediately lead the practitioner to discontinue the patient's extended-wear routine and change the patient to daily wear, something that can be done without refitting or dispensing new lenses. Also one can consider silicone hydrogel lenses, the new 30-day lenses (see the following text), for extended wear.

The patient is under some risk unless the fitter is prepared to provide careful monitoring. In addition, there are medicolegal implications for incorrect monitoring if serious problems arise. The most troublesome problem has been deposit formation and coating of the lenses. This not only interferes with vision but also increases the mass and alters the parameter of the lens and reduces its oxygen transmission, with attendant risks of corneal hypoxia. Deposits also add an immunoglobulin factor that may result in GPC and a red eye. Careful cleaning on a regular basis is an important factor in the satisfactory use of extended-wear lenses. With the current anxiety concerning acquired immunodeficiency syndrome (AIDS) in tears, hydrogen peroxide is an effective cleansing and disinfecting system. Apparently there also have been outbreaks of acanthamoebic infections. In this situation, thermal disinfection is the best method to destroy this organism.

Corneal hypoxia is a reality in aphakia, with the attendant hazards of neovascularization, diffuse corneal edema, and corneal alteration. A lens that is permeable for a myopic eye and that is 0.1 mm thick may show no permeability at an aphakic-level thickness of 0.35 to 0.50 mm.

Extended-wear lenses should be fitted with the flattest lens that will remain centered on the eye and that will provide good vision. A lens that may appear a little loose the first day may become tighter the next day because of dehydration. Thus a 24-hour examination is very important.

Acanthamoeba, a parasitic organism found in hot tubs, swimming pools, and contaminated distilled water, has been shown to cause serious eye infections in contact lens wearers (Figure 15.31). The amoebae adhere more readily to used contact lenses than to new ones. Homemade lens solutions and tap water are to be condemned as a care system. The lens case should be sterilized or replaced regularly. Cases can be microwaved for 3 minutes at 600 watts with water in the case and cap fitted loosely. Boiling will also work. Both microwave and boiling may distort some cases.

Acanthamoeba often causes permanent loss of vision. There are drugs that help to eradicate the organism, but the residual scarring is devastating to the eye.

Extended-wear lenses have come under greater attack because of reported cases of corneal ulcers directly related to their use. Some clinicians even advocate banning extended-wear soft lenses. Although the preponderance of medical opinion does not go that far, the following precautions should be taken:

1. Patients should be screened and those with corneal disease, dry eyes, allergies, or chronic blepharitis should not be fitted.
2. All new candidates should be day-adapted.
3. Patients should be educated about the need for hygiene procedures with respect to wearing of lenses.
4. Lenses should be worn preferably on a flexible-wear basis and disinfected at least once weekly.
5. The lenses should not be worn longer than 1 week continuously.
6. Follow-up examinations are essential. Patients should be seen at least twice a year by the ophthalmologist.
7. Any complications, such as a red eye or pain in the eye, should be reported immediately.
8. We advocate a hydrogen peroxide disinfecting and cleaning system for most extended-wear patients. This has been shown to kill the AIDS virus. Hydrogen peroxide needs long exposure to kill *Acanthamoeba*. This parasite requires heat or ultraviolet exposure to kill it.
9. It is recommended that any patient wearing extended-wear lenses be offered a form of disposable lenses or planned replacement lenses for added cleanliness.

With long-term use of extended-wear lenses or daily wear soft lenses, vacuoles and microcysts may occur in the epithelium of at least 40% of patients. This condition probably occurs because of prolonged low levels of cell death by hypoxia. It usually clears up after lens use is discontinued.

The sucked-on lens syndrome, reported by Wilson and others, involves a tight, unmovable lens that is associated with red eye. Its cause is still controversial but it may result from chemical changes that alter the steepness of the lens. It may be relieved by the use of alkaline drops such as balanced salts in solution.

New silicone hydrogel lenses (continuous wear)

Patients still want the convenience of safe vision around the clock and for extended periods. The new 30-day lenses fit in with busy and unpredictable schedules and eliminate the daily hassle of inserting, removing, and cleaning contact lenses, enabling wearers to lead a more normal life. Research has shown that approximately 38% of contact lens wearers worldwide are interested in a lens that they can sleep with for up to 30 nights without removal. These newer lenses:

*   Have a high oxygen transmission
*   Have a biocompatible lens surface
*   Have a low incidence of complications
*   Can be worn safely for up to 30 days with overnight wear

It is recommended to remove these lenses weekly, and clean, disinfect, and reinsert them the next day. These lenses are promoted as a safe and reliable alternative to LASIK surgery and provide at least six times more oxygen

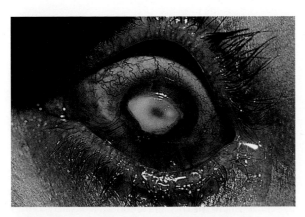

Figure 15.31 Corneal ulcer caused by *Acanthamoeba*.

than ordinary soft lenses. Patients want safety, good vision, comfort, affordability, and convenience. The practitioner, on the other hand, is interested in ocular health and the newer technology that is available. The fluorosilicone hydrogel material partially resists deposits and bacterial adhesions to the surface. A well-fitted lens does not show any edge lift and mucin balls are not created.

Available today are 30-day silicone hydrogel extended-wear (continuous-wear) lenses manufactured by Alcon (Night and Day lens) (Box 15.7) and by Bausch & Lomb (PureVision). Silicone hydrogel material has a high DK value and can be worn night and day on a continuous basis for up to 30 days. This eliminates care systems for storing lenses as well as possible hand contamination. These lenses meet the standards required for minimizing corneal edema in the morning.

The following is taken from the package insert for the Night and Day lens:

*"Night and Day and Air Optix 'Night and Day'®
Aqua (lotrafilcon A) soft contact lenses are made from
a lens material that is approximately 24% water and
76% lotrafilcon A, a fluorosilicone containing
hydrogel which is surface treated. Lenses may contain the
color additive copper phthalocyanine, a light blue
handling tint, which makes them easier to see when
handling."*

The following is taken from the package insert for the Bausch & Lomb PureVision lens:

*"The Bausch & Lomb PureVision® (balafilcon A)
Visibility Tinted Contact Lens is a soft hydrophilic
contact lens which is available as a spherical lens.
The lens material, balafilcon A, is a copolymer of a
silicone vinyl carbamate, N-vinyl-pyrrolidone, a
siloxane crosslinker and a vinyl alanine wetting
monomer, and is 36% water by weight when immersed
in a sterile borate buffered saline solution. This lens is
tinted blue with up to 300 ppm of Reactive Blue
Dye 246."*

Vistakon (Johnson & Johnson) has developed a silicone hydrogel (Acuvue Oasys), with hydraclear plus, which has a

DK/t value of 147. An advantage of this soft flexible material is its low *modulus,* which is a material's stress divided by its strain. It also has an ultraviolet (UV) blocker incorporated. It is recommended to be replaced on a 2-week basis and worn on a daily wear regimen. The following was taken from the instruction guide for the Acuvue Advance lens:

*"The lenses are made of a silicone hydrogel material
containing an internal wetting agent with visibility
tinted UV absorbing monomer. The AcuvueOasys
with hydraclear® Contact Lenses Visibility Tinted
with UV Blocker are tinted blue using Reactive Blue
Dye #4 to make the lens more visible for handling.
A benzotriazole UV-absorbing monomer is used to
block UV radiation. The transmittance
characteristics are less than 1% in the UVB range of
280 nm to 315 nm and less than 10% in the UVA
range of 316 nm to 380 nm for the entire
power range."*

This lens is also available in a toric design for astigmatism.

Table 15.2 compares the features of various silicone hydrogel lenses. The silicone hydrogel lenses are available in single vision, toric, and bifocal design.

Conclusion

The search for a lens that can be worn for prolonged periods was risky and adventurous. Today new plastics and better manufacturing techniques are available, although risk factors still are present with extended-wear lenses.

The fitting of the young myopic person with extended-wear lenses is much easier and more successful than that of the aphakic person because of the thinner lens centers, the healthier corneas, and the better tear film often found in the myopic individual. As a result of advances in cataract surgery and intraocular lenses, fitting aphakes with contact lenses is becoming a thing of the past.

DISPOSABLE LENSES

Lens technology has continued to advance so that disposable replacement regimens are available. This replacement modality is being recommended for 80% of fittings. These disposable lenses may be thrown away and replaced on a daily, weekly, or biweekly basis. With regard to the wear regimen (to differentiate from the replacement regimen) for our own patients, about 20% wear disposable replacement lenses on an extended-wear overnight basis, whereas 80% wear them on a daily wear basis.

The development of disposable replacement contact lenses has ushered in a new era in contact lens safety. Lenses such as the J&J Acuvue Oasys, B&L PureVision, Alcon Air

Table 15.2 Hydrogel silicone lens comparison

	Acuvue Oasys (J&J)	PureVision (B&L)	Air Optix Night and Day
Material	Galyfilcon A	Bafilcon A	Iotrafilcon A
Power range	+8.00 diopters (D) to −12.00 D	+6.00 D to −12.00 D	+8.00 D to −10.00 D
Diameter	14 mm	14 mm	13.8 mm
Base curve	8.4 and 8.8 mm	8.3[a] and 8.6 mm	8.4 and 8.6 mm
Center thickness	0.07 mm	0.07 mm	0.08 mm
Water content	38%	36%	24%
Oxygen transmissibility *DK/t*	147	110	175
Visibility tint	Yes	Yes	Yes
Ultraviolet (UV) blocking	Yes	No	No
Recommended replacement	2 weeks	30 days	30 days

[a]Low minus powers only.

Optix, and CooperVision Biofinity are designed to be replaced daily. Many additional brands are available on a disposable replacement basis with varying wear regimens. Consult a high-quality summary guide for a complete listing of these various brands with their different replacements and regimens.

Disposable replacement of lenses is a practical choice. A person can purchase two to four pairs of lenses at a time (3–6 months' supply) and discard them frequently.

Disposable lenses have the following advantages:

1. Clearer vision is obtained because clean lenses are introduced regularly.
2. The cost of lens-care solutions is greatly reduced.
3. There is minimal deposit formation.
4. Better compliance occurs because daily wear disposable lenses require minimal care compared with the cleaning routines necessary for regular soft lenses.
5. Loss or tearing of a lens is not as much of a problem because the wearer has a purse-size extra lens to carry and insert in emergencies.
6. Disposable lenses offer convenience for travel in that a small package is available, which ends the need to pack a great number of care-system bottles.
7. The incidence and degree of GPC are reduced.
8. The incidence of corneal infection is reduced.

Any disposable lens that is removed from the eye with the intent of reinserting it must be disinfected. It is our recommendation that all disposable lenses should be worn on a daily basis unless some occupational or other special reason requires extended wear.

On the negative side, the disposable system is more expensive than traditional lenses. Patients may skimp and save and try to wear lenses long beyond their recommended time.

The lenses are dispensed annually or semiannually, and the patient picks up new lenses periodically. Planned replacement, sometimes called programmed replacement, is often less expensive than disposable replacement simply because the lenses are not replaced as often. Intervals of between 3 weeks and 6 months are typical for a planned or programmed replacement regimen. Note that disposable replacement is really planned replacement on a regimen of 2 weeks or shorter.

With all disposable and planned replacement lenses, patient compliance in discarding the lenses regularly and adhering to care systems is necessary. Compliance is generally regarded as high because of less confusion about the proper solutions and their application. With the proliferation of disposable replacement lenses from many different manufacturers, wider power and parameter ranges are available to accommodate a greater number of patients.

Daily-wear disposable replacement lenses and planned replacement lenses are problem solvers for many patients with lens deposits, short lens life, and frequent damage to conventional lenses. The current disposable lenses stand up well to normal insertion and short-term removal.

There is now a significant pool of drop-outs from contact lens wear who can be reintroduced to a safe and more convenient system of soft lens wear.

INNOVATIONS IN DESIGN

Innovations are constantly appearing in the soft lens field, making old lenses and methods of cleaning and disinfecting obsolete. Soft lenses have become thinner and more

295

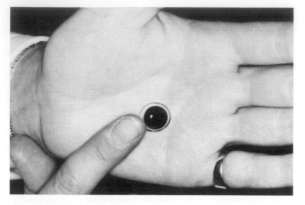

Figure 15.32 A blackened soft lens or iris print lens to cover cosmetically disfigured eyes.

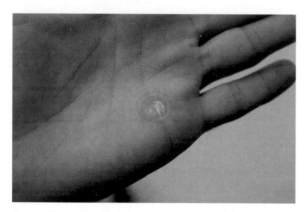

Figure 15.33 Iris print lens to enhance color of eyes.

durable. Their manufacturing techniques have become more automated and more reproducible.

Soft lenses are available in a variety of colors to cover cosmetically disfigured eyes (Figure 15.32). They may be used to occlude pupils for amblyopia and may be tinted red to correct color blindness. Slight handling tints are available for better identification of the lenses. Laser mark impregnation of size and power can be made directly on the soft lenses. Bifocal soft lenses are available for the presbyope. Lenses with dark irides and a clear central portion are available for albino or light-sensitive individuals. The rapidly expanding technology in daily and extended-wear lenses continues to enhance the practitioner's therapeutic armamentarium. UV-blocking lenses are becoming more common and disposable replacement, toric, iris-color-changing lenses are widely available (Figure 15.33). Cosmetic contact lenses include iris-color-changing lenses but also lenses with special designs (e.g., "cat eyes" and "circle lenses"). Some of these newer cosmetic lenses are being obtained without prescription, which can lead to misuse.

CONTACT LENSES IN INDUSTRY

The following statement by the Contact Lens Association of Ophthalmologists (CLAO) addresses the use of contact lenses in industry:

1. Contact lenses may be worn in industrial environments, in combination with appropriate industrial safety eyewear, except where there is likelihood of injury from intense heat, massive chemical splash, highly particulate atmosphere or where specific federal regulations prohibit such use.
2. Employees wearing contact lenses must be identified and known to their immediate supervisors and to the plant safety and medical personnel.
3. First aid personnel should be trained in the proper removal of contact lenses.
4. Employees whose central and peripheral vision can be increased by the wearing of contact lenses, as contrasted with spectacle lenses, should be encouraged to wear contact lenses in industry. Examples of such employees are those who have had a cataract removed from one or both eyes, those with irregular astigmatism from corneal scars or keratoconus, and those who are extremely near-sighted.
5. Employees must keep a spare pair of contacts and/or prescription spectacles in their possession on the job to avoid an inability to function should they damage or lose a contact lens while working.
6. Safety and/or medical personnel should not discriminate against an employee who can achieve visual rehabilitation by contact lenses, either in job placement or on return to a job category.
7. Safety and/or medical personnel should determine on an individual basis the wearing of spectacles or contact lenses in jobs that require unique visual performance. The Occupational Safety and Health Administration and the National Institute for Occupational Safety and Health recommendations must be considered.

SPECIAL OCCUPATIONS

People such as flight attendants, aircraft pilots, police, firefighters, and military personnel have special occupational requirements. For them, contact lenses may be a hazard because clear vision is necessary at all times. Flight attendants need to read warning labels, circuit-breaker labels, and controls; at the same time they must be able to see a small child at the rear of the airplane in case of an emergency. Similar good vision is required of police and firefighters. Contact lenses may be hazardous for these workers because of downtime, discontinuance of wear, loss or removal of the lenses, or other problems.

Downtime

Downtime can amount to as much as 10% to 15% of the wearing time. Contact lenses may have to be temporarily discontinued at critical moments.

1. Some individuals have difficulty with contact lenses because of allergies and sensitivity to smoke and other pollutants. Women who take birth control pills have diminished tear secretion and subtle changes in the cornea that make contact lenses difficult to wear.
2. Some individuals have recurrent conjunctival infections. Corneal ulceration can occur in 20 of 10,000 extended-wear contact lens users and 4 of 10,000 daily wear lens users.
3. Proper care and maintenance of contact lenses are important. Failure to follow directions and reliance on shortcuts, particularly during busy times, affect 75% of wearers. This can result in more contamination of the lenses.
4. Inflammation may be caused by cosmetic lotions in and around the eyes.
5. The carrying cases of contact lenses may harbor microorganisms.
6. A lens can alter its shape and consequently its fit so that it may become too tight or too loose.
7. Some contact lenses may chip or crack and may cause a corneal abrasion that requires removal and downtime. Breakage occurs in 4% to 5% of rigid contact lenses, and soft lenses may tear at a similar rate.
8. Fatigue plays an important role in the wearing of contact lenses. When fatigued, the wearer tends to stare, with reduced blinking time. This results in dehydration of the soft lens and irritation begins, often resulting in removal.

Discontinuance of wear

Situations occur, such as eye injury, during which the patient may have to discontinue contact lens wear for several months until the eye is healed. In this case the patient may have to rely on spectacles. Other reasons for discontinuance of wear include the following:

1. Warped rigid lenses may require discontinuance for several days to allow the cornea to restore its normal curvature.
2. Some people are more prone to infection with contact lens wear. This infection may cause severe ulceration and keratitis, resulting in several weeks of downtime.
3. Care systems may be time-consuming and cause an individual to discontinue using the lenses and revert to spectacles.
4. Many individuals are sensitive or become hypersensitive to the disinfectant solutions used for contact lens care and may be required to discontinue contact lens wear. Heat, hydrogen peroxide, and UV sterilization are alternatives.

5. Allergic conjunctivitis can occur in 1% to 5% of people who wear hard lenses and in at least 20% of those who use extended-wear soft contact lenses.

Loss or removal of the lenses

Loss of a lens is a common occurrence, particularly with rigid lenses.

1. Lenses can become lost during activity in certain occupations or sports.
2. Cigarette and pipe smoke can force the wearer to remove contact lenses.
3. In case of fire, smoke and toxic gases may become trapped behind the contact lens and irritate the eye, making removal necessary.
4. Foreign particles underneath a contact lens may scratch and irritate the eye, requiring removal of the lens.
5. Soft lenses dehydrate relatively quickly in low-humidity environments such as aircraft, which may necessitate their removal because of discomfort.

Problems with contact lenses

1. Contrast sensitivity in the everyday world is often reduced with contact lenses. In critical areas of visual function, this may become a hazard.
2. Scratches may occur on hard and soft contact lenses, which necessitates replacement of the lens to improve vision.
3. Debris may accumulate on the surface of the contact lenses as a result of mixtures of lipids and proteins. This can make the eye uncomfortable and impair vision.
4. Poor fitting can result in complications.

COMMON QUESTIONS AND ANSWERS

1. Should a contact lens be removed before evaluation with use of the air tonometer?
   Yes. The practitioner does not obtain reliable results of pressure unless the contact lens is removed before this measurement.
2. Should lenses be removed before a field test?
   No. The best visual acuity is required to perform a field test. If the lenses provide this, then the lenses may remain in the eyes.
3. How long should a contact lens be removed before an eye examination?
   If the examination does not involve a refraction, the contact lens need not necessarily be removed. The lens must be removed during the tonometric examination, however.

4. How long should a contact lens be removed before refraction?

To obtain a suitable refraction, a contact lens should be removed at least 24 to 48 hours before examination. This permits the corneal epithelium to regain its full corneal curvature and thus provide a suitable refraction. Sometimes epithelial edema is present, which clouds the refraction and produces an error in the refractive surface.

5. Can patients who wear contact lenses be considered for implant surgery?

Yes. The correct lenses provide no impairment to implant surgery. The use of biometry provides a new measurement for an intraocular lens that often will eliminate contact lenses.

6. Can contact lenses be used after refractive surgery?

Yes. The keratometer readings often are misleading. These patients should be fitted according to their original *K* readings. Soft lenses, if worn for any extended basis, provide some vascularization at the knee of the depression. Consequently, the patient should receive instructions for daily wear and minimal wearing times. Hard lenses are probably more suitable and will reduce any corneal toricity that may be present.

7. Can soft or rigid lenses be worn after implant surgery?

Yes. Usually, however, these are not required. On the other hand, in cases of higher astigmatism or residual refractive error, they may provide a very useful form of visual rehabilitation.

8. What are the major problems in care of contact lenses?

The most common problems are those caused by lack of compliance; that is, the patient does not follow the regimen given by the instructor. Because patients often become haphazard about lens care, care must be emphasized at almost every repeat visit. Reduced vision, discomfort, red eye, infections, and allergic responses are the problems that occur most frequently.

ROLE OF THE OPHTHALMIC ASSISTANT

A high percentage of the tasks in an efficient contact lens practice may be delegated to the ophthalmic assistant. Supplies and inventory of lenses add a dimension of expense to a practice that must be supervised and continually looked after. Unlike rigid lenses, soft lenses spoil and deteriorate once the vial has been opened unless cleaning and sterilizing routines are applied to trial sets and unopened vials. The ophthalmic assistant in a clinical contact lens practice often is responsible for maintaining inventory and helping in cost efficiency.

The following list indicates some of the duties of the ophthalmic assistant in a busy contact lens practice:

1. Maintain inventory and cost efficiency.
2. Handle insurance programs.
3. Provide instruction on lens care and handling.
4. Schedule appointments.
5. Make follow-up calls for drop-outs, particularly those prescribed extended-wear lenses.
6. Handle telephone calls.
7. Understand adaptive and abnormal symptoms.
8. Perform office cleaning of lenses.
9. Perform collections.
10. Order replacement lenses.

The assistant must become familiar with telephone communication with patients and in particular must be able to distinguish purely adaptive symptoms for both rigid and soft lenses from abnormal symptoms. Abnormal symptoms such as persistent red eyes, blurring of vision, excessive glare, and unusual discomfort require an emergency appointment with the ophthalmologist. When in doubt, assistants should exercise caution, turn the call over to someone more experienced, or schedule the patient for an examination. They should not assume responsibility for diagnosis on the telephone.

Questions for review and thought

1. Why is a soft lens so comfortable?
2. Describe a method of teaching a patient insertion and removal of a soft lens.
3. What are the advantages of soft hydrogel lenses compared with rigid lenses?
4. Review the fitting method of one type of soft lens.
5. How are soft lenses sterilized?
6. How are soft lenses cleaned?
7. How can you inspect and evaluate a soft lens returned by the patient?
8. Name some medical uses for the soft contact lens.
9. If the diameter of a lens is increased, is the lens made flatter or steeper?
10. How can you determine whether a soft lens is inside out?
11. Can fluorescein be used with a soft lens? Explain.
12. Which candidates are not suitable for soft lenses?
13. If the water content of a soft lens is increased, is its durability increased or decreased?

Self-evaluation questions

True–false statements

Directions: Indicate whether the statement is true **(T)** or false **(F).**

1. Soft lenses are better than rigid lenses in reducing glare and photophobia. **T** or **F**
2. Measurement of a soft lens is labeled in the fully hydrated state. **T** or **F**
3. Thin soft lenses are better for occasional wear such as sporting activities. **T** or **F**

Missing words

Directions: Write in the missing word in the following sentences:

4. Circumlimbal compression and injection are characteristic of a soft lens that has been fitted too _____.
5. Ultrathin lenses have _____ oxygen transmission compared with lenses of standard thickness.
6. Soft lenses worn in a dry environment should not be thin but be of _____ thickness to reduce dehydration.

Choice-completion questions

Directions: Select the one best answer in each case.

7. Soft lenses can be of great therapeutic value as a bandage lens. Which of the following conditions could benefit from a bandage soft lens?
   a. Bullous keratopathy
   b. Recurrent corneal erosion
   c. Keratitis sicca
   d. All of the above
   e. None of the above
8. Which of the following is true for present-day conventional extended-wear lenses for myopia?
   a. Difficult-to-handle lenses
   b. Loss factor common
   c. Deposit formation common
   d. Infection common
   e. Neovascularization
9. To maintain corneal integrity and proper cornea–lens relationship, the fit should exhibit:
   a. central touch.
   b. no movement.
   c. apical vaulting.
   d. three-point touch.
   e. slight edge lifting.

 Answers, notes, and explanations

1. **True.** Soft lenses reduce foreign body sensation and thus reduce the incidence of lens-induced photophobia. Also, the large optic zone eliminates the glare that can be experienced when light passes through the peripheral curves of a rigid lens or when the pupil dilates.
2. **True.** All soft lenses contain some percentage of water. The expressed parameters are measurements when the lens is fully hydrated. A lens tends to shrink and steepen as it dehydrates. In the manufacturing process of a soft lens, the measurements usually are made initially for the manufacture of the soft lens while it is still in the hard state. An allowance factor for the constant swelling of the material in the hydrated state is taken into consideration to arrive at the final dimensions of the required hydrated lens. The soft lenses are then measured in the fully hydrated state.
3. **True.** Thin and ultrathin lenses show better oxygen transmission and may be fitted larger and tighter and thus track with rapid movements of the eye. This reduces loss and prevents particles from getting under the lenses. This

can be a most useful feature in the stability of vision required for most sports.

4. **Tightly or steeply.** A lens that is too tight will show minimal or no movement and cause inadequate tear exchange under the lens, along with compression of the vessels at the limbus.
5. **Higher.** Oxygen permeability is a function of the material, whereas oxygen transmission also takes into account the thickness of the material. When any material thickness is reduced by 50%, the transmission of oxygen is doubled. Thus the thinner the lenses, the better is oxygen transmission through to the cornea.
6. **Standard.** In a dry environment the standard-thickness lenses perform better because they carry more water and permit greater evaporation before they become depleted of their water reservoir.
7. **d. All of the above.** These are but a few of a long list of indicators for the soft lens as a medical device in the therapeutic armamentarium against corneal disease processes.

A | Continued

8. **c. Deposit formation common.** Build-up of minerals, protein, and lipids is still the single main feature of contact lenses that are not cleaned on a daily basis. Although weekly or semimonthly cleaning routines are recommended for most patients with conventional extended-wear lenses, those who fail to follow this regimen often allow deposits to build up and cause spoilage of their soft lenses.

9. **d. Three-point touch.** The proper cornea–lens relationship for a soft lens involves slight central touch with touch of the lens at the periphery. For the smaller-diameter soft lenses, this peripheral touch may be at the limbus, whereas for the larger lenses this may be on the sclera. With each blink there is some movement of the lens and a small amount of tear exchange under the lens.

Chapter 16

Advanced techniques in soft and rigid contact lens fitting

Many ophthalmic assistants play an expanded role in contact lens delivery and thus require detailed knowledge of contact lenses. Although the changing and ordering of lenses may be beyond the scope of the ophthalmic assistant, an understanding of how to modify lenses and a review of abnormal symptoms and signs are not. This chapter highlights only some of the problems encountered; further information may be obtained from our textbook, *Fitting guide for rigid and soft contact lenses: a practical approach.* 4th ed. St Louis: Mosby, 2002.

ABNORMAL SYMPTOMS AND SIGNS

It is important to recognize purely adaptive symptoms and differentiate them from pathologic symptoms that could result in corneal damage. The ophthalmic assistant may be the first to hear of these symptoms and should alert the ophthalmologist to patients' complaints that might lead to serious corneal damage.

Flare or streaming of lights or glare from oncoming headlights may occur when the lens or the optical portion of the lens (optic zone) is too small. This symptom occurs because the pupil of the eye dilates at night or in a darkened room and the patient begins to have interference in his or her vision from the edge of the optic zone or the edge of the lens. It can be corrected by making the lens larger or by increasing the size of the optic zone.

Blurring of vision in daytime through the normal pupil may be a result of the lens riding too high or gravitating too low after each blink. This can be observed directly by watching the patient view a vision chart or distant object. The patient may respond by producing streaming opposite to the displacement of the lens (Figure 16.1). Lenses may ride high because of a high minus power and edge thickness that cause the lens to be lifted up by the upper lid. A small lens under a tight lid will also ride high. A lens that rides low may be too heavy because of thickness or because of high plus power or there may be insufficient edge thickness that will not permit the upper lid to grasp the lens and lift it. Redesigning the edge to provide proper compensation will permit the lens to center better. If this fails, smaller lenses may be required. Occasionally the lens will slide nasally or temporally because of an abnormally centered cornea. These lenses should be replaced with lenses of larger diameter or a larger optic zone.

Central corneal edema (Figure 16.2) with consequent blurring of vision occurs when there is insufficient oxygenation of the cornea brought about by poor tear exchange. The edematous area appears hazy on the slit-lamp microscope,

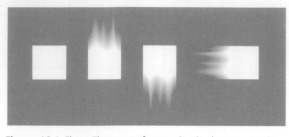

Figure 16.1 Flare. The zone of streaming is always opposite to the displacement of the lens. Such a lens requires recentering. Uniform flare indicates that the optic zone of the lens is too small.
(From Stein HA, Slatt BJ, Stein RM. Fitting guide for rigid and soft contact lenses: a practical approach. 4th ed. St Louis: Mosby; 2002.)

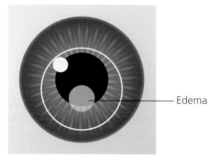

Edema

Figure 16.2 Corneal edema created by a contact lens.
(From Rosenthal P. International Ophthalmology Clinics 8:611, 1968.)

particularly if the light is shone off to the side of the area to be viewed so the area is illuminated from behind rather than directly. When the epithelial edema advances, some cells may die, causing central stippling, which will stain with fluorescein dye. The stippling may represent only a few small, discrete spots at the beginning, but the spots may increase in number as the condition progresses. If the condition progresses, *punctate staining* is said to occur. Patients who develop these objective signs will often complain of spectacle blur for some time after the lenses are removed. To correct this situation, the tear exchange must be improved. This can be done in the original rigid lens by:

- Blending the junctions of the curve better
- Flattening the peripheral curve
- Reducing the total diameter
- Reducing the diameter of the optic zone by increasing the width of the peripheral curve
- Fenestrating the lens

Corneal abrasion (Figure 16.3) may follow corneal edema caused by lack of oxygen, but may also result from too flat a lens rubbing on a portion of the cornea. Evaluation of the fit of the lens to indicate that the abraded area lies just under the touch area of the contact lens will determine whether the lens is rubbing the cornea and is too flat, too loose, or both. The excessive movement adds to the friction of the cornea and can be corrected with a new lens by:

- Increasing the rigid lens diameter
- Increasing the optic zone diameter
- Reducing the edge thickness
- Steepening the lens case curve
- Steepening the peripheral curve

Three o'clock and *nine o'clock staining* (see Figure 16.3) of the cornea with fluorescein refers to erosions at the 3 and 9 o'clock positions in the exposed portion of the palpebral fissure. It is usually believed to be a result of dryness because of inadequate blinking while wearing the contact lens, so that the small exposed portion of the cornea on each side of the lens becomes dry. This symptom is not usually seen with smaller and thinner lenses. Various methods such as a smaller, thinner lens; blinking exercises; or artificial tears may help eliminate this problem.

Insertion abrasions may result from improper or clumsy insertion. Abrasion causes either immediate pain or pain after removal of the lens. Further practice in insertion should be undertaken under observation of the instructor.

Foreign bodies trapped under the lens will show varying types of zigzag scratch marks on the cornea, which will stain with fluorescein. Common substances such as mascara and cosmetics may be the offending agents and should be used with caution.

Arc staining may occur either from poor insertion technique or most commonly from a sharp junction line between the central posterior curve and the intermediate or peripheral posterior curve. A proper blend is required.

Bubbles with staining occur when the lens is steep and there is too much sagittal depth to the lens so that air is trapped under the central curve. A flatter lens is required.

Blurring after reading may occur in the myope nearing the age of 40. The introduction of contact lenses requires a further accommodative effort and convergence that the patient cannot compensate for. Reading glasses may be required.

If the blur in the nonpresbyope occurs soon after insertion, it may be caused by the lower lid pushing the lens upward, thus causing poor centering of the lens in the reading position. This may be corrected by making the lens smaller.

If blurring occurs after prolonged reading, it may be the result of inadequate tear exchange and corneal anoxia. Concentrated reading reduces the blink reflex, induces staring, and consequently permits less tear exchange. A smaller lens, a flatter peripheral curve, or a material with a higher *DK* may alleviate this problem. For individuals who require prolonged reading activity, blinking exercises can be recommended.

Corneal warpage or induced astigmatism, both regular and irregular, can occur, resulting either from poorly fitting lenses that alter the corneal curvature or from chronic hypoxia of the cornea from overwearing the contact lenses. A complete reassessment of the fit is called for and possibly refitting in a more permeable material.

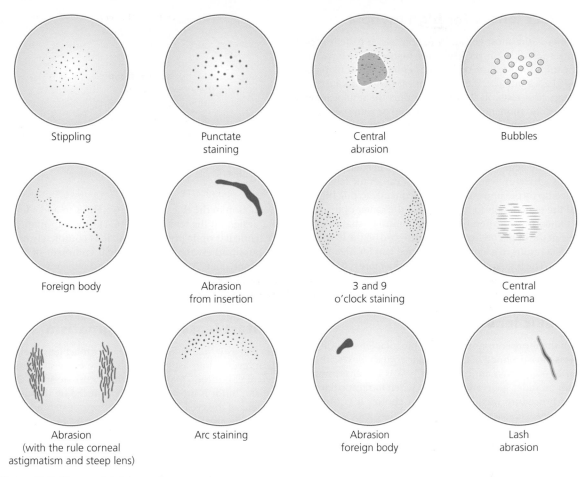

Figure 16.3 Abnormal staining patterns.

FOLLOW-UP KERATOMETRY

By performing keratometry on repeat visits, one can detect any molding or distortion of the cornea or induced astigmatism. One should record the difference in the *K* readings at subsequent visits. A notation such as *K* +1.25 + 0.50 indicates that the cornea has steepened by this amount in each meridian. Any changes over 1.00 diopter indicate that the wearing time should be reduced or the lens adjusted. Distortion of the mires also indicates that a change is needed.

SPECIAL LENSES

The methods of contact lens fitting for correction of the most common defects of the eye were described in Chapter 14. The techniques and devices available have proved highly successful for the majority of cases.

However, as with other natural systems, variations in the anatomy and physiology of the eye are broad. Thus for those defects associated with more extreme variations, corrective devices and methods must be custom-built to a highly sophisticated level. For example, patients with extremely high myopia (−6.00 diopters or greater) or aphakic patients (+8.00 diopters or greater) require modifications of the normal lens design because of an extrathick (myopic) or extrathin (hyperopic) peripheral edge of the corneal contact lens. Similarly, extreme cases of keratoconus require bicurvature lenses for effective apposition to the eye, whereas highly astigmatic cases require an asymmetric (nonspherical), nonrotating lens design. Special rigid lenses have been developed for a steepened apical characteristic of the cone in keratoconus. Many eye patients older than 40 years require bifocal lenses, and special lens systems with bifocal lens characteristics can be prepared for their accommodation. Certain pathologic cases requiring telescopic lenses also present a need for specially designed lenses.

Contact lenses for high myopia

Myopia is the most common reason why a patient seeks contact lenses. Contact lenses for high myopia have not only the added feature of cosmetic enhancement by replacing glasses but also increased optical benefit because the contact lens rests on the eye, and thus the retinal image is larger and more normal than it would be with spectacles. In addition, the high myope no longer has a visual field restricted by the edges of glasses and frames.

However, as the minus power of a contact lens increases, so does the edge thickness. This increase in edge thickness creates a base-up wedge effect, which causes the lens to be pulled up by the upper lid and consequently to ride high so that the patient fails to look through the center of the lens. To reduce the thickness of the edge, it must be shaved off to prevent the upper lid from tugging upward on the lens. This in effect results in a lenticular-designed lens for high minus powers. The higher the minus power, the more the anterior edge has to be reduced. Aspheric lens designs have thinner peripheral profiles.

Aphakic lenses

With the more common use of intraocular lenses, aphakic lenses have declined in use. Aphakic contact lenses are primarily used when an intraocular lens is not appropriate, or for an older-generation patient when intracapsular cataract procedure was the surgery of choice. It is obvious why intraocular lenses are preferred: they generally offer better vision and freedom from the daily handling of contact lenses. For an older adult who may have a hand tremor, lax eyelids, or a tear deficiency, this freedom from the hazards of contact lens wear is important. Yet not all cataract extractions are treated with intraocular lenses. Implants **may not be inserted** if any of the following occurs:

- Angle-closure glaucoma
- Recurrent iridocyclitis
- Any surgical contingency that makes the insertion of an intraocular lens hazardous

Thus knowledge of aphakic contact lenses should be acquired despite a definite downgrading of their importance in the management of a cataract patient.

Aphakic individuals require strong plus lenses. As the power of a plus lens increases, so too does its central thickness. This increase in central thickness creates a base-down wedge effect at the upper edge of the lens, thus the upper lid forces the lens downward. The high-plus lens is also heavy, which causes it to gravitate downward. One way of reducing the thickness and thus the weight of a high-plus lens is to keep the overall diameter of the lens very small. Unfortunately this does not solve the problem if the patient has large pupils or keyhole iridectomies, in which case the patient may be looking through the lens edge. A more practical way of fitting a high-plus lens with

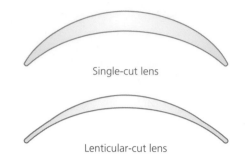

Figure 16.4 Single-cut and lenticular-cut lenses.

a reduction in the thickness and weight is to add a lenticular design on the lens (Figure 16.4). It is important that the lenticular optic portion of the lens completely covers the pupil, otherwise the patient will complain of blurry vision and glare. Another solution is to put a myopic edge finish on any high-plus lens, which will help the upper eyelid elevate the lens.

Contact lenses for astigmatism

Residual astigmatism occurs when a contact lens is placed on an eye and an astigmatic refractive error still results. Several conditions may contribute to this residual astigmatism, but it is most commonly induced by the crystalline lens of the eye (so-called *lenticular astigmatism*). If the amount is small, it will not significantly interfere with vision. If the amount of astigmatism is large, however, vision will be substandard unless one can compensate for this with the contact lens. Although this requires a complex type of lens, essentially a toric surface is ground on the front or back of the lens to prevent the lens from rotating, so that the toric surface is lined up with the axis of astigmatism. One must stop rotation of the lens by introducing a weight such as a prism ballast to the lens at the correct position.

Nonrotating lenses

Patients with a moderate or high degree of astigmatism will experience difficulties in wearing spherical contact lenses. Symptoms of blurred vision, excessive awareness of lens edge, and slipping of the lens off the cornea or even completely out of the eye will be encountered because of the rocking effect of the lens over the flatter meridian. Residual astigmatism, in which the cornea is spherical but the patient has a cylindric spectacle prescription, is another indication for nonrotating lenses. In these cases the astigmatism comes from the lens of the eye and it is necessary to add prism to the lens to stop lens rotation and to properly orient the cylinder over the correct optical axis.

Several types of nonrotating lenses have been designed.

Noncircular shapes

A *truncated* lens is really a circular lens in which the bottom or top portion, or both (double-truncated lens), has been cut off. The corners at the edge of the truncation are smoothed off. A double-truncated lens, although infrequently used, will tend to stabilize so that the flat portion lies adjacent to the upper and lower lid edges. If the edges are rounded off more, the lens assumes an oval shape, but this type of lens rotates frequently and thus negates the use for which it was intended. Rectangular and triangular lenses have been designed, but they have shown little practical value.

Toric curve lens

A lens may be cut so that it is not spherical on its back surface. It is called a *toric back curve lens* when it has two meridians of curvature on its back surface that are designed to conform somewhat to the two meridians of curvature of the front surface of the cornea. This lens is used to correct a high degree of astigmatism. When the lens is placed in the eye, it tends to align its curvature with that of the cornea. However, an optical problem of astigmatism may exist that may require the grinding of a toric surface on the front of the lens, the so-called *front surface toric lens*. These are used primarily to treat residual astigmatism in patients with spherical corneas. In some instances toric surfaces may be ground on both the front and back surfaces, the so-called *bitoric contact lens*.

Prism ballast lenses

When a prism is ground into a contact lens, the heavier base of the prism swings the lens around so that the heavier base rides low, attracted by gravity, and thus further rotation of the lens is eliminated (Figure 16.5). One can incorporate up to 3.00 diopters of prism in a lens to provide sufficient weight. In addition to preventing rotation, a prism may be used to create weight in a lens that tends to ride high or to reduce excessive lens movements. The weight of prism

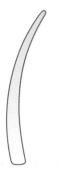

Figure 16.5 Prism ballast to provide weight and stop rotation of a lens.

ballast lenses and the thinner superior edge of the lens, which fits under the upper lid, provide stability and prevent rotation of the lens.

Correction of high astigmatism

Astigmatism may result from corneal surfaces of different radii or from changes in the lens of the eye. The latter is less common, but nevertheless does occur and accounts for residual astigmatism when corneal astigmatism has been fully corrected. It may also account for a very irregular corneal surface. Corneal topography is an excellent way of analyzing the corneal surface.

Keratometer readings provide a good index of the amount of corneal astigmatism present. Most spherical-based lenses are the first choice for fitting eyes with corneal astigmatism. Tear fluid readily fills in the interface and provides a good optical result in most cases. However, in some cases these lenses will not provide adequate tear interchange, rocking occurs, or poor staining is found. A back surface toric lens will be required that will conform to the corneal toricity. Diagnostic trial lenses may be a valuable adjunct. Frequently, changing the back surface to a toric surface causes induced or residual astigmatism; this must be corrected by grinding a toric surface on the front of the lens. This constitutes the so-called *bitoric lens*.

Toric soft contact lenses

A wide variety of toric soft contact lenses are on the market, and fitters must familiarize themselves with what is available on a lens-by-lens basis. Specific lenses are not discussed here because there are excellent fitting guides available from the manufacturers. Before choosing a specific lens, the fitter must make sure that the lens is available in parameters that match the patient's refractive error.

Some "off-the-shelf" toric lenses are available in a limited range of cylinders and axes. Manufacturers make lenses in the most commonly requested power ranges and these are available immediately. Most soft toric lenses are available in powers from −8.00 to +4.00 diopters, with cylinder powers of −0.75 to −2.50 diopters. Daily disposable toric lenses are available in limited cylinder power and axis. A diagnostic lens of the selected toric design must be evaluated on the patient's eye for fit and position of axis.

For "custom" work a fitting set must also be used. The fitting lenses are spherical designs with the diameters and orientation systems of the toric lenses that the patient will eventually wear. Toric lenses that can be fit in this manner are available in powers from −20.00 to +20.00 diopters, with axes of rotation available in 5-degree increments. A few manufacturers provide toric lenses made to order with even greater power and cylinder and with axes of rotation in 1-degree increments.

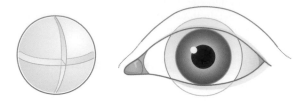

Figure 16.6 Double slab-off soft lens used to correct astigmatism. The lens is made thinner superiorly and inferiorly so that thinner portions tend to rotate and come to rest under the upper and lower eyelids.
(From Stein HA, Slatt BJ, Stein RM. Fitting guide for rigid and soft contact lenses: a practical approach. 4th ed. St Louis: Mosby; 2002.)

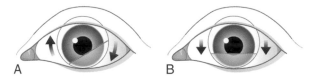

Figure 16.7 (A) Lens on immediate insertion. (B) The weighted portion, combined with the torsional effect of the eyelid muscles, rotates the lens to a stable position.
(From Stein HA, Slatt BJ, Stein RM. Fitting guide for rigid and soft contact lenses: a practical approach. 4th ed. St Louis: Mosby; 2002.)

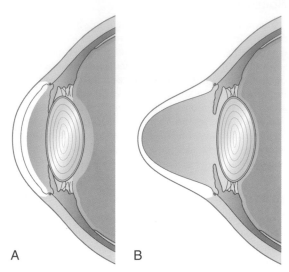

Figure 16.8 (A) Normal eye. (B) Keratoconus. Note thinning of the cornea as well as the forward protrusion.

Several design alternatives are used to maintain the orientation of toric lenses. *Double slab-off*, the creation of thin zones on the inferior and superior parts of the lens, allows lids to hold the lens in position (Figure 16.6). As with bifocal soft contact lenses, prism ballasting (Figure 16.7), periballasting, and truncation are also used to maintain orientation.

Toric lenses have *orientation* (or scribe) *marks* near the edge, some at the 3 o'clock and 9 o'clock positions, and others at the 6 o'clock position. The manufacturer can sometimes be verified by the marks or by the laser identification marks on the lens.

CONTACT LENSES FOR KERATOCONUS

Keratoconus is a forward bulging of the central cornea with irregular astigmatism (Figure 16.8). It usually begins in adolescence and progresses over the next several years. It is often bilateral, although one eye advances more than the other. Its cause is still unknown, but there is a strong hereditary feature.

This irregular astigmatism cannot be corrected by normal spectacles, but in the majority of cases vision can be satisfactorily corrected by contact lenses. In addition to vision correction, contact lenses tend to flatten and give symmetry to the cornea, although they do not change the progress of the disease. The apex of the cornea is very sensitive in early stages, giving rise to photophobia and lens-fitting problems, but in later stages the cornea becomes relatively insensitive (Figure 16.9).

The thinness of the cornea, ruptures in Descemet's membrane, and small apical tears may be detected in advanced cases by slit-lamp biomicroscopy, the hand keratoscope, or Placido's disc. Keratoconus is often associated with patients who have hay fever, atopic dermatitis, eczema, or asthma. Topography is often helpful (Figure 16.10).

A slit-lamp diagnosis is difficult to make in the early phase, whereas in the late stages the diagnosis becomes obvious with apical thinning, Fleischer's keratoconus ring, increased endothelial reflex, increased visibility of the nerve fibers, and scarring of Bowman's membrane. Keratometry is very helpful in the early phase of this disease because the mire images appear distorted and irregular. The two principal meridians are not at right angles to each other and the dioptric value of the readings is much higher than normal (48.00 diopters or higher). The range of the keratometer may have to be extended to accurately record the full corneal curvature. The addition of a 1.25-diopter lens over the front of the keratometer either by hand or by the special retention ring is most useful (conversion by means of a table is required for true *K* readings; Table 16.1).

Perhaps the best instrument for diagnosis of keratoconus in the early stages is the retinoscope, which reflects irregular light reflexes from the surface of the cornea with scissor-like movements. Dr. Joseph Baldone has described and popularized remote ophthalmoscopy as another valuable diagnostic tool. In this method an ophthalmoscope qualitates the red reflex.

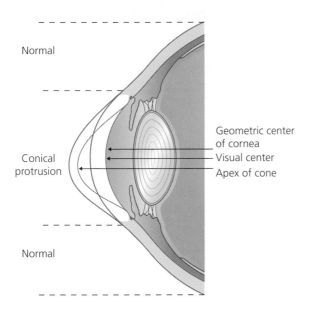

Figure 16.9 Keratoconus. Note the forward protrusion and thinning of the cornea.
(From Soper JW, Girard LJ. Special designs and fitting techniques. In: Girard LJ, editor. Corneal contact lenses. 2nd ed. St Louis: Mosby; 1970.)

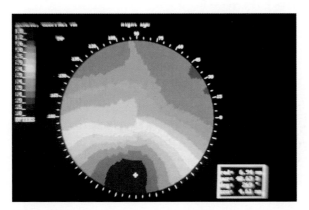

Figure 16.10 Topography indicating steepening inferiorly.

Corneal topographic analysis with the new computer-assisted keratovideoscopes offers a map-like correction of several thousand points of *K* readings on the cornea. This advancement has given us much more information than simple keratometry or corneoscopy. A more detailed explanation of topographic analysis of the cornea is presented later in the text. One of the main values of corneal topographic analysis by computer-assisted keratoscopy is the detection of early keratoconus.

The purpose of the contact lens is to cover the irregular astigmatism and the disordered anterior surface optics of

an ectatic cornea by providing a regular, spherical, optic surface before the eye. The lens does not retard the progression of the disease, which by itself may have long periods of natural remission; scleral, semiscleral, and corneal rigid lenses, as well as combinations of soft and rigid lenses and thick soft lenses, have been used in treating keratoconus.

Scleral lenses

The first scleral lenses were introduced in glass 125 years ago. Such lenses bridge the cornea by bearing on the sclera. Therefore, the corneal sensitivity is eliminated. Their diameter ranges from 15 to 25 mm. The tear reservoir between the lens and cornea masks all the corneal astigmatism and irregularities. Correcting the compromised cornea with scleral lenses has gained more popularity thanks to the advanced rigid gas-permeable (RGP) lens material, manufacturing technologies, and their great comfort.

Patients with corneal lenses may complain of occasional lens decantation, expulsion, or lens popping out during activities. Scleral lenses are mostly prescribed in case of corneal irregularity. Corneal irregularities can result from keratoconus, corneal surgery, trauma, or complications of other surgeries.

Scleral lenses vault over the cornea and rest on the sclera, providing good stability and centration. Patients with moderate to severe corneal irregularity and those who have previously failed in corneal RGP lenses are excellent candidates for scleral lenses. Scleral lenses may also be offered to patients with ocular diseases such as Sjogren's syndrome, Stevens-Johnson syndrome, and dry eye. Scleral lenses also could protect the compromised anterior ocular surface from exposure.

Scleral lenses were originally reserved for eyes with severe irregularity or surface diseases and were used only when other therapeutic options had been exhausted. Now the scleral lenses are being also marketed as an option for correction of uncomplicated refractive errors. Some of the current scleral lenses in the market are listed in Table 16.2.

There are three main components to scleral lens design: the optic zone, the transition zone over the limbus, and the landing zone on the sclera. Each zone is comprised of one or more curvatures, each of which has a defined diameter. The optic zone is the power center of the lens; it is designed to vault the cornea and protect its optical function. The transition zone raises and lowers the optic zone relative to the eye, and is vital to protect the limbal stem cells. The landing zone is the area in which contact between the lens and ocular surface is made. This contact must be done in a very controlled manner to prevent inflammation. Scleral lenses are designed to vault the cornea and limbus entirely and land solely on the sclera.

Table 16.1 Dioptric curves for extended range of keratometer

High power (with +1.25 lens over aperture)				Low power (with −1.00 lens over aperture)			
Drum reading	True dioptric curvature	Drum reading	True dioptric curvature	Drum reading	True dioptric curvature	Drum reading	True dioptric curvature
52.00	61.00	46.87	55.87	42.00	36.00	36.87	30.87
51.87	60.87	46.75	55.75	41.87	35.87	36.75	30.75
51.75	60.75	46.62	55.62	41.75	35.75	36.62	30.62
51.62	60.62	46.50	55.50	41.62	35.62	36.50	30.50
51.50	60.50	46.37	55.37	41.50	35.50	36.37	30.37
51.37	60.37	46.25	55.25	41.37	35.37	36.25	30.25
51.25	60.25	46.12	55.12	41.25	35.25	36.12	30.12
51.12	60.12	46.00	55.00	41.12	35.12	36.00	30.00
51.00	60.00			41.00	35.00		
		45.87	54.87				
50.87	59.87	45.75	54.75	40.87	34.87		
50.75	59.75	45.62	54.62	40.75	34.75		
50.62	59.62	45.50	54.50	40.62	34.62		
50.50	59.50	45.37	54.37	40.50	34.50		
50.37	59.37	45.25	54.25	40.37	34.37		
50.25	59.25	45.12	54.12	40.25	34.25		
50.12	59.12	45.00	54.00	40.12	34.12		
50.00	59.00			40.00	34.00		
		44.87	53.87				
49.87	58.87	44.75	53.75	39.87	33.87		
49.75	58.75	44.62	53.62	39.75	33.75		
49.62	58.62	44.50	53.50	39.62	33.62		
49.50	58.50	44.37	53.37	39.50	33.50		
49.37	58.37	44.25	53.25	39.37	33.37		
49.25	58.25	44.12	53.12	39.25	33.25		
49.12	58.12	44.00	53.00	39.12	33.12		
49.00	58.00			39.00	33.00		
		43.87	52.87				
48.75	57.75	43.75	52.75	38.87	32.87		
48.62	57.62	43.62	52.62	38.75	32.75		
48.50	57.50	43.50	52.50	38.62	32.62		
48.37	57.37	43.37	52.37	38.50	32.50		
48.25	57.25	43.25	52.25	38.37	32.37		
48.12	57.12	43.12	52.12	38.25	32.25		
48.00	57.00	43.00	52.00	38.12	32.12		
				38.00	32.00		
47.87	56.87						
47.75	56.75			37.87	31.87		
47.62	56.62			37.75	31.75		
47.50	56.50			37.62	31.62		
47.37	58.37			37.50	31.50		
47.25	56.25			37.37	31.37		
47.12	56.12			37.25	31.25		
47.00	56.00			37.12	31.12		
				37.00	31.00		

(Courtesy Bausch & Lomb)

Table 16.2 Current scleral lenses in the market

Company	Lens Name
Acculens	Maxim plus
Acculens	Comfort SL plus
Art optical	CO_2 clear progressive
Advanced vision technology	AVT
Alden	Zenelens
Blanchard	MSD
Blanchard	One fit
Essilor	Jupiter plus
Lens dynamics	Dyna semiscleral
Vally contax	Stable near

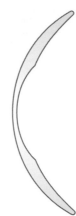

Figure 16.11 Soper cone lens for keratoconus.

Corneal lenses

It is controversial whether rigid corrective lenses should touch the apical cone lightly and rest on the peripheral cornea where there is little or no thinning or whether they should just clear the apex of the cone. Lenses fitted excessively flat eventually cause corneal abrasions. Minimal apical clearance of the cone has been advocated but this point of view does not represent the majority. Gas-permeable materials are the best choice for better maintenance of corneal integrity.

The majority of early to moderate cones exhibit a manifestation of the irregularity at or below the midline of the cornea. Because keratometric readings can be misleading, it is important to remember that the superior portion of the cornea may be relatively normal or much flatter than the K readings suggest. These early to moderate and some more advanced oval cones can be effectively fitted using spherical and aspherical designs that will align with the superior cornea. Diagnostic fitting and fluorescein evaluation are required to accurately fit rigid contact lenses over an irregular corneal surface. The fitter should not be alarmed at the slight to moderate inferior edge lift of the lens if it aligns well superiorly. The upper lid especially aids in holding the lens in position. It is not uncommon to fit an oval cone with irregular K readings in the 50.00-diopter range with a lens such as the Boston Envision, or Fluoroperm 90 with a base curve of 7.5 to 7.3 (45.00–46.25 diopters).

For more classic nipple-type cones, the Soper keratoconus lens can be of value. In our experience the Soper keratoconus trial lenses (Figure 16.11), combined with fluorescein assessment of their fit, have been a necessity in fitting these lenses. These trial lenses have a steep central base curve to permit the bulging of the cone and a much flatter peripheral curve. Ten lenses make up the trial set, extending from a central curve of 48.00 to 60.00 diopters, with increasing sagittal depth to accommodate an increasingly projecting cone (Table 16.3). There is a range of dioptric powers in the set to approximate normalcy for the average keratoconus patient. From the trial set, a lens is selected that has either a slight central touch or a slight vaulting at the apex.

Newer versions of the Soper design keratoconus lens with small modifications are available. The most current lens design is the Rose "K" design by Dr. Paul Rose of New Zealand. The design provides a smaller central optic area to fit over the cone with rapid flattening of the midperipheral curvature. The peripheral lens design consists of a series of computer-controlled curves to form an aspheric edge.

A global licensing agreement with UK-based UltraVision CLPL to market and sell KeraSoft soft contact lenses throughout the world, through the network of Bausch & Lomb laboratory channel partners, was announced in 2011. KeraSoft lenses, which have been awarded the UK's Queen's Award for Enterprise and Innovation, are a patented combination of the latest technologies in soft and silicone hydrogel materials using geometries from complex mathematics to offer comfortable wear and excellent vision. KeraSoft patented technology allows for custom-made contact lenses for irregular corneas and keratoconus.

The Boston Foundation for Sight can work with practitioners on difficult or advanced keratoconus cases and offers its prosthetic replacement of the ocular surface ecosystem (PROSE), which uses FDA-approved custom-made prosthetic devices to replace or support impaired ocular surface system functions that protect and enable vision. Information on PROSE is available on the Boston Foundation for Sight website (bostonsight.org).

Table 16.3 Soper cone diagnostic lens set

Sagittal depth (mm)	CPC	Power	Lens diameter (mm)	Thickness (mm)	Diameter of CPC (mm)
0.68	48/45	−4.50	7.5	0.10	6.0
0.73	52/45	−8.50	7.5	0.10	6.0
0.80	56/45	−12.50	7.5	0.10	6.0
0.87	60/45	−16.50	7.5	0.10	6.0
1.00	52/45	−8.50	8.5	0.10	7.0
1.12	56/45	−12.50	8.5	0.10	7.0
1.22	60.45	−16.50	8.5	0.10	7.0
1.37	52/45	−8.50	9.5	0.10	8.0
1.52	56/45	−12.50	9.5	0.10	8.0
1.67	60.45	−16.50	9.5	0.10	8.0
(Optional)	52/43	−8.50	8.5	0.10	7.0
	64/45	−20.00	8.5	0.10	7.0

Trial lens fitting

In the early phase of keratoconus, *K* readings are a guide to selecting a lens. As the condition develops, the mire image becomes irregular and the cone becomes steeper than 50.00 diopters so that the radius of curvature cannot be determined by ordinary keratometry. The only alternative is to fit the patient by diagnostic trial lens and fluorescein assessment.

The range of the keratometer can be extended to 61.00 diopters with an auxiliary +1.25 diopter lens. However, because of the disordered mires, problems in fixation and optic defects in the system, the results merely serve as a guide to trial lens selection. Fixation can be improved by using the viewing light of the topogometer; however, topography of the cornea provides the best making of the cornea to aid in keratoconus fitting.

A good fit should have a central touch of 2 to 3 mm centrally with a thin band of touch at the lens periphery, as determined by the fluorescein test. The three-point touch adds to the stability of the lens on the cornea and distributes the weight of the lens not only over the apex but also over other bearing areas. The peripheral touch area corresponds to the zone of the intermediate curve. The initial lens selected, using the *K* readings as a guide, should have a base curve flatter than *K*. Then, by using the fluorescein test, the examiner exchanges the lens until one is found that results in slight apical touch of 2 to 3 mm or 1 to 4 mm flatter than *K*. A light apical touch is desirable so that the lens can function as a pressure bandage on the thin, central, corneal apex (Figure 16.12). Overrefraction is then performed to arrive at the correct power.

ROLE OF CORNEAL TOPOGRAPHY

Contact lens fitting may be improved with the use of corneal topography. Corneal topography is covered in more depth in Chapter 40.

Piggyback and hybrid lenses

Piggyback lenses were introduced by Dr. Joseph Baldone for patients with irregular corneal astigmatism or keratoconus who could not tolerate a rigid lens. They consist of a soft lens carrier for comfort, with a rigid lens riding in the soft lens to add definition. The soft lenses have been modified to provide a donut groove. The diameter and wall height of the groove can be varied according to the needs of the patient. The following rules for fitting are simple:

1. Always evaluate the piggyback lens with the rigid lens in place.
2. Use the same disinfectant and storage solutions for both lenses.
3. The groove diameter when available should be 0.2 mm larger than the diameter of the rigid lens being used.

The Softperm lens was a successor to the Saturn II lens. It had a base curve of 7.1 to 8.1 mm. The lens was 14.3 mm in diameter and ranges from +6 to −13. This is used in contact lens management of keratoconus. The Softperm lens consisted of a hard styrene lens core or central button supported by a soft hydrogel lens skirt. The rigid lens button provides a clear, regular optical surface to yield

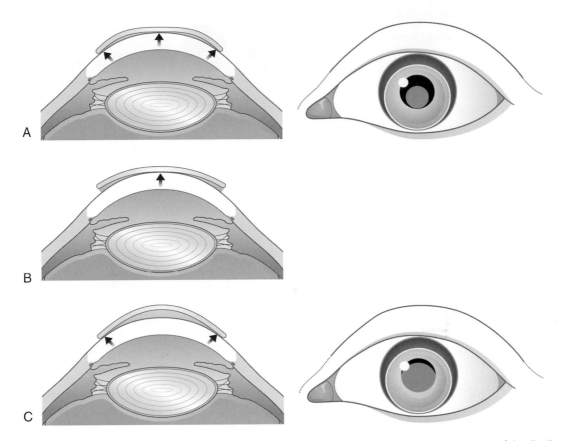

Figure 16.12 (A) Three-point fit. Apical touch to the cone plus peripheral touch. Ideal for keratoconus because of the distribution of weight of the lens. (B) Flat fit. Apical touch but poor centration because of rocking on the corneal cap and edge stand-off. (C) Steep fit. Two-point touch with an air bubble between the lens and the cone. The apical cone is cleared.
(From Stein HA, Slatt BJ, Stein RM. Fitting guide for rigid and soft contact lenses: a practical approach. 4th ed. St Louis: Mosby; 2002.)

good vision, and the soft lens flange gives the patient stability and comfort. With a keratoconus patient, in whom the shape and position of the cone button are unpredictable, stability of the lens fit is vital and use of the Softperm and Saturn II lenses has been discontinued. Clearkone Synerge hybrid lenses series are now produced. These lenses have higher *DK* values, have wider range or power availability, and have variety in the skirt curvature design. A broader range of irregular corneas are fitted with the SynergEyes lenses.

Thick-set lenses

For early to moderate keratoconus patients, Softk and Softk toric lenses have proven to be effective in correcting corneal irregularity. They are available in B-C 7.30 to 8.20 mm, with a diameter of 14.2 mm and water content of 67% with xylofilcon A material.

Bifocal contact lenses

Before fitting a patient with bifocal lenses, the practitioner would be wise to explore alternative solutions to the problem of presbyopia (Box 16.1). In early presbyopia the patient, particularly the hyperope, may be sufficiently able to accommodate with single-vision contact lenses.

However, some practitioners will put more plus in one or both lenses so that although distance vision is slightly blurred, the patient is still able to read at near. In addition to these methods, many patients are content to wear auxiliary spectacles for reading over their contact lenses. This is by far the simplest solution to the problem if the patient is not concerned with the cosmetic disadvantage of glasses.

Bifocal contact lenses are designed in the following two ways:

1. Those that provide alternating vision so the lens moves and permits the individual to see at times

Box 16.1 **Methods of fitting a presbyopic patient**

1. Reading glasses over contact lenses
2. Monovision
3. Bifocal contact lenses
   a. Segmented bifocal
   b. Annular bifocal
   c. Aspheric bifocal (Figure 16.13A)
   d. Diffractive bifocal (see Figure 16.13B)

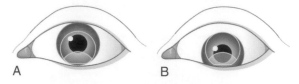

Figure 16.14 Action of a contact bifocal lens. (A) Vision through the distant portion. (B) The bifocal segment is pushed up for reading.
(From Stein HA, Slatt BJ, Stein RM. Fitting guide for rigid and soft contact lenses: a practical approach. 4th ed. St Louis: Mosby; 2002.)

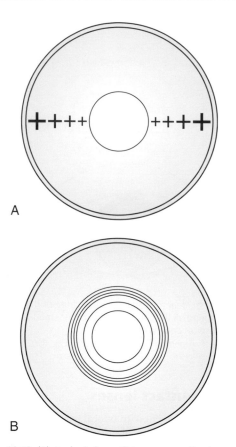

Figure 16.13 (A) Aspheric lens. Distance correction in center, increasing plus power toward the periphery. (B) Diffractive lens. Eschellettes in center provide the "add" for near vision.
(From Stein HA, Freeman MI, Stein RM. Contact lens fundamentals and clinical use. Thorofare, NJ: Slack Publishing; 1997.)

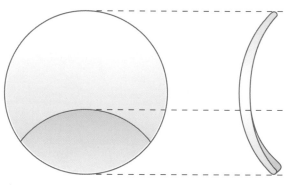

Figure 16.15 Fused bifocal lens.
(From Stein HA, Slatt BJ, Stein RM. Fitting guide for rigid and soft contact lenses: a practical approach. 4th ed. St Louis: Mosby; 2002.)

The simultaneous bifocal lenses have been designed in various ways. Most popular are those lenses in which the central optical zone of the lens contains the distance prescription and an outer peripheral ring contains the near prescription. This is called an *annular bifocal*. The lenses fit loosely, so the lower lid pushes the lens up to the reading portion when the eye looks down (Figure 16.16).

Another method is to construct the lens with the reading prescription in the center and the distance prescription in the outer ring. This is the central add type of bifocal contact lenses made by various manufacturers (Figure 16.17).

Alternating bifocals have been designed similar to the standard spectacle bifocal, with a stronger dioptric power segment below. These lenses must have a prism ballast or truncation to weight the lenses and prevent rotation. The segments on these bifocal contact lenses may be either fused or in one piece (Figure 16.18).

Of recent origin is a type of aspheric one-piece contact lens that provides a distance correction at the center, a reading correction off center, and an intermediate correction at midway points. This is available in both a soft lens and a rigid lens (variable focal lens; VFL) design (Figure 16.19).

The other soft lenses of multifocal designs are the reverse type of aspheric lenses such as the PS 45 and Unilens. These designs combine the maximum prescription in the center of the lens with progressively more minus as you move

through the distance portion and at other times through the reading portion
2. Those that provide simultaneous vision so the individual selects either distant or near vision

In principle, with the alternating design (RGP), when a patient looks down to read, the lower lid edge pushes up the near vision area of the contact so that it overlies the pupil (Figures 16.14 and 16.15).

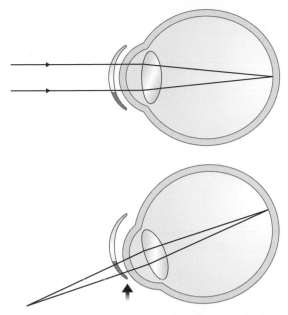

Figure 16.16 Bifocal contact lens. When the eye looks down, the lower eyelid moves the lens up to the reading position.

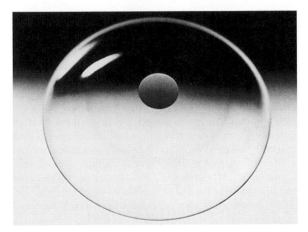

Figure 16.17 Central add bifocal contact lens.

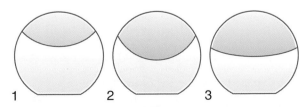

Figure 16.18 Variations in design of one-piece bifocal lens. 1, Standard lens design; 2, concave lens design: this lens affords greater side-to-side viewing for a near object; 3, flat lens design: this lens affords a wider sweep for distance vision. *(From Stein HA, Slatt BJ, Stein RM. Fitting guide for rigid and soft contact lenses: a practical approach. 4th ed. St Louis: Mosby; 2002.)*

away from the center. This helps to eliminate peripheral distortion at a distance, especially under low illumination.

All bifocal lenses are affected by ambient light. The most affected are those with either a central distance optical zone surrounded by a collarette of reading prescription or the opposite type in which the reading portion is central (Figure 16.20). Success in fitting a presbyope depends on the following conditions:

1. Suitable patient screening
2. Understanding of the strengths of each type of lens
3. Using the strengths of each lens to the best advantage for a particular patient
4. Good patient education and motivation
5. Enthusiasm of the fitter
6. An increased rate of success with the experience of the fitter

With well-motivated patients and knowledgeable, experienced, and enthusiastic fitters, the rate of success can be as high as 90%. It is recommended to carefully follow the manufacturer's fitting guide for their specific bifocal contact lens. Many companies provide fitting consultation services that can be very helpful to the practitioner.

Research since 1990 has been directed toward the aging baby-boomer population. The result is an explosion of bifocals, both soft and rigid, addressing this age group. Progressive-add designs are available with increased reading power. The Essential rigid bifocal from Blanchard (Figure 16.21) is an example, although most companies have their own version. The bifocal lenses of today have high success rates. With more designs on the way, fitting will be easier for both patient and practitioner. Bifocal contact lenses are available in a disposable replacement modality from a number of manufacturers including Bausch & Lomb (Soflens Multifocal, Pervasion multifocal), Johnson & Johnson Vision Care (Acuvue Oasys for presbyopia), and Alcon (Air optic multifocal). Toric multifocal soft contact lenses are manufactured by numerous companies. With changes in the field occurring quickly, practitioners are advised to review often a quality manufacturer's reference guide as a resource to available designs and materials. Some of these lenses are Essential soft toric multifocal by Blanchard, and Proclear topic multifocal by CooperVision.

Magnification with contact lenses

Patients with low visual acuity may benefit from contact lenses for two reasons. First, many visual defects may be a result of small corneal scars, which produce areas of irregular astigmatism. Rigid contact lenses overcome these surface irregularities of the cornea by providing a smooth tear film interface, which eliminates irregularities and can significantly improve vision. Second, visual improvement may be achieved by a telescopic system devised by a combination of a minus contact lens with high-plus glasses, which produces a magnified retinal image. This is the same

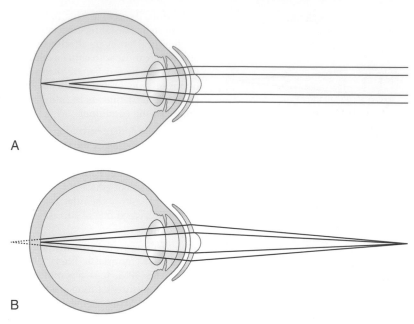

A

B

Figure 16.19 (A) Central add bifocal contact lens. Light from distant objects focuses on the retina; light from near objects is ignored. (B) Light from near objects focuses on the retina; light from distant objects is ignored.

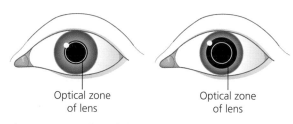

Optical zone of lens

Optical zone of lens

Figure 16.20 Ambient lighting affects the size of the pupil. A large dilated pupil may result in ghosting.

system found in standard opera glasses, which magnify four, five, six, and even seven times. The greater the magnification, however, the narrower is the field of vision, as can be appreciated when one looks through strong field glasses.

Contact lens combination with spectacles, such as a −30.00 diopter contact lens and a +20.00 diopter spectacle lens, provides a magnification of × 1.5 when there is 17-mm separation between the contact lens and spectacles. Often this magnification is a great help to the patient with markedly reduced vision. It certainly is a more pleasant and cosmetically better method than wearing only thick telescopic lenses. It is optically advantageous as well because in addition to the limited field of vision resulting from telescopic lenses, each time the patient turns his or her head there is a rapid movement of the visual field in the opposite direction. Also, many of the other disadvantages of magnification that appear with the use of thick telescopic lenses

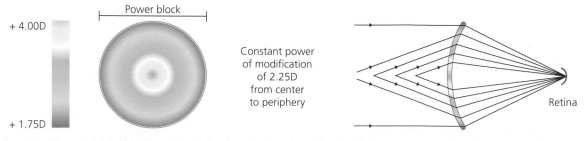

+ 4.00D

Power block

Constant power of modification of 2.25D from center to periphery

Retina

+ 1.75D

Figure 16.21 Essential rigid gas-permeable bifocal contact lens from Blanchard. *(Courtesy of Blanchard Contact Lens, Inc.)*

(such as making objects appear closer than they actually are) are removed or diminished through the use of contact lenses in combination with spectacles.

Orthokeratology

Orthokeratology is the reshaping of the cornea with rigid contact lenses for the correction of low myopia and astigmatism. The practice involves fitting a series of gradually flattening rigid lenses in progressive stages to reshape the cornea to a point where the myopia is corrected. When fitting lenses for orthokeratology, the first lens is fit approximately 1.00 diopter flatter than the flattest corneal curve. After a suitable wear time, varying from 2 to 8 weeks, the cornea should assume a flatter configuration across the apex. Subsequent lens fitting uses progressively flatter lenses to achieve the desired correction. Retainer contact lenses are then worn as necessary to stabilize and maintain the cornea's newly acquired shape. Initially, conventional design rigid lenses were used. Success rates were modest with these lenses because some corneas were unresponsive and some patients found orthokeratology to be uncomfortable.

Orthokeratology has undergone a recent resurgence fueled by a number of developments. New high-*DK* extended-wear rigid lenses are preferable to older lower-*DK* lenses for reshaping and contouring the cornea. Reverse geometry lens designs, initially conceived for the post-photorefractive keratotomy (PRK) cornea, have proven effective in orthokeratology. In addition, computerized corneal topography systems have been useful for fitting and monitoring the progressive reshaping of the cornea.

Numerous labs are investigating reverse geometry ortho-*K* designs for US Food and Drug Administration (FDA) approval. The FDA has approved the Contex OK lens for daily-wear orthokeratology. Although the FDA has warned that overnight ortho-*K* lens wear is risky, orthokeratology is permissible if the RGP extended-wear lens materials and reverse geometry lens design are specified. Some practitioners view orthokeratology as a nonsurgical alternative to excimer laser PRK for low myopia and astigmatism. Recent adverse situations have occurred with abrasions and corneal ulcers and have brought bad publicity to the technique of orthokeratology.

Corneal refractive therapy

This RGP lens design is based on the corneal topography for low myopes. The lens is used overnight to flatten the corneal surface by partial pushing of the epithelial cells to the periphery.

Corneal refractive therapy (CRT) is an FDA-approved contact lens corneal reshaping system used to reduce or temporarily correct myopia. The method was approved in June 2002 by the FDA for correction of up to −6.00 diopters of myopia with up to −1.75 diopters of cylinder. The *term corneal refractive therapy* is an FDA-approved indication and is in the public domain, whereas the acronym CRT is a registered trademark of Paragon Vision Sciences. CRT describes a method of correction for myopia by overnight wear of specially designed gas-permeable lenses that redistribute and compress the corneal epithelium such that central epithelial thickness is decreased and peripheral epithelial thickness is increased. The recognition of the epithelium results in redistribution of the refractive power of the cornea. The process is reversible when contact lens wear is discontinued.

The CRT process is achieved by the use of a specially designed 10.5-mm diameter contact lens with a central optic treatment zone, a midperipheral return zone and a peripheral landing zone. The four objectives in fitting contact lenses for corneal refractive therapy are to provide:

1. A base curve that will reshape the cornea to produce emmetropia or low hyperopia
2. Precise positioning of the base curve by configuration of the return zone depth
3. A landing zone that is tangential to the cornea in the midperiphery
4. Proper centration by coordination of the return zone depth, the landing zone angle and the overall diameter of the lens

Lens selection is guided by the patient's refraction, corneal curvature measurements, and confirmation of lens fit by evaluation of the fluorescein pattern beneath the contact lens. CRT is different from traditional orthokeratology in that refractive change is induced by reshaping of the corneal epithelium rather than the corneal stromal pattern.

Bandage lenses

Bandage lenses are soft contact lenses used for therapeutic purposes to enhance epithelial regeneration and corneal healing. They should provide sufficient oxygenation to the cornea to disturb corneal physiology only minimally. In addition, bandage lenses provide ocular comfort and act to protect the cornea from eyelids, eyelashes, and environmental conditions.

Therapeutic (bandage) lenses:

- Promote healing
- Provide splinting over lacerations, perforations, and wound leaks
- Provide comfort
- Protect the eye
- Improve corneal architecture and vision
- Act as a drug reservoir

Bandage lenses may be made of the following materials:

- Thin or high-water HEMA
- Silicone
- Collagen (12-, 24-, or 6-week lenses)
- Silicone hydrogel

The thickness of the lens affects the oxygen permeability. The thinner the lens, the greater is its oxygen permeability.

Bausch & Lomb pioneered the Plano T series, which has a water content of 38%. Since then, numerous other lenses have become available that provide greater oxygen permeability. Disposable replacement lenses are often used because they allow extended wear with good oxygen permeability. Focus Night & Day (ALCON), and Purevision (Bausch & Lomb) have very high *DK*. Collagen lenses that biodisintegrate in 24 to 48 hours or in 6 weeks provide good oxygen permeability.

MANUFACTURING AND MODIFICATION

RGP contact lens practitioners fall into three categories:

1. Those who make their own contact lenses from blanks
2. Those who order a finished lens or fit from an inventory system and then modify it depending on the fit and the requirements
3. Those who order finished lenses and return them to the laboratory for modification

An understanding of what can and cannot be done to RGP contact lenses is mandatory for a full understanding of contact lens technology. The ophthalmic assistant is well advised to spend some time in a contact lens laboratory, grinding and modifying at least a few lenses (Figure 16.22).

Today the majority of rigid contact lenses are lathe cut, rather than molded, in the following manner:

1. Buttons are cut from a rod of plastic that looks like a curtain rod.
2. The inside curve is then cut and polished. In this stage the lens is referred to as a semifinished blank.
3. The front surface is then cut and polished. This is now referred to as an uncut lens.
4. Intermediate and peripheral curves are applied.
5. The edge is then finished. This is now a completed lens.

Modifications of finished lenses

Note that many of the newer gas-permeable designs are not able to be modified in-office.

Diameter reduction

The diameter of a rigid lens can be reduced by means of a razor blade, knife, file, emery board, or sandpaper. The lens is mounted, concave side up, on a rotating spindle and the blade of the razor or knife is rocked back and forth on the edge. One must not allow the lens to overheat or scratch the front of the lens. The file and emery board are used mainly for small reductions in lens diameter. When a lens has been reduced, the intermediate peripheral curves and the edges must be applied and blended.

Blending (Figure 16.23)

Blending is done to smooth out the junction between the optic zone and the intermediate peripheral curve and between the intermediate and peripheral curves. When the transition zones are blended, a tool having a radius of curvature halfway between one curve and the next is used. The lens is held by a suction cup and rotated on the tool in the opposite direction to the tool rotation.

Edge shaping

If a lens has a secondary curve but no bevel, some edge shaping is usually necessary. The edge should be smoothly rounded by means of a file or razor blade. If the edge is relatively thick, it may be made thinner by means of a front surface bevel. Once the edge has been shaped, it is polished by means of a rag wheel, a felt disc, or a sponge.

Power change

Velveteen and a drum tool are used. The velveteen is first thoroughly soaked in water and then pulled over the sides

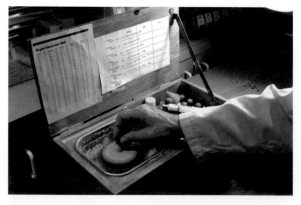

Figure 16.22 Modification unit for rigid contact lenses.

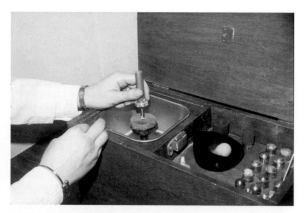

Figure 16.23 Polishing RGP contact lens.

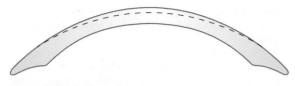

Figure 16.24 Adding minus power.
(From Stein HA, Slatt BJ, Stein RM. Fitting guide for rigid and soft contact lenses: a practical approach. 4th ed. St Louis: Mosby; 2002.)

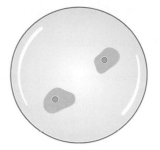

Figure 16.25 Fenestrations reduce corneal edema in a 1- or 2-mm zone around the aperture.
(From Stein HA, Slatt BJ, Stein RM. Fitting guide for rigid and soft contact lenses: a practical approach. 4th ed. St Louis: Mosby; 2002.)

of a drum tool and fastened tightly with rubber bands. A depression is formed in the tool. The lens is held by means of a brass lens holder or suction cup. To add plus power, the lens is held so that its convex surface is against the velveteen and is exactly centered on the tool. To add minus power, the lens is held so that the convex surface is against the velveteen at the outer edge of the tool. In either case the lens is rotated once or twice a full 360 degrees against the rotation of the tool (Figure 16.24).

Peripheral curve

A peripheral curve can be applied by the use of a tool having a radius of curvature of 12.25, 11.5, 10.5, or 9.5 mm. The lens is carefully mounted on the lens block so that it is not at an angle, or it is fixed by means of double-sided tape. The block is held perpendicular to the tool, concave side down, by a sharp-pointed pencil acting as a spindle. The polishing agent (such as X-Pal) is then applied to the surface of the radius tool. The lens is held so that the concave surface rests lightly against the tool, revolving at about 1500 rpm; the entire edge of the lens must touch the tool at the same time. Equal pressure should be exerted on all meridians of the lens.

Fenestration of rigid lenses

Small holes drilled through a contact lens permit better tear exchange and consequently better oxygenation of the cornea. This is also a remedy for moderately tight contact lenses. Practitioners vary as to whether one or several holes should be used or whether the lens should be completely redesigned. In any event, these holes should be no larger than 0.5 mm and the interior walls must be highly polished to prevent clogging with secretions and irritation to the cornea. The fenestrations, although they do not interfere optically, do have a tendency to allow warpage of a lens and to weaken its structure. They should lie over the area of corneal edema because they provide only a small amount of increased respiration to a very limited underlying area of the cornea (Figure 16.25).

Removing scratches

Care must be exercised when removing scratches from a rigid contact lens so as not to ruin its optics. In many cases a new lens is preferred to trying to remove scratches. When scratches are removed from the front surface of a lens, the lens is held with a suction cup or spindle against the velveteen-covered drum while the drum is rotated. As in other modifications of contact lenses, X-Pal is the polishing compound used.

Removing scratches from the inside (base curve) of a lens can be done by use of a convex-shaped tool and X-Pal as the polishing compound. The best method is to use a sponge tool to polish the concave side of the lens.

GAS-PERMEABLE LENSES

The gas-permeable polymer is a huge step forward in lens technology. The contact lens industry has not witnessed such an upheaval because the soft hydrogel lens was introduced.

Gas-permeable lenses are made from materials that permit oxygen and carbon dioxide to diffuse through the plastic. These materials also wet more easily than the ordinary rigid lens and thus permit the tears to flow better under them.

Gas-permeable lenses have become well established in clinical practice. They have replaced the conventional polymethyl methacrylate (PMMA) lenses because they offer all the advantages of a rigid lens but have fewer complications. Gas-permeable lenses are also safer and more comfortable than rigid lenses.

The scope of gas-permeable materials is widening. The materials available to date include the following:

1. Cellulose acetate butyrate (CAB)
2. Silicone
3. Combinations of various materials, which include:
   - silicone-PMMA (silicone acrylates)
   - PMMA-silicone-CAB
   - combinations of fluorocarbon-PMMA-silicone
4. Polystyrene

317

The attractive feature of these lenses is their oxygen permeability, expressed as *DK*.

$$\text{Oxygen transmissibility} = DK/T$$

where:

$D =$ the diffusion coefficient for oxygen movement in any substance

$K =$ the solubility constant for oxygen in that substance

$T =$ the thickness of the center of the lens

(Sometimes the letter L is used for thickness: DK/L.)

The oxygen permeability varies from lens to lens and according to the method used for measuring this factor. The silicone combinations, mixed with PMMA, have a high rating. The lenses with the highest oxygen permeability are those made of pure fluorocarbon or combinations of fluorocarbon and other proven contact lens materials.

The lens thickness of any given material must also be considered. The thicker the lens, the less permeable it is. Thus a lens that is made 0.1 mm thick has much greater permeability than one that is made for aphakia and is 0.5 mm thick.

Rigid lenses have been developed with a *DK* value of 140 and greater. This means greater freedom from the complications of corneal hypoxia, which permits the application of such high-*DK* lenses for extended wear. High-*DK* lenses are the lenses of choice for postcorneal grafts and keratoconus fitting (Table 16.4).

Table 16.4 Silicone-acrylate and fluorosilicone-acrylate data for rigid gas-permeable lenses

Lens name	Material	DK	Wetting angle
Boston II	Itafocon A (SA)	18.0	20
Boston IV	Itafocon B (SA)	26.0	17
Boston 7	Satafocon A (FSA)	73.0	33
Boston ES	Enflufocon A (FSA)	36.0	52
Boston EO	Enflufocon B (FSA)	82.0	49
Boston RXD	Itabisfluorofocon A	45.0	39
Boston Equalens	Itafluorofocon A (FSA)	71.0	26
Boston XO	Hexafocon A (FSA)	140.0	49
Boston EO Envision	Enflufocon B (FSA)	82.0	33
Boston Multivision	Enflufocon A (FSA)	31.0	n/a
Paragon HDS	Paflufocon B (FSA)	58.0	14.7
Paragon Thin	Paflufocon C (FSA)	29.0	12.8
Fluoroperm 30	Paflufocon C	30.0	12.8
Fluoroperm 60	Paflufocon B	60.0	14.7
Fluoroperm 92	Paflufocon A	92.0	16
Fluoroperm 151	Paflufocon A	151.0	42.0
Fluorex 700	Fluisifocon A	70.0	15.3
Latitude Multifocal	Telefocon B	43.5	n/a
Optacryl 60	Kolfolcon A	18.0	<25.0
Optimum Extra	Roflufocon C	100.0	<23.0
SGP II	Telefocon B	43.5	<30
Tyro-97	Hofocon A	97.0	23
PMMA		0.0	n/a

DK, diffusion coefficient for oxygen movement in lens material and the solubility coefficient of oxygen in the material; *FSA*, fluorosilicone acrylate; *PMMA*, polymethyl methacrylate; *SA*, silicone acrylate

Extended-wear rigid lenses

With higher *DK* values, the oxygen permeability of these lenses is sufficient to maintain corneal physiologic needs so that overnight wear is possible.

These lenses can be worn for extended periods, up to 2 weeks. Ptosis, variable vision, and lack of tolerance have been reported with RGP lenses, but not in alarming proportions.

Silicone-PMMA material

With the introduction of blends of material, the most popular has been the silicone-PMMA material often referred to as silicone acrylates. PMMA provides wetting, stability, and thinness; silicone provides oxygen permeability.

The better physiologic tolerance of these new plastics is a function not only of greater permeability but also of thermal conductivity. This is the ability of the plastic to allow heat to be dissipated through the lens so that the cornea has reduced oxygen demand. Clinically the role of heat in lens comfort is seen with skiers. Most skiers find their rigid lenses work best on the hill when temperatures are low and the oxygen demands of the cornea are reduced. Hot, aired office buildings are the worst for lens tolerance because they increase corneal oxygen demand.

Silicone-PMMA lenses are fitted 0.1 to 0.3 mm flatter than the flattest corneal meridian. This allows the lens to ride high under the upper lid. The decrease or elimination of lid impact between the edge of the lid and the edge of the lens accounts for the excellent comfort that these lenses offer. These lenses have a diameter from 8.5 to 9.5 mm, with occasionally large 11-mm lenses being prescribed.

The higher the silicone content, the higher is the permeability of these combination lenses. However, a higher silicone content also means a higher susceptibility to lipid and waxy deposits forming on their surface and a greater fragility of the lenses.

The silicone-acrylate material is the benchmark standard lens today (Box 16.2). In general, the advantages of silicone-based combinations include the following:

- Easier and faster adaptation
- Greater comfort
- Safety: oxygen deprivation of the cornea is a prime cause of PMMA complications, which include spectacle blur, change in the shape of the cornea, and lack of full-day tolerance. The acute oxygen deprivation resulting from hypoxia (the so-called *overwearing syndrome*) is extremely rare with gas-permeable lenses
- Wider application: because of their large size they are centered more easily than PMMA lenses. They are used to advantage in keratoconus, irregular corneal astigmatism, aphakia, and large degrees of corneal astigmatism from 3.00 to 5.00 diopters
- Better vision: the larger lens diameter results in a larger optic zone diameter (8.4–9.5 mm). This reduces glare from lights at night despite the healthy movement of the lens with blinking

Silicone-based combinations are a solution for chronic corneal edema in former rigid lens wearers. These lenses become a practical solution to refitting warped corneas from previously poorly fitting rigid lenses. They increase the wearing time of rigid lens wearers who can wear conventional lenses for short periods. They eliminate spectacle blur in rigid lens wearers. They are excellent for corneas with marginal function, such as with recurrent viral keratitis.

The drawbacks to these lenses include the following.

1. There is greater fragility than PMMA, which results in a tendency to chip or scratch. This is due largely to softness of the plastic.
2. There is a need for special lens solutions that are specific for these lenses to reduce the wetting angle and provide comfort.

Box 16.2 **Advantages and disadvantages of silicone-acrylate lenses**

Advantages	Disadvantages
Greater oxygen transmission	Softer than PMMA
Surface tension 40% higher than PMMA	Scratches and chips easily
Increased comfort and wearing time. Larger diameters mean a larger optic zone, which reduces annoying flare	Greater tendency to flex or warp than PMMA
Reduced spectacle blur	Deposit formation occurs
Design flexibility that allows for a large or small diameter in spherical or aspherical profiles	
Stable durable material	
Good wetting capability	

PMMA, Polymethyl methacrylate.

3. Special compounds such as X-Pal are required for modifying these lenses. For instance, these lenses must not be polished with compounds containing ammonia. Also they cannot be exposed to alcohols, esters, ketones, and chlorinated hydrocarbons because the material is more sensitive to them.

4. There is an increase in the frequency and severity of 3 and 9 o'clock staining. This is usually a result of thick edges and resolves itself when the edge profile is reduced to 0.06 mm or the lens is made larger.

Cellulose acetate butyrate

CAB was developed for photography by Eastman Kodak because it was less flammable than other materials. Although this plastic was created in 1938, it was not used for lenses until 1974.

The CAB lenses are fitted more steeply than conventional lenses because the material tends to flatten because of softness or even molding by the surface of the cornea. It is rarely used today because newer polymers have superseded it.

Fluorosilicone-acrylate lenses

The newest generation of RGP lenses comprises those that contain some form of fluorocarbon similar to the Teflon used in frying pans. The fluorocarbon component greatly increases the oxygen transmissibility of silicone-acrylate material. The lenses are lighter in weight, and an ultraviolet blocker may be added. Even the earliest fluorosilicone-acrylate (FSA)-type lenses have about double the DK/L of most silicone acrylates. Virtually all signs of clinical hypoxia are eliminated, thus increasing the extended-wear potential of rigid lenses. Deposit resistance is greater than any other soft or rigid lenses as a result of the Teflon or nonstick effect of the fluorocarbon (Box 16.3). The FSA lens design has flexibility that permits

---

Box 16.3 Advantages and disadvantages of fluorosilicone-acrylate lenses

Advantages	Disadvantages
High oxygen permeability	More flexible than SA
High deposit resistance	More brittle than SA
In-office adjustments possible	Glued-on syndrome may
Low wetting angle	occur (lens adhesion)
Lighter in weight than SA or PMMA	

PMMA, Polymethyl methacrylate; *SA,* silicone-acrylate.

---

larger or smaller diameters in both spherical and aspherical profiles.

Fitting FSA lenses usually requires a flatter base curve selection than when fitting silicone-acrylate materials. This compensates better for corneal cylinder correction and reduces the risk of "gluing on" or adhesion of the lens. (See Chapter 15 for additional information on FSA lenses.)

Pure fluorocarbon lenses

A pure fluorocarbon lens that contains no silicone or PMMA has been developed and manufactured by 3 M. The material has an extremely high DK, in the realm of 90. It is not brittle and is highly scratch-resistant.

HYDROGEL TINTED CONTACT LENSES

Tinted contact lenses have their role in many eye conditions. Their use over scarred corneas has been helpful in rehabilitating the individual and making the eye look cosmetically perfect. Tinted contact lenses have also had some use in patients with heterochromia. One lens is tinted to match the fellow eye. Tints may be used for cosmetic purposes or to make them easier to locate. Therapeutic applications of tinted lenses include scarred or opaque corneas, iris irregularities, iris coloboma, iridectomies, aniridia (absence of iris), fixed dilated pupil, photosensitivity resulting from albinism, and amblyopia.

We have treated two National Hockey League players who had eye injuries with widely dilated pupils and photophobia and who required tinted lenses. In one case, a star forward with the Chicago Blackhawks had an eye injury with a dilated fixed pupil that finally responded to diluted 1/64% pilocarpine. This caused an induced myopia of −6.00 diopters and he was unable to play hockey, a major disability. Because of the extreme glare reflecting from the ice, a very dark contact lens was provided and he is now able to play again.

Color enhancement lenses have been very popular. They make blue eyes bluer and green eyes greener. A retrospective study in patients we have fitted showed that aqua was preferred by 60%, green by 20%, blue by 15%, and the other colors by 5%. Also, *handling* tints were often used in the lenses of many of our patients for ease of identification.

Another use for cosmetic lenses is to alter the color of the eye, so that a brown-eyed patient can be made blue-eyed. CooperVision, Alcon, J&J, and the Narcissus Medical Foundation have good lenses in this area. Pupil size is very important because ambient light can have a major influence on the "tunnel vision" effect created by these lenses.

These color-altering lenses are also used for colobomas of the iris, where an opaque lens with a clear center can often give a very visually pleasing appearance.

The iris print method consists of placing an iris image on a dome of clear HEMA, producing an opaque tint. A dot matrix is placed on the front surface of the contact lens to alter the iris color of the wearer. The Toya Lens Company and CIBA Vision make a custom-designed tinted lens that is a combination of known and custom tinting. A sandwich process is involved that requires hand-painted or iris-printed images on HEMA plus lamination.

What affects a tint? Tints are often affected by noxious vapors and chemical agents; they may also be affected by aging. Some cleaning agents will bleach some lenses. Leaching of the lens dye out of the lens may be a problem with continual wear. Some companies have minimized this effect by burying the material deep in the lens or directly into the buttons before cutting.

Technology in contact lenses is moving forward. Blood glucose sensors may be introduced into contact lenses that may detect high and low sugars and may be of value in patients requiring a caregiver. Lenses may be impregnated with a sensor in the periphery of the contact lens to detect a rise in intraocular pressure (IOP). The contact lens as a drug delivery system, developed many years ago, may become a reality in the next decade.

Box 16.4 **Patients recommended for rigid contact lens wear**

1. Previous rigid contact lens wearers
2. Patients requiring sharp visual acuity
3. Patients with significant corneal cylinders over 1 diopter
4. Patients concerned with the cost of lens maintenance, replacement, and care
5. Patients requiring easy insertion and removal techniques
6. Patients with moderately dry eyes

RECOMMENDATIONS FOR SELECTION OF RIGID OR SOFT CONTACT LENSES

In some patients the presence of astigmatism or other conditions makes it difficult to choose between rigid and soft contact lenses. In others, this decision is made based on interaction with the patient. We currently recommend disposable soft contact lenses when the patient is suitable and powers are available. Throw-away soft lenses used on a daily or occasional-wear basis are also now available. Boxes 16.4 and 16.5 list some guidelines for rigid and soft contact lens wearers. Daily disposables come in nearly the same powers as regular disposables.

Box 16.5 **Patients recommended for soft contact lens wear**

1. Failed hard contact lens wearers
2. Intermittent or part-time wearers for social functions
3. Patients with small corneal cylinders desiring more comfort
4. Patients working in high-particle environments
5. Patients participating in sports, particularly body contact sports
6. Patients requiring therapeutic use
7. Specialized areas such as colored soft lenses, iris-changing lenses, and lenses for cosmesis

---

Questions for review and thought

1. When a male patient complains of blurring with his rigid contact lenses while in a movie theater, one physiologic mechanism occurs. How can this symptom be corrected?
2. What causes central corneal edema in a rigid contact lens wearer?
3. A female patient has been wearing rigid lenses successfully for several years, but recently she has been unable to wear them longer than 4 hours. What might be some sources of trouble?
4. What causes 3 and 9 o'clock position staining? How can it be corrected?
5. What is the value of repeat keratometry of contact lens wearers?
6. What is the value of fenestration of rigid contact lenses?
7. Why are keratoconus cases a special fitting problem?
8. If the keratometer cannot read a steep corneal radius, as occurs in keratoconus, how can the range of the keratometer be extended?
9. What types of lenses are available to correct presbyopia?
10. Bifocal lenses present a particular problem in obtaining a small additional reading power in a small lens. How are lenses designed so that the lower eyelids push them up when one looks down to read?
11. What is the principle behind using contact lenses for magnification as an aid for patients with limited vision?
12. What are the advantages and disadvantages of rigid gas-permeable lenses of the fluorocarbonated silicone-acrylate material?

Q Self-evaluation questions

True–false statements

Directions: Indicate whether the statement is true **(T)** or false **(F)**.

1. A thick, heavy plus lens will tend to ride high under the upper lid. **T** or **F**
2. Corneal molding or distortion can be detected by taking keratometric readings at repeat visits. **T** or **F**
3. Keratoconus fitting is the same as any other rigid lens fitting and may be approached in exactly the same manner. **T** or **F**

Missing words

Directions: Write in the missing word in the following sentences:

4. A front curve toric lens is held at its proper axis by means of a _____.
5. Spherical rigid lenses are usually the first choice for high degrees of _____ astigmatism.
6. Some bifocal lenses are fitted _____ so that the lower lid will push the lens up to the line of sight for near vision.

Choice-completion questions

Directions: Select the one best answer in each case.

7. If the keratometer cannot read a steep cornea, as in keratoconus, its range may be increased by which device?
   a. Placido's disc
   b. Soper cone lens
   c. INNS extension disc
   d. Fleischer's ring
   e. Prism ballast
8. To achieve better fitting characteristics with high refractive errors, what is the best design to incorporate into the lens?
   a. Lathe cut
   b. Wide flat peripheral curves
   c. Single cut
   d. Fenestrations
   e. Lenticular
9. What is the basic principle behind fitting high-minus contact lenses and wearing high-plus spectacle lenses over them?
   a. They overcome corneal surface irregularities.
   b. They create a telescopic system.
   c. They narrow the visual field.
   d. They magnify by −1.5.
   e. Cosmetically they are better than telescopic lenses.

A Answers, notes, and explanations

1. **False.** A thick heavy lens such as a high-plus lens tends to ride low because of its weight and the force of the lid on its thinnest portion, the edge. The use of lenticulation reduces the weight and thickness of the lens, thus enhancing its centering characteristics.
2. **True.** K readings taken at repeat visits are an excellent method of monitoring any corneal changes. If the K readings change, it may be important to modify or change the lens.
3. **False.** The cornea in keratoconus usually has a high degree of irregular astigmatism and the keratometer may be of very little value. Moderate to extreme cases may require fitting purely by trial lens evaluation.
4. **Prism ballast.** A front curve toric lens is held at its proper axis by means of a prism ballast. This thicker portion is ground into the lens at the time of manufacture. Gravity will hold the heaviest portion of the lens along the lower lid, stabilizing the cylindric correction.
5. **Corneal.** In general the corneal astigmatism is eliminated by the lens. However, certain fitting problems may indicate the need for a back surface toric lens.
6. **Loosely.** The peripheral ring that holds the near corrections rises slightly while the eye rotates downward, giving the proper alignment for the near vision.
7. **c. INNS extension disc.** The INNS extension disc enables a +1.25 lens to be placed over the keratometer face plate, extending its range of measurement by 9.00 diopters.
8. **e. Lenticular.** The lenticular design reduces thickness and weight of high-power lenses, thus giving better centering, comfort, and vision.
9. **b. They create a telescopic system.** The creation of a telescopic system that produces a magnified retinal image can be of great benefit to the patient with low visual acuity. The lens can overcome the corneal irregularities and thus cause the magnifying effect of the plus spectacles to give better acuity.

Chapter | **17** |

Dry eyes

Dry eyes is a condition in which there is insufficient lubrication of the cornea by a protective tear film layer. Dry eyes is a disorder caused by a tear deficiency or excessive evaporation, which results in damage to the ocular surface and is associated with ocular discomfort. Dry eyes (Lemp, 1995) is sometimes referred to as keratitis sicca or keratoconjunctivitis sicca, which is a common disorder affecting the cornea, bulbar conjunctiva, and inner portion of the lids.

The tear film plays a major role in the healthy integrity of the eye and the cornea for refractive surgery. More than 33 million Americans suffer discomfort from dry eyes. Women are twice as likely as men to develop this disorder, and estrogen supplements may increase dry eyes. Eye makeup may thin the oily layer of the tears.

Dry eyes may be a cornerstone cause of ocular surface-related disorders such as Sjögren's syndrome, persistent epithelial defects, neurotrophic keratopathy, recurrent corneal erosions, superior limbic keratitis, Stevens-Johnson syndrome, ocular pemphigus, and other ocular surface disorders as outlined in Box 17.1. Dry eyes is a fairly common condition caused by many factors and affects millions of people worldwide. It is more common in women and particularly postmenopausal. About 15% to 25% of the population is affected by dryness of the eyes. This increases significantly to 75% to 80% of contact lens wearers and patients immediately after surface laser (photorefractive keratotomy [PRK] or laser-assisted in situ keratomileusis [LASIK]).

THE TEAR FILM

The tear film lipid layer

The tear film lipid layer arises from the shallow reservoir of lipid at the lid margins and is spread onto the tear film with each blink. It has a mean thickness of 42 nm (15–157 nm) and plays a key role in retarding tear evaporation from the exposed ocular surface. Its deepest aspect is composed of polar lipids and some long-chain fatty acids, a few molecules thick, that interface with the aqueous subphase of the tear film. This represents about 5% to 15% of the total lipid composition. Some proteins and glycoproteins, such as lipocalins, lysozyme, and mucin, are thought to be intercalated with the lipid layer and enhance its stability.[25–30]

The aqueous layer

The aqueous layer forms the bulk of the tear film and contains salts and a large range of proteins derived from the lacrimal gland and conjunctiva. Proteins include growth factors such as epidermal growth factor and hepatocyte growth factor, important to the maintenance of the epithelium. There are also defense proteins, such as lysozyme, lactoferrin, surfactant protein-D, and trefoil peptide, concerned with innate immunity, and immunoglobulin (Ig) A, of lacrimal plasma cell origin, involved in adaptive immunity. Levels of these proteins may be decreased in dry eye disorders (DEDs), making the eye more vulnerable to infection. Additional proteins, such as albumin, normally present at low concentration are derived from the plasma and may be increased in DEDs as a result of inflammation caused by an increase in both vascular capillary permeability and that of the surface layer of the conjunctival epithelium.

The mucin layer

The goblet cells of the conjunctiva secrete a gel mucin into the tears, which interacts with the glycocalyx and performs a lubricating function between the lids and globe. This mucin layer may maintain wettability of the ocular surface where the glycocalyx is defective. It also traps shed epithelial cells, inflammatory cells, and debris to form a mucous thread within the lower conjunctival sac.

FUNCTION OF THE TEARS

The tear film has several functions. First, it is vital to the health and integrity of the underlying corneal epithelium. Corneal epithelium is responsible for clarity of vision and eye comfort. The anterior surface of the cornea is covered by the tear film, which is composed of an anterior lipid or oily layer, a middle aqueous or watery layer, and a posterior mucin or mucous layer (Figure 17.1).

The aqueous part of the tears arises from the main lacrimal gland and the accessory lacrimal glands. Drainage of tears works after blinking when tears flow through the lacrimal puncta to the canaliculus, then down to the lacrimal sac and through the nasolacrimal duct to the back of the nose.

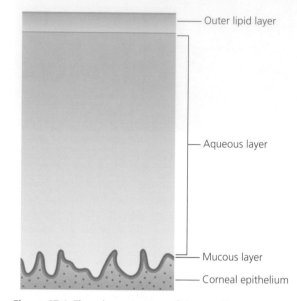

Figure 17.1 Three-layer structure of the tear film.

The optical quality and normal function of the eye for vision depend on an adequate supply of fluid covering the corneal surface

There are some subtypes of tears:

1. **Basal tears.** This is the major portion of tears that lubricate the cornea and protects from dust, bacteria, fumes, and foreign bodies.
2. **Reflex tears.** The eye responds spontaneously to onions, strong fragrances, spicy foods, and other irritants.
3. **Emotional tears.** A response to strong emotions.

TEAR FILM ASSESSMENT

The tear film has several functions (outlined in Box 17.1). The dry eye workup should include items listed in Box 17.2. The tear film is vital to the integrity of the cornea. It not only provides oxygen to the cornea when a contact lens is inserted, but also possesses lysozyme, an antibacterial

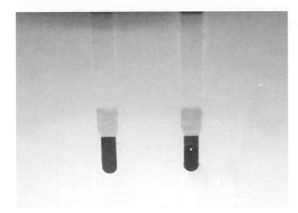

Figure 17.2 Rose bengal test. The red dye stains devitalized areas of cornea and conjunctiva.

(From Stein HS, Slatt BJ, Stein RM et al. Fitting guide for rigid and soft contact lenses: a practical approach. 4th ed. Elsevier Mosby; 2002.)

enzyme that inhibits bacterial proliferation in the eye. Normal tears are produced at a low volume of 1 µL per minute. The water-soluble components include proteins, inorganic salts, glucose, and oxygen. Aqueous tears form the middle layer of the tear film. This component is secreted by the lacrimal glands (Figure 17.2).

The outer layer is a lipid film over the aqueous layer. It is an oily layer secreted by the meibomian glands. Its function is to prevent evaporation of the tear film. Deficiencies in this section of the layer are uncommon. Studies have reported that evaporative dry eye, the most common cause of which is meibomian gland dysfunction, is the most common subtype of dry eye.

The inner layer lying against the corneal epithelium is the mucin film layer obtained from secretions of the goblet cells of the conjunctiva with some contribution from the surface cells of the cornea. Its purpose is to change the corneal epithelial hydrophobic surface to a hydrophilic surface on which aqueous tears can spread. Mucin deficiency can be encountered in such conditions: Stevens-Johnson syndrome, ocular pemphigoid, and alkali burns.

Patients with a tear deficiency are more prone to infections and often cannot be fitted comfortably with contact lenses. Serious problems can be anticipated.

Contamination of the tear film may be induced by rubbing of the eyes with unclean fingers or by consequence of high counts of bacterial skin and conjunctival flora, as found in acne rosacea and other skin disorders.

ROLE OF BLINKING

Poor blinking habits can create many symptoms of dry eyes. The front surface of the cornea becomes misty because of drying and lack of polishing by the lids and tear film, and vision suffers. Such a situation can create mild symptoms of burning and photophobia or create minor discomfort and an uncomfortable feeling when wearing a contact lens.

An equally disturbing event occurs when a patient does not have a full and upward Bell's response. In such a person, the eyes do not roll up and out; instead, they may not move or actually roll slightly downward. If the lids are not totally closed with sleep, the exposed corneas may show signs of dryness and desiccation. Such a person frequently wakes up in the morning with grittiness in the eyes. Poor blinkers and people with a poor Bell's response should not wear rigid lenses that require a good tear film.

A normal blink is executed by the pretarsal fibers of the orbicularis muscle. It is an automatic reflex movement. It should be distinguished from voluntary lid closure, which requires the action of the pretarsal, preseptal, and orbital segments of the orbicularis muscle. The latter is a much stronger action and is accompanied by Bell's phenomenon. Patients with blinking problems are frequently instructed in voluntary lid-closure movements.

The normal blink rate is quite variable. Approximately 15 to 18 blinks per minute is normal. Each blink lasts 0.3 second. The rate is higher for men than for women and is increased with emotional outbursts or anxiety states. With a poor or tired blinker, the rate may go down as much as 60%. This occurs frequently with reading, driving, or watching computer screens during the working day. People who have jobs that fatigue the normal blink response are best fitted with gas-permeable contact (GPC) lenses, which do not depend heavily on blinking to relieve corneal hypoxia.

Factors that affect the rate of blinking are thyroid disorder, stroke, facial palsy, Parkinson's disease, and antidepressants along with the side effects of several drugs. Occupational factors from staring may cause a slow blink rate and contribute to evaporation, for example, those watching video display terminals (Figure 17.3).

There are several ways of classifying dry eyes:

- By the cause, such as environmental (Figure 17.4)
- By their subtypes (see Figure 17.3)
- Keratoconjunctivitis sicca is any eye with some dryness
- Xerophthalmia: dryness caused by vitamin deficiency
- Special syndromes such as Sjögren's syndrome, a chronic autoimmune inflammatory entity in which dry eyes is often the principal symptom and dry mouth and parotid swelling is associated. As causative evidence becomes apparent, the classifications continue to change (Figure 17.5)
- Medication-induced: antidepressants, anticholinergics, decongestants, over-the-counter allergy drugs, oral contraceptives, sex enhancement drugs (e.g., Viagra)
- After PRK and LASIK
- High tear osmolarity (high salt in tears)
- Meibomian gland dysfunction (MGD). The concept of dry eye disease has changed over the past decade. It is now viewed as a disturbance of the tear film and ocular surface characterized by tear hyperosmolarity and tear film instability. These are closely related.

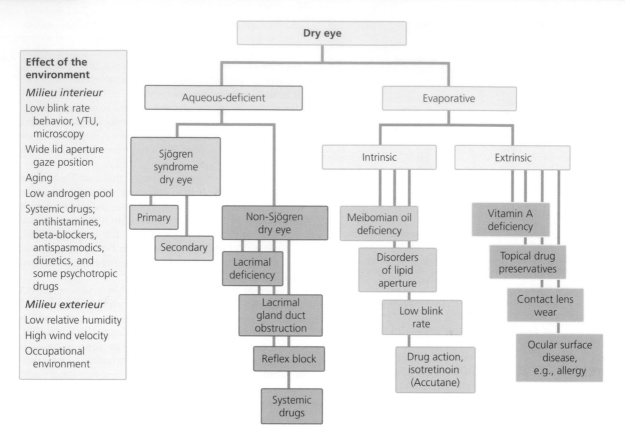

Figure 17.3 Major etiologic causes of dry eye. The box on the left illustrates the influence of environment on the risk of an individual to develop dry eye. The term *environment* is used broadly to include bodily states habitually experienced by an individual, whether it reflects their "milieu interieur" or is the result of exposure to external conditions that represent the "milieu exterieur." This background may influence the onset and type of dry eye disease in an individual, which may be aqueous-deficient or evaporative. Aqueous-deficient dry eye has two major groupings: Sjögren's syndrome dry eye and non-Sjögren's syndrome dry eye. Evaporative dry eye may be intrinsic, in which the regulation of evaporative loss from the tear film is directly affected, for example, by meibomian lipid deficiency, poor lid congruity and lid dynamics, low blink rate, and the effects of drug action, such as that of systemic retinoids. Extrinsic evaporative dry eye embraces those etiologies that increase evaporation by their pathologic effects on the ocular surface. Causes include vitamin A deficiency, the action of toxic topical agents such as preservatives, contact lens wear, and a range of ocular surface diseases, including allergic eye disease. Further details are given in the text.

(From Report of the International Dry Eye WorkShop (DEWS). The Ocular Surface, April 2007, Vol. 5, No. 2; www.theocularsurface.com; Copyright Elsevier. All rights reserved.)

Tear hyperosmolarity causes a variety of breakdowns in the structure and function of the tear film including causing inflammation, which damages the ocular surface.

TESTS FOR DRY EYES

The standard tests for dry eyes are cornea slit-lamp observation of the cornea, Schirmer's test (Figure 17.6) and BUT.

Ideally each patient should have the following:

The rose bengal test. Unlike fluorescein, this test identifies not only dryness of the cornea but also that of the conjunctiva. Rose bengal stains areas of devitalized tissue and cells that are damaged or unprotected by native mucoproteins. It may be administered by placing at least one or two drops of rose bengal solution or using the rose bengal filter paper test strips. With rose bengal, the staining in dry eyes is generally in the lateral margins of the cornea; in meibomianitis, this staining shows up at the superior and inferior margins (Figure 17.7).

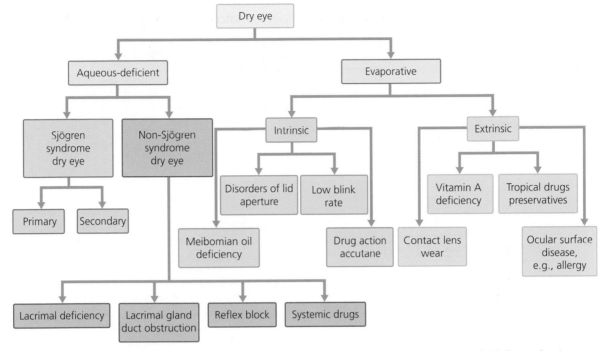

Figure 17.4 Etiologic classification of dry eye disease. The list *(bottom left)* illustrates the environmental risk factors for dry eye disease. The scheme indicates the etiologic classification of dry eye disease into aqueous-deficient or evaporative tear deficiency. *(Adapted from Krachmer et al., Cornea, 3rd ed., Mosby: Elsevier; 2010.)*

More recently lissamine green has been used for staining the conjunctiva. It should be read about 2 to 3 minutes after application and stains the same areas as the rose bengal but without the stinging.

Measurement of tear film break-up time (BUT). Instill some drops of fluorescein into the conjunctival sac. Observe the corneal tear film with the slit lamp. If the tear film breaks up in less than 10 seconds this is considered abnormal (Figure 17.8).

Corneal assessment for erosion is by slit-lamp examination. If the dryness is severe enough to cause pitting of the corneal epithelium, then dry eyes exists. There is a greater risk of infection because a portal of entry is created. Associated findings that do not prognosticate well for patients include blepharitis and chronic conjunctivitis. Corneal staining is, however, a relatively late manifestation of dry eye and many early cases of dry eye disease do not show staining.

i-Pen osmolarity system

The i-Pen is a portable handheld battery-operated unit that calculates and displays the tear film osmolarity. The unit includes a small display screen that shows the specific osmolarity.

i-Pen osmolarity test sensor

Each Single Use Sensor is a single-use, individually packaged sterile unit, designed to work in conjunction with the i-Pen. The Single Use Sensor does not contain chemicals or reagents.

Push the on/off switch message. You should hear a beep and the liquid crystal display (LCD) should display the i-Pen (Figure 17.9).

We are indebted to Dr. Michael Lemp and Dr. Linsy Farris for quantifying the role of tear osmolarity in dry eyes. Tear osmolarity can also be used to monitor the response to treatment. The TearLab osmolarity is thought to be the single most diagnostic test for dry eye. It also reflects the severity of the disease and can be used to monitor the response to treatment.

The tear osmolarity test quantifies the osmolarity of the tears in less than a minute. Developed by TearLab, the osmolarity value increases as the tear film because dryer eg the 1.The higher the value, the dryer the eye. This test is a modern tool to diagnose and to follow the response to the treatment of the dry eye to be sure the patient is getting better. By lowering the osmolarity level, one knows the treatment is helping.

How to perform the test

The TearLab Osmolarity System provides a quick and simple method for determining tear osmolarity using a 50-nL sample of tear fluid collected directly from the tear lid margin. To perform a test, insert a single-use, disposable test

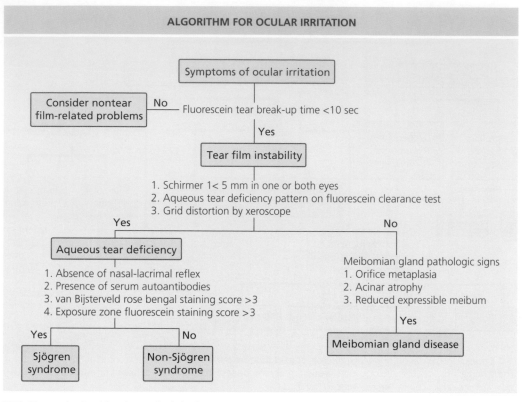

Figure 17.5 Diagnostic algorithm for ocular irritation.
(From Pflugfelder SC, Tseng SC, Sanabria O, et al. Evaluation of subjective assessments and objective diagnostic tests for diagnosing tear-film disorders known to cause ocular irritation. Cornea 1998.)

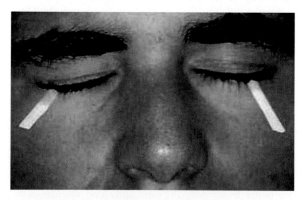

Figure 17.6 A Schirmer's test with and without a local anesthetic. Wetting of the paper strip 10 mm within 5 minutes is considered satisfactory.

card onto the pen and touch the tip of the pen to the tear fluid located above the lower eyelid (tear meniscus). After a successful collection, dock the pen in the reader and a quantitative tear osmolarity test result will be displayed

on the reader LCD. The total process, from tear collection to test result, takes less than 30 seconds. The TearLab Osmolarity System simplifies the tear collection process and leaves the diagnosis in the hands of the practitioner.

It should be noted that tear osmolarity should be tested in both eyes. Dry eye disease is a bilateral disease causing elevated tear osmolarity in both eyes. Because of the breakdown in the stability of the tear film, results in all tests tend to be variable with transient responses to environmental stress differing in each eye and in the same eye over time. This is in contrast to normal subjects in whom the tear osmolarity values in both eyes are close (less than 8 mosmol/L).

Values higher than 308 mosm/L (in the higher value eye) are indicative of dry eye disease; values from 316 to 327 are seen in moderate dry eye and values of 328 or higher are seen in severe dry eye. One should always take the higher of the two values and note the difference between the two eyes. Abnormally high differences (greater than 8 mosm/L) are confirmatory of dry eye disease. Both the higher individual eye values and the difference between eyes decrease and return to normal with effective treatment.

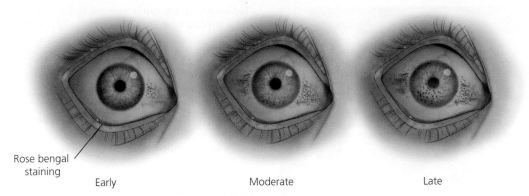

Rose bengal staining

Early   Moderate   Late

Figure 17.7 Rose bengal staining of cornea and conjunctiva.

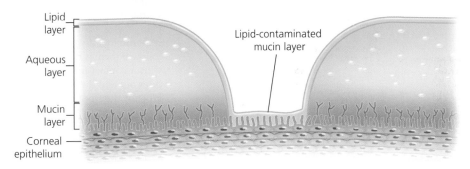

Lipid layer

Aqueous layer

Mucin layer

Corneal epithelium

Lipid-contaminated mucin layer

Figure 17.8 Measurement of tear film break-up time.

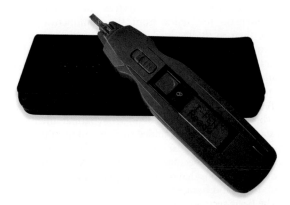

Figure 17.9 i-Pen Osmolarity System. The i-Pen is a portable handheld battery-operated unit that calculates and displays the osmolarity test result. The unit includes a small display screen that shows the osmolarity test result..3. i-Pen osmolarity test sensor.

Each Single Use Sensor is a single-use, individually packaged sterile unit, designed to work in conjunction with the i-Pen. The Single Use Sensor does not contain chemicals or reagents. Push the on/off switch message. You should hear a beep and the LCD display should display the i-Pen results.

Each Single Use Sensor is a single-use, individually packaged sterile unit, designed to work in conjunction with the i-Pen. The Single Use Sensor does not contain chemicals or reagents (Figure 17.10).

INSTRUCTIONS ON TAKING SAMPLES

- Seat the patient with head back and eyes upward toward the ceiling.
- Move the pen into place, then ask the patient to open the eyes.
- Lower the pen, allowing the bottom of the tip to come into contact with the lower eyelid and the line of moisture along the inner eyelid margin.
- Move the tip beyond the eyelashes near the corner of the eye.
- Press down lightly with the pen on the lower eyelid to collect tears.
- Fluid is collected at the bottom tip of the test card.
- Successful collection is indicated on the collecting pen by a light and a bell sound.

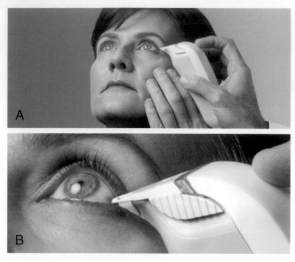

Figure 17.10 (A) Tear film osmolarity test using the TearLab osmometer. (B) Tip placed on tear film to capture tears. Do not touch white of eyes.

TEST FOR MEIBOMIAN GLAND DYSFUNCTION

Another test for dry eyes has been for meibomian gland dysfunction (MGD). A new instrument in use is the Lipi-View interferometer (TearScience) that quantifies the lipid layer of the tear film. It may be used with the LipiFlow device that increases the lipid layer of the tear film.

The normal eyelid contains 40 to 50 meibomian glands in upper and lower lids. They secrete an oily layer composed of lipids and proteins. These secretions prevent evaporation of the middle or aqueous portion of the tear film and prevent dry eyes. MGD results when this layer is low and evaporation of the tear film occurs, resulting in dry eyes. A diagnostic test and treatment for this deficiency are available (see following text).

TEAR PHYSIOLOGY

The tear film has several functions, outlined in Box 17.1. The dry eye workup should include items listed in Box 17.2.

The physiology of dry eyes has been shown to be caused by an inflammatory process on the conjunctiva. A drop consisting of cyclosporine (Restasis) in minimal concentration dose can effectively decrease this inflammation and increase the reflex from the conjunctiva to the brain, then to the lacrimal gland. This will increase tear production.

Lid hygiene is also an important factor and any inflammatory process of the meibomian glands may be reduced by proper cleaning and mediation to the lids.

GRADING OF DRY EYES

There are many grading systems for the severity of dry eyes. We use the grading system based on grading system from 1 to 4, in which grade 4 is the most serious (Table 17.1)

SYMPTOMS

Symptoms may be mild to severe, including blurring of vision, burning, scratchiness, grittiness, discomfort, or even pain. Excess tearing may occur as a reflex mechanism in response to a dry cornea. Depression of the individual may follow if there is no relief. Redness may occur (Box 17.3).

In a contact lens wearer the surface of the contact lens dries out and the vision becomes blurry as a result of wrinkling of the front surface (Figure 17.11).

PHYSIOLOGY

The physiology of dry eyes has been shown to be caused by an inflammatory process on the conjunctiva. A drop consisting of cyclosporine (Restasis) in minimal concentration dose (0.05%) can effectively decrease this inflammation and increase the reflex from the conjunctiva to the brain, then to the lacrimal gland. This will increase tear production.

Lid hygiene is also an important factor, and any inflammatory process of the meibomian glands may be reduced by proper lid hygiene and medication on the lids.

Tear formation is generally measured by Schirmer's test, in which a 35 × 5 mm strip of no. 41 Whatman filter paper or standardized paper is folded over the midportion of the lower lid. Generally if 10 mm or more of the paper from the point of the fold becomes wet in a 5-minute period, tear formation is considered to be normal. This test measures both reflex and basic secretion.

The basic secretion test is similarly performed, but only after a local an esthetic has been placed into the eye. This eliminates the reflex production of tears from the test and measures basal section.

The tear film has several functions, outlined in Box 17.1. The dry eye workup should include items listed in Box 17.2.

This tear film provides an exchange of oxygen and nutrients to the corneal epithelium. It also is a mechanism of rebuilding and removing debris and sloughed exfoliated cells and metabolites.

Table 17.1 Dry eye severity grading system

Dry eye severity level	1	2	3	4*
Discomfort, severity, and frequency	Mild or episodic; occurs under environmental stress	Moderate episodic or chronic, stress or no stress	Severe, frequent or constant without stress	Severe or disabling and constant
Visual symptoms	None or episodic mild fatigue	Annoying or activity-limiting episodic	Annoying, chronic or constant, limiting activity	Constant or possibly disabling
Conjunctival injection	None to mild	None to mild	+/−	+/++
Conjunctival staining	None to mild	Variable	Moderate to marked	Marked
Corneal staining (severity/location)	None to mild	Variable	Marked central	Severe punctate erosions
Corneal/tear signs	None to mild	Mild debris, ↓ meniscus	Filamentary keratitis, mucous clumping, ↑ tear debris	Filamentary keratitis, mucous clumping, ↑ tear debris, ulceration
Lid meibomian glands	MGD variably present	MGD variably present	Frequent	Trichiasis, keratinization, symblepharon
TBUT (seconds)	Variable	≤10	≤5	Immediate
Schirmer's score (mm/5 min)	Variable	≤10	≤5	≤2

*Must have signs *and* symptoms.
MGD, Meibomian gland dysfunction; *TBUT,* (fluorescein) tear break-up time.
From Behrens A, Doyle JJ, Stern L, et al. Dysfunctional tear syndrome. A Delphi approach to treatment recommendations. *Cornea* 2006; 25:90–97.

Box 17.3 **Symptoms of dry eye**

Scratchiness
Intermittent blurring
Dryness
No tears on crying
Mucoid discharge
Relief with tear substitutes
Discomfort or pain
Occasional burning and itching

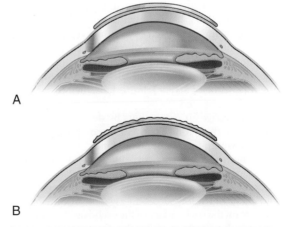

A

B

Figure 17.11 (A) Normal contact lens. (B) Dehydrated soft contact lens after exposure to a dry environment, causing blurred vision.

A severe dry eye condition is referred to as keratoconjunctivitis sicca. The quantity and the quality of tears play a major role in protecting the corneal epithelium. Contact lens wear is difficult because of discomfort and drying out of the contact lenses.

SJÖGREN'S SYNDROME

Sjögren's syndrome is a chronic autoimmune disease of both the lacrimal and salivary glands. The classic syndrome combines a dry eye, a dry mouth, and often an enlargement of the parotid gland. There may be associated rheumatoid arthritis or systemic lupus, polyarteritis nodosa, or mixed connective tissue disease. The condition affects females more than males. It becomes worse over the day. There is often a dry mouth and tongue. There may be a stringy discharge, redness, and blurry vision. The condition is often worse with wind and air conditioning. The ocular dryness in Sjögren's is caused by lacrimal hyposecretion from an inflammatory condition of the lacrimal gland.

MANAGEMENT OF THE DRY EYE PATIENT: TREATMENT

There are several approaches to treatment, depending on the severity of dry eyes. There are a large number of commercially available artificial tears in over-the-counter medications in almost every country. These are relatively inexpensive.

There are several drops that are thicker and more viscous drops that may be used such as gel forms. Prescription drops such as cyclosporine 0.05% (Restasis) may be used.

Many home remedies may be tried such as patching night and even daytime, flaxseed oil capsules, and using humidifiers to saturate the humidity in the house or office. Goggles with and without moisture packs may be tried. Treatments are often trial and error.

Recent trials with human serum, called autologous serum drops (ASD), have shown beneficial results in dry eye disorders and in Sjögren's syndrome (Box 17.4).

If these measures fail then silicone punctual plugs may be inserted in the lower and sometimes the upper puncta. These may be removable, or dissolvable (collagen) or permanent (silicone or acrylic). If this fails, then thermal cautery may be suggested.

Avoid excessive air movements by decreasing the speed of ceiling or oscillating fans. Warm compresses may be used to warm up the meibomian glands.

One newer treatment for dry eye introduced by TearScience attempts to restore meibomian gland function. In the past, treatment was applying warm compresses to the eyelid margins. The low success rate was because meibomian glands are on the back surface of the eyelids and the heat that was applied was directed to the front surface. A new

Box 17.4 Approaches to treatment—mild to severe dry eyes

1. Copious eyedrops, viscous or gels best. Ointments for bedtime. Alcon manufactures a common drop called Systane under a variety of subtypes, e.g., ultra, gels are best, balance vitamin, and makes an eye cleansing wipe as well
2. Warm eye compresses to stimulate the meibomian glands
3. Take in more water daily
4. Switch to preservative-free eye medication; more costly but more effective
5. Vitamins daily, particularly vitamins A and C
6. Humidifier: central or by bedside and in rooms
7. Take eye "breaks" every 20 to 30 minutes from reading or computer use
8. Flaxseed capsules, flaxseed powder, or fish oils
9. Protect eyes from wind and sun by wraparound sunglasses
10. Swim or ski goggles for bedtime use
11. Lid scrubs—with proper commercial eye cleansers—or baby shampoo
12. Patching at bedtime—alternate eyes
13. Restasis (cyclosporine 0.05%) 2 to 4 times daily
14. Punctal plugs temporary (collagen) or permanent (silicone)

[Box 17.4, Fig. 1 Punctal plug]

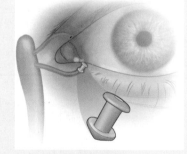

15. Punctal cautery upper and lower
16. Scleral silicone contact lenses
17. Secretagogues—oral pills that have cholinergic activity to promote tear flow by stimulating the salivary glands 2 mg pilocarpine (Salagen) is a cholinergic drug that stimulates secretory activity of the lacrimal gland. It can be used 2 to 4 times daily
18. LipiFlow meibomian gland treatment

treatment is available called LipiFlow, in which heat is applied to the back of the eyelid along with massage for 2 minutes. This device is designed to remove blockages in

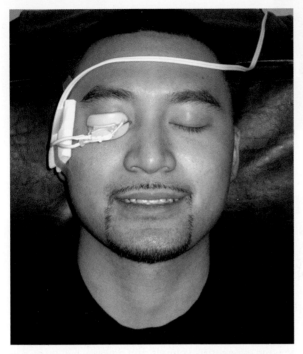

Figure 17.12 Meibomian gland treatment. LipiFlow treatment of meibomian glands to increase tear film of meibomian gland secretions.

the meibomian glands without injuring any of the structures of the eyelid or eye. A single treatment may last 12 to 24 months in restoring normal meibomian gland function and can be repeated (Figure 17.12).

SUMMARY

Dry eyes in minor or major ways is more common than reported, affecting a significant portion of the population worldwide. Dry eyes can be progressive and if left untreated can lead to more major problems with eye infection and reduced vision. As testing continues to be more available and treatment tends to be more successful, more effective managements for dry eye problems are becoming available to help the practitioner manage patients with this often chronic disorder.

More causes are continuing to appear such as environmental factors and drugs as well as side effects of newer drugs coming to light. Many of these precipitating causes can be avoided. New treatment modalities continue to appear and take their place as a benefit in increasing our therapeutic armamentarium for treating dry eyes.

A paper in June 2015 in *Cornea* offered some hope by the use of contact lenses loaded with lactoferrin that reinforces the tear film. There may be newer therapeutic approaches to patients with severe dry eye syndrome. On the horizon there have been a number of studies with nanowafers that have controlled release of moisture to add to the tear film and even cortisone. There is potential in these "on the eye" wafers to add a variety of drugs.

Efforts are continually being made to develop improved treatment programs for patients afflicted with dry eye disease. Many new products are been tried for dry eyes. At the time of writing, none except Restasis has been approved by the FDA in the United States. Better understanding of dry eyes and its pathophysiology will eventually lead to better medications to treat this common eye disorder.

FURTHER READING

Azari AA, Rapuno CJ. Autologous serum eye drops for the treatment of ocular surface disease. Eye and Contact Lens Review May 2015;41(3).

Lemp MA. Report of the national eye industry workshop on clinical trials in dry eye. CLAO J 1995;21:2212–32.

Report of the International Dry Eye WorkShop (DEWS). Ocul Surf April 2007;5(2). Copyright 2006 Ethis Communications, Inc. All rights reserved, www.theocularsurface.com.

Stein HS, Slatt BJ, Stein RM, et al. Fitting Guide for Rigid and Soft Contact Lenses: A Practical Approach. 4th ed. Elsevier/Mosby: St Louis; 2002.

Chapter | 18 |

Managing a contact lens practice

Harold A. Stein, Penny Pilliar, Lynn D. Maund, Korosh Nikeghbal

The clinical side of contact lens provision historically has been in selecting the correct lens and lens material design for an individual patient. The fitter must be knowledgeable about ocular physiologic responses and be able to solve problems.

However, in certain areas of the contact lens practice, contact lens practitioners must also learn about the business through experience, through continuing education programs, from colleagues, and through studying other types of business.

In this chapter we outline a dynamic approach to practice management for the contact lens practice. To succeed in the contact lens market, you should be knowledgeable about who the competitors are in your area and why they have or have not been successful.

There are many nontraditional channels via which the public can purchase lenses, such as mail order and mass merchandising. This is part of the competition for the professional contact lens fitter. Your practice focus should be on providing professional services based on your medical expertise. You should try to determine where your practice is located in the general milieu of other contact lens providers in the area. This relates to the specific city or specific region of the practice. Outline who the competition is, how you can differentiate yourself, and how you will succeed in a given market.

PATIENT MANAGEMENT

How to make patients happy

Making patients happy is not just good practice; it is also probably one of the best protections against lawsuits. The secret to making patients happy lies in developing good communication skills. Good communication skills start with an attitude of empathy and caring and of letting patients know directly and indirectly that they are important. This attitude is reflected not only by what a doctor says and does but what the office staff say and do and how psychologically comfortable the patient is made to feel in the office environment. There are a number of ways in which one can create an impression that the office does in fact care.

Minimize patient wait time

One of the key factors that affect a patient's overall rating of a practitioner is the time spent in the reception area (Figure 18.1). When possible, support staff should begin promptly with history taking, measurements, or contact lens instruction in advance of the appointment time with the practitioner. Waiting time is a major factor in patient dissatisfaction, which increases dramatically when waiting

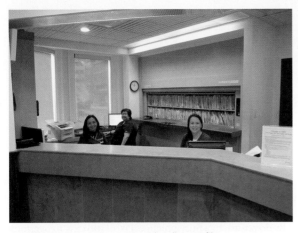

Figure 18.1 Reception area with adjacent files.

time exceeds 30 minutes. Office schedules cannot always be controlled, however, especially if there are added emergencies to deal with. Those doctors who are chronically behind schedule should take a close look at how bookings are made and try to prevent snarls in the schedule. If delays are unavoidable, patients should be told why they are waiting and how long the wait may be, to help minimize the aggravation. In addition, interesting diversions should be made available to help patients pass the time. These include video information or even a television set in the waiting room. Current magazines are not enough to compensate for long waiting periods.

Make patients feel important

The first contact the patient has with a doctor's office has to be courteous, respectful, and personalized. This can include little gestures of kindness, like the nurse asking after a recent baby, the receptionist asking for a preferred appointment time, or the doctor inquiring after an ailing family member or recalling some details of an earlier conversation.

It is also appropriate for both male and female doctors to stand up and shake a patient's hand when first greeting a patient. At the same time, consideration should be given to diverse cultural differences in the general population and a pleasant greeting may serve to convey empathy, friendliness, and concern. It is critical to convey information in a tone that is neither patronizing nor too technical so that the patient understands what the basic problem is and what is going to be done to help correct it.

The doctor and staff should have eye contact with the patient being examined. It is often offensive to older people if the doctor directs advice to a younger person who may have accompanied the patient. Patients are often reluctant to ask questions, and it is better to be on the side of too much rather than insufficient information. Finally, the doctor should not make patients feel that he or she is too busy to listen to their problems because that patient may not only go elsewhere, but also may be thoroughly dissatisfied and possibly become litigious.

Create space for comfort

Surprisingly small details, such as how the furniture is arranged, can make a difference in overall patient response. In an eye practice, a desk intervening between a patient and the doctor often represents a barrier to communication. It is much better to have a direct, closer interaction with the patient. Both intimacy and empathy are given a head start by placing the chairs near each other to eliminate any broad expanse of space between the doctor and patient.

Respect a patient's right to privacy

Any discussions with the doctor or other staff should be conducted privately so that a room full of strangers does not overhear details of diagnosis, treatment, fees, and payment arrangements. Particular attention may needs to be paid to the individual's Health Insurance Portability and Accountability Act (HIPAA) provisions.

Look the part

Look professional. People do not respond well to unkempt individuals. Patients expect the doctor and staff to be dressed in appropriate attire. Some offices allow business attire, whereas others adopt a uniform look that clearly differentiates the staff from patients.

Pay attention to detail

Unclean examining rooms make patients uneasy, especially when materials from previous examinations are clearly visible. Interruptions during an examination can be particularly annoying. A loud intercom system undermines privacy and may be considered disturbing and unprofessional. Small conveniences such as a coat rack in the waiting room, along with soothing decor, plants, current magazines, and art prints all help create the impression of a pleasant, welcoming environment and a caring doctor. Be sure that washrooms are tidied up and restocked once or twice daily.

Master communication skills

Conversation is an important factor in making or breaking the doctor–patient relationship. Here are a few tips.

1. *Be up-front.* Give information right at the beginning of the visit, not at the end.
2. *Be creative.* Use everyday language to explain what is wrong and how you are planning to correct it.

3. *Be personal.* Ask questions about the patients' family and social life so that they feel that they have not been forgotten from one visit to the next. Make notes on charts about a patient's interests and concerns for recall at future visits.

4. *Be caring.* A quiet professional tone conveys attentiveness.

5. *Be prepared.* If you have something that needs to be shared with a patient's family members, ask them to come in from the waiting room and share the information with them.

6. *Solicit patient feedback.* Confirm that what you have told the patient has been understood by asking the patient to relate the information back to you. This is particularly important when educating patients on care systems for contact lenses. Patients often leave the office without fully understanding all the steps involved with their contact lens care systems. Written information will make sure that the message gets across. Personalized handouts are an important and effective means to reinforce instructions and serve a quick reference for contacting the office and a means to refer friends.

7. *Be human.* Patients want human beings looking after them. It is perfectly acceptable to tell patients that you also feel badly when the news you have for them is bad.

Be fair in all matters of finance

Charge fairly for your professional services, but do not overcharge. Be fair in refunding patients who prove to be unsuited to contact lens wear. A clear statement of fees and partial refund in unsuccessful cases should be made initially. Always look at the situation from the standpoint of the patient. Maintain goodwill at all costs. By doing so you will help ensure a happy patient who will refer friends and family to the practice.

Patient information

The general information that a new patient has about contact lenses is often confusing and incorrect. The initial consultation should clear any misconceptions and answer all the questions. However, sensible handouts reinforce the answers to frequently asked questions and often answer other questions overlooked in the initial interview. Some of these pamphlets are available from manufacturers and from contact lens societies. They can, however, be customized for your own practice. Handouts are great practice builders and should be encouraged. In addition, video has significantly changed the communication system. Good videotapes and CDs are available on the care of contact lenses and they reinforce the spoken and written word. Additionally, abundant information is available online. Be prepared to address questions that patients may have about online information and direct them to trusted Internet sites.

Patient follow-up

It is most important that contact lens patients be adequately followed up. Lens patients require ongoing care. A number of satisfied lens wearers will simply forget to return for regular examination. However, lens patients require ongoing care. The rigid lens may warp, thus altering the corneal curvature, and the soft lens may become coated with protein, causing chronic anoxia of the cornea with vascular invasion. Routine appointments are preventive.

One may ask patients to return at regular intervals, but it is the responsibility of the practitioner to see that they actually do return. In a busy practice it is all too easy to overlook the drop-outs who do not return. Thus an effective recall system, by either phone or mail, is most important. Addresses and phone numbers may change, but a little detective work may greatly aid in locating patients, if for no other reason than to ensure that they obtain follow-up care either by the initial fitter or by another practitioner. We suggest that a patient agreement form be used, outlining the minimum follow-up requirements.

One may gear the recall system to a set time of year when all contact files are reviewed and those patients who have not returned are duly notified. Some practices use the birthday cross-reference or date of initial fit system by reviewing each chart during the month of the patient's birthday or date of initial fit, thus spreading the load over the year.

Disposable contact lenses permit a system of follow-up that is based on patients returning for their supply of additional lenses. It is important with disposable lenses that patients adhere to the prescribed replacement regimen and do not use the same lenses for too long in an attempt to save money. Computers can be invaluable in tracking patient contact lens replacement regimens.

A successful practice

Most professional offices cannot and do not advertise lenses at a discount price. Therefore, they are not widely known or chosen because they are not the cheapest purveyors of lenses. The only advantages of going to the doctor are his or her superior skills and willingness to take a personal interest in the patient's welfare. The following suggestions will help in achieving these aims:

1. *Minimize answering machines* during daytime office hours. Patients like to talk to a human being!

2. *Be selective.* Choose patients carefully. If a patient is contraindicated for contact lens wear, fully explain why this is so. The happy patient is your main source of advertisement.

3. *Inform your patient.* Information directly from the doctor and staff, along with office pamphlets, inform

the patient about possible problems and complications of contact lens wear and how to prevent them. Ongoing communication through newsletters and practice mailings helps reinforce this information.

4. *Be thorough.* Check tear film and lids and examine every facet of contact lens fitting so as to maximize your success rate.

5. *Emphasize safety.* Many patients think contact lenses are products like shoes or socks. A lens is a prosthetic medical device that requires expert supervision. In many countries, contact lenses are regulated by the government, and by law, require medical supervision.

6. *Follow up.* A follow-up service is essential. Many contact lens-induced problems are asymptomatic. The patient should be monitored carefully on an ongoing basis. The commercial way is to sell the contact lenses to the patient and then say good-bye. This should not be your way.

7. *Offer personal service.* Do special things for the patients such as providing free starter kits, solutions, and so on.

8. *Be current.* Attend lectures and seminars and read journals to stay up-to-date on developments in the field.

PLANNING

Developing a business plan is essential. You should sit down with pen and paper and describe your practice, how long it has been in operation, and the relevant legal structures. Check out available financing for promotion and advertising. A business plan should help you organize your goals, strategies, and activities. Place all this on paper because this increases your chance of making the contact lens practice more profitable. Putting pen to paper encourages you to commit to the strategies and share them with others who may be knowledgeable in this field. You should prepare key points and consider the allocation of resources and staff to various activities.

UNDERSTANDING YOUR ORGANIZATION

Describe who your current patients are and whom you would like to attract as patients. They may be from organizations, professionals, or businesses in your neighborhood. Develop your pricing strategy and your distribution methods. Ask yourself how you are promoting your contact lens practice. If you have companies or individuals within these companies that you would like to target, try to be placed on a "perk list" as a preferred business link.

Knowing the key individuals in a business or practice to contact is important to the development and expansion of your practice.

Actively consider how best your practice can thrive. You may decide to change contact lens vendors or even to relocate the practice to another part of the city or region.

FINANCES

Analyze the past 2 to 3 years of the balance sheet and income statement for the practice. In addition, it is a good idea to create some projections for cash flow. Monthly projections may be important if you are looking for financing from banks, and so on. These projections will serve as a basis for budgeting in the practice. There are many computer software packages for the business planning process. Most are inexpensive and useful.

Once you have a business plan, you can develop a marketing plan (see the following text).

Pricing policy in the contact lens practice

Two primary types of pricing policies are used in contact lens practices. One is a global fee encompassing all services provided to the patient. For example, practitioners can bundle lenses, care solutions, and follow-up care for disposable and frequent-replacement lenses for a set fee. The other pricing policy takes expenses into account by setting separate fees for examination, fitting, and services combined with retailing the contact lenses. This policy identifies specific costs to the patient.

When fitting custom contact lenses such as rigid gaspermeable (RGP) lenses, toric soft lenses, and other special lenses, a specified exchange warranty should be obtained from the manufacturer if possible. No matter how skilled the fitter, small modifications of the lens base curve, diameter, power, and axis and refit changes are needed for a successful fit.

An exchange warranty for RGP and custom toric lenses, as well as the security of being able to reorder as needed, is well worth the additional initial expense. Having the ability to reorder lenses without additional charges is a boon to practitioner and patient alike and emphasizes to the patient the individual professional care provided by your office.

Practitioners should research prices for products and disposable lenses. You also may be able to participate in a buying group. It is well worth researching alternative sources for the average 15% to 30% price discount that can be obtained. The highest-quality laboratory should be used for custom lens orders regardless of price.

Packaging care solutions with lenses is becoming popular as a valuable added service. Many contact lens starter kits are available from the major lens manufacturers. Some contain a contact lens case, contact lens disinfection solution, protein remover, a daily cleaner, and buffered saline. Others consist of a contact lens case and an all-in-one solution. Perhaps dispensing more than one starter kit of the same care system is useful to patients to accustom them to proper compliance.

Careful controls are necessary not only in researching lens sources but also when purchasing contact lenses and supplies for dispensing to patients. A bookkeeping system must be in place to keep up with the charges as well as credits on lenses returned. Either a manual system or a simple computer program is required to track these orders and credits.

Cost control

Maintaining your contact lens practice by following established business principles is essential to practice success. One such principle is the relationship between costs and gross sales. One rule of thumb is that the goods (contact lenses and care system) should amount to approximately 33% of gross sales. Salaries should amount to 25% and other costs should be approximately 17%. If the gross goes up, so too should the costs and vice versa. This leaves about 25% for profit and for future development and advertising. These ratios should be checked on a quarterly basis.

Performance bonuses

The fitter and some other staff may be encouraged by a performance bonus based on the contact lens practice revenue rather than salary increases.

Tracking finances

It is important to track the financial performances of a contact lens department as a separate profit center. Revenue should be incorporated with all expenses in the balance sheet. The more details one has, the better the analysis one can make of the practice. There is a direct relationship of cost of goods, salaries, and advertising to the gross revenue.

Track sales and sales data on a computer. Identify which are the top-selling contact lenses annually. Track the turnover of your lenses. Identify whether you have a proper mix of contact lens products—disposable, bifocal, and extended wear—for your patient clientele. Use computers if possible. Goods that sit on the shelf often represent lost revenue, so it can be helpful to create an inventory of the most commonly prescribed contact lens products. Stocks of trial and diagnostic sets should be maintained because these can be dispensed in an emergency situation to the patient. Identify the percentages of new fits, refits, and

replacements that are sold. Have service agreements in place for lens replacement programs.

MARKETING

Marketing is a very complex process that involves much more than paid advertising. Consider the following points:

1. How long is your database of patient records? Databases may be very important in marketing new products that become available from time to time.
2. What are the demographics and projected demographics for your market?
3. Review the marketing plan on a regular basis.
4. Where are you advertising? Think about dollars spent on advertisements in newspapers, radio, television, and in the Yellow Pages. Record from where new patients are coming.
5. What is your best market?
6. What is the best advertising budget as a percentage of your gross? It can be anywhere from 2% to 25%.
7. Create an ongoing newsletter program and use email.
8. Manufacturers have been known to share costs for advertising a new product. Explore this with your vendors.
9. Improve public relations by community involvement in your area such as soccer, basketball, giving talks in schools, and so on.
10. Develop a "thank-you" service to patients and to new fits. A handwritten thank-you letter might be suitable.
11. Have a recall system in place. Analyze your recall rate and percentage of returns.
12. Create a brochure for your practice for all new patients and for telephone shoppers.
13. Design a special appointment card to include telephone and fax numbers and email. If possible, have it designed.
14. Send someone in personally as a mystery shopper to your competitors. See how you match up.
15. Consider a patient satisfaction survey.
16. Professionally design a website detailing all the services provided by your office. Inquiries by email should be handled promptly.

Review your internal marketing, staff, and ambience of your practice. Examine your external marketing (e.g., advertising, direct mail, etc.). Build up patient loyalty to your practice.

A system should be devised to track the number of calls received by phone shoppers about pricing. It is important that staff have adequate training on how to discuss prices with phone shoppers, to maximize this source of new clients.

Actively participate in free trial lens programs offered by manufacturers. These may involve either new materials or new designs that become available. It may be convenient to offer mail-order free trial contact lenses to patients through email services. It is, however, in the long run better for them to pick up the lenses than to mail them out. This establishes better loyalty to the practice and relationships with the staff. However, it may be an option for a busy person. You could also provide a large number of lenses, such as a 6-month supply. It is important that you keep track of this and provide a reminder when the 6-month renewal is due. This is another opportunity for the patient to contact your office.

Consider whether you should bundle lenses and lens care products in an annual package. Some practices establish an "annual bundling" in which they include instructions, follow-up visits, lenses, and lens care products for 1 year.

Solutions and contact lenses can be purchased directly from manufacturers and forwarded to the patient. In this way the patient will know exactly in advance how much the yearly cost is for contact lens care.

It may be possible for you to offer the patient special payment plans, which may cement their relationship with your practice.

ADVERTISING

Advertising is a vital part of business planning. There are many ways to advertise. How do you differentiate your practice? Paper, television, and radio ads are expensive, require repeat ads for saturation, and are often beyond the means of a small practice. Websites are vital and effective in promoting special services in your practice. Professionally designed websites with search engines will ensure easy access by website browsers.

Advertising often can be shared with manufacturers, and you should take advantage of this. Direct mail is a powerful source of communication. Flyers can be attached to the local newspapers for special promotions. Newsletters can be personally drafted or commercially available newsletters can be used that permit your name and address to be inserted. Newsletters provide the individual contact lens wearer with information on topics such as new care systems and developments in contact lenses. They are not considered as junk mail if they are written well and can provide reliability and consistency for your practice recall system.

Remind all employees that patient loyalty is crucial to the survival of your practice. You do not want patients to look elsewhere. Phone calls or email can remind patients of prescheduled appointments or reschedule recall appointments.

Individuals calling to check prices and services can have a staff member answer all questions and follow up with a mailed or emailed patient brochure. The brochures may highlight specific subjects such as keratoconus and other disease processes and newer available treatments as well as emphasize the professional care your practice offers.

STAFF DEVELOPMENT

Pleasant and welcoming staff members are vital to your practice and its success. Most will interact with prospective patients and they can either gain or lose practice loyalty. Support staff often interacts more than the contact lens fitter by answering the telephone, scheduling appointments and answering queries or questions, recalling patients, or providing handy tips. This is a team effort.

Review goals and strategies with staff members regularly. Encourage teamwork in small, regularly scheduled staff meetings.

Try to encourage educational programs for the entire staff. The Contact Lens Society of America (CLSA), the Contact Lens Association of Ophthalmologists (CLAO), and the Joint Commission on Allied Health Personnel in Ophthalmology (JCAHPO) offer good courses that will help staff increase their expertise and become more knowledgeable in managing patients. Employee training is an investment in the practice's future. It is a good idea to have a staff development manual for the practice. This manual should be discussed annually with all staff members and updated and revised as needed.

Telephone answering is most important and is reviewed elsewhere in this textbook (see Chapter 6). All staff should have a 30- to 60-minute period every month to discuss areas of improvement.

THE CONTACT LENS PRACTICE STAFF

In a practice that includes contact lenses, the individual involved in fitting lenses is extremely important. This person's salary, along with those of other medical personnel, is probably the most costly business expense for an eye practice. Thus the practice must choose this individual with careful consideration. He or she must be innovative and knowledgeable about contact lens products and fitting techniques. In addition, this person must have sufficient skill to fit the complicated cases that are often seen in a professional practice, such as keratoconus and postsurgical patients. He or she must portray an image of competence so that patients have confidence not only in the individual but also in the practice. The ophthalmologist must also have confidence in the individual's ability to avoid or minimize complications of contact lenses and provide the best that modern care has to offer. Finally, this person must have excellent people skills such as patience and courtesy. In a practice that does not employ a contact lens specialist, the practitioner takes on this role.

In an efficient contact lens practice, each staff member should have specific responsibilities. The contact lens specialist is given the responsibility of fitting the contact lenses. Careful slit-lamp examination of the initial and subsequent fit, the adaptation status, and any complications during wear should be the primary concern of the contact lens specialist or practitioner. Another staff member should have training to instruct patients in insertion and removal techniques and provide excellent communication on wearing schedules and lens care. Ordering initial and replacement lenses and lens-tracking activities should be delegated to staff to encourage maximum efficiency.

Ordering and purchasing products for patients is the second most expensive office cost and needs to be handled efficiently to ensure profitability for the practice. The staff member who performs this task must be well trained, responsible, and thorough and must keep excellent records to keep costs down to a minimum.

OFFICE EQUIPMENT AND SPACE

Fitting contact lenses requires basic equipment such as the keratometer and lensmeter. Other equipment is useful, such as a Radiuscope to measure lenses and a corneal topography unit to aid in fitting and detecting irregular corneas. If available, video equipment for demonstration materials, such as patient education and training films, is also useful. A specific area must be established in the office for handwashing and for training in lens insertion and removal. An area is also needed for storage of trial lenses and solutions and for eventual storage of a contact lens inventory. Supplies should be easily accessible.

Trial lens-fitting sets

In a practice, there is a need to have a selection of trial RGP lenses, soft toric design lenses, and soft disposable lenses available. Traditionally, manufacturers simplified the fitting process by supplying a variety of trial lenses to determine fit, comfort, and vision. More than 25% of the population has astigmatism greater than 1.00 diopter that may require toric or RGP lenses. There can be charges associated with trial sets that are not minimal, however, especially if two or three trial sets of RGP and soft toric trials are required. A large number of keratoconus patients in a practice may dictate the need for keratoconus trial lens sets.

Our office experience suggests that the fitting of soft lenses and RGP lenses with trial lenses will suffice in most cases. Only a small percentage of cases require a custom trial lens.

Contact lens inventory and ordering

The ability to fit and deliver suitable contact lenses on the same day is essential to building a successful practice. This requires a contact lens inventory and a system for reordering. Fitting custom products such as standard toric soft lenses and other special lenses has become a necessity, but maintaining a contact lens inventory makes sense. Patients often desire instant service; in addition, disposable lenses require an inventory so that patients can obtain replacement lenses on demand.

All practitioners maintain a small inventory of their favorite soft disposable lenses so that patients may leave with the lenses at their initial fitting and training. However, the growth of relatively inexpensive courier services allows rapid delivery of contact lenses from the manufacturer to a practice. One can receive initial or replacement contact lenses in 1 or 2 days. Patients are also pleased to know they can obtain lenses promptly either in person or by shipment. In our practice, the cost of courier service is often borne by the individual who orders the lenses.

The ongoing cost of maintaining an inventory and ordering lenses should be of major concern to the contact lens practitioner. Replacements for inventory lenses must be ordered, and although bulk orders often will reduce shipping costs, custom ordering will be needed for many patients. Inventory lenses should be kept in locked storage cabinets. Maintenance of the inventory stock should be the responsibility of one staff member, who also keeps the keys to the storage cabinets.

ONGOING CARE

Ongoing care for contact lens patients is essential. Patients should be advised that regular checks are a valuable deterrent to contact lens problems and essential for ocular health. This care over the years distinguishes your practice and builds loyalty.

Lid care

Lid scrubs are useful for many individuals with meibomianitis, chalazions, and other inflammatory disorders of the eyelid. Many companies sell these in individual packages like hand wipes (e.g., Lid Care, Ocusoft, Ocusoft Plus, and Lid and Lash); we have found the last of these to have minimum sting and longer-term coating on the eyelids. These wipes are also recommended for removal of make-up. Patients are instructed to put a warm compress on the eyelids followed by a sterile scrub of the lash line. Starting samples are often given; this enhances patient loyalty.

Chapter | **19** |

Visual fields

When determining the visual field the perimetrist attempts to make a two-dimensional map of a patient's entire area of vision. Normally in everyday living we do not place much importance on the width of our vision, the emphasis being directed on seeing clearly straight ahead. However, those people who have lost much of their peripheral field are just as incapacitated functionally as those who have lost much of their central field. Try rolling up two sheets of paper and placing them before your eyes so that you are basically looking through two large-diameter straws. Although you can see directly ahead clearly, it is very difficult to walk through a room without bumping into the furniture.

The circumference of the visual field depends on many factors. Obviously, the field of vision needed for seeing a mosquito flying about would be different than for seeing a jumbo jet. Thus the size of an object is important in referring to the dimensions of the seeing area. Also the ability to perceive at the sides is not as great when the visibility is poor, as opposed to when it is clear; therefore, illumination is an important factor in mapping the field of vision. The state of adaptation of the eye, whether light-adapted or dark-adapted, although not a critical factor, influences the measurable size of the visual field area.

These factors are objective and can in all instances be controlled by the perimetrist. The difficulty in qualitative or quantitative perimetry is not in assessing the factors of size, illumination, and adaptation but in assessing the patient. Perimetry depends entirely on obtaining an accurate and rapid subjective response. How does one compare the replies of a 72-year-old belligerent, slightly confused patient who has recently had a stroke to those of an intelligent 25-year-old woman with no cerebral disease? Because it is difficult to evaluate such factors as reaction time, fatigue, and general health, what is done and noted in every case is a simple evaluation (good, fair, or poor) of the patient's cooperation and reliability.

Although perimetry is not an exact science because it is entirely dependent on the subjective replies of the patient, the visual field for a given reliable patient should be reproducible. Many methods have been devised for estimating visual fields. We discuss only those methods that have survived the tests of time and their applications and limitations.

PRELIMINARY PROCEDURES

A general statement should be recorded about the patient's visual behavior. If it is noted that the patient tends to bump into objects located on either the right or left, a right- or left-sided total loss of visual field (homonymous hemianopia) may be present.

Visual acuity, with and without glasses, should be noted before taking a visual field. As a rule it can be stated that the poorer the patient's visual acuity, the larger is the test object that must be used to plot an accurate visual field. The manner in which the patient responds to visual acuity testing should be recorded. If the patient appears to see only the last three letters of all the lines on the chart, a loss of one-half of the visual field may be present.

Color vision should be checked, especially if colored test objects are going to be used.

The purpose of the visual field examination should be noted so emphasis can be given to specific areas. Such instruction must come from the ophthalmologist, who has made a complete ocular examination and a tentative diagnosis. For instance, for a patient with papilledema, the tangent screen might be thoroughly explored, with particular attention paid to the state of the blind spots, as opposed to the patient with retinitis pigmentosa, in whom a ring scotoma might be anticipated.

FACILITIES FOR FIELD TESTING

Ideally every office or clinic should have a visual field room that is quiet and out of the way of the normal practice traffic. This room should be of simple design so that distraction is kept to a minimum. Approximately 7 footcandles of illumination (see Chapter 3) are necessary for adequate visual field tests if the test apparatus does not contain its own light source.

Realistically, most offices do not have special visual field quarters because of the cost involved and lack of available space. Similarly, the equipment used varies from place to place. Although it is helpful to have the best ophthalmic equipment, the room and equipment always take a subordinate position to the skill and ingenuity of a competent perimetrist. If the patient understands what is expected and has rapport with the examiner, adequate perimetry can be performed.

CONFRONTATION TEST

Of all methods of perimetry, the confrontation test is the most widely used because it requires no special facilities or equipment and can be performed in the home, on bed-ridden patients, and in hospitals. This is essentially a screening test. Any pathologic condition discovered requires a more sophisticated test when possible to determine the exact nature of the visual defect.

In this test the examiner compares the range of the patient's field with his or her own, which is presumed to be normal. The examiner stands facing the patient at a distance of approximately 2 feet (60 cm). Opposite eyes are occluded; that is, the patient's left eye is covered while

the examiner closes his or her right eye. Each of them then fixes the exposed eye of the other. The examiner moves a finger or a white test object, such as a small hatpin mounted on a handle, from the extreme periphery midway between examiner and patient and notes when it comes into the field of view; the patient and examiner should see it simultaneously (Figure 19.1). The test is best performed while the patient's back is to the light and the background behind the examiner is uniform and dark.

All four quadrants of the visual field should be tested and two different approaches should be used in each quadrant. If any defect is indicated or suspected, the field should be accurately mapped and recorded with the perimeter and tangent screen. When vision is extremely poor, a small penlight may be used for a rough test.

A modification of this test is to have the patient count fingers. While one eye is occluded, the examiner brings in from the periphery one, two, or three fingers and asks the patient to count the number of fingers brought in from each quadrant.

The confrontation test is an excellent method of screening patients and, if used skillfully, can be surprisingly accurate. It may be the only method of examining children, people who cannot read, and the cognitively challenged. With children, a small article of interest such as a brightly colored plastic toy may be used as a test object. The preservation of a field in a particular area is indicated when the child makes a quick glance at the object of interest detected in the peripheral field. Finally, when fixation is lost or essential vision is grossly impaired, this method may be more valuable than a more refined technique. For example, in a patient with a cataract, the accurate perception and projection of light or a hand in all four quadrants may be the only method of determining retinal function.

However, this should be regarded only as a rough test, and failure to demonstrate a field defect does not imply a normal field. Defects of large size may easily be missed by this method.

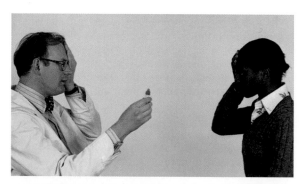

Figure 19.1 Confrontation test. A test object is brought in from the periphery to the seeing area.
(Reproduced from Spalton D, Hitchings R, Hunter P. Atlas of clinical ophthalmology. 3rd ed. St Louis: Mosby, 2004; with permission.)

PERIMETERS

Many perimeters are constructed in such a manner that the eye is at the center of rotation of a hemisphere that has a radius of curvature of 33 cm. Some perimeters consist of an arc of a circle that is rotated, and the test object is moved either manually or mechanically along this arc from the periphery toward the center. The more elaborate perimeters, such as the Goldmann perimeter, are constructed from a half shell, in which the test object is projected (Figure 19.2). In this type of perimeter, the intensity of the illumination of the test object be controlled and the patient's fixation can be continually checked by a viewing device behind the perimeter.

Before use, the Goldmann perimeter should be aligned and calibrated as follows:

1. Level the instrument so that the projector arm will swing back automatically into the protected position on the sphere when the instrument is not being used. Insert the chart paper and position the vertical and horizontal lines with the V-notch on the frame. If a fixation light projector is used, the chart is positioned 5 degrees from the center line.
2. Use the 15-degree position to the right and left for examination when the central scotoma device is indicated.
3. Adjust the telescope so that the reticule and the patient's eye are clear and in plain focus. Proper

adjustment of the light within the sphere and of the projected target is most important. Position the recording arm at the 70-degree mark on the chart. This allows you to lock the projector arm in the proper position by pushing the centering pin on the operator's side into the socket on the upper left side of the instrument. When the arm is locked in, light from the projector will fall onto the light meter.

4. Position the size and brightness control levers to the far right. Turn the instrument on and the room lights off. Turn the appropriate control knob and adjust to a reading of 1000 apostilbs on the light meter.
5. Set the gray filter level to the 0.0315 position. This produces an illumination of 31.5 apostilbs.
6. Interpose the white photometer shade between the projected light and the light meter.
7. At this point look at the photometer screen through the cut-out on the opposite side of the sphere. Match the sphere's brightness to the brightness on the photometer shade or screen by moving the diaphragm up or down. To achieve reliable and accurate fields, calibration of the instrument should be performed before each examination, but from a practical standpoint once monthly is adequate. You are now ready to proceed with the visual field test.

When the visual field has been mapped out on a perimeter, the following notations should be made: (1) the size of the test object, which can vary from 1 to 25 mm, (2) the test

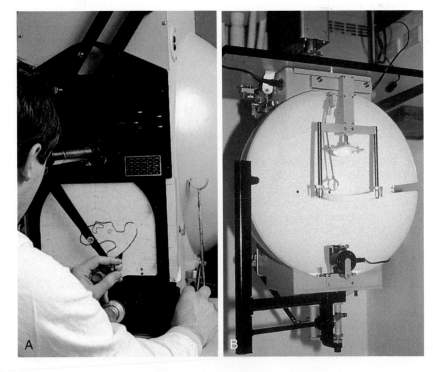

Figure 19.2 (A), (B) Goldmann spherical projection perimeter, an excellent apparatus for both peripheral and central fields. *(Reproduced from Spalton D, Hitchings R, Hunter P. Atlas of clinical ophthalmology. 3rd ed. St Louis: Mosby, 2004; with permission.)*

A

B

distance, which is always 330 mm in a perimeter, (3) the color of the test object, and (4) the cooperation and reliability of the patient.

MEASURING A FIELD ON THE PERIMETER

Just before the actual perimetric examination, the patient should be told in detail what is expected during this test. It is essential that the patient be comfortable, relaxed, and alert. Glasses are not required. The patient is brought to the perimeter and his or her chin is set on the chin rest. The chin should be placed comfortably on the rest so that the patient's face is held vertically and not tilted to one side. One eye is covered. The other eye, situated in the center of the arc, fixes on the white fixation target at the center of the perimeter around which the arc revolves.

The size of the test object chosen depends on the accuracy of the patient's fixation and reaction time. If the patient is young and alert and has 20/20 vision, the examination is begun with a 1- or 2-mm white target (I-2-e or I-3-e on the Goldmann perimeter). However, if the patient is confused and suffers with early stages of dementia, or has dementia, and has vision no better than 20/200, it would probably be best to use a 10 mm, 20 mm, or even larger test object (III-4-e) as the initial stimulus. The test object is always brought in from the periphery toward the center (from the nonseeing to the seeing area). The test object should be brought in slowly so that the time lag from the patient's response to the mark of the examiner will not be great. In many instances the ophthalmologist will request a perimetric examination to be performed with certain test targets. These different targets show characteristically larger fields with the larger target. In follow-up visits it is important to reuse the same targets to show any regression or progression of the field changes. The different targets show a different-sized field at a common illumination and distance; each of these completed mappings of a single target size and brightness is called an *isopter*. The ophthalmologist will inform the ophthalmic assistant which isopters are desired.

The patient should be taught to buzz or tap when the stimulus is seen. Conversation during the test should be kept to a minimum because it only serves to distract the patient and cause head movement.

Ideally 24 meridians should be tested. The normal physiologic response to an object in the peripheral field is to turn the eyes toward it. When the field of vision is charted, this normal response has to be suppressed because fixation by the patient must be rigidly maintained on the central target. Therefore, it is imperative to observe the patient's fixation at all times. In some of the more elaborate perimeters a viewing system at the back of the shell enables the examiner to constantly watch the patient's eyes during the entire examination.

Field testing is taxing. Accuracy depends on the subject's accurate and quick response. It should not be laborious because prolonged visual field testing will tire a patient and cause erroneous results. Drooping eyelids or eyeglass frames interfering with a clear view of the test object can cause these erroneous results.

Errors in field testing can occur on the part of either the patient or the examiner. Errors attributable to the patient may include following the test object rather than maintaining proper fixation, tilting the head or moving the chin off the chin rest, not understanding the test or being generally uncooperative, responding slowly, most often done by mentally challenged patients with low visual acuity or obvious field defects, and physical, mental, or psychologic handicaps. Errors attributable to the examiner may include poor patient instruction, too-rapid movement of the test object, incorrect monitoring of the patient's fixation, poor or inaccurate marking of the chart, and poor or incorrect adjustment of the perimeter.

CHARTS

The visual field chart is merely a permanent record of the patient's responses at tangent screen and perimeter examinations. The best type of tangent screen chart is that in which both fields are represented on a small pad that can be fastened to the patient's record so that the whole picture of the patient's visual status can be seen at a glance. The right eye and left eye should be indicated and the chart should be as the patient sees the visual field; that is, the field for the right eye is on the right side of the chart. A notation should be made of the patient's name, the date, and the examiner's name. In addition, the size and color of target used, the corrected visual acuity, the pupillary size, and the patient's cooperation and reliability should be noted.

An isopter is the map of the circumference of a visual field determined by a test object of a certain size, with the patient at a certain distance from the tangent screen or perimeter. The isopter, as indicated on the visual field chart, should be noted as a fraction, the numerator indicating the size of the test object used in millimeters, and the denominator indicating the distance of the patient from the field chart in millimeters. Thus the fraction 5/1000 indicates to anyone what test object was used and at what distance in millimeters.

SPECIAL PERIMETRIC TECHNIQUES

Visual field screening

Visual field screening is a good method for rapidly determining the presence or absence of a field defect. It is useful as a preliminary procedure in offices or in testing large groups, such as military personnel or students.

Automated visual fields

The automated perimeter or visual field plotter is a quick, randomized test to determine field defects (Figure 19.3). A complete discussion of automated visual field equipment is found in Chapter 19.

Indications of a field defect include the following:

1. Two or more adjacent test spots that were missed at a single test intensity
2. A single spot missed at two or more stimulus intensities
3. Marked contraction of the visual field

The automated suprathreshold screener is extremely useful for preliminary visual field testing because it does not take up the amount of time required for the Goldmann perimeter (Figures 19.4 and 19.5). Those patients examined in the office whose responses to the Amsler grid (see following text) are questionable or who reveal constriction during finger confrontation tests should be examined by the automated screener. If results are normal, generally no further testing is required. If defects are found during the automated screener test, however, then more detailed visual field examination must be done, with particular attention paid to the areas having defects as noted on the automated screener.

There are other models of visual field screeners, all using these principles.

Amsler grid

The Amsler grid was devised to detect abnormalities in the central 20 degrees in the field of vision. This chart consists essentially of vertical and horizontal lines with a central white fixation dot. The squares on the grid are 5 mm in size and subtend an angle of 1 degree at 30 cm. The Amsler chart is of greatest value in detecting small areas of macular or perimacular edema in which visual distortion is a prominent sign (Figure 19.6).

To use the Amsler grid one looks at the central black dot one eye at a time while covering the other eye. The illumination should be good and the patient should wear reading glasses if required. Any areas that appear blurred, missing a grid pattern, or wavy lines should be noted. Home Amsler grids are available. One can rotate the grid card 90 degrees to capture more of the horizontal periphery.

The following series of questions should be asked while the patient is viewing the central white spot:

1. Is the center spot visible? If not, a central scotoma may be present.
2. While viewing the center, can you see all four sides? If not, an arcuate scotoma or a cecocentral scotoma may be present.
3. Do you see the entire grid? Are there any defects? If any areas are absent, then a paracentral scotoma may be present.
4. Are the horizontal and vertical lines straight and parallel? If not, then metamorphopsia is present. The parallel lines may bend inward, indicating micropsia, or bend outward, indicating macropsia.

Figure 19.3 Assessing fields with the Humphrey Visual Field Analyzer.

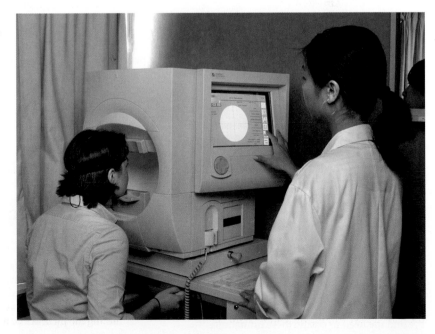

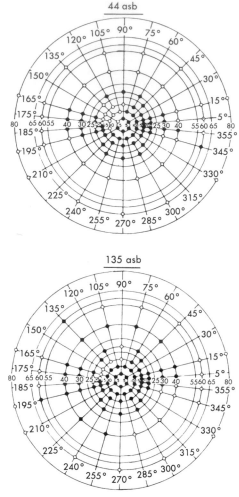

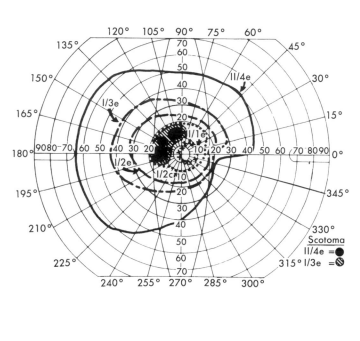

Figure 19.4 Goldmann *(left)* and suprathreshold *(right)* field plots in a patient with glaucoma.

NORMAL VISUAL FIELD

The normal visual field is determined by the size of the test object and the distance at which the test was made. With a 3-mm white target on a perimeter of a 330-degree radius, the average peripheral limit is about 95 degrees outward, 75 degrees downward, 60 degrees inward, and 60 degrees upward (Figure 19.7). If the size of the target is increased, the temporal limit can be pushed outward to about 110 degrees. In many cases allowances have to be made for the contours of the face. Especially to be considered during field testing is the loss of field caused by the projection of the brow and nose. If the visual field is taken without making allowances for these contours, the field is called a relative visual field. The absolute field is obtained by rotating the eye and the head to escape these limitations.

The blind spot marks a physiologic blind area of the retina. It corresponds with the entrance of the optic nerve to the posterior pole of the eye. This blind spot is located about 12 to 15 degrees to the outside of the fixation point and about 1.5 degrees below the horizontal meridian. It measures approximately 7.5 degrees high and 5.5 degrees wide.

PATHOLOGIC DEFECTS IN THE VISUAL FIELD

Pathologic field defects resulting from derangement within the optic nerve or its extensions to the occipital lobe of the brain cause a loss of vision but not a sensation of blackness. Only field defects that arise from disturbances in front of the retina, such as those caused by a vitreous or macular

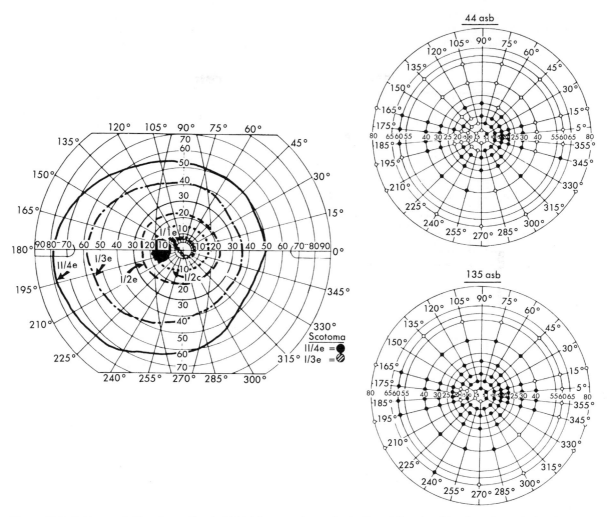

Figure 19.5 Goldmann *(left)* and suprathreshold *(right)* screens in a patient with nutritional amblyopia and a central scotoma.

hemorrhage, result in awareness of something black before the eyes. The distinction between the two is subtle. In disorders of the brain, the patient complains of the effects of the field loss but not of any particular sensation associated with this loss. With retinal disease the patient will complain of both types.

Field defects are classified according to those that emanate from the periphery of the field and those that originate from within the confines of the field itself.

Scotoma

The scotoma is an area of partial or complete blindness within the confines of a normal or relatively normal visual field. Within a scotoma the vision is more depressed than in the area of visual field surrounding it. When the depressed area of a scotoma expands into the periphery of the field, it is said to have "broken through."

Scotomas may be divided into the following types:

1. *Central*, which involves the fixation area and is always associated with a loss of visual acuity (Figure 19.8)
2. *Pericentral*, in which the fixation area is relatively clear and the field immediately surrounding it is deficient
3. *Paracentral*, in which the area of depressed visual field is to one side of fixation (Figure 19.9A). These scotomas also may be denoted as to their position: whether they are nasal or temporal to the fixation point
4. *Cecal*, which involves the area of the normal blind spot (Figure 19.9B)
5. *Nerve fiber bundle scotoma.* This is also referred to as an arcuate, Bjerrum, or comet type of scotoma (Figure 19.9C). This type of lesion extends around the

fixation point from the blind spot in an arc and ends typically on the nasal field with a sharply demarcated border. It can occur either above or below the blind spot. In some instances it is not even attached to the blind spot, but seems to issue from it (Figure 19.10).

The intensity of a scotoma varies from absolute blindness to a minimum detectable loss of visual acuity. If there is complete blindness to test objects of all sizes, the scotoma is absolute. If the area involves loss of only the smaller test objects, it is referred to as a relative scotoma.

CONTRACTION OF THE VISUAL FIELD

Contraction usually occurs as an area of blindness emanating from the periphery of the field toward the center. If the contraction affects only one part of the field, it often is referred to as a *sector defect*. Sector defects bounded by vertical diameters of the field are hemianopic defects. The term *hemianopic* is used to indicate a defect occupying half of the visual field; invariably it is a bilateral defect. A hemianopic defect is homonymous right or left when the corresponding half of both eyes is affected (Figure 19.11). In this instance there is total blindness in the temporal field of one eye and the nasal field of the other eye. The vertical dividing line between the seeing and the nonseeing portion of the field is midline. When a quadrant of each field is affected, a quadrant hemianopia or quadrantanopia is present (Figure 19.12). A bitemporal hemianopia is a visual field

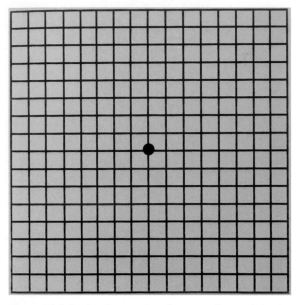

Figure 19.6 Amsler chart used to detect small central visual field defects and distortions of the central visual field.

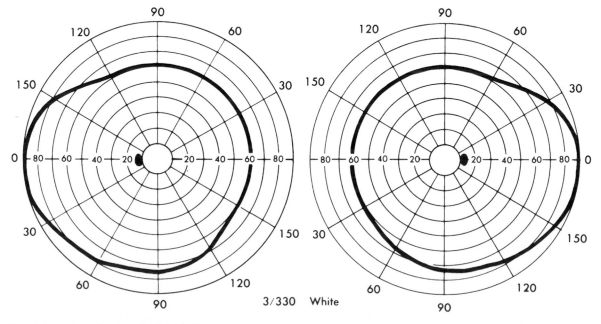

3/330 White

Figure 19.7 Normal perimetric visual field.

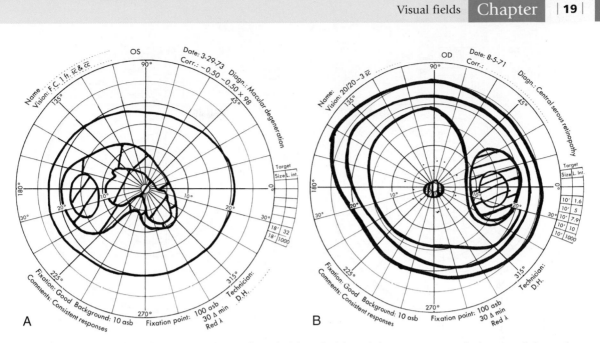

Figure 19.8 (A) A central absolute scotoma, kinetically and with static. (B) A relative scotoma centrally (note small depression on static).

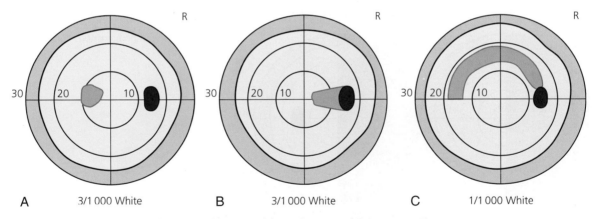

Figure 19.9 Kinetic perimetry. (A) Paracentral scotoma. (B) Cecal scotoma. (C) Arcuate, or Bjerrum, scotoma.

defect in which part or all of each temporal field is depressed (Figure 19.13). The defect may vary from the slightest depression of the upper temporal portion of the field to complete blindness in each temporal field.

A congruous homonymous hemianopic defect is one in which the defect in the two fields is superimposable; that is, completely identical. In this instance when the examiner maps the visual field of one eye, its margin will be identical to the visual field of the other (Figure 19.14).

HYSTERICAL VISUAL FIELD

In some instances defects of the visual field are functional rather than organic; that is, they are caused by disturbance of the patient's emotional status or malingering rather than by disease of the retina or its visual pathways. In this instance the most common field of vision seems to be narrowed down to only 10 to 20 degrees in diameter. If the patient is free of any organic disease, a tubular

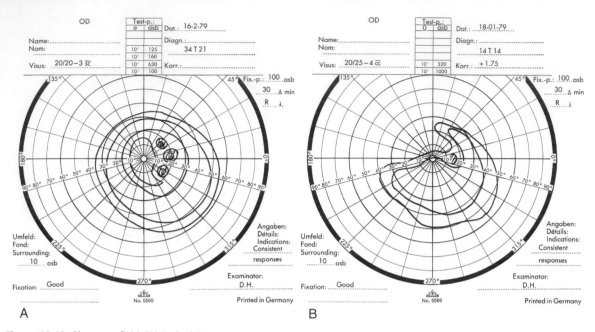

Figure 19.10 Glaucoma field. (A) Early. (B) Late.

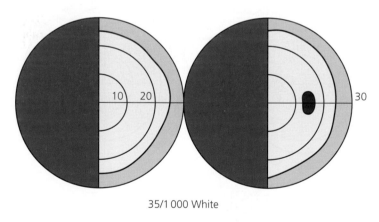

35/1 000 White

Figure 19.11 Left homonymous hemianopia.

defect should indicate, or at least give rise to suspicion, that the patient has hysterical or malingering fields (Figure 19.15).

The presence of such a functional defect can easily be checked by moving the patient back another meter from the tangent screen and doubling the size of the test object. By doing this the visual angle of the field remains the same, but the diameter of the field on the tangent screen should double in size. If the diameter remains the same at 1 and 2 meters, a nonorganic cause should be strongly suspected.

If the diameter of the visual field increases as it should, organic visual loss must be considered. In this case the differential diagnosis of tubular fields includes vitamin deficiency, retinitis pigmentosa, and glaucoma.

With hysterical or malingering patients the size and shape of the field defect can be suggested by the examiner. Other field defects frequently noted with this type of situation are the spiraling field and the star-shaped field. With retinitis pigmentosa, the patient has true tunnel vision. Driving a car with this type of field restriction is hazardous (Figure 19.16).

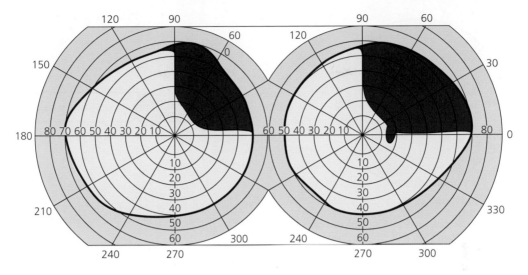

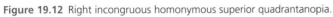

Figure 19.12 Right incongruous homonymous superior quadrantanopia.

Figure 19.13 Bitemporal hemianopia.

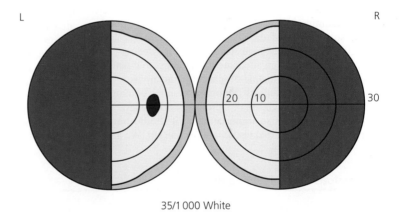

35/1 000 White

Figure 19.14 Left congruous homonymous hemianopia.

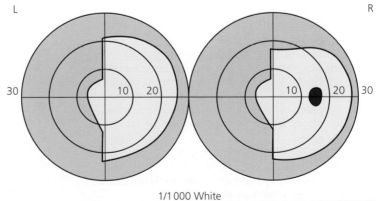

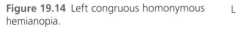

1/1 000 White

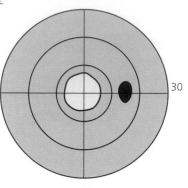

L

30

3/1 000 White

Figure 19.15 Tubular, or hysterical, field. The size of the field remains unchanged when testing at 1 or 2 meters.

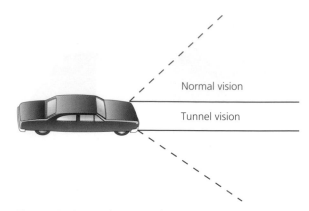

Normal vision

Tunnel vision

Figure 19.16 Tunnel vision, with gross construction of the visual field as is found in retinitis pigmentosa. Driving is hazardous.

SUMMARY

The assessment of the visual field is vital to any complete ocular examination. It is of paramount importance in diagnosing lesions of the visual pathway, retinal lesions, and glaucoma. It is the mainstay of deciding whether glaucoma therapy has been adequate for an individual patient, because the entire principle of glaucoma therapy is to prevent loss of visual field. Its importance cannot be emphasized strongly enough. Many professionals believe that visual field testing is so important that it should be performed only by a trained visual field technician. We are in total agreement with this principle. We do believe, however, that the ophthalmic assistant, if properly trained to do a meticulous examination, can perform a valuable service in visual field testing as a preliminary examination. The final interpretation of the visual field must always be done by an ophthalmologist because only the physician can correlate the results of the visual field test with the patient's problem and the signs obtained on physical examination.

Instruction in visual field examination is best done by demonstration. Competence in visual field testing requires experience. The ophthalmic assistant should take every opportunity to perform routine normal visual field examinations to become familiar with the best techniques of visual field testing.

Questions for review and thought

1. What is an isopter?
2. If a tangent screen examination is recorded as 3/1000, what do the numerator and denominator stand for?
3. What are the pitfalls to avoid in obtaining a good visual field?
4. In a field examination when should the patient's spectacles be removed? When should they be left on?
5. Outline a method of performing the confrontation test.
6. Screening devices are rough guides to detecting possible defects. If a defect is found, what further examination is required?
7. If you find a defect during the tangent screen examination, how do you outline the size, shape, and density of the area?
8. What is the value of the Amsler grid?
9. How can you detect a hysterical field?
10. A lesion in the right side of the brain may show a defect on which side of the visual field?
11. Defects such as a retinal detachment in the lower half of the retina are evident in which part of the visual field?
12. In detecting a defect in the peripheral field, would you be more likely to use the tangent screen or the perimeter?
13. What effect does illumination have on the size of the visual field?
14. A patient who has nystagmus frequently sees better when turning the head in one direction. Is head turning permissible during a field test?
15. What is the field defect that may arise from pressure on the optic chiasm?
16. Contraction usually occurs in one or both eyes as an area of blindness emanating from the periphery. How can you determine whether the field is contracted?
17. The eye with the best vision should always be tested first to obtain an idea of the reliability of the patient. Why?
18. Is the blind spot located nasally or temporally in the visual field? Is it more prominent in the lower or upper field?
19. Patients with macular disease complain of inability to see clearly straight ahead but retain good peripheral vision. What type of field would be found?

Self-evaluation questions

True–false statements

Directions: Indicate whether the statement is true (**T**) or false (**F**).

1. Static perimetry is performed by presenting test points of increasing brightness. **T** or **F**

2. Static perimetry is accomplished with stationary targets with variable brightness in the test targets. **T** or **F**

3. The fixation area of the field is the first to be affected in glaucoma. **T** or **F**

Missing words

Directions: Write in the missing word in the following sentences:

4. A bitemporal defect always suggests a defect in the _____.

5. Static or profile perimetry uses projected light spots in which the luminance is increased by measured increments of light until the patient signals that the stimulus is _____.

6. The visual field defect most commonly found in hysteria is the _____.

Choice-completion questions

Directions: Select the one best answer in each case.

7. The following conditions cause a ring scotoma.
   a. Retinitis pigmentosa
   b. Glaucoma
   c. Normal-tension glaucoma
   d. Vitamin A deficiency
   e. All of the above

8. Tobacco amblyopia usually is caused by:
   a. smoking pipes and cigars.
   b. smoking cigarettes.
   c. common use of chewing tobacco and snuff.
   d. smoking marijuana.
   e. none of the above.

9. The most common visual field defect in patients with optic neuritis is:
   a. an enlarged blind spot.
   b. peripheral contraction of the field.
   c. a sector defect.
   d. a central scotoma.
   e. a centrocecal scotoma.

 Answers, notes, and explanations

1. **True.** The light is held stationary (static) and the illumination is varied until it can be seen by the patient.

2. **True.** Most perimeters have an attachment that enables the perimetrist to choose a meridian on the visual field to discover the retinal sensitivity along a particular meridian. It is used to best advantage to plot out a field defect picked up by a screening device or with conventional kinetic (moving targets) perimetry. Initially, 1-second flashes of subthreshold intensity are used, and these are increased or decreased until a profile of the field defect is uncovered. Any defect in the field of vision is delineated as an area of reduced light sensitivity.

3. **False.** The nerve fiber bundles first affected usually are 5 to 15 degrees away from fixation. The first defect appears as small isolated scotomas that become larger and denser, eventually fusing to form the sweeping arcuate scotoma. Typically these field defects follow the pattern of the nerve fiber bundle and end abruptly at the horizontal raphe. The raphe corresponds to the 180-degree axis on the field chart. The other early field defect is the nasal step. In fact, the very last areas to be afflicted by glaucoma in the visual field are fixation and a small temporal island of vision.

4. **Chiasm.** The only area in the visual system that can produce bitemporal defects is the chiasm. The chiasm is largely composed of crossed nasal fibers, which accounts for the loss of temporal fields of vision. The most common sources of compression of the chiasm are the pituitary gland and its congenital remnants and the hypothalamus. In adults, a tumor called chromophobe adenoma of the pituitary is the most likely cause of chiasmal compression, whereas in children the craniopharyngioma, derived from the congenital remnant of the pituitary, is frequently the major source of chiasmal distress. Other lesions that can affect the chiasm include meningiomas, aneurysms, and compression from a swollen third ventricle of the brain. Bitemporal hemianopias are pathognomonic for chiasmal interference, but the causes of such disturbances are myriad.

5. **Visible.** With static perimetry, the stimulus is not moved but rather increased from zero to visibility. Static perimetry is regarded as being somewhat more accurate than the kinetic method, but is less flexible. A major advantage of kinetic perimetry is that it is less time-consuming.

A Continued

6. **Tubular field.** The key to a hysterical field is that the field loss is the same size regardless of the distance of the test object from the patient's eye, be it 1 or 2 meters. The tubular field is remarkably constant in size, shape, and steepness or margin. It is commonly found in military personnel attempting to escape duty or in children, where it is a device to avoid stress at home or at school. Hysteria should be separated from malingering, which is a conscious simulation of visual loss and in which the field defect is used for monetary gain. The malingerer overstates the case and the hysterical person seems indifferent to the disability. The malingerer is often a person involved in litigation regarding a motor vehicle accident or an industrial mishap. The hysterical patient is cooperative and reliable. The malingerer is snarly, hostile, and afraid to be uncovered. This individual will often not complete a test, complaining of lights, headaches, and watering of the eyes. The discovery of a hysterical patient requires wit, shrewdness, and ingenuity. With the malingerer, the patient views the examiner with hostility and suspicion. The examiner must not only be creative in field testing but also be careful lest the patient turn against the perimetrist.

7. **e. All of the above.** Retinitis pigmentosa is a bilateral condition, passed from one generation to another, that causes night blindness and patchy visual loss in a ring pattern in the midperipheral areas of the visual field (around 15–45 degrees from fixation). Eventually the rings expand and grow denser until the patient is looking through tunnels of vision. The clinical progress of vitamin A deficiency is often indistinguishable from that of retinitis pigmentosa. With glaucoma it is quite common to encounter a double arcuate scotoma that arises from the blind spot and arches above and below the fixation to meet in the nasal field as a ring scotoma. The fact that the blind spot is always involved in the ring serves to distinguish it from retinitis pigmentosa. Also, the halves of the ring are rarely symmetric, so there is an overlap at the horizontal meridian. Dr. Stephen Drance suggests that the basic disorder of low-tension glaucoma is really caused by an ischemic process of the optic nerve head. Certainly the field defects are similar.

8. **a. Smoking pipes and cigars.** The most common cause of bilateral centrocecal scotomas from tobacco is pipe and cigar smoking. Most cases develop in older adult men who smoke frequently and use a dark strong leaf. Scotomas are rare in cigarette smokers but have been reported in snuff inhalers and those who chew tobacco. They appear to be a more common condition in northern England and Scotland and are not encountered with great frequency in North America because of different smoking habits.

9. **d. Central scotoma.** The central scotoma is the most common defect of optic neuritis because of the predilection of these lesions for the pupillomacular bundle of nerve fibers. Perhaps the most common cause of such optic nerve lesions is multiple sclerosis. Retrobulbar neuritis that creates central scotomas occurs in at least 50% of all cases. It is usually unilateral, although bilateral involvement does occur. The scotoma is most commonly central, but other forms can occur, such as paracentral, pericentral, annular, or centrocecal. The scotomas are variable and may be present one day and absent on another.

Chapter | 20 |

Automated visual field testing

Richard P. Mills

A dramatic revolution has occurred in perimetry. The way visual fields are tested and mapped is significantly different now. In the past the standard of excellence revolved around the manual Goldmann perimeter and the perimetrist. The visual field was plotted (see Figure 20.1) after a lengthy examination during which both kinetic (moving) targets and static (stationary) targets were presented in random fashion. Technicians required extensive training and, perhaps more important, considerable patience to perform this task accurately. If prior tests were available, they were carefully studied before testing to minimize testing time and to make sure that the results "made sense." Results became subject to bias of the previous test findings. Testing strategies also contributed to the problem of bias because of the selection and omission of areas of the visual field to be tested.

The problems with test results changed with the use of the microprocessor and the computer. At first glance it seemed too easy. The computer was capable of performing the tedious task of testing by presenting targets in a random fashion, analyzing the results, and printing a map of the visual field. Unfortunately, not all the problems were solved

immediately. Automated perimeters were expensive, test strategies were slow to evolve, and data were difficult to understand and interpret. Many of the software and hardware problems have been solved and the automated testing process has been standardized. Kinetic testing has been almost exclusively replaced by static techniques because the latter are more easily automated. Infrared and mosaic video cameras now monitor fixation. Patient consistency is constantly evaluated during the test by catch trials designed to elicit false-positive and false-negative responses.

In spite of these advances, perimetry remains a subjective test. The entire process depends on the patient's ability to concentrate and respond to the test stimulus. The key person interfacing between the patient and the computer is the technician. It is his or her responsibility to ensure that the patient understands the test and that the testing process runs smoothly. It is also the responsibility of the technician to ensure that fixation remains aligned, that the patient is given a break, and that he or she is reinstructed if fatigue is observed. No automated perimeter available today has eliminated the need for a technician to administer the test and monitor its quality in real time. In this chapter the technician's duties are outlined and, when appropriate, suggestions given to make the task easier and more relevant to the patient's needs.

DIFFERENCES BETWEEN MANUAL AND AUTOMATED PERIMETERS

Both manual and automated perimetry ultimately perform the same function: they test the field of vision, but they do so in different ways. Manual devices highlight moving (kinetic) targets to map out the visual field (Figure 20.1A)

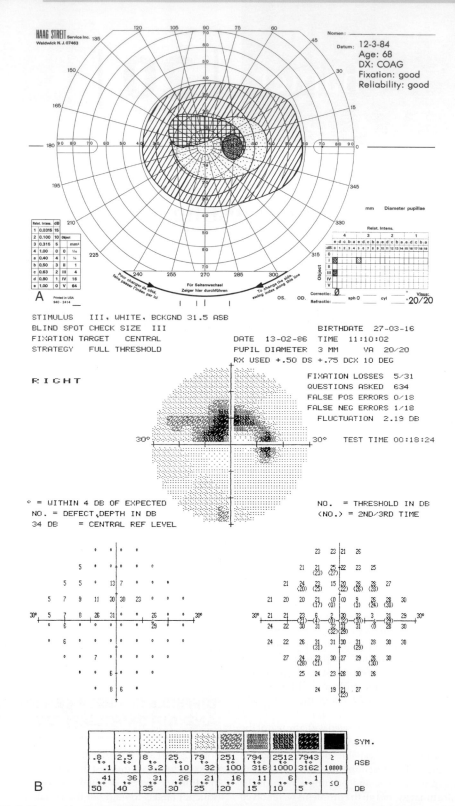

Figure 20.1 (A) Goldmann kinetic visual field. (B) Patient examined with use of Humphrey visual field (static technique).

and spend less time exploring the field with stationary or static techniques, whereas automated devices depend on static techniques almost exclusively (Figure 20.1B).

The best way to describe static perimetry is to contrast it with the more familiar kinetic perimetry. The analogy of the visual field to an island of vision sitting amid a sea of blindness is a useful one (Figure 20.2). The highest point near the center of the island corresponds to the area of greatest visual sensitivity (for the fovea of the retina). As a person moves toward the water's edge, the sensitivity falls to zero. In other words, the farther away from the area of greatest visual sensitivity a person is, the brighter a light target must be to be seen. At the water's edge, in the analogy, not even the brightest target can be seen.

The task of perimetry is to map the island of vision. The problem is that the island is enshrouded in a fog bank (Figure 20.3), and indirect methods of mapping it are required.

Kinetic testing can be likened to airplanes flying toward the visual island at different altitudes (Figure 20.4). If we know the altitude at which the planes fly and if we record the coordinates of each "crash site" of many planes flying at the same altitude, then we can draw an "isopter" line connecting the points. With several isopters, the shape of the island unfolds.

There are disadvantages with kinetic techniques. Flat sections of the island are hard to map unless we use many closely spaced isopters. In a similar fashion, hollowed-out valleys in the interior portion of the island are hard to identify, and we are often dependent on our luck in choosing the proper airplane altitude, or isopter, to detect its presence (Figure 20.5).

Static perimetry uses an entirely different method of visual field exploration. Continuing the analogy, instead of flying airplanes at a known altitude into the island, parachutes are dropped onto the island from above,

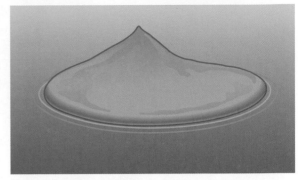

Figure 20.2 Traquair's island of vision in a sea of darkness.
(From Mills RP. Automated perimetry, part I. Am Intraocular Implant Soc J 1984;10:347.)

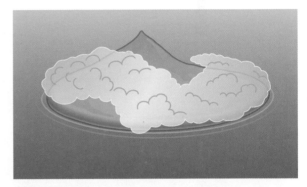

Figure 20.3 Island of vision enshrouded in fog.
(From Mills RP. Automated perimetry, part I. Am Intraocular Implant Soc J 1984;10:347.)

Figure 20.4 Kinetic mapping of the visual field.
(From Mills RP. Automated perimetry, part I. Am Intraocular Implant Soc J 1984;10:347.)

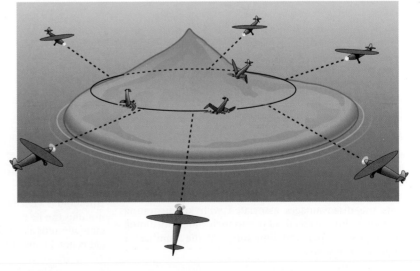

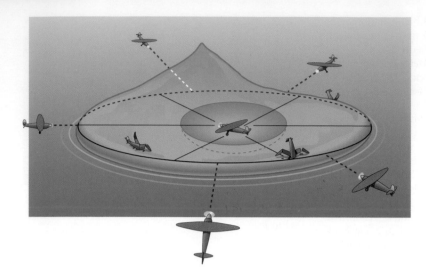

Figure 20.5 Limitations to kinetic perimetry.
(From Mills RP. Automated perimetry, part I. Am Intraocular Implant Soc J 1984;10:347.)

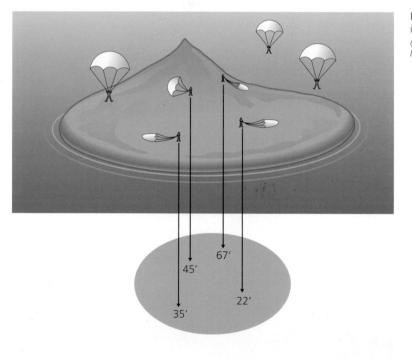

Figure 20.6 Static mapping of the visual island with parachutes.
(From Mills RP. Automated perimetry, part I. Am Intraocular Implant Soc J 1984;10:347.)

and the altitude where each parachute lands is recorded. Once enough parachutes have landed, a topographic map of the island can be created because the coordinates of each parachute are known (Figure 20.6). This circumvents the disadvantages associated with kinetic-testing techniques, but this method is extremely time-consuming and imposes a practical limitation on the number of points to be tested.

UNDERSTANDING THRESHOLD

Threshold is a relative term and represents the level where a stimulus can be seen 50% of the time. This means that the same stimulus also will be missed 50% of the time. Threshold is not an absolute number; rather it is a mathematical approximation described by the sigmoidal curve (Figure 20.7). As the brightness of the stimulus increases, the likelihood of detecting it becomes higher and higher. This percentage of seeing the stimulus does not approach 100% until it is brighter than threshold. In the example illustrated, a stimulus of 55 brightness is seen half of the time. When the stimulus is increased to 59 brightness, the likelihood of seeing it is 95%, yet it is still missed 5% of the time.

Accurate approximation of threshold requires multiple tests of the same points. Single-test determinations may inaccurately reflect the true threshold based on multiple determinations. For similar reasons, stimuli that are clearly suprathreshold still may be missed on chance alone.

The same variability affects kinetic testing when the patient responds to the same moving target at different eccentricities on multiple presentations. Not only is target illumination a consideration, but so too is the actual target motion. The threshold level of seeing a moving test object reflects the patient's ability to detect movement (Figure 20.8A). Therefore, it may be stated that kinetic testing is affected by threshold considerations, but in different ways than static testing (Figure 20.8B), and visual fields from kinetic and static perimeters cannot be directly and consistently compared.

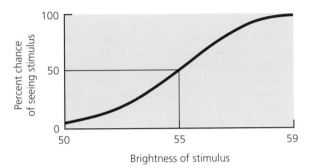

Figure 20.7 Determination of threshold.
(From Mills RP. Automated perimetry, part I. Am Intraocular Implant Soc J 1984;10:347.)

THRESHOLD TESTING

In threshold testing the actual threshold level for each point tested is measured. Starting with a stimulus brighter than calculated normal threshold, the automated perimeter gradually reduces illumination in 4-decibel (dB) steps until it is no longer seen. At that point the computer brightens the stimulus in smaller 2-dB steps until the stimulus is seen again.

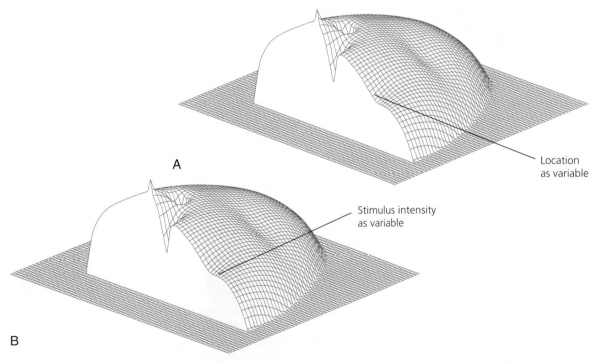

Location as variable

Stimulus intensity as variable

Figure 20.8 (A) Kinetic perimetry: the test variable of stimulus movement. (B) Static testing: the test variable of stimulus intensity.
(From Choplin NT. Octopus perimetry: a meaningful approach to interpretation. Interzeag AG, Koeniz, Switzerland; 1985.)

Using the 4-to-2 staircase technique, the threshold level is crossed at least twice, and the true threshold level is estimated efficiently. Newer algorithms, such as Humphrey's SITA Program, use a testing strategy incorporating a similar but even faster approach.

Swedish Interactive Thresholding Algorithm

The newest computer program for visual field testing, the Swedish Interactive Thresholding Algorithm (SITA), uses an interactive strategy. The program saves time by posing "smart questions." This is accomplished by testing threshold points starting close to the predicted threshold level. If the patient responds in the anticipated manner, thresholding more than once, if at all, is not required because additional information gained by "double" thresholding adds little value. However, if a patient has a condition in which the actual threshold value is not the value predicted, each subsequent location testing will be affected. Thus the computer can start testing adjacent locations incorporating a different starting level (brightness) based on the patient's earlier interaction.

An additional feature of this program is the approach used to interpret patient reliability. Earlier programs used the catch "trial" technique to evaluate fixation errors, false-positive errors, and false-negative errors. This required additional time. Careful research has shown that the patient's response time between seeing a light stimulus and clicking a response button can provide similar information concerning patient reliability. There is a window of time (measured in milliseconds) when a patient should respond to a stimulus. The timing of a patient's response gives information about reliability. If, for example, a patient responds too early to a stimulus, this is a false-positive error because there are physiologic limitations to the interval between seeing a stimulus and physically commanding the hand to click the response button.

To save time, the threshold level start points may be calculated from either prior threshold tests or stored age-corrected normal information. If neither is available, four primary points, one in each quadrant of the field, are tested twice, and the overall level of the hill of vision and then the threshold start point level are extrapolated from these four threshold points.

FREQUENCY DOUBLING TECHNOLOGY

New techniques continue to evolve to solve the problems of making automated perimetry quicker and less of an ordeal. The speed issue is an important one, especially when perimetry is required for screening purposes. A new perimeter, which tests the visual field using a technique called frequency doubling technology (FDT), is capable of screening the central 20 degrees in less than 1 minute per eye with excellent detection ability. This equipment flickers a grid of bars. By varying the brightness of the grid, the visual field can be measured using a suprathreshold or even a threshold strategy. A more sophisticated perimeter using FDT threshold strategy is called Matrix FDT, and is marketed by Zeiss Meditec.

UNITS OF MEASURE

Goldmann perimetry uses an alphanumeric code to denote target illumination. Each letter step from *a* to *e* represents 0.1 log unit (1 dB) brighter in illumination, and each number step from 1 to 4 is a 0.5 log unit (5 dB) change in intensity. Roman numerals from I to V indicate stimulus size changes and not variation in brightness. Because most automated threshold perimetry uses only intensity and not size changes, the automated devices use a different unit of measure, that is, decibels. The advantages of the Goldmann code are enhanced in decibel nomenclature with its direct logarithmic scale. For example, a 20-dB light source seems 10 times brighter than a 10-dB stimulus.

Unfortunately not all manufacturers have adopted the decibel scale. Some have continued to use the apostilb (asb) notation, which is nonlogarithmic, whereas others have adopted the decibel notation. Compared with log units, the two scales are inversely related (Figure 20.9). Note that 0 dB on the automated devices corresponds to

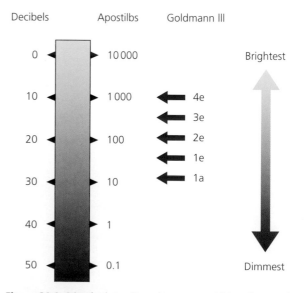

Figure 20.9 Stimulus intensity scales compared (Humphrey and Goldmann equivalent).

(From Haley MJ. The field analyzer primer. San Leandro, CA: Allergan Humphrey; 1986.)

the maximal stimulus intensity, and 0 asb on the nonlogarithmic scale refers to absolutely no illumination. To add to the confusion, not all automated perimeters produce the same absolute levels of target brightness or use the same level of background illumination. The Octopus perimeters use a dimmer background level of illumination (4 asb) and therefore do not need to produce a target stimulus brighter than 1000 asb. The Humphrey perimeters adopted the traditional Goldmann level of background illumination (31.5 asb); thus they produce a maximum stimulus of 10,000 asb. Other perimeters, such as the Dicon, have several different options for background illumination and use light-emitting diodes (LEDs) for targets instead of a projected target source.

Some perimeters have a maximum stimulus brightness of 1000 asb, and others have the capability to produce 10,000 asb stimuli. Because each machine is different, it is important for both the technician and the physician to understand what units of measure are used and the breadth of the scale. In one automated perimeter the brightest possible stimulus, which is 0 dB, corresponds to 10,000 asb, whereas in another 0 dB corresponds to 1000 asb.

AUTOMATED PERIMETRY: BASIC RULES OF TESTING

Before the test

Preparing the patient

One of the greatest sources of error is the patient's not knowing what to expect. Even the most experienced kinetic perimetry patient will produce erratic results on static testing unless some education is provided. Therefore, the patient must be provided with a rulebook to the game. Many perimeter manufacturers make this job easier by providing a script for the ophthalmic assistant to read, accessed by using the "patient instruction" command on the monitor. Testing seems to be less traumatic if the patient can anticipate what will occur. For example, we know that threshold-testing strategy projects stimuli that are visible only half the time. This means that the informed patient should expect to miss about half the presented stimuli.

The operator should share the importance of good fixation by letting the patient know about the telescope or video monitor. Often simply telling the patient about the television monitor that the operator watches during the test will minimize fixation losses. If the patient complains of burning or watering of the eye, an artificial tear can be comforting.

Remember, do not neglect to patch the other eye!

Finally, the operator must determine whether the patient is fresh and alert. If not, the examiner should consider rescheduling the test to minimize any patient wait in the office and ask whether the patient has a preference for a morning or afternoon appointment. It is surprising how well people know themselves and prefer to schedule a visual field test at their best times.

Using best-corrected vision

Another source of frustration and error is not incorporating the proper refractive correction. The visual acuity in each eye should be checked separately before testing, and the patient's medical record should be consulted for the most recent refraction. If one is not available, the technician performs refractometry (if allowed) unless the vision is 20/20. A good rule of thumb is to repeat the refraction if the visual acuity has dropped two lines or more since the last visual field.

Determining the proper trial lens to use

1. Ignore any cylinder less than 1.00 diopter and instead use the spheroequivalent. (Add +0.25 sphere for each +0.50 cylinder ignored.)
2. Calculate lens power for *near!* This depends on the patient's age and degree of cycloplegia. Not all perimeter bowls have a 33-cm depth, so one must consult the manual provided by the manufacturer (Table 20.1).
3. Adjust the lens holder to barely clear the eyelashes (Figure 20.10).
4. Use narrow-rimmed trial lenses (Figure 20.11).
5. Remove the lens correction for testing the periphery outside the central 30 degrees.

Having carefully recorded the patient's best visual acuity and incorporated this refraction with the proper trial lenses for near, the examiner must check pupil diameter to ensure that it is adequately dilated. Small pupils artificially induce a constricted or narrow visual field, which will return to

Table 20.1 Guide for calculating proper near add using a perimeter with a bowl depth of 33 cm

Age	Add for perimetry
30–39	+1.00
40–44	+1.50
45–49	+2.00
50–54	+2.50
Older than 55	+3.00
Dilated/pseudophakic/aphakic	+3.00

Courtesy of Humphrey Instruments with modification.

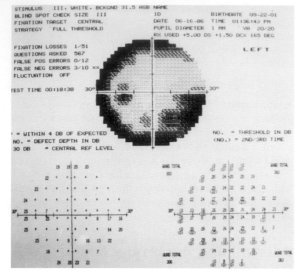

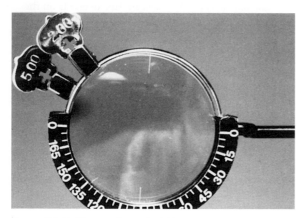

Figure 20.10 Automated visual field with pseudoperipheral field defect created by lens holder and lens positioned too far from eye.

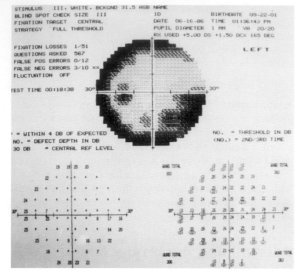

Figure 20.11 Narrow-rimmed trial lens.

normal proportions once dilated. Cataracts or corneal scars dramatically affect the field if the pupil is small. Optimal pupil diameter is 2.5 mm or larger.

It is important to check for droopy or ptotic eyelids capable of impinging on the superior portion of the field. Taping the eyelid up with adhesive or paper tape is permissible.

Preparing the perimeter

Compared with the manual Goldmann perimeter, for which calibration of the light source and background illuminating light is supposed to be performed daily, the newer automated devices are easy. Most are programmed to automatically self-test and check calibration once the power switch is turned on.

A thorough database must be completed before starting the test on a patient. Each machine differs slightly, but most require the patient's name, including middle initial, birth date, visual acuity, lenses used for the test, and pupil size. The technician must avoid the temptation to skip over this step. It is crucial to record the information properly for interpretation and analysis of test results.

The machine is placed in a dimly lit room away from distracting noise. An adjustable, motorized table seems like a luxury at first, but the benefits are obvious. Comfortable and proper alignment for the entire procedure is important (Figure 20.12). Comfortable chairs for both patient and technician are needed.

During the test

The patient should not be left alone. Automation has not and never will eliminate the need to have a technician present during the entire test. A 12- to 20-minute field test can seem like an eternity, and fatigue is a common complaint. If you do not believe this, try a field test on yourself. What you will discover firsthand is that the technician feedback is important and encouragement is very helpful.

Monitoring fixation

This is a tedious task, but very important. Different fixation devices are integrated into different field machines; some use the manual method with a telescope, others use miniaturized infrared video monitors. Neither method is perfect and without its problems. It is important that the technician viewing the monitors have patience and skill.

The technician's role changes dramatically once the person is behind the controls of an automated perimeter. It is tempting for the technician to disengage completely from the test. No one will know. As long as the perimeter keeps marching along and the patient keeps on pressing the buzzer, no one can really determine how attentive the technician really was. The computer does not know if the technician is really monitoring fixation. Yet much like a pilot, the perimetrist constantly needs to scan the control panel, interpret information, and make adjustments. For example, pleasant 91-year-old Mrs. Johnson looks as if she is dozing off for a nap. This is understandable inasmuch as the test has taken nearly 18 minutes and is almost complete. It is important to stop the test, arouse Mrs. Johnson, encourage her that the test is nearly completed, and perhaps even give her a brief break before finishing. Once done, it is equally important to note on the hard copy printout that Mrs. Johnson fatigued easily.

Choosing the best strategy

Initially the task of choosing the proper and best testing strategy is puzzling to both physician and technician.

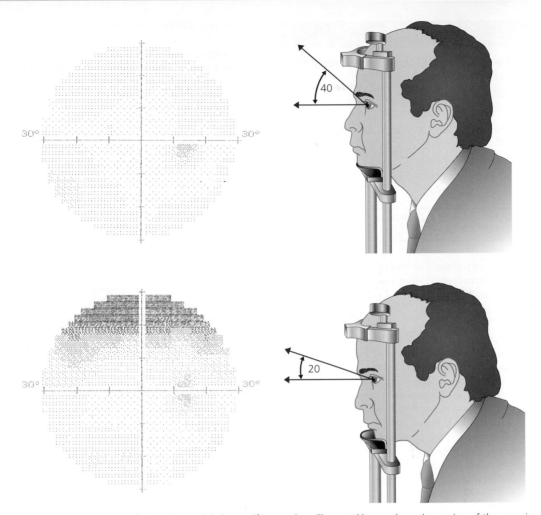

Figure 20.12 Proper positioning of the patient minimizes artifacts such as illustrated here, where depression of the superior visual field is exaggerated because of incorrect patient alignment.
(From Anderson DR. Perimetry: with and without automation. St Louis: Mosby; 1987.)

Many options are available: screening or threshold, and short or long.

Two important precepts are important to recognize. One is that experience has dictated that only a handful of test strategies will be used on a regular basis. Glaucoma patients almost uniformly require a threshold 24-degree central field. For the Humphrey Field Analyzer it is the 24-2 program, and for the Octopus 500E it is the 38 or G1 program.

The second precept is to determine what question the field test is expected to answer. The test could be part of a large population-screening study, or it could be looking for a specific problem: chloroquine maculopathy, for example. In most cases the physician will need to answer this question to direct the test and the choice of strategy.

Box 20.1 is a guide that we have created and used. This can be a starting place to establish a set of criteria for a visual field protocol. The technician whose particular instrument is not listed can review the possible testing programs and select the most similar ones available to fulfill individual needs.

Monitoring the test

Fixation

Different machines monitor fixation differently, but generally, fixation is recorded in a similar fashion: the number of fixation losses is relative to the number of fixation checks.

Some perimeters retest those spots evaluated just before the fixation loss, whereas others simply note the loss and beep, and then continue with the test.

False positives

This is a measure of the patient's understanding of the test. A false-positive error occurs when a patient thinks the light stimulus is one at a time when it is not projecting. Often a click of the shutter opening is heard just before the light stimulus is flashed on. Patients may respond to the click and not the light. To evaluate this potential source of error, the computer randomly clicks open the shutter but does not turn on the light. If the patient responds to the noise, then a false-positive response is indicated. The more frequent the number of false-positive errors encountered, the less valid are the visual field results.

False negatives

This parameter attempts to quantify the patient's alertness during the test. During the test program, the computer retests spots where the stimulus was previously seen. The retesting uses the brightest possible illumination. Thus if the patient does not respond to the brighter light, then the assumption is made that at that particular point the patient was not alert to respond. Again, a high ratio of false-negative responses indicates a potentially serious problem with test reliability.

ANALYSIS SOFTWARE AND PRINTOUTS

Proper interpretation of the visual field results on a patient is key to effective diagnosis and treatment. Modern automated perimeters have a variety of important tools to help the physician in this task. The technicalities of how these tools function is beyond the scope of this chapter, but it is important that the perimetrist be able to print the reports that the doctor will require. Protocols incorporating the various reports should be developed for each office.

In all cases, it is important that patient data be entered correctly because the computer uses the patient's name (exact spelling) and birth date to identify prior visual fields from the computer memory, and to compare the patient to an average patient of similar age stored in the perimeter database.

Each perimeter has its own menu of reports, but generally these fall into two categories: single-field analysis and visual field progression analysis. The examples provided are from the Humphrey Field Analyzer family of perimeters manufactured by Zeiss Meditec.

Single-field analysis

This standard printout (Figure 20.13) has demographic and test-specific information in the top section. Six visual field maps are arranged on the left side. The patient fixation point is located at the intersection of the vertical and horizontal lines. The top row contains a numeric printout of the threshold values at each tested point and a gray scale where darker color indicates worse vision. The middle row contains numeric comparisons to the normal age-corrected database. The bottom row shows the probability of normality at each tested point, darker squares indicating poorer vision relative to the normal database. In the box at the right, the present single-field test result is compared with past visual field tests on the same patient to flag possible progression (worsening) of the visual field over time.

Visual field progression analysis

On this summary printout (Figure 20.14), the most recent visual field is located on the four maps at the bottom: the gray scale on the left, followed to the right by the probability plot, a numeric comparison to the patient's baseline, and the progression analysis referred to earlier. The top row contains the two baseline fields on the patient. These could be the first two fields, or a different pair of baseline fields, as described in the following. The baseline fields have their respective probability plots to the right of the gray-scale maps. In the middle is a graph of the visual field index (VFI), as the patient has aged. In this example, the patient has been rapidly deteriorating over a decade. The scale of the VFI is from 0 to 100, so in a rough sense it represents the percentage of the visual field that the patient has remaining.

The perimetrist must ensure that the baseline examinations chosen by the machine represent an accurate representation of the patient's field at baseline. For example, one of them could have been obtained on a "bad day," and this one should be replaced by a more typical field (perhaps the next one). Another reason for changing the baseline fields is when the patient has glaucoma surgery,

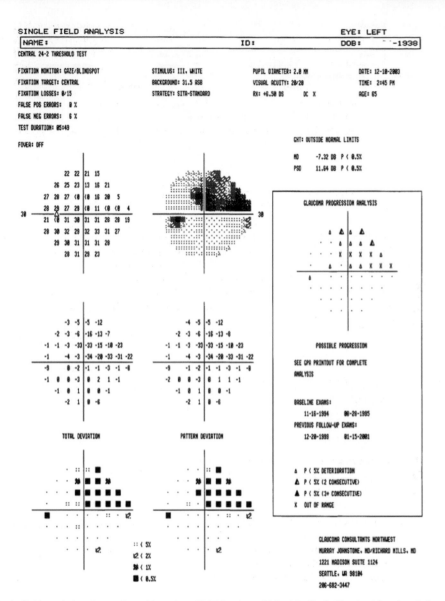

Figure 20.13 Single-field analysis printout from Humphrey Field Analyzer (Zeiss Meditec). (See text for description.)

and the ophthalmologist is interested in determining progression from that point onward. In that event, one should use the two fields just after the patient's surgery date.

SUMMARY

It should be apparent that automated perimetry is here to stay. The power of the computer to perform redundant and complex tasks frees the perimetrist to perform better visual field tests than before. The key component is not the computer or sophisticated software programs; rather, the key component continues to be the technician. Initial fears that computers would eliminate the need for a qualified ophthalmic assistant or technician are unfounded. There is no computerized perimeter currently available with enough artificial intelligence to replace the well-trained and knowledgeable perimetrist. The role of the perimetrist is continuing to evolve as the automated perimeter eases many aspects of testing. As this occurs, the attention of the technician is now directed toward other areas. In

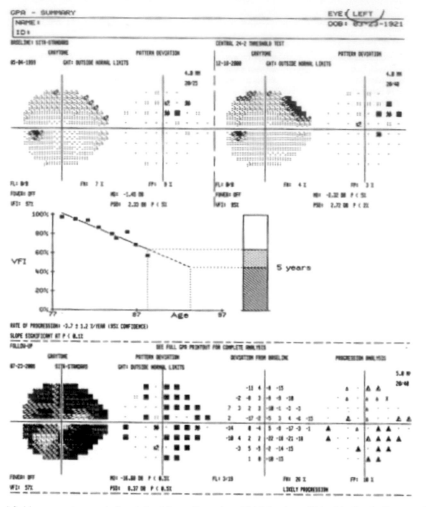

Figure 20.14 Visual field progression analysis printout from Humphrey Field Analyzer (Zeiss Meditec). (See text for description.)

particular, the perimetrist has more time for guiding and encouraging the patient through the testing procedure.

Automated perimeters can be as useful and reliable as manual perimeters used by skilled technicians. Many clinicians believe that automated fields may be even more reliable than manual field examinations in that an important variable is eliminated, that is, the visual field technician. For patients whose attention span or understanding is weak, however, manual perimetry may be required. Such

patients as older adults, children, and those with decreased levels of consciousness, ptosis, or posture abnormalities may be suitable candidates for manual perimetry.

In the recent past, many new automated perimeters have appeared in the marketplace and have been valuable in suprathreshold and threshold static perimetry, with detection rates as high as 90% to 98% and false-positive findings of only 5% to 10%. Interpretation of field test results requires careful analysis for proper diagnosis.

Chapter | **21** |

Ocular injuries

The ophthalmic assistant and associated allied personnel in ophthalmology should have knowledge about the prevention of eye accidents and the first-aid therapy of trauma in industry as well as at home. Reports from the National Society for the Prevention of Blindness reveal that ocular injury is responsible for 5% of all blindness in children of school and preschool age. Many athletic activities, including racquet sports, boxing, and hockey, carry the risk of visual casualties. Industrial eye injuries are virtually a daily occurrence in every ophthalmologist's office and in every emergency center of a hospital.

The escalation of traumatic eye injuries is partly attributable to the progress achieved in the field of transportation, to the development of potentially dangerous consumer home products and children's toys, and to advancements in industrial mechanization, without corresponding advances in personal safety devices. Only in large industrial plants have safety programs been inaugurated to detect visual disabilities and to prevent eye accidents. From the industrial safety organizations have sprouted the Wise Owl clubs in the United States, now numbering 26,000. Members are employees who have had one or both eyes saved from a serious injury by the use of protective lenses.

Despite rigid precautionary safety measures, however, eye accidents will continue to occur because of carelessness, chance, and the tendency of people to ignore the safety measures provided for them.

This chapter deals with first-aid therapy of eye injuries and preventive measures to help reduce the loss of vision from trauma.

DIAGNOSIS OF OCULAR INJURY

The diagnosis of an eye injury can be made by a careful history of the injury in relation to the time and type of injury. A history of discomfort and reduction in vision may indicate the severity of injury. Objective signs require careful external examination that includes comparison with the unaffected eye. Pressure should never be exerted in separating the eyelids, but the upper lid should be pushed up against the bone under the eyebrow and the lower lid depressed with pressure only on the bone of the cheek below. All injuries to the globe, until proved otherwise, should be examined as if the globe has been ruptured. If magnification is required, a × 2 loupe or slit-lamp microscope can detect areas of damage not otherwise discovered.

CONJUNCTIVAL AND CORNEAL FOREIGN BODIES

Despite the many anatomic and physiologic protective factors around the eye, nearly everyone at one time or another has had a foreign body in the eye. In most instances the ensuing tearing and blinking of the lids have been sufficient to dislodge the irritant. It is when these natural mechanisms fail to remove a foreign body that one has to have it located and removed (Figures 21.1 and 21.2).

When a foreign body has lodged in the cornea, examination should always begin by determining the patient's best-corrected visual acuity of the injured eye with glasses on or with the addition of a pinhole disc if the vision is reduced. In this way any preexisting visual impairment will not be attributed to the trauma and removal of the foreign body. In taking the history, the examiner should attempt to ascertain the source of the fragment, because the type of foreign body will influence the amount of tissue destruction and rate of repair. Particles of copper and brass are notoriously more irritating to the eye than are iron and steel. High-velocity foreign bodies—that is, those catapulted by hammering, chiseling, or lathing—are prone to penetrate the cornea deeply, or even to perforate it, as opposed to the wind-blown particle that embeds itself in the superficial corneal epithelium.

It usually is expedient to place two or three drops of a local anesthetic, such as proparacaine hydrochloride (Ophthaine, Ophthetic) or tetracaine hydrochloride

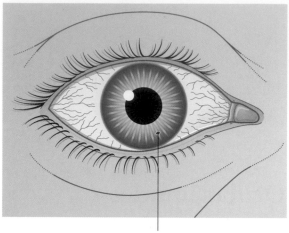

Foreign object

Figure 21.2 Redness, foreign body sensation, and photophobia occur in the presence of a corneal foreign body.
(From Stein HA, Slatt BJ, Stein RM. A primer in ophthalmology: a textbook for students. St Louis: Mosby; 1992.)

(Pontocaine), into the lower conjunctival sac to facilitate surface anesthesia. This makes the patient more comfortable and allows the examiner to scrutinize the injured eye with ease. The best instrument for examining the cornea is the slit-lamp microscope because it offers simultaneously high magnification and strong focal illumination. A useful alternative is an ordinary electric light or flashlight placed about 30 inches (75 cm) from the patient and slightly below the level of the eyes. The light can then be brought into focus on the eye by means of a condensing lens. Magnification is obtained with the use of jewelers' loupes or other types of binocular magnifying glasses.

If a foreign body cannot be seen, a strip of fluorescein paper can be placed in the eye to stain the surface of the cornea because foreign bodies become visible when surrounded by the stain. If the foreign body has become dislodged by the patient's blinking and tearing, the fluorescein will stain the resultant corneal defect. In many cases the cornea will show many surface scratches and the foreign body will be located on the undersurface of the upper or lower lid. Routinely, an examination of the palpebral conjunctiva lining both the upper and lower lids should be performed. Inspection of the conjunctiva lining the lower lid is carried out simply by depressing the lower lid. The undersurface of the upper lid is examined by everting it. The patient is asked to look down while the eyelashes are grasped and pulled over a glass rod, toothpick, or tightly wound cotton swab (Figure 21.3). Alternatively, this examination can be accomplished by everting the upper lid over a transilluminator or muscle light. The foreign body is usually revealed as an opaque speck in the red glow of the lid tissue.

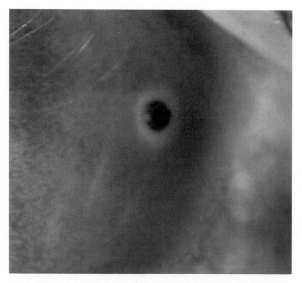

Figure 21.1 Metallic foreign body of the superficial cornea with surrounding cellular infiltration.
(From Kanski J, Bowling B. Clinical ophthalmology—a systematic approach. 7th ed. Edinburgh: Saunders; 2011.)

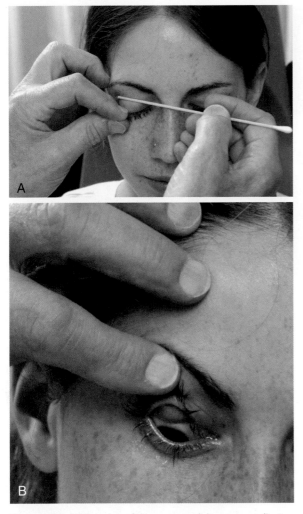

Figure 21.3 (A) Eversion of the upper eyelid over an applicator. (B) Identification of foreign body on underside of eyelid.

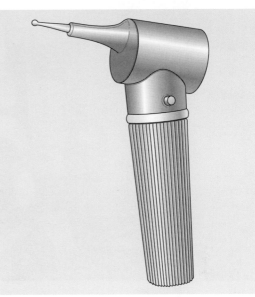

Figure 21.4 Rotating burr for removal of deeply embedded corneal foreign bodies and rust rings.

The treatment of corneal foreign bodies is total removal. A superficial foreign body often can be dislodged by a gentle stream of saline solution delivered from an irrigator, or it can be wiped off by a tightly bound cotton toothpick swab. If these measures fail, the foreign body must be lifted from its base by the use of a corneal spud or burr (Figure 21.4), preferably under magnification by a slit-lamp microscope (Figure 21.5).

After 6 to 8 hours a metallic foreign body may form a rust ring in the corneal tissue. This rust spot is much more difficult to remove because it becomes adherent to the surrounding corneal stroma. The tenacity of the rust is so great that often the corneal spud will only fragment the rusted spot. In such cases it is wise to have a corneal burr on hand to remove the rust ring completely. Small dental drills make excellent corneal burrs. Some ophthalmologists advocate patching an eye that has a rust ring for approximately 24 hours because the slight necrosis of the tissue that results enables easier extraction.

Once the foreign body has been removed, a patch is placed over the affected eye. Adhesive tape applied firmly is used to keep the patch tight against the eyelid. The purpose of the patch is to immobilize the eyelid, thus allowing the corneal epithelium to regenerate without irritation from a moving eyelid. It is important that the patch remain firm to keep the eyelid from blinking. The patient should be advised to avoid excessive eye movements. If the tape securing the patch becomes loose, the patient should be told to refasten it. Most corneal defects treated in this manner will be adequately repaired within 24 hours. However, if the foreign body is organic (e.g., a fingernail, a piece of wood, or a piece of paper), corneal repair may take as long as 3 or 4 days. Most ophthalmologists use antibiotic drops or ointment before applying an eyepatch.

A corneal foreign body should be treated as an ocular emergency. It is desirable, but not mandatory, that the foreign body be removed as soon after the mishap as possible. If there are extenuating circumstances, however, such as the ophthalmologist's being involved in surgery, the injured eye should receive some antibiotic drops and be firmly patched until the patient is seen. It is imperative, however, to relieve the patient's symptoms. The discomfort of a corneal foreign body can be intense. Satisfactory relief of pain can be obtained with over-the-counter medications such as acetaminophen (Tylenol) or ibuprofen (Advil). The patient should never be given a local anesthetic ointment or drops to take home because local anesthetics only interfere with wound healing and mask complications.

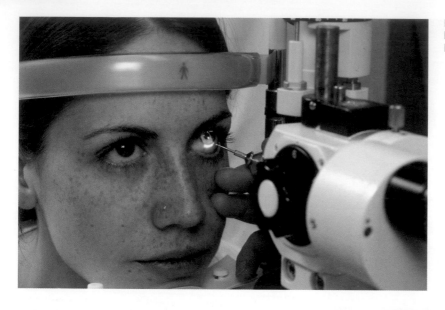

Figure 21.5 Removal of foreign body under magnification of the slit-lamp microscope.

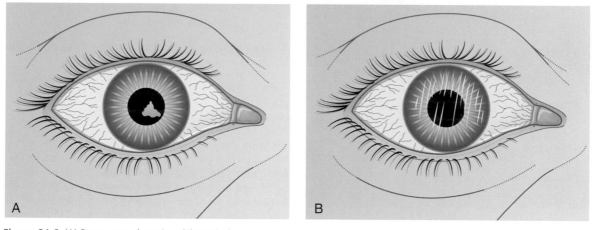

Figure 21.6 (A) Deep corneal erosion. (B) Vertical corneal scratches from foreign body under upper lid.

If the foreign body becomes dislodged by forceful and frequent blinking and the profusion of tears, the patient may still feel that something is in the eye. This is because injury to the cornea, whether it is caused by inflammation, a foreign body, or an abrasion, yields the same symptom: a foreign body sensation.

Conjunctival foreign bodies do not, as a rule, give rise to pain or discomfort in the eye. If they lodge in the bulbar conjunctiva, they usually are easily visible because of the white background of the underlying sclera. Exceptions that are not visible are chips of glass and plastic from a broken contact lens. Superficial conjunctival foreign bodies are removed either by the application of a moistened cotton-tipped applicator or by gentle irrigation with saline solution. Occasionally forceps may be required if there is blood around the foreign body; the ophthalmic assistant should be aware that penetration of the eye may have occurred.

Corneal abrasions

Corneal abrasions are superficial scratches and erosions of the cornea (Figures 21.6 and 21.7). They are found after corneal foreign bodies have been removed, either spontaneously or with treatment. They are most commonly found after injuries caused by paper, fingernails, wires, and so forth. A corneal abrasion, unless it is large, cannot be seen with the naked eye. Patients with a corneal abrasion complain of a foreign body sensation of the eye. Often these patients are seen by a nurse or a friend and told that there is nothing in their eye and as a result they suffer until they are finally seen by the ophthalmologist. Any patient who

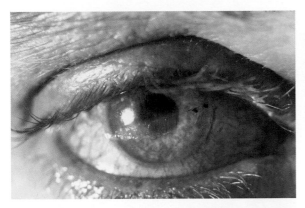

Figure 21.7 Corneal abrasion as a result of thermal burn from hair curler.

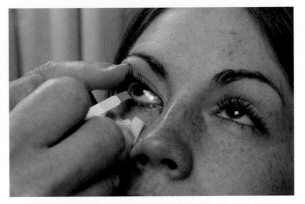

Figure 21.9 Application of moistened fluorescein paper strip. Some practitioners find the lower cul-de-sac easier to use.

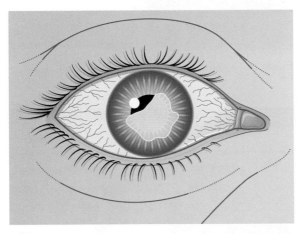

Figure 21.8 Corneal abrasion is characterized by ciliary injection and an epithelial defect (which stains with fluorescein). *(From Stein HA, Slatt BJ, Stein RM. A primer in ophthalmology: a textbook for students. St Louis: Mosby; 1992.)*

2. The patient should be warned that discomfort in the eye may occur an hour or two after office treatment. This is the length of time that the local anesthetic given in the office usually remains effective. If a feeling of irritation continues, the patient should be instructed to take a pain-relieving drug.

3. The patient should be told not to remove the patch until instructed. Medication other than some general analgesics should not be given. The patient also should be told that it is best to return home and rest. Movements of the cheeks, such as in talking, only serve to loosen the patch and free the eyelid. A blinking lid causes pain and removes the regenerated epithelium.

4. The rate of healing depends on the area of the tissue injured, the amount of tissue devitalized, the presence or absence of infection, and the nature of the injuring agent.

INTRAOCULAR FOREIGN BODIES

Intraocular foreign bodies constitute a surgical emergency. Often the site of penetration is not visible externally (Figure 21.10). The ophthalmic assistant should not make a judgment on the gravity of a foreign body injury on the basis of the eye's external appearance.

Because the severity of the intraocular damage depends on the size, shape, and composition of the foreign body, the assistant should attempt to obtain an accurate description of the nature of the type of metal embedded. Often it is possible to ascertain the source of the fragment. This is very important because the success of the operative procedure depends to a large extent on whether the fragment is magnetic. The patient should be reassured that everything possible will be done, but should not be promised a full recovery of the eye because eyes injured by foreign bodies,

complains of a foreign body sensation of the eye should be seen. Fluorescein strips should be placed in the eye (Figures 21.8 and 21.9) to stain the area of the corneal defect, and the eye should be examined with magnifying glasses. Corneal abrasions are treated by firm patching for 24 hours. The larger the abrasion, the more time it takes to heal. A bandage contact lens may minimize pain. This is the case after laser photorefractive keratotomy (PRK).

Aftercare of patients with superficial injuries

The following points summarize the aftercare of a patient with a superficial corneal and conjunctival injury:

1. Arrangements should be made to have the patient driven home.

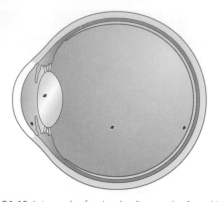

Figure 21.10 Intraocular foreign bodies can be found in a variety of sites: in the anterior chamber, lens, vitreous, or retina. *(From Stein HA, Slatt BJ, Stein RM. A primer in ophthalmology: a textbook for students. St Louis: Mosby; 1992.)*

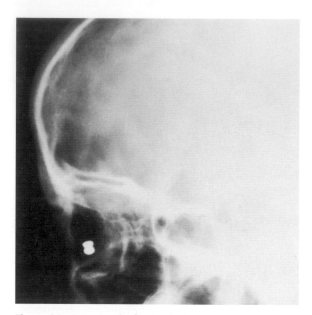

Figure 21.11 Intraocular foreign body. Air pellet entry into the globe.

particularly those lodged in the posterior pole (i.e., in the retina or vitreous), often do poorly.

One can serve the patient best by making sure that this type of injury is seen by the attending ophthalmologist immediately. Relatives should be notified and the hospital, particularly the operating room personnel, should be informed of the emergency. Transportation to the hospital should be arranged so that the patient is not kept waiting in the office. The patient's eye should be patched, primarily to prevent infection and prevent the patient from causing further damage to the eye by rubbing it or by cleaning it with a dirty handkerchief.

The ophthalmic assistant should always be aware of the possibility of the presence of an intraocular foreign body. Intraocular foreign bodies usually are high-velocity small missiles and should be suspected in accidents in which striking, grinding, or cutting force is applied to metal. Fast-moving particles may penetrate the eye without producing any pain, discomfort, or gross visible signs and yet still may cause severe damage to the eye. Figure 21.11 shows an air pellet in the eye that passed through the upper eyelid.

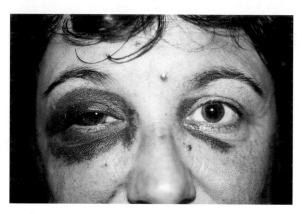

Figure 21.12 Contusions of the eyelids with ecchymosis. *(From Kanski J. Clinical ophthalmology, 8th edn. Oxford: Elsevier/Mosby.)*

CONTUSION OF THE EYELIDS: BLACK EYE

A black eye is the result of an injury to the orbital margin or eyelids from a blunt object, such as a fist (Figure 21.12). The appearance of a black eye is quite alarming to the patient because of the large extravasation of blood underneath the skin. A patient with this type of injury should be seen immediately because examination of the globe is easiest in the period following the injury. After 1 or 2 hours the lids become so swollen and taut that examination of the underlying eye becomes very difficult. The orbital rim should be palpated to make sure there are no broken chips.

Treatment of a black eye is the application of cold compresses in the immediate phase to reduce the swelling and further bleeding and use of local analgesics to relieve the pain. Usually within 5 to 7 days the swelling subsides and the hematoma changes in color, gradually fading away as the blood decomposes underneath the skin. Although a black eye is quite innocuous, the secondary contusion to the globe can cause considerable disruption within the eye. The effects of contusion to the globe include traumatic hyphema, dislocated lens, vitreous hemorrhage, and tears in the choroid and retina.

A black eye also may be associated with a broken nose because the bones between the orbit and the nose are extremely thin. Consequently, an abnormal communication (fistula) may arise between the nose and the soft tissues of the lids. When the nose is blown, air may be forced under the pressure into the lids, causing swelling and the development of a curious crackling feeling under the skin. Because there is a risk of spreading infection from the nose into the orbit and eyelids, the patient should be instructed not to blow the nose forcefully.

Frequently a blow to the lids and globe is sufficiently strong to cause a blow-out fracture of the orbit. The muscles on the inferior surface of the globe (the inferior rectus and inferior oblique muscles) may become incarcerated in the defect in the floor of the orbit and the eye cannot be elevated. The patient complains of diplopia, especially when looking up. X-rays are required. These cases are treated surgically by freeing the wedged muscles and placing an implant of bone or plastic over the fracture site. The results of surgical repair are best when the patient is treated early.

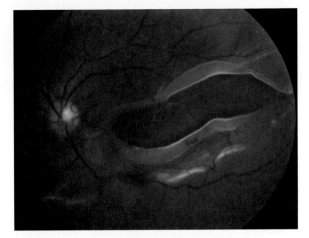

Figure 21.13 Large retinal tear with associated retinal detachment.
(From Kanski J, Bowling B. Clinical ophthalmology—a systematic approach. 7th ed. Edinburgh: Saunders; 2011.)

CONTUSIONS OF THE GLOBE

Contusions of the globe may be caused by an explosive force, such as an air blast, a blow to the bony orbit, or direct injury to the eye itself. Initially the effects of a blow to the eye can be disastrous because perforation of the globe, with prolapse of the intraocular contents, vitreous hemorrhage, retinal detachment, and rupture of the choroid may occur as an immediate complication. If the hemorrhage is confined to the anterior chamber, it is called a hyphema. If the hemorrhage involves the posterior chamber as well as the anterior chamber, it is sometimes called a black-ball hemorrhage. In the event that the initial injury to the eye appears to be minimal, loss of vision can result from complications occurring later, for example glaucoma, cataract, and sympathetic ophthalmia.

Sometimes the retina may be affected. Any shadow, floaters, or loss of vision should be investigated because tears in the retina, retinal detachment, or vitreous hemorrhage may have occurred (Figures 21.13 to 21.15).

Early complications

Early complications of contusion injuries include subconjunctival hemorrhage, hyphema (hemorrhage into the anterior chamber) (Figure 21.16), iris involvement (iridodialysis or separation of the iris at its base), tears of the sphincter muscle and iritis, glaucoma secondary to iritis or hyphema, dislocation of the lens, vitreous hemorrhage, retinal tears, detachment and hemorrhage, choroidal rupture, scleral rupture, and avulsion of the optic nerve.

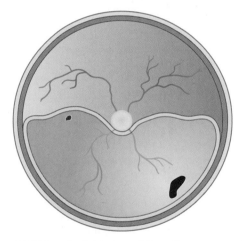

Figure 21.14 In retinal detachment the retina appears white when elevated. If the macula is detached, the central vision will be diminished.
(Adapted from Stein R, Stein H, editors. Management of ocular emergencies. 5th ed. Montreal: Mediconcept; 2010.)

Of the early complications, injury to the anterior segment of the eye is the most frequent because it receives the greater proportion of the force of injury. Frequently the injuries to the eye are multiple, the most common of which are tears either at the root or at the pupillary margin of the iris combined with a hyphema (Figure 21.17).

Late complications

Late complications of contusions of the globe include glaucoma, which may appear many years after the original injury (called angle-recession glaucoma), sympathetic

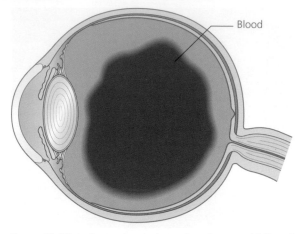

Figure 21.15 A vitreous hemorrhage that obscures visibility of the fundus.

(Adapted from Stein R, Stein H, editors. Management of ocular emergencies. 5th ed. Montreal: Mediconcept; 2010.)

ophthalmia, cataract, band keratitis, and phthisis bulbi (shrunken and disorganized eyeball).

Of the late complications, sympathetic ophthalmia is most feared. It occurs in the uninjured eye when the injured eye has had extensive damage to the iris and ciliary body. Sympathetic ophthalmia takes at least 2 weeks to appear, being most common 2 months after injury. It may even take 6 to 12 months before it manifests. The early symptoms of this condition are slight pain, photophobia, lacrimation, disturbances in accommodation, and diminution in vision in the unaffected eye. This condition often leads to extensive loss of vision, and even blindness, despite treatment with steroids. For this reason many surgeons enucleate a blind, disorganized, injured eye within 2 weeks of the injury to avoid this dreaded complication of sympathetic ophthalmia. Enucleation after 2 weeks has no prophylactic value once the condition has commenced.

PENETRATING EYE INJURIES

Recognition of penetrating injuries is most important because prompt treatment may result in complete or partial recovery of vision. However, the examiner must be very careful not to press on the globe in trying to separate the eyelids. If blepharospasm exists and the eye does not open readily, it is best to leave the problem alone until the ophthalmologist arrives. Any medication instilled in the eye to relieve pain and blepharospasm should be administered only on the instruction of the attending physician and the medication should have proper dating and be sterile.

Identification of a penetrating eye injury may be made by the following:

1. Black or brown uveal tissue showing through the white sclera
2. Iris protruding from the lips of a laceration of the cornea
3. Flat anterior chamber with collapse of the front portion of the eye
4. Irregularly shaped pupil
5. Any localized tears or holes in the iris
6. Purulent or cloudy material within the eye

The management of a penetrating eye injury is beyond the scope of an ophthalmic assistant. It will depend on the nature and severity of the injury, as well as its site. The ultimate concerns are the restoration of the functional capability of the injured eye to see again and protection of the normal fellow eye from sympathetic ophthalmia.

LACERATIONS OF THE LIDS

Lacerations of the lids should be seen immediately. A delay of 6 to 8 hours in repairing a lid laceration may result in

Figure 21.16 Hyphema or hemorrhage in the anterior chamber. (A) Front view. (B) Side view.

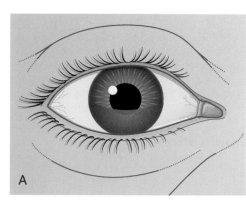

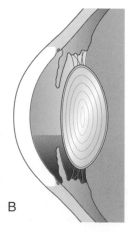

A   B

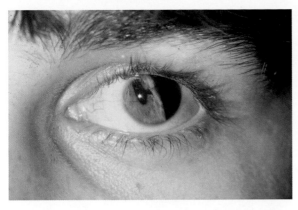

Figure 21.17 Iris sector loss with iridodialysis from globe injury. Double vision and cosmetically poor appearance.

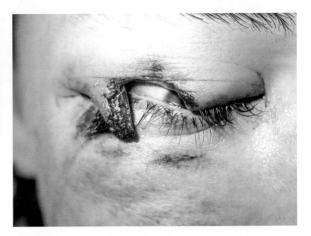

Figure 21.18 Vertical laceration of the upper eyelid.
(From Nerad J, Carter K, Alford M. Oculoplastic and reconstructive surgery. In Rogers AH, Duker JS, editors. Rapid diagnosis in ophthalmology. St Louis: Mosby; 2008.)

serious infection. A wound is considered contaminated if it does not close within 6 to 8 hours after injury. Early surgery enables the surgeon to restore the tissues to their original position with greater accuracy than can be achieved if retraction and swelling of the tissues have been allowed to develop. Normally the ophthalmologist prepares the patient by administering an injection of a broad-spectrum antibiotic and some tetanus toxoid or tetanus antiserum. The ophthalmic assistant should keep these materials on hand for such a contingency.

Lacerations of the eyelid are caused by explosive injuries, deflected high-velocity metal or wood, blunt objects such as the dashboard or steering wheel of a car, and careless play with knives, especially in children. Lid lacerations can involve any site on the upper or lower eyelid. In the upper eyelid the major structure that is disrupted by a large, through-and-through laceration is the levator palpebrae superioris muscle (Figure 21.18). Damage to this muscle and its subsequent retraction may result in posttraumatic ptosis. In the lower eyelid the delicate canaliculus on the medial aspect of the lower eyelid may be severed. Permanent tearing will result unless accurate apposition of the cut ends is immediately performed (Figure 21.19). Other complications of lid lacerations include notched lid margins, entropion, and ectropion.

In all major wounds to the lids or globe, the ophthalmic assistant can best serve the patient by immediately patching the eye and notifying the attending ophthalmologist of the mishap immediately. This action stops bleeding and prevents infection.

FRACTURES OF THE ORBIT

Direct injury to the eye, as from a blow, a golf ball, or a piece of equipment, may result in a fracture of the orbital rim or wall (Figure 21.20). Two types of fractures may

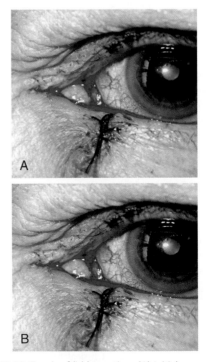

Figure 21.19 Repair of lid laceration. (A) Initial approximation of the tarsal plate with an absorbable suture and lid margin with a silk suture. (B) Completed repair.
(From Nerad J, Carter K, Alford M. Oculoplastic and reconstructive surgery. In Rogers AH, Duker JS, editors. Rapid diagnosis in ophthalmology. St Louis: Mosby; 2008.)

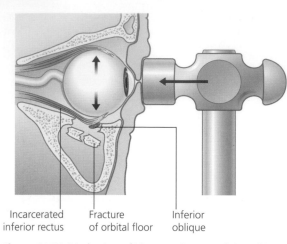

Figure 21.20 Mechanism of blow-out fracture of the orbit. A blow on the eye causes internal pressure on the delicate floor of the orbit, resulting in a fracture. The inferior oblique and inferior rectus muscles may herniate into the maxillary sinus below.

Incarcerated inferior rectus   Fracture of orbital floor   Inferior oblique

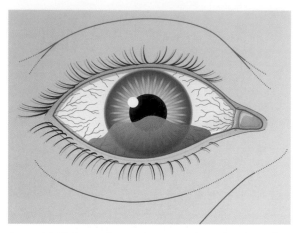

Figure 21.21 Depending on the type and severity, signs of chemical injury may include conjunctivitis, superficial punctate keratitis, epithelial defects of the cornea and conjunctiva, blanching of blood vessels, and necrosis of tissues.
(From Stein HA, Slatt BJ, Stein RM. A primer in ophthalmology: a textbook for students. St Louis: Mosby; 1992.)

occur. One type involves the bony rim of the orbit, along with part of the wall of the orbit, and is usually readily detected by x-ray film. A less commonly detected fracture is a blow-out fracture of the orbital floor. Any direct blow to the eye may drive the globe back into the orbit, where a sudden transfer of pressure to the thin orbital wall occurs. The weakest part of the orbital wall fractures relatively easily because the walls are adjacent to air-containing sinuses and are not supported by heavy fluids or tissue. Whenever a black eye is seen, a blow-out fracture of the floor of the orbit should be suspected, particularly if diplopia occurs in any direction of gaze. The diplopia is a result of entrapment of the inferior muscles that support the globe. Muscle-balance testing, along with x-ray tomograms of the floor of the orbit, will bring this defect to light. Surgical repair of an orbital fracture depends on the computed tomography (CT) scan findings (see Chapter 40) or the clinical signs during the subsequent few days, or both. Surgery is indicated if there is soft tissue entrapment.

CHEMICAL INJURIES

Alkali injuries often are more severe than acid injuries, because acids tend to coagulate tissue and inhibit further penetration into the cornea. Clinical findings of chemical injury vary with severity of the injury: a mild injury is characterized by conjunctivitis, superficial punctate keratitis, and an epithelial defect of the cornea and conjunctiva; a severe injury exhibits blanching of limbal blood vessels and opacification of the cornea (Figure 21.21).

Acids

The acids used extensively in industry are sulfuric, hydrochloric, nitric, and acetic. In small quantity, either as fumes or as a fine spray, these acids can cause injury to the eye. The injury is not as severe as alkali, with redness, watering, and irritation of the lids and conjunctiva occurring (Figure 21.22). With repeated or prolonged exposure, small erosions on the surface of the cornea may result. A copious splash of an acid can produce an extensive burn of the face and eyelids, in addition to serious local damage to the eye itself. Acid burns are frequently complicated by glass injuries as a result of flasks and bottles bursting. These injuries arise particularly in laboratories associated with industries, schools, research establishments, and universities.

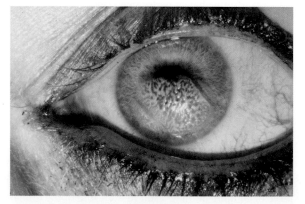

Figure 21.22 Acid burn of the cornea.

Alkalis

Sodium, potassium, ammonium, and calcium hydroxide are the common alkalis involved in industrial burns. In general, alkali burns are more serious and penetrate the eye more deeply than do acid burns. In the home, ammonia is a common cause of corneal burns because it is used extensively as a cleaning agent. It also is used in domestic refrigerating apparatus. Calcium hydroxide, or lime, burns are perhaps the most common alkali burns to the eye. These may occur whenever cements, mortars, whitewash, and plaster are used. The severity of lime burns is related to the fact that the alkali becomes adherent to the corneal and conjunctival tissues and produces chemical reactions between its products and the tissue proteins.

First-aid care

Because the degree of damage done to the cornea or conjunctiva is directly proportional to the concentration of the chemical at the time of injury and to the duration for which the chemical is in contact with the eye, it is vitally important to dilute the chemical and to start therapy as soon as possible. Water is the most nearly universal solvent; it is also the most universally available cleansing liquid in industrial establishments. It should be used abundantly and quickly. If there are no special irrigating facilities available, the patient's eye should be irrigated with water in a pail, glass, or any other available container. The personnel in charge of first aid should separate the lids to overcome the lid spasm and to allow the water to irrigate the conjunctiva and cornea. Separation of the lid is difficult to maintain and is best accomplished by using a paper towel and pressing the lids on the bony prominences above and below the eye. For alkali burns this irrigation should be continued for at least 20 to 30 minutes until arrangements have been made to transport the patient to an ophthalmologist (Figure 21.23).

If the industrial plant has many chemical injuries, thus constituting an occupational hazard of this particular plant, a sterile wash fluid should be kept on hand. This can be distilled water, physiologic saline solution, or Ringer's solution. In other situations the sterility of the water is of secondary importance to the effectiveness of water as a diluent and an irrigator. Irrigators that may be found in an industrial plant include jet-stream drinking fountains and safety showers (Figure 21.24).

The use of neutralizing or buffered solutions to counteract the specific effects of the injurious chemicals has virtually been abandoned today. The reason for this is that the delay in discovering the proper buffer has been regarded as a greater disadvantage than the advantage obtained by having a direct counteracting chemical. Further, if the irrigation is sufficient, neutralization is usually unnecessary.

Second-stage emergency care

Once the patient has been seen by the industrial nurse or the ophthalmic assistant, the patient's vision should be tested to assess the degree of damage. In many cases the amount of lid swelling, pain, and redness is of such magnitude that a visual acuity assessment is not possible. The industrial nurse or ophthalmic assistant should place two or three drops of a suitable topical anesthetic in the eye to relieve the pain and lid spasm. Irrigation with sterile saline solution is continued if the previous attempts have been unsatisfactory.

While this is being done, information should be obtained as to the nature of the chemical involved in the accident, its concentration, the method of the injury, and the duration of probable exposure. The upper and lower fornices should be thoroughly examined with a bright focal illumination for solid particles. These particles, if present, should be removed with a wet cotton-tipped applicator. Because of the copious tearing and lid spasm, it may be difficult to visualize the palpebral conjunctiva for embedded

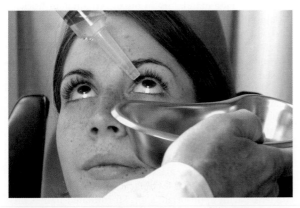

Figure 21.23 Irrigation for chemical burn of the eye.

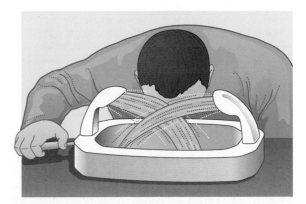

Figure 21.24 Irrigation of the eye by a jet fountain.

particles. To obtain better exposure, the lids should be pinioned against the orbital margin with a dry cotton cloth rather than with the fingers, which tend to slip. An alternative method would be to evert the upper lid over a retractor.

Particles of calcium hydroxide, mortar, or plaster often adhere tenuously to the conjunctival or corneal tissue despite irrigation with water. In such instances the offending particles have to be manually removed or irrigated with a 0.01 molar solution of ethylenediaminetetraacetic acid (EDTA).

It is imperative that any patient with an injury caused by alkalis, strong acids, or any other chemicals known to produce severe ocular injury be seen by an ophthalmologist after emergency eye care has been given. It is helpful if the ophthalmic assistant or industrial nurse can give the ophthalmologist a summary of the events that transpired, including the patient's visual acuity, the nature of the injury, the concentration of the offending agent, the chemical involved, the duration of chemical exposure, and the emergency therapy initiated. The patient should not be sent back to work without the consent of the ophthalmologist. Small particles of alkali that can be visualized only by using a slit-lamp microscope may still be embedded in the cornea. Also, damage to the cornea and conjunctiva may continue for some time after the accident has occurred. If the ophthalmologist is delayed and the patient cannot be seen immediately, the ophthalmic assistant should bandage the injured eye firmly after placing a few topical anesthetic drops on the conjunctival sac. The assistant should also attempt to calm the patient during the period of stress, but should not attempt to make any prognosis regarding recovery. This is the prerogative of the ophthalmologist.

Personal protection against chemical eye hazards

Many plants have rigid safety controls for the handling and transport of dangerous chemicals. There are safety engineering systems for designing clear-air ventilation, segregating hazardous material from the rest of the plant, and designing automatic equipment for the handling of toxic materials in closed or semiclosed systems. The employee is best protected by some type of eye safety glass if the plant uses chemicals in abundance.

INJURIES CAUSED BY SPORTS

Eye protection in sports is an issue that affects everyone. A number of sports contribute to injuries that involve the eye and the adjacent tissues (Figures 21.25 and 21.26). In 1970 and 1971, there were 543 injuries in two seasons of Canadian hockey, in which 63 eyes were blinded. Most of these were caused by hockey sticks raised above the shoulder during the game. Since that time, certified face protectors attached to a certified helmet have become

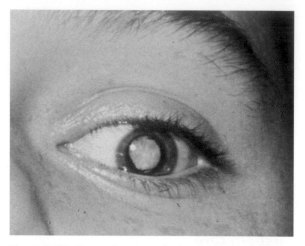

Figure 21.25 Traumatic cataract from tennis ball injury.

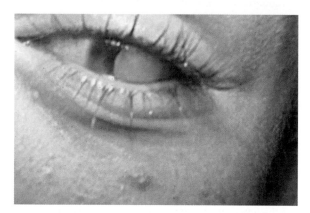

Figure 21.26 Dislocated cataract lens into anterior chamber from squash racquet injury.

mandatory for most minor hockey players in Canada and the United States and are voluntary for professional hockey players. In Canada, ocular trauma decreased by 90% after certified full-face protectors attached to the headgear were made mandatory in organized amateur hockey.

Annually in the United States there are more than 600,000 eye injuries related to sports and recreational activities; 40,000 of these require emergency department visits. Most injuries occurring in school-aged children are sports-related, and eye injuries are the leading cause of blindness in children. Baseball/softball is the leading cause of sports-related eye injuries in children 14 years and younger, and basketball is the leading cause in youths 15 years and older. A listing of sports-related eye injuries by age is shown in Table 21.1. More than 90% of eye injuries can be prevented by the use of appropriative protective eyewear. Protective eyewear includes safety glasses and goggles, safety shields, and eye guards designed for a particular sport. Polycarbonate lenses with appropriate sports-formulated frames provide the best eye protection for many sports, are 10 times more impact-resistant than other plastic lenses, and do

Table 21.1 Sports-related eye injuries by age

Activity	Estimated injuries*	Ages 0 to 14	Ages 15+
Basketball	6,307	1,789	4,518
Water and pool activities	5,505	2,510	2,995
Guns—air, gas, spring, and BB	2,397	1,265	1,132
Baseball/softball	2,100	1,154	945
Football	1,726	686	1,040
Bicycles	1,483	271	1,212
Soccer	1,338	229	1,109
Health club—exercise, weightlifting	1,325	318	1,007
Fishing	1,183	476	708
Table or air hockey	1,180	1,025	154
Racquet sports	1,048	405	643
Ball sports, unspecified	741	380	361
Golf	729	6	723
All-terrain vehicles (4 wheels)	653	260	392
Sports and recreational activity, not elsewhere classified	582	199	383
Winter sports	558	180	378
Volleyball	415	186	22
Playground equipment, not specified	404	404	0
Scooters, skateboards, go-carts	365	155	210
Swings or swing sets	358	226	132
Trampoline	331	233	98
Boxing, wrestling	319	6	313
Totals Top 22 Categories	**31,047**	**12,363**	**18,682**

Based on statistics provided by the US Consumer Product Safety Commission, Directorate for Epidemiology; National Injury Information Clearinghouse; National Electronic Injury Surveillance System (NEISS).
Product Summary Report—Eye Injuries Only—Calendar Year 2014.
Table source: Prevent Blindness. Reproduced by permission of Prevent Blindness.
*Totals may not equal due to rounding.

not adversely affect vision. Ordinary perception glasses and "street wear" frames, contact lenses, and sunglasses do not protect against eye injuries. Safety goggles need to be worn over them. BB guns should be avoided and darts should be played with safety goggles.

INJURIES CAUSED BY RADIANT ENERGY

Ultraviolet radiation

The most common radiation injury encountered results from the absorption of ultraviolet by the cornea. The ultraviolet light of the sun is absorbed mainly by the atmosphere. Except in high altitudes or on exceptionally clear days, the ultraviolet content of the sun seldom exceeds 1% or 2%. Sunlight reflected from the sea, snow, or bright sand, however, may contain 4% to 6% ultraviolet light, and such reflections constitute a greater ultraviolet light hazard than the sun itself. Industrial and domestic sources of ultraviolet rays include the carbon arc lamp, the arc used in welding, and sunlamps used for tanning. The ultraviolet rays from these sources may be reflected and that reflection, as well as direct viewing, may be a source of injury.

With ultraviolet burns to the cornea there are no immediate symptoms, but a few hours later the recipient's eyes begin to water and feel gritty. Later, as the symptoms progress, the foreign body sensation becomes extreme and the patient is in a great deal of pain. Tearing, congestion of the globe, and marked photophobia (inability to tolerate light) occur. Staining of the cornea with fluorescein reveals slight pitting of its surface, which is caused by erosion of the superficial epithelium.

Before commencing therapy, the ophthalmic assistant should attempt to record the patient's visual acuity. The ocular examination is facilitated by placing an anesthetic agent in the patient's eyes, which relieves the distress and enables the patient to cooperate for the ensuing eye examination. Patching the eyes for 24 hours is usually sufficient to allow the cornea to heal completely. However, during that time the patient may experience a great deal of discomfort. One hour or so after leaving the ophthalmologist's office, the patient may have a recurrence of symptoms because the local anesthetic wears off. The patient should be warned that a scratching sensation and pain may occur at home. Most ophthalmologists provide the patient with pain-relieving medication. The patient is best advised to rest as much as possible with both eyes closed under the patches for 24 hours.

When the patches are removed the next day, the condition has usually cleared. The patient should be told, however, that some blurring of vision and sensitivity to light may remain for a week or so after the accident. The patient also should be advised to wear protective lenses against ultraviolet radiation in the future.

Infrared rays

The most common infrared calamity to the eye is an eclipse burn to the retina. This follows direct observation of a total eclipse of the sun. The effect of this injury to the retina is a marked reduction in visual acuity that is permanent. Ordinary protective devices such as tinted glass, Polaroid lenses, and the usual filters are of no value in protecting against this hazard. Direct viewing of eclipses should be avoided.

X-rays

X-rays are of very short wavelength, shorter than ultraviolet radiation and considerably shorter than the visible violet end of the spectrum (see Figure 3.4). Exposure to x-rays can produce many ocular complications, including glaucoma, cataracts, necrosis of the skin, loss of lashes, and iritis. Great care has consequently been taken, in the clinical use of x-ray exposure about the eye, to protect the patient from excessive dosage and the hospital staff from unnecessary exposure to dangerous radiation. As a result, the incident rate of eye complications among x-ray and radium workers is extremely low.

PREVENTION OF TRAUMATIC INJURIES TO THE EYE

Prevention in industry

At present the only effective area where safety measures have significantly reduced the number of ocular injuries is in industry. Most industrial safety programs revolve around four categories:

1. The detection of ocular disabilities before placement of workers in specific jobs
2. The wearing of protective goggles, visors, or masks
3. The education of workers in eye safety
4. The correct diagnosis and early treatment of eye injuries.

The use of safety glasses has been of greatest importance inasmuch as the glass itself becomes a protective shield for the eye. Although ordinary glasses for street wear and industrial glasses may look alike, the similarity ends there. The difference between the two types of lenses and frames is vast.

Regular street glasses, for example, can shatter easily into the eye. In contrast, industrial safety lenses are thicker and hardened so that they resist, without shattering, the impact of a standard steel ball dropped onto their surface (see Figure 13.20). The best safety glasses are made of polycarbonate plastic. The frames of safety glasses also are of different construction. In addition to being flame-resistant, they are designed to retain the safety lenses under heavy impact.

Contact lens wear may be hazardous in the fume- and chemical-laden environments of some industries. Contact lens wear, however, should not be considered a deterrent to employment in most industries. In some industries contact lens wearers must wear protective goggles as well, as a protection against flying missiles.

Prevention at home

Industrial safety lenses should be used when work or hobbies involve lathing, chiseling, grinding, or hammering. The hazard to the eye is even greater than in industry, because home lighting conditions are not always optimal and built-in safety guards are not always found in home machinery.

Children in particular should not be allowed to wear glasses that will shatter. Every pair of glasses given to a child should serve as a shield for the eyes. Safety glasses available include case-hardened lenses, tempered glass, and plastic lenses. Industrial glasses with industrial frames also serve as an excellent protective shield for the child. A sturdy frame, although not a requirement for safety, is an appreciated asset to the family who must repair frames frequently.

FIRST-AID CARE BY THE OPHTHALMIC ASSISTANT

1. Never place a miotic or mydriatic agent in an eye that has been injured.
2. Never put pressure on the globe when trying to separate the eyelids.
3. Never place any ointment in the eye before it has been seen by the ophthalmologist. It only makes the subsequent examination more difficult.
4. Never send a patient back to work who has pain in the eye, loss of vision, or congestion of the globe. Such a patient should be seen by the ophthalmologist first.
5. Never attempt to reassure the patient with a cheery prognosis. It may be wrong.
6. Do not attempt to use any ophthalmic instruments on an eye, especially corneal spuds, burrs, or curets.
7. When you are in doubt, patch the eye and call for help. The only exception to this rule occurs with a chemical burn of the eye. This must be irrigated immediately.
8. Keep accurate accounts and records of all injuries occurring in the office or clinic. The first step in the prevention of ocular trauma is to obtain statistics of their frequency, their mode of occurrence, and the type of activity being pursued at the time of the accident.
9. Never evaluate the severity of an ocular injury by its external appearance. Superficial injuries are often more painful than deep, penetrating ones.

10. Be prepared. All emergency drugs, trays, and instruments should be available, sterile, and ready to use for any contingency. It also is important to have a blood pressure cuff, oxygen, epinephrine (Adrenalin), and meperidine (Demerol) in the office in case a severe accident occurs and general systemic complications ensue.

COMPUTED TOMOGRAPHY SCANS (ALSO SEE CHAPTER 40)

CT scanners, which were developed in Great Britain in 1972, convert x-ray pictures into digital computer codes to make high-resolution video images. The computer graphics are similar to those used to reassemble pictures transmitted from distant space probes. Depicting bone structures in fine detail, CT scans also can show small differences between normal and abnormal tissues. CT scans are used for diagnostic purposes in the detection of orbital and lacrimal gland masses and of intraocular and orbital foreign bodies, as well as the exclusion of fractures of the orbital bones.

Foreign body injuries often result in a blood-filled eye that does not permit ophthalmoscopic viewing. Plain x-ray studies demonstrate only iron-containing foreign bodies and do not allow the physician to determine whether the foreign body is within or behind the globe. A CT scan demonstrates most foreign objects, which enables the examiner to localize the foreign body accurately. Figure 21.27 shows a CT scan that demonstrates a foreign body, as well as air and a vitreous hemorrhage, in the left globe.

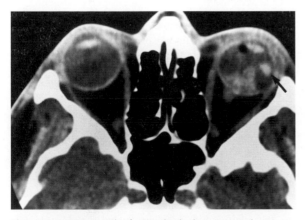

Figure 21.27 Intraocular foreign body demonstrated on computed tomography (CT) scan. The black area within the eye represents air that entered at the time of penetration by the intraocular body.

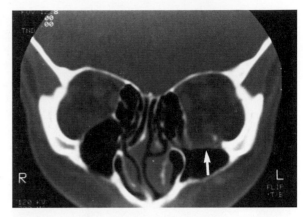

Figure 21.28 Orbital floor fracture demonstrated on computed tomography (CT) scan.

After a blow to the eye, patients can have diplopia and a restriction in motility because of an orbital bone fracture. The most common bone to be fractured is the orbital floor. Figure 21.28 shows a CT scan with a coronal view that demonstrates an orbital floor fracture with herniation of the inferior rectus into the underlying maxillary sinus.

MAGNETIC RESONANCE IMAGING

Magnetic resonance imaging (MRI) is a revolutionary diagnostic imaging technique that uses a strong magnetic field, a radiofrequency pulse, and the energy emission of hydrogen nuclei (protons). Unlike x-ray studies and CT scans, MRI does not use ionizing radiation; therefore, patients are free from the dangers of radiation exposure.

MRI often detects subtle differences between tissue structures. This is represented on film as a change in black and white density. Figure 21.29 depicts an MRI scan that demonstrates the normal anatomy of the brain and eye. The various structures of the brain can be appreciated in exquisite detail. Figure 21.30 demonstrates an enlarged lateral rectus muscle of the right eye. The patient was found to have an inflammatory condition that resolved rapidly with a short course of systemic steroids. Unlike CT scanners, bone does not appear in MRI; therefore, the detection of orbital fractures is not an indication for its use. Also, because of the strong magnetic field, patients with intraocular foreign bodies should not have MRI scans performed for fear that the foreign bodies may be magnetic. This can result in significant ocular injury if the foreign body is pulled through ocular structures, such as the retina or lens. Because of the ability of MRI to depict soft tissues in high contrast, it has proved effective in ophthalmology for imaging orbital and lacrimal gland lesions.

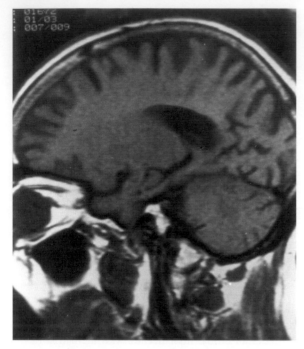

Figure 21.29 Magnetic resonance imaging (MRI) scan that shows the fine details of brain and orbit.

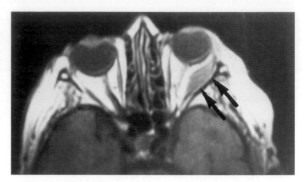

Figure 21.30 Enlargement of lateral rectus muscle on magnetic resonance imaging (MRI) scan.

Although MRI is an exciting field, it also is an expensive one. The equipment, which consists of a huge electromagnet, a radiofrequency generator, and a computer for evaluation, costs about $1 to $2 million. The equipment must be kept in a room completely insulated from external radiofrequencies, adding another three-quarters of a million dollars to the cost. MRI has become a major part of the imaging armamentarium and has proved to be as great a tool to modern medicine as the x-ray.

Questions for review and thought

1. Sympathetic ophthalmia occurs in the fellow eye after a serious injury to one eye. For how many weeks should one be on guard for this dreaded complication?

2. Name the anatomic structures that may be cut in a through-and-through vertical laceration of the upper eyelid.

3. How can rust rings of the cornea best be handled?

4. What is the term used for blood in the anterior chamber? How does it occur after injuries?

5. What is the term used for tears of the iris from its root?

6. A patient is hit directly in the eye by a golf ball. Name the damage that can result.

7. What is the first-aid treatment by the ophthalmic assistant when the eye is perforated by a knife and before the patient can be seen by the ophthalmologist?

8. After grinding or chiseling accidents, the examiner must always be alert for the possibility of intraocular foreign bodies. How may they be detected?

9. After an emergency, it is important to check the patient's vision. Occasionally other procedures, such as irrigation, take precedence but in general it is wise to assess visual acuity. Why?

10. The most common type of cut results from a twig, fingernail, or piece of paper scratching the cornea. The immediate symptoms may be severe. What is the purpose of fluorescein and how does it help determine the extent of the damage?

11. Injuries to the eye frequently result in a form of traumatic iritis. What are the symptoms of such an injury?

12. After lime burns to the eye, plaques of lime may adhere to the undersurface of the upper eyelid. How can the upper eyelid be everted?

13. Distortions of the iris and softness of the eye are signs that the eye has been perforated. The ophthalmic assistant must be careful to avoid any manipulations. What is the first-aid treatment?

14. A mother calls and informs you that her young son was injured in the right eye by a tennis ball. When she looked at the eye, the pupil was red instead of black and the child could not see with the eye. What would you suspect?

15. Which foreign substance is apt to be more injurious to the eye: iron, steel, or copper?

16. The industrial nurse telephones saying that an employee has spilled a strong chemical in his eyes. What is your instruction to the nurse?

Q Self-evaluation questions

True–false statements

Directions: Indicate whether the statement is true **(T)** or false **(F)**.

1. Alkali burns are more serious than acid burns of the cornea. **T** or **F**
2. Sympathetic ophthalmia usually causes blindness in the fellow eye after an injury to one eye. **T** or **F**
3. Corneal abrasions are often painful. **T** or **F**

Missing words

Directions: Write in the missing word in the following sentences:

4. Blunt injuries may result in an intraocular hemorrhage. This hemorrhage, when confined to the anterior chamber of the eye, is called a _____.
5. Hemorrhage in the eye is called a *black-ball* hemorrhage when it is present in both the anterior and the _____ chambers.
6. A patient has had an intraocular lens inserted and receives a blow to the eye. The lens is knocked into the vitreous. The intraocular lens is said to be _____.

Choice-completion questions

Directions: Select the one best answer in each case.

7. Which of the following is not an ocular injury?
   a. Corneal abrasion resulting from fingernail injury to cornea
   b. Painless loss of vision in one eye over a period of 3 months
   c. Loss of vision after hammering a nail
   d. Splashing caustic soda in the eye
   e. Double vision following a blow to the eye.

8. A squash ball injury to the eye may result in damage to:
   a. the lids.
   b. the lens.
   c. the retina.
   d. the bony wall.
   e. all of the above.

9. Penetrating injuries to the eye do not usually result in damage to:
   a. the cornea.
   b. the lens.
   c. the iris.
   d. the retina.
   e. bone.

A Answers, notes, and explanations

1. **True.** Alkali burns can be devastating to the cornea because they continue to penetrate through the corneal thickness. Chemicals persist even after copious washing for 10 minutes; thus irrigation should be continued for at least 20 to 30 minutes. Because alkalis continue to penetrate and destroy the cornea, a vascular response is created in which vessels grow into the cornea and preclude any possibilities for a successful corneal transplant later. Acids, on the other hand, precipitate the underlying layer and inhibit the progression of the acid into the cornea and the eye. Whereas acids may turn the outer corneal layer immediately white, the epithelium falls off and a new coat of epithelium regrows and leaves the cornea transparent. Thus alkali burns are much more severe and require prolonged attention by copious irrigation.

2. **False.** Sympathetic ophthalmia is a rare occurrence that follows an ocular injury to one eye, resulting in involvement of the uveal tissue of the fellow eye. It is not common, however, and its onset may be prevented or delayed by the systemic use of cortisone. However, eyes that are damaged beyond any hope of repair or restoration of visual function often are considered for enucleation to minimize this risk factor.

3. **True.** Corneal abrasions are often painful because of exposure of the corneal nerves. The epithelium has been denuded from an area of the cornea, leaving the corneal nerve endings exposed. A firm pressure bandage minimizes the exposure of these nerve endings and provides a smooth contour for new epithelium to rapidly heal over a corneal abrasion. Topical anesthetics and ointments inhibit the growth of epithelium over a corneal abrasion, and consequently their use should be minimal in the treatment of corneal abrasions.

4. **Hyphema.** Hyphema is an intraocular hemorrhage confined to the anterior chamber. When small it pools inferiorly, but if the hemorrhage continues it may fill the anterior chamber and cause blood staining of the cornea. This is often irreparable and leads to loss of vision. It is most important for people with hemophilia to be aware of this tendency and to prevent further bleeding. Hyphema frequently follows a blunt injury, and there may be recurrent bleeding 3 or 4 days after the initial injury. Consequently, the patient often is hospitalized and bed rest is prescribed, with one or both eyes bandaged.

A Continued

5. **Vitreous or posterior.** When a black-ball hemorrhage occurs, with blood in the anterior and posterior chambers of the eye, there is a grave prognosis in that the reabsorption of the hemorrhage from the posterior chamber or vitreous is often slow when hemorrhage becomes mixed with vitreous. If this is unresolved, a vitrectomy may be required to restore vision.

6. **Dislocated.** Intraocular lenses always carry the danger that trauma can dislocate them posteriorly and anteriorly. Consequently, their use in children is still somewhat hazardous. This is particularly so in children involved in competitive sports. These lenses are loosely attached and do not have the firm fixation of a normal lens, which is retained by the natural zonular ligaments.

7. **b. Painless loss of vision in one eye over a period of 3 months.** This usually is a medical problem caused by a number of medical conditions that result in visual decrease. The other areas are all injuries that result from trauma.

8. **e. All of the above.** A squash ball injury may cause ecchymoses of the lid or a dislocation of the lens of the eye. It may result in contrecoup injury involving the posterior globe and lead to a tear of the choroid or a retinal detachment. The small ball may strike the eye directly and result in a blow-out fracture of the orbit. Racquet injuries, particularly those incurred while playing squash, may be prevented by the use of special squash glasses. With their proper use, the incidence of eyeball damage has decreased considerably.

9. **e. Bone.** Any injury that penetrates the globe may perforate and injure all the structures within the globe and may cause damage to them. No particular tissue is spared. The corneal injury is often the least destructive and can be repaired with either suturing or, in small lacerations, a soft bandage lens. Lens injuries, however, may result in cataracts or may cause dislocation backward into the vitreous. In these cases the lens may have to be removed. Iris injury may result in tearing of the iris from its root or in a portion of the iris being exposed outside the globe, requiring surgical removal. The retina may be damaged by tears, resulting in retinal detachments. Bone, however, is usually damaged by blunt injuries, and sharp instruments tend to carom off the bone into the soft tissues and particularly into the globe.

Chapter | 22 |

The urgent case

The decision as to whether a patient requires an immediate examination is important and it rests heavily on the shoulders of the ophthalmic assistant. Without previous medical training and amid the noisy clatter of the outer office or clinic, the assistant must be prepared to screen the incoming calls and decide in a period of 30 seconds or less which patient has a complaint that could be symptomatic of an ocular emergency.

With industrial or traumatic injuries, this decision can be discharged rapidly and with authority. Obviously a patient who has suffered a flash burn of the cornea or a laceration of the eyelid cannot be kept waiting until there is an open appointment. On the other hand, each patient who calls to make an appointment has some ocular problem that is causing some real or functional derangement of vision. The high myope with lost glasses is just as incapacitated as is the individual who has suffered an episode of acute chorioretinitis. Both patients cannot see. The only difference between the two situations is that the myope has a static problem that can be solved the moment spectacles or contact lenses are received, whereas chorioretinitis is a progressive problem that must be stopped before serious damage has occurred.

When patients are screened, a system of priority must be established that can be exercised rapidly and efficiently. In this section, instead of merely cataloging the diseases that constitute an immediate threat to an eye, we discuss their symptoms and signs and attempt to assemble them into a meaningful classification. As with all classifications, the purpose is to provide an orderly way of thinking about a particular symptom or disease. It is impossible to cover all situations. Professionals cannot blame patients for not presenting "textbook" problems, but with some flexibility they can realize that exceptions will occur. We favor, in cases of doubt, erring on the side of caution and providing an appointment rather than letting the single "functional patient" with a flashing-lights symptom silently extend a retinal hole or tears to a full retinal detachment while patiently awaiting that cherished appointment 3 months hence.

OCULAR EMERGENCIES

True emergencies (therapy should be instituted within minutes)

1. Chemical burns of the eye
2. Central retinal artery occlusion (Figures 22.1–22.3)
3. Penetrating injuries of the eye (Figure 22.4)
4. Sudden loss of vision

Urgent situations (patients should be seen the same day)

1. Acute narrow-angle glaucoma (Figure 22.5)
2. Corneal ulcer (Figure 22.6)
3. Corneal foreign body
4. Corneal abrasion

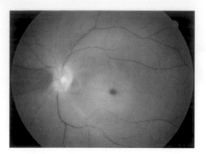

Figure 22.1 Recent central retinal artery occlusion with a cherry-red spot at the macula.
(From Kanski J, Bowling B. Clinical ophthalmology—a systematic approach. 7th ed. Edinburgh: Saunders; 2011.)

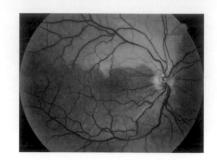

Figure 22.2 Superior branch retinal artery occlusion caused by an embolus at the disc with ischemic whitening of the superiortemporal retina.
(From Kanski J, Bowling B. Clinical ophthalmology—a systematic approach. 7th ed. Edinburgh: Saunders; 2011.)

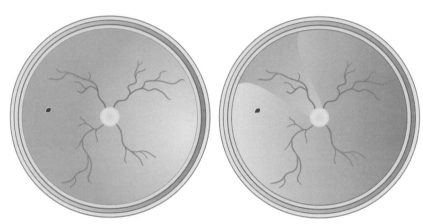

Figure 22.3 Ischemic whitening of the retina is indicative of a central retinal artery occlusion *(left)* or a branch retinal artery occlusion *(right)*.
(Adapted from Stein RM, Stein HA. Management of ocular emergencies. 5th ed. Montreal: Mediconcept; 2010.)

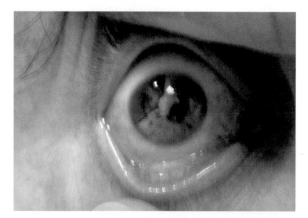

Figure 22.4 Tennis ball injury causing severe damage to the eye.

5. Acute iritis (Figures 22.7 and 22.8)
6. Retinal detachment
7. Hyphema (hemorrhage in the eye)
8. Lid laceration
9. Blow-out fracture of the orbit
10. Temporal arteritis

Semiurgent situations (patients should be seen within days)

1. Optic neuritis
2. Ocular tumors
3. Protrusion of an eye
4. Previously undiagnosed glaucoma
5. Old retinal detachment.

URGENT CASE: TO BE SEEN WITHIN THE HOUR

Sudden loss of vision in one eye without pain

This symptom in an adult usually means a central retinal artery occlusion, a central retinal vein occlusion, a vitreous hemorrhage, or a massive retinal detachment. A retrobulbar neuritis causes a loss of central vision, but side vision (peripheral vision) usually remains intact. All these conditions require immediate examination and early therapy and therefore belong to the category of the urgent situation.

Elevated intraocular pressure

Ciliary injection   Mid-dilated pupil

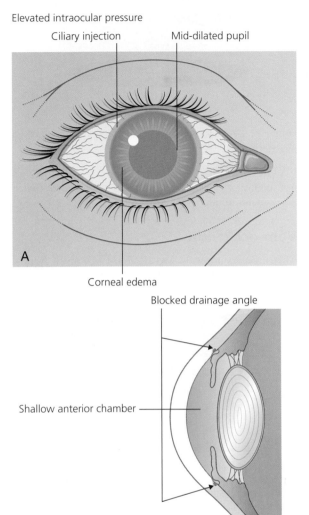

A

Corneal edema

Blocked drainage angle

Shallow anterior chamber

B

Figure 22.5 Glaucoma. (A) Acute angle-closure glaucoma.
(B) Acute angle-closure glaucoma. The trabecular meshwork is
covered by the root of the iris.
*(A, from Stein RM, Stein HA, Slatt BJ. Ocular emergencies: a practical
approach to management. Montreal: Medicopea; 1990.)*

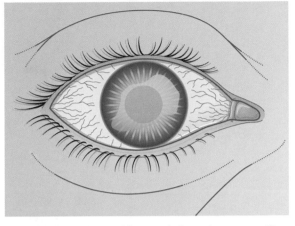

Figure 22.6 In patients with corneal ulcers, the cornea will
have a whitish infiltrate with an overlying epithelial defect
that stains with fluorescein.
*(From Stein HA, Slatt BJ, Stein RM. A primer in ophthalmology: a textbook
for students. St Louis: Mosby; 1992.)*

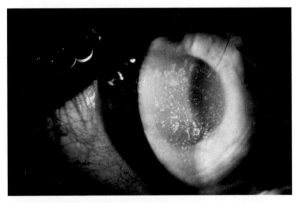

Figure 22.7 Iris with cellular debris on the cornea.

Central retinal artery occlusion is the most urgent in
terms of time. If this artery remains occluded for 2 to
4 hours or more, the involved eye most likely will go blind.
If sight is to be salvaged, the ophthalmologist must attempt
to dislodge the occlusion in the central retinal artery to a
more peripheral branch. Only minutes should be allowed
to elapse between the initial event and the onset of therapy.
Not only must the patient be on hand but the emergency
drug and instruments must be ready, prepared, and sterilized for immediate use. In some cases the ophthalmologist
may institute treatment up to 48 hours after the onset of
symptoms even though the prognosis for any vision restoration is very poor.

The other conditions mentioned also require early treatment, but this can be measured in hours rather than
minutes. On the basis of symptoms, the patient with a central retinal artery occlusion cannot be differentiated from
the patient with a vitreous hemorrhage or retinal vein
thrombosis. Therefore *any patient who complains of sudden
loss of vision in one eye is an emergency case* and requires
fire-alarm respect.

It is true that the ophthalmic assistant may experience
many false-positive cases and believe that he or she is gaining a reputation as an alarmist. A patient may state that
vision in one eye is lost, whereas examination reveals that
vision was merely blurred. However, one good result in a
potentially serious case is worth the feeling of chagrin in
finding 10 false-positive cases.

Some patients may lose sight in one eye insidiously and
make this appalling discovery quite suddenly. This can occur
in glaucoma patients who quietly lose sight in one eye and

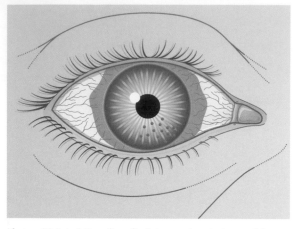

Figure 22.8 In iritis, ciliary flush is prominent, the pupil is constricted, and slit-lamp examination reveals keratic precipitates.
(From Stein HA, Slatt BJ, Stein RM. A primer in ophthalmology: a textbook for students. St Louis: Mosby; 1992.)

then casually rub their good eye, only to discover that they are momentarily blind. Therefore, the discovery of blindness in one eye may be sudden but the inciting sequence of events leading to this state can be chronic. This type of case must be added to the list of false-positive ocular emergencies.

Options for therapy by the ophthalmologists for central retinal artery occlusion include (1) increasing the blood oxygen content to the eye by using vasodilators, pentoxyphyline, inhalation of carbogen, hyperbaric oxygen, or sublingual isosorbide dinitrate; (2) reducing intraocular pressure and thereby increasing the retinal artery perfusion or helping dislodge the embolus by ocular massage, anterior chamber paracentesis, intravenous acetazolamide, intravenous mannitol, or topical antiglaucoma medications; (3) reducing retinal edema by intravenous methylprednisolone; (4) lysing or dislodging the clot by Nd:YAG laser embolectomy; and (5) assisting in thrombolysis of the embolus by intraarterial or intravenous thrombolysis.

The ophthalmic assistant should always be prepared for a central retinal artery occlusion by consulting, in advance of the need, with the ophthalmologist to determine which instruments, medications, inhalants, and supplies the ophthalmologist wishes to have readily available to institute rapid therapy in the event of a patient presenting with a central retinal artery occlusion (Figure 22.9).

Chemical injuries to the eye require prompt attention. As soon as the patient arrives at the office, the ophthalmic assistant should institute initial therapy, which consists irrigating the eyes with water or saline for approximately 30 minutes. This is done to wash away any chemicals that still have the potential to cause ocular damage. The visual prognosis as a result of chemical injuries must initially be guarded because the full effects of the injury may not be appreciated for several weeks.

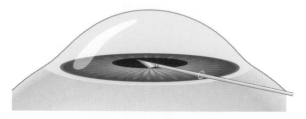

Figure 22.9 Anterior chamber tap to promote lowering of intraocular pressure in central retinal artery occlusion.

Sudden loss of vision in both eyes is a rare event and does not require any degree of sophistication to realize that it also constitutes an ocular emergency.

Vein occlusion

A significant and acute loss of vision can result from a central retinal vein occlusion (CRVO) (Figure 22.10) or a branch retinal vein occlusion (BRVO) (Figure 22.11). In

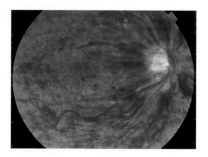

Figure 22.10 Recent nonischemic central retinal vein occlusion with venous tortuosity and dilation, and extensive flame-shaped hemorrhages.
(From Kanski J, Bowling B. Clinical ophthalmology—a systematic approach. 7th ed. Edinburgh: Saunders; 2011.)

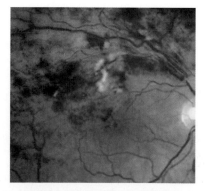

Figure 22.11 Major superior branch vein occlusion with flame-shaped and blot hemorrhages, a few cotton wool spots, and venous tortuosity.
(From Kanski J, Bowling B. Clinical ophthalmology—a systematic approach. 7th ed. Edinburgh: Saunders; 2011.)

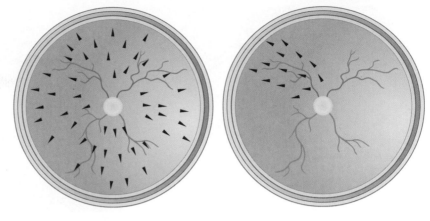

Figure 22.12 Scattered superficial hemorrhages are indicative of central retinal vein occlusion *(left)* or branch retinal vein occlusion *(right).* *(Adapted from Stein RM, Stein HA. Management of ocular emergencies. 5th ed. Montreal: Mediconcept; 2010.)*

CRVO the hemorrhages are located primarily at the posterior pole but may be seen throughout the fundus (Figure 22.12). In BRVO the hemorrhages are located in the distribution of the occluded vein (see Figure 22.12).

The intraocular pressure may be elevated, inasmuch as patients with vein occlusions often have a higher incidence of glaucoma. Fluorescein angiography may be performed to determine the extent of retinal ischemia or macular edema. Panretinal laser photocoagulation is indicated if the retina shows significant ischemic changes. This prevents the neovascularization of the anterior chamber angle, which can lead to glaucoma. In BRVO, focal laser photocoagulation may improve visual acuity and may be indicated for chronic macular edema. If neovascularization does occur, then focal laser photocoagulation may resolve the neovascular tufts and prevent vitreous hemorrhage.

URGENT CASE: TO BE SEEN THE SAME DAY

Painful red eye

Painful red eye, with or without a concomitant decrease in visual acuity, is a symptom complex that deserves immediate attention. Four conditions usually are responsible for a painful red eye:

1. Acute glaucoma (a congested, tense eyeball caused by sudden blockage of the aqueous outflow)
2. Acute conjunctivitis (inflammation of the outer eye) (Figure 22.13)
3. Acute iritis (inflammation of the inner eye)
4. Acute keratitis (which generally is caused by a corneal infiltrate or ulcer)

Diagnostic investigation may be required in cases of acute iritis because this condition may be an incident in the course of a general body disorder. In particular, the ophthalmologist may want to investigate for tuberculosis, syphilis, sarcoidosis, arthritis, and other diseases.

After an attack of angle-closure glaucoma, the patient is treated with a number of pressure-lowering drugs before either a laser or surgical iridectomy. The following drugs should be kept on hand for emergency treatment: acetazolamide, 250 mL in oral and injectable form; glycerin or isosorbide; pilocarpine 2%; timolol 0.5%; and meperidine hydrochloride (Demerol) or an equivalent pain-relieving drug.

Keratitis or corneal inflammation is not commonly present as an isolated entity. It may result from a preexisting conjunctivitis or may be the initiating cause of a secondary iritis. Among the causes of a painful eye, *herpes simplex keratitis* warrants special mention (Figure 22.14). It is commonly diagnosed as a simple conjunctivitis because the eye is red, is sensitive to light, and has a watery discharge. The patient experiences a gritty sensation of the eye that actually decreases in severity as the condition becomes worse. If the eye is left untreated, many complications can develop, including corneal scarring, secondary iritis, and glaucoma. In the more severe cases, the late corneal

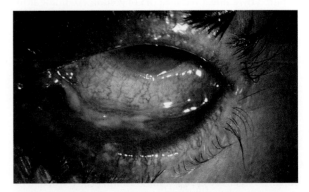

Figure 22.13 Acute bacterial conjunctivitis. Inflammation of the conjunctival lining caused by streptococcal infection.

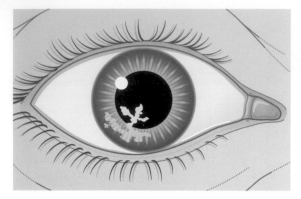

Figure 22.14 Dendritic pattern of herpes simplex keratitis on the cornea.

scarring can be so extensive as to warrant a corneal transplant to restore vision. Early treatment in the form of antiviral drops (for example, trifluridine or idoxuridine [IDU] or debridement of the involved corneal epithelium may reduce the frequency of these late complications. The ophthalmic assistant must always keep this condition in mind when presented with a seemingly innocent and common case of simple conjunctivitis.

Swollen eyelid

The most alarming aspect of an acutely swollen eyelid is the cosmetic disfigurement of the face, which causes the patient to believe that some terrible malady of the eye is present. In fact, the most common cause of acute lid swellings is an infection of the tiny sweat and oil glands emptying into the margin of the lids. The patient with an infection of a sweat gland, commonly known as a stye, usually exhibits diffuse swelling of the lid, with a tiny raised nodule on the lid margin that denotes the actual site of involvement.

Inflammation of the meibomian or oil glands results in an internal hordeolum that also can result in diffuse lid swelling. On eversion of the lid, however, the site of infection is denoted by a linear red area of congestion extending from the lid margin vertically across the tarsus along the full extent of the meibomian gland. With time an internal hordeolum may resolve and the infection may become walled off by the formation of a capsule in the tissues of the lid. The patient then has a firm lump that can be felt through the skin surface of the eyelid. This lump, or *chalazion,* is an eruption of the contents of the meibomian glands into adjacent tissues that results in a granulomatous response with a cystic change. If the initial infection is minimal, a chalazion may develop without any history of a swollen lid (Figure 22.15).

Another cause of acute swelling of the eyelid is an *insect bite.* With insect bites the swelling of the eyelid tends to be so severe that the eyelid cannot be opened. Occasionally the site of the bite is visible as a tiny raised red mark on the surface of the eyelid.

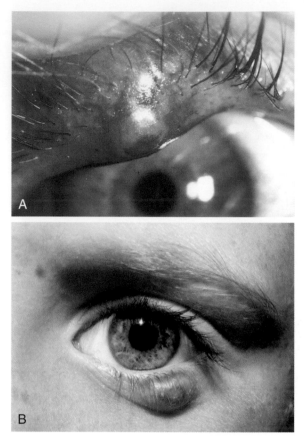

Figure 22.15 A meibomian cyst (chalazion) develops from a blockage of one of the meibomian glands in the tarsal plate. Clinically it presents in the acute stage as a red, tender swelling within the tarsal plate of the upper or lower eyelid (A). This either resolves completely or leaves a firm nodule (B). *(Reproduced from Spalton D, Hitchings R, Hunter P. Atlas of clinical ophthalmology. 3rd ed. St Louis: Mosby; 2004, with permission.).*

Allergic reactions also may give rise to diffuse, painless swelling of the eyelids. The allergy may be a result of eyedrops, skin creams, perfumes, mascara, or environmental causes (e.g., dust, molds, and pollen). Most allergic reactions tend to be bilateral and are often accompanied by uncomfortable itchiness.

Flashes of light

Flashes of light coming across the field of vision often are a forerunner of a *retinal detachment* (Figure 22.16); therefore, the patient with this symptom should be seen promptly. In this condition, however, time is not quite as critical a factor; often days or a week can pass between the formulation of such a diagnosis and the initiation of therapy.

Although flashes of light are a dangerous symptom, they occur in other conditions besides retinal detachment.

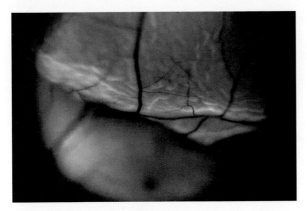

Figure 22.16 Retinal detachment superiorly.

Patients with *migraine* often experience a "lightning flash" that flickers on and off for 20 to 30 minutes before onset of the headache. Also vitreous detachment, an innocuous and common event in middle-aged or older adults, also may appear in a similar fashion. Although it is important, the symptom of flashes of light does not possess the urgency of an emergency condition, which is usually associated with pain or loss of vision. Its association with an impending retinal detachment, however, is so constant that it does merit recognition as a symptom of paramount importance. Patients with this symptom in one eye should undergo wide dilation to permit a complete examination of the retina for a retinal tear and associated retinal detachment (Figure 22.17).

Double vision or lid droop

Any person older than 5 years will see double if a single extraocular muscle becomes weak or paralyzed. The eye

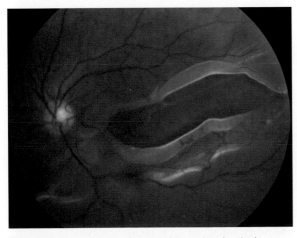

Figure 22.17 Large retinal tear with associated retinal detachment.
(From Kanski J, Bowling B. Clinical ophthalmology—a systematic approach. 7th ed. Edinburgh: Saunders; 2011.)

may be turned in (*esotropia:* Figure 22.18) if a lateral rectus muscle is paralyzed, or turned out (*exotropia:* Figure 22.19) if a medial rectus muscle is paralyzed. *Hypertropia* occurs if there is paralysis or weakness of any of the muscles that move the eye up or down (Figure 22.20). The symptom of double vision is of grave importance because it occurs as a result of disease within the brain itself, the nerves going to the extraocular muscles, or the muscles themselves. Among the more serious conditions that produce double vision are brain tumors, aneurysms, myasthenia gravis, and strokes.

The lid is primarily held open by the action of the levator palpebrae superioris, which is innervated by the same nerve that supplies many of the extraocular muscles of the eye. Weakness of the levator muscle results in lid droop, or *ptosis*. The significance of an acquired lid droop has the same gravity as the onset of double vision.

TEMPORAL ARTERITIS

Temporal arteritis (also called giant cell arteritis or cranial arteritis) is a condition caused by chronic inflammation of the large and medium arteries of the head that can result in an inadequate supply of oxygen to areas of the head and brain. It is an autoimmune disorder in which the body's immune system mistakenly attacks normal healthy cells and tissues causing inflammation. Temporal arteritis often affects the temporal arteries of the head, but can also affect other arteries throughout the body. Temporal arteritis can cause a wide variety of symptoms that can affect the eyes, head, face, and the body in general. Though a relatively uncommon disorder, it is the most frequent cause of inflammation of the blood vessels. It is more common in people older than age 50, and it affects women more often than men.

Symptoms of temporal arteritis can include blurred vision; reduced vision; double vision or sudden permanent loss of vision in one eye; throbbing headache, especially on one side of the head (usually in the temple) or back of the head; tenderness in the scalp and temple areas; facial pain; jaw pain with chewing; fatigue; weakness; and a general ill feeling.

The diagnosis of temporal arteritis includes a physical examination with emphasis on the head to determine whether there is any tenderness of the arteries. In addition certain blood tests can be useful in the diagnosis. These tests include a hemoglobin and hematocrit, erythrocyte sedimentation rate (ESR), C-reactive protein, and a liver function test. A high sedimentation rate is often diagnostic. Although these blood tests can be helpful in diagnosis, their results are not enough for a definitive diagnosis. To make a definitive diagnosis, a biopsy of the artery that the ophthalmologist suspects is affected needs to be performed. This can be done as an outpatient procedure.

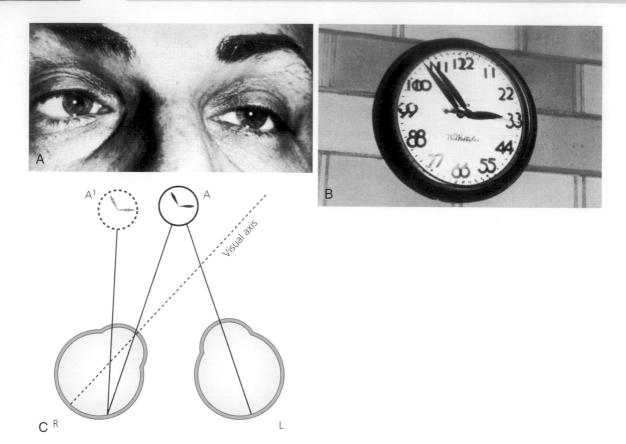

Figure 22.18 (A) Esotropia. The right eye is turned in because of paralysis of the right lateral rectus muscle. (B) Horizontal diplopia. The patient sees two clocks side by side. (C) Image of the clock falls on the macula of the left eye and a point on the retina nasal to the macula of the right eye. The projection of the image of the clock is displaced horizontally to A^1 and is on the same side as the turned eye.

Other tests that may be used in making a diagnosis include a computed tomography (CT) scan and magnetic resonance imaging (MRI).

If temporal arteritis is suspected, treatment should begin immediately, even if test results have not yet confirmed the definitive diagnosis because, if the temporal arteritis is allowed to continue untreated, it can cause serious and potentially life-threatening complications including blindness and stroke. Therefore, if the diagnosis is suspected and the results are pending, oral corticosteroids need to be prescribed immediately. Aspirin to treat the musculoskeletal symptoms also may be recommended. The typical course of treatment lasts for 1 to 2 years.

PRIORITY CASE: TO BE SEEN WITHIN DAYS

In the priority group the patients concerned are not involved in an ophthalmic emergency, but symptoms

may herald an acute emergency, cause immediate functional loss, or indicate a chronic and serious derangement within the eye or brain. Again, our approach is based on the patient's symptoms.

Halos around lights

The symptom of seeing halos around lights is caused by the formation of droplets somewhere in the optic media that break up white light into its spectral components. The rainbow seen after a storm has a similar explanation, being formed by suspended droplets of rainwater, which spectrally divide light. In the eye the most common cause of seeing halos around lights is related to the formation of mucous deposits on the surface of the conjunctiva, which occurs in association with chronic conjunctivitis, allergies, and ocular irritations. Early cataracts, if cystic spaces form in the lens, also can produce this symptom. However, the phenomenon of seeing colored halos around lights has its major importance as an impending sign of acute angle-closure glaucoma. In an eye predisposed to this

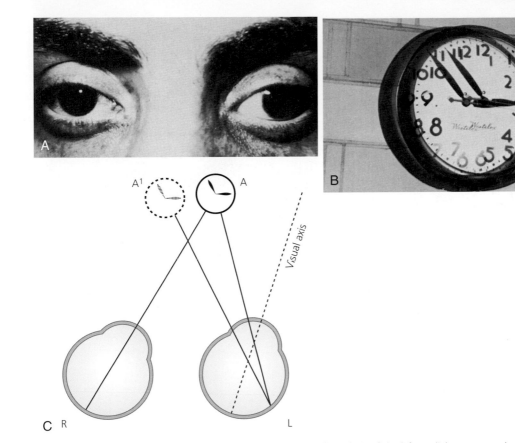

Figure 22.19 (A) Exotropia. The left eye is turned out because of paralysis of the left medial rectus muscle. (B) Horizontal diplopia. The patient sees two clocks side by side. (C) Image of the clock falls on the macula of the right eye and a point on the retina temporal to the macula of the left eye. The projection of the image of the clock is displaced horizontally to A^1 and is on the side opposite to the turned eye.

condition, elevations in ocular tension occur that are insufficient to cause an acute attack but high enough to allow edema fluid to form in the stroma of the cornea.

The episodes of seeing colored rings around lights usually are transient. They are commonly associated with some blurring of vision and some ocular discomfort. Often, these "small attacks" of intermittent elevations of ocular pressure are so mild that the patient does not seek advice on their account. The symptom of seeing colored rings around lights is a small problem as far as the patient is concerned.

Headaches

Headaches usually are prominent among the reasons for which patients are referred. The causes of headaches in or about the eye are numerous. They can include such varied conditions as sinusitis, tooth abscess, migraine, hypertension, and brain tumor. They also appear as a symptom of chronic anxiety and tension and of oculomotor disturbances. Of all the causes of headaches, ocular dysfunction is quite low on the list.

Ocular headaches usually appear after prolonged periods of close work or after performing other tasks that require visual concentration, such as driving or watching movies or television. The pain is mild and is not associated with such symptoms as nausea, vomiting, or muscular weakness. It is usually relieved by rest, vacations, and so on. The site of the headache can be virtually anywhere in the cranium, but most often the headaches appear in or behind the eyes, around the eyes, or in the temporal regions. Commonly the patient with an ocular headache has recently changed activities, thereby becoming bothered by uncorrected refractive errors or disturbances in oculomotor balance. For example, such a patient often has decided to finish a university degree at night, been promoted to a desk job, or returned to the workforce. Part of the discomfort may be visual, but the factors of anxiety in doing unfamiliar activities, in forced concentration, and in learning can be of significance as well.

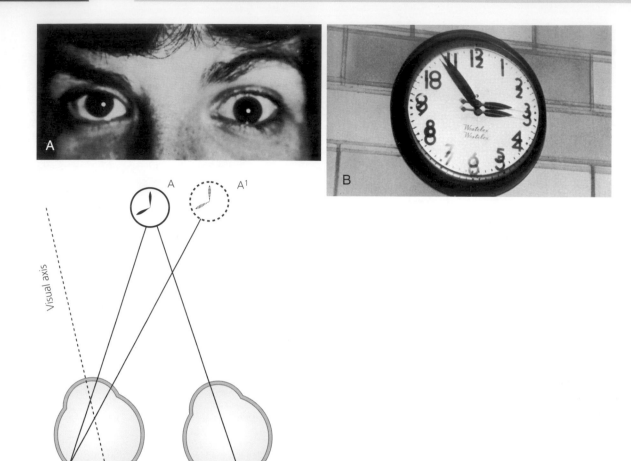

Figure 22.20 (A) Right hypertropia. The right eye is turned up because of paralysis of the right inferior rectus muscle. (B) Vertical diplopia. The patient sees two clocks, one above the other. (C) Image of the clocks falls on the macula of the left eye and a point above the macula on the right eye. The projection of the image of the clock is displaced inferiorly to A^1.

The types of headache that should be included in the category of the priority case are nonocular because they may be indicative of serious neurologic or systemic disorder. Headaches not related to the eyes may:

- Occur at any time and be so severe as to awaken the patient during the night
- Be associated with other systemic symptoms, such as nausea, vomiting, fainting spells, drowsiness, or stiffness of the neck
- Be preceded by an aura of flickering lights and jagged lightning flashes lasting 15 to 20 minutes (an aura often precedes a migraine headache)
- Be throbbing in nature and occur in clusters
- Be aggravated by the position of the head or movements of the body.

In practice, one should be aware that a headache may be a serious symptom and give the patient with consequential associated findings priority treatment. (Many brain tumors are first noticed in ocular assessment.)

Lost or broken spectacles

Although lost or broken spectacles appear to be a minor problem, this can be a disabling event to the patient. A myope of −3.00 to −4.00 diopters without correction may not be able to see better than 20/200 and legally may be considered blind. The patient with a considerable refractive error who has lost his or her spectacles can be totally incapacitated. The high myope cannot drive a car, the presbyope cannot read, and the patient with high astigmatism cannot do either activity. For these patients, improving vision with glasses can be as dramatic, satisfying, and rehabilitating as any other form of therapy involving drops or surgery.

Gradual loss of sight in quiet eyes

Gradual loss of vision occurs in conditions in which a progressive deterioration develops without obvious external signs of ocular disease. In children this symptom is generally caused by uncorrected refractive errors. Once the child receives spectacles, the difficulty with vision is improved for a time. As the child grows, the refractive status constantly changes until physical maturity is reached. These changes are particularly prone to occur in myopia. Once the age of 19 or 20 years is reached, the growth of the eye is complete and changes in vision are less likely to be caused by errors of refraction. A quiescent period supervenes for about 20 to 25 years, and then most people find that focusing at near becomes difficult and the era of the presbyope is ushered in. Again, a reduction in the ability to see, this time at near, occurs and the presbyopic patient's reading glasses must be strengthened from time to time.

Apart from uncorrected refractive errors, the most common pathologic causes of painless progressive loss of vision are cataracts and macular degeneration. They occur most commonly in older adults, but are by no means restricted to this group. The patient with a cataract sees as though looking through a frosted window or gazing at something through a piece of paper. Objects appear hazy because of irregular refraction of light and are dim because some of the light is reflected by the opacities in the lens and does not reach the interior of the eye. Often the cataract patient complains of photophobia or sensitivity to light, because the retina cannot adequately adapt to the vagaries of illumination coming through a semiopaque lens. Most cataracts are bilateral, but their development may be asymmetric, so that a patient may have a moderate reduction of vision in one eye and a severe visual loss in the other. It is only when the cataract becomes mature or totally opaque that vision drops to the point of mere light perception and projection. Most people who have access to a medical center have their cataracts removed before the cataracts become mature. In areas where medical facilities are not available, cataracts are a leading cause of blindness.

The patient with macular disease has difficulty seeing clearly straight ahead because of destruction of this most vital region of the retina. Macular disease may be slow or acute in onset. Often it is bilateral, but rarely do both eyes become involved simultaneously. Central vision is lost and the patient usually cannot see looking straight ahead. Side vision or peripheral vision, however, is intact so that patients afflicted with this problem can still navigate through a room without bumping into things even though their visual acuity is 20/200 or less. To envision what a patient with macular disease sees, close one eye, place your thumb close to your open eye in your line of vision and look at a framed picture hanging on the wall. You will find that all you can see is the frame on the surrounding wall; the picture is blotted out.

SUMMARY

The task of screening or triaging patients on the telephone is difficult and a heavy responsibility for the ophthalmic assistant. It would be impossible even for a well-trained ophthalmologist to adequately screen large numbers of patients through a conversation that lasts only minutes. The only method of solving this problem is to make errors of inclusion rather than exclusion. Far better to reward the functional patient with a bit of eye time than to turn away the patient with a serious but treatable organic problem.

Every patient who calls an eye doctor's office believes he or she has an important, serious problem that requires immediate attention. Even though all complaints do not fall under the category of urgency or priority, they should not be minimized and dismissed as trivial. Patience and understanding are required in the handling of all patients. Discretion must be used to ferret out the urgent patient.

Questions for review and thought

1. A patient telephones, complaining of sudden loss of vision in one eye. What are the possible causes? When should the patient be seen?

2. Severe pain in an eye, accompanied by nausea and vomiting, is often an indication of what condition? How should the telephone receptionist handle such a call?

3. When a patient calls complaining of redness of one or both eyes, what is the common differential diagnosis? What are the common characteristics that differentiate types of red eyes?

4. What is the significance of flashes of light?

5. What is the significance of sudden onset of double vision?

6. Compose a list of possible causes of headaches.

7. A patient calls in and says that her baby scratched her eye. What advice would you give her?

8. What advice would you give an ophthalmic assistant who gives medical advice over the telephone?

9. A patient has been hit by a fist and has a simple black eye. Should that patient be seen the same day? Why?

10. A high myope loses his glasses. Is the problem urgent?

Q Self-evaluation questions

True–false statements

Directions: Indicate whether the statement is true **(T)** or false **(F).**

1. A central retinal artery occlusion can be salvaged if seen within 2 hours. **T** or **F**
2. Pain in the eye represents a severe corneal malady. **T** or **F**
3. A chalazion of the upper lid can cause a loss of vision. **T** or **F**

Missing words

Directions: Write in the missing word(s) in the following sentences:

4. A person who has an esotropia has the displaced image on the _____ side.
5. A headache that is preceded by flashing lights for 15 minutes is invariably a _____ headache.
6. The most common cause of halos around lights is _____.

Choice-completion questions

Directions: Select the one best answer in each case.

7. Patients with cataracts:
   a. have better distance vision than near vision.
   b. develop better near vision than distance vision.
   c. have variable vision depending on the time of day.
   d. see better at night.
   e. see better with miotics.
8. The most common cause of headaches is:
   a. eyestrain.
   b. sinusitis.
   c. migraine.
   d. stress-anxiety-depression (SAD).
   e. hypertension.
9. Flashes of light can indicate:
   a. syneresis of vitreous.
   b. migraine.
   c. retinal detachment.
   d. a blow to the back of the head.
   e. all of the above.

A Answers, notes, and explanations

1. **False.** A true central retinal artery occlusion rarely can be salvaged. Usually 20 minutes is all that the retina can take without oxygen before permanent damage sets in. It is unusual for the diagnosis and treatment to be done that fast once the incident occurs. Sometimes the occlusive plug fragments and lodges in a branch so that the entire retina is not destroyed. The typical fundus picture is that of a retina drained of blood; thus the retinal arteries are narrow and the macula appears red because of the choroidal blush. The glowing epithet, cherry-red spot, applied to the condition of the macula does not really do justice to this blinding event.

2. **False.** Pain in the eye is commonly corneal and can be caused by anything from a foreign body in the cornea to herpes simplex keratitis. The pain of iritis, and especially of acute glaucoma, however, is far more severe than corneal pain.

   Naturally everyone with pain in the eye should be seen right away. If the eye is fiercely red and the vision is hazy, the worst should be suspected. If the patient states that the pain occurred suddenly and reveals that the pupil is dilated, the assistant can almost start booking the hospital for an acute glaucoma admission.

3. **True.** Any mass, nodule, or lump on the upper lid can cause a slight ptosis of the lid and a flexure of the cornea by compression. It is like pressing on a balloon: the top goes in and the sides go out. The eye is not as flexible as a balloon, but alteration in the corneal curvature does occur. The radius of curvature becomes steeper and more toric in shape. Visual loss of one to three lines on the Snellen chart is common.

4. **Same.** Because the eye is turned in, the nasal side of the retina is exposed to the object of regard. The projection is straight ahead and the false second image is beside the real one and located on the same side as the paralyzed muscle.

5. **Migraine.** Migraine is characterized by the following:
   - A family history of headaches
   - An aura lasting 15 to 20 minutes consisting of light flashes, off-and-on signals, and loss of visual field
   - Precipitation of the headache by stress, drugs, birth control or diet pills, or trauma
   - A tense, commonly compulsive personality
   - Onset in young adults, although it can occur in childhood

| **A** | **Continued** |

6. **Mucous deposits on the cornea.** A halo is caused by the presence of water droplets breaking up white light into its colored components. Its most sinister cause is acute glaucoma, in which episodes of corneal edema occur. Other causes of corneal edema, however, can produce halos.

   The most common causes are mucus droplets on the cornea in association with chronic conjunctivitis, atopic conjunctival allergies, and ocular irritations. Cigarette smoke, pollution, and dry office buildings are a common source of ocular irritation, mucus production, and halo formation. Thus the assistant should not panic over halos.

7. **b. Develop better near vision than distance vision.** Patients with cataracts often see poorly in the distance but still manage to read. This occurs because the hardening of the lens of the eye increases the index of refraction of the eye. This is the reason why the elderly get "second sight."

8. **d. Stress-anxiety-depression (SAD).** Problems of living are the most common cause of headaches. It is the so-called tension headache that is so endemic. Eyestrain rarely causes a headache. Further, the eye is a sensory organ, a fact that cannot be overlooked. Anybody with persistent headaches should have a physical examination to rule out hypertension, sinusitis, or a neurologic disorder.

9. **e. All of the above.** Flashes of light are a dangerous symptom for the patient to report. The most urgent condition that it might indicate is a retinal detachment, which requires immediate surgery. Other symptoms to be worried about in association with flashes of light include a veil over the affected eye, a shower of spots before one eye, and loss of vision or distortion of vision in the same eye.

   Migraine is sometimes a puzzle. On occasion patients have the flashes of light for 15 minutes but no headache.

   Syneresis of vitreous is a result of the liquefaction of a part of the vitreous. The remaining gel-like vitreous bumps into the retina whenever the eyes move. The impact of the vitreous against the retina causes flashes of light.

Chapter | 23 |

Common eye disorders

Perhaps the most interesting part of an ophthalmologist's professional life is the challenge presented in diagnosing diseases of the eye. It is toward this end that his or her training has been directed, first as a medical doctor, then as a specialist. Although refraction seems to occupy much of an ophthalmologist's time, it is merely a step in the process of defining disease.

For the ophthalmic assistant the study of disease processes can only aid in making the examination of the eye more rewarding. Despite the assistant's limitations in training and instrumentation, there are many common eye disorders seen daily that should be appreciated. The function of this chapter is not to make diagnosticians out of ophthalmic assistants, but to enrich their career through the study of the various disorders that are commonly seen.

CONJUNCTIVA

The conjunctiva commences at the lid margin, lines the inner surface of the lids, forms a cul-de-sac, and then lines the surface of the eye itself, becoming circumferentially attached to the cornea at the limbus. It is translucent, moist, and membranous; has a rich vasculature; and is kept supple by the tear film.

Hyperemia

Hyperemia, or redness, of the conjunctiva is perhaps the most common condition seen. Everyone gets red eyes at one time or another. The offensive redness is caused merely by dilation of the normal vascular channels in the conjunctiva. It can result from such transitory and innocuous events as exposure to dust, wind or air pollutants, fatigue, excessive reading, exposure to strong light or heat, poor ventilation, excessive dryness, and even the moderate consumption of alcoholic beverages. Many people equate red eyes with infection or inflammation and become alarmed. It is for this reason that proprietary medications "to get the red out" are so successful with their in-depth media advertising. Many people think that by getting the red out they are nipping a disease process in the bud, as well as removing a socially unacceptable disorder.

Transitory redness of the eyes requires no treatment because it is not a disease. People who find some relief with the use of eyewashes or astringent drops get only a temporary abatement of their symptoms and become addicted to eye-whitening drops for the rest of their lives. When the medication wears off, the conjunctival vessels have a tendency to dilate again, so that the redness becomes more prominent than before: the so-called rebound reaction.

Subconjunctival hemorrhage

Subconjunctival hemorrhage is caused by a ruptured conjunctival blood vessel. It usually produces an irregular red patch because of pooling of blood under the conjunctiva (Figure 23.1). Its appearance is particularly gruesome and alarming because it is accentuated by the white of the sclera (Figure 23.2). Invariably, a collection of blood, like any other bruise under the skin, spreads and seems

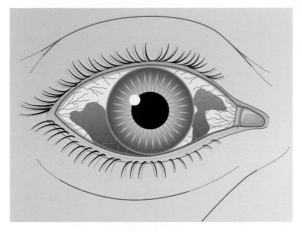

Figure 23.1 A ruptured vessel with blood accumulation in the subconjunctival space is diagnosed as a subconjunctival hemorrhage.
(From Stein HA, Slatt BJ, Stein RM. A primer in ophthalmology: a textbook for students. St Louis: Mosby; 1992.)

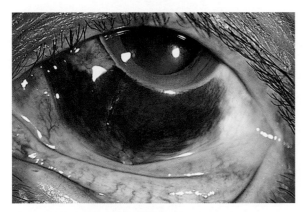

Figure 23.2 Subconjunctival hemorrhage.

to enlarge as the blood is disseminated. Eventually the blood pigment breaks down to its component parts until it is absorbed. This process can take anywhere from 7 days to 3 weeks, depending on the size of the hemorrhage.

Subconjunctival hemorrhage occurs most often in older adult patients with diabetes or hypertension, but commonly no cause can be found. A predisposing cause appears to be events that produce a sudden rise in venous pressure, such as coughing, straining, lifting, sneezing, or vomiting. There is no required treatment for this condition, which is entirely innocuous, other than reassurance. Occasionally a subconjunctival hemorrhage is part of a general bleeding disorder, but it must be emphasized that such an event is rare. Patients should be sent to their family doctor to rule out high blood pressure and diabetes. Cold compresses on the first day followed by warm compresses may speed up recovery.

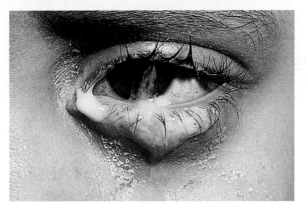

Figure 23.3 Purulent conjunctivitis.

Conjunctivitis

Conjunctivitis is an inflammation of the conjunctiva characterized by redness of the conjunctiva, swelling, a discharge that can be watery or purulent, and congestion of the tissues (Figure 23.3). The patient commonly complains of a burning or grittiness of the eyes. Characteristically, the discharge accumulates during sleep, and its resultant drying on the lashes makes the lids difficult to open in the morning. Usually the lids have to be bathed to open the eyes.

Conjunctivitis may have an *infectious, allergic, or toxic* cause. The most common infectious agents are viruses, bacteria, and chlamydial organisms. A virus is the most common cause of conjunctivitis. Unlike bacterial or chlamydial conjunctivitis, the discharge is characteristically watery. Adenovirus is the most common viral conjunctivitis. Certain serotypes of this infectious agent may be responsible for epidemic keratoconjunctivitis (EKC) or pharyngoconjunctival fever (PCF). EKC is highly contagious and often is associated with epidemic outbreaks in a localized area. This disease is characterized by conjunctival and corneal involvement. PCF differs from EKC in that patients usually exhibit symptoms of a sore throat just preceding or at the time of their ocular symptoms.

Staphylococcus aureus is the most common cause of *bacterial conjunctivitis.* The organism is also responsible for such common conditions as boils or impetigo of the skin. Gonococcal conjunctivitis can be a severe infection resulting in blindness if appropriate treatment is delayed. The disease can be seen in newborns, who contact the organism while traveling through the birth canal. The sequelae of neonatal conjunctivitis can be so devastating that it is mandatory in most countries for either antibacterial drops or 1% silver nitrate to be placed into the lower conjunctival sac of all newborns immediately after birth. Gonococcal conjunctivitis also can be seen in adults and is characterized by a significant purulent discharge. These patients and their sexual contacts need to be evaluated for a venereal disease that was probably the source of the conjunctivitis.

Haemophilus influenzae, another bacterial organism, can cause pinkeye, especially in children.

Chlamydial conjunctivitis can be caused by inclusion conjunctivitis or trachoma. The disease is characterized by a red eye and often a mucoid discharge. Inclusion conjunctivitis is the more prevalent of the two in North America and occurs in newborns and young adults. Trachoma is a more severe disease that can give rise to extensive scarring of the lids, conjunctiva, and cornea. It is epidemic in some parts of the world, such as North Africa, the Middle East, and South Asia, where poor hygiene, poor sanitation, deficient diets, and crowding are the norm. It is a major cause of blindness in the world.

The features that distinguish acute conjunctivitis, acute iritis, and acute glaucoma are shown in Figure 23.4 and Table 23.1. In cases of acute conjunctivitis, antibiotic drops should never be administered before the patient is seen by the ophthalmologist. Smears and cultures may be required in selected cases, especially in patients with *ophthalmia neonatorum* (conjunctivitis of the newborn), membranous conjunctivitis (diphtheria), and purulent conjunctivitis (gonococcal).

Allergic conjunctivitis is basically a hypersensitivity reaction (Figure 23.5). It may occur as a component of hay fever or as an independent ocular allergy. There may be large formations of papules or cobblestones under the eyelid. At times the conjunctivitis may be an allergic response to an invading organism, such as the tuberculosis, protein, or staphylococcal bacillus. Contact allergies to drugs are a common occurrence and one of the main reasons why an inflammation can progress despite copious applications of medication. Neomycin and sulfur preparations are particularly sensitizing. Many pharmaceutical agents are available to bring relief. Agents such as cromolyn, lodoxamide, olopatadine, naphazoline/antazoline, and a corticosteroid may be helpful.

Chemical conjunctivitis often is seen in the summer and is caused by irritation from chlorine in swimming pools. It also may occur in industrial workers after exposure to irritating fumes.

Evidently the treatment of conjunctivitis depends on identifying its cause and applying the appropriate therapy. Local antibiotic drops that are effective for a bacterial conjunctivitis would obviously be of no value for a viral infection.

In most offices the diagnosis of conjunctivitis is made largely on clinical grounds and, if serious enough, enhanced with laboratory studies. For example, in a membranous conjunctivitis caused by diphtheria, swabs are taken from the discharge for a smear preparation, and samples are cultured for growth identification and drug sensitivity. Routine cultures and sensitivity tests are rarely done because the time lag in obtaining the results of such investigation does not warrant the delay in treatment. When the conjunctivitis is potentially serious, the ophthalmologist will do appropriate laboratory investigations, but will

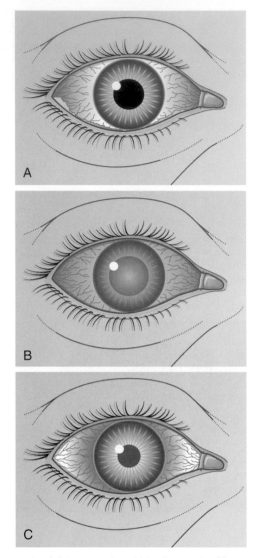

Figure 23.4 (A) Acute conjunctivitis, characterized by discharge, injection greater in the fornix, clear cornea, and pupil normal in size. (B) Acute glaucoma, characterized by tearing, extreme injection of entire eye, hazy cornea, and pupil that is dilated, oval, and fixed to light. (C) Iritis, characterized by absent discharge, circumcorneal injection, clear to slightly hazy cornea, and small pupil.

institute therapy first. If the trial of therapy does not work, it can later be altered when the precise etiologic agent has been identified and the exact drug to which it is sensitive has been determined.

Episcleritis

Episcleritis is characterized by a salmon-pink hue of the superficial layer of the eye, with involvement of the

Table 23.1 Differential diagnosis of common eye disorders

Factor	Acute conjunctivitis	Acute iritis	Acute glaucoma
Pain	None to grittiness or foreign body sensation	Moderate to severe	Severe
Discharge	Watery or purulent	None	Tearing only
Sensitivity to light (photophobia)	Mild	Severe	Moderate
Cornea	Bright and clear	Clear or hazy	Hazy
Pupil	Normal	Constricted or small	Dilated, oval, fixed to light
Intraocular pressure	Normal	Usually normal	Elevated

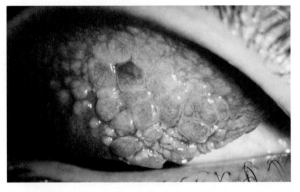

Figure 23.5 Vernal conjunctivitis. Note cobblestone formation of upper tarsus when lid is everted.

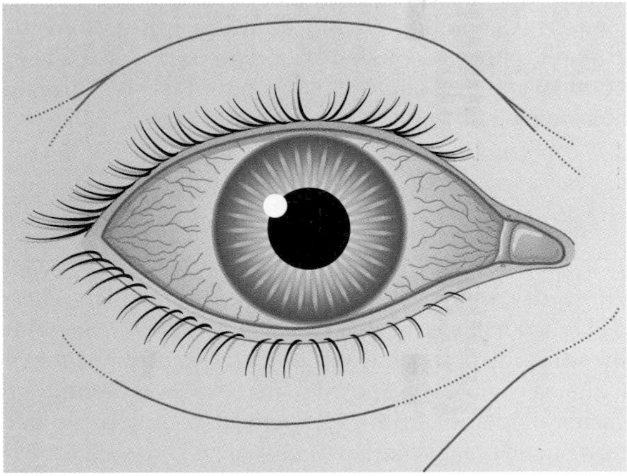

[Figure 23.6 illustration]

Figure 23.6 Sectorial episcleritis is characterized by a salmon-pink color of the conjunctival and episcleral tissues. *(From Stein HA, Slatt BJ, Stein RM. A primer in ophthalmology: a textbook for students. St Louis: Mosby; 1992.)*

conjunctiva and episclera (Figure 23.6). At least one-third of the lesions are tender to touch. Simple episcleritis may be sectorial in 70% or generalized in 30% of patients. In nodular episcleritis, the nodules that form are movable with a cotton-tipped swab, unlike nodular scleritis.

Pinguecula/pterygium

A *pinguecula* is a triangular, wedge-shaped thickening of the conjunctiva, usually found encroaching on the nasal limbus. If it invades the cornea, it is then referred to as a *pterygium* (Figure 23.7). These lesions appear as yellowish or white vascularized masses. They are common in tropical climates where people spend a great deal of time outdoors and are exposed to sunlight and the harmful effects of ultraviolet light. Pingueculae usually do not cause symptoms. Occasionally they may cause some irritation, or may be a cosmetic blemish. Treatment with artificial tears, vasoconstrictors or, rarely, surgical excision may be indicated.

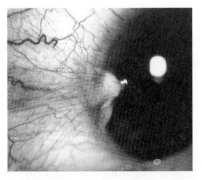

Figure 23.7 Pterygium actively invading the cornea.

401

Pterygia can occasionally extend across the cornea and eventually encroach on the visual axis and cause loss of vision. If there is documented evidence of growth, or if the lesion is close to the visual axis, then surgical excision is indicated. Unfortunately there is a high incidence of recurrence; thus surgical removal is commonly combined with mitomycin application, beta-radiation, or even excimer laser surface ablation to minimize recurrence. Amniotic membranes and mucous membranes have been grafted in place and introduced to reduce recurrence. They may be available from companies in sterile packs.

Conjunctival nevus

A *nevus* is a benign neoplasm that appears on the conjunctiva at birth or in early childhood. The most common appearance is that of a flat, slightly elevated brown spot. It usually becomes pigmented late in childhood or in adolescence. It is uncommon for a nevus to become malignant. This condition should be differentiated from the acquired pigmented lesion that can occur by the age of 40 to 50 and that can, with growth, turn into a malignant melanoma.

CORNEA

The cornea, which forms the anterior one-sixth of the globe and functionally is the main refracting surface of the eye, is the structure most vulnerable to injury or inflammation. It is almost completely exposed so that it receives the brunt of chemical injuries to the eye, foreign bodies, particulate matter, and organisms that can invade it from such contiguous sources as the conjunctiva and the lacrimal sac. It is avascular tissue, which means that it is robbed of the defense mechanisms that normally are marshaled against any inflammatory insult elsewhere in the body. The corneal epithelium provides a strong barrier against bacterial invasion. The integrity of this surface is best appreciated by applying fluorescein to its surface and noting any defects in the integrity of this layer by staining and the accumulation of fluorescein pools.

Keratoconus

Keratoconus is a developmental abnormality in which the cornea progressively becomes thinned centrally and bulges forward in a conical fashion (Figure 23.8). It is usually bilateral and occurs more often in females than in males. Keratoconus is often found in patients who have hay fever, atopic dermatitis, eczema, or asthma.

It creates irregular corneal astigmatism that defies correction by ordinary spectacles. Rigid contact lenses, and sometimes a piggyback of soft and rigid lenses (see Chapter 16), have been used to correct the visual defect. If the patient is

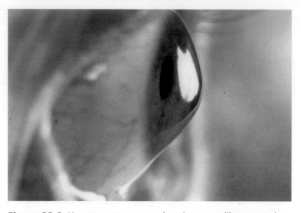

Figure 23.8 Keratoconus cornea showing cone-like protrusion. *(From Levin L, Albert D. Ocular disease: mechanisms and management. Philadelphia: Saunders/Elsevier; 2010.)*

unable to be fitted properly with contact lenses because of high irregular astigmatism, keratoplasty is necessary to restore vision.

Keratoconus can be detected by *Munson's sign.* This is observed when the examiner has the patient look down and notes from above the indentation of the lower lid by the cone of the cornea. The diagnosis may be made by slit-lamp examination; by the keratometer or retinoscope, which shows the presence of irregular corneal astigmatism; or by use of a keratoscope, computerized videokeratography, or Placido's disc, which reflects the images of disordered and irregular concentric circles on the surface of the cornea. Topographic analysis (see Chapter 40) with the pentacam is now the most popular method to detect keratoconus.

Corneal cross-linking has become a popular technique in the treatment of keratoconus. Cross-linking with ultraviolet light and riboflavin drops often arrests the progress of keratoconus and keractesia. (For more information see Chapter 37.)

Herpes simplex keratitis

Herpes simplex keratitis is a common corneal inflammatory disorder created by the herpes simplex virus, which is the offending agent of the common coldsore. The first exposure to herpes simplex virus in 90% of cases results in subclinical, usually mild, disease. Characteristically the young child is infected by salivary contamination from an adult who has labial herpes. The incubation period is 3 to 9 days. The clinical features of herpes simplex are both ocular and nonocular. The symptoms are relatively mild and consist of an irritating foreign body sensation, mild tearing with no frank pus or purulent discharge, and some haziness of vision accompanied by sensitivity to light. The classic herpes lesion is the dendritic figure, which when stained with fluorescein reveals a branchlike erosion of

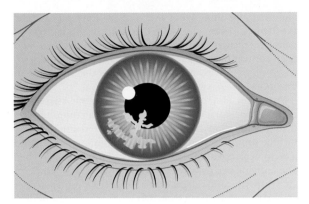

Figure 23.9 Dendritic figure, typical of herpes simplex keratitis.

the cornea, as a single lesion or as multiple disturbances (Figure 23.9).

The virus will remain dormant in the sensory nerves to the face, where it can be aroused by a variety of precipitating factors including emotional stress, trauma, menstruation, sunlight, or the use of either local or systemic steroid drugs. When aroused, the virus will travel down the sensory nerves to the face, lids, conjunctiva, and cornea to produce a recurrence of the disease. These recurrences may be frequent, adding insult to each previous episode, so that reduction of vision over the years is a common complication. If only the epithelium is involved, no scarring occurs. However, the inflammatory process commonly extends deep down toward the stroma, which heals with vascular proliferation from the limbus and results in corneal scarring.

This condition can be a diagnostic danger because it appears to be a simple conjunctivitis. Many patients treat themselves or are treated by their family physician with antibiotics for several days before arriving in the ophthalmologist's office. Local antibiotics are of no value in this condition because it is caused by a virus. In many instances, self-medication severely aggravates the condition because many antibiotic preparations are coupled with steroids, which cause the virus to proliferate even more, thus ensuring the spread of the ulcer and further necrosis of tissue.

The treatment of herpes keratitis is instillation of trifluridine (Viroptic) drops or application of idoxuridine (IDU) (Stoxil) or vidarabine (Vira-A) ointment. The cornea heals in 7 to 14 days in approximately 85% of cases. Some ophthalmologists prefer to remove the offending virus by scraping off the diseased epithelium. This can be done at the slit lamp with a dull blade.

Other forms of the disease include the following:

1. *Gingivostomatitis.* Symptoms are fever, malaise, and lymphadenopathy, along with sore throat.
2. *Pharyngitis.* Often pharyngitis occurs with vesicles on the tonsils.
3. *Cutaneous disease.* This usually manifests as type I, which occurs above the waist, or type II, below the waist. The disease is seen in wrestlers and rugby players.
4. *General infection.* Type II infection, which is more common than type I, is characterized by fever, myalgia, extensive vesicular lesions, and inguinal and pelvic lymphadenopathy.

Recurrent herpes simplex

The virus develops a symbiosis with human beings. Any of the previously mentioned precipitating factors (trauma, fever, etc.), which provoke viral shedding and the immunologic functions, may be causative factors in episodes of recurrence. The trigeminal ganglion is a reservoir for the type I disease. The virus has a 50% recurrence rate over 5 years and may be highly localized in the lymph nodes, chin, eyes, and genitals. Cultures usually are unnecessary because this is chiefly a clinical diagnosis.

Superficial punctate keratitis

Superficial punctate keratitis consists of fine erosions in the corneal epithelium that can be diagnosed by means of the slit lamp and fluorescein staining. These lesions are common and can be seen in dry eye conditions, infections such as adenovirus and herpes simplex, and chemical injuries. Treatment varies, depending on the cause of the superficial punctate keratitis.

Herpes zoster ophthalmicus

Herpes zoster ophthalmicus (HZO) is caused by the varicella virus, which causes chickenpox in children. In the adult it is ushered in by a severe neuralgic type of pain, which usually includes the upper lid and extends upward beyond the brow to envelop the forehead through the scalp almost to the vertex of the head. After the pain a vesicular eruption of the skin usually occurs and the skin surface becomes swollen, red, and heavily blistered (Figure 23.10). The severe pain and vesicular phase lasts approximately 2 weeks. With healing, the skin often is pockmarked with deep, pitted scars and sensitivity to normal sensation is depressed. The incidence of HZO is 10% of all herpes zoster infections. HZO is frequently seen by an ophthalmologist first.

The virus has a predilection for dermatomes T3–L3, but the most common site is the trigeminal nerve. Cutaneous lesions of herpes zoster are histopathologically identical to varicella but have a greater inflammatory reaction, which can cause scarring. The dermatome pattern of herpes zoster may occur in three sites supplied by branches of the trigeminal nerve:

- The ophthalmic nerve distribution (V_1), where it occurs 20 times more frequently than at the V_2 or V_3 sites.

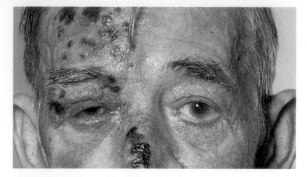

Figure 23.10 Herpes zoster ophthalmicus.
(Reproduced from Spalton D, Hitchings R, Hunter P. Atlas of clinical ophthalmology. 3rd ed. St Louis: Mosby; 2004, with permission.)

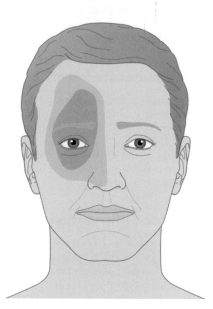

Figure 23.11 Herpes zoster ophthalmicus is characterized by vesicular skin eruptions in the distribution of any of the branches of the trigeminal nerve.
(From Stein HA, Slatt BJ, Stein RM. A primer in ophthalmology: a textbook for students. St Louis: Mosby; 1992.)

Frontal involvement is the most common, including the upper lid, forehead, and superior conjunctiva, which are supplied by the supraorbital and supratrochlear branches (Figure 23.11). Alternatively, herpes zoster may spread to the lacrimal and nasociliary area, which supplies the cornea, iris, ciliary body, and tip of the nose.
- The maxillary nerve distribution (V_2)
- The mandibular nerve distribution (V_3)

The virus may affect none, any, or all of these branches.

If the tip of the nose has a vesicular eruption, it usually means that the nasociliary nerve has been affected

and that the underlying eye also will be affected by the herpes zoster virus. This occurs in about 50% of patients. Ocular disturbances include superficial and deep corneal ulcers, iritis, secondary glaucoma, and even paralysis of an extraocular muscle in the minority of instances.

Treatment may include the use of systemic steroids to decrease the scarring and pain that are so common after the inflammation has subsided. Ocular treatment may include topical steroids to decrease the inflammation and a cycloplegic agent to make the patient more comfortable. The antiviral agents acyclovir sodium (Zovirax), famciclovir (Famvir), and valacyclovir (Valtrex), administered in an oral form, have been shown to be effective in shortening the course of disease in herpes zoster.

The use of the herpes zoster vaccine (Zostavax) is becoming popular. Almost all adults older than 50 years may be susceptible to the virus. The vaccination has been shown to reduce not only the disease but also the postherpetic neurology that follows.

Marginal corneal ulcers

Marginal corneal ulcers are usually secondary to inflammation caused by the toxin of *S. aureus* combined with cells and other mediators involved in the body's immunologic response. Ulcers are extremely painful, and most patients believe that they have a large foreign body in their eye. There is marked redness around the eye, and usually a white infiltrate extends from the limbus into the substance of the cornea for 2 to 4 mm. At times the cornea is ulcerated over the surface, but the epithelium may also be intact. The discharge is scant and usually watery.

Because this condition has an immunologic basis, it responds well to antibiotic-steroid medication. Other less common causes of marginal ulcers include nonimmunologic bacterial infections, herpes simplex, and inflammation secondary to a variety of systemic diseases, such as rheumatoid arthritis.

Recurrent corneal erosion

The typical history of recurrent corneal erosion is abrasion of the cornea by a fingernail, a branch of a tree, the edge of a piece of paper or cardboard, or any other organic agent. The actual injury heals temporarily but a few days, weeks, or even months later the person experiences a complete recurrence of signs and symptoms of the original injury, but does not have any recollection of having reinjured the eye. Invariably the symptoms occur in the morning and are thought to be caused by opening the eyes or by the trauma of rubbing the eyes, which removes the area of freshly healed epithelium on the cornea. The disorder is disabling because of the recurrent pain and is somewhat baffling because the features of the disorder are not evident between attacks. The symptoms may last anywhere from 30 minutes to several hours or several days.

The use of hypertonic drops during the day and ointment at night is helpful in dehydrating the corneal epithelium, which makes it less likely to slough off. If this is unsuccessful, a therapeutic soft contact lens can be tried. Another treatment modality is the technique of anterior stromal puncture, in which a fine needle is used to make multiple puncture marks in the anterior third of the cornea. This technique decreases the recurrence rate by forming stronger bonds between the epithelium and the underlying tissue. One may also debride the corneal epithelium in the local area.

EYELIDS

Certain anatomic features of the lids affect the manner of lid response. For instance, the skin of the lid, unlike that in the rest of the face, is extremely thin, loosely attached, and devoid of thick connective tissue and a fatty layer. Therefore, any inflammatory swelling may cause the skin of the lid to balloon out and look puffy, whereas the weight of the collection of fluid is commonly sufficient to cause ptosis. The lid margins contain the openings of the meibomian glands (oil-secreting glands), as well as small sweat glands (Moll's glands). It is easy to understand why people who put eyeliner on their lid margins get recurrent cysts. They do so by obstructing the orifices of these tiny glands with cosmetic pigments.

The cilia or eyelashes are strong, short, curved hairs arranged in two or more closely set rows. They are longer and more numerous on the upper lid than the lower. They have a protective effect, eliminating debris from the eye except when they themselves are caked by debris of a heavy mascara brush.

Chronic inflammation of the lid margins results in thickened, heavily vascularized lids. At times lashes fall out and, even worse, grow aberrantly. Instead of curving out, they turn in to rub against the sensitive cornea, creating erosions and even ulcerations.

Normally the upper lid just covers the upper millimeter or so of the cornea, whereas the lower lid skirts at its lower level. If the sclera is visible either above or below the cornea, it suggests either retraction of the lids or protrusion of the eye, which might be seen in hyperthyroidism, orbital inflammation, or a tumor.

If the lid droops more than 1 to 2 mm over the cornea, the eye seems smaller by virtue of narrowing the palpebral fissure. This condition, called *ptosis*, is caused by the weakness of the muscles that elevate the upper lid (Müller's smooth muscle or the levator palpebrae superioris muscle).

Epicanthus

Epicanthus is a common congenital variation in young white children. A vertical fold extends from the upper lid over the medial angle of the eye and the caruncle (Figure 23.12). Epicanthus makes the eyes seem closely set together, and many parents and general practitioners mistake this condition for strabismus. Invariably the condition is self-correcting with the growth of the root of the nose and the face. In Asians this variation persists throughout adult life. Surgical procedures that eliminate this fold to make the eyes look rounder or more like those of Westerners are popular in Japan.

Entropion

An *entropion* is an in-turning of the lids; usually one of the lower lids is affected. The spastic type is more common in old age than in youth. Its major disability is created by irritation of the cornea by in-turned lashes (Figure 23.13).

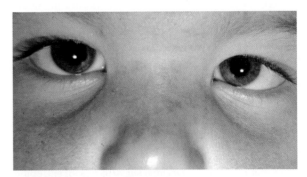

Figure 23.12 Epicanthic folds.
(From Kanski J, Bowling B. Clinical ophthalmology—a systematic approach. 7th ed. Edinburgh: Saunders; 2011.)

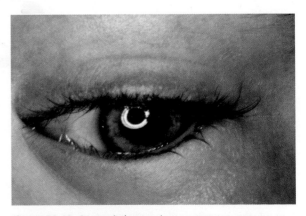

Figure 23.13 Congenital entropion.
(From Kanski J, Bowling B. Clinical ophthalmology—a systematic approach. 7th ed. Edinburgh: Saunders; 2011.)

The inversion of the lid margin is caused by a spasm of the orbicularis oculi, the washer-like muscle under the skin of the lid. The spasm closes the eye. This muscle spasm is often induced by ocular inflammation or irritation. In an older adult it is easy for a spastic muscle to turn in on an atonic lid. A more severe form of entropion is caused by scarring, which can follow inflammation of the conjunctiva such as in ocular pemphigus, trachoma, lacerations of the lid, and chemical burns of the eye with attendant scarring. Again, surgery is required to remedy the condition.

The treatment of entropion is generally surgical, although temporary relief can be obtained by drawing the skin of the lower lid down toward the cheeks by means of adhesive tape. The surgery is safe, simple, and effective and is usually performed with the patient under local anesthesia.

Ectropion

In *ectropion* the lid suffers a loss of tone and flops away from the eye (Figure 23.14), so that the conjunctiva lining the inner surface of the lid becomes exposed, irritated, and thickened. It occurs primarily in older adults and is aggravated by attendant tearing as a result of aversion or stenosis of the punctum. The wiping away of tears from the lower lid makes the lower lid droop further, setting up a vicious cycle of tearing and progressive ectropion. Exposure of the conjunctiva causes burning and irritation and predisposes the eye to secondary inflammation. Again, the most common type is a result of senile atrophy of the lid structures, which causes the lids to stray outward. Scarring also can produce the same defect and is caused by the same conditions that create *cicatricial entropion*. This type of entropion is a mechanical defect of the lids that can be remedied only by surgery.

Ptosis

In unilateral ptosis there is a conspicuous droop of the upper lid and the opening of one eye seems smaller than the other (Figure 23.15). Commonly the lid fold is absent or smooth on the affected side. It is evident when the individual has to look up, because the lid on the affected side does not move upward with the globe compared with the opposite normal side. If both lids are involved, a child will develop a characteristic head posture with the head thrown back and the upper lids elevated as a compensatory mechanism to raise the drooped eyelids.

Treatment of the condition is invariably surgical. It is directed toward shortening the levator palpebrae superioris muscle, the primary elevator of the lid. Resection of a section of this muscle and advancement of its insertion strengthen it and increase its leverage.

In congenital ptosis it is often bilateral.

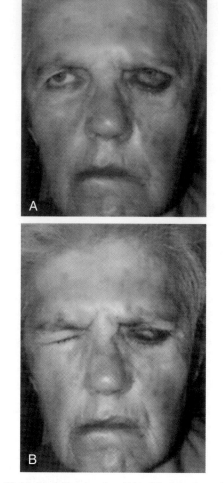

Figure 23.14 Paralytic ectropion. (A) Left facial palsy and severe ectropion. (B) Lagophthalmos.
(From Kanski J, Bowling B. Clinical ophthalmology—a systematic approach. 7th ed. Edinburgh: Saunders; 2011.)

Exaggerated blink activity

Exaggerated blink activity is a common condition seen especially in children. The sole feature is the presence of conspicuous, repetitive blinking motions of the lids, called *myokymia*. Invariably the ocular examination reveals the presence of normal eyes. The rapid reflex blinking is thought to be the mechanism by which anxiety and restless motor activity are released in a young child. It clears up on its own, so parents are best advised to ignore this self-limiting condition, which disappears more rapidly if it is ignored. Constant attention to these repetitive blinking motions only increases the child's anxiety.

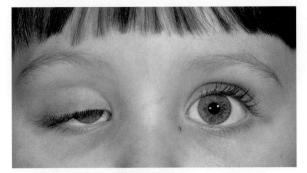

Figure 23.15 Simple unilateral congenital ptosis.
(From Hoyt C, Taylor D. Pediatric ophthalmology and strabismus. 4th ed. Philadelphia: Elsevier/Saunders; 2013.)

A corollary to reflex blinking in the adult is tremor of the orbicularis oculi muscle. Many adults complain of a fine lid flutter that is like a current going through the lower lid. Other than the annoying spontaneous twitch, it does not cause any other symptoms. The condition is usually caused by a mixture of tension and fatigue and disappears on its own. Rarely, however, it can be caused by serious conditions such as Parkinson's disease, multiple sclerosis, and hyperthyroidism.

Blepharochalasis and dermatochalasis

Blepharochalasis is a condition that often drives middle-aged individuals to the plastic surgeon. It is caused by recurrent swelling of the upper lids and appears most prominently in the morning. The continuous stretching of the skin of the upper lids and the accumulation of edema cause the skin to lose its tone and hang lifelessly as a redundant fold or curtain over the upper lids. One disability is that it interferes with the application of eye make-up to the lids. In extreme cases it can even weigh on the lashes, creating a sensation of heaviness and ocular fatigue. It may cause restriction of the upper field of vision. At times this condition is accompanied by the protrusion of fat from behind the eye through the orbital septum just under the skin. These fat pads most prominently appear on the medial side of the upper lids and on the lower lids as rather large, unattractive mounds.

This condition is mainly, but not entirely, cosmetic and can be remedied surgically by removing the excess skin and the fat and repairing the septum so that further protrusion of the retroorbital fat cannot occur.

Although blepharochalasis is largely innocuous, occasionally it is a manifestation of thyroid disease, kidney disorder, severe allergic reaction, or angioneurotic edema. This condition should be differentiated from dermatochalasis, which is predominantly an involutional aging change. Dermatochalasis is a result not of recurrent edema, but of loss of elastic tissue and relaxation of the fascial bands that connect the skin and underlying orbicularis muscle.

Trichiasis

In *trichiasis*, instead of being directed outward, the lashes turn in toward the eye, causing irritation and sometimes erosion and ulceration of the cornea. Often there are irregular rows of lashes. Trichiasis may be a result of scarring of the lid, which can be caused by previous injury, chemical burns of the lids, and severe lid inflammations. Simple epilation of the offending cilia is really a palliative measure, because the lashes tend to regrow aberrantly. If only a few lashes are irritating, their base can be cauterized by electrolysis. In more severe cases a freezing technique applied to the base of the cilia, referred to as *cryosurgery*, or surgical reconstruction of the lid margin may be necessary to remove the aberrant lashes that rub against the conjunctiva or cornea and cause the irritation.

Blepharitis

Blepharitis is a common chronic inflammation of the lid margin. Patients usually complain of a sandy or itchy feeling of their eyes, especially in the morning. There is usually redness, as well as a thickening and irregularity of the lid margins. The disease may occur at any age. The two most common types of chronic inflammation of the lids are *staphylococcal blepharitis* and *seborrheic blepharitis*. Seborrhea is a common cause of dandruff. Telltale diagnostic patches of seborrheic involvement in such patients are commonly seen in the medial aspect of the brows, the forehead, and sometimes behind the skin of the ear or on the nose. The base of the eyelash is usually caked with a greasy type of scale that comes off easily, leaving an intact lid margin.

At times the blepharitis can be infective in origin; when this is the case, it is invariably a result of *S. aureus*. The lid margins become ulcerated and congested and adhesive exudate forms on the base of the follicles and on the lid margin. When the scale is removed, it always reveals an ulcerative defect on the lid margin. The ulcerative type of blepharitis is more serious because if the inflammation reaches down to the base of the follicles it can cause permanent scarring, with either loss of lashes or misdirection of lash and regrowth with accompanying trichiasis. Also, the cosmetic consequences are undesirable because the lids become thickened, heavily vascularized, and unattractive.

An uncommon pathogen is the *Demodex* mite. Demodex increases with age and is fairly common after age 60. Once the mite lodges in the skin it moves to the eyelashes and can be seen with the slit-lamp microscope. Once demodex gets out of control, blepharitis follows. The adult version of demodex folliculorum is the most resistant to treatment. Lid hygiene is most important

Essential blepharospasm

Essential blepharospasm is a condition in which the individual is severely handicapped by spastic closure of the eyes along with severe sensitivity (photophobia) to light. Closing the eyes every few seconds renders the individual virtually blind. By being closed a great deal of a patient's waking hours, the patient is seriously handicapped. Remedies range from special tinted glasses (fl-41), sedatives, and mild tranquilizers to botulinum toxin (Botox) injections. The last is used to paralyze the orbicularis oculi muscle that surrounds the eye and reduce the spasm. If this does not relieve the spasm, then surgical myomectomy of the orbicularis may be performed.

External hordeolum (stye) and internal hordeolum

A *stye* or *external hordeolum* is an acute suppurative inflammation of small sebaceous glands on the lid margin, the *glands of Zeis*, which empty their secretion into the hair follicles of the cilia. An internal hordeolum is an acute inflammation of the sebaceous glands that reside in the tarsal plates: the meibomian glands. In the early stages of the inflammation, the affected gland becomes swollen and the lid becomes red and edematous. An abscess forms with a small collection of pus, which usually points at the apex of one of these glands. Unless the suppuration is opened, the discomfort can be considerable. The inflammation generally results from invasion by bacterial *S. aureus*. It is a common affliction of young adults, but it can occur at all ages, especially in patients with blepharitis.

Treatment consists primarily of hot compresses to rupture the gland in the early stage. If this is unsuccessful, the ophthalmologist can incise and drain the hordeolum or inject local steroids into the lesion in the hope of bringing about its resolution.

Chalazion

A *chalazion* is a chronic inflammatory granuloma of the large meibomian glands embedded in the tarsus of the lid. Multiple chalazia can occur in the upper or lower lids. Unlike the infectious causes of the internal and external hordeolum, chalazia are the result of a sterile process. Initially the orifice of the meibomian gland becomes occluded by a small inflammatory swelling and the accumulated sebum ruptures the gland, creating a granulomatous type of inflammatory reaction in the lid itself. The lid becomes swollen, painful and inflamed until eventually the inflammatory reaction is walled off and a cyst forms (Figure 23.16). If the cyst is large and thickly walled, it must be opened surgically and evacuated with a curet and blunt dissection.

Occasionally the injection of localized steroids into the lesion may obviate the need for surgical drainage. Sometimes, in the early stages, hot compresses rupture the

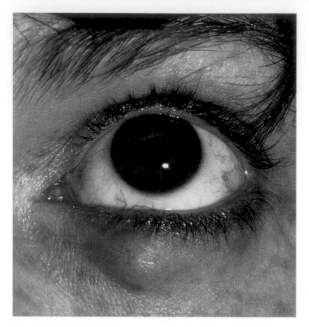

Figure 23.16 Chalazion.
(Reproduced from Spalton D, Hitchings R, Hunter P. Atlas of clinical ophthalmology. 3rd ed. St Louis: Mosby 2004; with permission.)

chalazion and can effect resolution of the inflammation. Many times the patient comes to the ophthalmologist with a nonpainful, localized swelling of the lid after the inflammation has subsided. The lesion may be surgically excised.

One must differentiate from other benign and malignant growths as listed in the following text. Traditional medical treatments include warm compresses, lid massage, lid scrubs, and topical steroids. A reduced cholesterol diet may minimize future chalazion and meibomianitis.

Tumors of the lid

Milia

Milia are small, white, slightly elevated cysts of the skin with a pedunculated apex. They can create a cosmetic blemish when they appear in crops.

Xanthelasma

Xanthelasma are yellowish fatty deposits, or plaques, that occur in the upper and lower lids on the medial side. The condition is largely cosmetic, but it may indicate a more serious lipid disorder because it represents a deposit of circulating cholesterol or other lipids. The deposits can be destroyed or removed by trichloroacetic acid, carbon dioxide snow, or surgery. The purpose of removing xanthelasma is strictly cosmetic.

Carcinoma

Eyelid tumors account for 5% to 10% of skin cancers. The most common malignant growth of the lid is the *basal cell carcinoma* (BCC) (Figure 23.17). This carcinoma accounts for 90% of cancers of the eyelid. Exposure to UV radiation is the main cause, although there is a hereditary component. It rarely metastasizes, but can recur. Eyelid reconstruction or grafts are uncommon unless the tumor is very large.

It usually appears on the lower lid near the inner canthus or on the lateral side of the lower lid, and finally and least commonly on the upper lids. The tumor typically has a raised ulcerated surface. Its margin is pearly white and despite the appearance of tissue destruction, it rarely causes any symptoms. If it is treated early with either radiotherapy or surgery, a complete cure can be effected. The tumor is invasive if it is not treated and tends to spread directly to the tissues surrounding it.

Squamous cell carcinoma (SCC) is more malignant and can spread throughout the body. It must be entirely removed. Excisional biopsy is sometimes the only way to differentiate BCC from SCC.

Seborrheic keratosis (senile verruca)

This is one of the most common lesions involving the eyelid skin. It appears as a well-defined, small, elevated, brown to brownish-black lesion on the eyelid, much like a button flush on the skin surface. It is benign but may be surgically removed for cosmetic reasons.

Keratoacanthoma

This is a benign lesion but, because of its rapid growth, it is often mistaken for a malignancy. It grows rapidly but reaches maximum size in 6 to 8 weeks. There may be spontaneous regression, but it is usually excised.

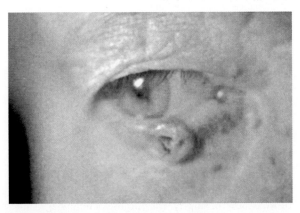

Figure 23.17 Basal cell carcinoma of eyelid.

Molluscum contagiosum

These are waxy, raised nodules, often with an umbilicated center. The lesions are caused by a member of the pox virus group. Toxic debris released from the lesion into the tears may give rise to a chronic conjunctivitis. The lesion usually has to be surgically excised. Other treatments include cauterization, cryotherapy, and laser.

LACRIMAL APPARATUS

Acute dacryoadenitis

Acute dacryoadenitis is an inflammation of the lacrimal gland that causes pain and discomfort in the upper outer portion of the orbit and swelling of the lid laterally. Eversion of the upper lid reveals a swollen, reddened gland on its lateral surface. Mumps and infectious mononucleosis are the usual systemic causes of this condition.

Lacrimal gland enlargement

Mass lesions of the lacrimal gland may manifest in a variety of ways. They may be painful or painless, they may be palpable and they may be associated with swelling of the lid and ptosis. Enlargement of the lacrimal gland can be caused by tumor formation, such as the mixed tumor, adenoid cystic tumor or lymphoma, or by a granulomatous inflammation.

Tearing (Box 23.1)

Tearing may be the result of lacrimation, which is excessive tear formation of the lacrimal gland, or it may be caused by *epiphora*, which is defective drainage of tears. Lacrimation may result from psychologic stimuli (e.g., grief or depression), from irritation of the eye by wind or dust, or from irritative inflammatory disorders of the conjunctiva, cornea, or lids. These causes of lacrimation usually are self-evident and desist once the stimulus has stopped.

Persistent tearing, with overflow onto the cheek, is usually caused by obstruction somewhere in the lacrimal drainage system from the punctum situated on the medial

Box 23.1 **Tear film function**
1. Hydrates and protects the ocular surface
2. Reduces friction on blinking
3. Enhances oxygen to the cornea
4. Removes waste and cell debris
5. Protects against infection

409

aspect of the lower lid to the nasolacrimal duct. The patency of tear elimination can be tested in several ways. Fluorescein solution 2% instilled in the conjunctival sac normally disappears within 1 minute. A cotton swab placed in the nasal passages can usually prove the patency of the system, as it becomes stained with fluorescein. Irrigation of the lacrimal system with saline solution is less physiologic, but can at least demonstrate that tears will flow from the punctum to the nasolacrimal duct and empty into the nasal passages. If there is obstruction of the nasolacrimal canal, the tears forced through the lower canaliculus will reflux out through the upper punctum. This reflux of tears through the upper punctum is plainly visible. An additional point is that the person being tested will not taste the saline solution, which should be coming through the nose. Another test of tear function uses saccharin solutions placed in the conjunctival sac. If tears are being eliminated, 1 or 2 minutes later the patency is proved by the patient indicating the taste of something in the throat.

It is also important to note the presence of apposition of the lower lid against the globe. Tearing can occur if the lower lid is not in contact with the globe, as can be seen with medial ectropions.

Regardless of the cause, the treatment of tearing caused by defective drainage is largely surgical. No one has ever died from a bit of tearing; thus the decision to operate depends on the distress of the patient created by the mechanical reflux of tears and the association of secondary infections.

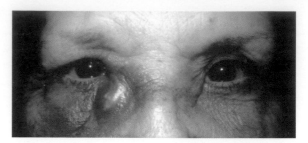

Figure 23.18 Dacryocystitis. Note the marked swelling over the lacrimal sac.

Dacryocystitis

Dacryocystitis, an inflammation of the lacrimal sac, is indicated by an inflammatory swelling at the site of the sac. This inflamed swelling is seen as a visible red lump just below the caruncle overriding the inframedial aspect of the orbital bone (Figure 23.18).

Sometimes pressure over the sac causes pus or mucoid material to regurgitate through the punctum. This condition usually results from the effects of stricture of a nasolacrimal duct arising from chronic inflammation, usually of nasal origin. Obstruction of the lower end of this duct can be caused by the presence of a nasal polyp and extreme deviation of the septum, or by a marked congestion of the inferior turbinate. Surgery, called *dacryocystorhinostomy* (DCR), is required to establish a new canal for the tears, thus preventing stagnation.

Questions for review and thought

1. Describe the typical contact conjunctival allergic response to neomycin.
2. What is a nevus? What type should cause concern?
3. What is a xanthelasma plaque? Does it have any significance?
4. What influence do cortisone drops have on the herpes simplex virus?
5. Keratoconus affects the cornea and is revealed by a forward protrusion of the globe. Why does it impair vision?
6. What are the external signs and symptoms that distinguish herpes zoster ophthalmicus?
7. What would you see if you stained the eye of a patient who has two marginal corneal ulcers with fluorescein? What is the usual cause of such ulcers?
8. What glands lie in the eyelid and what are the conditions called when they become inflamed?
9. What causes repeated blinking in childhood?
10. Describe the typical picture of chronic blepharitis.
11. What is the treatment for a stye?
12. What causes persistent tearing?
13. What virus that produces cold sores on the lips can also cause a severe keratitis? What is the typical pattern of infection that it produces on the cornea?
14. Name three causes of purulent conjunctivitis of the newborn.
15. What is a basal cell carcinoma? Where is it usually located with respect to the lids? How is it treated? What is the prognosis after treatment?

Q Self-evaluation questions

True–false statements

Directions: Indicate whether the statement is true **(T)** or false **(F)**.

1. Large cobblestones under the eyelid often are seen in vernal conjunctivitis. **T** or **F**
2. A pterygium is a vascular invasive area on the cornea. **T** or **F**
3. Keratoconus results in scarring and irregular curvature of the cornea. **T** or **F**

Missing words

Directions: Write in the missing word in the following sentences:

4. The virus that causes a dendritic pattern of the cornea is called _____.
5. When herpes zoster ophthalmicus involves the eye, the tip of the _____ is usually involved and blistered.
6. A fingernail injury to the cornea may result in recurrent _____ of the cornea a few months later.

Choice-completion questions

Directions: Select the one best answer in each case.

7. Ptosis or blepharoptosis is a drooping of the upper lid caused by a paralysis of:
   a. the levator palpebrae superioris muscle.
   b. Müller's muscle.
   c. the orbicularis oculi.
   d. a or b.
   e. none of the above.
8. A subconjunctival hemorrhage may occur in which of the following conditions?
   a. Trauma
   b. Blood disorders
   c. After sneezing
   d. Perforating injury of the globe
   e. All of the above.
9. Abrasion of the cornea is not caused by:
   a. entropion resulting from scarring of the conjunctiva.
   b. entropion resulting from spasm of the orbicularis.
   c. trichiasis.
   d. dacryocystitis.
   e. contact lenses.

A Answers, notes, and explanations

1. **True.** Although cobblestones or large papules on the undersurface of the eyelid are typically seen in vernal conjunctivitis, they may also occur in a number of allergic conditions. In addition, giant papillary conjunctivitis is seen with the use of both rigid and soft contact lenses, secondary to protruding corneal sutures and in poor-fitting ocular prostheses. It is believed in these cases to be caused by an allergic response to some protein constituent that builds up on the contact lens.

2. **True.** A pterygium is a locally invasive area that extends across the cornea and eventually may interfere significantly with vision. Once removed, there is a significant incidence of recurrence and each removal increases the risk of further recurrence. A number of surgical procedures have been advocated to try to overcome the recurrence rate of pterygia.

3. **True.** Keratoconus is marked by a cone-shaped protrusion of the cornea, resulting in irregularity of the spherical surface of the cornea. The cornea develops an irregularity that can no longer be corrected by spectacle lenses and requires correction by contact lenses. There are many microbreaks in the extremely thin cornea, resulting in scar formation and even hydrops of the cornea. Each small break in the cornea becomes devastating to the homogeneous regularity of the cornea and results in further scarring and reduction in vision.

4. **Herpes simplex.** The herpes simplex virus most commonly forms a dendritic pattern, usually in the central or paracentral area of the cornea. However, there is no set manner by which it manifests in the eye. It may appear as a conjunctivitis or may extend deeply into the stroma of the cornea and become a necrotic central ulcer that fails to heal. However, the dendritic pattern, which represents an involvement of the corneal epithelium, is the most typical manifestation of the herpes simplex virus.

5. **Nose.** When the tip of the nose is affected the ciliary ganglion is involved, through which the nasociliary branch of the fifth or ophthalmic nerve courses. Serious ocular damage can often be predicted if the tip of the nose is involved.

6. **Erosion.** Often any abrasion of the cornea by objects such as paper or a fingernail that involves the corneal epithelium also interferes with the basement membrane sufficiently to result in inadequate attachment of the epithelium to the basement membrane. During the night the epithelium becomes relatively edematous. In the morning, on awakening, there is a tendency to dislodge the epithelium that is not firmly attached to the underlying basement

A Continued

membrane. This results in the typical symptoms of recurrent corneal erosion, with all the irritation and foreign body reaction that were present during the original injury.

7. **d. a or b.** The levator palpebrae superioris muscle may be affected in this condition, as occurs in most congenital ptoses and in many of the acquired paralytic ptoses. If Müller's muscle is paralyzed, such as occurs in Horner's syndrome with paralysis of the sympathetic nerve, a slight ptosis is present.

8. **e. All of the above.** Whereas a subconjunctival hemorrhage is often harmless, it is important to be aware that it may be an ominous sign of a small perforating wound of the globe from a sharp flying missile. Thus radiologic studies and further detailed examination of the interior of the eye with a well-dilated pupil become important. In addition, the examiner should rule out medical conditions such as blood disorders, hypertension, diabetes, and so on that may be responsible for a subconjunctival hemorrhage.

9. **d. Dacryocystitis.** Dacryocystitis does not cause abrasions of the cornea. Contact lenses result in the most serious type of abrasions of the cornea, either by incorrect insertion or by overwear syndrome. Trichiasis, or an abnormal row of eyelashes, may result in a constant irritation and abrasion of the corneal epithelium. Entropion also may result in irritation of the cornea by eyelashes.

Chapter | 24 |

Common retinal disorders*

As an ophthalmic medical assistant or technician, it is important to have a fundamental understanding of the common retinal disorders in clinical practice that are not seen on external examination. Detection of retinal disorders requires ophthalmoscopic examination. Although this

*Contributed by Efrem D. Mandelcorn, MD, FRCSC, DBO; Peng Yan, MD, FRCSC; Tina Felfeli BSc, and Arielle R. Brickman.

assessment is not within the domain of an ophthalmic medical assistant or technician, patients may ask questions of any member of the ophthalmic team to which they entrust the safety and security of their eyes. Therefore, this chapter discusses some of the most common retinal disorders.

The clinical evaluation of the retina includes refraction, ophthalmoscopy (both direct and indirect), visual fields for peripheral and central vision, color vision assessment, dark adaptation studies, electroretinography, ultrasonography, and fluorescein angiography.

RETINAL ARTERY OCCLUSION

Retinal artery occlusion occurs when the central retinal artery is obstructed by an embolus or thrombus. This in turn results in retinal nonperfusion, where the nine layers of the retina undergo ischemic necrosis, leading to a sudden and painless loss of vision in the affected eye.

If the condition is seen within 30 minutes, there is a possibility of reperfusion by dilating the retinal arterioles to allow the embolus to dislodge and move into the peripheral circulation. Irreversible damage to the sensory retina occurs after approximately 90 minutes of nonperfusion.

The diagnosis is based on the retinal finding of the classic *cherry-red spot*. The retina becomes gray from swelling or edema because the retina loses its normal transparency. The blood vessels become attenuated and segmented (Figure 24.1). Ischemia changes the entire transparent nerve fiber layer of the retina gray except the foveal region, which is absent of the nerve fiber layer. Consequently, the background in the fovea remains its normal red color from the underlying choroidal vascular supply, leading to the

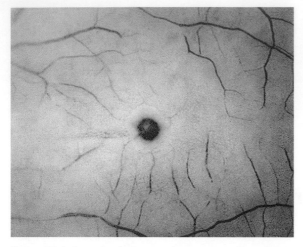

Figure 24.1 Central retinal artery closure, acute. Note the graying in the macular area and the cherry-red spot.

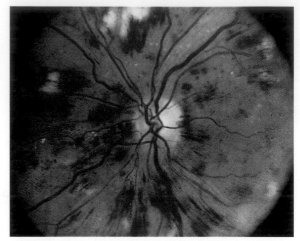

Figure 24.3 Central venous occlusion. Note multiple hemorrhages and distended vessels.
(Courtesy of Mount Sinai Hospital, Toronto, Canada.)

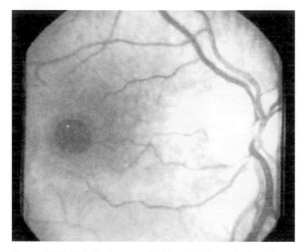

Figure 24.2 Hole in the macula. Note the "punched-out" reddened area.

appearance of a cherry-red spot. The usual prognosis is total and permanent loss of light perception in the involved eye (Figure 24.2).

RETINAL VEIN OCCLUSION

Central retinal vein occlusion (CRVO) is generally caused by a thrombus in a central retinal vein. Conditions associated with an increased risk of retinal vein occlusion include diabetes, hypertension, polycythemia, glaucoma, and any other condition that causes stasis of blood flow.

Because CRVO is a painless cause of vision loss, patients may not be immediately aware of the onset of the condition. The profound loss of vision may not be detected until the patient "discovers" it by rubbing or closing the good eye.

On ophthalmoscopic examination, the entire retina may be covered with superficial hemorrhages that appear flame-shaped (Figure 24.3). There may be scattered cotton-wool spots, which are microinfarcts of the retinal nerve fiber layer. The retinal veins appear dilated and tortuous distal to the site of occlusion. The macula is usually edematous, and this leads to cystoid macular edema with loss of vision. If a branch of the vein is involved, only one sector of the retina will be affected, so the vision may or may not be affected. The prognosis for visual recovery is significantly better with a branch vein occlusion than with a central vein occlusion.

The most dreaded complication is neovascular glaucoma, which can result in a blind eye with severe pain that may eventually be managed by enucleation. With ischemia, there is proliferation of new blood vessels that can occur on the iris and extend over the trabecular meshwork, resulting in obstruction of aqueous outflow and elevated intraocular pressure, hence the term neovascular glaucoma.

Once the diagnosis of a CRVO is made, a fluorescein angiogram is usually performed to determine the degree of retinal ischemia. If there is significant ischemia, laser photocoagulation to all peripheral ischemic retina (i.e., panretinal) can be performed. This is thought to destroy areas of ischemic retina that are thought to be responsible for producing a chemical mediator that leads to neovascularization, the formation of new blood vessels. Although the initial studies looking at laser photocoagulation in the treatment for CRVO demonstrated no beneficial effect, more recent studies (CRUISE, COPERNICUS, and GALILEO) have demonstrated that the use of intravitreal ranibizumab, an anti-vascular endothelial growth factor (VEGF) inhibitor, results in rapid and sustained improvements in visual acuity and central foveal thickness for patients with macular edema secondary to CRVO.

Similarly, if there is macular involvement in branch vein occlusions (BVOs) (see Figure 24.3), vision will be affected. Studies involving BVOs have demonstrated that if vision has been decreased for more than 3 months and fluorescein angiogram shows a leakage of fluid in the macula, laser photocoagulation in a sector distribution can improve the visual prognosis. The risk of neovascular glaucoma is generally less of a concern with BVOs.

More recent studies (BRAVO and VIBRANT) have shown that monthly injections of anti-VEGF improved both visual acuity and central foveal thickness in patients with macular edema secondary to BVO.

Patients with venous occlusive disease should have a general medical evaluation to rule out diabetes, hypertension, or blood dyscrasias. The ophthalmologist must evaluate the nonaffected eye to rule out glaucoma, which is commonly associated with vein occlusions.

DIABETIC RETINOPATHY

Diabetic retinopathy is a prominent cause of vision loss around the world. Diabetic retinopathy affects more than 350 million individuals worldwide, particularly between the ages of 20 and 70 years, with an estimated 10,000 new cases of blindness annually in the United States. These numbers are projected to continually increase with the increased prevalence of diabetes mellitus. Fortunately, a number of clinical trials (DCCT and UKPDS) have demonstrated a significant reduction in ocular complications with aggressive control of blood glucose and hemoglobin A_{1c} (Hb A_{1c}) levels.

Diabetes may have a juvenile or adult onset. Generally the incidence of diabetic complications increases with the duration of the disease. Complications may include systemic and ocular problems. Systemic complications include peripheral nerve disease, kidney disease, and vascular problems that can result in peripheral neuropathy and poor wound healing. Ocular manifestations of diabetes are categorized into nonproliferative and proliferative diabetic retinopathy.

Early nonproliferative diabetic retinopathy includes the presence of microaneurysms (small vascular buds), dot and blot hemorrhages, and lipid exudates from a serous leakage of the retinal vessels (Figure 24.4). Preproliferative retinopathy is characterized by cotton-wool spots, irregular dilatation of retinal veins, and intraretinal microvascular

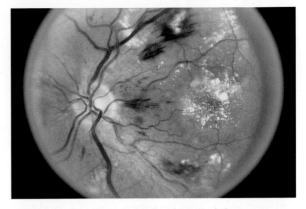

Figure 24.4 Diabetic retinopathy. The retinal changes occur predominantly at the posterior pole with microaneurysms and "dot and blot" hemorrhages, and hard exudates occur in the macular area.

abnormalities (IRMAs), which are abnormal capillaries within the retina as a result of ischemia. Proliferative diabetic retinopathy is defined by the presence of abnormal blood vessel formation, that is, neovascularization on the optic disc, the surface of the retina, or the iris. These fragile aberrant blood vessels are easily ruptured, causing recurrent vitreous hemorrhage. New formation on the iris, with extension over the trabecular meshwork, can lead to neovascular glaucoma.

Ocular treatment modalities for diabetic retinopathy depend on the stage of the disease and the absence or presence of a variety of complications. If neovascularization is present, then panretinal photocoagulation is the treatment of choice. Approximately 2000 to 3000 photocoagulation spots are applied with an argon laser, essentially destroying the ischemic retina, which is thought to be the source of vasoproliferative factors. This reduces and often resolves the neovascularization. If vision is decreased by macular edema, photocoagulation of leaking microaneurysms in the macular area has been shown to improve vision. If the patient has a nonclearing vitreous hemorrhage, or if there are fibrovascular bands producing a tractional retinal detachment, a pars plana vitrectomy is the surgical procedure of choice. The vitrectomy infusion suction and cutting instruments are introduced over the pars plana, and the vitreous hemorrhage is removed and replaced with saline. The tractional bands are also cut and released, allowing the retina to reattach to its normal position.

Multiple studies have implicated VEGF as the main culprit in the pathogenesis of diabetic retinopathy and diabetic macular edema. The retina becomes ischemic as a result of capillary damage from diabetes. Ischemic areas of the retina release VEGF and other chemical factors, resulting in proliferation of abnormally formed blood vessels. These abnormal blood vessels are fragile and may leak (causing macular edema), bleed (causing vitreous hemorrhage), and eventually form fibrovascular scar and traction, ultimately causing tractional retinal detachment and blindness. After decades of clinical trials, the use of recombinant antibodies specifically targeting VEGF not only restore the integrity of the blood–retinal barrier, minimizing serum leakage, but also dramatically improve vision in the majority of patients with diabetic macular edema. The three most commonly used anti-VEGF medications are: bevacizumab (Avastin), ranibizumab (Lucentis), and aflibercept (Eyelea). Multiple pivotal studies (RESTORE, READ2, RISE/RIDE, DA VINCI, VIVID AND VISTA) and results released by the Diabetic Retinopathy Clinical Research Network (DRCR. net) demonstrate that intravitreal anti-VEGF blocks the effects of VEGF and significantly improves vision loss from diabetic macular edema.

The management of diabetes requires a coordinated effort between health care providers including the ophthalmologist, general practitioner, endocrinologist, and dietitian. Although technologic advances have been beneficial, diabetic retinopathy remains one of the leading causes of blindness in North America.

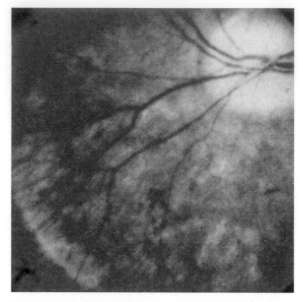

Figure 24.5 Retinitis pigmentosa. Attenuated arterioles, bone spicule pigment formation in the periphery, and waxy pallor of the optic disc.

RETINITIS PIGMENTOSA

Retinitis pigmentosa (RP) is a complex hereditary disorder that has a variable pattern of transmission. It can be passed on as a sex-linked trait or as an autosomal dominant or recessive trait. Although there are various subtypes of RP, the most classic symptoms of this condition include nyctalopia (difficulty seeing in dim illumination) and progressive loss of peripheral visual field. There are various subtypes of RP, and depending on the nature of the condition and its duration, RP may be mild or may progress to cause severe blindness.

Not all cases of RP result in severe loss of vision or visual field; some cases remain stable for a lifetime.

The diagnosis can often be made with direct visualization of the fundus using ophthalmoscopy. The following findings are characteristic features:

1. Bone spicule-like pigment debris in the midperiphery of the retina (Figure 24.5)
2. Retinal vessel attenuation
3. Tubular visual fields
4. A waxy pallor of the disc
5. Posterior subcapsular cataract

Occasionally a patient is found with typical symptoms but no retinal pigment dispersion. An electroretinogram (ERG) will show the depressed rod function, despite the absence of characteristic retinal changes.

Night blindness also may be caused by vitamin A deficiency, syphilis, and glaucoma. At times, RP may occur with other disorders, including deafness, metabolic abnormalities, and mental retardation.

At this time there is no specific treatment for this disease. Treatment with 15,000 International Units per day of vitamin A palmitate has been suggested. It is important to elicit a genetic tree from the patient so that genetic counseling may be undertaken. It is also imperative to follow the patient's progress. This is done to treat any complications that may occur and to ensure that the patient does not feel that the situation is hopeless. Many causes of RP are mild and either do not appear to progress or do so quite slowly. People who develop the disease in their first decade are worse off than those who develop RP in their 40s or 50s.

There are RP foundations in many states and provinces. Patients should be directed to these groups for counseling, assurance, and a line to new therapies.

RETINOPATHY OF PREMATURITY

Retinopathy of prematurity is a proliferative vascular disease occurring in premature infants exposed to high concentrations of oxygen soon after birth. The fibrovascular proliferation can lead to retinal detachment or a white retrolental membrane (a fibrovascular membrane behind the lens of the eye). The disease is usually bilateral and, in severe cases, can cause blindness.

Prevention of this disease is of the utmost importance. The pediatrician should try to use the lowest oxygen level that is compatible with good neonatal care. An eye examination should be done on all premature infants, especially those with a complicated course and who received significant oxygen therapy. Careful follow-up examinations should be performed to rule out any fibrovascular proliferation. Treatment of retinopathy of prematurity may include observation for spontaneous regression, cryosurgery (CRYO-ROP study), laser photocoagulation (ET-ROP study), intravitreal anti-VEGF therapy (BEAT-ROP study), vitrectomy, or retinal detachment surgery.

RETINOSCHISIS

Retinoschisis is the abnormal splitting of the retina's neurosensory layers. The partial-thickness split occurs in the outer plexiform layer in degenerative retinoschisis and nerve fiber layer in X-linked juvenile retinoschisis (XLJR). Associated with the retinoschisis, there may be occasional partial-thickness inner or outer retinal hole formation. Degenerative retinoschisis is a condition that usually occurs in the peripheral retina and therefore rarely affects central vision. This condition occurs in 3% of the population and almost never leads to a retinal detachment. Hereditary XLJR, however, is an X-linked recessive disorder, primarily affecting young males. Unlike the degenerative form, hereditary juvenile retinoschisis commonly affects central vision as a result of central foveal schisis, in addition to the peripheral retinal schisis.

RETINAL BREAKS

Retinal breaks may take the form of holes or tears. A *retinal hole* is often the result of an atrophic process that leads to a full-thickness defect of the retina. If it occurs in the macula it can cause permanent loss of vision to 20/200 or less. A different type of hole or tear can be produced when vitreous detachment, a degenerative process, pulls off a small piece of retina in the retinal periphery. If the operculum, or the everting lip of retinal tissue, is still attached to the retina, a *retinal* tear is produced. If the operculum is free from the retina, a hole is produced (Figure 24.6).

Most retinal tears and holes occur in the periphery of the retina and detection requires a fully dilated pupil and visualization with an indirect ophthalmoscope (see Figure 24.3). Retinal tears should be treated by applying laser photocoagulation around the tear or hole, allowing scar tissue formation and thereby preventing the possible entry of liquefied vitreous through the tear, leading to a retinal detachment. The use of the laser in this setting is analogous to spot-welding, preventing liquefied vitreous from peeling the retina off the underlying retinal pigment epithelium. Retinal holes in which the patient has recently

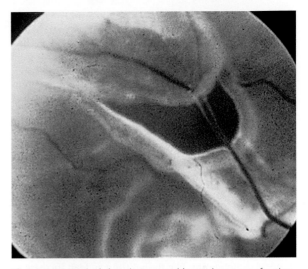

Figure 24.6 Retinal detachment and horseshoe tear of retina.

exhibited symptoms of flashing lights or floaters, or in those who had previous retinal tear or detachment, should be treated with laser photocoagulation.

Vitreous hemorrhage

Vitreous hemorrhage is characterized by a hazy view of the fundus with a reduced or altered red reflex. The most common causes are posterior vitreous detachment, proliferative diabetic retinopathy, retinal vein occlusion with neovascularization of the retina, retinal tear without detachment, retinal detachment, macroaneurysm of the retina, and trauma.

Workup for vitreous hemorrhage

Ophthalmology referral is recommended. A B-scan ultrasound should be performed to rule out an associated retinal detachment or mass lesion such as a malignant melanoma.

Management of vitreous hemorrhage

The majority of vitreous hemorrhages resolve spontaneously in a few weeks to months. Vitrectomy may be indicated after a few months in a nonclearing vitreous hemorrhage and should be combined with laser photocoagulation if there is an associated retinal tear or neovascularization.

RETINAL DETACHMENT

Retinal detachments usually are rhegmatogenous (retinal tear-induced). Three things are required for a retinal detachment to occur: the presence of a retinal hole or tear, liquefied vitreous (which can get under the sensory layers of the retina and "peel off the retina"), and traction. The force of traction can be secondary to minor trauma or even by eye movement.

In axial myopia, which is characterized by a large axial length, there is a greater tendency for peripheral vitreoretinal degenerative changes such as lattice degeneration and atrophic holes, and thus a higher incidence of retinal detachment. Axial myopia is often characterized by a posterior staphyloma, a tilted optic disc with a temporal conus, and a high refractive error (6.00 diopters or greater).

Holes or tears are usually treated using laser or cryotherapy if detected early. It is important to carefully screen patients at risk for retinal tear by asking them if there is a family history of retinal detachment; these patients are more at risk.

A retinal tear may be detected at the time of routine assessment (Figure 24.7). Common visual symptoms include spontaneous flashes that are often described as camera- or lightening-like flashes, or a sudden increase in floaters. The floaters may be caused by small broken blood vessels that liberate free red blood cells, which in turn cast shadows on the retina. The patient may, however, have no symptoms, which may delay their detection. With the onset of retinal detachment, patients will seek medical attention because of a persistent shadow or curtain that slowly expands in the affected eye. Vitreous traction is the major cause of retinal tears and almost always occurs spontaneously. Although trauma to the eye does cause vitreous traction, it is not the most common cause.

At times the retina can be detached and no holes found. This could be the result of trauma or inflammation. The most sinister cause of a nonrhegmatogenous retinal detachment is a malignant melanoma.

A retinal detachment warrants immediate repair, especially in the case of retinal detachment. The goal of treatment is to identify the holes or tears to be sealed using either laser or cryotherapy. There are various surgical approaches to

repairing retinal detachment depending on the pathology and mechanism, but the most common approaches include pars plana vitrectomy to relieve any vitreous traction as well as laser or cryotherapy to seal off the offending hole or tear. Sometimes a scleral buckle may be necessary to indent the globe to bring the detached tissues into proximity and to reduce tractional forces. The liquefied vitreous that has accumulated beneath the retina is often drained during surgery so that the retina will lie flat.

Most retinal detachment repair procedures are successful with good visual prognosis (more than 90% of routine cases) when patients present early, before the macula becomes involved. If the macula becomes detached, a reduction in the final visual acuity is more likely to occur. Visual recovery often takes 6 to 12 months after surgery.

CENTRAL SEROUS CHORIORETINOPATHY

Central serous chorioretinopathy (CSR) is a type of serous retinal detachment involving the macula but is unassociated with a retinal tear or hole. Serous detachment of the macula is more common in males than in females and typically occurs in younger patients (25–50 years of age). There appears to be a strong association between stress, type-A personality trait, and steroid use with the development of this disorder.

Patients often complain of blurred vision and commonly describe distortion of vision with loss of color perception. Objects often appear curved, darker in color, and smaller.

Fluorescein angiography typically shows a leakage point in which fluid passes from the choroid, through a defect in the retinal pigment epithelium, to a location beneath the retina. Most cases clear spontaneously within 3 months, and therefore require no specific therapy. Treatment may be indicated in cases with prolonged visual loss or, with signs of degenerative changes. Treatment options include laser photocoagulation to seal the defect in the pigment epithelium or photodynamic therapy (PDT) with good efficacy.

CHANGES IN THE RETINA FROM CONCUSSION

Commotio retinae (Berlin's "edema")

Commotio retinae is secondary to blunt trauma to the eye, resulting in a shockwave effect that disturbs the vitreous and the retina. With sufficient force, blunt trauma to the eye can result in misalignment of the outer segments of

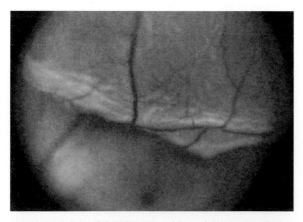

Figure 24.7 Retinal detachment. Folding of the retina, which is in focus anteriorly.

the photoreceptors in the retina without any edema. The whitish appearance around the macula is a result of structural changes of the photoreceptors. With time the whitish appearance resolves and mild pigmentary changes of the retina can be seen on funduscopic examination.

Retinal hemorrhages

Retinal hemorrhages may be in front of the retina (preretinal), under the retina (subretinal), or within the retina (intraretinal).

Some common causes of retinal hemorrhages include hypertensive retinopathy, diabetic retinopathy, age-related macular degeneration, central retinal vein occlusion, Valsalva retinopathy, posterior vitreous detachment, and macroaneurysm. Birth injury is a cause of traumatic retinal hemorrhage of the newborn. Child abuse or shaken baby syndrome is another cause of retinal hemorrhages.

Retinal detachment

Although retinal detachments are uncommon immediately after trauma, patients with retinal injury must be followed closely because of the increased risk for retinal detachment months or even years after the injury.

FOREIGN BODY IN THE EYE

The degree of damage from an intraocular foreign body depends on the mechanical disruption of tissue, as well as the chemical composition of the foreign object within the eye.

A foreign body composed of relatively pure copper (greater than 90%) can cause a massive inflammation. Copper in a concentration of 70% to 90% will cause *chalcosis*, with the deposition of copper in intraocular structures leading to cataracts and glaucoma. If the foreign body is an alloy of copper in a concentration of less than 70%, it rarely will cause any intraocular problems.

Gold, silver, platinum, aluminum, and glass are chemically inert and do damage only by traumatic disruption of the ocular tissue.

A retained iron foreign body can cause siderosis bulbi. Iron is toxic to the retina and other ocular tissues. An intraocular foreign body containing iron should be removed to prevent sensory retinal toxicity and profound loss of vision as indicated by a flat or extinguished ERG. The trabecular meshwork can also be affected, which can result in glaucoma. These changes can be observed for months to years after the accident. If the foreign body is removed at an early stage, the entire process of siderosis bulbi may be prevented.

Iron injuries are common. Fortunately, metallic foreign bodies are magnetic. This makes their surgical removal somewhat easier. Most retained ocular foreign bodies are

a result of industrial accidents. The best treatment is prevention, which means the use of polycarbonate safety goggles or facemask.

SOLAR MACULOPATHY (ECLIPSE BURNS OF THE RETINA)

Direct sun gazing or looking directly at an eclipse, even if only for seconds, can result in a macular burn. The macula will appear mottled with subtle retinal pigment epithelium changes after the initial injury. With time, a macular hole can result, with permanent decrease in vision.

There is no absolute safe way to protect children against such mishaps. The best treatment is prevention. Either abstain from sungazing or exercise caution by wearing proper eye protection when observing an eclipse. There is, however, no guarantee of patient compliance, especially with young children.

AGE-RELATED MACULAR DEGENERATION

Age-related macular degeneration (AMD) is the leading cause of severe central vision loss in people older than 50 years in developed nations. The risk of developing some form of AMD increases with age, and by age 75 the risk approaches 40%. There are two types of AMD: nonexudative (atrophic) AMD (85%–90% of AMD) and neovascular (wet) AMD (10%–15% of AMD). Severe visual loss from AMD usually occurs in neovascular AMD. With increased life expectancy, the number of patients with visual impairment from AMD is projected to increase by more than 50% by 2030.

Common risk factors for AMD include age, positive family history, smoking, hyperopia, light iris color, hypertension, elevated serum cholesterol, female gender, and cardiovascular disease.

A variety of clinical conditions are labeled *age-related macular degeneration*. The clinical findings may include the following:

1. *Absent foveal reflex.* This is the most subtle of changes. The architecture of the fovea is slightly altered so that the reflex of the foveal pit is not seen.
2. *Pigment mottling.* These macular changes are caused by scattered areas of clumping and atrophy of the retinal pigment epithelium.
3. *Drusen.* These are small, yellowish-white lesions located between the retinal pigment epithelium and Bruch's membrane. They are a common aging change and a predisposing factor to splitting of Bruch's membrane, which can lead to neovascularization from the choroid.

4. *Subretinal neovascularization.* These new vessels can leak serum or blood and cause a serous or hemorrhagic detachment of the pigment epithelium, resulting in a dramatic decrease in vision. When the blood has not broken through the retina, it may appear as a black mass and simulate a malignant melanoma. If these new vessels are detected early and confirmed with a fluorescein angiogram, laser treatment can be used to try to destroy the abnormal vessels and prevent subsequent leakage.

5. *Disciform degeneration of the macula* (Figure 24.8). If serum or blood leaks into the macula, the healing process can lead to gliosis, which leaves a flat grayish white scar. This scar results in permanent loss of central vision, but the peripheral field of vision is left intact. Degenerative changes also can occur if the pigment epithelium undergoes atrophy, which leads to death of the photoreceptors and a decrease in vision.

Unfortunately for most patients with atrophic AMD, no treatment has so far proven helpful. Multicenter randomized clinical trials (AREDS 1 and 2) demonstrated the benefit of micronutrient supplements (500 mg vitamin C, 400 iu vitamin E, 10 mg lutein, 2 mg zeaxanthin, 80 mg zinc, 2 mg copper) in AMD and vision loss. The results showed that patients with intermediate AMD or advanced unilateral AMD had a 25% reduction of vision loss, and a significantly reduced risk of progression to advanced AMD.

Because most older adults with bilateral disciform degeneration have a visual acuity often reduced to 20/200 or less, referral for low vision rehabilitation should be considered.

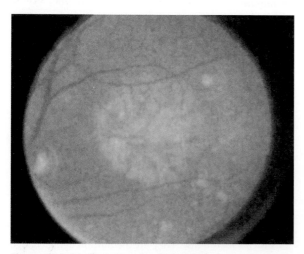

Figure 24.8 Disciform macular degeneration.

Classification

AMD is classified into two clinical entities: atrophic (dry) and exudative (wet).

Atrophic AMD

Atrophic AMD comprises approximately 85% of all patients suffering from AMD and is responsible for 10% to 20% of cases of blindness caused by this disease. Vision loss tends to be gradual and the severity of vision loss is determined by the number, size, morphology, and location of drusen in the macula, as well as the amount and location of associated retinal pigment epithelium (RPE) atrophy. Drusen size can be categorized as small (<63 μm), intermediate (63–124 μm), or large (<125 μm). Small, hard drusen are at low risk of progression to advanced AMD, especially when in small numbers (e.g., <5). Intermediate and large drusen and confluent drusen are signs of more advanced AMD that could progress to exudative AMD. Pigmentary clumping is often associated with drusen. Noncentral geographic RPE atrophy is an indicator of more advanced atrophic AMD. Maculae with at least one large druse and/or extensive intermediate drusen are more likely to develop RPE atrophy. In patients with advanced atrophic AMD, up to 43% of eyes progress to exudative AMD within 5 years.

Exudative AMD

Exudative AMD comprises approximately 15% of all patients suffering from AMD, yet is responsible for 80% to 90% of cases of blindness caused by this disease. Vision loss tends to be rapid—over days to months—and is determined by the amount of subretinal and intraretinal blood, lipid, and fluid, and resultant submacular scarring. The conventionally accepted pathophysiology involves proliferation of abnormal new blood vessels in the choroid that leads to the development of a choroidal neovascular membrane (CNVM). This penetrates through Bruch's membrane into the sub-RPE and subretinal space. Exudation, hemorrhage, and fibrovascular scarring damage and destroy paramacular photoreceptors, resulting in severe central visual loss.

An alternative pathophysiologic process called retinal angiomatous proliferation (RAP) that can also result in severe central vision loss is included in the exudative AMD category. In RAP, capillary proliferation begins in the paramacular region within the deep capillary plexus of the retina. Neovascular proliferation proceeds anteriorly as well as posteriorly. Posterior proliferation eventually invades the subretinal space, and a subretinal neovascular membrane and a serous RPE detachment are formed. Further proliferation causes vessels to invade the choroid to form a CNVM. Vessels proliferating anteriorly form an anastomosis with the retinal circulation. Thus a chorioretinal anastomosis is formed. The end result appears clinically and angiographically similar to, and is often indistinguishable from, AMD where neovascularization begins in the choroid rather than the retina. The two entities may respond differently to available treatment modalities at different stages of their development.

Clinical presentation

Patients older than 55 years, presenting with blurred or distorted vision, should be suspected of having AMD. Other symptoms may include difficulty in reading or difficulty with vision under conditions of limited illumination. Patient assessment should include age of onset, duration of symptoms, location of distortion/paracentral scotomata, and degree of contrast sensitivity loss. Risk factors for AMD should be reviewed, including age, gender, light iris color, family history, coronary artery disease, hypertension, hypercholesterolemia, history of smoking, and prolonged ultraviolet light exposure. Patients with a fair complexion are at a higher risk of developing exudative AMD; females have twice the risk for its development over their male counterparts and smokers are at six times the risk. Patients should be asked about medications that could have an adverse effect on macular function (e.g., chloroquine derivatives, phenothiazines, and tuberculosis medications).

The ocular examination

The ocular examination should establish the presence of decreased vision and rule out any refractive error as the underlying cause, by either refraction or pinhole visual acuity.

Amsler grid testing should be performed for all AMD assessments because it is simple to perform and, if positive, can help direct attention to a specific area during the fundus examination. If significant lenticular opacity is present, macular function testing with laser interferometry or a potential acuity meter may help determine how much vision loss is secondary to cataract versus macular pathology. A visual field assessment is recommended to rule out concomitant peripheral visual field loss or neurologic causes for central vision loss. If available, Pelli-Robson contrast sensitivity charts are quick and reliable for evaluating and following visual function in AMD. Examination of the macula should be performed using biomicroscopy with a biconvex indirect (60.00–90.00 diopters) or Hruby lens. Although the image is inverted, good stereopsis is achieved. During macular biomicroscopy, the size, location, and morphology of drusen should be noted. Pigmentary clumping and areas of geographic RPE atrophy also should be noted because they may be indicators of more

advanced atrophic AMD. Subretinal blood, lipid, or fluid is a suspicious sign for the presence of a CNVM. Direct ophthalmoscopy fails to provide stereopsis and is inadequate to properly assess the macula in AMD. The best optical view of the macula can be achieved with a macular contact lens. This, however, requires topical anesthesia and viscous fluid to eliminate the air–cornea interface. The viscous fluid can interfere with the quality of photography/angiography if these are to be performed shortly after examination.

Patients with acutely decreased vision, Amsler grid distortion, and clinically evident subretinal blood, lipid, or fluid require an urgent referral to a retina specialist for optical coherence tomography (OCT) or fluorescein angiography assessment. The algorithm for determining the best course of action to reduce vision loss in a patient with CNVM is based on interpretation of fluorescein angiography and OCT. Both imaging modalities can help the retinal specialist to determine whether the patient would benefit greatly from thermal laser, photodynamic therapy with Visudyne, an anti-VEGF injection, or should simply be followed with periodic observation.

Natural history

In the natural history of AMD, several factors are associated with the progression of atrophic to exudative AMD. Eyes with large and/or extensive intermediate drusen or noncentral geographic atrophy are most likely to progress to CNVM. If one eye has already developed subfoveal CNVM, there are major prognostic factors for vision loss in the fellow eye, secondary to the development of a CNVM. These factors are based on the type of late AMD documented in the first eye and include more than five drusen, large soft drusen, pigment clumping, and systemic hypertension. As the number of risk factors increases, the risk of developing exudative AMD in the fellow eye approaches 90%.

Diagnostic evaluation

The following tests are valuable in determining and staging the presence of AMD.

Amsler grid

The Amsler grid is an excellent monocular macular function test to determine the presence of macular pathology. Each 5-mm square on the grid subtends a visual angle of 1 degree when the chart is held at 30 cm. Therefore, the entire chart tests 10 degrees on either side of fixation, in both horizontal and vertical meridians.

Amsler grid testing should be performed before pupil dilation and applanation tonometry. With their reading glasses on, patients should be asked to cover one eye and concentrate on the central dot on the grid. If all lines are visible without distortion and all boxes are observed to be present, then the testing result is considered to be normal and the fellow eye is tested. If the patient notices distortion, blurring, or paracentral scotomata, these should be recorded on the grid and stored in the chart. They may be useful for future comparison to document progression or regression of disease.

Fluorescein angiography

Fluorescein angiography is the gold standard for assessing retinal and choroidal circulation in AMD. After performing color fundus photographs, sodium fluorescein dye is injected intravenously. The dye is excited by light from the camera flash passing through a blue excitatory filter. The 490-nm wavelength of the blue light is absorbed by the fluorescein molecules in the choroidal circulation and then the retinal circulation. The dye is stimulated to emit a yellow-green light (530 nm), and this passes back to the camera through a yellow-green barrier filter, blocking reflected blue light, and allowing the fluorescence to be photographed. Photographs are taken as the dye transits through the choroidal and retinal circulation. Drusen may fluoresce, RPE atrophy is demonstrated as window defects, and choroidal neovascularization (CNV) leaks dye and hyperfluoresces. CNV is interpreted and classified by its leakage pattern. Classic CNV is seen as an area of bright, well-demarcated hyperfluoresence identified in the early phase of the angiogram, with progressive dye leakage into the overlying subretinal space in the late phase of the angiogram.

Indocyanine green

Indocyanine green (ICG) angiography is an important diagnostic adjunct in the evaluation of CNVM in AMD. ICG is a tricarbocyanine dye that absorbs light at 790 to 805 nm and has a peak emission at 835 nm, which is in the infrared spectrum. It is injected intravenously, and digital infrared videoangiography is used to photograph the retinal and choroidal vasculature. ICG is 95% plasma bound and therefore remains largely intravascular, facilitating visualization of the choroidal vasculature. ICG can be visualized through thin blood, serous fluid, and pigment. In conjunction with fluorescein angiography, it can better delineate the full extent of a lesion in patients with occult or minimally classic CNVM. This translates into better diagnosis and improved treatment success and reduced rates of retreatment.

ICG is safe for general use and is less toxic than sodium fluorescein. It contains approximately 5% iodine by weight and is removed by the liver. ICG is therefore contraindicated for patients with iodine or shellfish allergies or significant liver disease.

Optical Coherence Tomography

During the past decade, OCT has become a fundamental tool for diagnosis and management of various ophthalmologic conditions including AMD. This is a noninvasive optical diagnostic imaging modality that allows for in vivo cross-sectional tomographic visualization of retinal microstructures at resolutions as small as 1 to 3 μm. Retinal imaging in vivo could be correlated with histopathologic findings. OCT is an important tool used to determine CNVM activity by detecting subtle changes in retinal thickness including evidence of intraretinal or subretinal fluid. Many studies include the use of OCT imaging in treatment decision making for patients with exudative AMD (see Chapter 36).

Clinical Treatment

Atrophic AMD

Fluorescein angiography is often not necessary in the case of atrophic (dry) AMD, which is diagnosed based on clinical examination with or without an OCT. Patients with atrophic AMD should be given an Amsler grid for self-monitoring at home. They should be reminded to wear their reading correction and to perform the test under consistent lighting conditions. Patients should be instructed to call the office if they notice a significant change in Amsler grid lasting more than 3 days. Urgent reassessment should be provided and, if exudative AMD is suspected, urgent referral to a retina specialist is warranted. Patients should be counseled to eat a diet rich in vegetables. Reducing dietary fat intake also may be helpful.

Nonsmoking patients with extensive intermediate drusen (63–124 μm), at least one large druse (>125 μm), noncentral geographic atrophy in one or both eyes, or advanced AMD or vision loss as a result of AMD in one eye, may benefit from micronutrient supplementation as reported in AREDS (both AREDS 1 and 2 studies). AREDS 2 demonstrated that among patients with intermediate AMD or unilateral advanced AMD, daily dietary supplements (500 mg vitamin C, 400 iu vitamin E, 10 mg lutein, 2 mg zeaxanthin, 80 mg zinc, 2 mg copper) lowered the risk of macular degeneration progression to an advanced stage and the rate of moderate vision loss of more than three lines of visual acuity. However, these supplements were not found to be beneficial in healthy or minimal AMD patients. AREDS formulations and vitamin supplements are not a cure for AMD, and will not restore vision.

Smokers are at a higher risk of developing lung cancer if they take beta-carotene. There is no agreement about how long a smoker must stop smoking before safely taking beta-carotene, but the consensus is to avoid beta-carotene in smokers or ex-smokers because of the potential increased cancer risk. Patients with AMD also may benefit from ultraviolet protection by wearing wrap-around sunglasses whenever outdoors in daylight.

Exudative AMD

Patients suspected of having exudative AMD require further investigation. Fluorescein angiography is the diagnostic test of choice for assessing exudative AMD because it provides information regarding the location, composition, and extent of the lesion. Laser photocoagulation therapy has been used for extrafoveal or juxtafoveal classic CNVMs that are well demarcated, although this treatment is now rarely implemented. CNVMs that are subfoveal may benefit from PDT with Visudyne, depending on baseline visual acuity, lesion composition, and size. The Treatment of Age-Related Macular Degeneration with Photodynamic Therapy (TAP) study demonstrated a statistically significant beneficial effect of PDT with Visudyne versus placebo for subfoveal lesions that are predominantly classic, with baseline visual acuity 20/40 to 20/200.

The Verteporfin in Photodynamic Therapy (VIP) trial demonstrated a clinically significant treatment benefit of PDT with Visudyne on visual function for patients who had occult without classic subfoveal CNVM and a demonstrated recent progression of disease.

Eyes with baseline visual acuity less than 20/50 and lesion size less than four disc areas had the best results. There was no statistically significant treatment benefit of PDT with Visudyne demonstrated for eyes with minimally classic subfoveal CNVM. For predominantly classic lesions or occult with no classic lesions that are juxtafoveal, photodynamic therapy with Visudyne should be considered when the lesion is so close to the foveal center that conventional thermal laser photocoagulation would likely extend under the center of the foveal avascular zone.

Since 2006 the majority of clinical trials have focused on VEGF, a chemical expressed during early stages of AMD, which induces neovascularization, vascular permeability, and lymphangiogenesis. There has been a paradigm shift in the treatment of AMD since 2006, when the results of two pivotal clinical trials, MARINA and ANCHOR, demonstrated significant visual improvement after monthly intravitreal injections of ranibizumab for the treatment of exudative AMD. Previous treatments using laser photocoagulation or PDT only demonstrated a decrease in visual *loss*, but ANCHOR and MARINA also manifested an impressive visual gain in almost 40% of patients. Both ANCHOR and MARINA studies also demonstrated sustainability of visual outcome with almost 80% to 90% of patients maintaining or improving vision after 24 months. Ranibizumab received US Food and Drug Administration (FDA) approval in July 2006 for the treatment of wet AMD.

Ever since MARINA and ANCHOR demonstrated visual benefit with monthly intravitreal injections, multiple studies have been published in an attempt to demonstrate an equal visual benefit with reduced frequency of injections (PIER, EXCITE, SUSTAIN, PRONTO). Current treatment protocols vary among specialists, from monthly injections to an OCT-guided treatment regimen.

The three most commonly used anti-VEGF agents are bevacizumab (Avastin), ranibizumab (Lucentis), and aflibercept (Eyelea). Both ranibizumab and aflibercept have received FDA approval for the treatment of wet AMD. Bevacizumab, an anti-VEGF agent approved by FDA in 2004 for the treatment of metastatic colorectal cancer, however, has been used off-label for wet AMD. Both bevacizumab and ranibizumab are made by Genentech. The fundamental difference between bevacizumab and ranibizumab is that bevacizumab is a full-sized immunoglobulin with two antigen-binding domains, whereas ranibizumab is an immunoglobulin fragment with only one antigen binding site. Ranibizumab is significantly more expensive than bevacizumab. The Comparison of AMD Treatments Trial (CATT) and Inhibition of VEGF in the Age-Related Choroidal Neovascularization (IVAN) study compared head-to-head bevacizumab and ranibizumab in the treatment of wet AMD. The 2-year results demonstrated that bevacizumab and ranibizumab had equivalent effects on visual acuity when administered according to the same schedule.

The newest member of the anti-VEGF family is aflibercept (Eyelea), a longer-acting anti-VEGF agent with equal efficacy as ranibizumab in the treatment of wet.

Given the multifactorial and complex nature of wet AMD that includes inflammation, angiogenesis, and fibrosis, a combination therapy using anti-VEGF and PDT may be an alternative treatment option to combat this condition.

Finally, for patients with bilateral end-stage AMD, trials are underway to investigate visual prostheses (Second Sight Argus) and various implantable intraocular devices (miniaturized telescope) for visual rehabilitation. In conclusion, new approaches to AMD and rapidly evolving technology are changing the way AMD is assessed and managed. Exciting new treatment modalities will help us meet the challenge of this devastating disease and improve the quality of life for patients with AMD.

OCULAR MANIFESTATIONS OF COMMON SYSTEMIC DISEASES

Retinal examination often reflects the status and severity of various systemic conditions. These are reviewed in the following text (Figures 24.9–24.13).

Hypertension

Patients with high blood pressure, or malignant hypertension, may be diagnosed by the ophthalmologist. Elevated

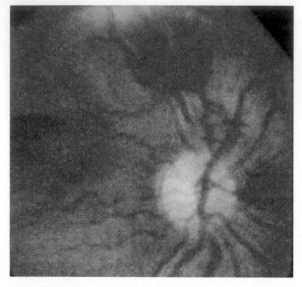

Figure 24.9 Acute myelogenous leukemia. Note the blotches of hemorrhage.

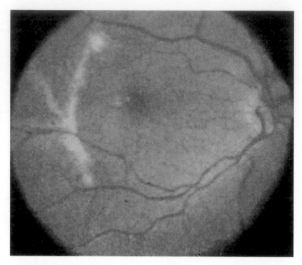

Figure 24.11 Choroidal tear. A white scar follows contusion of the globe, resulting from rupture of the choroid.

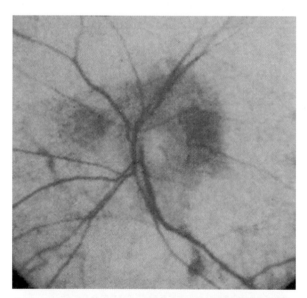

Figure 24.10 Ophthalmic metastasis from breast cancer in the right eye showing elevation of the peripheral retina.

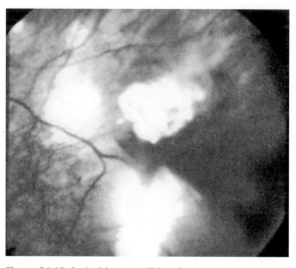

Figure 24.12 Retinoblastoma. This is the most common retinal tumor in children, manifested by large white lesions in the posterior pole of the eye.

blood pressure may be asymptomatic and can present with early microvascular damage and retinal vascular changes.

In the early phase of hypertensive retinopathy, the only manifestation may be an attenuation of the retinal arterioles. This narrowing may be uniform, as found in older people, or focal, which may occur in a younger person.

In older adults the changes may be mild as the retinal vessels become thicker, with a dulling of the light reflexes on the retinal arteriole surface. At the area of crossings, the retinal arterioles may appear to compress the underlying veins and cause banking or *arteriovenous nicking* of the underlying blood column.

Younger patients with severe hypertension (malignant hypertension or eclampsia in pregnancy) may display a florid type of retinopathy with flame-shaped hemorrhages, exudates, cotton-wool spots, and marked narrowing of the retinal arterioles.

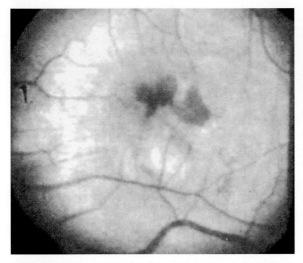

Figure 24.13 Choroideremia. Hereditary atrophy of the vascular choroid reveals a white underlying sclera. The retina is also affected. It usually leads to blindness.

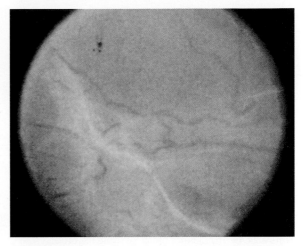

Figure 24.14 Sickle cell retinopathy. Note the retinitis proliferans with underlying traction retinal detachment inferiorly.
(Courtesy of Mount Sinai Hospital, Toronto, Canada.)

The most ominous sign is edema, or swelling, of the optic disc.

Sickle cell disease

Sickle cell hemoglobinopathies are most common in patients of African and Mediterranean ancestry. The disorder is hereditary. The normal hemoglobin in the red cell is replaced by the sickle hemoglobin (hemoglobin S), which assumes an abnormally rigid sickle-like shape under various circumstances. The rigid sickle cells have difficulty passing through blood vessels, which often result in vascular occlusion (vasoocclusive crisis).

Retinal changes are common in this disease (Figure 24.14). Early stages of sickle cell retinopathy include retinal hemorrhages and small retinal arteriole occlusions. As the retina becomes progressively more ischemic, neovascularization occurs on the surface of the retina—leading to retinal and vitreous hemorrhages—and preretinal membranes. Comma-shaped capillaries in the conjunctiva are part of the general vascular pattern. The final stages of sickle cell retinopathy, like proliferative diabetic retinopathy, are neovascularization and associated tractional retinal detachment.

Thyroid disorders

Ocular disease can be seen in patients with hyperthyroidism (excessive thyroid activity), hypothyroidism (depressed thyroid activity), and even euthyroidism (normal thyroid function after successful treatment for hyperthyroidism).

People with hyperthyroidism tend to have a rapid pulse, shortness of breath, and weight loss. Those with hypothyroidism show a deceleration of activity and may be dull mentally with a low voice, reduced pulse rate, dry skin, and weight gain.

Patients with a thyroid disorder and specific eye findings have a condition referred to as Graves' disease. The etiologic factors of this condition are thought to be immunologic. A variety of tests can be used to diagnose a thyroid condition: serum thyroxine, triiodothyronine (T_3) resin uptake, thyroid autoantibodies, thyrotropin-releasing hormone (TRH), and T_3 assay.

The ocular manifestations of Graves' disease include the following:

1. Lid lag. This is one of the earliest findings. When the patient looks down, the lid tends to lag behind the downward moving eye.
2. Lid retraction. The lids may leave a clear white space between the lid margins, both upper and lower, and the limbus.
3. Exophthalmos or protrusion of the eye (Figures 24.15 and 24.16). Using either the Hertel or Krahn exophthalmometer, the degree of protrusion can be measured. It is usually between 20 and 28 mm of exophthalmos. The forward displacement of the globe is caused by an increase in the bulk of ocular muscles and orbital fat swelling. A computed tomography scan will document the swollen extraocular muscles.
4. Exposure keratitis. Lid retraction and proptosis lead to exposure of the cornea and a consequent drying effect.
5. Motility disturbance. Limitation of eye movements can ensue because of direct involvement of the extraocular muscles. The cellular infiltration of these muscles can lead to fibrosis, with a resultant tethering effect on their function. The muscles most commonly

425

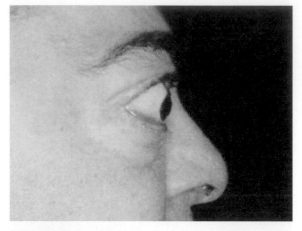

Figure 24.15 Thyroid exophthalmos. Note the ocular protrusion and lid retraction.

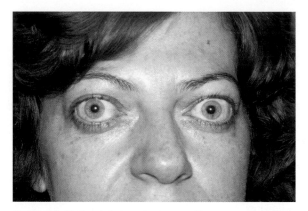

Figure 24.16 Exophthalmos in Graves' disease.

affected, in descending order of frequency, are the inferior rectus, medial rectus, superior rectus, and lateral rectus.

6. *Disc edema.* Flow through the optic nerve can be slowed by orbital compression. This can lead to disc edema. The swollen nerve is commonly a prelude to optic atrophy with a permanent visual loss.

Management of Graves' disease involves both the internist, to treat and manage the thyroid condition, and the ophthalmologist, to deal with the ocular complications. Guanethidine (10%) eyedrops often are helpful in reducing the lid retraction, which is cosmetically disfiguring. The lid retraction also can be aided surgically by cutting Müller's muscle and a section of the levator palpebrae superioris.

Exposure keratitis can be managed by the liberal use of lubrication in the form of artificial tears and ointment. Therapy is indicated if the orbital congestion causes a decrease in either color vision or central vision, or a defect on visual field testing. Therapy may consist of systemic

steroids, orbital radiation, or an orbital decompression (removing a wall of the orbit) to reduce the severe orbital pressure. If double vision results, muscle surgery can be used to relax the muscles and align the eyes.

INFECTIOUS DISEASES OF THE RETINA AND CHOROIDS

Toxoplasmosis

Toxoplasma gondii is a protozoal parasite that can cause chorioretinitis of the eye. Congenital toxoplasmosis secondary to intrauterine infection is the more severe form because it is bilateral and involves the macula so there is often considerable visual loss.

In the active stage the affected retina looks gray and edematous with overlying vitreous haze. Once the active phase resolves, chorioretinal atrophy occurs, and eventually a toxoplasmosis chorioretinal scar forms with a ring of pigmentation around a whitish center.

Ocular toxoplasmosis is mostly a clinical diagnosis based on the appearance and location of chorioretinal scar. Infrequently, ocular cultures may be required for polymerase chain reaction (PCR) analysis and culture. A variety of serologic tests can be done to document whether the patient has ever been exposed to toxoplasmosis. The inherent problem in the serology result is that at least 50% of the population has been exposed to this organism; hence the only valuable result is a negative blood test. Active infection in immunocompromised and pregnant patients or those with active infections near the optic disc or macula should be aggressively treated with systemic antibiotics. Alternatively, intravitreal clindamycin is another option for those who cannot take systemic antibiotics.

Histoplasmosis

Histoplasma capsulatum is a fungus that is commonly responsible for significant ocular morbidity. The infection is most prevalent in certain areas of the United States and Canada, including states in the Mississippi and Ohio river valley. The fungus is carried on the feathers of pigeons and chickens, as well as bat droppings. Once inhaled, the fungus can disseminate through the bloodstream. Most ocular infections and visual symptoms occur years after the initial infection. The clinical hallmarks of ocular histoplasmosis include "punched-out" chorioretinal scars, peripupillary scarring, absence of vitreous inflammation (no vitritis), and subretinal neovascular membranes (Figure 24.17). Most patients remain asymptomatic until they develop CNVM, like AMD, which can result in permanent vision loss. If the new vessels are detected early, laser photocoagulation, PDT, or anti-VEGF therapy may improve the visual prognosis.

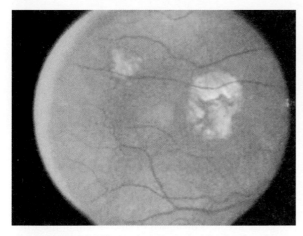

Figure 24.17 Histoplasmosis. Discrete localized areas of chorioretinitis are caused by *Histoplasma capsulatum*, an endemic organism common in certain parts of North America (e.g., Arizona).
(Courtesy of Mount Sinai Hospital, Toronto, Canada.)

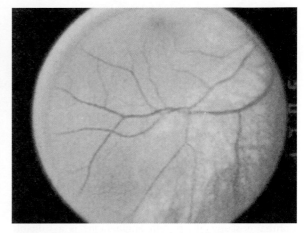

Figure 24.18 Benign melanoma of choroid. There is an elevated lesion in the fundus, which is often, but not always, pigmented.

MALIGNANT MELANOMA

Melanoma, although rare, is the most common intraocular malignant neoplasm found in the adult human eye. This tumor is 15 times more prevalent in white than in African Americans, is more common in males than in females, and is often detected in the fifth and sixth decades of life.

Clinical symptoms may be absent unless the macula is involved, with a resultant decrease in vision or if there is an overlying retinal detachment with visual field loss. Diagnosis is based on indirect ophthalmoscopy with scleral depression, slit-lamp examination, and gonioscopy to examine the anterior segment of the eye for signs of tumor involvement; A- and B-scan ultrasonography; and fluorescein angiography. The tumor appears as a greenish brown choroidal mass that in an advanced state may assume a mushroom shape if the tumor breaks through Bruch's membrane (Figures 24.18 and 24.19). The characteristic ultrasound findings include low internal reflectivity, spontaneous vascular pulsation, acoustic hollowness, and the classic mushroom-shaped choroidal mass. Based on the Collaborative Ocular Melanoma Study (COMS), the incidence of tumor spread beyond the eye is 25% at 5 years after initial treatment. The most common sites of tumor spread are the liver, lung, and bone. Therefore, all patients require metastatic evaluation before definitive treatment of intraocular melanoma, which includes full physical examination, liver function test, chest x-ray, and abdominal ultrasound.

A variety of treatment modalities can be offered based on tumor size and location. The COMS classified posterior uveal melanoma as small, medium, and large based on

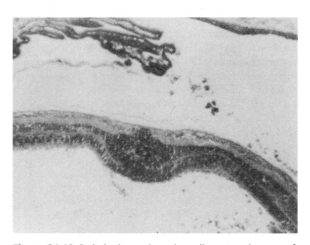

Figure 24.19 Pathologic specimen in malignant melanoma of choroid. Note the elevation of the retina. Often it creates a retinal detachment without holes (nonrhegmatogenous).

tumor thickness and base diameter, and investigated various treatment options for each. For small tumors, less than 2.5 mm in thickness, observation with sequential fundus photographs and A-scan ultrasonography to detect growth is the recommended choice. For medium choroidal melanoma (2.5–10 mm apical height), treatment options include standard enucleation, or iodine (I^{125}) brachytherapy (radioactive plaque). For larger tumors (>10 mm apical height), management is enucleation. Long-term results of radiation therapy are not well known. Because of these uncertainties, the patient and the clinician are often faced with a difficult decision regarding the most appropriate management.

The prognosis with and without treatment cannot be given with certainty. Even after enucleations, spread of the tumor has been reported 20 years after the diagnosis has been made. Once the tumor has spread outside the eye, the survival period is usually 6 months. New developments in the field of immunology, in which cells are created to attack specific tumor cells, may eventually lead to an improvement in survival.

RETINAL IMAGING MODALITIES: FLUORESCEIN ANGIOGRAPHY

Fluorescein angiography has become a widely used imaging technique to study retinal circulation, and diseases involving the retina and choroid since the late 1950s. Although the retina is readily visible by direct and indirect ophthalmoscopy, fluorescein angiography is a valuable adjunct to these methods of clinical examination, offering valuable information on the retinal and choroidal vasculature and circulation.

Fluorescein angiography is made possible by the unique chemical and physical properties of fluorescein, which is an inexpensive, nontoxic, highly fluorescent compound first synthesized by Adolf von Baeryer in 1871. It is available in concentrations of 5%, 10%, and 25%. Fluorescein emits light after excitation. After absorbing blue light (465–490 nm), fluorescein subsequently emits yellow-green light (520–530 nm), which requires relatively minor modification in existing fundus cameras to perform angiography. The test can be performed with minimum discomfort to the patient.

Fundus photography in rapid sequence after intravenous injection of fluorescent dye provides information about the flow characteristics in the retinal vasculature, as well as fine details of the retina and choroid that may not be appreciated by other means. These details depend on anatomic features of the retinal and choroidal vessels and retinal pigment epithelium. Normal retinal vessels are impermeable to the dye. This characteristic allows a clear picture of the retinal vessels and assessment of their functional integrity inasmuch as leakage from any retinal vessel is abnormal. Because the fine vessels of the choroid (the choriocapillaries) leak fluorescein dye and the normal retinal pigment epithelium is a barrier to both the passage of the dye and its fluorescence, it is possible to use the technique of fluorescein angiography to study diseases that affect the retinal pigment epithelium.

Intravascular fluorescein is normally prevented from entering the retina by the intact retinal vascular endothelium (blood–retinal barrier) and the intact retinal pigment endothelium. Defects in either the retinal vessels or the pigment epithelium will allow leakage of fluorescein, which can then be studied by either direct observation or photography. For good results, appropriate filters are needed to excite the fluorescein and exclude unwanted wavelengths. The peak frequencies for excitation lie between 465 and 490 nm, and for emission between 520 and 530 nm.

Fluorescein has proved to be a safe diagnostic agent, the most common side effects being nausea and vomiting. However, occasional allergic and vagal reactions do occur, so oxygen and emergency equipment must be readily available when angiography is performed. Patients should also be warned that the dye will temporarily stain their skin and urine; in the average patient this lasts no more than a day.

ICG has been used in recent years, either alone or with fluorescein, to obtain better films of choroid neovascularization. The technique of dye administration is as follows:

1. The patient is seated comfortably at the fundus camera with one arm extended and the forearm exposed.
2. Fluorescein dye is drawn into a 10-mL syringe. A 21-gauge needle is then used to enter a vein in the arm. Care should be taken to ensure that the needle is in the vein by drawing back blood and injecting just a slight amount of dye. It is important to make sure that the dye does not extravasate from the vein because this may be painful and can cause local necrosis.
3. Before injection of the main bolus of dye, red-free photographs usually are taken. This can be done with the appropriate filter in the fundus camera.
4. The dye is injected into the patient's arm fairly rapidly so that the entire volume of dye is injected in about 2 seconds.
5. Photographs are taken at moderately rapid intervals (about one each second) immediately following injection of the dye. After the dye has filled the retinal vessels in one eye, pictures are taken of the fellow eye. In most instances it is helpful to photograph both eyes so that the fellow eye can be used for comparison and as a control.

There is a mild degree of morbidity inherent in this method. Some patients have transient nausea and occasional vomiting 30 to 60 seconds after the injection of the dye. Vomiting usually can be avoided by reassuring the patient. Hives and asthmatic symptoms occasionally may develop, which can be treated by oral or intravenous administration of diphenhydramine hydrochloride (Benadryl) or cortisone.

A number of fluorescein angiographic phases are recognized (Figure 24.20). After intravenous injection into the antecubital vein, the dye reaches the ocular circulation in approximately 10 to 15 seconds. In the *prearterial phase* the choroidal vessels fill and one can discern a patchy hyperfluorescent "choroidal flush." In the *arterial phase*, which is 1 second later, the retinal arterioles fill. The dye then flows into the capillaries and from there into the veins. When there is partial venous filling (i.e., *laminar flow*), the *arteriovenous phase* is recognized. When the veins are filled with fluorescein, this is the *venous phase*. The dye is distributed throughout the blood (*recirculation phase*) 3 to 5 minutes after injection, and early leakage and staining

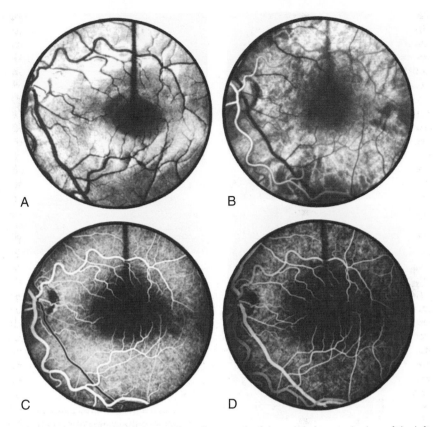

Figure 24.20 Normal fluorescein angiogram. (A) A red-free photograph of the ophthalmoscopic view of the left macula. (B) In this retinal arterial-filling phase of the fluorescein angiogram, there is patchy filling of the choroid. Large choroid vessels can be seen in some areas. The central retinal artery has begun to fill. (C) In the early retinal arteriovenous phase, the choroid has completely filled with a diffuse and even fluorescence. The retinal arteries fluoresce; the retinal veins show laminar flow. (D) In the later arteriovenous phase or recirculation phase, fluorescence has begun to fade from the choroidal and retinal vascular circulations.
(From Schatz H, Burton TC, Yannuzzi LA et al. Interpretation of fundus fluorescein angiography. St Louis: Mosby; 1978.)

occur during this period. The *elimination phase* can be observed between 30 and 60 minutes after injection.

Damage to the endothelium of retinal capillaries or the retinal pigment epithelium causes leakage into and beneath the retina. Diagnostic patterns include defects of the pigment epithelium (which act as windows to the underlying choroidal fluorescence), accumulation of dye between choroid and retina (e.g., serous detachment), staining within the retina (secondary to leakage from retinal capillaries), interference with visualization of choroidal fluorescence (by exudates, pigment, or hemorrhage), obstruction to filling (arteriole or venous occlusion), and abnormal vessels (e.g., neovascularization).

Figure 24.21 shows the presence of dye leakage into the macula. This is associated with a decrease in vision and is consistent with the diagnosis of cystoid macular edema. This condition may be seen after any type of intraocular surgery, most commonly after cataract extraction, or it

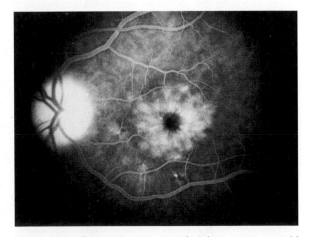

Figure 24.21 Fluorescein angiogram that demonstrates cystoid macular edema.

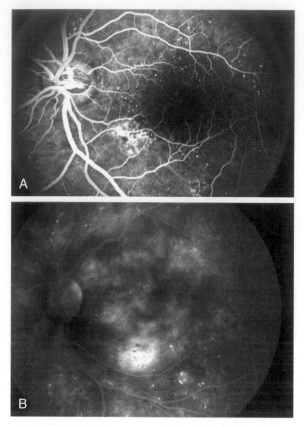

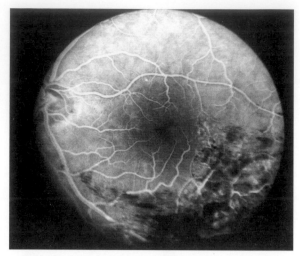

Figure 24.24 Fluorescein angiogram of a branch retinal vein occlusion.

Figure 24.22 (A) Fluorescein angiogram of a diabetic fundus. (B) Later angiogram phase of the same diabetic fundus. Areas of hyperfluorescence represent leakage of fluid into the macula.

may be a consequence of an inflammatory condition of the posterior segment that causes leakage of the macular vessels.

Figure 24.22A shows a diabetic fundus with microaneurysms, which appear as punctate areas of hyperfluorescence. A later stage of the angiogram (Figure 24.22B) shows significant leakage of dye into the macula, which accounts for the decrease in vision.

Figure 24.23 is an angiogram of a central retinal vein occlusion. One can appreciate the tortuous retinal veins, hypofluorescent areas that represent scattered hemorrhages, and hyperfluorescent areas that are a result of leakage from the vessels. This is in contrast to Figure 24.24, which is an angiogram of a branch retinal vein occlusion that shows blockage of the choroidal fluorescein by blood in a sector distribution. The patient has decreased vision as a result of macular edema from vessel leakage. Laser photocoagulation can be performed to improve the visual prognosis.

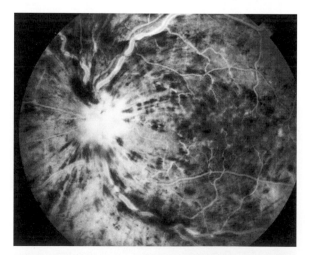

Figure 24.23 Fluorescein angiogram of a central retinal vein occlusion.

Questions for review and thought

1. Discuss the possible eye involvement of diabetes mellitus.
2. What is the use of the laser in ophthalmology?
3. What is the clinical picture of someone who has had a central retinal artery occlusion?
4. What symptoms suggest a retinal detachment?
5. What are the retinal findings that suggest retinitis pigmentosa?
6. What is retinopathy of prematurity? What is its cause?
7. An individual has a metallic foreign body that perforates the eye and enters the posterior chamber. What possible eye involvements may there be?
8. What are the clinical manifestations of hyperthyroidism?

 Self-evaluation questions

True–false statements

Directions: Indicate whether the statement is true (**T**) or false (**F**).

1. Retinopathy of prematurity occurs in one eye of premature infants exposed to high concentrations of oxygen. **T** or **F**
2. Every retinal hole should be sealed with either laser beam or cryosurgery. **T** or **F**
3. Drusen of the retina rarely cause any loss of vision. **T** or **F**

Missing words

Directions: Write in the missing word in the following sentences:

4. Central retinal vein occlusion can cause _____ 3 months after the event.
5. Diabetic retinopathy is more prevalent amongst patients with poorly controlled diabetes and those who have had a diagnosis for at least _____ years.
6. Retinitis pigmentosa causes _____ field defect in the early stages.

Choice-completion questions

Directions: Select the one best answer in each case.

7. Retinal detachments are common:
   a. in high myopes.
   b. after contusion.
   c. with malignant melanomas.
   d. with retinal tears with an operculum.
   e. in all of the above.
8. Central serous retinopathy is a disease of:
   a. adults older than 65 years.
   b. individuals between 25 and 50 years.
   c. females.
   d. African Americans.
   e. absent symptoms.
9. Central retinal artery occlusion usually is caused by:
   a. a tumor of the optic nerve.
   b. a thrombus.
   c. an embolus.
   d. glaucoma.
   e. carotid artery stenosis.

A **Answers, notes, and explanations**

1. **False.** Retinopathy of prematurity is a bilateral disease occurring in infants born before 36 weeks of gestation or weighing less than 4.2 pounds at birth and having a history of significant oxygen therapy. These infants develop three signs: peripheral neovascularization (especially on the temporal periphery), vitreous bleeding, and retinal detachment. Infants exposed to high doses of oxygen should be examined with the indirect ophthalmoscope before discharge from the hospital and every 2 months until the condition is considered stable. The treatment of this condition is still not satisfactory despite the use of lasers, cryotherapy, vitamins C and E (tocopherol), and encircling retinal buckles. The most serious complication of retinopathy of prematurity is retinal detachment, which may not be evident until the age of 10 to 20 years. The difficulty in evaluating treatment of this condition results from the fact that many infants have a spontaneous regression.

2. **False.** Every break or retinal hole should not be sealed with laser beam or cryosurgery. Many retinal holes are not through-and-through or do not have an operculum or lip developed through traction. It is true, however, that in many retinal detachments a retinal break develops. A hole in the retina permits the accumulation of fluid between the

A Continued

pigment layer of the retina and the anterior nine sensory layers of the retina. The subretinal fluid that accumulates acts as a wedge between the retinal layers, and further detachment results. Most retinal holes occur in the extreme periphery of the retina. They are quite common and most do not lead to detachment. If a retinal hole is found with a break in the retina, with evidence of traction or a serous wedge, these breaks are treated. Although most retinal holes do not cause a retinal detachment, most detachments (>85%) reveal multiple holes.

3. **True.** Drusen of the choroid are basically excrescences of Bruch's membrane of the choroid. They appear as yellow deposits in the posterior pole of the retina, sometimes surrounded by a collarette of retinal pigment. Unless associated with macular degenerative phenomena, these drusen usually are harmless. Drusen of the optic nerve are another matter. They consist of hyalin or calcium, and these deposits take up and compress tissue in the optic nerve. Field defects are common and may be varied depending on the size of the drusen, their location, and their development. In addition to causing visual field defects, drusen may simulate the appearance of papilledema or swelling of the optic nerve head. Typically drusen are glistening pearl-like bodies, which, when visible, are seen in the surface of the optic disc. When they are buried, the disc is heaped up and its margins are blurred.

4. **Neovascular glaucoma.** Central retinal vein occlusion can cause a severe, intractable glaucoma within 3 months after the venous occlusion. The vascular ischemia of the venous occlusion causes neovascularization at the level of the retina and iris. In the retina, macroaneurysms and vascular buds appear. These can create retinal hemorrhage and lead to retinal detachment. In the iris the vascular proliferation can sew up the angle structures with fibrovascular tissue. This leads to a permanent angle-closure type of glaucoma that cannot be satisfactorily treated medically or surgically. The term *hemorrhagic glaucoma* is a misnomer because it is not the presence of the blood in the anterior chamber that causes the glaucoma. It is caused by the growth of active fibrovascular bands that invade and occlude the angle structures.

5. **15.** Diabetic retinopathy is a major cause of blindness in North America. Initially the retinopathy was thought to be a straight function of duration. Those with diabetes for 15 years or longer were the most susceptible to the disease. The duration factor is still valid inasmuch as it is uncommon to see diabetics of 25 years without some form of retinopathy. That is not to say that long-term diabetics invariably go blind, but they show a few microaneurysms, perhaps some neovascularization of the retina, or turgid retinal veins. In addition to duration, most researchers believe that hyperglycemia by itself is toxic and proper control is important to minimize the disease. For years this point was contentious but appears now to be settled.

Another area of dispute is the relationship of age to retinopathy. It was believed that maturity-onset (40 years or over) diabetics were free of the complications of retinopathy. This is definitely not true. Approximately 20% of maturity-onset diabetics develop retinopathy. When this occurs, it usually is more severe than in the juvenile diabetics. Some physicians believe that the division of juvenile diabetes and maturity-onset diabetes should be abolished and replaced by insulin-dependent and noninsulin-dependent disease. Insulin-dependent diabetics are more prone to retinal complications of this disease.

6. **Tubular or signet ring.** Retinitis pigmentosa can cause tubular field defects. Such defects in the visual field also can be caused by syphilis, glaucoma, quinine poisoning, eclampsia, and, on occasion, hysteria. The diagnosis of this disease can be made by observing the bone spicule pigment deposits in the retina at the level of the midperiphery. Also, an ERG can reveal the flat electrical response of the rods, which is abolished under dim light. There usually is a family history of the disease. This may not be obvious because the disease can be transmitted as a dominant, recessive, or sex-linked type of hereditary pattern. Occasionally vitamin A deficiency can be uncovered, and this plus nutritional disorders, although rare in industrialized countries, may mimic retinitis pigmentosa. At present there is no cure for this disease. In many patients the evolution of this disease may be slow, thus blindness may not occur in all afflicted patients.

7. **a. In high myopes.** The typical high myope has a tilted disc with an oblique entry of the optic nerve though the sclera, an elongated eye sometimes with a large posterior staphyloma, and a stretched vascular system for both the retinal and the choroidal circulations. As a result, through vascular ischemia, retinal holes (some leading to retinal tears and subsequent detachment) are common. A retinal tear with an operculum is merely a large retinal tear with a lip or edge that is everting. Such tears cannot be sealed by laser therapy and represent a further stage in the development or evolution of a retinal detachment. A malignant melanoma can cause a detachment by virtue of this solid mass derived from the choroid pressing forward from behind and pushing the retina anteriorly. Diagnostically the melanoma is one of the few instances in which a retinal detachment may be present without a retinal hole or tear. Injury also may cause retinal detachment as a result of the underlying presence of blood, edema fluid, and inflammatory debris. Injury is not the major cause, however, of most retinal detachments.

8. **b. Individuals between 25 and 50 years.** Central serous retinopathy is a disease of young people. At times it may be related to stress or a prolonged period of anxiety or to an allergic reaction to drugs, vapors, or chemicals, but commonly it has no antecedent of any kind. The person invariably is made aware of the problem because of blurred

A Continued

and distorted vision. Lines appear curved, at times with missing pieces in the center, and color vision is depressed or darker in hue. The patient's symptoms are pathognomonic of this condition. However, support for the diagnosis can be made by the Amsler grid or by looking for the telltale macular blister, which usually is clinically evident. Often the condition improves without any drug or device. Angiography of the retinal and choroidal circulation should be done because simulating conditions include a small macular melanoma, histoplasmosis, hematoma, and an effusion of a hemangioma.

9. **c. An embolus.** Central retinal artery occlusion is invariably a result of an embolus from an atheromatous plaque of the carotid artery. It is commonly a mixture of fatty debris, platelets, and fibrin and appears as a glistening yellow plaque at the head of the optic nerve in the central retinal artery. At times, nothing is found at this location but fragments of the embolus may be visible in the retinal circulation. Such an event invariably causes blindness unless heroic measures such as ocular paracentesis or heavy massage of the globe are undertaken within 5 minutes. Such patients should receive the benefit of a neurologic investigation to direct attention to the carotid artery on that side, which also may be stenosed or compromised by the presence of an atheromatous ulcer in the wall of the vessel. Patients with this disease often worry about a similar event occurring in the other eye. Of course, it is possible, because atheroma in a person usually is not limited to a single vessel but is present more or less in all large blood vessels. Statistically the chances of such a catastrophe being bilateral are extremely remote and highly improbable.

FURTHER READING

Age-Related Eye Disease Study 2 (AREDS2) Research Group, Chew E, Clemons T, SanGiovanni J, Danis R, Ferris 3rd F, et al. Secondary Analyses of the Effects of Lutein/Zeaxanthin on Age-Related Macular Degeneration Progression: AREDS2 Report No 3. JAMA Ophthalmol 2014; 132(2):142–9.

Age-Related Eye Disease Study 2 (AREDS2). Study design and baseline characteristics. AREDS2 Report No.1. Ophthalmology 2012;26:26.

Age-Related Eye Disease Study Research Group. A randomized, placebo-controlled, clinical trial of high-dose supplementation with vitamins C and E, beta carotene, and zinc for age-related macular degeneration and vision loss: AREDS report No. 8. Arch Ophthalmol 2001;119(10):1417–36.

Berkow JW, Flower RW, Orth DH, Kelley JS. Fluorescein and Indocyanine Green Angiography: Technique and Interpretation. In: Ophthalmology Monograph 5. 2nd ed. San Francisco: American Academy of Ophthalmology; 1997.

Branch Vein Occlusion Study Group. Argon laser scatter photocoagulation for prevention of neovascularization and vitreous hemorrhage in branch vein occlusion. Arch Ophthalmol 1986;104(1):34–41.

The Branch Vein Occlusion Study Group. Argon laser photocoagulation for macula edema in branch vein occlusion. Am J Ophthalmol 1984; 98:271–82.

Bressler NM. Photodynamic therapy of subfoveal choroidal neovascularization in age-related macular degeneration with verteporfin: 2-year results of 2 randomized clinical trials—TAP report 2. Arch Ophthalmol 2001; 119:198–207.

Brown DM, Campochiaro PA, Singh RP, et al. Ranibizumab for macular edema following central retinal vein occlusion: six-month primary end point results of a phase III study. Ophthalmology 2010 Jun; 117(6):1124–33.

Brown DM, Campochiaro PA, Singh RP, et al. CRUISE Investigators. Ranibizumab for macular edema after central retinal vein occlusion: 6-month primary end point results of a phase III study. Ophthalmology 2010;117: 1124–33.

Brown DM, Campochiaro PA, Singh RP, Li Z, Gray S, Saroj N, et al. Ranibizumab for macular edema following central retinal vein occlusion: 6-month primary end point results of a phase III study. Ophthalmology 2010 June;117(6):1124–33 e1. Published online 2010 April 9.

Brown DM for the COPERNICUS Study Investigators. Intravitreal aflibercept injection of central retinal vein occlusions: 2-year results from the COPERNICUS Study. Am Acad Ophthal 2012;155(3):429–37.

Brown DM, Kaiser PK, Michels M, et al. Ranibizumab versus verteporfin for neovascular age-related macular degeneration. N Engl J Med 2006 Oct 5;355(14):1432–44.

Brown DM, Kaiser PK, Michels M, et al. ANCHOR Study Group. Ranibizumab versus verteporfin for neovascular age-related macular degeneration. [1-year results of the ANCHOR Study]. N Engl J Med 2006; 355(14):1432–14444.

Busbee BG, Ho AC, Brown DM, et al; for the HARBOR Study Group. Twelve-month efficacy and safety of 0.5 mg or 2.0 mg ranibizumab in patients with subfoveal neovascular age-related macular degeneration [published online ahead of print January 23, 2013]. Ophthalmology. http://dx.doi.org/10.1016/j.ophtha.2012.10.014.

Campochiaro PA, Heier JS, Feiner L, et al. Ranibizumab for macular edema following branch retinal vein occlusion: six-month primary end point results of a phase III study. Ophthalmology 2010 Jun;117(6):1102–1112e1 Epub 2010 Apr 15.

The Central Vein Occlusion Study (CVO). Baseline and early natural history report. Arch Ophthalmol 1993; 111(8):1087–95.

The Central Vein Occlusion Study (CVO). Natural history and clinical management of central retinal vein occlusion. Arch Ophthalmol 1997; 115(4):486–91.

The Central Vein Occlusion Study Group. Evaluation of grid pattern photocoagulation for macular edema in central vein occlusion. Ophthalmology 1995;102:1425–33.

Clinicaltrials.gov. Diabetic Retinopathy Clinical Research Network. Comparative Effectiveness Study of Intravitreal Aflibercept, Bevacizumab, and Ranibizumab for DME. ClinicalTrial. gov Identifier NCT01627249

Cryotherapy for Retinopathy of Prematurity Cooperative Group. Cryotherapy for Retinopathy of Prematurity: ophthalmological outcomes at 10 years. Arch Ophthalmol. 2001;119(8): 1110–1118.

Diabetes Control and Complications Trial Research Group. Progression of retinopathy with intensive versus conventional treatment in the Diabetes Control and Complications Trial. Ophthalmology. 1995; 102 (4):647–661.

Diabetic Retinopathy Clinical Research Network (DRCR.net), Beck RW, Edwards AR, Aiello LP, Bressler NM, Ferris F, et al. 3-year follow-up of a randomized trial comparing focal/ grid photocoagulation and intravitreal triamcinolone for diabetic macular edema. Arch Ophthalmol 2009;127(3):245–51.

The Diabetic Retinopathy Study Research Group. Photocoagulation treatment of proliferative diabetic retinopathy. Clinical application of Diabetic Retinopathy Study (DRS) findings, ERS report no. 8. Ophthalmology. 1981; 88(7):583–600.

Diener-West M, Earle JD, Fine SL, et al. The COMS randomized trial of iodine 125 brachytherapy for choroidal melanoma, III: initial mortality findings. COMS report no. 18. Arch Ophthalmol 2001;119(7):969–82.

Do DV, Nguyen QD, Boyer D, Schmidt-Erfurth U, Brown DM, et al. DA VINCI Study Group. One-year outcomes of the DA VINCI study of VEGF Trap-Eye in eyes with diabetic macular edema. Ophthalmology 2012;119:1658–65.

Do DV. Intravitreal aflibercept injection (IAI) for diabetic macular edema (DME): 12-month results of VISTA-DME and VIVID-DME. Paper presented at: the 2013 Annual Meeting of the American Academy of Ophthalmology; November 16-19, 2013; New Orleans, LA.

Early Treatment for Retinopathy of Prematurity cooperative Group. Revised indications for the treatment of retinopathy of prematurity: results of the Early Treatment for Retinopathy of Prematurity randomized Trial. Arch Ophthalmol 2003; 121(12):1684–94.

Ferris FL, Davis MD, Clemons TE, et al. Age-Related Eye Disease Study (AREDS) Research Group. A simplified severity scale for age-related macular degeneration: AREDS report no. 18. Arch Ophthalmol 2005; 123(11):1570–4.

Hawkins BS. Collaborative Ocular Melanoma Study group. The collaborative Ocular Melanoma Study (COMS) randomized trial of pre-enucleation radiation of large choroidal melanoma: IV. Ten-year mortality findings and prognostic factors. COMS report no. 24. Am J Ophthalmol 2004; 138(6):936–51.

Heier JS, Brown DM, Chong V, VIEW 1 and VIEW 2 Study Groups, et al. Intravitreal aflibercept (VEGF Trap-Eye) in wet age-related macular degeneration. Ophthalmology 2012; 119(12):2537–48.

Holz FG, Roider J, Ogura Y, et al. VEGF Trap-Eye for macular oedema secondary to central retinal vein occlusion: 6-month results of the Phase III GALILEO study. Br J Ophthalmol 2013;97(3):278–84.

Imamura Y, Fujiwara T, Margolis R, Spaide RF. Enhanced depth imaging optical coherence tomography of the choroid in central serous chorioretinopathy. Retina 2009; 29(10):1469–73.

IVAN Study Investigators, Chakravarthy U, Harding SP, Rogers CA, Downes SM, Lotery AJ, et al. Ranibizumab versus bevacizumab to treat neovascular age-related macular degeneration: 1-year findings from the IVAN randomized trial. Ophthalmology 2012; 119(7):1399–411 Epub 2012 May 11.

Kiernan F, Mieler WF, Hariprasad SM. Spectral-domain optical coherence tomography: a comparison of modern high-resolution retinal imaging systems. Am J Ophthalmol 2010; 149(1):18–31.

Kreissig I, ed. Primary Retinal Detachment: Options for Repair. Berlin: Springer-Verlag; 2005Williams GA, Aaberg Jr. TM. Primary Retinal Detachment: Options for Repair. Berlin: Springer-Verlag; 2005. In: Ryan SJ, Hinton DR, Schachat AP, Wilkinson CP, editors. Techniques of scleral buckling. 4th ed. Retina3: Philadelphia: Elsevier/Mosby; 2006. p. 2035–70.

Lalwani GA, Rosenfeld PJ, Fung AE, et al. A variable dosing regimen with intravitreal ranibizumab for neovascular age-related macular degeneration: year 2 of the PrONTO Study. Am J Ophthalmol 2009;148(1):43–58.

Lim JW, Kang SW, Kim YT, et al. Comparative study of patients with central serous chorioretinopathy undergoing focal laser photocoagulation or photodynamic therapy. Br J Ophthalmol 2011;95(4):514–7.

Machemer R, Aaberg TM, Freeman HM, Irvine AR, Lean JS, Michels RM. An updated classification of retinal detachment with proliferative vitreoretinopathy. Am J Ophthalmol 1991;112(2):159–65.

Macular Photocoagulation Study (MPS) Group. Argon laser photocoagulation for neovascular maculopathy: 5-year results from randomized clinical trials. Arch Ophthalmol 1991; 109:1109–14.

Martin DF, Maguire MG, Fine SL, et al. Ranibizumab and Bevacizumab for Treatment of Neovascular Age-Related Macular Degeneration: 2-Year Results: Comparison of Age-related Macular Degeneration Treatments Trials (CATT) Research Group. Ophthalmology 2012;119(7):1388–98. http://dx.doi.org/10.1016/j.ophtha. 2012.03.053.

Mintz-Hittner HA, Kennedy KA, Chuang AZ. BEAT-ROP Cooperative Group. Efficacy of intravitreal bevacizumab for stage 3 + retinopathy of prematurity. N Engl J Med 2011; 364(7):603–15.

Mitchell P, Gillies MC, Larsen M, Staurenghi G, Holz FG, Katz TA, et al. Intravitreal Aflibercept for the Treatment of Diabetic Macular Edema: Evaluating the Impact on Diabetic Retinopathy. Invest Ophthalmol Vis Sci 2015;56(7):3146.

Nguyen QD, Brown DM, Marcus DM, et al. Ranibizumab for diabetic macular edema: results from 2 phase III randomized trials: RISE and RIDE. Ophthalmology 2012;119:789–801.

Nguyen QD, Shah SM, Khwaja AA, Channa R, Hatef E, Do DV, et al. READ-2 Study Group. Two-year outcomes of the Ranibizumab for Edema of the Macula in Diabetes (READ-2) study. Ophthalmology 2010; 117(11):2146–51 Epub 2010 Sep 19.

Ober MD, Yannuzzi LA, Do DV, et al. Photodynamic therapy for focal retinal pigment epithelial leaks secondary to central serous chorioretinopathy. Ophthalmology 2005; 112(12):2088–94.

Palmer EA, Flynn JT, Hardy RJ, et al. Incidence and early course of retinopathy of prematurity. The Cryotherapy for Retinopathy of Prematurity Cooperative Group.

Ophthalmology 1991; 98(11):1628–40.

Regillo CD, Brown DM, Abraham P, et al. Randomized, double-masked, sham-controlled trial of ranibizumab for neovascular age-related macular degeneration: PIER Study year 1. Am J Ophthalmol 2008 Feb; 145(2):239–48.

Rosenfeld PJ, Brown DM, Heier JS, et al. Ranibizumab for neovascular age-related macular degeneration. N Engl J Med 2006 Oct 5;355(14):1419–31.

Rosenfeld PJ, Brown DM, Heier JS, et al. Ranibizumab for neovascular age-related macular degeneration. [2-year results of the MARINA study]. N Engl J Med 2006;355(14):1419–31.

Scott IU, Ip MS, Van Veldhuisen PC, et al. SCORE Study Research Group. A randomized trial comparing the efficacy and safety of intravitreal triamcinolone with standard care to treat vision loss associated with macular edema secondary to branch retinal vein occlusion: the Arch Standard Care vs Corticosteroid for Retinal Vein Occlusion (SCORE) study report 6. Ophthalmology 2009; 127(9):1115–28.

Soo Y, Cheng Y, Haller JA, Campochiaro PA, Clark WL, Boyer DS, et al. Intravitreal aflibercept for macular edema following branch retinal vein occlusion: The 24-week results of the VIBRANT study. Ophthalmology 2015;3:538–44.

UK Prospective Diabetes Study Group (UKPDS). Tight blood pressure control and risk of macrovascular and microvascular complications in type2 diabetes: UKPDS 38. Br Med J. 1998; 317(7160):703–713.

Verteporfin in Photodynamic Therapy Study Group. Verteporfin therapy of subfoveal choroidal neovascularization in age-related macular degeneration: 2-year results of a randomized clinical trial including lesions with occult with no classic choroidal neovascularization—Verteporfin In Photodynamic Therapy (VIP) report 2. Am J Ophthalmol 2001; 131:541–60.

Wilkinson CP. Evidence-based analysis of prophylactic treatment of asymptomatic retinal breaks and lattice degeneration. Ophthalmology 2000; 107(1):12–8.

Chapter 25

Glaucoma

Michael S. Berlin, Harold A. Stein, Daniella Lent-Schochet, Christine Quach, Zijie Cai

CHAPTER CONTENTS

The ophthalmic technician is a critical member of the glaucoma patient management team. Responsibilities integral to the ophthalmic technician's role in the care of patients with glaucoma include:

- Identifying factors that may be indicative of glaucoma when taking a patient's history
- Performing key tests to define the glaucoma patient's status
- Aiding in glaucoma patients' treatment by teaching them about their condition, demonstrating treatment techniques (such as applying eyedrops), and monitoring their compliance and treatment efficacy in preventing progression
- Assisting in the preoperative preparation and especially in the postoperative care of glaucoma surgical patients

Each one of these aspects is essential to the complete care of the glaucoma patient.

An understanding of what glaucoma is, what glaucoma does to the eye, and what we can do about it enables the technician to become a key component of this glaucoma patient management team. It is the ophthalmic technician who has the potential to effect a positive outcome in the prognosis of glaucoma patients. More than 60 million people worldwide are afflicted by glaucoma. There are countless millions in whom glaucoma has not been diagnosed. For every person blinded by glaucoma, there are at least six individuals who have lost useful vision in one eye[1].

CLASSIFICATION

Glaucoma is a localized ocular disease characterized by optic nerve cupping and visual field loss, and is usually associated with elevated intraocular pressure (IOP). The hallmark of glaucoma is a progressive optic neuropathy. Risk factors for glaucoma include:

- Elevated IOP
- Family history of glaucoma
- African American or Hispanic ancestry
- Diabetes
- Myopia
- Trauma to the eye
- Advanced age

Glaucoma falls roughly into five classifications (Table 25.1).

1. *Primary open-angle* or *chronic glaucoma.* This condition is thought to arise from a progressive outflow obstruction in the trabecular meshwork of the anterior chamber angle structures, with a subsequent increase in IOP. It is insidious and symptomless, initially causing loss of the peripheral visual field but often undetected until significant irreversible loss has occurred. Most cases of glaucoma fall into this group.

2. *Secondary glaucoma.* Secondary glaucoma can be of either the open-angle or the narrow-angle type. The

Table 25.1 Types of glaucoma

Type	Cause	Symptoms	Comments
Primary open angle	Gradual blockage of drainage channel; pressure builds slowly	Gradual loss of side vision; affects side vision first	Progresses very slowly and is a lifelong condition; considered the "thief in the night"
Secondary	Injury, infection, tumors, drugs, or inflammation, which causes scar tissue growth, blocking the drainage channel	Gradual loss of side vision; affects side vision first	May progress slowly; similar to chronic open-angle glaucoma
Angle-closure glaucoma	Total blockage of drainage channel; sudden increase in pressure	Nausea, blurred vision, severe pain, halos around lights	A medical emergency because permanent blindness occurs rapidly without immediate treatment
Congenital (infantile)	Fluid drainage system abnormal at birth	Light sensitivity, excessive tearing, enlarged eyes, cloudy cornea	Must be treated soon after birth if vision is to be saved

elevated IOP results from a specific disease within the eye, such as iritis, uveitis, venous obstruction in the eye, or tumor, which interferes with aqueous flowing out of the eye. It may occur after trauma or may follow neovascularization in the anterior chamber, as may occur with diabetes. Different types of secondary glaucoma include pigmentary, exfoliative, and uveitic glaucoma.

3. *Angle-closure glaucoma.* In this condition there is a sudden marked increase in IOP caused by mechanical obstruction of angle structures of the eye near the root of the iris (see Figure 2.15). Vision is blurred rapidly, the eye becomes red, and the patient complains of excruciating pain and often halos.

4. *Congenital* or *infantile glaucoma.* This condition is also referred to as *buphthalmos* (ox eye) because the soft infantile eyeball distends as a result of the elevated IOP and becomes noticeably enlarged (Figure 25.1).

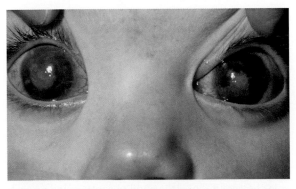

Figure 25.1 Congenital glaucoma. Note enlarged eyes and corneal scarring from ulceration
(From Krachmer JH, Palay D. Cornea atlas. 3rd ed. Philadelphia: Elsevier; 2014.)

5. *Normal-tension glaucoma.* Patients with this condition have IOP within a normal range but continue to lose field of vision. This condition is often vascular in origin, associated with other vasculopathy and often caused by systemic hypotension while sleeping.

PRIMARY OPEN-ANGLE OR CHRONIC GLAUCOMA

Primary open-angle glaucoma (POAG) is a chronic progressive bilateral disease. It most often develops in middle life or later. The onset is gradual and without external signs or symptoms. It has been determined that 3 million Americans have POAG.

The cause of this disorder is obstruction of the outflow of aqueous humor at the trabecular meshwork. Most cases of POAG are caused by an inability of aqueous fluid to leave the eye and not by an overproduction of aqueous fluid (Figure 25.2).

Because there are often no symptoms until the disease is far progressed, POAG is most often discovered during routine eye examinations or screening examinations, when the patient is found to have elevated IOP or an excavated optic nerve. The diagnosis of this condition usually depends on three objective signs—abnormal cupping of the optic disc (Figures 25.3 and 25.4), typical changes in the visual field, elevated IOP—and other diagnostic tests (Box 25.1).

Ocular hypertension

In contrast to POAG, some people have high IOP but do not show any changes in their optic discs or visual fields. These are individuals whose nerve can tolerate higher than normal IOPs without apparent damage. Some

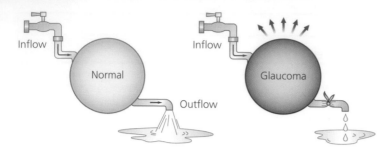

Figure 25.2 Obstruction of aqueous outflow causes an elevation of intraocular tension.

ophthalmologists believe they may be preglaucomatous or "glaucoma suspects." However, ophthalmic personnel label this condition *ocular hypertension* to avoid using terms that might needlessly upset and worry patients. The term *ocular hypertension* creates a convenient category, without a gloomy label, for keeping patients under close observation. Actually most of these people will live most of their lives without needing therapy. However, they must remain under observation because some individuals in this group are at greater risk of developing preventable glaucomatous changes in their optic disc and field. Topical ocular hypotensive medication is effective in delaying or preventing the onset of POAG in individuals with elevated IOP. Clinicians should consider initiating treatment for individuals with ocular hypertension who are at moderate or high risk for developing POAG.

At one time people older than 40 years with pressures greater than 21 mm Hg were considered to have glaucoma and were treated on the basis that field loss would inevitably follow. However, clinical evidence has shown that whereas an estimated 10 million Americans older than age 40 have pressures greater than 21 mm Hg, only 0.3% of the same population have detectable visual impairment. Of those with ocular hypertension, 10% have field loss and another 4% will develop field loss during the 5- to 10-year follow-up.

Therapy for those with ocular hypertension is not without risk. Therapy may restrict a healthy person to a schedule requiring medication one to three times daily, limiting the patient's ability to manage daily activities or interfering with systemic medication or systemic conditions. For these reasons the decision to treat this group of patients with elevated IOP is a judgment call dependent on the perceived threat to vision. Thus ocular hypertension is often treated by watchful waiting.

SECONDARY GLAUCOMA

Secondary glaucoma occurs as a result of an additional pathology within the eye. Because in essence there are two diseases in the eye—the precipitating cause and the glaucoma—the condition is often more difficult to treat. Secondary glaucomas include secondary open angle, reviewed in this section and secondary angle closure, reviewed under Angle-Closure Glaucoma, in the following text.

Causes of *secondary open-angle glaucoma* include pigment or protein accumulation in the drainage structures, iritis, cyclitis, and trauma and rarely invasion of the trabecular meshwork by tumors of the iris, ciliary body, and choroid.

Pseudoexfoliative (or exfoliative) glaucoma

Exfoliative glaucoma is caused by the accumulation of an insoluble protein in the drainage channels or other structures of the eye resulting in higher pressures than in patients with other types of glaucoma. The abnormal protein is often found in the lens epithelium, trabecular meshwork, iris, ciliary processes, conjunctiva, and periocular tissue. This condition is common among those of Scandinavian descent and seems to be related to a gene abnormality. It rarely occurs in patients younger than age 50.

Traditional IOP-lowering medications may be less effective in patients with exfoliative glaucoma, thus requiring additional therapy such as argon laser trabeculoplasty (ALT) or selective laser trabeculoplasty (SLT).

Pigmentary glaucoma

Pigmentary glaucoma occurs when iris pigment granules flake into the aqueous humor or other structures such as the trabecular meshwork and clog the drainage channels of the eye. This condition tends to occur at a younger age, usually in the 20s or 30s, and in near-sighted patients. It is more common in men than in women.

Patients are often treated with drops such as a prostaglandin or a beta-blocker because these drops have a relatively low incidence of side effects and are well tolerated in younger patients. Miotics can be used to treat pigmentary glaucoma because it causes the pupil to constrict and prevents the iris from rubbing against the lens, thereby preventing release of pigment onto the surrounding structures. However, miotics often cause blurred vision and require more

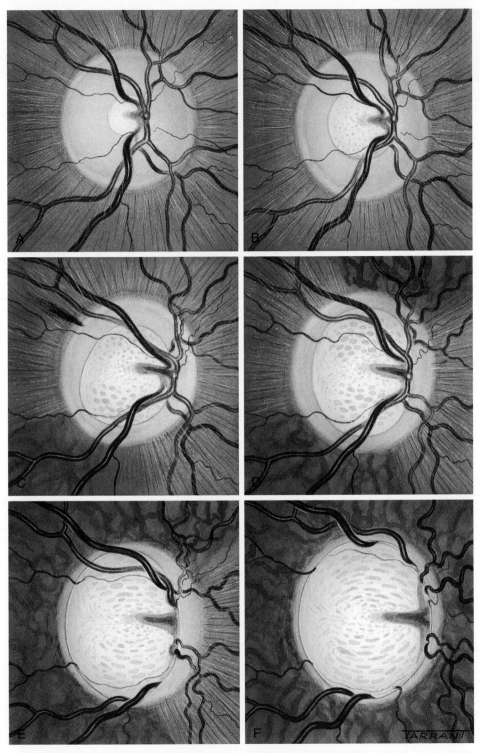

Figure 25.3 Progression of optic nerve damage. (A) Early (B) Moderate and (C) Advanced cupping.

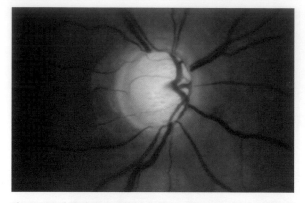

Figure 25.4 End-stage glaucomatous cupping.
(From Kanski J. Clinical ophthalmology: a systematic approach. 5th ed. Oxford: Butterworth-Heinemann; 2003, with permission.)

Box 25.1 **Diagnostic tests for glaucoma**

Intraocular pressure: tonometry
Gonioscopy
Central corneal thickness
Structural: optic nerve

- Stereo disc photography
- Nerve fiber layer thickness (optical coherence tomography [OCT])
- Ultrasound biomicroscopy (UBM)
- Confocal scanning ophthalmoscopy (Heidelberg retina tomograph)
- Retinal nerve fiber layer assessment (GDx VCC)

Functional: visual fields (see Chapter 19)

- Standard automated perimetry ([SAP] white on white)
- Short-wave automated perimetry ([SWAP] blue on yellow)
- Frequency doubling technology (FDT)

---

frequent dosing, thus limiting their use. Other options include laser iridotomy and argon laser trabeculoplasty or selective laser trabeculoplasty.

Neovascular glaucoma

Neovascular glaucoma is a severe form of secondary glaucoma. It is associated with the proliferation of vessels in the anterior chamber angle. The blood vessels generated through neovascular glaucoma are abnormal, and when new blood vessels form in the anterior chamber angle the aqueous outflow can be compromised. Typically the three most common conditions responsible for neovascular glaucoma are diabetic retinopathy, central retinal vein occlusion, and carotid artery obstructive disease.

Neovascular glaucoma is often treated with panretinal photocoagulation, which has been shown to reduce anterior segment neovascularization. Traditional IOP-lowering medications also can be used to lower the pressure, as well as trabeculectomy and aqueous drain implants.

Traumatic glaucoma

Traumatic glaucoma refers to any injuries to the eye that result in glaucoma. Blunt trauma, such as a direct injury to the eye or a blow to the head, usually as a result of sports, can cause an accumulation of blood and debris that clogs the drainage channels. In this case glaucoma medications can be used to control eye pressure, and surgery may be necessary. In most cases the elevated eye pressure is temporary.

When a penetrating eye injury occurs, such as by a sharp instrument, it can cause the eye to become swollen and bleed, leading to elevated eye pressure. Additionally drainage channels can be blocked by damaged tissue and scarring. Ocular trauma is often treated by topical corticosteroid therapy as an initial treatment to minimize permanent tissue damage and scarring.

Glaucomatocyclitic crisis

Glaucomatocyclitic crisis is a condition with self-limited recurrent episodes of markedly elevated IOP with mild idiopathic anterior chamber inflammation. It is most often classified as secondary inflammatory glaucoma.

In 1948, Posner and Schlossman first recognized glaucomatocyclitic crisis and described the features of this syndrome. For this reason the entity is often termed Posner-Schlossman syndrome (PSS).

Most commonly, a "crisis" presents with slight discomfort. The patient may be pain-free even though the IOP is quite elevated. The patient may report blurred vision or halo vision if the IOP is high. A history of attacks of blurred vision lasting several days, which recur monthly or yearly, is usual. IOP is usually elevated in the range of 40 to 60 mm Hg.

The favored initial treatment for PSS is a combined regimen of a topical nonsteroidal antiinflammatory drug (NSAID, e.g., diclofenac) and an antiglaucoma drug such as timolol or dorzolamide. Prostaglandins are often avoided initially. Surgery is never indicated.

PRIMARY ANGLE-CLOSURE GLAUCOMA

Angle-closure glaucoma may be primary or secondary. Primary angle-closure glaucoma constitutes approximately 10% of all glaucoma cases and occurs in about 5% to 10% of the older adult population. In the general population a higher incidence of angle-closure glaucoma occurs in association with shallower anterior chambers. Angle-closure glaucoma shows increased incidence among Asians and Inuits and is less common among African Americans.

Patients with this disorder have essentially normal but often short (hyperopic) eyes with a shallow anterior chamber and a narrow entrance into the angle. Such crowding of the angle structure tends to occur more often in hyperopia and increases as the patient becomes older. The narrowing is mainly caused by the increased size of the crystalline lens as a cataract forms, which tends to push the entire iris diaphragm forward, narrowing the endocorneal angle of the anterior chamber to less than 20 degrees, thus enabling the term *narrow angle*.

A common trigger mechanism that brings about closure of a critically narrowed angle is dilation of the pupil. Pupil dilation relaxes the iris and causes its tissue to bunch up toward the base of the iris, thereby effectively blocking the angle outflow structures. Also, dilation of the pupil may relax the periphery of the iris sufficiently so that the pressure in the posterior chamber exceeds that in the anterior chamber, resulting in further forward displacement of the iris and crowding of the angle structures. If the pupillary border of the iris is bound down (as a result of inflammation) to the anterior lens capsule, or if the pupil is blocked by a prolapsed vitreous body, a pupillary block mechanism exists. This may lead to bowing of the iris, or iris bombé (Figure 25.5). In this situation the pupil is blocked so that the aqueous pressure from the posterior chamber bows the iris forward, thus blocking the angle of the anterior chamber and preventing fluid outflow.

An attack of acute angle-closure glaucoma can become fully developed within 30 to 60 minutes. The abruptness of the onset is so characteristic that a presumptive diagnosis of acute angle-closure glaucoma can virtually be made over the telephone. The attack commonly begins under conditions that lead to pupillary dilation, for example, conditions of dark adaptation (movie theaters), fear, or emotional arousal. Such attacks are often precipitated by dilation during an eye examination.

The pain can vary from a feeling of discomfort and fullness around the eyes to a severe, referred pain that can radiate to the back of the head or down toward the teeth. With severe pain the patient may be prostrate and nauseated and may even vomit. Vision is usually reduced and patients often report seeing halos as the result of a cloudy edematous cornea.

Certain drugs can also precipitate an attack, the most common being cyclopentolate and tropicamide. Other often used medications that can precipitate an attack are epinephrine derivatives. These drugs are frequently agents in common hay fever remedies, and the package insert indicates their contraindication in glaucoma; however, the phenylephrine derivative drugs are usually safe in open-angle glaucoma.

Examination reveals that the eyelids and conjunctiva are edematous and congested, especially around the limbus. The cornea appears steamy and hazy because of epithelial edema, which results from aggregations of tiny water droplets in the superficial layers of the cornea. The iris itself appears dull, gray, and patternless because of the edema. The pupil is typically middilated and may be oval. It does not respond normally to light. The IOP is often extremely high, in the range of 40 to 60 mm Hg or higher.

This type of ocular catastrophe is preceded in nearly half of cases by premonitory self-limiting episodes of aching blur, lasting a few hours each time and occurring with increasing frequency before an acute attack. Also, the patient may report seeing halos or rainbows around lights, which are caused by the slight edema of the cornea in these premonitory periods. These halos, although not pathognomonic of glaucoma, are most significantly related to this disease and are caused by dispersion of light by the epithelial edema. They are typically composed of two colored rings: an inner blue-violet ring and an outer yellow-red ring (Figure 25.6). Between attacks, little or no abnormality may be noted.

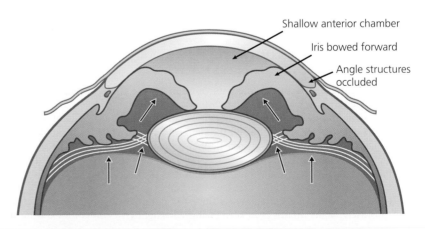

Figure 25.5 Pupillary block glaucoma. The pressure in the posterior chamber exceeds that of the anterior chamber. The iris is bowed forward (iris bombé) and occludes the angle structures. Without treatment the iris becomes permanently adherent to the angle structures and intractable secondary glaucoma ensues.

Shallow anterior chamber

Iris bowed forward

Angle structures occluded

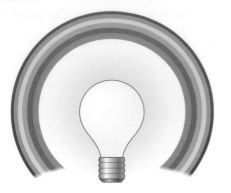

Figure 25.6 Halos around lights. This is a prominent symptom in angle-closure glaucoma. These colors are related to the spectral colors of light through water droplets in the cornea.

The halos caused by subacute attacks can be distinguished from the permanent halos caused by lens opacities by placing a stenopeic slit across the line of vision. A glaucoma halo remains intact but with diminished intensity behind the slit, whereas a lenticular halo is broken up into segments that revolve as the slit is moved. The halos that are sometimes caused by conjunctival debris can be swept away by movements of the lid.

Secondary angle-closure glaucoma occurs as a result of an underlying pathologic etiology.

The conditions that can lead to *secondary angle-closure glaucoma* are:

- Iritis or uveitis
- Lens dislocation
- Lens swelling
- Scar tissue or peripheral anterior synechiae between the iris and the trabecular meshwork
- Posterior synechiae to the lens
- Blockage of drainage channels by the accumulation of "flaky" protein or iris pigment

The most common cause of anterior synechiae is chronic angle-closure glaucoma and the most common cause of posterior synechiae is chronic, severe iritis.

CONGENITAL GLAUCOMA

Congenital glaucoma is an extremely uncommon disease. It is estimated that an average ophthalmologist is unlikely to see more than one new case of congenital glaucoma in 5 years of practice. Despite its rarity, the signs and symptoms of the disease are so characteristic that a diagnosis should not be missed.

Often the parents are aware that their baby has something wrong with the eye in the first few weeks or months of life. The child appears extremely sensitive to light and tears profusely. Many infants even keep their eyelids tightly closed most of the day to avoid the light. However, it is the corneal haziness caused by the corneal edema that makes most parents suspect that something is wrong with the child's eyes. Because the eyeball tissue is distensible in early infancy, the increased IOP causes progressive enlargement of the infant's eye and cornea. Most infant corneas measure less than 10.5 mm in horizontal diameter. A measurement greater than 12 mm is considered diagnostic of congenital glaucoma. These eyes, hazy and enlarged, appear so abnormal that the term *buphthalmos* has been commonly applied to designate this condition (see Figure 25.1).

It is important that any child with a symptom of tearing is seen immediately because the earlier glaucoma is diagnosed and brought under control, the better is the prognosis. In most cases tearing is caused by a blocked tear duct, but the ophthalmic assistant should always be aware of the possibility of congenital glaucoma.

DIAGNOSIS

Screening and aids in diagnosis

Screening for glaucoma

A comprehensive screening program consisting of tonometry, optic disc examination, and screening perimetry, although costly, helps detect and initiate early treatment to prevent vision loss. Screening programs that involve a single tonometer reading are inadequate because they miss many glaucoma patients. The over-referral rate of screening by pressure measurement alone is enormous, ranging from 10% to 30%, which means that large groups of patients undergo costly follow-up examinations. Also, some glaucoma cases are missed: low-tension glaucoma, diurnal variations in which higher pressures are not found during office visits, and angle-closure glaucoma in which the pressure may be normal between attacks. Usually the IOP criterion for a glaucoma referral is 21 mm Hg. Because structural damage precedes functional change, screening test results are vastly improved if one includes an inspection of the optic disc. This usually requires the services of an ophthalmologist or well-trained technician.

Open-angle glaucoma

In suspected cases of open-angle glaucoma in which the pressure is borderline and the disc is equivocal in appearance, the ophthalmologist may resort to provocative tests to determine the presence or absence of glaucoma.

Normally the IOP is greatest in the early morning and lowest during the day. This diurnal variation in the IOP seldom exceeds 3 or 4 mm Hg. However, in a glaucomatous patient it may exceed 7 to 8 mm Hg. In this test ocular tension measurements are taken throughout the day and sometimes during the night, noting times when the IOP is found to be highest. A drawback is that it is costly and time-consuming because the patient must be hospitalized for a full 24-hour diurnal test to be performed. Often checking a patient's pressures over the course of a day is adequate to find fluctuation, or bringing the patient back for pressure checks at various times in the day on subsequent visits can assist in determining large diurnal IOP variations.

Observation over time is the most widely used method of following glaucoma. In suspected cases patients usually are told that they have borderline glaucoma or that glaucoma is suspected and they are asked to return to the office on three or four occasions during the year. On these occasions the pressures are measured, the optic discs are examined, and the visual fields are tested. The ophthalmologist basically looks for an alteration in any one of these three parameters to confirm the diagnosis or determine the adequacy of control. The patient may show a pattern of gradually increasing pressures, increase in cupping of the disc, or an early glaucomatous field defect, which is an indication of the need to initiate or increase treatment.

Angle-closure glaucoma

The shallow-chambered, narrow-angled eye should be identified by a routine eye examination. The observer can easily see the convex iris diaphragm by illuminating the limbal area with a flashlight and noting the proximity of the iris periphery to the cornea. If there is any doubt as to whether the angle is narrowed, mydriatic drops such as cyclopentolate (Cyclogyl) or homatropine should not be used because they can, in such an eye, induce an attack of acute angle-closure glaucoma. It must also be emphasized that the finding of normal pressure by tonometry before dilation is no guarantee that this type of glaucoma will not ensue. The only method of assessing such an eye is by examination of the angles themselves with the use of the gonioscope.

Many tests provoke an angle-closure attack and therefore confirm the diagnosis of angle-closure glaucoma. The *dark room provocative test* is the time-honored method of revealing this condition. In this test the patient is kept in a dark room for 60 to 90 minutes, and the ocular pressure is subsequently measured. A rise of 8 mm Hg or more is considered a positive reaction. Unfortunately this test is not specific for predicting future angle-closure attacks and, although useful, is not relied on as much as the mydriatic test.

The *mydriatic test* for angle-closure glaucoma consists of instilling one or two drops of a weak-acting mydriatic agent, such as phenylephrine (Neo-Synephrine) 2.5%, into the conjunctival sac. Again, an 8 mm Hg rise in pressure by the end of 1 hour is considered a positive reaction in which gonioscopy confirms that the angle has narrowed and possibly closed during the period of pressure elevation.

Tonometry

Measuring IOP, or *tonometry*, is an essential part of all eye examinations for adults and children. The reason is simple:

routine tonometry can assist in detecting undiagnosed glaucoma. Glaucoma affects an estimated 3.5% of adults between the ages of 40 and 80, and the prevalence increases in individuals older than age 70; in fact, some investigations have found elevated IOP (greater than 21 mm Hg) in as many as 6.5% of normal individuals and 80% of untreated glaucoma patients.[1]

Because eye pressure measurement is such an important parameter to record, most ophthalmologists instruct their personnel to perform tonometry. It therefore behooves the ophthalmic assistant to understand the basic techniques and underlying physiologic principles of tonometry and to become comfortable, competent, and knowledgeable with it.

Eye pressure is not measured directly. It is simply not practical or safe to place a needle in the eye and record the actual IOP. Instead, the pressure is determined noninvasively. Noninvasive devices work via either an indentation or an applanation principle. Each method has advantages, as well as limitations, which are outlined in the following text.

The accuracy of either technique is limited by the physical properties of the cornea. During the actual measuring process, an indenting apparatus deforms the cornea more than an applanating one. Therefore, more aqueous fluid, normally in the anterior chamber of the eye between the cornea and the iris, is displaced by indentation. The displaced aqueous ultimately distends the other structures inside the eye. These intraocular structures have an inherent elastic property that resists distension; that is, the eye does not expand like a balloon, but rather its natural elastic qualities maintain a constant volume. Because the volume does not change, the pressure inside the eye must change. Thus the IOP as measured by indentation is "falsely" elevated. This phenomenon is well known, and calibration charts formulated to compensate for this abnormal false elevation of pressure are readily available.

The applanation technique differs from the indenting technique by displacing a lesser amount of fluid. Therefore, applanation tonometer-induced IOP elevation is a less significant concern but becomes a significant concern when corneal thickness is greater or lesser than the average for which the applanating device is calibrated. This is the major reason that many ophthalmologists believe applanation techniques are more accurate than the indentation procedure.

Applanation tonometry

In applanation tonometry the cornea is flattened and the flattened area is measured, or a specific known area is flattened and the amount of force needed to flatten this area is measured. (The word *applanation* originates from the Latin *planare* or *ad planare,* meaning "to flatten.") The higher the IOP (the harder the eye), the smaller the flattened area is, assuming that the same pressure is used for flattening each time tonometry is performed.

Applanation tonometry eliminates some of the errors inherent in indentation tonometry. Indentation tonometry creates pressure forces in the indented ocular wall and these forces act against the plunger of the tonometer. In addition, during indentation tonometry the considerable weight of the tonometer itself artificially raises the IOP. However, in applanation tonometry the pressure forces that are created in the applanated ocular wall are lying in the plane of applanation and oppose each other; thus they cancel each other for all practical purposes. Also in applanation tonometry the artificial increase of the IOP during tonometry caused by the weight of the tonometer is minimal. Another common source of error of indentation tonometry is underestimation of the IOP in eyes that have low "ocular rigidity," such as the eyes of myopes. Applanation minimizes this error.

Goldmann applanation tonometer

The Goldmann applanation tonometer, the most commonly used tonometer, enables a reliable measurement of IOP to within ±0.5 mm Hg. This tonometer, because it flattens or applanates the cornea and does not indent it, gives accurate information about the pressure in the undisturbed eye. Scleral rigidity can be disregarded because less than 0.5 mm of volume is displaced. It also causes little increase in pressure, so that minimal massage effect is produced by repeated measurements that might lower the pressure. A plastic tip is attached to a sensitive balance mounted on the slit lamp (Figure 25.7). This small tip is designed to minimize both the "inward" pull from the liquid tear film on the cornea and the "outward" push from the elastic cornea. The volume of displaced fluid inside

the eye is so small that any variation in ocular rigidity can be ignored. When the circular tip with a 3.06-mm diameter is used to applanate the cornea, no significant elevation of eye pressure is created.

One disadvantage of the Goldmann applanation tonometer is its lack of portability. However, handheld applanation tonometers have been devised. Other disadvantages are that the technique requires training for successful use. In addition, corneal distortion associated with conditions such as scarring or high astigmatism creates difficulty in obtaining reliable endpoint measurements. Corneal abrasions are always a potential hazard if the assistant is too aggressive during the pressure reading or if any underlying corneal problem is present. Infection is a potential risk as well, thus cleaning the tip or single-use tips are necessary.

The method of applanation tonometry is as follows: A drop of a local anesthetic solution is placed into the lower conjunctival sac. Then a drop of fluorescein from a fluorescein strip (small strips of filter paper impregnated with fluorescein) is instilled into the eye. Combination drops, which include both an anesthetic and fluorescein, are available. After the drop is instilled, the patient's head is positioned at the slit-lamp microscope with the chin on the chin rest and forehead pressed firmly against the headrest.

Once the cornea is in focus, the appropriate blue filter is used and the slit diaphragm is opened completely. In the beam the whole surface of the patient's eye should glow (fluoresce) in a bright greenish yellow. The blue light should be approximately 45 to 60 degrees to the side of the tonometer and should illuminate the front end of the prism head. The low magnification is used on the slit-lamp microscope.

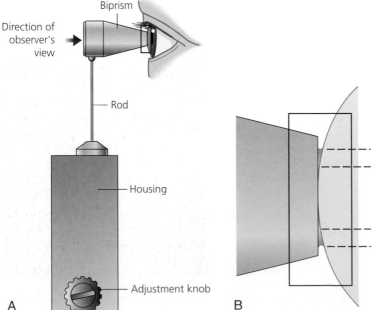

Figure 25.7 Goldmann applanation tonometry. (A) Basic features of tonometer, shown in contact with patient's cornea. (B) Enlargement of (A) shows tear film meniscus created by contact of biprism and cornea. *(From Shields MB, editor. Textbook of glaucoma. 4th ed. Baltimore: Williams & Wilkins; 1998.)*

Biprism

Direction of observer's view

Rod

Housing

Adjustment knob

A

B

The patient's lids must be open and unblinking. It is necessary to avoid any contact between the tonometer and the lid margin or lashes because this contact only induces further blinking. The patient is instructed to look straight ahead or at some target device attached to the slit lamp or the examiner's ear to ensure fixation. Once the patient is ready, the tonometer, with the measuring drum set at 1 g (1 on the dial), is brought forward by the joystick of the slit lamp until it comes into contact with the center of the cornea.

Looking through one eyepiece of the microscope, the examiner sees, at the moment of contact, a bright yellow-green spot that quickly separates into two bright yellow-green semicircular arcs as the tonometer is moved slightly farther forward. These arcs should be in sharp focus and of equal circumference both above and below the horizontal dividing line. Any necessary correction should be made by the control lever or the height adjustment control on the slit lamp. The calibrated drum on the side of the tonometer is then turned toward higher numbers corresponding to increasing force of applanation. As this occurs, the two semicircular arcs move until they overlap, the inner edge of the upper semicircle becoming aligned with the inner edge of the lower semicircle (Figure 25.8). This

is the desired endpoint at which the reading is taken from the drum.

The reading obtained is multiplied by 10 to convert the number to equivalent millimeters of mercury of IOP. Therefore, 1 on the drum is equal to 10 mm Hg. It is best to take at least two readings from each eye to obtain an average value. If the values obtained on two successive readings are approximately the same, the technique is probably adequate.

Checking the calibration of the Goldmann applanation tonometer

Applanation tonometers should be calibrated for accuracy by the use of a central weight regularly. For the Goldmann tonometer, a short rod of measured weight is attached to the balancing arm of the tonometer and the rod set at 0, 2, and 6 respectively. At each measure the measuring drum should be placed at the corresponding stop. At each stop the tonometer head should move only ±0.05 g (0.5 mm Hg) of these settings (Figure 25.9).

The applanation tonometer consists of a plastic removable tip that contains a prism. This tip has a flat anterior surface, which is brought into contact with a fluorescein-stained tear film of the cornea, which it displaces to the periphery of the contact zone until a surface of known and constant size, 3.06 mm, is flattened. The prism within the tip splits the image of this 3.06 mm circle into two semicircles. The inner border of the semicircles, when they are touching, represents the line of demarcation between the cornea flattened by applanation and the cornea not flattened. Thus this is the endpoint of the measurement of an applanation circle of 3.06 mm. This tip is connected to a spring device that allows measurement of the amount of pressure needed to flatten the cornea and is regulated by a knob on the side that has markings of this amount of pressure. The knob can regulate the spring tension to produce a force that is between 0 and 8 g. Once the inner semicircles are touching following turning the knob to apply adequate pressure to flatten the cornea, this number is read from the knob's outer ring.

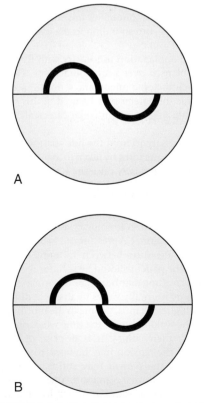

A

B

Figure 25.8 (A) Split half circles at beginning of applanation. Intraocular pressure is read when the inner half circles touch one another (endpoint), as shown in (B).

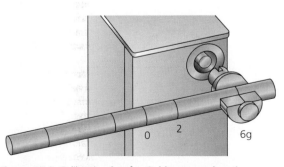

Figure 25.9 Calibration bar for Goldmann applanation tonometer.

Errors in Goldmann tonometry

1. If the fluorescein ring is too wide (Figure 25.10), too much fluorescein may have been instilled. In this case a small tissue can be used to absorb excess fluorescein and the procedure repeated. Alternatively, the measuring prism may not have been cleaned of previous fluorescein. A wide band results in an erroneous high reading.

2. If the fluorescein band is too narrow (Figure 25.11), evaporation of the stained tear layer during protracted measurement has occurred. The reading on the drum will be lower than normal. The patient should be told to blink several times and the measurement repeated.

3. The two semicircles may not be on the middle field (Figure 25.12). The patient may have moved slightly or the chin rest may not be properly adjusted; thus the fluorescein rings are not two exact semicircles because of incorrect centering of the tonometer head. This produces a considerably elevated IOP. The slit lamp should be adjusted up or down to obtain two exact semicircles.

4. If the patient's head is not pressed firmly against the forehead bar, there may be intermittent contact of the

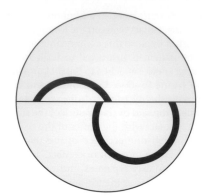

Figure 25.12 Unequal semicircles caused by incorrect centering of the tonometer head.

prism with the cornea, resulting in apparent pulsations of the fluorescein rings. However, note that the normal cardiac cycle pulsation can be seen as pulsation of the rings.

5. With a spherical or near-spherical cornea, measurement can be made in any meridian. However, if astigmatism greater than 3.00 diopters exists, the flattened area becomes elliptical rather than circular. In this instance the tonometer prism head should be set with the axis corresponding to the axis of the minus cylinder.

6. Standard applanation tonometry with fluorescein cannot be used over a soft contact lens. The MacKay-Marg tonometer, a pneumatic tonometer, or an electronic tonometer may be used in this situation.

7. Breath-holding or a tight collar can create a false high reading.

8. If it is necessary to hold the lids apart with the fingers and thumb, care must be taken to avoid pressing on the globe; this will falsely raise the IOP.

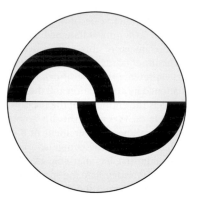

Figure 25.10 Too much fluorescein has been instilled.

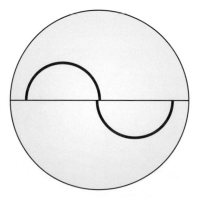

Figure 25.11 Too narrow a fluorescein band caused by too little fluorescein or evaporation of fluorescein.

Evaluating the pressures

If the pressure is found to be more than 21 mm Hg with the Goldmann applanation tonometer measurements, the eye is considered abnormal. A pressure of 21 should be regarded as borderline. Pressures between 18 and 21 are generally normal, but the patient should be seen for repeated examinations. This reading may be unsafe in corneas that are thin.

The pressure normally varies in an eye at different times of day. It is highest in most people in the morning and lowest during the waking hours, the time when ophthalmologists conduct their clinics. It is because of this diurnal variation that the tension may be borderline or less than borderline and the patient may still have glaucoma. In addition to the diurnal variation, there are other low-tension glaucomatous states in which the pressure recordings may be normal or even below normal and the patient may still have clinical evidence of the disease. Although applanation tonometry is the best method of discovering the most characteristic risk factor for glaucoma, it is not an infallible test, for the reasons mentioned.

As mentioned, elevated IOP without demonstrable damage to the optic nerve and without visual field changes is called *ocular hypertension*. These cases require relentless and meticulous repeated observations.

The monitoring of glaucoma requires an ongoing evaluation of pressure, optic disc assessment, and visual field change.

Hints for tonometry use

1. *Educate the patient.* Less anxiety is created if the examiner tells the patient that the tonometer tip will touch the tear film instead of saying the tip will actually touch the eye.
2. *Instill topical anesthetic.* Again, tell the patient what to expect: "This drop may feel cold or may even sting for a few seconds." Tell the patient to dab the eye with tissue paper, and to avoid rubbing or wiping the eye. After the anesthetic is given, touch the conjunctiva with a strip of fluorescein-impregnated paper. A drop of a combination topical anesthetic–fluorescein mixture such as Fluress can be used.
3. *Alignment.* Place the patient's chin on the rest and press the forehead against the headband. The patient's eyes should be open. Ask the patient to stare straight ahead and not at the blue slit light.
4. *Slit lamp and tonometer alignment.* Set the magnification on low (this is much easier to use). Position the tonometer with the plastic tip centered and position the light so that the tonometer tip is as brightly illuminated as possible—usually a 45-degree angle between the light and tip. Do not forget to use the blue filter! Remember, if corneal astigmatism is greater than 3.00 diopters, set the tip corresponding to the axis of the minus cylinder of the astigmatism (Figure 25.13).

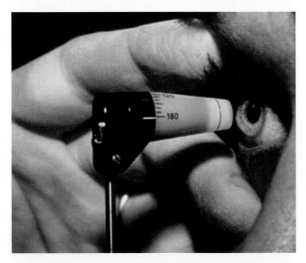

Figure 25.13 Markings on the tonometer head for alignment with high cylinders.

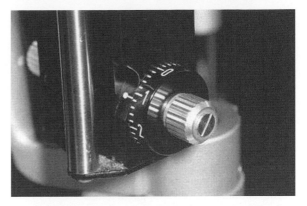

Figure 25.14 Tonometer scale is adjusted to align inner edges of the two fluorescein arcs on the cornea.

Move the slit lamp toward the patient, with the joystick held back. Once 3 to 5 mm away from the cornea, slowly advance the slit lamp forward with the joystick. At this point the examiner can look through the left eyepiece and begin to see a faint purple semicircle created by the reflected corneal image of the prism tip. These arcs will touch each other just before the tip actually touches the cornea.

5. *Align tonometer mires.* Just as the tip touches the cornea, two bright green semicircles appear. If this does not happen, pull the joystick back, recheck both patient and tonometer alignment, wipe the tip, and start again. If the semicircles are slightly out of line, alignment can be adjusted without repositioning the slit lamp.
6. Proper measurement depends on the two arcs being sharply focused, symmetric, and bright. Rotate the dial on the tonometer scale until the inner edges of the two arcs exactly align (Figure 25.14). To calculate the IOP, multiply the scale reading times 10. Pulsatile movements of the mires can be frustrating as the examiner tries to carefully touch the two inner edges together. A setting halfway between the two extreme pulse pressures will provide the truest pressure measurements.

Perkins handheld applanation tonometer

The principle of this instrument is the same as that of the Goldmann applanation tonometer, in that an applanating surface is placed in contact with the cornea and that force applied is varied until a fixed diameter of applanation is achieved. In the handheld instrument, the Goldmann doubling prism tip is mounted on a counterbalanced arm and the change in force is obtained by rotation of a spiral spring. The instrument operates on two AA batteries, and a tiny light bulb underneath the doubling prism gives off a cobalt blue glow. The instrument can be used in any position and need not be held vertically. The patient can be sitting or lying flat.

The method of use is as follows: The eye is anesthetized with one drop of a fluorescein solution (Fluress).

The tonometer should be held so that the thumb rests on the thumb wheel, controlling the spring. The light is switched on by turning the thumb wheel until the scale reading is above 0 and the filter holder is adjusted to illuminate the end of the doubling prism, when the latter is at approximately its midpoint of travel, which is the position used for measurement.

The instrument has a forehead rest that can be used when the tonometer is positioned on the patient's cornea. It is easier to hold the tonometer obliquely, with the handle slanted away from the patient's nose. Care should be taken that the prism is not touching the lids, in which case the readings obtained will be invalid.

The doubling prism is applied to the center of the patient's cornea, with the scale reading 1. Semicircles of fluorescein should now be visible through the viewing lens; force is adjusted by turning the thumb wheel until the inner margins of the semicircles coincide. The tonometer is then removed from the eye and the reading noted. The reading is multiplied by 10 to give the tension in millimeters of mercury. The usual method is to repeat the reading for each eye twice and, if elevated, to take three readings.

If the semicircles appear large and are not reduced by altering the force of the spring, the tonometer has been pushed too close to the eye. Withdrawing it slightly will bring the prism within the range of free movement.

Electronic applanation tonometer

Electronics represents the final adaptation of the applanation principle and is best represented by the MacKay-Marg tonometer or the Electro Medical Technology tonometer. With this technique, as the tip is applied to the eye, the pressure flexes an ultrathin membrane. This pressure is indirectly transmitted to a force transducer. The pressure waveform is converted into electrical impulses proportional to the applied pressure and recorded on a graph with a thermal stylus. This original device is no longer available, but several miniaturized versions that function on similar principles have been developed and appear accurate and reliable.

Other applanation tonometers

Several lightweight, portable, handheld tonometers are available. One of them, the Tono-Pen (Figure 25.15), is a pen-like instrument that permits repeated accurate reading by applanation. It is a very useful instrument that incorporates its own battery power supply and digital readout and provides both an IOP reading and an indicator of the reliability of the value. The results correlate well with the Goldmann tonometer, although it slightly overestimates low IOPs and underestimates high IOPs. It can take measurements in an eye with an irregular or edematous cornea or through a soft contact lens in a variety of clinical settings because the area of applanation is much smaller than with the Goldmann applanation tonometer. Also available are applanation tonometers that can measure the IOPs

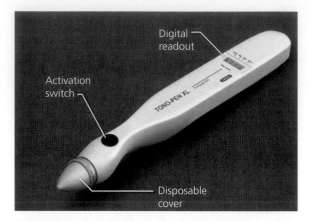

Figure 25.15 The Tono-Pen XL to measure intraocular pressure. *(From Thomsen TW, et al. Measurement of intraocular pressure: Tono-Pen technique. © Copyright 2011 Elsevier Inc.)*

through use of an operating room microscope. This operating room device allows the surgeon to estimate whether the IOP is high, medium, or low at the end of intraocular surgery. Another is the AccuPen, a handheld tonometer that uses high-resolution, real-time waveform analysis to provide accurate IOP measurements. It uses gravity offset technology, which requires less calibration compared with other handheld tonometers. The user enters the central corneal thickness and the AccuPen creates an adjusted IOP.

Icare tonometer

The Icare rebound tonometer uses a tiny plastic-tipped, single-use probe surrounded by a magnetic field. A magnetic coil "fires" the probe forward onto the cornea, creating a very small applanation region. The time it takes the probe to return to its resting position is indicative of the IOP. The contact time is so brief that often no anesthetic is used.

Dynamic contour tonometer

The dynamic contour tonometer (DCT) is a digital tonometer that provides a direct transcorneal measurement of IOP. This tonometer is based on the principle that, by surrounding and matching the contour of a sphere, the pressure on the outside equals the pressure on the inside. In the DCT, the tip of the probe matches the contour of the cornea. A pressure transducer built into the center of the probe measures the outside pressure, which should equal the inside pressure, and the IOP is recorded digitally. The DCT eliminates the systematic errors inherent in other tonometers, such as the influence of corneal thickness and rigidity.

Indentation tonometry (Schiøtz tonometry)

Although Schiøtz tonometry has been largely replaced by applanation, it remains useful for general practitioners, hospitals, and less affluent countries.

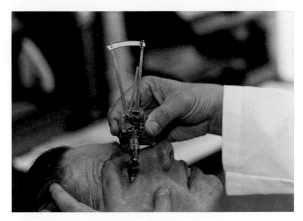

Figure 25.16 Measurement of intraocular pressure with Schiøtz tonometer. Note that the lids are pinioned against the bony orbit by the examiner's fingers.

The Schiøtz tonometer has been used historically for the detection and determination of IOP because it is convenient to use, portable, fairly reliable, and low in cost. It is not dependent on batteries, electricity, or a slit-lamp biomicroscope.

When the Schiøtz tonometer is used, the patient is usually placed in a recumbent position and asked to look up at a fixation point directed vertically above (Figure 25.16). The corneas are anesthetized with a topical anesthetic such as proparacaine. If the blinking motion is excessive, the examiner may pinion the lids against the margin of the orbit with his or her fingers, taking care not to press on the globe itself. The tonometer is allowed to rest on the patient's cornea, and the extent to which the plunger of the tonometer indents the cornea is, indirectly, a measure of IOP. The greater the distance the plunger indents the cornea, the softer is the eye or the lower the IOP. This is recorded on a scale on which the reading reflects the excursion distance of the plunger. If the eye is soft, as the Schiøtz tonometer plunger moves, the recording needle moves farther along the scale located at the top of the tonometer. The higher the scale reading, the lower the eye pressure. Conversely, minimal excursion of the plunger suggests that the eye is firm and the IOP high.

The indicator on the tonometer points to the scale readings of the tonometer. Converting from scale readings with Schiøtz tonometry to millimeters of mercury requires a conversion table or graph (Table 25.2). This is usually supplied with the instrument. This chart converts plunger excursion into IOP (millimeters of mercury), which is designated P_o, the true eye pressure before the tonometer is placed on the cornea. Once the tonometer rests on the eye, an abnormally high pressure is created and this is often referred to as P_1.

Intuitively the ophthalmologist realizes that significant limitations are present when indentation or Schiøtz tonometry is performed. The possibility of false readings deserves special mention. Schiøtz tonometry raises pressure inside the eye by indenting its surface. The tonometer weight is sufficient not only to double the IOP but also to displace a significant volume of aqueous in the anterior chamber. This point is important because any variation in ocular rigidity or scleral elasticity could lead to an inaccurate pressure reading (Figures 25.17 and 25.18).

Several clinical situations exist in which the Schiøtz tonometer can give such erroneous information. For example, a child's eye is usually quite elastic. This distensible quality is important when the amount of growth that occurs in a child's early years is taken into consideration. The eye's elastic property means the eye wall (cornea plus sclera) has a low ocular rigidity. This is where the Schiøtz tonometer may provide inaccurate results.

Indentation or Schiøtz tonometry counts on a predictable change in the eye wall elasticity. If an unexpected change occurs, the anticipated movement of the indenting plunger will be altered and an expansion in the eye wall size will occur instead. This problem may occur with highly myopic (near-sighted) patients, who commonly have a low ocular rigidity because the sclera is thinner and stretched. When a Schiøtz tonometer is used, the elasticity of this myopic eye does not resist the "normal" shift in aqueous fluid. The anticipated tonometer-induced (P_1) pressure rise is blunted and an erroneous low IOP reading is recorded. These errors may be reduced by making two measurements, each with a different weight, such as the 5.5- or 10-g weight, on the tonometer. When a difference of 3 mm or more is found, an error involving scleral rigidity should be suspected. Nomogram charts are available to calculate the IOP from a scale that compensates for different scleral rigidity.

In recording pressures, the heavier weights must be used when higher pressures are recorded. For routine use, the 5.5- and 7.5-g weights are adequate. With the 5.5-g weight a finding of 3 units or less on the scale indicates the need for further investigation for glaucoma. In all instances, if the IOP is high or even suspect, the patient should be checked by applanation tonometry.

Thus glaucoma should be suggested in any patient with an applanation reading of 21 mm Hg or more, a reading of 3 scale units or less using Schiøtz tonometry, and a family history of glaucoma, because there is a high percentage of glaucoma (approximately 30%) among patients with a family history of this disease.

The Schiøtz tonometer requires a great deal of maintenance to ensure that its parts are working properly. The applanation tonometer, being a simpler design, does not require the same type of constant care. Before its use, the Schiøtz tonometer should be checked by placing it on the zero test block provided, to make sure that the indicator properly comes to rest at zero. Scale readings of 3 or less are not reliable. If the scale reading is too low, a heavier weight should be used. The commonly used weights are 5.5, 7.5,

Table 25.2 Calibration scale for Schiøtz tonometers

Tonometer reading	Pressure (mm Hg)				Tonometer reading	Pressure (mm Hg)			
	5.5 g	7.5 g	10 g	15 g		5.5 g	7.5 g	10 g	15 g
0.0	41.5	59.1	81.7	127.5	10.0	7.1	10.9	16.5	29.6
0.5	37.8	54.2	75.1	117.9	10.5	6.5	10.0	15.1	27.4
1.0	34.5	49.8	69.3	109.3	11.0	5.9	9.0	13.8	25.3
1.5	31.6	45.8	64.0	101.4	11.5	5.3	8.3	12.6	23.3
2.0	29.0	42.1	59.1	94.3	12.0	4.9	7.5	11.5	21.4
2.5	26.6	38.8	54.7	88.0	12.5	4.4	6.8	10.5	19.7
3.0	24.4	35.8	50.6	81.8	13.0	4.0	6.2	9.5	18.1
3.5	22.4	33.0	46.9	76.2	13.5		5.6	8.6	16.5
4.0	20.6	30.4	43.4	71.0	14.0		5.0	7.8	15.1
4.5	18.9	28.0	40.2	66.2	14.5		4.5	7.1	13.7
5.0	17.3	25.8	37.2	61.8	15.0		4.0	6.4	12.6
5.5	15.9	23.8	34.4	57.6	15.5			5.8	11.4
6.0	14.6	21.9	31.8	53.6	16.0			5.2	10.4
6.5	13.4	20.1	29.4	49.9	16.5			4.7	9.4
7.0	12.2	18.5	27.2	46.5	17.0			4.2	8.5
7.5	11.2	17.0	25.1	43.2	17.5				7.7
8.0	10.2	15.6	23.1	40.2	18.0				6.9
8.5	9.4	14.3	21.3	38.1	18.5				6.2
9.0	8.5	13.1	19.6	34.6	19.0				5.6
9.5	7.8	12.0	18.0	32.0	19.5				4.9
					20.0				4.5

and 10 g. It is extremely important not to switch the 5.5-g weight from one Schiøtz tonometer to another because these weights are calibrated to the individual instrument. The lower the scale reading, the higher the pressure is in terms of millimeters of mercury.

In day-to-day use it is important that the tonometer be kept clean so that the plunger moves freely and the curvature of the footplate is not altered by foreign material. Cleanliness is maintained by disassembling the parts and washing the well of the instrument using a pipe cleaner or a brush moistened with alcohol or ether. The other parts, such as the plunger itself, are cleaned with a cotton cloth and alcohol.

Most ophthalmologists do not sterilize their tonometer. If desired, however, the base of the instrument can be sterilized by using a flame or burner, gaseous sterilization chamber, or small disposable rubber caps (Tonofilms) applied over the base of the instrument. Some ophthalmologists house the tonometer in an ultraviolet sterilizer. If possible, tonometry should be avoided on infected eyes as prevention against spread of the infectious organisms.

Concern has been raised regarding tonometry and the potential transmissibility of infectious diseases, especially the acquired immunodeficiency syndrome (AIDS) virus (human immunodeficiency virus [HIV]) and the hepatitis virus. Although the AIDS virus has been isolated in the tears of patients with known AIDS, the infectivity of the virus through tears appears low because there are no known instances in which the virus has been transmitted in this manner. The concern about transmissibility, however, has led to recommendations for the sterilization of contact tonometer tips. It is recommended that gloves be used when high-risk patients are examined, especially if the examiner has scratches or skin lesions on the hands.

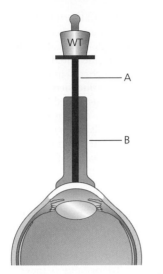

Figure 25.17 Principle of indentation tonometer. (A) Plunger to indent cornea. (B) Frame resting on cornea.
(From Reinecke R, Stein H, Slatt B. Introductory manual for the ophthalmic assistant. St Louis: Mosby; 1972.)

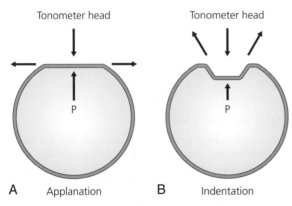

Figure 25.18 Comparison of applanation and indentation tonometry. (A) In applanation tonometry the cornea is flattened and the pressure is distributed evenly on each side; the pressure measurement is very close to that of the undisturbed eye. (B) Indentation of the cornea causes buckling of the ocular coats because of the oblique distribution of pressure.

Instruments contacting the external eye surfaces should be wiped clean and disinfected with either hydrogen peroxide 3% for 10 minutes or a 1:10 dilution of liquid bleach (5000 parts per million). Bleach may remove the printed markings on the plastic tonometer tip. Ethanol or isopropanol 70% is an effective disinfectant, but both agents will discolor the plastic and create a haze on its surface.

Patient preparation

The patient should be comfortable, well anesthetized with drops (proparacaine), and relaxed. Fixation should be maintained on one spot. Coughing, breath holding, and wandering eye movements make pressure recordings inaccurate. The most common error in Schiøtz tonometry results from the patient's squeezing the lids together, thus either preventing the easy application of the tonometer to the cornea or gripping it like a vise. In such situations, the lids should be manually opened by the examiner without any pressure on the globe. At the same time, the patient is asked to open his or her mouth and take a deep breath. This last maneuver serves to distract the patient and also takes advantage of a primitive reflex that prevents forceful closure of the lids with the mouth held wide open.

Comparison of the Schiøtz tonometer and the applanation tonometer

1. The Schiøtz tonometer indents the cornea, whereas the applanation tonometer flattens it.
2. The Schiøtz tonometer is portable; the conventional applanation tonometer is not. The Tono-Pen applanation tonometer is also conveniently portable.
3. The Schiøtz tonometer measures the amount of corneal indentation produced by a given weight; the applanation tonometer measures the amount of force required to produce a constant corneal flattening.
4. The Schiøtz tonometer raises the IOP because of indentation and the weight of the instrument itself; the applanation tonometer exerts only a small force on the cornea.
5. The Schiøtz tonometer may give an inaccurate measure because of the distortion of ocular coats. The footplate of the instrument is shaped to the average corneal curvature, but most patients' corneas are not exact fits. This poor fit introduces errors. Readings with the applanation tonometer are relatively independent of the rigidity of the ocular coats and are unaffected by corneal curvature variations.
6. Because of the buckling of the cornea and the resultant displacement of aqueous humor by the Schiøtz tonometer, second and third readings may be slightly lower as a result of massage of aqueous humor out of the eye. This does not occur with the applanation tonometer.
7. The Schiøtz tonometer measures tension with the patient in the recumbent position, whereas the conventional applanation tonometer measures tension with the patient in the sitting position. The new handheld applanation tonometer can be used with the patient in any position.
8. The Schiøtz tonometer can be used for tonography; the applanation tonometer cannot.

Noncontact tonometers

These tonometers measure IOP without coming into contact with the eye (Figure 25.19). Essentially, an air pump blows a calibrated jet or puff of air onto the cornea,

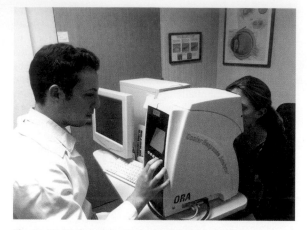

Figure 25.19 American Optical noncontact applanation tonometer. A jet of air flattens the cornea and pressure is recorded electronically.

flattening and thereby applanating it. It works on the principle of an interval timer, measuring the time it takes from the generation of the puff of air to the point at which the cornea is exactly flat; this time (usually about 3 ms) can be related directly to the IOP. Infrared light and detectors determine when the cornea is flat, at which point the timing device stops. It takes less time for the puff of air to flatten a soft eye than it does a hard one and hence an accurate relationship between time and IOP can be established. Digital readout numbers indicate the pressure in millimeters of mercury. This is an excellent screening device that can be used by the ophthalmic assistant; its regular use ensures a fair degree of accuracy in screening. However, the air puff tonometer tends to err slightly on the high side, so positive results (high pressures) should be rechecked with another tonometer such as a Goldmann tonometer. The noncontact tonometer is ideal as a scaling tool because it eliminates contact with the cornea and therefore any threat of abrasion, infection, or topical anesthetic reactions. The major drawback is the cost of the instrument. Examples of noncontact tonometers include the Pulsair tonometer, the Reichert Pneumatonometer, and the Reichert Ocular Response Analyzer.

Home use tonometers are also being introduced for patients to monitor their pressures at home. The accuracy of current models is not comparable to office-based devices.

Ocular response analyzer

The ocular response analyzer (ORA) is a recently developed device that uses bidirectional applanation to determine three calculated values: a Goldmann-correlated IOP, corneal "hysteresis," and "excess ocular pressure." It has been proven that "hard" corneas tend to cause an artificially high IOP, whereas "soft" corneas do the opposite. For this reason, the ORA records two applanation events: one while the cornea is moving inward and the other while it is

moving outward. This bidirectional applanation allows for the calculation of a value called *corneal hysteresis,* which relates to the influence that corneal rigidity has on the IOP. The average hysteresis measured is typically 5 mm Hg. Those measurements higher than this value indicate stiffer corneas, whereas lower values denote softer corneas. By calculating the IOP and hysteresis, the ORA can analyze what the intraocular pressure would be without the influence of the corneal thickness. This excess ocular pressure (EOP) is a value determined without the influence of corneal rigidity and may be a better indicator of the true IOP.

Tonography

Tonography is a technique to measure the outflow facility of an eye (i.e., how easily aqueous exits). It is based on the principle that pressing on an eye lowers the IOP. This effect is rapid in a normal eye, but occurs much more slowly in a glaucomatous eye. Tonography is indentation tonometry maintained over time (usually 3 minutes) to measure the "massaging" effect of a tonometer to express fluid from the eye. The measurement of outflow facility is a means of measuring the increased resistance to aqueous outflow, common to most open-angle glaucoma. Tonography is rarely used in client practice today, but offers the ophthalmologist three important pieces of information: the P_o or the IOP in the undisturbed eye, the flow of aqueous into the eye, and the C value or facility of outflow. The P_o:C ratio has been found to be helpful. A P_o:C ratio greater than 140 usually means a diagnosis of glaucoma in 90% of cases.

Water-drinking test

The water-drinking test used to be popular but has fallen out of favor because of a lack of specificity. Briefly, a rise in ocular tension of 8 to 10 mm Hg after the rapid ingestion of 1 quart of water suggests glaucoma. A negative reaction does not rule out this condition. This test was often coupled with tonography because the number of positive reactions is very high in the combined test.

Gonioscopy

Gonioscopy is a clinical technique used to examine the structures of the anterior chamber angle. With this technique one can differentiate between the two major types of glaucoma: open-angle and angle-closure glaucoma.

Normally light rays coming from the anterior chamber angle are reflected back into the anterior chamber, preventing the visualization of the angle. A lens in contact with the cornea is used to alter the optical surface and enable visualization of the angle structures.

Two major types of lenses are used in gonioscopy: a "direct" goniolens and an "indirect," mirrored lens (Figure 25.20). The *direct goniolens* is used primarily for infants, and is applied with the patient in the supine position. A viscous preparation

Figure 25.20 Scheie's gonioscopic classification of the anterior chamber angle, based on the extent of visible angle structures. (A) Root of the iris. (B) Ciliary body band. (C) Scleral spur. (D) Trabecular meshwork. (E) Schwalbe's line.

(From Shields MB, editor. Textbook of glaucoma. 4th ed. Baltimore: Williams & Wilkins; 1998.)

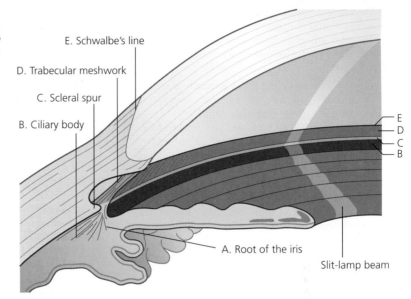

E. Schwalbe's line

D. Trabecular meshwork

C. Scleral spur

B. Ciliary body

A. Root of the iris

Slit-lamp beam

such as methylcellulose is placed between the lens and the cornea. The gonioscope is held in one hand and the light source in the other. This type of goniolens is also useful for surgical procedures on angle structures, such as goniotomy. In indirect gonioscopy the light rays are reflected by mirrors in the contact lens (the *gonioprism*). The mirrors are usually inclined at an angle between 55 and 65 degrees. Frequently some mirrors are tilted at a steeper angle to permit examination of the peripheral retina (Figure 25.21).

In the four-mirrored lens, each of the mirrors is tilted at 64 degrees to permit examination of the angle without rotating the lens. Such lenses may be applied to the tear film directly or with methylcellulose. Several gonioscopic lenses are pictured in Figure 25.22.

The technique of using the goniolens is as follows. A topical anesthetic is applied to the eye and with some goniolenses, goniolens gel is applied to the lens to optically couple the lens to the cornea. With other goniolenses the patient's tear film is adequate to optically couple the lens. The lens is applied directly with the lids held apart. Examination of the angle is performed with the slit-lamp biomicroscope. Once the examination is over, the lens should be cleaned with warm water and soap, then wiped gently with alcohol and allowed to air dry before placing it away. Never

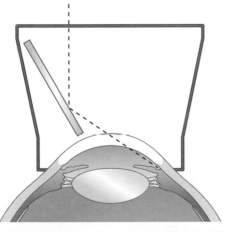

Figure 25.21 Indirect goniolens. A beam of light is deflected into the opposite angle of the anterior chamber by a mirror that is angled 55 to 65 degrees.

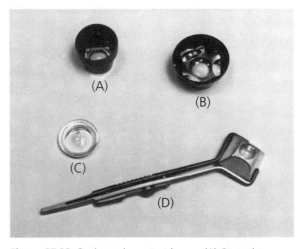

Figure 25.22 Gonioscopic contact lenses. (A) One-mirror Goldmann. (B) Three-mirror Goldmann. (C) Koeppe. (D) Handheld Zeiss.

(From Stamper RL, Lieberman MF, Drake MV. Becker-Shaffer's diagnosis and therapy of the glaucomas. 8th ed. St Louis: Mosby Elsevier; 2009.)

place a recently alcohol-wiped lens onto a patient's cornea because this would damage the corneal epithelium.

The normal anterior chamber angle as seen through gonioscopy reveals the following structures from posterior to anterior:

1. *The ciliary body band.* The band is usually gray or dark and depends on the level above the iris insertion. It is a little wider in people who are myopic.
2. *The scleral spur.* This is seen as a prominent white line between the ciliary body band and the trabecular meshwork. Fine pigmented strands crossing the scleral spur may frequently be visible. These are the iris processes.
3. *Trabecular meshwork.* This is a pigmented band just anterior to the scleral spur. The appearance of the trabecular meshwork is variable. Usually it gathers pigment as an age-related change. The color is anywhere from tan to a dark brown that may be irregular and more mottled in appearance.
4. *Schwalbe's line,* which demonstrates the meeting of corneal endothelium and trabecular meshwork at the internal junction of cornea and sclera. This is viewed as a fine ridge just anterior to the trabecular meshwork.

Figure 25.23 shows the gonioscopic anatomy of a normal adult anterior chamber angle, showing the gonioscopic appearance and cross-sectional appearance.

Oblique flashlight illumination, with the light coming from the temporal side of the eye, gives a fairly accurate evaluation of the depth of the anterior chamber. With a deep chamber the entire iris is illuminated. If the iris is bowed forward, its distal portions beyond the pupil are in the shadows.

Gonioscopy is still the most valued technique used to evaluate the anterior chamber angle. Most of these evaluations are concerned with the angular width of the angular recess. This is largely based on the extent of the angle structures that can be visualized. Angles are recorded according to a grading system. The Shaffer grading system is based on angularity and uses a number system from 0 to 4, with grade 4 being wide open (Figure 25.24). The Scheie system is based on the anatomic structures of the angle and also uses a number system from 0 to 4. However, the system is the opposite of the Shaffer system, with grade 4 as narrow (Table 25.3).

Pupillary dilation plus gonioscopy provides the most thorough basis for confirmation of angle-closure glaucoma. After the pupil of one eye is dilated with a weak mydriatic agent, tonographic examination is performed in dim light. A decrease of 25% to 30% in the facility of outflow, if coupled with gonioscopic evidence of angle closure, is considered a position reaction.

A negative provocative test reaction certainly does not rule out the possibility of the patient's ever having an angle-closure glaucoma attack. The most important diagnostic investigation into this condition is the use of gonioscopy (see Figure 25.22 and Table 25.3). If the angles are unduly narrowed despite negative provocative test reactions, the patient should be observed closely or preventive laser iridotomy performed.

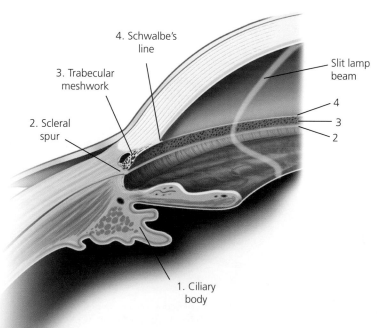

4. Schwalbe's line

3. Trabecular meshwork

2. Scleral spur

1. Ciliary body

Slit lamp beam

4

3

2

Figure 25.23 Gonioscopic anatomy of normal adult anterior chamber angle showing gonioscopic appearance *(right)* and cross-section of corresponding structures *(left)*. (1) Ciliary body band. (2) Scleral spur. (3) Trabecular meshwork. (4) Schwalbe's line.

(Modified from Shields MB, editor. Textbook of glaucoma. 2nd ed. Baltimore: Williams & Wilkins; 1987.)

Figure 25.24 Shaffer classification of anterior chamber angle, based on angular width of angle recess.

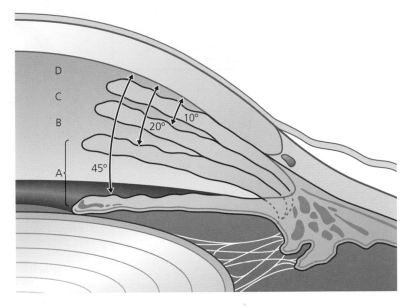

Angle width/Grade	Numeric Grade*
(A) → 4	4
(B) → 3	3
(C) → 2	2 or 1
(D) → 1	Slit or closed

*These grades are assigned to various portions of the angle.

Table 25.3 Classification of angles based on gonioscopic appearance (Scheie's classification)

Classification	Appearance
Wide open	All angle structures seen
Grade I narrow	Difficult to see over the iris root
Grade II narrow	Ciliary band obscured
Grade III narrow	Posterior trabeculum hazy
Grade IV narrow	Only Schwalbe's line visible

Modified from Shields MB, editor. Textbook of glaucoma. 3rd ed. Baltimore: Williams & Wilkins; 1991.

Corneal thickness

The role of corneal thickness is being assessed today. In understanding the patient's actual IOP, thin corneas may place patients under greater risks. Corneal thickness or pachymetry is measured by a pachymeter. Conventional pachymeters are devices that display the thickness of the cornea, usually in micrometers, when the ultrasonic transducer touches the cornea. Newer generations of ultrasonic pachymeters work by way of corneal waveform (CWF). With this technology the user can capture an ultrahigh definition echogram of the cornea. Pachymeter measurement should be performed on all glaucoma patients and suspects. It is known that thinner corneas, such as in patients who have had laser refractive surgery, may give a false lower IOP value by standard Goldmann applanation tonometry.

It has been suggested that in thin corneas the tonometer readings should be corrected to account for the inherent measurement errors (Table 25.4). For example, if a patient has a corneal thickness of 445, which is not uncommon following laser refractive surgery, one must add a factor of 7 mm Hg to the measured IOP. These correction tables are not reliably accurate and should be used only as guides.

On the other hand, a thicker than normal cornea decreases the risk. Basically this means that if corneas are thin, one may have to initiate treatment earlier because the true IOP is higher than initially recorded.

Structural: optic nerve

Examination of the optic disc

Inspection of the optic disc is key to diagnosing glaucoma. Because of an abnormal IOP, the cumulative effect of sustained pressure results in atrophy of the retinal ganglion cells and of the optic nerve at its exit from the eye, called the optic *disc* (Figures 25.25 and 25.26). These changes consist of "cupping" and "pallor" of the optic disc. *Cupping*, which is usually manifested on the temporal aspect of the optic disc, results in the central retinal vessels dipping down over a saucerized edge at the margin of the disc, instead of crossing it smoothly. With glaucomatous atrophy, the central disc also may appear pale.

Glaucoma specialists follow the course of changes in the optic disc at regular intervals by several techniques: by drawing or photographing the disc and noticing changes over time and by using devices to scan the optic disc or the nerve fiber layer of the retina, which contains the axons that travel from the ganglion cells in the inner retina to comprise the optic nerve. These axons terminate in a part

Table 25.4 Corrected IOP for corneal thickness

Corneal thickness (μm)	Correction value (mm Hg)
445	+7
455	+6
465	+6
475	+5
485	+4
495	+4
505	+3
515	+2
525	+1
535	+1
545	0
555	−1
565	−1
575	−2
585	−3
595	−4
605	−4
615	−5
625	−6
635	−6
645	−7

Courtesy of Sonogage.
Correction values according to corneal thickness of 545 μm.
Arithmetic mean of corneal thickness in healthy subjects: 545 μm (Doughty and Zaman, 2000).
IOP, Intraocular pressure.
Calculation based on data of Ehlers et al. (1975). Modified from Stodtmeister (1998).

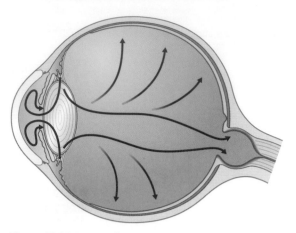

Figure 25.25 Increased pressure causes excavation of optic disc.

the edge of the optic disc are other important indicators of damage to the neural tissue. Normally the cups are symmetric; significant asymmetry can indicate glaucoma. When the neural rim becomes severely atrophied, the retinal vessels crossing the sharpened rim are acutely angulated at the edge of the disc. The ultimate course in this process is advanced glaucomatous cupping, in which all the neural rim tissue is eventually lost. This is seen as a pale white disc with thinning of all the vessels at the sharp margin of the disc.

Evaluation of the optic cups requires practice (Figure 25.27). Normal variations include large discs with large cups but normal numbers of nerve fibers passing through and tilted discs, often associated with myopia. Atrophy of the sclera near the disc and hereditary "colobomas" or notches of the optic nerve, with loss of optic neural tissue, can mimic variations of the normal appearance of the optic cup and may confuse the examiner. These discs may appear cupped and yet be normal.

Because of the difficulties of evaluating progressive glaucomatous optic neuropathy by direct observation, use techniques such as serial photography and scanning devices (such as optical coherence tomography [OCT] and the Heidelberg retina tomograph [HRT]) that attempt to measure objective change to detect structural change caused by glaucoma before functional changes such as visual field loss are detected. These better enable one to compare the appearance of the optic disc and nerve fiber layer at one visit with that at another time. Stereo photographs can be taken by shooting two photos in sequence by using prisms that create two pictures. Devices for optic disc imaging can provide reliable images of the depth of the cupping. By repeating the imaging, one can detect subtle changes in the disc and a computer can provide an analysis of these changes.

The nerve fiber layer

The nerve fiber layer—the layer of axons that travel from ganglion cells in the inner retina through the optic nerve

of the brain called the *lateral geniculate*. The fibers going through the optic nerve are called the *neural rim*. The depression in the center of the optic disc is termed the *optic cup*. The ratio of the cup to the disc is used to follow the progress of changes in the optic nerve head. There is a very large variation of the cup-to-disc ratio in the normal population; however, the documentation of progressive cupping is one of the most important clinical findings in glaucoma. The optic cup normally has a horizontal oval shape. Thus the detection of vertical elongation suggests glaucoma. Notching, pallor, and small hemorrhages at

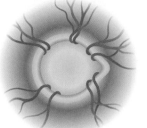
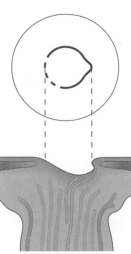

A

cup-to-disc ratio: >0.5

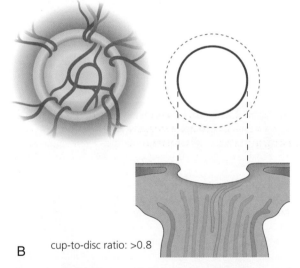

B   cup-to-disc ratio: >0.8

Figure 25.26 (A) Diagram of moderately cupped disc. Dotted line indicates a sloping edge; solid line, undetermined edge of the cup. (B) Diagram of markedly cupped disc.
(From Stamper, RL. Becker-Shaffer's diagnosis and therapy of the glaucomas. 7th ed. St Louis: Mosby; 1999.)

to terminate in the lateral geniculate—is damaged early in glaucoma; 25% to 40% of these nerve fibers can be lost in an eye that appears to maintain a normal visual field. The damage can be seen as a wedge-shaped sector loss of nerve fibers crossing the retina to end at the optic nerve. Injury to the nerve fiber layer can be observed long before visual field defects are seen. Therefore, objectively monitoring structural changes in the thickness of the nerve fiber layer and in the cupping of the optic disc by means of these devices enables earlier detection of change in glaucoma and

allows physicians to better monitor their therapeutic effects to prevent the irreversible tissue and vision loss of glaucoma.

Stereo photography

Stereoscopic photographs of the fundus can be obtained by taking successive photographs and altering the optical axis of the camera between exposures. Several different methods for altering the optical axis exist, including rotating the camera, shifting the camera laterally, moving the patient's fixation, and altering the direction of the optical system by a prism that creates two pictures. Using a prism has the advantage that a change in the direction of the light pathway can be made rapidly, thereby enabling the photographer to match up the images in intensity of illumination and focus. An additional advantage is that throughout the procedure the patient's fixation and the camera remain stationary. It is helpful that the patient's eyes are dilated. With the prism in one lateral position, the image is focused and taken. The prism is then rotated to the opposite lateral position to give a beam separation of 3 to 5 mm. The two pictures may be viewed manually with a stereoviewer or by a computer monitor through goggles using three-dimensional (3-D) software.

Optical coherence tomography (for additional information see Chapter 39)

Optical coherence tomography (OCT) is a technique for obtaining subsurface images of translucent or opaque materials at a resolution equivalent to a low-power microscope. It is effectively "optical ultrasound," imaging reflections from within tissue to provide cross-sectional images. OCT provides tissue morphology imagery at much higher resolution (better than 10 µm) than other imaging modalities such as magnetic resonance imaging (MRI) or ultrasound. This noncontact test is usually performed by the ophthalmic assistant and can be accomplished in minutes. OCT scans frequently can be performed with undilated pupils, some as small as 3 mm.

OCT delivers high resolution because it is based on high-frequency light rather than lower-frequency sound or radio waves. An optical beam is directed at the tissue, and a small portion of this light that reflects from subsurface features is collected. Note that most light is not reflected but rather scatters. The scattered light has lost its original direction and does not contribute to forming an image but contributes to *glare*. Using the OCT technique, scattered light can be filtered out, completely removing the glare.

The proportion of reflected light that is not scattered can then be detected and used to form an image in, for example, a scanning OCT system. The physics principle allowing the filtering of scattered light is optical coherence. *Only* the reflected (nonscattered) light is coherent. In the OCT instrument, an optical interferometer is used in such a manner as to detect *only* coherent light. Essentially the

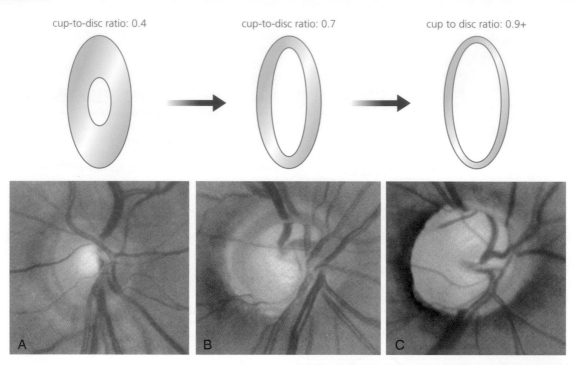

cup-to-disc ratio: 0.4   cup-to-disc ratio: 0.7   cup to disc ratio: 0.9+

A   B   C

Figure 25.27 Progressive cupping or increasing cup-to-disc ratio in the right eye in glaucoma. Cup-to-disc ratio: 0.4=normal disc (A). Cup-to-disc ratio: 0.7 with vertical elongation= moderate glaucoma (B). Cup-to-disc ratio: 0.9+ = severe glaucoma (C).

interferometer strips off scattered light from the reflected light needed to generate an image. In the process, depth and intensity of light reflected from a subsurface feature are obtained. A 3-D image can be built up by scanning.

The technique is limited to imaging about 3 mm below the surface in biologic tissue because at greater depths the proportion of light available without scattering is too small to be detected. No special preparation is required, and images can be obtained "noncontact" or through the cornea. The penetration depth of 3 mm allows images of the optical disc and of the anterior chamber, both of value in the evaluation of glaucoma.

The colors in Figure 25.28 are meant to represent how reflective a tissue is. The more reflective tissue is represented as red, orange, and white, whereas greens, blue, and black are less reflective. The retinal nerve fiber layer (RNFL) and retinal pigmented epithelium (RPE) are represented as red landmarks on an OCT. The RNFL is always thickest as you get closer to the nerve head.

The printout of the RNFL and optic nerve head disc cube 200 × 200

The scan pattern is a 6 × 6 mm cube consisting of 200 lines of 200 two-dimensional A-scans. This densely packed cube has 30 μm between slices. The 1.73-radius circle is automatically placed and centered around the optic nerve and is used to calculate the thickness of the RNFL around the optic nerve. Because a cube is captured, additional

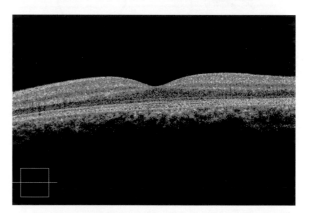

Figure 25.28 High-definition optical coherence tomography (OCT) enables interpretation of retinal layers. Significant for glaucoma is monitoring the thickness of nerve fiber layer.

information is gathered throughout the cube and not just at the calculation circle.

The RNFL thickness map displays patterns that represent retinal nerve fiber thickness within the 6 × 6 mm cube. The colors correlate to a micrometer scale in which white, red, and orange have thicker micrometer values than do blue and green. In glaucoma there can be diffuse loss of RNFL and a wedge or slit defects. This graphic representation does not contain metrics that compare to a normative database (Figure 25.29). Studies have suggested that OCT assessment

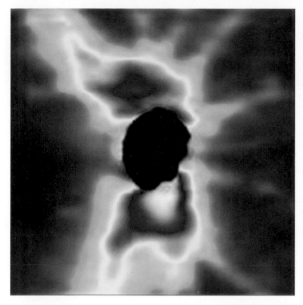

Figure 25.29 The retinal nerve fiber layer (RNFL) thickness map displays patterns that represent retinal nerve fiber thickness within the 6 × 6 mm cube.

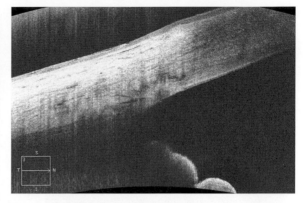

Figure 25.30 Normal wide angle between iris and cornea.

of RNFL thickness abnormalities may assist in the diagnosis of early glaucoma because thinning of the RNFL demonstrable by optical coherence tomography (OCT) may be detected before visual field defects become manifest. In one study up to 35% of eyes examined had an abnormal average RNFL thickness 4 years before visual field loss and 19% of eyes showed abnormal results 8 years before any noticeable field loss.[2] Future improvements in OCT imaging may enable earlier diagnosis of glaucoma, even before visual field defects have developed; however, both objective disc evaluations, like OCT, HRT and photography, and VF monitoring are the best means of detecting glaucoma and monitoring potential progression.

Anterior segment OCT

To visualize the anterior chamber OCT is a helpful tool for viewing the angle and cornea. It is also helpful for patient education for understanding an open, narrow, and closed angle (Figure 25.30).

Heidelberg retina tomograph

The HRT is a confocal laser ophthalmoscope that allows for topographic analysis of the posterior segment of the eye, especially the optic nerve head. A laser light scans the retina in 24-ms sequential scans, starting above the retinal surface, then capturing parallel images at increasing depths. A 3-D representation is created from the layering of optical section images from different locations of the focal plane. Then a topographic figure is produced, consisting of more than 65,000 local measurements of the retinal surface

height. The image is color-coded, with dark colors representing elevated structures and light colors signifying depressed areas. Images are aligned and compared using software for both individual examinations and for detecting change between examinations. Comparison of images taken over time enables a computerized determination of glaucomatous progression.

When applying the technology to glaucoma, the HRT takes data from a 3-D stack of tomographic images of the optic nerve and RNFL, aligns the images, and computes a 3-D topographic map of the surface of the retina. This map is analyzed for signs of glaucomatous damage.

The HRT scans the retina in 24 ms, faster than most voluntary and involuntary eye movements. Each scan is composed of 384 × 384 pixels for a total of 147,456 data points covering a 15-degree area of the retina.

The software aligns images within and between examinations, using anatomic features (such as blood vessel patterns) and other image characteristics to align them (Figure 25.31). Good image analysis requires both high-quality images (fast scanning) and image alignment. To construct a single examination, the software aligns a stack of individual scans.

Pictor

The Pictor is a handheld portable camera with four imaging modules, two of which are for eye examinations. The retinal module is used for fundus imaging and the anterior module is used for exterior ophthalmic imaging. To take an image in the retinal module, the patient looks straight ahead at a target behind the assistant or at the assistant's ear. The camera approaches the patient's eye from 4 inches away until a reflection of the fundus is visible. The still image created can be transferred to a computer for viewing. The images allow the ophthalmic assistant and ophthalmologist to view the optic disc, macula, and retinal vasculature and screen for abnormalities.

Ultrasound biomicroscopy

High-frequency ultrasound biomicroscopy (UBM) provides high-resolution in vivo imaging of the anterior

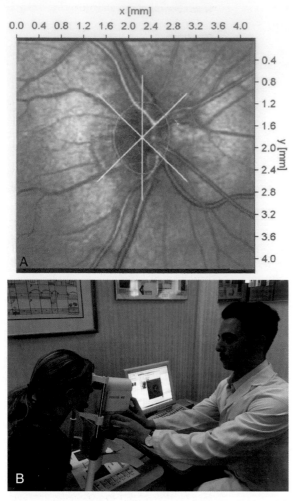

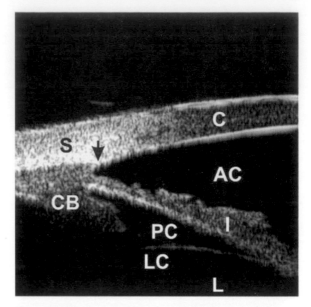

Figure 25.32 Ultrasound biomicroscopic appearance of a normal eye. The cornea (C), sclera (S), anterior chamber (AC), posterior chamber (PC), iris (I), ciliary body (CB), lens capsule (LC), and lens (L) can be identified. The scleral spur *(black arrow)* is an important landmark to assess the morphologic relationships among the anterior segment structures.

Figure 25.31 Heidelberg retina tomograph II optic disc scan (A). Procedure obtaining an HRT image (B).

segment in a noninvasive fashion. In addition to the tissues easily seen using conventional methods (i.e., slit lamp), such as the cornea, iris, and sclera, structures including the ciliary body and zonules, previously hidden from clinical observation, can be imaged and their morphology assessed. Pathophysiologic changes involving anterior segment architecture can be evaluated qualitatively and quantitatively.

The technology for UBM is based on 50- to 100-MHz transducers incorporated into a B-mode clinical scanner. Higher-frequency transducers provide finer resolution of more superficial structures, whereas lower-frequency transducers provide greater depth of penetration with less resolution. The commercially available units operate at 50 MHz and provide lateral and axial physical resolutions of approximately 50 μm and 25 μm, respectively. Tissue penetration is approximately 4 to 5 mm. The scanner produces

a 5 × 5 mm field with 256 vertical image lines (or A-scans) at a scan rate of eight frames per second.

The image acquisition technique is similar to traditional immersion B-scan ultrasonography. To maximize the detection of the reflected signal, the transducer should be oriented so that the scanning ultrasound beam strikes the target surface perpendicularly. Figure 25.32 is a UBM picture of a normal eye.

Functional: visual fields

Glaucomatous field defects arise as a consequence of damage to the nerve fiber layer and the optic disc. Field defects do not occur in glaucoma if the disc is normal. In most instances the ophthalmologist can predict the location of the field defect by noting the portion of the disc that is excavated. For example, if the pathologic cupping and atrophy are found on the lower outer pole of the disc, as occurs in most early cases of glaucoma, the field defect will be found in the upper nasal region.

The types of field defects to be expected in glaucoma are as follows:

1. Enlargement of the normal blind spot.
2. *Nerve fiber bundle defect.* This type of defect is curved and arches from the blind spot around the central fixation point in the area between 10 and 20 degrees. It usually ends in a very sharply demarcated border on the horizontal line. The nerve fiber

bundle defect is a prototype of glaucomatous field defects.

3. *Baring of the blind spot.* Baring of the blind spot is an arcuate or partial nerve fiber bundle defect emerging from the blind spot.

4. *Nerve fiber bundle defect or Bjerrum's arcuate scotoma.* This defect is a complete type of nerve fiber bundle defect emanating from the blind spot, arching over central fixation, and ending on the horizontal line. In its early stages this defect may not be attached to the blind spot and may extend only partway around the macular region.

5. *Nasal depression of the field.* This type of defect may appear quite early in glaucoma and later merges with a nerve fiber bundle defect to create an area of considerable visual loss.

The presence of typical glaucomatous field defects is virtually diagnostic of glaucoma, irrespective of the IOP. The treatment of glaucoma is directed principally toward avoiding further field loss, not merely reducing IOP. If a patient is under treatment and the pressure has been maintained at a satisfactory level, visual fields should be examined approximately two or three times a year. It is important in field testing to use an adequate-sized test object; many glaucoma patients cannot see well because they have cataracts. The examiner should use the smallest detectable stimulus that can be seen temporal to the blind spot.

The last area of visual field loss in glaucoma is the central vision area. Thus the wave of darkness that comes from the blind spot first surrounds the central area, extends to the periphery, and leaves the individual at the end stage of the disease looking clearly straight ahead through a long tunnel of darkness, so-called *tunnel vision* (Figure 25.33).

Changes of the optic nerve head often precede detectable visual field loss. It has been estimated that almost half of the near fibers of the disc have to be lost before reproducible early field defects can be found. The correlation between optic nerve changes as noted by alterations of the disc and changes in visual function as detected by visual field assessment is usually parallel. If the correlation is not there, then one has to look for other sources of visual field changes such as other defects or disturbances of the optic nerve, retina, or even farther along the optic neural pathways in the brain.

Techniques of perimetry

Because perimetry is discussed in Chapter 19, the following points highlight only its importance in glaucoma.

Kinetic perimetry involves moving the test object from a nonseeing area to a seeing area, whereas *static perimetry* involves the use of stationary test objects presented at random. The points at which the patient fails to recognize the spot of light are noted.

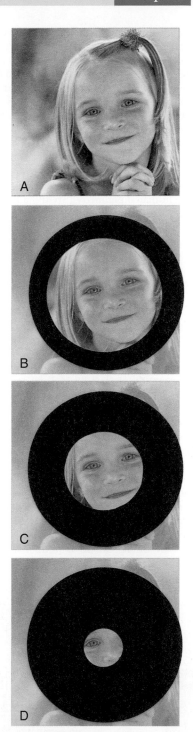

Figure 25.33 Progressive constriction of visual field caused by advancing, irreversible glaucoma damage. Normal vision (A). Progressive constriction of visual field (B–D).

Threshold static perimetry measures the intensity thresholds of visual acuity of the individual points within the field of vision. This is accomplished by gradually increasing the target light on the subthreshold intensity and recording the level at which the patient first recognizes the target. The process also can be approached from the other direction, that is, decreasing from the suprathreshold level and recording the lowest value found.

Static perimetry has been shown to be more sensitive than kinetic perimetry at detecting early glaucomatous field defects. Most commonly, white targets are presented on a white background (white-on-white; WOW). In short-wavelength automated perimetry (SWAP), a blue target is presented on a yellow background. SWAP often can identify earlier field loss than WOW.

Cataracts can also cause visual field defects. In one study of 90 eyes with open-angle glaucoma and cataracts, 41% had a partial or complete scotoma reversed after the cataract was removed. Reduced ocular clarity from other causes such as corneal scarring also may affect and reduce the visual field. A miotic pupil may depress central and peripheral threshold retinal sensitivity and exaggerate field defects.

The correction of myopia with glasses is not required with the use of a 300-mm perimeter unless the refractive error exceeds 3.00 diopters. With high myopia, refractive scotomas may appear that can be confused with glaucomatous field defects. Usually they are eliminated with appropriate correction of the refractive error. Astigmatic errors should first be corrected before visual field tests unless they are less than 1.00 diopter. Increasing age also causes a reduction in retinal threshold sensitivity.

Psychologic factors may depress the visual field and create false pockets of visual field loss. The field test is definitely influenced by the state of the patient's alertness, anxiety, calm, and degree of cooperation. A lack of familiarity with the test and heightened tension about performing well often lead to a poor first-test result, which invariably improves on the second or third visual field test. This improvement is not a reflection of a change in optic nerve status; rather, it is a result of familiarity with the test and better response to the visual stimuli.

The frequency doubling technology (FDT) field technique works by flickering a coarse pattern of vertical dark and bright bars at a very high frequency. The advantages of the FDT are that it is a compact, transportable perimeter with tolerance to refractive errors and rapid test times.

The tangent screen is almost a historic relic of visual field testing. It suffers from the drawbacks of monitoring fixation and is limited by variations in background lighting. No visible record is automatically elicited, the area is strictly limited to the central 30 degrees, and the screen does not reveal the peripheral field where early glaucomatous defects may appear.

Approaches to glaucoma field testing

There are two approaches to glaucoma field testing. The first is a screening technique to detect the presence of a glaucoma field defect. The second is to measure accurately the breadth, depth, and density of the field defect so that it can be appropriately charted on subsequent dates to ascertain any progressive loss of field.

The goal in visual field testing for glaucoma is the earliest detection of visual field changes. Historical methods include the Goldmann perimeter, a technician-driven kinetic perimeter, which maps the size and shape of scotomas by means of both central threshold targets and peripheral targets and reveals glaucomatous defects with a high probability. However, the most commonly used perimeters today are the Humphrey field analyzer (Figures 25.34 and 25.35), a static perimeter that is automated, monitors fixation, and is less technician-dependent than the Goldmann perimeter. However, by the time visual field loss is detected by standard automated perimetry, substantial structural

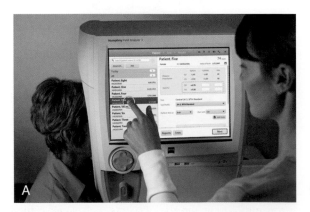

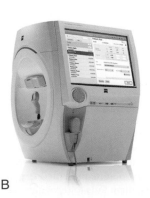

Figure 25.34 Touchscreen programming of Humphrey Field Analyzer 3 (A). Humphrey Field Analyzer 3 (B).
(Courtesy of Carl Zeiss Meditec, Inc., Dublin, CA.)

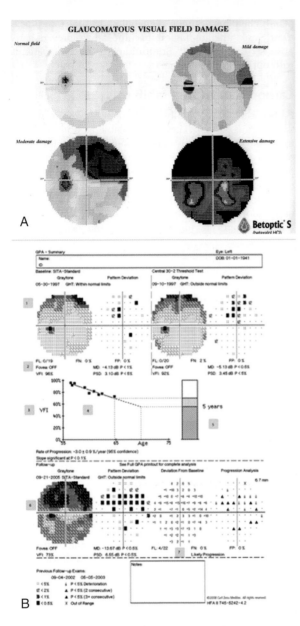

Figure 25.35 Typical visual field progression due to glaucomatous optic neuropathy demonstrated per automated perimetry (A). Humphrey perimetry offers several printouts to assist in documenting and monitoring progression (B). *(Courtesy of Alcon; https://www.alcon.com)*

damage may exist. For this reason, also in use is the Humphrey FDT visual field instrument, which provides suprathreshold screening tests that identify early visual field loss. Short-wavelength automated perimetry may also detect functional loss earlier.

TREATMENT

Open-angle glaucoma cannot be cured, but it can be adequately controlled so that further loss of visual function does not occur. Increased IOP is the primary modifiable risk factor for the progression to blindness in open-angle glaucoma; therefore, reduction in IOP constitutes the principal goal of treatment. Every patient with cupping of the optic disc and visual field changes should be treated. Glaucoma therapy traditionally consists of topical medication, oral medication, laser procedure, and conventional surgery. Additionally, recent advancements in microinvasive glaucoma surgeries have diversified treatment options for qualifying patients.

The decision of when to treat and whom to treat is based on multiple factors that include medication effects, side effects, and costs; ability of the patient to comply with medication regimen; surgical risk–benefit issues; and quality of life issues. In glaucoma therapy the goal is to buy time and delay the effects of a progressive, potentially blinding disease.

In every clinic or office, there is usually a large group of patients who have ocular hypertension. These are patients with ocular pressure values greater than 22 mm Hg, but who maintain normal discs with no detected visual field loss. The decision as to whether this type of patient should be actively treated requires individual consideration. These cases of suspected or borderline glaucoma frequently can be followed without treatment for many years. If follow-up examinations are difficult to obtain or if the ophthalmologist has poor rapport with the patient, the patient may be treated earlier.

Medical therapy

Glaucoma can usually be adequately controlled with topical medication. The past three decades have seen the development of numerous effective drops for glaucoma: prostaglandins, beta-blockers, alpha agonists, and topical carbonic anhydrase antagonists. Prostaglandin analogs, used once daily, are generally the first agents to be used, followed by nonselective beta-blockers to treat open-angle glaucoma. The nonselective beta-blockers affect both beta-1 and beta-2 receptors and have the potential to cause serious cardiovascular and pulmonary side effects. They may be contraindicated in patients with actual or suspected compromised cardiovascular or pulmonary function because they can cause cardiac arrhythmias, bradycardia, or bronchospasm. Depression, dizziness, and impotence are well-recognized complications of beta-blockers.

Certain older topical medications such as pilocarpine contain benzalkonium chloride (BAK) as a preservative, which has a toxic effect on the cornea, particularly if used frequently during the day. Patients with some corneal toxicity may do better by switching to more costly preservative-free topical solutions. Combination therapies are also available. An advantage of combination drops is convenience and often improved adherence.

Pharmaceutical agents commonly used by class

Prostaglandins

Prostaglandins increase the outflow of the aqueous humor through the trabecular meshwork and the uveoscleral routes. Examples of these agents are bimatoprost (Lumigan RC), latanoprost (Xalatan), travoprost (Travatan Z), and tafluprost (Taflotan). Ocular side effects that have been observed include conjunctival hyperemia, ocular itching, and tearing. Prostaglandins have been reported to cause changes to pigmented tissue and adipose tissue. The most frequent reported changes have been increased pigmentation of the iris, eyelids, and increased pigmentation, growth of eyelashes, and sunken orbits. These changes may be permanent. BAK preserved, SofZia preserved, Polyquad preserved, and nonpreserved formulations are available.

Beta-adrenergic blocking agents

Beta-adrenergic blocking agents decrease aqueous secretion. Examples of these agents are betaxolol hydrochloride (Betoptic S and generic preparations), carteolol hydrochloride (Ocupress and generic preparations), levobunolol hydrochloride (Betagan and generic preparations), metipranolol (OptiPranolol and generic preparations), timolol (Betimol), timolol maleate (Timoptic, Timoptic XE gel, and generic preparations). Beta-adrenergic blocking agents used in ocular therapy may affect beta-adrenergic sites throughout the body with systemic effects including slowing cardiac rates, lowering blood pressure, and exacerbating asthma and obstructive airway disease. Timolol maleate (Timoptic) solutions of 0.25% and 0.5% concentration are used once or twice daily, depending on the severity of the glaucoma. Timolol maleate and levobunolol hydrochloride (Betagan) have minimal side effects and can be used for most patients except those with asthma, cardiopulmonary disease, heart failure, or second- to third-degree heart block. Betaxolol hydrochloride (Betoptic S) is a more selective beta-blocker with apparently fewer cardiovascular side effects and similar potency. This selectively affects only beta-1 receptors. Betaxolol hydrochloride, a cardioselective beta-blocker, has a significantly lesser effect on the respiratory system and can therefore be used in some patients with respiratory diseases.

Alpha-2 selective agonists

Alpha-2 selective agonists reduce aqueous humor production and increase uveoscleral outflow. Examples of these agents are apraclonidine (Iopidine) and brimonidine (Alphagan P and generic preparations). Apraclonidine is mostly used in argon laser trabeculoplasty to prevent early postlaser spikes in IOP. Brimonidine is used for patients with open-angle glaucoma.

Carbonic anhydrase inhibitors

Carbonic anhydrase inhibitors decrease the production of the aqueous humor. They are available as both oral and injectable systemic agents and as topical agents. Examples of topical agents are brinzolamide (Azopt) and dorzolamide hydrochloride (Trusopt). These have been developed to be used two or three times daily. They can be used in addition to other medications. Side effects include a bitter taste and headaches. Other side effects of the topical agents include superficial punctate keratitis and ocular allergic reactions.

Examples of systemic agents are acetazolamide (Diamox and generic preparations), methazolamide (Neptazane and generic preparations) and dichlorphenamide (diclofenamid [Daranide, Oratrol]). Although oral acetazolamide is effective in lowering IOP, it is used rarely and sparingly because of its side effects. Many patients develop tingling in their fingers and toes, diarrhea, nausea, loss of appetite, and general malaise. Other side effects of systemic carbonic anhydrase inhibitors include paresthesias, gastrointestinal problems, and sodium and potassium depletion. Severe but rare side effects include renal stones, Stevens-Johnson syndrome, and blood dyscrasias. Patients sensitive to sulfa may be allergic to Diamox, a sulfa derivative. The systemic agents most commonly supplement other topical agents used to treat glaucoma.

Combination drops

Combination drops are another option for patients who require more than one therapy to manage their pressure. These combinations include two different classes of agents, for example timolol maleate and dorzolamide hydrochloride (Cosopt) is a combination of a beta-blocker and carbonic anhydrase inhibitor. Other examples of combination medications include brimonidine tartrate and timolol maleate (Combiga), and brinzolamide and brimonidine (Simbrinza suspension).

Miotics

Miotics (parasympathomimetic agents) are rarely used as a topical therapy for glaucoma but have historical importance. They act by mimicking the action of acetylcholine on parasympathomimetic postganglionic nerve endings in the eye. Examples of these agents are carbachol and pilocarpine hydrochloride. Miotics also are used to control accommodative esotropia. However, pilocarpines and epinephrine derivatives have been used less commonly in recent years, because of their required frequency as well as their well-known ocular surface complications.

Sympathomimetics

Sympathomimetics, also rarely used, improve the aqueous outflow within the eye and to a smaller extent uveoscleral output. Examples of these agents are dipivefrin hydrochloride (Propine and generic preparations) and epinephrine hydrochloride (Epifrin).

Hyperosmotic agents

Hyperosmotic agents produce an osmotic gradient between the intraocular fluid and the blood, decreasing IOP by causing ocular fluids to move from the globe into the bloodstream. These agents are used in the acute treatment of angle-closure glaucoma and rarely in intraocular surgery when IOP is very high. Examples of these agents are oral glycerin, oral isosorbide (Ismotic), intravenous mannitol (Osmitrol), and intravenous urea (Ureaphil). Side effects of hyperosmotic agents include cardiovascular overload, urinary retention and headaches, nausea, and mental confusion.

Adherence with medication

A medication regimen should be as simple as possible. It has been estimated that anywhere from 20% to 40% of patients prescribed medication for open-angle glaucoma miss some or all of their drop dosages. Those who were asked to instill three times a day were more likely not to use the drops than those told to use them twice a day. Other disturbing factors that lead to relative noncompliance or poor compliance are side effects of the medication, such as miosis and loss of focusing accuracy with pilocarpine, as well as failure to understand that the treatment preserves the visual field and the acuity already present. In many instances these patients do not believe they are sick, especially if no other disease is present, and are reluctant to undertake a treatment of medication when they have only the physician's pronouncement that they need it.

Office-based laser treatments

Argon laser trabeculoplasty

Laser treatment of the trabecular meshwork has been effective in controlling open-angle glaucoma and obviating the need for invasive surgery in many patients. The actual procedure involves treating the mid- to anterior portion of the trabecular meshwork with a thermal laser. A gonioprism is used to position the light into the trabecular meshwork. Approximately 80 to 100 spots of 50 µm size are equally spaced over 180 degrees of the angle. Often, the remainder of the angle will be treated at a later time.

The argon laser trabeculoplasty reduces the IOP. Although the exact mechanisms are unknown, IOP most likely lowers secondary to both mechanical and biologic effects. Although the success rates vary for different types of open-angle glaucoma, there does appear to be a relationship between laser success and a patient's age and degree of trabecular meshwork pigmentation. In some patients laser therapy is used as a first-line treatment. However, laser therapy is often an adjunct to medical therapy and does not ensure that medications may be stopped.

Selective laser trabeculoplasty (Figure 25.36)

A less thermal laser treatment for managing patients with open-angle glaucoma, SLT is an improvement over argon

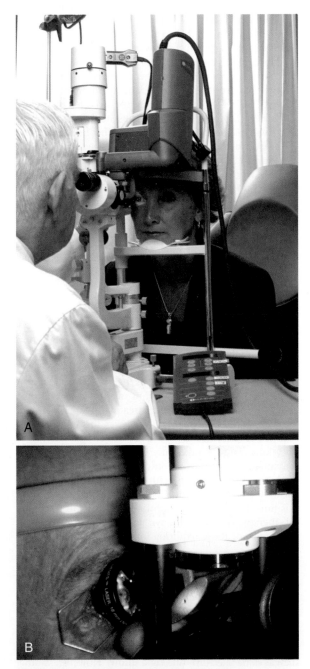

Figure 25.36 Patient undergoing Selective Laser Trabeculoplasty (SLT) (A). Gonio lens use for SLT may be performed with or without an additional eyelid speculum (B).

laser trabeculoplasty (ALT). Selective laser trabeculoplasty (SLT) is a q-switched, 532-nm laser and has a 200 μm spot size. This procedure uses a very short laser pulse to irradiate and selectively target pigmented cells in the trabecular meshwork, thought to work by triggering a biologic response that stimulates an increase in the drainage of aqueous humor to ultimately reduce IOP within several weeks postprocedure. SLT has a distinct advantage in that it is less thermal; adverse scarring or damage to adjacent tissues is avoided with this treatment so the technique may potentially be repeated if necessary.

Although the use of prostaglandins has decreased the need for laser therapy, laser therapy may eliminate or at least reduce drop dependency, which can prove costly to patients. SLT often can eliminate the need for drops and the issue of compliance with drops in the management of glaucoma, especially when used as first-line therapy.

SLT has proven beneficial in early-stage treatment and has become a primary option for open-angle glaucoma patients who cannot tolerate or who are noncompliant with medical therapy. It is effective for those who have undergone prior argon laser treatments and may not interfere with the success of future surgical interventions. In fact, SLT may postpone or even preclude the need for additional medications or incisional surgery, thereby reducing the overall expense associated with treatment. An additional advantage of SLT to ALT is that significantly less TM scarring occurs such that later MIGS procedures are possible.

When to treat

Newly diagnosed patients should be treated as early as possible to reach and consistently maintain a low IOP to reduce the risk of progression. Most clinicians initiate glaucoma therapy with medications before laser therapy is attempted. There has been a shift in thinking toward the use of laser therapy as an initial treatment, especially since the availability of the SLT laser. Laser therapy does not require compliance and is virtually free of significant complications from the procedure itself. It is performed on an outpatient basis during an office visit and requires no hospital stay. A rare problem with this treatment is a possible rise in IOP occurring in the first weeks after laser therapy. At this time, however, most ophthalmologists still use medical therapy first and reserve laser treatment for poor responders or those requiring long-term oral therapy.

Surgery for glaucoma

Common therapeutic regimens for the treatment of glaucoma are most often medications followed by office lasers (SLT and ALT) and then, reserved for patients in whom these attempts at controlling IOP to prevent permanent vision loss are not adequate, invasive surgical procedures such as trabeculectomy and tube shunts. However, another option has become available; it is surgical but far less traumatic than trabeculectomy or tube shunts. This group of

surgical procedures is microinvasive glaucoma surgery (MIGS) and is likely to become more common, replacing some medication therapies and some of the more invasive surgical therapies.

Surgery has historically been used only if the patient continues to lose visual field despite attempts by the ophthalmologist to provide maximally tolerated medical- and office-based laser therapy. This usually means that the ophthalmologist has been unable to effectively lower the IOP with the most potent drugs available, either singly or in combination, or the patient is not compliant with medication use. Newer surgical procedures such as MIGS, which are Schlemm's canal procedures, enable outflow restrictions to be bypassed within the eye. This is achieved by improving flow from the anterior chamber into Schlemm's canal instead of making a full-thickness hole in the sclera. Thus the surgical treatment of glaucoma, especially with MIGS, may come to be performed earlier in the course of the patient's glaucoma conditions as the risks of surgery and postsurgical eye conditions are significantly decreased with newer techniques and technologies.

Surgery may come to be performed earlier in the course of the patient's glaucoma condition as the risks of surgery and postsurgical eye conditions are significantly decreased with newer techniques and technologies.

Many types of invasive surgical procedures are performed for open-angle glaucoma. They are essentially fistulizing operations, that is, they attempt to create an opening between the anterior chamber and the subconjunctival space with and without implant devices (tube shunts, e.g., Ahmed, Molteno, and Baerveldt) or between surgically prepared layers of the sclera ("subscleral," "nonpenetrating," or suprachoroidal stent filtering procedures). In all glaucoma surgeries, the actual operation is a small part of the care that guarantees a successful outcome. Postoperative management is critical to successful glaucoma surgery. Recognizing and controlling postoperative complications is key. Hypotony, wound leaks, fluid shifts within the eye, infection, and inadequate pressure control are conditions often managed in the short-term postoperative period as the patient's wound healing is modulated to enable eventual controlled IOP lowering. Long-term risks include a more rapid progression of cataract and an ongoing risk for infection (e.g., endophthalmitis), the onset of which requires emergency attention and management.

Unlike cataract surgery, in which patients expect to see well within a short time postoperatively, glaucoma patients must understand that their surgery is not to improve current vision, but to preserve their vision over the long term. Immediately after glaucoma surgery, vision may be slightly worse than preoperatively, and patients will often need an eventual change in their glasses prescription. Because cataract and glaucoma often occur in the same older adult population, combined glaucoma and cataract surgery may be performed.

Glaucoma surgical procedures are being performed less often today because of the adequacy in most instances of medical management. However, if untreated or inadequately treated, *absolute glaucoma* with complete blindness and markedly elevated pressure in an eye is still a tragic entity.

Key to the success of all glaucoma surgery is the postoperative time period in which wound-healing modulation is necessary and stabilizing IOP is paramount. Teamwork among the surgeon, the technician, and the patient is essential to ensure successful outcomes of glaucoma surgical procedures.

MIGS

MIGS are novel methods for treating glaucoma that may replace or decrease the need for medications and may replace or delay the need for more invasive surgical procedures. MIGS include various methods of increasing aqueous outflow via device implantation or physiologic tissue alteration, such as excimer laser trabeculostomy (ELT), Trabectome, and iStent. Clinical trials are being conducted with these and several other MIGS devices. MIGS have the ability to provide a safe alternative to traditional medications, especially in early or midstage glaucoma patients who are not able to comply with more traditional medication therapies. Although many of these new MIGS are in clinical trials, their use in treating glaucoma is likely to increase.

Excimer laser trabeculostomy (Figure 25.37)

Excimer laser trabeculostomy (ELT), an innovative glaucoma laser treatment based on laser-assisted in situ keratomileusis (LASIK) technology, is a minimally invasive outpatient procedure that effects a significant and long-lasting reduction in IOP without causing healing or

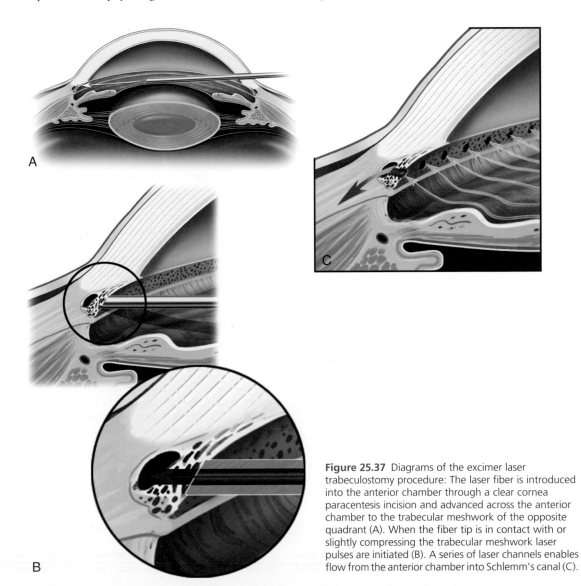

Figure 25.37 Diagrams of the excimer laser trabeculostomy procedure: The laser fiber is introduced into the anterior chamber through a clear cornea paracentesis incision and advanced across the anterior chamber to the trabecular meshwork of the opposite quadrant (A). When the fiber tip is in contact with or slightly compressing the trabecular meshwork laser pulses are initiated (B). A series of laser channels enables flow from the anterior chamber into Schlemm's canal (C).

scarring. This MIGS procedure, which is sometimes referred to as LASIK of the trabecular meshwork, enables an essentially nonthermal creation of channels in the trabecular meshwork, to significantly reduce outflow resistance. A 308-nm xenon chloride excimer laser is used because of its precision and effectively nonthermal laser/tissue interaction properties. Unlike the use of thermal lasers that evoke healing responses at and adjacent to the treatment sites as a result of collateral tissue disruption and subsequent inflammatory responses, the ELT laser creates outflow channels from the anterior chamber into Schlemm's canal with far less collateral damage, thus enabling longevity of these outflow channels. ELT surgery is performed as an outpatient procedure under local anesthesia (i.e., topical, peribulbar, or retrobulbar).

ELT enhances aqueous outflow without the creation of a filtering fistula or bleb, instead using Schlemm's canal as the conduit to increase outflow. A small excimer laser probe is inserted into the anterior chamber of the eye via a clear corneal incision and placed against the trabecular meshwork. Small channels are ablated, passing through the trabecular meshwork into Schlemm's canal, bypassing the increased resistance of an obstructed trabecular meshwork. For patients with open-angle glaucoma and cataracts, ELT can be combined with cataract surgery to generate a greater reduction of IOP than either cataract or ELT surgery alone.

Extensive data have shown that the IOP-lowering and medication-reducing effects of ELT are maintained at least over a 5-year period. Although approved in Europe, ELT therapy is awaiting US Food and Drug Administration (FDA) approval for use in the United States.

Trabectome

The Trabectome is a microsurgical device that enables an ab interno removal of a strip of trabecular meshwork and inner wall of Schlemm's canal, termed "ab interno trabeculotomy" through microelectrocautery under gonioscopic control. A mobile console provides infusion, aspiration, and electrosurgical energy. The instrument includes a triangular ceramic-coated footplate, the point and body of which are sized to fit into and act as a guide within Schlemm's canal. A cautery is positioned so as to receive and thermally ablate angle tissues. Infusion during ablation helps decrease heat-related damage to adjacent tissues, and aspiration through the instrument's shaft removes tissue debris. The instrument allows surgeons to reduce IOP without shunts or mechanical implants. The procedure enhances outflow of aqueous from the anterior chamber through increased access to Schlemm's canal; however, the thermal effects often limit efficacy over time and because of the size of the openings created, hyphema is a significant undesirable side effect.

iStent (Figure 25.38)

The iStent is an L-shaped, titanium trabecular microbypass stent that is often implanted in conjunction with cataract

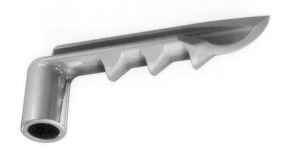

Figure 25.38 iStent is designed to create a patent bypass through the trabecular meshwork to facilitate physiologic outflow and thus lower intraocular pressure (IOP). *(Courtesy of Glaukos Corporation; http://www.glaukos.com.)*

surgery. The iStent is designed to create a bypass through the trabecular meshwork to facilitate physiologic outflow and thus lower IOP. It is the smallest medical device known to be implanted into the human body, with a length of 1 mm and a bore diameter of 0.12 mm. To achieve adequate lowering of IOP, often at least two iStents must be implanted. Side effects include misplacement and occasional dislodging.

Canaloplasty

Canaloplasty achieves a reduction in IOP without the many complications associated with trabeculectomy. Canaloplasty's goal is to improve outflow by circumferentially catheterizing and viscodilating Schlemm's canal along its entire length with the use of a flexible microcatheter. The placement of an intracanalicular tension suture within Schlemm's canal distends the trabecular meshwork inward, acting to stent the canal open. Unlike trabeculectomy, a hole is not created in the eye to achieve drainage, thus there are fewer risks compared with trabeculectomy. However, there is also less efficacy of IOP lowering.

Invasive glaucoma surgical procedures

Trabeculectomy (Figure 25.39)

Trabeculectomy, also called *filtration surgery*, is a surgical procedure used in treating glaucoma to relieve IOP by removing part of the eye's trabecular meshwork and adjacent structures in the drainage angle of the eye. It is the most common glaucoma surgery performed and allows drainage of aqueous humor from within the eye to underneath the conjunctiva, where it is absorbed. This outpatient procedure is most commonly performed under monitored anesthesia care using a retrobulbar block or peribulbar block or a combination of topical and subTenon's (Tenon's capsule) anesthesia. Occasionally sedation or general anesthesia is used.

During a trabeculectomy an eyelid speculum is used to enable exposure of the patient's eye. An initial pocket is

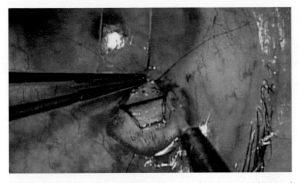

Figure 25.39 A trabeculectomy showing the removal of part of the eye's trabecular meshwork and adjacent structures in the drainage angle of the eye.

created under the conjunctiva and Tenon's capsule, and the wound bed may be treated for several seconds to several minutes with mitomycin C or with 5-fluorouracil (5-FU, 50 mg/mL). With a sponge, surgeons generally use 0.1 mg/ml to 0.4 mg/ml of mitomycin C, but when injecting it, a lower concentration of 0.05 to 0.1 mg/ml is used because of the direct injection into Tenon's layer. These chemotherapeutic agents inhibit fibroblast proliferation and thereby help prevent failure of the filter bleb as a result of scarring. A partial-thickness scleral flap with its base at the corneoscleral junction is then made after careful cauterization of this flap area, and a window opening to access the anterior chamber is created under the flap with a surgical punch to remove the remaining portion of the sclera, Schlemm's canal, and the trabecular meshwork to enter the anterior chamber. Because of the fluid egress, the iris may partially prolapse through the sclerostomy and is usually therefore partially removed (this procedure is called an *iridectomy*). This iridectomy also prevents future blockage of the sclerostomy opening by iris. The scleral flap is then sutured loosely back in place with several sutures in a manner to carefully allow

adequate egress of aqueous and maintain adequate IOP. The conjunctiva is then closed in a watertight fashion and tested to be leak-free at the end of the procedure.

Complications associated with trabeculectomy are intraoperative and postoperative bleeding, shallow anterior chamber, hypotony, choroidal detachment, cataract formation, suprachoroidal hemorrhage, and bleb-related endophthalmitis. On average, 10% of trabeculectomy surgeries fail each year (Figure 25.40). Common risk factors of trabeculectomy are infection, vision loss, bleb leak, bleb scarring, hypotony, cataract, and the need for subsequent surgery. At 2.5 years the probability of bleb-related infections is 1.5%. The major risk factors for infectious complications of filtering blebs are leaks, thin/avascular blebs, the use of antimetabolites, and blepharitis/conjunctivitis.[3] All trabeculectomy patients must be taught to carefully monitor their postsurgical eye for any sign of redness or discharge and immediately inform their ophthalmologist. When detected and treated early, blebitis can be prevented from becoming endophthalmitis, with inherent risks of blindness prevented.

Tube shunts (Figure 25.41)

Tube-shunt surgery involves placing a flexible tube covered by eyebank sclera, cornea, or pericardial tissue to prevent erosion with an attached drainage plate in the eye to help drain fluid (aqueous humor) from the eye. Like trabeculectomy, its aim is to create a filtering bleb more posterior than a traditional limbal trabeculectomy, which often closes from scarring. Glaucoma tube-shunt surgery may be needed in patients with glaucoma that is not controlled by medications or laser treatment. It is useful either after failure of previous trabeculectomy surgery or in certain types of glaucoma in which traditional trabeculectomy surgery would almost certainly fail. Examples of such patients are those with neovascular glaucoma and patients who have corneal transplants.

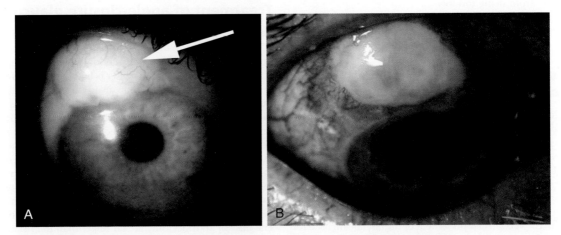

Figure 25.40 The newly formed bleb (*arrow*) after trabeculectomy (A). An infected bleb (bleibitis) (B).

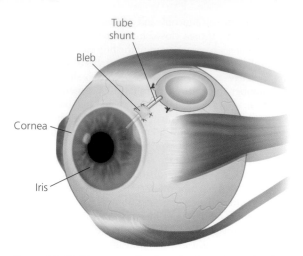

Figure 25.41 Glaucoma tube shunt implantation. Tube-shunt surgery involves placing a flexible tube covered by eyebank sclera, cornea, or pericardial tissue to prevent erosion with an attached drainage plate in the eye to help drain fluid (aqueous humor) from the eye.

During the first few weeks after surgery, a bleb of fibrous tissue and collagen forms around the plate of the implant. The thickness of the bleb determines the rate at which aqueous flows out of the anterior chamber of the eye. The excess aqueous fluid is shunted through the tubing of the implant, and passes through the space that develops between the bleb and the plate. By diffusion, the fluid flows into the capillaries, where it exits the eye and enters the general circulation. The IOP is lowered as a result of this increase in outflow. The device is partially visible behind the upper eyelid after the surgery.

The types of implants used in glaucoma surgery fall into two categories: nonvalved (e.g., Molteno, Baerveldt) or valved implants (e.g., Ahmed). Restrictive implants have valves to limit fluid flow in one direction and prevent the IOP from being too low.

The major complications of tube-shunt surgery are bleeding, double vision, retinal detachment, IOP too high or too low, and corneal decompensation.

Cyclophotocoagulation and cyclocryopexy

Cyclophotocoagulation and cyclocryopexy are used to treat the ciliary processes with thermal laser radiation or freezing, respectively, to create scar tissue in the ciliary body to reduce the production of aqueous humor and thus lower the IOP. Cyclophotocoagulation can be performed either by transscleral cyclophotocoagulation (TCP) or endoscopic guidance cyclophotocoagulation (ECP). ECP allows the surgeon to view the area through an endoscopic camera, which aids in the very precise placement of the laser beam used for treatment of individual ciliary processes.

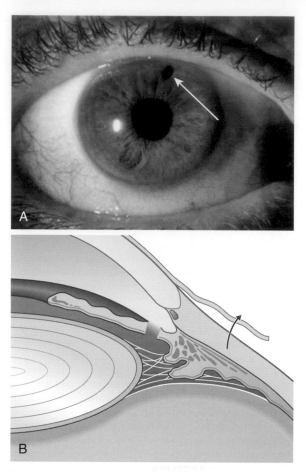

Figure 25.42 Peripheral iridotomy (A) eliminates pupillary block (B).

(B, From Shields MB, editor. Textbook of glaucoma. 4th ed. Baltimore: Williams & Wilkins; 1998.)

Treatment of angle-closure glaucoma

The procedure of choice is laser iridotomy (Figure 25.42). A peripheral iridotomy is accomplished to relieve the pupillary block and allow the anterior chamber to deepen. A thermal or photodisruptive laser is used to create a small opening in the iris, which creates an additional pathway for fluid to flow. The procedure is curative if the attack has not caused adhesions between the iris and the angle structures. An iridotomy should be performed eventually in both eyes of patients with narrow angles because it has been shown that 50% to 70% of patients with angle-closure glaucoma in one eye will have an attack in the fellow eye within 5 to 10 years despite miotic treatment. For this reason most surgeons prefer to do a prophylactic iridectomy on the healthy eye to avoid the hazards of acute-closure glaucoma. The risks of an iridectomy are far lower than the risks of a second angle-closure attack.

Medical therapy for angle-closure glaucoma is used only as a prelude to laser iridotomy. The purpose is to reduce the pressure and eliminate the corneal edema so that an effective laser procedure can be accomplished with greater safety and ease.

If the attack is not aborted early, permanent scar tissue can result in secondary glaucoma and vision can be permanently affected by damage to the optic nerve.

Acetazolamide (Diamox) or methazolamide (Neptazane), carbonic anhydrase inhibitors, are used to temporarily lower the IOP. Acetazolamide may be given orally, intramuscularly, or intravenously. Beta-blockers such as timolol, levobunolol, and betaxolol work in concert with carbonic anhydrase inhibitors to lower IOP. Miotic agents are used to mobilize the iris away from the peripheral angle.

In addition, various hypertonic solutions have been used to gain a more prompt and rapid reduction of IOP. The agents most commonly used today are mannitol, given in a dose of 1 to 2 g/kg of body weight (intravenously over 30–60 minutes), and glycerin, given in a dose of 1.5 g/kg of body weight (orally). Usually 1.5 to 2 ounces (32–55 g) of glycerin is mixed with orange juice or lemon juice to avoid nausea caused by the sweet taste of the glycerin. Because the use of such agents can cause wide fluctuations in systemic blood pressure and in electrolyte balance, patients must be monitored closely during and after the use of these agents.

The ophthalmic assistant should be familiar with angle-closure glaucoma because it constitutes a true ocular emergency. The abruptness of its onset is its most obvious clue. The patient may complain of intense eye pain, redness, or blurred vision. The pain can be so severe that the patient may experience headaches, nausea, or vomiting. There may have been earlier symptoms of pain and blurred vision lasting 15 to 30 minutes and then subsiding over a period of several months. This is because the acute rise in pressure subsided between pressure rises.

On examination, the dilation of the pupil fixed to light, combined with a steamy (clouded) cornea, is its most imposing sign. Such patients must be examined as soon as possible. Because treatment should begin as soon as the diagnosis is made, the ophthalmic assistant should keep all the medications for the treatment of this condition available for immediate use.

MANAGEMENT OF THE PATIENT BY THE OPHTHALMIC ASSISTANT

The ophthalmic assistant is a critical part of the patient care team assisting the patient through the regimens of glaucoma diagnosis and compliance with therapy. It is imperative that patients be educated about their condition and the importance of being seen at regular intervals to maintain control of their disease. They should also be encouraged to interact with questions about diagnosis, progression, and their therapeutic options. Usually the ophthalmologist designates when the next appointment should take place, but the ophthalmic assistant must remind the patient of the importance of these follow-up examinations. If a particular patient with glaucoma has been remiss in keeping appointments, the patient should be contacted and informed about the dangers of ignoring ongoing monitoring.

At each visit, reminders should be given to patients about the exact time of administration of their drops and the methods of placing them into their eye. Adherence with instructions is a critical component of care in preventing vision loss from glaucoma. Glaucoma medications are best instilled by depressing the lower lid and placing the drops in the lower fornix. If this procedure is difficult, the patient should be instructed to lie down and place the drops directly over the cornea. To minimize systemic absorption and side effects of topical drops, patients are taught techniques of closing the eye without blinking for a full minute after each drop and of punctal occlusion (blocking the tear ducts at the inner canthus with a fingertip covered by a tissue as the drop is instilled and the eyelid closed) (Figure 25.43). Certain drops, such as Xalatan, should be kept out of sunlight and heat. The patient should be instructed in the management and care of medications,

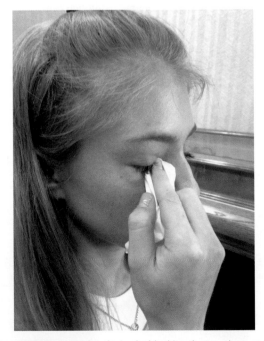

Figure 25.43 Punctal occlusion by blocking the tear ducts at the inner canthus with a fingertip covered by a tissue as the drop is instilled and the eyelid closed.

discarding medications that are out of date or might have been contaminated by mishandling.

It is helpful if patients are given a card stating that they have glaucoma and indicating their medications. Patients should know the names of their drugs, the dosage, and the frequency of application. The card is invaluable for patients who lose their medication, especially during travel. Also, if the patient becomes involved in an accident, the attending physician will be in a better position to evaluate the consequences of the injury if he or she is aware of the cause of unusual ocular findings.

In many instances patients have unusual ideas regarding the nature of glaucoma. Some believe they have an incurable disease leading to blindness or that they will become invalids because of glaucoma. Glaucoma patients should be reassured that by teaming with their caregivers to maintain good control, there is no reason why vision or visual fields should ever be compromised. Patients also should know that there is little or no evidence that limitations of activities, diet, alcohol, movies, television, reading, driving, and so forth alter the control of their glaucoma. They should be encouraged to enjoy a normal lifestyle.

SUMMARY

Glaucoma is one of the most common treatable ocular diseases, second only to cataract. Although early diagnosis and proper management remain the responsibility of the eye care professional, the ophthalmic assistant plays a key role in patient understanding, management, and especially adherence to the treatment regimen. The ophthalmic assistant must be aware of the signs and symptoms of acute angle-closure glaucoma, and should understand that glaucoma is treatable and blindness preventable when patients control their condition on a daily basis. Because vision lost to glaucoma is irreversible, the importance of early detection should be stressed. It is the ophthalmic assistant's duty to help glaucoma patients understand the nature of their disease as well as the therapeutic regimens necessary for management. It is also the ophthalmic assistant's duty to encourage adherence, especially because glaucoma, in a similar manner to systemic hypertension, presents without symptoms and is therefore easily ignored by patients.

Recent and ongoing innovations have provided ophthalmologists and their patients improved techniques and technologies for diagnosing and monitoring glaucoma. New scanning devices can detect optic nerve abnormalities and narrowing angles earlier. Potential neuroprotective agents that may slow the progression of glaucoma independent of controlling the IOP, which is today's standard of treatment, are being evaluated. This research, as well as new classes of IOP-lowering medications, long-acting sustained-release medications, stem cell research, gene therapy, antioxidant therapy, and vasoactive medications further increase the likelihood of even more successful management of glaucoma. In addition, self-test devices for monitoring IOP and "home" visual field tests will soon become available, enabling patients to better monitor and manage their glaucoma with improved efficiency. The ophthalmic assistant's ultimate goal of providing early glaucoma detection, patient education, and a well-monitored treatment plan is becoming increasingly more viable with the advent of new medications, microsurgical techniques, automated diagnostic devices, home monitoring, and increased patient awareness.

Questions for review and thought

1. What causes angle-closure glaucoma?
2. List the classic symptoms that might suggest angle-closure glaucoma in a patient telephoning the office for an appointment.
3. What are the classic signs of angle-closure glaucoma?
4. Outline the medical treatment for an acute attack of angle-closure glaucoma.
5. What causes open-angle glaucoma?
6. What are the classic signs of damage from open-angle glaucoma?
7. What is the principle of applanation tonometry? How is applanation tonometry performed?
8. Discuss the usefulness of handheld applanation tonometers.
9. Outline visual field changes that may occur in open-angle glaucoma.
10. Outline a plan for the medical therapy of open-angle glaucoma.
11. Why does the eye enlarge in congenital glaucoma?
12. What causes pupillary block glaucoma and how does this mechanism come about?
13. Why does the eye enlarge in congenital glaucoma?
14. List ways to promote patient compliance with medications and proper drop instillation.

Q   Self-evaluation questions

True–false statements

Directions: Indicate whether the statement is true **(T)** or false **(F).**

1. Patients with acute angle-closure glaucoma complain of halos or rainbows around lights. **T** or **F**
2. Primary angle-closure glaucoma occurs more commonly in males than in females. **T** or **F**
3. All patients with a high IOP (greater than 21 mm Hg) have glaucoma. **T** or **F**

Missing words

Directions: Write in the missing word in the following sentences:

4. In children with congenital or infantile glaucoma, distension of the eyeball is referred to as _____.
5. _____ is the most common cause of posterior synechiae.

Choice-completion questions

Directions: Select the one best answer in each case.

6. Chronic open-angle glaucoma is *not* characterized by:
   a. raised IOP.
   b. sudden loss of vision associated with excruciating pain.
   c. slow erosion of the visual field.
   d. slow progressive loss of visual acuity.
   e. cupping of the temporal aspect of the optic disc.

7. Which of the following are provocative tests available for the diagnosis of primary angle-closure glaucoma?
   a. Miotic test using pilocarpine
   b. Mydriatic test using hydroxyamphetamine
   c. Dark room provocative test
   d. Pupillary dilation plus gonioscopy
   e. All of the above

8. Which of the following field defects is *not* commonly seen in patients with chronic open-angle glaucoma?
   a. Nerve fiber bundle defect
   b. Loss of central vision (central scotoma)
   c. Paracentral scotoma
   d. Nasal depression
   e. Peripheral constriction

A   Answers, notes, and explanations

1. **True.** The halos around lights are caused by corneal edema. Light is dispersed by the droplets of fluid in the corneal epithelium and the halos are typically composed of two colored rings: an inner blue-violet ring and an outer yellow-red ring. Halos are not pathognomonic of glaucoma. They also may occur in patients with cataracts (nuclear sclerosis) and excess conjunctival debris.

2. **False.** Primary angle-closure glaucoma occurs more commonly in females, particularly those more than 50 years of age. Patients with this disorder have essentially normal eyes with the exception of a shallow anterior chamber and a narrow entrance into the angle. In addition, these patients are usually hyperopic and have a "smaller eye" than normal. Crowding of the angle structures tends to increase as patients become older because of an increase in the size of the lens, which pushes the iris diaphragm forward.

3. **False.** *Glaucoma* is a term applied to a diverse group of ocular disorders characterized by an elevation of IOP to a level capable of producing damage to the ocular structures, the most important being the optic nerve head. About 2% of people older than age 40 have an increased IOP, but only 0.5% have raised IOP and field loss. Patients with an increased IOP and no field loss are referred to as having *ocular hypertension.* About 5% to 10% of these patients

may develop field loss with time and should be carefully observed. Some physicians treat ocular hypertensive patients, in anticipation of eventual nerve damage. Some physicians may treat these patients if the pressure reaches levels greater than 25 to 30 mm Hg. There is a group of patients who develop field loss with an IOP less than 21 mm Hg. These patients may have a compromised blood supply to the optic nerve head. In this group an IOP of 18 mm Hg may produce damage, and these patients are said to have normal tension (or low tension).

4. **Buphthalmos.** If increased IOP is present in an infant's eye, there is a progressive enlargement of both the eye and the cornea. This can result in a huge eye, which is referred to as *buphthalmos* or ox eye. If pressure does not become elevated until after the age of 3 years, the eye usually resists distension. In infants, an increasing corneal diameter is a very significant sign of uncontrolled glaucoma. The enlarged cornea usually is associated with tears in Descemet's membrane. The stretching results in myopia and irregular corneal astigmatism.

5. **Iritis.** Iritis is inflammation of the iris and behaves like inflammation anywhere else in the body. Posterior synechiae form as a result of the iris becoming adherent to the lens or vitreous in an aphakic eye. As a result, the aqueous cannot enter the anterior chamber and is forced to

A | Continued

accumulate behind the iris, which is pushed forward, resulting in blockage of the outflow. At the same time there is an increase in IOP, and secondary angle-closure glaucoma results. This cycle of events may be prevented by treating patients with iritis with antiinflammatory agents and mydriatics. If secondary angle-closure glaucoma occurs, a surgical or laser peripheral iridectomy should be performed so that the aqueous can bypass the pupillary pathway and enter the anterior chamber from the posterior chamber.

6. **b. Sudden loss of vision associated with excruciating pain.** The main purpose of this question is to emphasize the fact that chronic open-angle glaucoma is insidious in onset, and routine IOP should be performed on patients to detect this condition. Acute angle-closure glaucoma is characterized by a sudden marked rise in IOP. The vision is lost rapidly, the eye becomes red, and the patient complains of excruciating pain.

7. **e. All of the above.** An eye with a narrow angle should be investigated to determine its actual capacity to occlude.

There are many provocative tests available for diagnosing primary angle-closure glaucoma. Answers b, c, and d are often used. The pilocarpine provocative test may be used in narrow-angle glaucoma patients with closure and elevated pressure to rule out the possibility of an open-angle glaucoma component. In addition, pilocarpine constricts the pupil and may cause an increase in pupil block and hence precipitate an attack of acute-angle closure.

8. **b. Loss of central vision (central scotoma).** Central vision is classically spared in patients with chronic open-angle glaucoma. These patients may have a markedly constricted visual field (so-called tunnel vision) with good central visual acuity. The visual acuity may even be 20/20 with extensive loss of visual field. The last area of involvement of visual field in glaucoma is central vision. Loss of central vision, so-called central scotoma, causes profound loss of visual acuity with a relatively full peripheral field. Central scotomas are seen classically with disorders of the optic nerve, for example, optic neuritis secondary to demyelinating disorders.

ACKNOWLEDGMENTS

Dr. Michael S. Berlin and Dr. Harold Stein gratefully acknowledge the assistance and expertise of Christine Quach, Daniella Lent-Schochet, and Elias Saba in creating this chapter.

REFERENCES

1. Tham YC, Li X, Wong TY, Quigley HA, Aung T, Cheng CY. Global prevalence of glaucoma and projections of glaucoma burden through 2040: a systematic review and meta-analysis. Ophthalmology 2014;121 (11):2081–90.

2. Kuang TM, Zhang C, Zangwill LM, Weinreb RN, Medeiros FA. Estimating lead time gained by optical coherence tomography in detecting glaucoma before development of visual field defects. Ophthalmology 2015;122 (10):2002–9.

3. Taken from aao.com.

Chapter 26

Uveitis

Thellea K. Leveque, Russell N. Van Gelder

INTRODUCTION

"Uveitis" refers to the group of eye conditions defined by the presence of intraocular inflammation. The middle pigmented layers of the eye—the iris, ciliary body, and choroid—are collectively called the uvea, from the Latin word, *uva* (grape) for its round shape and dark color. The suffix, *itis* is of Greek origin, meaning "inflammation" (Figure 26.1).

In modern ophthalmology uveitis is used as an umbrella term to encompass a diverse group of autoimmune and infectious diseases of the uvea, retina, retinal vessels, optic nerve head, sclera, and cornea. Inflammation of these structures can cause an abnormal accumulation of white blood cells in the anterior chamber (anterior uveitis), vitreous cavity (intermediate uveitis), or retina and choroid (posterior uveitis). Often multiple structures may be involved. When all three regions are involved, the condition is considered a panuveitis. Infiltration of the cornea or sclera can cause opacity, redness, or thinning (Figure 26.2). Depending on the location and type of inflammation, patients may experience eye redness, pain, light sensitivity, blurred vision, or floaters. Over time, untreated inflammation may lead to complications such as tissue swelling, scarring, cataract, or glaucoma, which can result in permanent vision loss (Figure 26.3).

Uveitis accounts for between 5% and 20% of blindness in the United States and Europe, and up to 25% of blindness in the developing world.[1] In Western countries, in different studies uveitis is found to affect between 15 and 100 per 100,000 people per year,[2,3] and may be responsible for up to 30,000 new cases of legal blindness annually in the United States.[4] Uveitis can affect patients at any age; many forms may have a female predominance. In about half of patients, the age of onset is in the third or fourth decade of life, making uveitis one of the ocular diseases with an important socioeconomic effect.[5] In 25% to 50% of cases, there is an associated underlying systemic disease. The etiologic factor in more than 30% of uveitis cases is unknown.[5,6]

Only with prompt identification and complete and proper treatment can the ophthalmic team mitigate damage and preserve vision. Even low levels of asymptomatic smoldering inflammation are capable of inflicting permanent vision loss over time. Additionally the treatments used in uveitis can cause significant ocular and systemic side effects, requiring ongoing monitoring. In no other subspecialty of ophthalmology are the patient's medications, exposures, medical history, and current symptoms so critical to diagnosis and treatment. As the front line to the patient, the ophthalmic assistant has a key role to play in gathering patient information and initial examination data. This information not only will alert the physician to the possibility of a uveitic disease, but also help narrow the differential diagnosis, ask appropriate follow-up questions, and choose the most appropriate therapy.

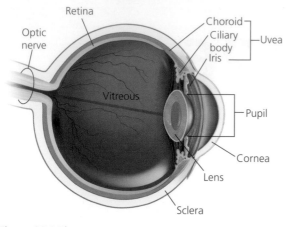

Figure 26.1 The uvea.

CLASSIFICATION OF UVEITIS

In 2005 a panel of experts formed the Standardization of Uveitis Nomenclature (SUN) Working Group in order to define a set of common terms to classify uveitis.[7] Uveitic diseases are organized by primary site of inflammation: anterior, intermediate, posterior, and panuveitis. The SUN system also provides nomenclature to describe the character and severity of uveitis (Table 26.1).

The character of the uveitis is ascertained by taking a thorough history of the present illness. The uveitis may occur suddenly or gradually (insidious onset). It may resolve relatively quickly or it may persist for months to years. A summation of these characteristics can help define what is called the "course" of uveitis: whether it is acute,

recurrent, or chronic (Table 26.2). Other descriptive categories frequently used include unilateral versus bilateral involvement, solitary retinal/choroidal lesions versus multifocal lesions, and others.[8]

The inflammatory activity of uveitis is defined by the degree of circulating white blood cells seen on physical examination. A high-magnification, bright, obliquely aimed 1×1 mm slit-lamp beam is focused on the space between the cornea and the iris. The number of individual white blood cells floating in this anterior chamber space is counted to grade the degree of anterior chamber cell on a 1 to 4 scale. The phenomenon of white blood cells floating in the anterior chamber is said to look like specks of dust floating in a sunbeam. Typically the anterior chamber should look completely black, or optically empty. If this space is cloudy, it represents protein extravasation from a damaged blood–aqueous barrier. This physical examination finding, called flare, can be a marker of disease severity or chronicity. The appearance of flare is often likened to that of headlights in the fog (Figure 26.4). Grading systems for vitreous inflammation are more complex, often focusing on the degree of obscuration of fundus details. The degree of vitreous cell and haze is also graded on a 1 to 4 scale. Scleritis is categorized as either anterior (e.g., diffuse, sectorial, nodular, or necrotizing) or posterior.

Causes of uveitis

Ocular inflammatory diseases may be limited to the eye, or have systemic manifestations. They may be caused by infectious or noninfectious etiology. Certain uveitic diseases have a predilection for the young or for the old, for a particular anatomic section of the eye, or for unilateral or bilateral disease. Entering the patient encounter with basic knowledge of some of the causes of uveitis can give new

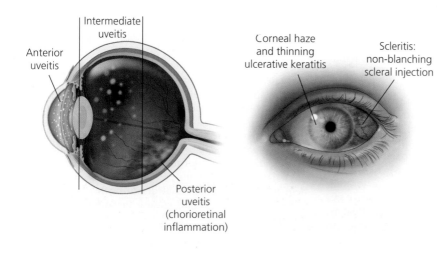

Figure 26.2 Uveitis includes anterior, intermediate, and posterior uveitis, panuveitis, scleritis, and keratitis.

Figure 26.3 Examples of uveitis complications that may result in vision loss. (A) Scleral perforation (B) Uveitic glaucoma (C) Posterior synechiae, iris nodules (D) Intraocular lens complications (E) Uveitic cataract with corneal opacity, band keratopathy (F) Optic disc edema (G) Retinal scar (H) Cystoid macular edema.

(A, from Tarabishy AB, et al. Survey of Ophthalmology. vol 55, issue 5, pp 429–44; 2010. B, from Bowling B. Glaucoma. In: Kanski's clinical ophthalmology, Chapter 10, 305–394. ©2016. C, E, F, from Bowling B. Uveitis. In: Kanski's Clinical Ophthalmology, Chapter 11, 395–465. ©2016. D, from From Afredo, A. Explantation of intraocular lenses in children with juvenile idiopathic arthritis–associated uveitis. In: Journal of Cataract and Refractive Surgery. Volume 35, Issue 3. Copyright © 2009 ASCRS and ESCRS. G, From Vasconcelos-Santos DV. Ocular Toxoplasmosis. In: Yanoff, M. and Duker, J. Ophthalmology, 4th edn. © 2014 Elsevier Inc. H, From Witmer, MT, Kiss, S. Cystoid Macular Edema. In: Yanoff, M. and Duker, J. Ophthalmology, 4th edn. © 2014 Elsevier Inc.)

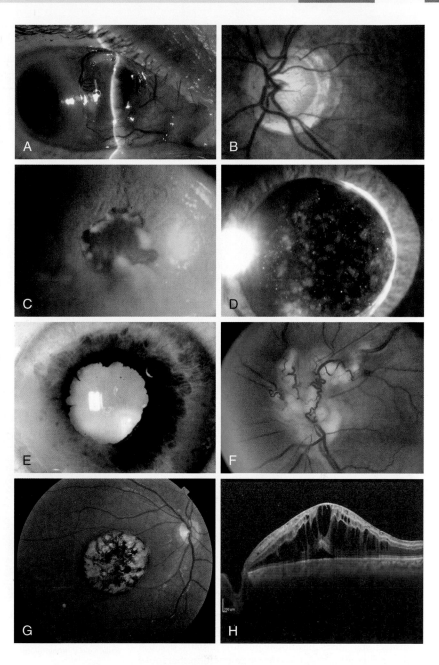

importance to patient responses to health and symptom questions when uveitis is suspected.

Infectious diseases that can enter the eye to cause uveitis include viruses, such as the herpesviruses that cause cold sores and shingles; bacteria, such as syphilis, tuberculosis, or Lyme disease; fungi, such as *Candida* (usually from contamination in the setting of indwelling intravenous [IV] lines in hospitalized patients, or IV drug users); and parasites, such as the tiny intracellular toxoplasmosis organism transmitted from undercooked meat or exposure to cat feces.

Inflammatory causes can be linked to systemic autoimmune diseases, such as juvenile idiopathic arthritis, multiple sclerosis, ankylosing spondylitis, and sarcoidosis, or they can be isolated to the eye, as is the case with sympathetic ophthalmia and birdshot chorioretinitis. Blunt trauma, occult penetrating trauma, or a retained intraocular foreign body can cause chronic intraocular

Table 26.1 The SUN Working Group anatomic classification of uveitis

Type	Primary site of inflammation*	Includes
Anterior uveitis	Anterior chamber	Iritis Iridocyclitis
Intermediate uveitis	Vitreous	Pars planitis Posterior cyclitis Hyalitis
Posterior uveitis	Retina or choroid	Focal, multifocal, or diffuse choroiditis Chorioretinitis Retinochoroiditis Retinitis Neuroretinitis
Panuveitis	Anterior chamber, vitreous, and retina or choroid	

In Albert DM, et al. Albert & Jakobiec's principles & practice of ophthalmology. 3rd ed. Philadelphia: Saunders; 2008. Adapted from Jabs DA, Nussenblatt RB, Rosenbaum JT. Standardization of uveitis nomenclature for reporting clinical data. Results of the First International Workshop. Am J Ophthalmol 2005;140(3):509–16.
SUN, Standardization of Uveitis Nomenclature.
*As determined clinically. Adapted from the International Study Group anatomic classification.

Table 26.2 The SUN Working Group descriptors of uveitis

Category	Descriptor	Comment
Onset	Sudden Insidious	
Duration	Limited Persistent	≤3 months' duration >3 months' duration
Course	Acute	Episode characterized by sudden onset and limited duration
	Recurrent	Repeated episodes separated by periods of inactivity without treatment ≥ 3 months in duration
	Chronic	Persistent uveitis with relapse in <3 months after discontinuing treatment

In Albert DM, et al. Albert & Jakobiec's principles & practice of ophthalmology. 3rd ed. Philadelphia: Saunders; 2008. Adapted from Jabs DA, Nussenblatt RB, Rosenbaum JT. Standardization of uveitis nomenclature for reporting clinical data. Results of the First International Workshop. Am J Ophthalmol 2005;140(3):509–16.
SUN, Standardization of Uveitis Nomenclature.

inflammation. In rare cases uveitis can be caused by an inflammatory reaction to certain systemic medications. Finally, some cancers such as lymphoma can mimic or "masquerade" as uveitis, with deposition of abnormal white blood cells in various structures of the eye. See Table 26.3 for a more complete list of uveitis causes.

APPROACH TO THE PATIENT WITH UVEITIS

In clinical practice, distinguishing between infectious and noninfectious causes may not be possible initially, because both can present with intraocular inflammation that looks highly similar (e.g., white spots on the choroid caused by a tuberculosis infection or by an autoimmune sarcoidosis infiltration). Instead, the type of uveitis is categorized as described in the previous section: how does it behave and where is it located? Much like providing a description of a criminal to a forensic sketch artist, a good description creates an image that can then be cross-referenced against known suspects. In this scenario, the suspects are the known causes of uveitis, each of which with its own typical set of clinical characteristics. Matching the forensic sketch with the correct suspect (making the correct diagnosis) is

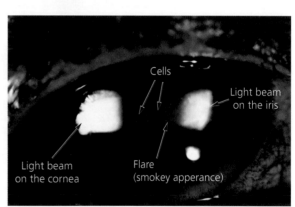

Figure 26.4 Clinical appearance of anterior chamber cell and flare at the slit lamp.
(From Witmer, MT, Kiss, S. Cystoid Macular Edema. In: Yanoff, M. and Duker, J. Ophthalmology, 4th edn. © 2014 Elsevier Inc.)

aided by obtaining a review of systems and performing diagnostic tests such as labs or imaging.

For example, a recurring uveitis that suddenly affects the anterior chamber of one eye could fit the description of ocular herpes simplex or that of anterior uveitis associated with a genetically associated inflammatory arthritis (HLA-B27 arthritis or ankylosing spondylitis). A review of systems that reveals morning low back stiffness and a blood test showing a positive marker for the gene, HLA-B27 allows us to pick the right suspect from the line-up.

Table 26.3 Selected causes of uveitis

Noninfectious	Infectious
With systemic disease	**Viral**
Systemic lupus erythematosus	Herpetic (HSV, VZV, CMV, EBV)
Sarcoidosis	Fuchs heterochromic iridocyclitis (rubella)
Systemic vasculitis	Measles virus
Juvenile or rheumatoid arthritis	West Nile virus
Behçet's disease	**Bacterial**
Inflammatory bowel disease (Crohn's/ulcerative colitis)	Syphilis
Ankylosing spondylitis, psoriatic arthritis, HLA-B27 diseases	Tuberculosis
Without systemic disease	Cat scratch disease (*Bartonella henselae*)
Vogt-Koyonagi-Harada (VKH) syndrome	Lyme disease (*Borrelia burgdorferi*)
Sympathetic ophthalmia	Brucellosis
Inflammatory chorioretinopathies (white dot syndromes)	Rickettsial diseases (e.g., Rocky Mountain spotted fever)
Drug induced	**Fungal**
Rifabutin	*Candida* species
Cidofovir	*Aspergillus* species
Osteoporosis drugs (bisphosphonates)	Histoplasmosis
Select antibiotics: sulfonamides, fluoroquinolones	**Parasitic**
Select topical drops: brimonidine, prostaglandin analogs	Toxoplasmosis
Trauma	Toxocariasis
Blunt trauma	Diffuse unilateral subacute neuroretinitis (DUSN)
Occult foreign body or ruptured globe	Onchocerciasis (river blindness)
Masquerade	
Primary intraocular lymphoma	
Metastasis to eye from extraocular cancer site	

CMV, Cytomegalovirus; *EBV*, Epstein-Barr Virus; *HSV*, Herpes Simplex Virus; *VZV*, Varicella Zoster Virus.

History

"Listen to your patient. He is telling you the diagnosis."

—William Osler, MD (1849–1919),
"Father of Modern Medicine"

Eye symptoms

Patients with anterior uveitis are likely to complain of redness, light sensitivity, decreased vision, or pain. They may notice a change in the size or shape of their pupil if there is scar tissue formation (posterior synechiae). Patients with intermediate or posterior uveitis are more likely to describe blind spots, floaters, or flashes instead of redness or pain. Ask the patient how long the symptoms have lasted, if they occurred suddenly or gradually, whether they have occurred previously, and whether they are in one or both eyes.

Medical history

Obtaining a complete medical, family, and social history is critical to the evaluation of the patient with uveitis. Emphasis on personal or family history of autoimmune, inflammatory, or infectious diseases is useful. Additionally, understanding a patient's comorbid conditions is necessary when considering local ophthalmic or systemic medications. Smoking can make uveitis worse. IV drug use or unprotected sex can increase risk of certain bacterial and viral causes of uveitis. Occupations or hobbies involving the handling of animals increase the risk of certain zoonotic infections. Infectious uveitis has been linked to exposure to household pets or travel to countries with high levels of endemic infections. A complete list of medications, including recent changes or additions can reveal use of a prescription drug known to cause uveitis (including rifabutin, pamidronate, or certain newer chemotherapy drugs such as ipilimumab). A history of ocular trauma or surgery can cause uveitis in some cases.

Review of systems

A variety of systemic symptoms can be manifestations of diseases also known to cause uveitis. Skin changes such as peeling, redness, or loss of pigment can be seen in conditions such as lupus, sarcoidosis, vasculitis, HLA-B27 arthropathies, syphilis, or Vogt-Koyonagi-Harada (VKH). Joint pain, swelling, or stiffness is another common feature of certain autoimmune diseases. Bloody diarrhea can be seen in inflammatory bowel disease, neurologic changes in multiple sclerosis, oral and genital ulcers in Behçet's disease, cold sores or shingles in herpetic uveitis, and fevers or lethargy in a variety or infectious and noninfectious uveitic diseases. Most uveitis specialists have a questionnaire specific to the investigation of social, behavioral, and symptomatic clues to the cause of uveitis (Table 26.4).

Table 26.4 Example uveitis patient questions

Symptoms	Exposures
Oral or genital ulcers	Sexually transmitted diseases
Cold sores	Dogs, cats, or other pets at home
Ringing in ears	Farm animal exposures
Weight gain or loss	Raw meat consumption
Numbness, tingling, weakness	Unpasteurized milk, unwashed fruits and vegetables
Bowel or bladder incontinence, blood, frequency	Tick bites, mosquito bites
Skin rashes, spots, or depigmentations	Tuberculosis (TB) risk factors: travel to endemic areas, homelessness, incarceration
Joint pains or arthritis	Intravenous drug use
Shortness of breath	

Physical examination

"I have made a discovery…by means of which it is possible to see the dark background of the eye…."

—Hermann von Helmholtz (1821–1894), inventor of the ophthalmoscope

The ophthalmic technician is uniquely poised to acquire front-line physical examination data. The visual acuity, refractive state, intraocular pressure, pupils, confrontational fields, and extraocular motility are key components in evaluating the patient with uveitis. Identification of scleral redness (injection), corneal epitheliopathy, endothelial deposits (called keratic precipitates), and anterior chamber cell and depth are examination findings that may have a direct effect on what the doctor chooses as the next best step (gonioscopy, assessment of corneal sensation, endothelial cell counts, instillation of eyedrops, etc.). Table 26.5 lists uveitis physical examination signs that may be seen by the ophthalmic technician at the initial slit-lamp examination. It also includes a section describing how certain physical examination signs may be altered by the instillation of office drops commonly used for diagnosis (tetracaine/proparacaine, phenylephrine, and fluorescein sodium).

Ancillary clinic tests and laboratory workup

"As to diseases, make a habit of two things—to help, or at least, to do no harm."

—Hippocrates (460–370 BC), "Father of Western Medicine"

There is no single standardized workup for uveitis. That said, syphilis, sarcoidosis, and tuberculosis have protean uveitic manifestations, and these entities should be considered early and often in the uveitis workup. Generally speaking, laboratory testing should be used to detect infectious diseases that cannot be identified by the clinical presentation or systemic diseases with an effect on the patient's health.[9]

Based on patient demographics and uveitis characteristics, the following diagnostic testing may be appropriate: for suspicion of tuberculosis, interferon gamma release assay (IGRA) (QuantiFERON-TB Gold In-Tube or T-SPOT.TB test), or tuberculin skin testing; for sarcoidosis, chest x-ray (CXR) or chest computed tomography (CT) scan, with limited utility of blood tests angiotensin converting enzyme and lysozyme; for syphilis, treponemal (*Treponema pallidum* immunoglobulin G [IgG] enzyme-linked immunoassay [EIA] test, Treponema pallidum particle agglutination assay [TPPA] test, and FTA-ABS test) and nontreponemal tests (rapid plasma reagin [RPR] and venereal disease research laboratory [VDRL]); serum antibody testing for IgM and IgG may be appropriate when there is suspicion for toxoplasmosis, *Bartonella*, herpesviridae, Lyme disease and others; for systemic vasculitides

Table 26.5 Examination pearls for the ophthalmic technician

Anterior scleritis	• Painful, purplish red "violaceous" hue of the sclera that does not blanch with the instillation of phenylephrine dilating drops
Anterior segment inflammation	• Dot-like clusters of white blood cells on the corneal endothelium called keratic precipitates (KP) • Irregular pupil shape caused by iris adhesion to the lens called posterior synechiae (PS) • Scarring of the peripheral iris to the cornea, resulting in a shallow anterior chamber called peripheral anterior synechiae (PAS) • Anterior chamber cell and flare, or white cells in a layer, called hypopyon
Corneal defects, thinning, or clouding	• Branch-like epithelial defects and reduced corneal sensation may be seen in herpetic keratouveitis • Peripheral cloudiness or thinning may be features of peripheral ulcerative keratitis • Subepithelial calcium deposits, called band keratopathy
Intraocular pressure (IOP)	• IOP may be elevated in viral uveitis, otherwise it is often low in other forms of uveitis
Fluorescein sodium eyedrops	• Instillation causes a green haze in the anterior chamber, which can alter the grading of flare
Phenylephrine eyedrops	• Instillation causes vascular constriction and pupil dilation. Can reduce the degree of conjunctival/episcleral redness, and can cause release of pigmented cells from the iris into the anterior chamber
Tetracaine or proparacaine eyedrops	• Instillation may cause mild redness, may cause or exacerbate punctate epitheliopathy, eliminates the ability for the physician to test for corneal sensation

and collagen vascular disease, cANCA (antiproteinase 3), pANCA (antimyeloperoxidase), antinuclear antibody test, with the addition of rheumatoid factor for scleritis and ulcerative keratitis; for tubulointerstitial nephritis and uveitis syndrome (TINU), urinalysis, and urine beta-2 microglobulin, with renal biopsy when indicated.

Adjunctive testing with lumbar puncture and brain imaging may be useful in determining neurologic involvement when warranted by clinical suspicion. Immune system compromise from human immunodeficiency virus (HIV) can alter the appearance of uveitis. Additionally the differential diagnosis broadens in the context of the potential for unexpected opportunistic infections.

In-office diagnostic imaging is often useful in further classification of the clinical features of uveitis. Color photos of the anterior segment are useful in tracking the progress of scleritis, corneal processes, or iris scarring. Ultrasound biomicroscopy (UBM) and anterior segment optical coherence tomography (OCT) can be useful in detailed assessment of the iridocorneal angle or interaction between the iris and the lens. Color fundus photographs may be helpful in documenting the degree of vitreous haze and extent and progression of chorioretinal lesions. B-scan ultrasound can be useful in quantifying the degree of vitritis, choroidal thickening, or retinal traction or detachments.

OCT is useful in refining posterior segment disease location and characteristics. Optic nerve atrophy or focal nerve fiber layer loss may be seen as long-term sequelae of hypertensive uveitis, papillitis, or occlusive vasculitis at the nerve head. Disc edema may be seen in many types of panuveitis. Diffuse retinal thickening, cystoid edema, selective layer loss, or inflammatory deposits are common features of many forms of panuveitis. OCT is also critical in the diagnosis of choroidal neovascular membrane and subretinal scarring, complications of many types of posterior uveitis.

Fundus autofluorescence (FAF) is another noninvasive retinal imaging modality that highlights lipofuscin accumulation within the retinal pigment epithelium (RPE). Increased FAF is expected in the presence of increased RPE metabolic activity, and decreased FAF in the setting of loss of photoreceptors or the RPE. It has applications for many types of posterior uveitis, including white dot syndromes, VKH disease, and infectious uveitis.[10]

Fluorescein angiography (FA) and indocyanine green angiography (ICG) are specialized forms of posterior photography that rely on IV injection of the fluorescent molecules fluorescein sodium and indocyanine green dye, respectively. The molecular characteristics and emission spectrum make fluorescein useful in assessing retinal and to a certain extent, choroidal, vessels and structures. ICG is a large iodine-based molecule that remains within choroidal vasculature and is useful in highlighting choroidal circulation and choroidal inflammatory lesions, and should not be given to patients with iodine or shellfish allergy.

TREATMENT OF UVEITIS

"If it's wet, dry it. If it's dry, wet it. If in doubt, use steroids...."

—A satirical medical school saying

Corticosteroids are a class of fast acting, powerful antiinflammatory medications used frequently in the treatment of noninfectious uveitis. They may be used locally in the eye in the form of eyedrops, periocular and intraocular injections, or slow-release implantable pellets that may be injected or surgically implanted. Typically, eyedrops are used for certain types of anterior and intermediate uveitis but do not have good enough depth of penetration to treat posterior segment manifestations of uveitis. Systemic steroids may be administered intravenously or orally to treat severe disease or posterior manifestations of disease.

Ophthalmic and systemic side effects of steroids are significant. In the eye they may cause ocular hypertension and cataract. Systemic corticosteroids may cause multiple side effects, including weight gain, insomnia, mood changes, bone thinning, muscle weakness, infection risk, diabetes, and hypertension. The risks posed by untreated uveitis must be weighed against the risks posed by steroid treatments. Unilateral uveitic diseases without systemic manifestations are the best candidates for local therapy. Systemic treatment is mandatory when there is a significant systemic disease component. Many patients receive combination local and systemic therapy.

Infectious diseases are typically treated with the appropriate antibiotic, antifungal, antiviral, or antiparasitic agent. Once the infectious etiology is controlled, adjunctive steroid-based therapies may be used with caution.

Recognizing the need to reduce steroid exposure has led to a large body of work detailing the safety and efficacy of steroid-sparing medications for patients requiring chronic immune-modulating therapy. These agents are commonly grouped into the categories of antimetabolites (methotrexate, azathioprine, or mycophenolate mofetil), T-cell inhibitors (cyclosporine, tacrolimus, sirolimus), alkylating agents (cyclophosphamide, chlorambucil), and biologic agents (infliximab, adalimumab, rituximab, among others).

Surgical therapy may be required to treat uveitic cataract (cataract surgery), uveitic glaucoma (glaucoma drainage devices), and certain forms of intermediate and panuveitis (vitrectomy). Unless the surgery is an emergency, the uveitis should be well controlled for at least 3 months in order to prevent uveitis exacerbation from the surgical insult.

 ### Case examples

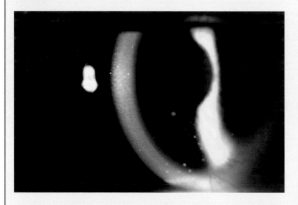

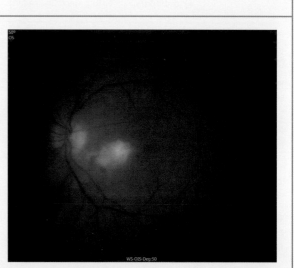

Case 1. Glaucomatocyclitic crisis Posner-Schlossman syndrome (anterior uveitis)

Unilateral, limited, recurrent unilateral anterior uveitis associated with small round keratic precipitates seen in the image. The patient has minimal discomfort, and intraocular pressure spikes to 40 to 50. A viral etiology such as cytomegalovirus (CMV), or other herpesviridae has been proposed. Treated with topical steroids and ocular antihypertensive drops. Consideration of antiviral medications.

Case 2. Behçet's disease (panuveitis)

Sudden onset of a central blind spot in the setting of mild redness and light sensitivity in a 41-year-old Japanese male with oral and genital ulcers. Examination shows a relatively quiet eye with a small hypopyon, vitritis, and a branch retinal artery occlusion (white retinal infarct shown in the image). Clinicians perform a careful review for other systemic involvement. Treated with systemic steroids and long-term immunosuppression.

Continued

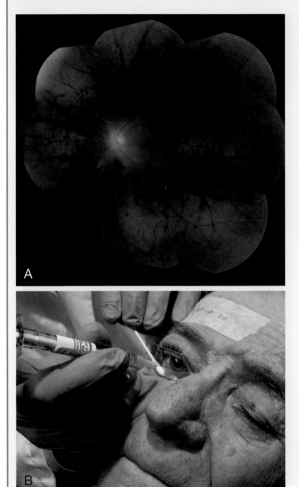

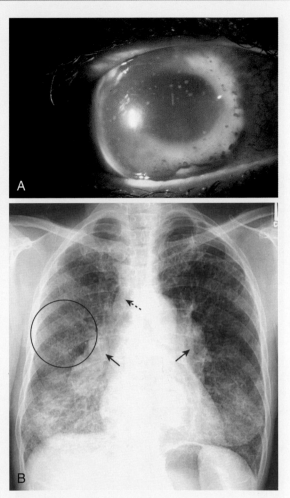

Case 3. Acute retinal necrosis (panuveitis)

Sudden-onset unilateral redness, light sensitivity, decreased vision, and pain in the left eye of an otherwise healthy 67-year-old patient. Examination reveals elevated IOP, with anterior and intermediate uveitis and a rapidly progressive peripheral retinitis with occlusive retinal arteriolitis, shown in the image. Vitreous tap is positive at 10^6 copies/mL of varicella zoster virus (VZV). Treatment is with local and/or systemic antivirals with adjunctive corticosteroids.

(B, From Intravitreal injections. Bhavsar, AR., Surgical techniques in ophthalmology: Retina and Vitreous Surgery, 133–143. Philadelphia: Saunders; 2009.)

Case 4. Sarcoid uveitis (variable presentation)

Bilateral chronic iridocyclitis in a 55-year-old African American female with large greasy-appearing keratic precipitates shown in the slit-lamp image. Chest x-ray shows bilateral hilar lymphadenopathy, as shown by the arrows. Treatment varies with disease severity and other organ system involvement. Treatment is with steroids and immunomodulatory therapy.

(A, from Nussenblat R, Whitcup S. Uveitis: fundamentals and clinical practice. 4th ed. Philadelphia: Mosby; 2010. B, from Herring, W. Learning radiology: recognizing the basics. 3rd ed. Philadelphia: Saunders; 2009.)

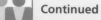 Continued

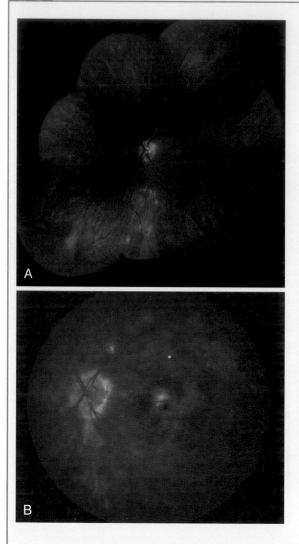

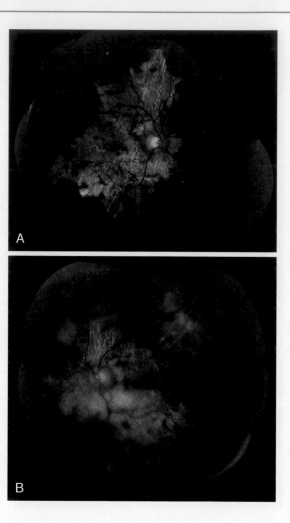

Case 5. Birdshot chorioretinopathy (panuveitis)

A 60-year-old white female with insidious onset of bilateral floaters and photopsias. Dilated funduscopic examination reveals multiple yellow choroidal spots (noted in the image), panuveitis, and cystoid macular edema. Retinal vasculitis noted on fluorescein angiography. Blood test positive for HLA-A29. Treat with slow-release local steroids or systemic immunomodulation.

Case 6. Serpiginous chorioretinopathy (posterior uveitis)

A 40-year-old white male with bilateral rapidly progressive field constriction, absent anterior, and vitreous inflammation with a negative uveitis workup. Dilated funduscopic examination reveals nearly confluent, atrophic chorioretinal lesions with serpent-like borders. Treated with systemic immunomodulation.

Continued

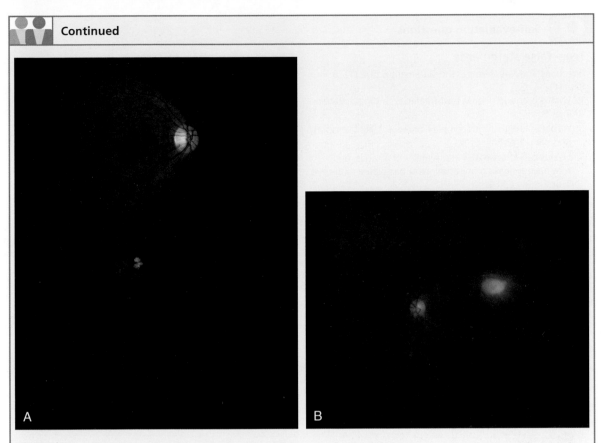

A

B

Case 7. Toxoplasmosis reactivation (panuveitis)

Insidious onset of redness, pain, floaters, and decreased vision in the left eye of a 12-year-old girl born in Brazil. The right eye has an inactive scar. The images show that the right eye has an inactive scar, and the left has panuveitis with a fluffy white patch of retinochoroiditis. Toxoplasmosis serum IgG is positive. Treatment with short-term antibiotic therapy and adjunctive corticosteroids.

Questions for review and thought

1. What is uveitis?
2. Can you identify some of the vision-threatening complications of untreated uveitis?
3. Why is it important to carefully classify and describe uveitis?
4. What are some of the broad categories that cause uveitis?
5. What are some of the symptoms that typify anterior uveitis? Intermediate and posterior uveitis?
6. What are some reasons to take a careful medical family and social history?
7. What role does the technician play in gathering physical examination data?
8. Why is there no single set of laboratory tests specific to the uveitis workup?
9. What is the role of corticosteroid therapy in uveitis? Why is it good, and why is it bad?
10. How do we decide when to treat systemically or locally?
11. When is surgery indicated in the treatment of uveitis?

Q Self-evaluation questions

True–false statements

Directions: Indicate whether the statement is true **(T)** or false **(F).**

1. Uveitis is an eye disease best treated with topical steroids. **T** or **F**
2. All patients with uveitis complain of redness, light sensitivity and pain. **T** or **F**
3. Uveitis can affect males and females of all ages, and may have systemic manifestations or be isolated to the eye. **T** or **F**

Missing words

Directions: Write in the missing word in the following sentences:

4. Cellular deposits on the corneal endothelium are called _____.
5. _____, or iris adhesions to the anterior lens capsule, may cause pupillary irregularities.
6. Because sympathetic ophthalmia affects the anterior, intermediate and posterior eye segments, it is best classified as _____.

Choice-completion questions

Directions: Select the one best answer in each case.

7. Which of the following is *not* typically included under the umbrella term "uveitis"?
   a. Retinitis
   b. Intermediate uveitis
   c. Scleritis
   d. Conjunctivitis
8. Which of the following is true regarding the workup, diagnosis and treatment of uveitis?
   a. The patient history is typically not important in the diagnosis of uveitis.
   b. Most uveitis patients should get the same set of laboratory tests and in-office imaging studies to aid in diagnosis.
   c. Topical and systemic steroids are effective, safe, and have few side effects.
   d. None of the above
9. Which of the following is *not* a known cause of uveitis?
   a. Parasite infection
   b. Autoimmune disease
   c. Primary open-angle glaucoma
   d. Certain medications
   e. Eye trauma

A Answers, notes, and explanations

1. **False.** Uveitis is an eye disease best treated with topical steroids. Uveitis refers to a diverse group of inflammatory eye diseases. Topical steroids are a common treatment but are inadequate to treat posterior segment disease, uveitic disease with systemic manifestations, or uveitic disease with an infectious etiology.
2. **False.** All patients with uveitis complain of redness, light sensitivity, and pain. Most patients with anterior uveitis describe some combination of redness, light sensitivity, decreased vision, and pain. However, patients with intermediate or posterior uveitis may have a painless, quiet eye with floaters and/or photopsias. Sometimes uveitis has no symptoms.
3. **True.** Uveitis can affect males and females of all ages, and may have systemic manifestations or be isolated to the eye. The wide diversity of patient features and of disease manifestations is part of what makes the diagnosis of uveitis challenging and exciting. The inflammatory chorioretinopathies ("white dot syndromes") are more likely to affect young myopic females. The panuveitis with occlusive vasculitis of Behçet's disease is more likely to affect individuals with ancestry in southern Europe, the

Middle East, and central Asia. Children suffer from the severe anterior uveitis of juvenile idiopathic arthritis. A detailed description of the characteristics of the patient and of the uveitis allows the diagnostician to choose the right uveitis suspect from the lineup.

4. **Keratic precipitates.** These are cellular deposits on the corneal endothelium.
5. **Posterior synechiae,** or iris adhesions to the anterior lens capsule, may cause pupillary irregularities.
6. **Posterior uveitis.** Because sympathetic ophthalmia affects the anterior, intermediate, and posterior eye segments, it is best classified as posterior uveitis.
7. **d.** Uveitis is an umbrella term used to describe inflammatory diseases of the deep inner coat of the eye known as the uvea: the iris, ciliary body, and choroid. Because adjacent structures are often involved, uveitis has grown to include inflammatory diseases of the retina, cornea and sclera. It is categorized into anterior, intermediate, and posterior disease, with the posterior component being retinitis or choroiditis. Inflammation of the conjunctiva is not deep enough to be considered part of the uveitis family.

A   Continued

8. **d.** As discussed in question 3, the patient history is critical because it may reveal symptoms, exposures, or diagnoses that contribute to our understanding of the nature of the uveitis at hand. There is no single laboratory workup for uveitis. Most uveitis is diagnosed on clinical grounds, with laboratory tests used to detect infectious diseases that cannot be identified by the clinical presentation, to detect systemic diseases with an effect on the patient's health, or to ensure the absence of unrelated underlying infectious disease before initiating an immunosuppressive regimen. Topical and systemic steroids are effective, but they may have dangerous side effects. In the eye they cause cataract and glaucoma. Systemically there are many side effects including insomnia, blood glucose abnormalities, mood changes, and weight gain.

9. **c.** Parasitic infections may cause diffuse unilateral subacute neuroretinitis (DUSN), toxoplasmosis retinochoroiditis, toxocariasis granulomas, and others. Autoimmune diseases such as Behçet's, or the HLA-B27-associated spondyloarthropathies and many others have well-described ophthalmic manifestations. Cidofovir, rifabutin, and others can cause uveitis. Blunt or penetrating ocular trauma can cause inflammation. Rarely a penetrating injury to one eye can cause a cascade of inflammation that results in uveitis in the fellow eye (sympathetic ophthalmia). Primary open-angle glaucoma does not cause uveitis.

REFERENCES

1. de Smet MD, Taylor SR, Bodaghi B, et al. Understanding uveitis: the impact of research on visual outcomes. Prog Retin Eye Res 2011;30(6):452–70.

2. Gritz DC, Wong IG. Incidence and prevalence of uveitis in Northern California; the Northern California Epidemiology of Uveitis Study. Ophthalmology 2004;11 (3):491–500 discussion.

3. Acharya NR, Tham VM, Esterberg E, et al. Incidence and prevalence of uveitis: results from the Pacific Ocular Inflammation Study. JAMA Ophthalmol 2013;131(11):1405–12.

4. Nussenblatt RB. The natural history of uveitis. Int Ophthalmol 1990; 14(5–6):303–8.

5. Suttorp-Schulten MS, Rothova A. The possible impact of uveitis in blindness: a literature survey. Br J Ophthalmol 1996;80(9):844–8.

6. Rothova A, Suttorp-van Schulten MS, Frits Treffers W, Kijlstra A. Causes and frequency of blindness in patients with intraocular inflammatory disease. Br J Ophthalmol 1996;80(4):332–6.

7. Jabs DA, Nussenblatt RB, Rosenbaum JT. Standardization of uveitis nomenclature for reporting clinical data. Results of the First International Workshop. Am J Ophthalmol 2005;140(3):509–16.

8. Dunn JP. Uveitis. Prim Care 2015; 42(3):305–23.

9. Jabs DA, Busingye J. Approach to the diagnosis of the uveitides. Am J Ophthalmol 2013;156(2):228–36.

10. Samy A, Lightman S, Ismetova F, et al. Role of autofluorescence in inflammatory/infective diseases of the retina and choroid. J Ophthalmol 2014;2014:418193.

Chapter 27

Examination of the newborn, infant, and small child

Alex V. Levin

Ocular examination of a newborn, infant, or small child presents unique challenges that require special techniques and particular knowledge of the normal variations in eyeball anatomy and function of this age group. Children may be unable or unwilling to participate voluntarily in the examination. The ophthalmic assistant must also remember that the child's caretaker is an integral part of the "patient team." Attention to the needs of both parent and child is essential for obtaining the desired information.

APPROACH TO PARENT AND CHILD

Children are unique patients in that they are almost always accompanied by a caretaker who is their advocate, communicator, and guardian. The parent must be enlisted as a positive participant in the child's eye examination. In taking the ocular history, it is also important to distinguish between the parental concerns and the child's symptoms that led to examination. Sometimes the parent may have observed a visual behavior that is of concern. In other situations the parent may not have observed a problem that was noted by the referring pediatrician or family physician. One must never underestimate the value of parental observations, which should be noted on the patient's chart even if they contradict the physician's observation that initiated the referral. This is particularly important in assessing a baby who is thought to have poor vision or blindness. The first question should be, "Do you think your baby sees?" Although some parents may deny that their baby's sight is poor, most will make an accurate assessment of the baby's ability to see objects and people, in particular the face of the parent during feeding. The parental assessment provides a most valuable piece of information.

Although it is important for ophthalmic assistants to introduce themselves to the parents, a self-introduction directly to the small child is also recommended. The child's individuality must be recognized and honored. Young children need to know that they have some control over the examination environment. They are often scared, unsure, or even tearful and combative. The initial introduction and conversation with the child may determine the success or failure of the remainder of the examination. Before conversing with the parents, the assistant can chat with the child about issues unrelated to the visit, inquiring about the youngster's age, siblings, pets, or a toy the child is clutching. Ask what game the child is playing on his or her tablet or smart phone and have the child demonstrate. Notice what is on the child's T-shirt, unusual jewelry, or a book he or she may be reading. If a teenager looks bored or unhappy, try to break the ice with some humor about the teen not wanting to be there. These comments often provide valuable reassurance to the child that the examiner has true interest and concern for the child's well-being.

It is usually harmless to allow younger children to gain some feeling of control over this unfamiliar environment by asking if they want to sit alone or on the lap of a particular parent, allowing them to explore the room and touch equipment, and allowing them to play with toys or siblings in the room while the interview with the parent proceeds. It is essential for the ophthalmic assistant to have several toys available to distract the younger child both before and during the examination.

The assistant can make the examination a game by constantly carrying on a playful banter while presenting the child with tasks, and toys. Banter about more mature matters such as sports, dating, and extracurricular activities can even keep the teenager engaged. For younger and more fearful children, it is important to glean as much information as possible without touching the child. Often one can assess eye movements, pupillary reactions, external ocular anatomy, and even visual acuity with only the most minimal physical contact. When the child is asked to answer questions or perform visual tasks, such as visual acuity testing or binocular vision testing, one should always be positive when responding to the child's answer even if that answer is incorrect. If the child makes a mistake, one can simply say "good job" and move on to the next letter. Undermining a child's confidence by indicating a poor performance on a visual test may decrease compliance with the examination. It is also helpful if the examination is conducted without external interruptions such as answering telephone calls or the movement of people walking in and out of the room. Because children in the younger age groups or older children with developmental challenges have very short attention spans, the examination must be conducted swiftly, in good humor, and with minimal extraneous distractions.

If the child becomes tearful or uncooperative, it often is best to back off and either undertake an unrelated conversation or ask the child how he or she would like to proceed. For example, some children prefer to hold the penlight or direct ophthalmoscope themselves. They can hold the instrument along with the assistant who is conducting the examination. It may be helpful to perform part of the examination on the parents or the child's toy (e.g., a teddy bear) in a mock fashion to demonstrate that it is painless before carrying out that step of the examination on the child.

Children have certain biologic needs that must be satisfied if an optimum examination is to be completed. If an infant appears cranky, one might inquire if the parent believes that the child needs to feed. Quite a bit of information can be obtained while the child is being examined during a feeding. A pacifier or favorite toy also should be allowed because it may increase the child's level of comfort and security. Interruptions for diaper changes and visits to the washroom must be permitted. If a sibling's behavior is distracting, the examiner can turn attention to that child and invite him or her to participate in the examination.

For example, a sibling can be asked to flip the switch when the lights are being turned on and off or to hand the examiner toys and tools that are being used.

VISION ASSESSMENT

Assessment of the visual acuity in neonates and infants is often limited to ascertaining whether vision is absent, present, or within normal limits for their age and equal in both eyes. Visual fixation is present at birth. The best visual target for the neonate is the human face. Normal infants should smile responsively and briefly follow a stimulus by 2 months of age. In the second and third months of life, infants develop the ability to follow a target beyond the midline, although it may not be until the fourth month that they can follow completely from one side over to the other (180 degrees). When the examiner presents an infant with a target, it is important to use a silent toy to ensure that any following or responsive behavior that is observed results from visual rather than auditory stimuli. High-contrast (black and white) targets are particularly helpful.

Children who are blind or have very poor sight often have wandering, purposeless, dysconjugate eye movements or nystagmus. The presence of nystagmus at birth, however, does not necessarily imply complete blindness. If a child has very poor sight, it is important to note if there is a response to light (light perception [LP]). One can look for the "eye-popping reflex" by abruptly turning off all illumination in the room. A sighted baby or infant will demonstrate a reflex opening of the eyes. When the lights are then turned on abruptly, both eyes should close. Even premature babies should respond to a bright light. If the child's eyes are closed, the bright light can be shone through the closed eyelid and a reflex contraction of the eyelid and surrounding muscles should be seen.

More formal technical tests are available to better quantify an infant's visual acuity, such as preferential-looking tests, and graded optokinetic nystagmus (OKN). The visual evoked potential (VEP) is a test designed to measure the ability of the occipital cortex in the brain to register a response to visual targets of increasingly difficult resolution by placing electrodes on the scalp that sense the passage of visual information from the eyeballs to the brain. The OKN drum (Figure 27.1) will elicit nystagmus in anyone capable of seeing the stripes on the rotating drum. Preferential-looking techniques (Figure 27.2) rely on the ability of an infant to distinguish between and favor a target that is variably different in terms of resolution (e.g., black-and-white stripes) compared with a bland gray target. The electroretinogram (ERG) is used to assess whether the retina is functioning in a child who is apparently blind or has poor sight. This test does not, however, measure visual acuity.

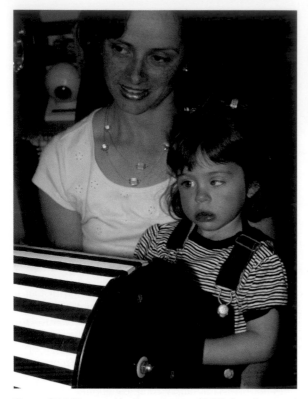

Figure 27.1 The optokinetic nystagmus (OKN) drum is rotated in front of the patient, inducing nystagmus in any patient who is neurologically normal and sighted. Note that this child has a crossed (esotropic) left eye. She is viewing with her preferred right eye.
(Photograph by Leslie MacKeen.)

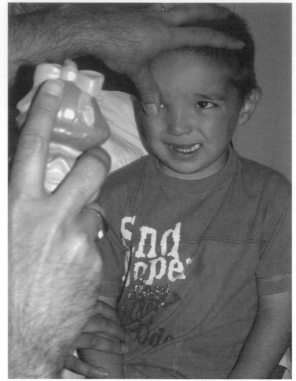

Figure 27.3 The examiner covers the child's right eye while showing a toy for fixation. If the child has better vision in the right eye, he may become visibly upset or attempt to remove the examiner's thumb, indicating that the preferred eye is being covered. When the unpreferred eye is covered, the child may show no reaction at all.
(Photograph by Leslie MacKeen.)

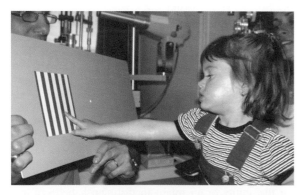

Figure 27.2 Preferential-looking technique. Given the ability to distinguish between the stripes and the other side of the board, the child indicates the striped target. As the stripes get closer together, they become more difficult to distinguish from the homogeneous gray side, and the striped target becomes less preferred.
(Photograph by Leslie MacKeen.)

If a significant difference exists in the visual acuity between the two eyes, the small child will object to the examiner covering the better eye. Although the eye can be covered by a piece of tape, the examiner's hand, or a commercially available occluder paddle, just using one thumb may be less frightening (Figure 27.3). The child may become visibly uncomfortable or may attempt to remove the obstruction only when the better-seeing eye is covered. This test is best performed while presenting the child with a target of interest such as a bright toy. A differential response on the covering of either eye is a critical sign of a difference in vision between the eyes.

The visual acuity in infants and preverbal children is usually recorded as central steady maintained (CSM) or good steady maintained (GSM). This indicates that the eyeball fixates with the fovea straight along the visual axis, nystagmus does not occur in the straight-ahead position, and there is no preference for either eye. If an eye is clearly unpreferred (i.e., not seeing as well as the other eye), but is otherwise straight and steady when it is fixating a target, the examiner may record the child's vision as CSNM: central, steady, but not maintained. Vision is not central when the patient appears to be fixating on a target although the eyeball is not pointing directly at what is being presented (eccentric fixation).

As children approach 3 to 5 years of age, they begin to be able to participate more voluntarily in the assessment of their visual acuity. Several types of charts that can be projected or posted for use in more formal visual acuity testing are listed in Box 27.1. The method chosen must be consistent with the child's developmental level and skills. For example, projected pictures (Allen pictures, Figure 27.4) are a good test for a child who does not yet know letters. One might show the pictures to the child up close and ask that the figures be identified so that the examiner is aware of what interpretation the child gives to these somewhat abstract diagrams. For example, the birthday cake may be called a "bag of french fries" and the telephone a "butterfly." As long as the examiner knows what the child calls that picture, testing can proceed. At distance, even normally sighted children may have difficulty seeing pictures smaller than the 20/30 line.

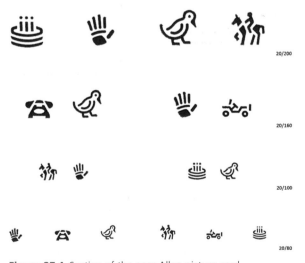

20/200

20/160

20/100

20/80

Figure 27.4 Section of the near Allen picture card. *(Courtesy of the Franel Optical Supply, Apopka, FL.)*

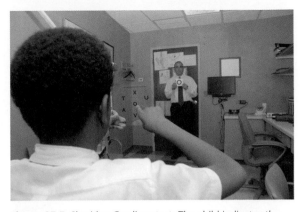

Figure 27.5 Sheridan-Gardiner test. The child indicates the letter on the card that is being presented by the examiner. *(Photograph by Jack Scully.)*

The use of recognition letter charts (Snellen letters) should be reserved for those children whose ability to identify letters is verified in advance by the parent. For children in the intermediate stage in which they recognize some of their letters, the Sheridan-Gardiner (Keeler, London, England) and HOTV tests may be helpful because they allow the child to match letter cards held by the examiner or projected letters with a cue card the child holds (Figure 27.5). This approach also gives shy children more confidence and allows them to guess letters they might otherwise not feel secure enough to guess at orally. Children in these young age groups are often afraid of being wrong and, even with the greatest encouragement, will not read letters that they really are able to see. This underscores the constant need for building the child's confidence by indicating that the answer given is correct even when it is not. The tumbling E chart also can be used for children who do not recognize their letters. This test can, however, be difficult for small children to interpret because they may not know left from right and they may have trouble indicating with their hands in which direction the tumbling E is pointing, particularly when they are between 4 and 6 years old, the age range when handedness normally develops. At this age, they are almost always able to use other methods, rendering the tumbling E unnecessary.

When the visual acuity is tested, one eye must be covered at a time. Children will unconsciously make every effort to use their better eye if there is a difference between the visual acuity in their two eyes. Therefore, the occlusion of one eye must be absolute. Children should never be allowed to hold their hand over their eye or to handhold a plastic occluder paddle. They may look around the occluder or look through tiny holes between their fingers, which can actually create a pinhole effect and improve the vision in the covered eye. It is recommended that 2-inch (5 cm)

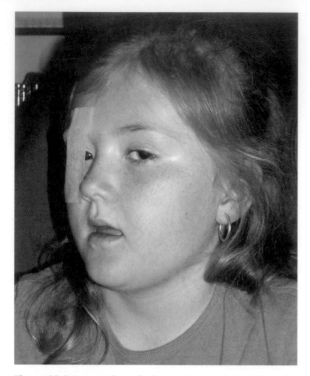

Figure 27.6 Incorrectly applied paper tape occlusion allows the child to visualize the chart with the better right eye by peeking between the tape and the bridge of the nose.
(Photograph by Leslie MacKeen.)

paper tape be applied over the eye to effect complete occlusion. Children must be observed constantly throughout the visual acuity examination to be sure that they are not peeking between the tape and their skin (Figure 27.6). This can be accomplished either by the use of a "cheater's mirror" placed behind the child, which allows the examiner to view the projected target behind them while still facing the child, or by having the examiner stand next to the chart at the end of the examination lane while viewing the child and indicating which letters are to be read. If a child objects to the covering of one eye by tape, the examiner can hold a +5.00 or greater spherical lens in front of the eye not being tested. In most children this sufficiently blurs that eye so that the child is actually viewing with the eye that does not have a lens in front of it even though both eyes are open. Having the parent use a hand to cover the child's eye invites the same problems as having the eye covered by the child's hand. If there is no other option, make sure the parent uses the palm rather than fingers to occlude the eye. If the child completely resists any form of intervention, ask him or her to read the chart with both eyes open and record the binocular vision.

To accommodate the child's short attention span, it is helpful to have the child identify only a few letters from each line. Most children have normal vision, so it may be advisable to start at the 6/9 or even 6/6 line rather than start at the top of a chart and work the child down through many lines of letters/pictures, which may lead to a loss of the child's attention and artificially poor results. It may be helpful to ask the parent to remain silent during this examination, because distracting comments such as "you can do better" may serve to undermine a child's honest effort at good performance.

Remember, some children just are not ready to perform formal visual acuity testing. It is more important to forgo this part of the examination when one senses that the child's cooperation is being lost than to persist and develop a negative relationship with the child that would make the remainder of the examination difficult. Instead of a numerical acuity, one can revert to the CSM method described earlier.

Vision of 6/9 is considered acceptable up to grade 1, after which vision of 6/6 is expected on vision testing. If not, an explanation must be sought. That explanation may be poor compliance with testing if nothing else is found on examination. This conclusion, however, should be reached only after a complete ophthalmic examination has ruled out the presence of refractive error or anatomic problems. Ancillary testing may be requested by the ophthalmologist. A repeat visual acuity test performed later at a subsequent visit within a few months with a more confident and comfortable child also may be successful.

In most clinical situations it is not necessary to test the near vision of children because it can be assumed that the remarkable accommodative abilities of young children allow for normal near vision in almost every child. Assessment of near vision is necessary only when there is subnormal ($<6/18$) distance vision in the better eye or a specific complaint about near vision. In the former situation, near vision should be tested with both eyes open simultaneously. If the vision is normal at near but abnormal at distance, one might suspect that the child is either nearsighted (myopic) or simply noncompliant with distance vision testing. In children who clearly have very poor vision at distance, the knowledge of the maximum near vision with both eyes open allows for proper educational intervention at school.

In children with nystagmus, the vision also should be tested with both eyes open, as well as with one eye fogged with a +5.00 sphere. Completely occluding one eye may make the nystagmus worse (latent nystagmus). Sometimes the visual acuity with both eyes open is better than with either eye individually. Some children with nystagmus may hold their head in an abnormal position while viewing straight ahead (Figure 27.7). This abnormal position should be allowed because it is used unconsciously to help dampen the nystagmus (null point).

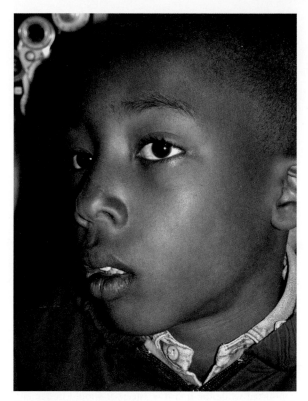

Figure 27.7 This child has nystagmus. When his eyes are in left gaze the nystagmus is least (null point). Therefore, he turns his face to the right when looking straight ahead so that his eyes are in left gaze. This keeps his nystagmus to a minimum and allows for better vision.

(Photograph by Leslie MacKeen.)

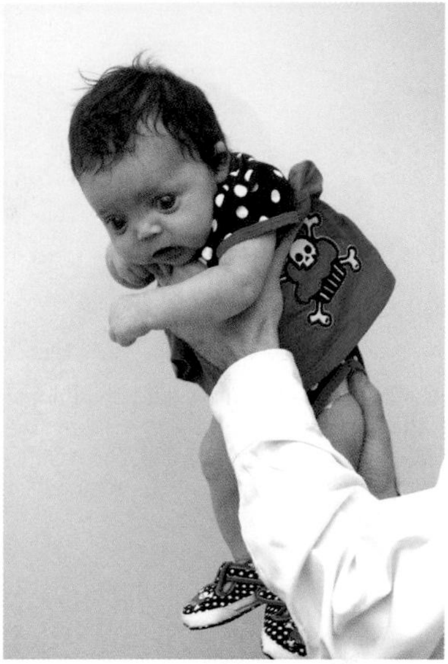

Figure 27.8 By holding a newborn or young infant at a 45-degree angle with one hand on the baby's chest and the other on the buttocks, the baby's eyes will usually open when the buttocks are jiggled. Note that this child has very large eyes as a result of congenital glaucoma.

(Photograph by Jack Scully.)

EXTERNAL EXAMINATION

The anatomy of the eyelids, lashes, conjunctiva, cornea, and anterior segment should be no different from that of a normal young adult, except for size. Visualization of these structures, however, may be difficult because of the challenges with compliance or cooperation. In infants and newborns, eye opening can often be achieved by holding the child in the position demonstrated in Figure 27.8. Sometimes it is necessary to restrain a child in a supine position (Figures 27.9 and 27.10) and insert a lid speculum (Figure 27.11). To obtain magnification, one can look through the direct ophthalmoscope, using it as a handheld magnifier by dialing in the black or green "plus" numbers and getting progressively closer to the child. With the young children, this can be turned into a peek-a-boo game to allow the examiner to get close enough to visualize the front of the eye.

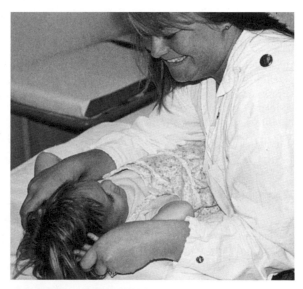

Figure 27.9 Technique for restraining a small child. The parent or ophthalmic assistant leans over the child's abdomen while holding the child's hands next to the temples to immobilize the head.

(Photograph by Leslie MacKeen.)

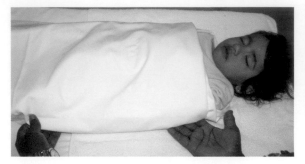

Figure 27.10 Technique for restraining an infant. The child is wrapped in a towel with her arms at her sides. The parent or ophthalmic assistant can then lean over the child's abdomen while controlling the child's head at the temples.
(Photograph by Leslie MacKeen.)

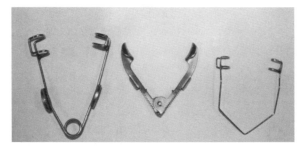

Figure 27.11 Pediatric eyelid speculums.
(Photograph by Leslie MacKeen.)

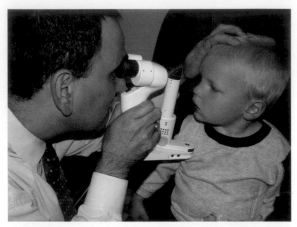

Figure 27.12 Examiner using handheld slit lamp.
(Photograph by Leslie MacKeen.)

If more magnification is desired, the adult slit lamp can be used even for a small infant by holding the child in a horizontal position as the chin is placed on the chin rest. When doing this, it is important that the examiner be "in position," with all the necessary adjustments to the slit lamp already made for proper visualization, because the child may quickly become uncomfortable and tearful. A handheld slit lamp is invaluable for examining infants and small children (Figure 27.12).

Pupils

The examination of a child's pupils is conducted in the same way as for adults. It is sometimes difficult, however, to obtain the distance fixation required to eliminate the normal miosis that occurs when a person focuses on a near target. To do this, many pediatric ophthalmologists have animated toys or movies on the far wall of their offices that can be controlled by a foot pedal. This distracts the child to the distant target while the pupils are being tested. One can even play a "magic game" by turning the child's nose while secretly stepping on the pedal that activates the toy or movie. Children then think that they can control the toy with their nose. This keeps them sufficiently amused while

the examination continues. This trick is also useful for the examination of ocular motility and alignment.

The pupils should normally respond to light at birth, although the pupillary light reaction may be sluggish until the baby is 1 to 2 months old. The pupils of infants are relatively small compared with those of adults. In addition, because the eye examination of an infant may at times be conducted while the infant is asleep, it should be remembered that during sleep pupils are physiologically constricted. The consensual pupillary reaction is present at birth.

The red reflex is the yellow-orange-red reflection sometimes seen in the pupil in photographs. It can be elicited by looking through the direct ophthalmoscope while standing about 3 feet (1 m) away and keeping the face in focus while illuminating both eyes. The reflex should be equal in both eyes. This test plays an important role in the screening of newborns and infants for intraocular abnormalities, in particular a form of hereditary childhood eye cancer (retinoblastoma). A white reflex (leukocoria) may be the first sign of this potentially fatal tumor that is very curable if detected early. The presence of a black reflex (absent red reflex) may indicate an abnormality in the eye such as cataract or vitreous hemorrhage that is blocking the light reflex. A falsely absent red reflex may be caused by the small pupils of newborns and infants that may not allow enough light in to create the reflex. In this situation the testing should be repeated after pharmacologic dilation. The red reflex can also be used to assess pupil size, symmetry, position, and roundness.

INSTILLATION OF EYEDROPS

Eyedrops are feared by most children with the same vigor that they object to receiving injections. In fact, some children will immediately ask "Am I getting drops?" when they walk into the room for their eye examination. Although one should never lie to a child, one might defer the answer to that question by saying, "Let's talk first and then decide."

Once the time comes for the instillation of eyedrops, the child must be informed, but it is preferable to wait to do so as the child is being positioned for this procedure. The child can be held securely in the parent's arms in a cradled position as if receiving a bottle or breast for feeding. The parent should be responsible for restraining the child's hands while the examiner controls the child's head and eyes. It is preferred that the child be told that the drops are going to sting. Well-meaning attempts by parents to alleviate a child's fears by indicating that "this won't hurt" should be corrected by saying that the drops might be painful for approximately 15 to 20 seconds or one can tell the child to count to 10 as a means of distraction. Lying to the child can seriously undermine compliance and trust. It can be helpful to instill first a drop of topical anesthetic (proparacaine or tetracaine), immediately followed by the dilating drops. The onset of action of these topical anesthetics is quite rapid, which helps to lessen the painful sting of the mydriatic drops. Before eyedrops are instilled, the parents should be informed about the number of drops that are to be given and their purpose.

Relaxation of the pupillary sphincter and the ciliary muscles that govern accommodation can be much more difficult in children, particularly if they have heavily pigmented brown irides. Although different examiners may vary in their selection of mydriatic agents, it is usually safe to use some combination of phenylephrine 2.5% and tropicamide 1% or cyclopentolate 1% in all children except premature babies. Children who are corrected age before 36 weeks' gestation or those born small for gestational age at full term may require more dilute solutions of mydriatic agents, in particular cyclopentolate 0.5%.

A repeat instillation of drops may be necessary if the pupils do not dilate well, particularly in premature babies and darkly pigmented children. A full 20 to 30 minutes should be given for adequate paralysis of accommodation to occur. If there is any concern on the part of the ophthalmic assistant that a given child should not receive the standard eyedrop regimen, then instillation should be deferred until consultation with the ophthalmologist or pediatrician is sought. In particular, newborns and infants with hypertension, heart problems, seizures, or respiratory problems may require an alteration in the usual regimen.

Some children do not respond adequately to the eyedrops used in routine eye examination, or they may require stronger cycloplegic agents for assessing far-sightedness (hyperopia) particularly as it relates to esotropia (accommodative esotropia). In these situations a prescription may be given by the physician for atropine drops (0.5% for children younger than 1 year, 1% for children older than 1 year) to be used twice daily for 3 days before a repeat

examination. Parents should be cautioned to monitor their child for signs of atropine toxicity such as fever and redness (flushing). Although this protocol is generally safe, parents must be cautioned to keep this medication locked away because ingestion by a toddler or small child could be fatal.

When the child returns to the examination room for dilated eye examination, it is often helpful to begin that segment of the examination by announcing that no more drops will be necessary. If the discovery is made that the initial drops were insufficient, the examiner should adhere to the basic principle of being honest with pediatric patients, and perhaps prescribe the atropine drop regimen for home use before another visit rather than break the promise and instill drops again.

REFRACTION

Newborns, infants, and small children cannot participate in analysis and refinement of their refractions by sitting behind the phoropter and indicating which lenses give them better vision. Rather, the examiner uses the retinoscope and handheld lenses, as described elsewhere in this book, to determine the child's refractive error.

Most infants and small children are far-sighted, although glasses usually are not required because the strong accommodative power of their eyeballs allows them to self-correct for their hyperopia. Higher degrees of far-sightedness, however, can lead to esotropia (crossed eyes) and amblyopia (subnormal vision development). Likewise, myopia in the newborn and infant may be functional because their visual world is almost completely at near. Higher degrees of near-sightedness, however, may lead to ocular misalignment and amblyopia. Different ophthalmologists have different thresholds for the prescription of glasses. Contact lenses may be used in babies and small children with extremely high refractive errors or surgical aphakia after cataract extraction. Ophthalmic assistants can play an important role in teaching parents how to insert and remove contact lenses in their children.

RETINA AND OPTIC NERVE EXAMINATION

Examination of the posterior segment of the eyeball through the dilated pupil in an infant or young child is essentially identical to that for an adult and requires the use of an indirect ophthalmoscope. In certain situations, however, it may be difficult to open the eyelids sufficiently to allow an adequate view. This may be best accomplished by the use of pediatric specula, which are commercially available (see Figure 27.11). They are placed after the child has been restrained and a topical anesthetic applied. In some situations, examination under general anesthesia is necessary.

Although various commercially available papoose boards can be used, it usually is most reassuring and comfortable for the child to be restrained by having an adult, preferably the parent, leaning comfortably across the child's chest while holding the child's hands on either temple to keep the head still (see Figure 27.9). The reassuring voice of a parent can often be quite helpful. Newborns and infants can be restrained by wrapping a towel or blanket around the child's arms and trunk (see Figure 27.10). Some parents may feel quite uncomfortable about watching a speculum being placed into the eye. The examiner should explain the procedure first, giving the parents the option of staying, turning away, or stepping out of the room. The examination is virtually painless, but quite scary for a small child. Immediately after the examination is complete, the child should be allowed to seek solace in the parent's arms.

For older children who may sit cooperatively in their parent's lap, the introduction of the large and unusual indirect ophthalmoscope headpiece can be frightening. The ophthalmic assistant or examiner might reassure the child by giving this hat a silly name such as a space hat or allow the parent to be examined first. Once the child knows that this imposing instrument is safe, cooperation may be enhanced.

Although the macula may not be completely developed in the first few months of life, the intraocular anatomy of a newborn and infant appears otherwise identical to that of an adult.

COMMON PEDIATRIC DISORDERS

Amblyopia

Approximately 2% to 4% of all children have amblyopia. Because the visual system continues to develop through the first decade of life, any abnormality (e.g., unequal refractive error, ptosis, strabismus, cataract) that makes one eye less favored than its fellow eye may cause the brain to prefer one eye. In doing so, the brain begins to neglect the visual development of the unfavored eye, causing its vision to become "lazy." Patching the good eye and correcting the underlying defect (e.g., glasses for anisometropia, surgery for ptosis) force the brain to use the unfavored eye and redevelop the vision properly. The ophthalmologist will also decide the number of hours per day that the child should patch. Research has shown that patching may even be effective into the early teen years, but compliance may be difficult because of cosmetic concerns and teasing at school. In some scenarios instilling atropine (atropine penalization) daily or weekly into the better eye can blur that eye sufficiently to allow the brain to redevelop vision in the amblyopic eye. Ongoing follow-up is essential to assess the progress of the amblyopic eye and to ensure that the patch or atropine is not causing impairment of vision in the better eye (occlusion amblyopia).

Strabismus

Any misalignment of the eyes is called strabismus. When one or both eyes are crossed, the condition is called esotropia (see Figure 27.1). Some infants develop a form of severe crossing called infantile esotropia, whereas other children do not develop esotropia until later in childhood. Crossing of the eyes caused by uncorrected hyperopia is called accommodative esotropia. Prescribing glasses to "do the work" instead of the focusing muscles inside the eye (ciliary muscles) keeps the eyes straight, although they will still cross with the glasses off. If the crossing is particularly prominent when the child reads, bifocals may be prescribed.

Children with uncorrected near-sightedness may have an eye that drifts out (exotropia). If one eye is too high, it is called hypertropia. If an eye is too low, the term is hypotropia. Intermittent misalignment of the eyes, particularly intermittent exotropia, is common and within normal limits up to 3 to 4 months of age and occasionally for longer. Most forms of strabismus that persist beyond infancy require eye muscle surgery, an outpatient procedure. This topic is covered in more detail elsewhere in this book.

Nasolacrimal duct obstruction

Many infants are born with an incompletely developed nasolacrimal drainage system such that the duct does not open completely into the nose. Sometimes referred to as blocked tear ducts, this unilateral or bilateral disorder is usually characterized by crusting on the eyelids, especially on waking, and by tearing and discharge in the absence of conjunctival injection. More than 95% of cases resolve spontaneously with the use of massage. One to four times daily, a finger is placed over the lacrimal sac, between the medial canthus and the nose, and pressure is applied posteriorly to compress the sac and send pressure down the duct. Some ophthalmologists may also prescribe topical antibiotics if the discharge is copious or the conjunctiva inflamed. If symptoms persist after 3 months of proper massage and the child is more than 1 year old, surgical probing to open the duct may be considered. Some ophthalmologists practice in-office earlier probing, although others believe the usual spontaneous resolution of the condition should be allowed and probing conducted only if the symptoms and signs persist beyond 1 year, at which time general anesthesia is usually preferred for the procedure.

Retinopathy of prematurity

During development of the fetus, the retinal blood vessels are brought into the eye with the developing optic nerve and then grow progressively to reach the peripheral retinal edges by the end of gestation. If a baby is born prematurely, before the vessels have finished growing, the process may be abruptly halted, leaving the vessels to form an abnormal demarcation zone between their premature termination point and the more peripheral nonvascularized retina.

The vessels may grow abnormally (neovascularization) and cause distortion (macular drag) or detachment of the retina. This very serious disorder may result in blindness. Premature infants, especially those born at 32 weeks or less and weighing less than 2.6 pounds (1200 g), are regularly screened by ophthalmologists for this problem, which often can be treated successfully using retinal laser therapy. Age and weight thresholds for screening may vary in different locales.

Cataracts and glaucoma

Although uncommon, these disorders deserve mention because they are potential causes of blindness. They may be present at birth or develop at any time during childhood. Cataract may first be discovered by the presence of a white opacity in the pupil or by an abnormal red reflex test conducted by the primary care physician. Glaucoma in newborns and infants is often characterized by an enlarged (see Figure 27.8) hazy cornea, epiphora, and photophobia. Urgent surgery is often required for both disorders. Although intraocular lenses are being used with increasing regularity for older children with cataracts, in the first 1 to 2 years of life rehabilitation is still often accomplished with aphakic spectacles or contact lenses that the parents learn to insert and remove for the child. Many of the same drops and medications used to treat adult glaucoma may be used in children, although infantile glaucoma often requires unique surgical procedures (goniotomy or trabeculotomy) that open the trabecular network. The antiglaucoma medications brimonidine and apraclonidine should be avoided in the first year of life.

Questions for review and thought

1. What techniques can you use to reassure a frightened child during the examination?
2. What are the normal developmental visual milestones for a newborn and infant?
3. What factors should you use when deciding which chart is most appropriate for testing vision in a child?
4. What is the red reflex test?
5. How can a child be restrained safely?
6. What might happen to a child who is far-sighted if glasses are not prescribed?
7. What options are available to treat amblyopia?
8. What drops usually are used to dilate a baby's eyes for examination?

Q Self-evaluation questions

True–false statements

Directions: Indicate whether the statement is true (T) or false (F).
1. Atropine 1% eyedrops should be used to dilate the pupils of a 6-month-old baby. **T** or **F**
2. Most babies are near-sighted. **T** or **F**
3. Children with nystagmus see better when one eye is covered. **T** or **F**

Missing words

Directions: Write in the missing word in the following sentences:
4. The type of strabismus more often associated with hyperopia is _____.
5. The abbreviation used to record the visual assessment of a preverbal child with no nystagmus who has good straight-ahead fixation with the right eye and equal vision in both eyes is _____.
6. Two tests that are useful in assessing visual acuity when a child is just learning letters are the _____ and _____ tests.

Choice-completion questions

Directions: Select the one best answer in each case.
7. Before instilling eyedrops in a child, the parent and patient should be informed that:
   a. the drops will sting.
   b. a certain number of drops will be given.
   c. the drops are given to make the pupils dilate.
   d. the child should be cradled securely and lovingly in the parent's arms.
   e. all of the above.
8. Quantitative tests of visual acuity include all of the following except:
   a. Snellen letters.
   b. visual evoked potential (VEP).
   c. electroretinogram (ERG).
   d. Allen pictures.
   e. preferential looking.

Q Continued

9. All of the following statements about the newborn are true except:
   a. visual fixation should be present.
   b. intermittent strabismus may be present.
   c. hyperopia may be present.
   d. the pupils do not react to light.
   e. an equal and symmetric red reflex should present.

10. The blind or very poorly sighted infant:
    a. may have wandering eye movements.
    b. may have nystagmus.
    c. may have dysconjugate eye movements.
    d. may still show normal "eye-popping reflex."
    e. may have all of the above.

A Answers, notes, and explanations

1. **False.** Atropine 0.5% eyedrops should be used in children younger than 1 year old to avoid systemic complications such as irritability, flushing, and fever. Atropine is not used routinely as the primary in-office method to dilate pupils.

2. **False.** Most babies are hyperopic in the first few years of life. Myopia becomes more common after 5 to 6 years old.

3. **False.** When one eye of a child with nystagmus is covered, the amplitude of the nystagmus in the uncovered eye may increase. This is called latent nystagmus. Visual acuity may worsen. It is preferable to test the visual acuity of children with nystagmus by fogging the untested eye with a +5.00 sphere. This prevents latent nystagmus. Visual acuity with both eyes open, while allowing the child to adopt any preferred anomalous head position, is also important.

4. **Accommodative esotropia.** When children use their inherent mechanisms of accommodation to correct for their hyperopic refractive error, a reflex crossing of the eyes may occur. By giving hyperopic spectacles to do the work instead of the eyeball, this esotropia may be corrected.

5. **CSM or GSM** (central [or good], steady, maintained). The child fixates in the straight-ahead position (central), with an eye that does not have nystagmus (steady) but with apparently equal vision relative to the other eye (maintained).

6. **Sheridan-Gardiner, HOTV matching, or Allen pictures.** In the first two tests the child is holding a cue card that allows him or her to match projected letters or letters held by the examiner, thus providing some extra support if the child is not completely comfortable with verbalizing letter recognition. Picture recognition is also an option for a child who does not know letters.

7. **e. All of the above.** The parent must be completely informed about the instillation of eyedrops. The drops are painful for only 15 to 20 seconds, particularly if a topical anesthetic is given before the mydriatic agents. Each ophthalmologist may have an individual regimen of dilating drops. That regimen should be explained to the parent, who can then provide support by restraining the child in a comfortable fashion.

8. **c. ERG (electroretinogram).** The ERG is a quantitative and qualitative test of retinal function but it does not give information about visual acuity. Visual acuity is a foveal function. The ERG is a test of the entire retina, which masks specific assessment of the small foveal area. The multifocal ERG can better assess foveal function, but still does not measure acuity.

9. **d. The pupils do not react to light.** Although the pupillary reactions of a neonate may be sluggish, constriction to a bright light normally should be observed at full-term birth. At birth some visual fixation to a large object or light should be present, although the eyes may be intermittently misaligned. Intermittent exotropia is the most common form of strabismus in neonates. Most newborn babies are hyperopic. In all babies an equal and symmetric red reflex should be seen, although the relatively miotic newborn pupil may make this test difficult.

10. **e. All of the above.** Infants who are blind or very poorly sighted often manifest wandering, purposeless, dysconjugate eye movements or true nystagmus. The presence of nystagmus, however, does not necessarily indicate that the child is blind. Some children with congenital nystagmus may have surprisingly good vision. The eye-popping reflex may still be seen in poorly sighted children, although it is absent in children who are completely blind. It is a normal infant reflex in children with at least light perception. It disappears approximately 3 to 4 months after birth.

Chapter | 28 |

Maintenance of ophthalmic equipment and instruments

The maintenance of ophthalmic equipment and instruments often becomes the responsibility of one person in the office. Someone may be more technically adept to take on this responsibility. Simplified instructions on care and maintenance are noted in the following text.

It is important that adequate supplies of replacement bulbs be maintained and that everyone be familiar with the different bulbs required for each of the available pieces of equipment. Lists of the required bulb for each piece of equipment should be made and posted. If batteries are required, a suitable battery supply should also be maintained. If the batteries are the rechargeable type, they should be charged fully the first time. They can be recharged to the same full capacity on each recharging, which should take place on a regular basis. Handles usually contain rechargeable batteries that require nightly recharging in a battery well. All equipment should be kept covered with dust covers supplied by the manufacturer.

APPLANATION TONOMETER

Calibration of the applanation tonometer is important, and it should be checked approximately every 2 months or sooner with regular use. Tonometers are always supplied with a calibration bar. The most common applanation tonometer is the Goldmann tonometer. Applanation tonometers may be checked for accuracy by the use of a central weight. For the Goldmann tonometer, a short rod of measured weight is attached to the balancing arm of the tonometer and the rod set at 0, 2, and 6. At each measure, the measuring drum should be placed at the corresponding stop. At each stop, the tonometer head should move only 0.05 to 0.1 g of these settings (Figure 28.1).

To be specific, follow these guidelines.

1. To check at drum position zero (0), insert the measuring prism at measuring position −0.05. The zero mark on the measuring drum is set one line width below the index. When the pressure arm, with prism in position, is gently pushed, it should move freely between the two stops and return toward the stop on the examiner's side (Figure 28.2). At measuring position +0.05, the zero mark on the measuring drum is set one line width above the index. As this procedure is followed, the pressure arm should move toward the patient's side.

2. Check at drum position 2. For this check the control weight is used. Five circles are engraved on the weight

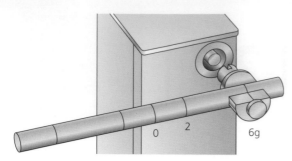

Figure 28.1 Calibration bar for Goldmann applanation tonometer.

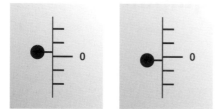

Figure 28.2 Calibrating Goldmann applanation tonometer at position 2. The tonometer head should move only 0.05 to 0.1 g from zero.

bar. The middle one corresponds to drum position zero, the two immediately to the left and right are position 2, and the outer ones are position 6. One of the marks on the weight corresponding to drum position 2 is set precisely on the index mark of the weight holder. Holder and weight are then fitted over the axis of the tonometer so that the longer part of the weight points toward the examiner (Figure 28.3).

3. At drum positions 1.95 and 2.05 (graduation mark 2 on measuring drum set one line width below or above the index), the pressure arm should return from the area of free movement to the corresponding stop.

4. The check at drum position 2 is the most important and should be carried out frequently because the measurement of intraocular pressure in this range is of particular importance.

5. Check at drum position 6 in the same manner. The corresponding checking points are 5.9 and 6.1. The graduation mark 6 on the drum is offset by half an interval below or above the index.

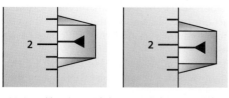

Figure 28.3 Calibration with larger weight toward the examiner. Balance should show scale variation no greater than zero.

The applanation tonometer consists of a plastic prism with a flat anterior surface and a diameter of 7 mm. This prism is brought into contact with a fluorescein-stained tear film of the cornea, which it displaces to the periphery of the contact zone until a surface of known and constant size of 3.06 mm is flattened. The inner border of the ring represents the line of demarcation between the cornea flattened by applanation and the cornea not flattened. The measuring drum can regulate the tension to produce a force between zero and 8 g.

NONCONTACT TONOMETER

Calibration of the noncontact tonometer is important. The use of the logic circuits in the instrument, which are necessary to measure and record intraocular pressure, enables the operator to check the calibration of the pneumatic-electronic network by the following procedure:

1. Turn the instrument to on (red dot).
2. Remove the objective cap and wait 30 seconds for warm-up.
3. Depress the trigger switch-display at 68.
4. Push the power switch knob and set it at D.
5. Depress the trigger switch-display at 47 + 1.

Triggering is repeated several times 8 to 10 seconds apart. The display must not change more than +1 count. There must be no source light indicator (SLI) light in any of the tests. During the check of calibration, the display number has no quantitative significance; its repeatability must be the concern. The number displayed is a specially selected equivalent to a critical check at approximately 20 mm Hg, with twice the resolution that is used in the actual intraocular pressure (IOP) measurement.

The noncontact tonometer is sturdily constructed and normally requires little care to keep it operationally perfect. Protecting the equipment against dust is important to maintain it in good working order. It is recommended that the supplied dust covers be used.

Bulb replacement

Target illuminator bulb

1. Always disconnect the instrument from its source of electrical power.
2. Remove the instrument top by unscrewing two screws with a 3/32 hex wrench.
3. Free the bulb holder by loosening the set screw, marked B, with a 1/16 hex wrench.
4. Pull out the bulb holder.
5. Remove the bulb by unscrewing the knurled retainer ring.
6. Replace the bulb with a no. 12419 bulb and wipe the bulb clean of fingerprints.

7. To adjust for maximum and even target illumination, view the red-dot target through the objective orifice and adjust the bulb holder on axis with the power on. Tighten the set screw.

8. Replace and secure the instrument cover to protect against dust.

Source light indicator

If replacement is ever necessary, it should be made only by a qualified service technician. An authorized American Optical distributor should be contacted.

Fixation lamp

To replace the fixation bulb, the center joint is separated by pulling apart. The screw base bulb (no. 11583) is exposed for replacement.

Chin rest

The chin rest is easily removed by twisting it 90 degrees, then pulling up. It is made of a durable material that can be sterilized (maximum 250°F [121°C]) or washed in soap and water or alcohol.

Paper chin rests also are available.

Headrest cushions

Headrest cushions are wiped clean with alcohol. They also may be replaced.

Eyepiece and objective

1. The exposed surfaces of the eyepiece and objective should be kept free of dust, fingerprints, and smudges. The lens surfaces should be dusted occasionally with a camelhair brush.

2. The alignment target, as viewed by the operator, may become blurred by accumulation of grease from eyelashes on the annular aperture of the objective. Clean the annulus with a dry cotton-tipped stick.

3. After prolonged service or use in a dusty or humid environment, the inside surface of the objective should be cleaned. Remove the objective by unscrewing it counterclockwise and dust the surface with a brush or, if necessary, wipe it clean with a dampened tissue paper before reassembly.

LENSMETER

The lensmeter requires little maintenance. The eyepiece should always be adjusted for each technician using this instrument. Operators should focus or adjust the eyepiece to their eye.

If the lensmeter has a prism compensator, which is located just under the eyepiece, the compensator should always be set on zero to ensure you obtain the correct reading. (For further details see Chapter 8.)

KERATOMETER

We shall use the Bausch & Lomb keratometer as an example. When not in use, or at least overnight, the keratometer should be kept covered with the dust cover supplied with the instrument.

1. Dirt on the daylight-blue filter sometimes causes smudges in the mire imagery. The filter can be removed easily and cleaned by removing the two screws that hold the lamp housing to the body of the instrument.

2. When carbon deposits begin to form on the lamp bulb, the mire imagery will be diminished. If this occurs, a new bulb should be used in the instrument.

3. The lower part of the lamp housing is removed easily for the insertion of a new bulb. To replace the bulb, rotate the instrument by turning the set until the lamp housing is away from the central carriage. The base can be removed by loosening the two screws on the sides of the lamp housing. In replacing the base, one must take care to see that the base rests squarely on the shoulder of the housing; otherwise that part will not clear the carriage when it is rotated back into position.

4. There is also an attachment that can be used for checking keratometer measurements. This attachment comes complete with bracket and three test ball bearings with specific radii. To calibrate, use a spherical test ball of known radius of curvature inserted in a holder. When the correct radius of curvature of the test ball is obtained, the accuracy of the keratometer can be confirmed. If the keratometer is out of alignment, it should be repaired by a trained professional.

SLIT-LAMP BIOMICROSCOPE

The slit lamp is an important instrument. All personnel who use it should make a habit of keeping it covered with a dust cover when it is not in use.

1. When changing bulbs, be sure the instrument is unplugged. Also always remember to wipe off all fingerprints on the bulb to extend its life.

2. If the slit lamp will not operate, replace bulbs even if they appear to be in good condition. If the slit lamp does not light when a new main bulb is installed, check contacts on the bulb cap and remove any dirt with a small file or knife. If the slit lamp still does not operate, check all electrical connections to make sure

that all wires are plugged into the transformer and that the main power cord is plugged in. Also check for a faulty fuse in the transformer.

3. The Haag-Streit and copies are the only slit lamps with mirrors that require cleaning. Removal of the mirror is easiest when the microscope and illuminator are well separated and the latter is inclined by approximately 10 degrees or more. Grasp the narrow shank of the long mirror and pull upward. The small mirror, which has no shank, is more difficult to grasp; therefore, the point of a pencil should be used to get the mirror started on its way out. The mirror should then be dusted and sprayed with a glass cleaner. Wipe clean with cotton balls or some other material that will not scratch the surface, using a downward stroke. Repeat until dry.

4. If the slit lamp becomes difficult to move with the joystick, clean the joystick pad with a cleaning solution. If slit-lamp movement still continues to be difficult, apply a thin coat of three-in-one oil or sewing machine oil to the pad.

PHOROPTER (FIGURE 28.4)

All personnel should make it a habit to keep the phoropter protected with a dust cover when not in use. Alcohol should not be used on any part of the phoropter.

1. The semipermanent face shields furnished with the phoropter are made of white nylon. This material can be washed with soap and water, soaked in alcohol, or boiled in water.

2. All lenses should be kept clean and free of dust and fingerprints. Do not put a finger in the sight aperture to check lens placement. Fingerprints on the lenses make refraction difficult. Cleaning of dust on enclosed lenses can be done with an ear syringe. The back lenses are the retinoscopy lens, polarizing lens, red lens, and Maddox rod. These are the only lenses that may be cleaned by office personnel; a glass cleaner and cotton-tipped swabs are used. The phoropter should be sent to an authorized repair shop every 2 years for preventive maintenance and lens cleaning.

3. Because the cross cylinder and the rotary prism are not enclosed, it is advisable occasionally to wipe each one carefully with lens tissue to remove dust.

Green's refractor

The Green's refractor (see Chapter 10) should be protected with a dust cover when not in use. Alcohol should not be used on any part of the refractor.

1. Face shields, which can be purchased from a local supplier, should be replaced after each patient use.

2. The only lenses that can be cleaned in the office are the retinoscopy lens and the +0.12 diopter lens. These are

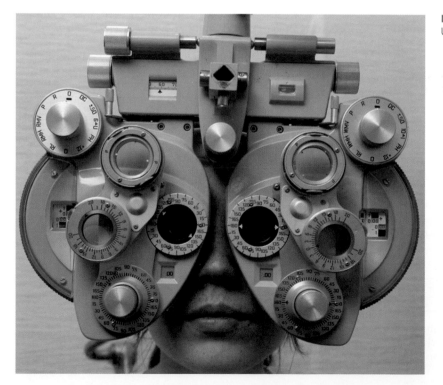

Figure 28.4 American Optical Ultramatic Phoropter.

located in the shutter disc and may be cleaned with a glass cleaner and cotton-tipped swabs. These two lenses become dirty because they are in the back of the refractor where patients' eyelashes may come into contact.

3. Because the cross cylinder and the rotary prism are not enclosed, it is advisable occasionally to wipe each one carefully with lens tissue to remove dust.

4. Do not put a finger in the sight aperture to check lens placement. Fingerprints on the lenses make refraction difficult.

5. Removing dust from the internal lens may be done by blowing with an ear syringe. It is not recommended, however, for self-cleaning of the internal lens.

6. The Green's refractor should be sent to an authorized repair department for preventive maintenance and lens cleaning every 2 years.

PROJECTOR

The vision screen projector requires little care. Occasionally the glass slides and the lenses in the focusing tube should be wiped with a soft clean cloth. Best results are obtained if the cloth is dry because any moisture can cause streaks that will be projected onto the screen.

1. Do not remove lenses from the objective barrels. The refractor can be easily cleaned because the entire inner lamp house is removable.

2. When it is not in use, switch off the instrument to conserve the life of the lamp and prevent burning it out prematurely. It is desirable to keep several spare bulbs on hand to ensure always having a lamp of correct voltage and proper filament center.

Projection slide

Water or any other substance should not be sprayed on the slide. Wet substances can slip between the lenses and destroy the slide. Only the slide is cleaned by rubbing lightly with a camera lens tissue.

Cleaning the projector screen

The projector screen has a high reflectance characteristic. It is, however, susceptible to damage from abrasive scratches and fingerprints.

1. Periodic cleaning of the screen is advised. Simply use a mild detergent solution, wiping the screen surface gently with dampened absorbent cotton.

2. Fingerprints are normally removed by the recommended cleaning procedure. Scratches, however, cannot be removed and the screen does not lend itself to refinishing.

Replacing the lamp

Warning: Projector must be off for a few minutes before proceeding with lamp replacement!

To replace the lamp, push the small aluminum button on the side of the instrument. This releases the catch and allows the outer lamp house to swing back, exposing the inner lamp house. To remove the inner lamp house, pull the top back until the spring clips have disengaged, then lift out. The lamp is then entirely exposed and can be removed from the socket by a downward pressure, at the same time turning the lamp until it is free of the bayonet slide.

Caution: The lamp socket and reflector are factory-adjusted and should not be disassembled.

Projection front-surface mirrors

Front-surface mirrors have silvering on the first or front surface. They are cleaned by spraying a glass cleaner in small amounts on the mirror, stroking downward with a cotton ball (do not rub back and forth) and disposing of the cotton ball. The process is repeated until the mirror is dry.

Patient viewing mirror

The patient viewing mirror is cleaned like any other mirror (except the front-surface mirror). Most viewing mirrors are not front surface; they are plate glass with rear silvering. A front-surface mirror is identified by touching the mirror surface with an object such as a pen or pencil. If the end of the object touches the reflection in the mirror, it is front surface.

Chapter 29

Aseptic technique and minor office surgery

ASEPTIC TECHNIQUE

Aseptic technique in the office or hospital is an attempt to prevent infection by the elimination of microorganisms. Ophthalmic surgery demands maximum asepsis, particularly in operations involving the globe itself. Microorganisms that gain access to the interior of the eye can multiply and cause irreparable damage, often resulting in blindness. Aseptic technique demands:

- Proper sterilization of all instruments
- Sterilization of the skin adjacent to the operative site
- Sterilization of the hands of both the operator and the assistant
- Use of sterile solutions and ointments during and after the operation

For the most part, the following discussion of aseptic technique will be oriented toward ophthalmic surgery in the office.

Disinfection of eyelid skin

Office surgery for conditions involving eyelid skin requires carefully applied skin antiseptics (Table 29.1). (Spray packs of antiseptics are contraindicated.) Care must be taken that none of the antiseptic material enters the eye. This may be done with careful application by cotton applicators soaked in such solutions as tincture of iodine 2%, povidone-iodine (Betadine), Ioprep, alcohol, and cetrimonium bromide. It also may be done by scrupulous scrubbing of the area with hexachlorophene (Phisohex) or green soap. Betadine and alcohol are available in large presoaked swabs.

Scrubbing (degerming of hands)

For many minor office procedures, scrubbing may be unnecessary if both the operator and the assistant adhere to a "no-touch" technique. In this technique the tops of the sterile instruments are never touched by hands or laid down in a nonsterile area.

The skin of the hands contains normal bacterial inhabitants, as well as many transient microorganisms with which the individual may recently have come into contact. It is virtually impossible to scrub the hands sufficiently to get rid of all normal inhabitants, but the use of gloves overcomes this handicap. We tend to use powderless gloves, because particulate matter (e.g., starches) of powder can have a damaging effect in the eye.

Scrubbing with a brush degerms the hands by the removal of bacteria, and the dilution of the bacteria content is achieved by rinses and the use of antiseptic skin agents that are bactericidal. Before scrubbing, the fingernails should be cleansed with an orangewood stick. The various antiseptic agents available have their own scrubbing time, which should be followed rigidly. The fingers and nails should be carefully scrubbed and all hidden recesses of the hands scrupulously cleansed.

Instillation of eye medication

Eye medication easily can become contaminated by incorrect instillation. There is a right and a wrong way to instill

Table 29.1 Skin preparations and disinfecting solutions

Classification	Manufacturer	Type of bactericide
Tinctures		
Tincture of iodine 2%		Iodine-alcohol
Alcohol 70%		Alcohol
Zephiran chloride	Winthrop	Quaternary ammonium compound + alcohol
Merthiolate	Eli Lilly & Co	Sodium ethylmercurithiosalicylate + alcohol
Aqueous preparations		
Merthiolate	Eli Lilly & Co	Sodium ethylmercurithiosalicylate
Zephiran chloride	Winthrop	Quaternary ammonium compound
Hexachlorophene scrubs		
Gamophen	Arwood	Hexachlorophene
Septisol	Vestal	Hexachlorophene
Phisohex	Winthrop	Hexachlorophene
Iodophors		
Ioprep	Johnson & Johnson	Iodophor
Wescodyne	West	Iodophor
Betadine	British Drug Houses	Iodophor

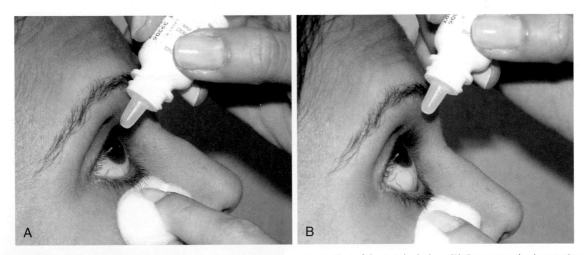

Figure 29.1 Instillation of eyedrops. (A) Incorrect method; note contamination of dropper by lashes. (B) Correct method; note tip of dropper held free of globe and lashes.

eye medication both before and after minor office surgery (Figure 29.1). With the patient's head tilted back, the dropper, dropper bottle, or ointment tube should be held about half an inch (1.25 cm) from the eye before the release of medication. When corneal anesthesia is required, the patient should be asked to look down so that the cornea will be completely covered by the medication. It is important that the tip of the dropper or dropper bottle never touches the eye or eyelid. Contamination will result, in which case the dropper and medication should be discarded. Alcohol and alcohol-type solutions must never enter the eye. They are damaging to the corneal epithelium.

Sterility of ophthalmic solutions

The sterility of eye solutions is desirable not only because of the obvious danger of ocular infection, but also because contaminated solutions may prove toxic and irritating to the eye. The sterilization of ophthalmic solutions may be performed effectively by pouring through bacterial filters. The addition of a preservative, such as chlorobutanol or benzalkonium chloride, aids in preventing contamination.

The ophthalmologist's office should have solutions that are well prepared and contain an added preservative. They should be kept in small bottles, never in large stock sizes. Individual-dose sizes are commercially available in disposable plastic containers. In addition, one must be careful about contamination of the eyedropper, particularly if it has touched an infected eye. If contamination is suspected, the solution should be discarded. One solution notorious for harboring microorganisms, particularly *Pseudomonas aeruginosa*, is fluorescein. However, fluorescein is available in dried sterile strips that are safe to use.

All solutions that enter the eye should be of the nonpreserved type (e.g., lidocaine 1% [Xylocaine], vancomycin). All solutions that are applied to an open wound should be made up fresh through micropore filters (e.g., mitomycin).

Disinfection of tonometer prism

Every tonometer prism should be cleaned and disinfected before use. The main purpose of this is to prevent the spread of infection from patient to patient, especially of the viruses that cause epidemic keratoconjunctivitis and acquired immunodeficiency syndrome (AIDS).

The Goldmann application tonometer prism is best cleaned and disinfected by soaking in 1:10 sodium hypochlorite solution (bleach) or 3% hydrogen peroxide. Some practices use 70% isopropyl alcohol soaks or wipe with an alcohol pad. After disinfecting, the prism should be rinsed in running water and dried. Detailed instructions are available on the manufacturer's website.

Several handheld applanation tonometers are available (e.g., TonoPen). These require a special sterile rubber cover for each individual.

MINOR OFFICE SURGERY

Ophthalmologists vary in the amount and type of office surgery they perform. Such factors as the availability of outpatient facilities in a nearby hospital, the time spent at the hospital by the physician, the physical layout of the physician's office, and the presence of a trained and efficient ophthalmic assistant influence the decision whether to perform surgical procedures in the office or in the hospital outpatient department. When adequate physical facilities and a trained assistant are available, many minor procedures can be performed in the ophthalmic office in a special sterile operating room. Age may be a consideration for choice of patient.

Of fundamental importance is the general sterility of the area in which the surgical procedure is to be performed. Maintenance of adequate cleanliness and dusting of the surgical area should be performed regularly. The area should be segregated from the routine patient flow as much as possible. An office operating room will not achieve the same high standard of sterility that is found in a hospital operating room. Such factors as a separate scrub area, elimination of all street clothing, shoe covers, air filtration, and positive-pressure operating rooms are not generally found in an office minor-procedure operating room. In an office that one enters without a mask, airborne bacteria may remain active for hours. In all offices emphasis must be placed on adequate sterilization of instruments, combined with personal measures to ensure that there is reasonable cleanliness and sterility in the surgical area.

Careful and complete cleanliness of instruments must precede all efforts at sterilization. It is useless to place a blood-stained curet into an antiseptic solution, heat oven, or autoclave because these dirty instruments can never be thoroughly sterilized. Scrupulous cleansing with a fine nailbrush or toothbrush and careful inspection of the instruments are essential. This inspection is done most efficiently with magnifying lenses or loupes. The cleansing may be done in soapy water or with one of the many detergents available. Protein enzyme solutions are available to remove blood and tissue debris from the instruments. Instruments with moving parts should be lubricated periodically or dipped into surgical instrument milk. After these instruments are carefully rinsed, they are sterilized (Figure 29.2).

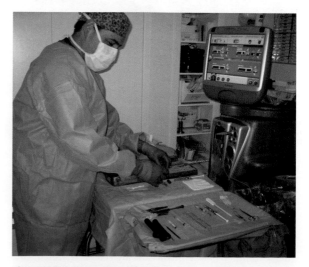

Figure 29.2 Preparation of a sterile instrument tray.

Sterilization of the instruments may be performed by one of the methods outlined previously. Small autoclaves are available for office use. They have their own timing device and will sterilize within 5 minutes. Disinfection of the patient's skin is performed for many lid procedures by applying an antiseptic solution such as iodine, povidone-iodine (Betadine), or benzalkonium chloride.

The surgeon and the ophthalmic assistant should observe all rules of cleanliness, particularly for the more advanced procedures that may be performed in the office. Before handling sterilized instruments, the ophthalmic assistant should scrub, preferably with hexachlorophene soap. Gloves may be required for some of the minor operations. Powderless gloves are preferred. Assistants should not use nail polish or wear hand or wrist jewelry when assisting during minor office procedures. Masks and caps are often not necessary for most minor office procedures. More extensive operations, however, such as pterygium removal and plastic surgery on the eyelid, may require surgical care comparable to the standards used in a first-class hospital operating room. Minor surgery is often performed under magnification with loupes (Figure 29.3).

Safety considerations

Defibrillator apparatus should be available in a conspicuous place (Figure 29.4). All staff should be trained on this in association with regular cardiopulmonary resuscitation (CPR) courses.

Instruments and surgical materials for ophthalmic procedures

The following surgical instruments may be required in minor office surgery: forceps, scissors, needle holders, clamps, curets, scalpels and blades, and lacrimal instruments and cannulas. The numerous individual variations of these instruments depend on the surgeon's choice.

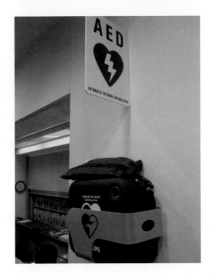

Figure 29.4 An automatic external defibrillator should be visible in a conspicuous place.

Forceps

Forceps are used to grasp small tissues for either removal or suture insertion. The teeth of these instruments vary from 0.12 to 0.5 mm. The jaws may be rounded, flat, or serrated. Some forceps, called tying forceps, have no teeth. Others, called epilation forceps, also have no teeth and are used to remove eyelashes. Thus both tooth and nontooth forceps often are available in the office (Figure 29.5).

Scissors

Scissors may be blunt or sharp, curved or straight. They may have spring action or direct action.

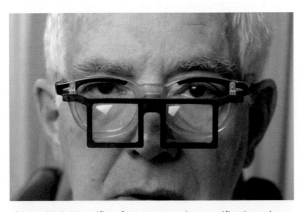

Figure 29.3 Magnifiers for stereoscopic magnification when performing office surgery.

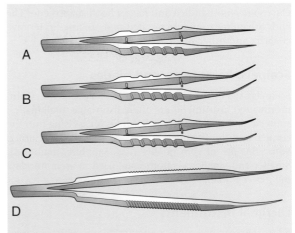

Figure 29.5 Forceps. (A) Colibri 0.12 mm. (B) Capsulorrhexis. (C) Tying. (D) 0.5-mm teeth.

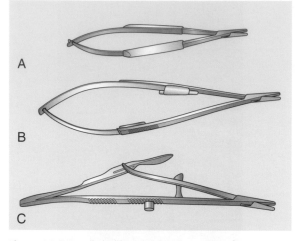

Figure 29.6 Needle holders. (A) Small needle holder. (B) Medium-sized needle holder. (C) Large needle holder.

Needle holders

Needle holders hold suture needles and provide good control for inserting needles. Some of these instruments are nonlocking, some locking; some handles are spring-loaded. Some needle holders for larger-size needles have a thumb release (Figure 29.6).

Clamps

Clamps used in ophthalmic surgery may be round, with a guarded plate behind to provide hemostasis during removal of chalazia. Other clamps are used to hold eyelids during surgery, as well as to create hemostasis.

Curets

Curets are slim-handled and have a bowl-shaped end. The ends are either round or serrated and are used to remove chalazia and other small cystic material.

Scalpels, keratomes, and blades

Scalpels used by the physician depend on preference. Commonly used instruments are often disposable small blades, some angled blades, some keratomes for incising into the cornea, and the Bard-Parker scalpel used for skin cutting. Some tips are of gem quality (e.g., sapphire, diamond). Smaller and smaller keratomes are used to accommodate the newer foldable lenses.

Lacrimal instruments

A lacrimal set consists of a punctum dilator, which enlarges the punctum; a sterile medicine glass to hold sterile saline solution or an antibiotic solution; and a disposable syringe

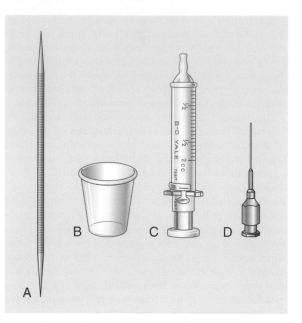

Figure 29.7 Lacrimal set. (A) Punctum dilator. (B) Sterile medicine glass to contain either sterile normal saline solution or an antibiotic solution. (C) Syringe. (D) Lacrimal needle.

with a blunt lacrimal cannula. The last introduces a solution into the canaliculus (Figure 29.7).

Corrosion of stainless steel instruments

What is known as "'stainless steel'" may contain a wide range of metals. These always include iron and chromium, but the alloy may also contain carbon, nickel, sulfur, tungsten, manganese, molybdenum, and other elements. Chromium imparts the stainless quality to the metal and the more chromium present, the more resistant it is to corrosion. Carbon provides hardness to the metal but reduces the corrosion-resistant effect of chromium. Special hardening processes are used by different manufacturers to try to produce a hardened instrument with low corrosion properties. Polishing also reduces the corrosive effect, but some areas such as the knurled handles cannot be polished very well and consequently are the first to suffer corrosion.

The most common causes of corrosion are inadequate cleaning and drying after use, overlong exposure to sterilizing solutions, or too corrosive a sterilizing solution. The most important factor that causes corrosion is inadequate cleaning so that particles of material remain on the surface.

Fortunately, many sharp instruments today are available in disposable form. Where available, these usually are preferred because a sharp instrument is guaranteed every time.

Procedures

Chalazion surgery

A chalazion is caused by an obstruction of a meibomian gland of the eyelid. Because of this blockage, the gland becomes distended and ruptures, the oily contents being liberated into the substance of the lid. This results in a granulomatous inflammatory reaction that subsides spontaneously in some cases, but in other cases appears to remain as a chronic nodule on the eyelid (Figure 29.8). The nodule may be removed under the eyelid through a vertical conjunctival incision or, occasionally, externally through the skin.

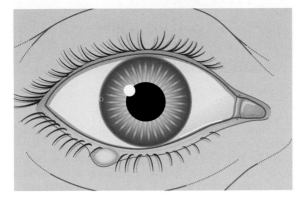

Figure 29.8 Chalazion of the lower eyelid.

The ophthalmic assistant's help is essential in:

- Arranging the patient comfortably in the operating chair
- Anesthetizing the eye adequately with topical anesthetic drops
- Setting out the syringe and needle with the local anesthetic for infiltration into the eyelid
- Setting out a sterile towel with the instruments required
- Securing hemostasis by applying pressure directly at the operative site after chalazion removal
- Preparing the dressing, which usually consists of an antibiotic ointment and a firmly applied eye pad

The instruments required for the chalazion operation are shown in Figure 29.9.

Eyepatch application

An eyepatch must be applied correctly if it is to perform the necessary function of preventing further bleeding and an accumulation of lid edema (Figure 29.10). After the instillation of an antibiotic ointment, a recommended method is to immobilize the eyelid through pressure by applying an eye pad doubled in half over the site of the chalazion, applying a second eye pad over this pad, and fixing the pad firmly by small ½-inch (1.25 cm) strips of adhesive tape in an overlapping fashion, taking care that the hair is not involved in any way in the adhesive. Sometimes double pads are used if there is a concern about bleeding.

Figure 29.9 Chalazion set. (A) Chalazion clamp. (B) Scalpel. (C) Curet. (D) Fine scissors. (E) Fine forceps.

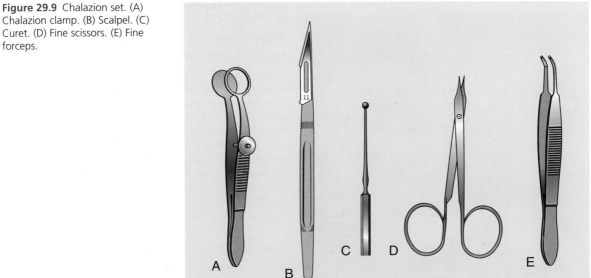

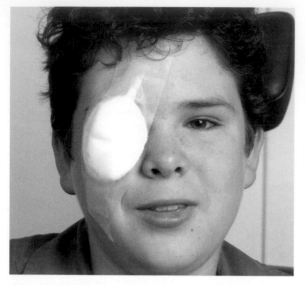

Figure 29.10 Eyepatch. Note that the patch is angled away from the mouth to prevent interference with eating.

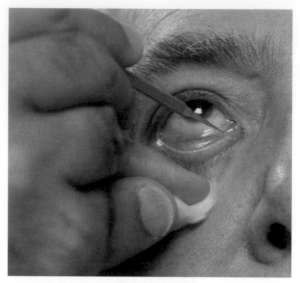

Figure 29.12 Dilation of the punctum.

Tear duct irrigation

Epiphora, or watering of the eye, is a common condition, especially affecting older patients. This condition may result from a blockage of the nasolacrimal passage (passage of the tears from the punctum to the back of the throat). One important test to determine the site of blockage is washing out or irrigating the nasolacrimal passageway (Figure 29.11).

In most cases, disposable syringes are used. However, carefully cleaned and sterilized reusable syringes may be used. The latter are most often used in parts of the world where cost is a factor and labor is inexpensive. Lacrimal instruments are best sterilized by using a dry heat oven.

Normally the upper and lower puncta are small and do not admit a lacrimal needle or probe. The punctum dilator is used to enlarge the orifice of the punctum to permit the lacrimal needle to enter the lacrimal canaliculus (Figure 29.12). Many ophthalmologists prefer to use an antibiotic solution for irrigation in case the lacrimal passageways are traumatized.

Fluorescein test to determine lacrimal function

A simple test to determine the patency of the lacrimal passageway is performed by placing 1 or 2 drops of fluorescein into the conjunctival sac, with the patient's head bent forward. If there is no obstruction to flow, then the fluorescein will drain into the nose within 30 seconds. A test that indicates good patency consists of placing a dried cotton swab in the nose to see whether the stain is present. Occasionally the fluorescein will drain to the back of the throat and the stain can be found by having the patient cough and deposit the stained sputum into a tissue. The fellow eye can be checked at the same time with use of rose bengal stain.

Tear duct probing

In cases of complete blockage of the nasolacrimal passage, either constant watering (epiphora) or sometimes a combination of watering with an infection of the lacrimal sac

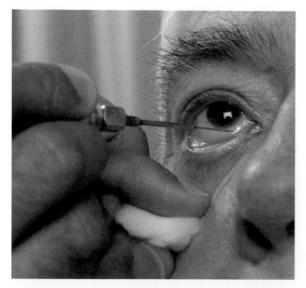

Figure 29.11 Irrigation of nasolacrimal duct.

(dacryocystitis) may be found. This is particularly common among newborn infants.

Many ophthalmologists prefer to perform this procedure at the hospital with the patient under general anesthesia. When a general anesthetic is used, it should be just sufficient to allow the patient to retain the swallowing reflex. The ophthalmologist can observe whether the irrigation is successful and prevents fluid from entering the patient's lungs.

With adults, the probing of tear ducts may be performed with the use of a topical anesthetic (such as proparacaine or tetracaine) combined with local infiltration of anesthetic. The injectable anesthetic may be combined with some hyaluronidase to increase the spreading effect throughout the tissues. Further anesthesia may be achieved by irrigating a small amount of proparacaine or tetracaine through the punctum. It is important that the patient be relaxed and comfortable because sudden movement of the head may cause damage to the eye or produce a false passage in the lacrimal apparatus. The instruments required for probing are shown in Figure 29.13.

Ziegler cautery

Ziegler cautery refers to thermal, or heat, cauterizing of the lower eyelid to either invert or evert it (Figure 29.14). This procedure is used more commonly for spastic senile entropion (turning inward of the eyelid) but it also may be used for ectropion (turning outward of the eyelid). This

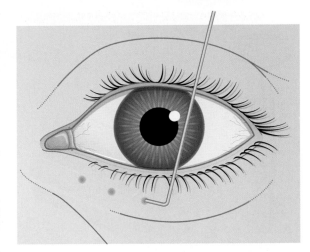

Figure 29.14 Correction of entropion by Ziegler cautery.

operation has particular value for an older adult patient with a spastic entropion. The instruments used are shown in Figure 29.15.

Electrolysis

A method used to permanently remove lashes from the eyelid margin by applying heat to the base of the hair follicle is known as electrolysis. It is used to treat congenitally

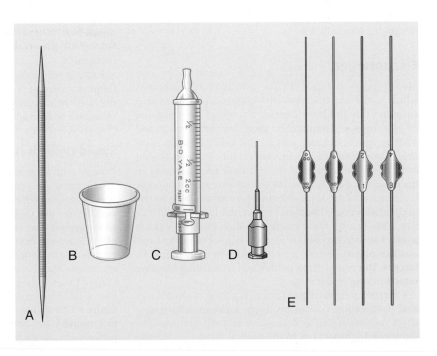

Figure 29.13 Tear duct probing set. (A) Punctum dilator. (B) Medicine glass. (C) Syringe. (D) Lacrimal needle. (E) Series of probes usually ranging from 00 to 2 wire size.

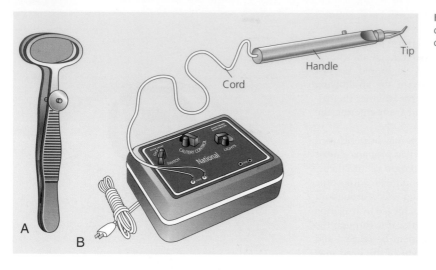

Figure 29.15 Instruments for Ziegler cautery. (A) Large chalazion or lid clamp. (B) Fine thermal cautery.

aberrant lashes, trichiasis, and postoperative and posttraumatic conditions that result in the turning of the lashes toward the cornea.

Anesthesia is performed by direct infiltration of anesthetic into the base of the lashes. The hyfrecator with a fine needle is inserted along the pathway to the root of the lash. Magnification is essential in this procedure to see the tiny orifices through which the hairs emerge. Epilation is complete after the hyfrecator has been turned on for a few seconds and the lash can be removed without pulling. Cryotherapy is another useful method of permanently destroying hair follicles.

Electrosurgery

Electrosurgery is based on the principles of diathermy, which is the amplification of high-frequency alternating currents. This produces heat as a result of the resistance of the tissues. Frequencies used are between 2 and 4 MHz, which includes part of the radiofrequency spectrum. Because of this, as a precaution these currents should not be used with individuals who have pacemakers or in the presence of any flammable or explosive gases or liquids.

A number of modes of electrosurgery are available for use in ophthalmology. The most familiar mode is wet field cautery. This is a bipolar cautery in which electrical current passes between two points in a wet field of saline and creates hemostasis. The two points are usually the two tips of a forceps. This is one of the methods of coagulating bleeding vessels during ocular surgery.

Fulguration or spark gap current is a form of electric current. Fulguration current produces a potent dehydrating effect on tissues that is destructive and self-limiting. The spark must jump across to the tissues, thereby producing a charring or carbon effect on the tissues. This procedure can coagulate heavy bleeders or destroy bases of tissue to prevent such things as recurrences of carcinoma.

A fully filtered current is a continuous flow of a high-frequency current that results in a nonpulsating flow of current. This produces a smooth cutting flow with a minimal amount of heat and tissue destruction. This type of current is ideal for cutting.

Fully rectified current produces a minute, but perceptible, pulsating effect that can, under certain conditions, reduce the efficiency of the cutting while producing some lateral heat. A benefit is that this heat can produce coagulation of the tissue surfaces and provide effective hemostasis.

Partially rectified current is an intermittent flow of high-frequency current. Because it is partially rectified, it produces more hemostasis and seals off bleeders. This type of current is commonly used in eyelid surgery.

Eyelid growth removal

Patients with large growths of the eyelid may require hospital surgery for removal of the growth under adequate operating room conditions. However, many small papillomas, benign melanomas, verrucae, and other small lesions of the eyelids may be carefully and safely removed in the office. Specimen bottles that contain formaldehyde should be available from the local pathology laboratory so that the specimens may be stored and microscopically examined. Many of these lesions on the eyelid may be removed and the base cauterized. Others may require sutures. Figure 29.16 shows the instruments that are required and that should be available when eyelid procedures are performed.

Figure 29.16 Eyelid growth removal set. (A) Scalpel. (B) Fine forceps. (C) Fine scissors. (D) Needle holder. (E) Fine suture.

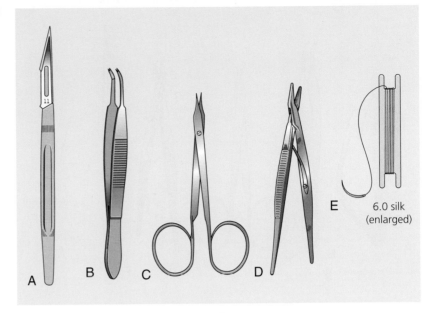

E 6.0 silk (enlarged)

Pterygium removal

A pterygium is a fibrovascular membrane that extends from the medial aspect of the bulbar conjunctiva and invades the cornea (Figure 29.17). It tends to be progressive and in time can make its way to the central portion of the cornea and interfere with vision. Pterygia are most common in southern climates where people have greater exposure to ultraviolet light, which appears to promote growth. In northern areas, people who have outdoor vocations, such as farmers, sailors, and postal workers, are most prone to develop this growth.

The purpose of pterygium removal is to excise the membrane before it can significantly interfere with vision. Because this operation requires incision into the cornea as well as the conjunctiva, scrupulous cleanliness, disinfection of the patient's skin and the surgeon's hands, and sterilization of the instruments are required. The anesthesia is usually provided by topical drops, either alone or combined with subconjunctival injection. Placing the patient in a horizontal position is the preferred method for the surgical removal of the pterygium. Application of mitomycin solution is often helpful in preventing recurrence. Amniotic membrane graphs are used for recurrences. The instruments for a pterygium procedure are shown in Figure 29.18.

Xanthelasma lesion removal

Xanthelasma lesions are yellowish and subcutaneous and are found on the inner aspect of the upper and lower eyelids (Figure 29.19). They are normally bilateral and progress slowly. These lesions tend to form an arc in both the upper and lower eyelids and are often associated with high serum cholesterol levels. Xanthelasma lesions are removed for cosmetic purposes only, because these deposits have no invasive properties. Despite removal, however, they tend to recur. Smaller lesions may be removed by the application of a chemical such as trichloroacetic acid. Larger xanthelasma deposits require surgical removal. Excision is usually quite simple, requiring excision of the skin and the underlying subcutaneous tissue. Instruments required for removal of xanthelasma lesions are shown in Figure 29.20.

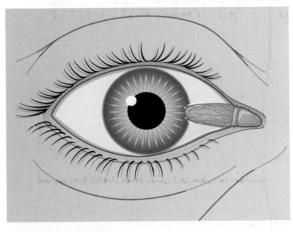

Figure 29.17 Pterygium.

513

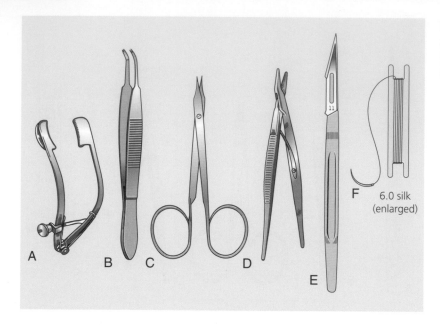

Figure 29.18 Pterygium set. (A) Eyelid speculum. (B) Fine forceps. (C) Fine scissors. (D) Needle holder. (E) Bard-Parker scalpel or angled superblade. (F) Fine suture.

F   6.0 silk (enlarged)

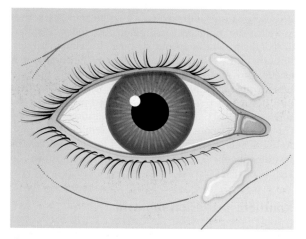

Figure 29.19 Xanthelasma.

COMPLICATIONS DURING AND AFTER OFFICE SURGERY

The ophthalmic assistant must be alert for complications that may arise after surgery. The assistant may be the closest at hand and in a position to render immediate first aid for the following conditions that may arise: fainting, central nervous system stimulation, respiratory emergencies, allergic reaction, and drug reaction.

Fainting

Fainting is a common occurrence in office surgery. The patient who faints should be placed in a head-down position, with the head lower than the heart. This may be done by tilting the head forward between the knees or tilting back the operating table or chair. Ophthalmic personnel should be sure that there is an adequate airway present and that a tight collar is loosened. Aromatic spirits of ammonia or smelling salts may be administered to encourage breathing by reflex stimulation.

Central nervous system stimulation

A patient may show signs of great excitability, tremors, or even convulsions. This may be the result of cocaine or other drug toxicity. The patient should be placed head down, ensuring that the airway is not restricted by collars or ties, and given reassurance. The ophthalmologist should be contacted immediately if not already available. The ophthalmologist may consider giving intravenous sedation. Epinephrine should be on hand.

Respiratory emergencies

If any difficulties arise in breathing, such as shallowness or decreased respirations, the patient must be watched carefully. Oxygen may be administered by a small portable oxygen unit, which must be readily available. If artificial resuscitation becomes necessary, mouth-to-mouth

Figure 29.20 Xanthelasma set. (A) Scalpel. (B) Fine forceps. (C) Fine scissors. (D) Needle holder. (E) Silk or nylon suture.

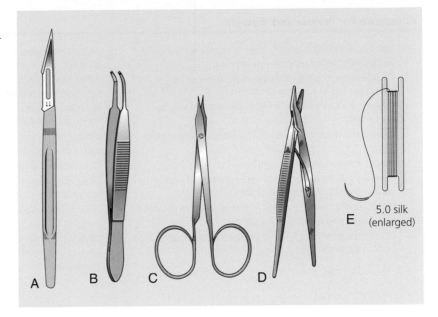

5.0 silk (enlarged)

resuscitation is the treatment of choice. See Chapter 49 on cardiopulmonary resuscitation for more detailed information.

Allergic reaction

Severe allergic reactions or idiosyncratic reactions may occur, with resultant edema of the respiratory passages. This may require mouth-to-mouth resuscitation, oxygen therapy, and intravenous cortisone.

Drug reaction

The ophthalmologist should be immediately alerted to any signs of a drug reaction. He or she may elect to control the reaction by the use of drugs such as epinephrine (Adrenalin) or cortisone.

An important rule for the ophthalmic assistant is to have the following available at all times in an easily visible and accessible place:

- Oxygen
- Epinephrine (Adrenalin)
- Sterile syringes with needles
- Meperidine (Demerol)
- Barbiturates
- Intravenous cortisone
- Spirits of ammonia or smelling salts
- A scalpel

The assistant should allow a routine time to periodically check for current dating on supplies.

SUMMARY

An outline of effective aseptic technique and methods of dealing with instruments and layouts for office surgical procedure has been presented. The ophthalmic assistant who has been given this challenging responsibility must become familiar with the basic routine of the ophthalmologist. The assistant will then become a necessary and invaluable aid in the smooth performance of these minor surgical procedures and will derive a great deal of personal satisfaction from the work.

Questions for review and thought

1. What is meant by asepsis? When is aseptic technique of particular importance in eye surgery?
2. Outline ways in which the operative field may be contaminated at the time of surgery.
3. Outline ways in which wound contamination may be prevented.
4. Discuss the methods by which skin may be prepared for surgery.
5. How are tonometers sterilized?
6. How are eye medications rendered sterile and how is contamination of such medications avoided?
7. What are the main functions of the ophthalmic assistant with respect to minor office surgery?
8. List several minor ophthalmic procedures commonly performed in the office.
9. Discuss the procedure for nasolacrimal irrigation in an adult.
10. What instruments should be set out for the surgical removal of a chalazion?
11. What are general complications that may result from minor office surgery?
12. What emergency supplies should be on hand to deal with such complications?
13. How would you handle a patient who faints in the office?
14. What instruments are available for removing a corneal foreign body?
15. What is the purpose of an eyepatch after a corneal abrasion?
16. What is the advantage of fluorescein strips over solutions?
17. What reactions may occur after injection of a local anesthetic?

Q Self-evaluation questions

True–false statements

Directions: Indicate whether the statement is true **(T)** or false **(F).**

1. In office practice, fluorescein in paper strip form is preferable to the large solution form of 2% fluorescein. **T** or **F**
2. Ophthalmic solutions are always sterile. **T** or **F**

Missing words

Directions: Write in the missing word(s) in the following sentences:

3. A technique that results in absence of microorganisms is called _____ technique.
4. Excitability, tremors, and convulsions are indications of _____ stimulation.
5. An agent that may be used to relieve immediate serious allergic reactions to drugs is _____.

Choice-completion questions

Directions: Select the one best answer in each case.

6. Which of the following is not necessary for a chalazion procedure?
   a. Scalpel blade
   b. Curet
   c. Forceps
   d. Speculum
   e. Clamp
7. Which of the following is incorrect? Tear duct irrigation for epiphora may be used to identify:
   a. blockage of the punctum.
   b. stenosis of the canaliculus.
   c. blockage of the nasolacrimal duct.
   d. ectropion.
   e. presence of a stone in the lacrimal sac.

A Answers, notes, and explanations

1. **True.** Fluorescein in large bottle solutions can easily become contaminated, particularly with *Pseudomonas aeruginosa*, and consequently one may be introducing a new organism into the eye. Paper strips are far safer for office use. However, individual sterile dropper units are available and, although these are relatively expensive, they may also be used.

The technique of applying fluorescein paper is to wet the fluorescein strip with saline solution or touch the wet conjunctiva so that a thin film of fluorescein will spread over the corneal surface. Any defect in the epithelial cells will be stained by fluorescein and become more easily visualized. It is advisable in record keeping to make a sketch of the staining area on the patient's record for later comparison

A Continued

and to follow the progress of healing. This may become important in recurrent corneal abrasion to identify the site of initial injury.

2. **False.** Although manufacturers provide preservatives such as chlorobutanol, thimerosal, ethylenediaminetetraacetic (EDTA), and benzalkonium chloride to prevent the solutions becoming contaminated, there is no fail-safe method. Once a bottle has been opened and used on any patient, organisms can enter the solution and not be destroyed by the preservative. The longer the bottle remains on the shelf of the ophthalmic office, the more likely this is to occur.

   As a consequence, safeguards for ophthalmic drugs should be put into action once the bottle has been opened. These bottles should not remain on the shelf for any length of time. Second, when introducing drops into the eye, one should avoid contaminating the tip of the bottle or the tip of the eyedropper by touching the lashes or eyelid of the individual receiving the drops. If contamination is suspected, the solution should be discarded.

3. **Aseptic.** Aseptic technique refers to a method of surgery in which there is an absence of all living microorganisms. This technique involves sterilization of instruments, disinfecting the skin of the patient and the hands of the operator, and the use of sterile solutions, drapes, and medications so that nothing reaching the operative site has any microorganisms that will cause contamination.

4. **Central nervous system.** Some drugs reach the central nervous system and induce this type of excitability, tremors, or convulsions. Cocaine may be such an offending agent.

5. **Epinephrine (Adrenalin), cortisone.** Both agents may be used in certain situations to relieve an acute anaphylactic reaction in which the body responds adversely to some drug. Both of these agents should be kept on hand and be readily available for such emergencies.

6. **d. Speculum.** A chalazion clamp is usually satisfactory for holding the lid and creating hemostasis during the procedure. Chalazion clamps can be small or large and can be selected to suit the size of the chalazion.

7. **d. Ectropion.** The diagnosis of ectropion is usually made from external examination and does not require probing or tear duct irrigation to identify the problem. However, these procedures might identify any stenosis of the canaliculus that might have occurred as a result of the ectropion.

   In other situations, such as occlusion, stenosis, or presence of a stone of the lacrimal sac, there will be a resistance on irrigation of the nasolacrimal system.

Chapter | 30 |

The operative patient

Those involved with patient care for operative patients should be familiar with the preoperative and postoperative routines for management of the eye patient. Such a patient must feel secure that the case is being dealt with professionally from the time the decision is made to have surgery until postoperative management is complete. A single error, such as giving the patient the wrong date of surgery, will only increase the patient's anxiety and undermine his or her confidence in the physician. Operative routines should be well explained so that at each phase the patient knows exactly what to expect.

This chapter deals with the total management of the patient's care before surgery and during the postoperative period.

ARRANGEMENTS FOR THE OPERATION

The person who makes the booking and arrangement of admission to the appropriate hospital or surgical center has been delegated a great deal of responsibility (Figure 30.1). Each operative procedure involves a dislocation in the patient's life. The patient will be required to take time off from work, school, or homemaking and to make arrangements for someone to fill his or her place in the performance of regular duties. Therefore, it is helpful if the patient is asked beforehand which date is most convenient to schedule the necessary surgery.

In addition to scheduling time for surgery according to the convenience of the patient, the ophthalmic assistant should prepare the surgical schedule according to the convenience of the surgeon. The assistant must know the duration of each operative procedure so that a surgical schedule will not be unreasonably crowded, as well as the number of surgeries the ophthalmologist can perform and follow each week without creating a strain.

The ophthalmic assistant often may be responsible for obtaining a properly signed consent form. It is important that this be reviewed carefully with the patient and all questions answered. Three types of operative bookings require special attention: emergency admission, urgent admission, and elective admission.

Emergency admission

The emergency patient is one who experiences a serious ocular or periocular calamity, usually from trauma, and because of the nature of the condition must be treated by surgery without delay. This type of patient does not have the time to adjust psychologically to the onset of the illness or to the necessary treatment. This patient usually is anxious, agitated, often confused, and commonly in a great deal of pain as well as emotionally disturbed because of the loss of vision. Because the patient cannot be psychologically prepared for surgery, prime attention is focused on the orderly transfer of the patient from the office to the hospital's emergency room. None of the details of the transfer should ever be left to the patient. Relatives or friends should be called and transportation

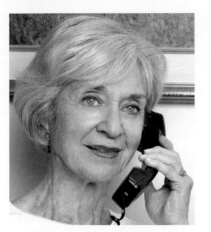

Figure 30.1 Correct bookings are important to patient, hospital, and surgeon.

to the hospital or surgicenter area arranged through them. They can also, at a later date, bring the patient's personal articles and take care of the patient's personal commitments. If in a hospital, the emergency room should be notified to anticipate the patient's arrival so that delay will not be incurred because of the number of routine admissions. It is helpful to note the patient's room number and visiting hours for family and friends. Each hospital has its own regulations regarding visiting time, duration of visits, number of relatives admitted per visit, and visiting by children. Thus the ophthalmic assistant should understand the rules for visitors.

The most common ocular emergencies that require surgical intervention are lacerated globes and eyelids, intraocular foreign bodies, acute glaucoma, and intraocular hemorrhage.

Urgent admission

The urgent patient is one whose problem requires special consideration because of the patient's condition. Such a patient requires priority admission because the problem cannot be tolerated for an unlimited time. For example, the patient with a retinal detachment is best treated as soon as the detachment is discovered. If, however, the hospital is overcrowded and immediate admission is not possible, the patient should be placed on the urgent list on a day-to-day basis.

The patient with an urgent problem should always be available and prepared to enter the hospital on a day-to-day basis. Patients in this category should be called regularly so that they do not feel they are languishing forgotten at home.

Other conditions that may be classified as urgent disorders are chronic glaucoma, orbital tumors, dislocated lenses, uveitis, and temporal arteritis.

Elective admission

The patient with an elective problem has an ocular disorder that is chronic and slowly progressive and that will not significantly deteriorate by a delay in admission to a hospital or surgicenter. The patient has ample time to be fully briefed on the duration of the hospital stay and the expected postoperative convalescence. It is helpful if patients of this type are prepared for surgery by giving them some of the available literature on their particular condition. A personal letter from the doctor may be welcomed. Pamphlets and videotapes on glaucoma, strabismus, and cataracts explain the nature of these disorders and the purpose of operative therapy.

Operative booking schedule

To ensure that all arrangements with the patient and the surgicenter or hospital are secure, the ophthalmic assistant should have a plan to follow on each operative case. Our plan has been for the ophthalmic assistant to record a number of essential points before a patient is considered to be booked and awaiting surgery:

- Date of admission
- Type of bed if any required
- Date and time of operation, with type of anesthesia
- Date the patient was notified by telephone
- Date of letter sent requiring confirmation
- Confirmation by the patient

A bright red reminder slip is affixed to the front of every surgical chart.

It is helpful to provide a pamphlet as a response to the numerous questions that have been asked regarding modern cataract surgery and today's hospitalization procedures. Patients should be advised that this surgery is not a frightening procedure, but will actually turn out pleasant for them. Box 30.1 is an example of such a pamphlet.

The date of admission often is the day of outpatient surgery. It may, however, be the evening before surgery if the patient requires hospitalization. If such a condition is not under complete control, surgery may be hazardous to the patient. A medical consultation may be necessary to ensure that the patient does not have any infections, cardiac irregularities, uncontrolled diabetes, hypertension, or other medical disorders.

Operative time and date must be carefully integrated with the surgeon's schedule so that there is no duplication of this time by office appointments or other commitments. Patients with infection such as dacryocystitis always should be placed last on the operative schedule. The ophthalmic assistant should be familiar with the length of time required for the surgeon to complete a procedure. Additional time should be set aside during the time of surgery for changeover of instruments and materials between patients.

Box 30.1 **What to do before and after cataract surgery (handout to patient)**

Be sure to bring your insurance details with you.

If you are currently taking medication, please bring these to the hospital with you. A nurse will inquire about all the medication you are taking.

Obtain a good night's sleep before admission to hospital.

Shampoo your hair the night before entering hospital.

Women: Please do not wear makeup, particularly mascara and facial preparations.

Do not wear or bring valuable jewelry.

Special relaxing medication may be given to you on the morning of surgery.

For local anesthesia

Eyedrops and occasionally a small local freezing injection may be given to you just before surgery.

In the operating room you may see the usual lights and sterile equipment and a special microscope. You will not see anything of the surgery during the operation.

Surgery lasts about 15 minutes. Soon after, you will be able to sit up in bed.

After cataract surgery you may have a bandage over only the operative eye. This will be removed soon after surgery and no eye bandage need be worn.

A small plastic shield may be placed over the eye at bedtime to prevent unconscious rubbing of the eye when asleep.

You will be out of bed soon after surgery.

Although you need not restrict your movements after surgery, please be careful of heavy lifting and excess bending.

Avoid bright window sunshine. If bright, wear sunglasses.

On the first night there may be some discomfort. If so, take a mild pain-killing pill.

On discharge you will be given a two-page list of do's and don'ts.

24 hours to 2 weeks after surgery

Go back to normal activities using caution. If you have pain, call the office. You may bend over gently to put on shoes. You may read and watch TV as you wish. You can do anything you were doing before surgery with the following exceptions:

- No contact sports
- Avoid getting water in eye while swimming
- No swinging of golf clubs; however, chipping and putting should be safe
- No strenuous exercise
- You may wash your hair gently, or go to the beauty parlor, but avoid getting water in the eye.

Just remember to use common sense!

After 2 weeks

You can function as you had before surgery and it is hoped, with much better vision. Medication may be stopped soon after this point.

Common symptoms after surgery

The following common symptoms may occur after surgery and should not cause alarm:

- Light sensitivity, especially to sunlight; be sure to use dark glasses.
- Don't be surprised if color perception is improved with your operated eye.
- Mild irritation, redness, itchiness, or watery eye may occur for the first several days following surgery.
- Your vision may be fuzzy for several weeks. Patients vary as to the time required before their vision returns.
- There may be some bruising around the eyelids or the side of your head, which will soon fade.
- A small amount of residue may collect in your eyelids or the corner of your eye on awakening in the morning. (This is most likely caused by eyedrop residue.)

You should report any sudden onset of severe pain, loss of vision, or marked redness in the operated eye.

The decision whether to use local or general anesthesia is most important in booking the operating room. It is preferable if procedures that require general anesthesia are scheduled to follow each other so that the anesthetist's time is more efficiently used.

As soon as arrangements for the operative time and date have been completed, the patient should be notified by telephone to be sure that the time is suitable. Occasional adjustments may have to be made for illness, holidays, work, and special requests of the patient. A well-run ophthalmic practice, emphasizing goodwill, permits some latitude in this direction, depending on the urgency of the problem.

For previous retinal surgery

Often more conservative instructions may apply for cataract surgery:

1. Preoperative assessment is often scheduled directly or emailed.
2. Aspirin and other blood thinners should be stopped 1 week before surgery if possible.
3. Only the one eye having surgery will be patched.

Our practice has been to follow the telephone call with a confirming letter outlining the date and time of admission to the hospital and requesting confirmation by return call or letter. The purpose of having the patient provide a return call or letter is to ensure that the date of surgery is suitable and that the patient's schedule has been altered accordingly.

The confirmation should always be double-checked and those patients who have not confirmed should be contacted.

A simplification of this routine may be followed when the patient has outpatient surgery. With outpatient surgery today, blood tests and physical examinations are arranged ahead of time. The patient may be asked to return to the office to pick up blood test forms. In addition, intraocular lens implant power will be required for all cataract procedures. An A-scan, or intraocular lens (IOL) Master, may be performed at this time if it has not been performed before. These measurements are usually performed on both eyes at the same time. In some cases a B-scan may be required if the cataract is dense and the practitioner wishes to view the vitreous cavity and the status of the retina. Other investigational tests may be performed. Visual aids are available for demonstration purposes (Figure 30.2).

Patients may be asked to have a physical check-up and a report from their doctor.

Consent form

Today consent forms are mandatory for all surgical procedures, whether minor procedures, such as yttrium-aluminum-garnet (YAG) laser iridotomy or capsulotomy, or major procedures such as cataract removal, laser-assisted in situ keratomileusis (LASIK), photorefractive keratotomy (PRK), or other refractive procedures.

The contents of a proper consent form are outlined in Box 30.2. The patient should carefully review and understand this material. The surgeon should personally review

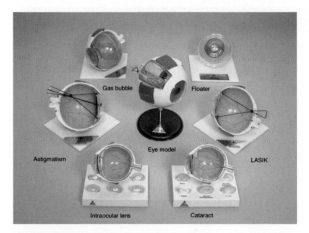

Figure 30.2 Visual aids, such as eye models, are available for demonstration purposes.
(Courtesy of Gulden Ophthalmics, Elkins Park, PA, USA.)

Box 30.2 **Contents of informed consent document**
1. Risks of procedure
2. Benefits of procedure
3. Complications
4. Alternative treatments
5. Explanation of procedure
6. Advantages of one procedure over another
7. Significant issues (e.g., bilateral versus sequential)

significant risks, note these in the medical record, and permit the patient to ask questions. Duly signed consents onsite have been challenged in the courts!

We provide a simplified form that is mailed to patients. This permits them to discuss it at home. They bring this form back in and can ask questions of the ophthalmic assistant or surgeon. The ophthalmic assistant double-checks that the signed form is available before patients come for surgery. In some cases and in some centers, a more detailed consent and acceptance is indicated, supported by video explanation.

PREPARING THE CHILD AND PARENT FOR SURGERY

The child who is about to enter the hospital will have a great deal of apprehension. If this is the second or third hospital visit, the child's apprehension may have been increased by previous experiences. For many children this will be the first experience away from their parents in strange surroundings.

Some hospitals have facilities for admission of the mother to the same room so that she may stay with the child the night before surgery and the night after. This is good practice because it diminishes the child's sense of insecurity and abandonment. If dual admissions are not possible, the child should be admitted to a room with other children where the child would feel more comfortable. The child may be terrified if placed with a sick adult given to groaning or erratic behavior.

It is important that the child be given some explanation about the purpose of the visit to the hospital and the routines to be expected. Virtually every hospital requires some preliminary investigations, including a chest x-ray, urinalysis, hemoglobin determination, and temperature reading. The child should be told that a few simple painless tests will be performed the day before surgery. The child should be informed by the parent that he or she will go to sleep and, on awakening, will find a bandage over one eye.

The parent should be instructed as to the time of discharge and the necessary office visits that may be required afterward. A fully informed parent will be a cooperative parent after surgery.

PREPARING THE ADULT FOR MAJOR OCULAR SURGERY

It is necessary to have the patient who will be undergoing surgery in the best physical and emotional condition to avoid any complications. The ophthalmic assistant should endeavor, when possible, to relieve the patient's anxiety and apprehension. Fostering cooperation and confidence is all-important in the patient's psychologic approach to the operation.

The patient should be told how to find the admitting department of the hospital and what documents may be required for entry. The patient should leave all valuables at home. The ophthalmic assistant should call the hospital before the patient's admission to ensure that the accommodation the patient desires is available. If changes are necessary, the patient should be told beforehand, rather than at the admitting desk.

Alterations in the patient's personal habits may be necessary in the pre- and postoperative periods. The patient who is a heavy smoker should be asked to abstain for at least 1 week preoperatively and during the immediate postoperative period, because a smoker's cough can easily cause disruption of the delicate operative wound. The patient who is taking aspirin or anticoagulants should be asked to refrain from doing so for at least 1 week before surgery to avoid excessive bleeding (Box 30.3).

On discharge from the hospital the patient will need to have medication. If the patient is unable to perform the task personally, prior arrangements should be made for a spouse or partner, nurse, or member of the family to instill the medication.

Restrictions have gradually been lightened in the past few years as a result of smaller-incision surgery and better wound architecture. Thus today the patient can return home immediately and carry on normal activities with little restriction.

EYE SURGERY

The patient contemplating eye surgery is beset with many misgivings and fears about the amount of suffering that will be endured and the possibility of losing sight permanently. As opposed to the internal organs of the body, the patient has some concept of the eye and therefore is more likely to develop anxieties. The patient knows where the eyes are, what they are used for, and that they are extremely painful to touch with a hair, let alone a sharp scalpel. In contrast, a patient who is going to have a gallbladder removed usually has, at best, a remote idea of the location of this structure and certainly no concept of its function because the body appears to carry on with or without a gallbladder. The patient with an ocular problem that requires surgery consciously fears damage to the eye and knows full well the consequences of removal.

Because ocular surgery is often dramatic, in that near-blind people are given sight, it is often the subject of much attention in the popular and lay press, in current magazines, and on television. Much of this medical information

---

Box 30.3 Guidelines for patients having cataract surgery

- You will be required to have an intraocular lens (IOL) measurement.
- Continue to take all medications prescribed for you.
- Because you will have a topical or local anesthetic, you may eat a light meal.
- Wear a short-sleeved shirt or blouse that buttons in the front with loose-fitting sleeves.
- Do not wear undershirts or long underwear.
- Do not wear pantyhose. Wear socks or knee-highs and loose-fitting pants.
- Do not wear eye makeup or nail polish.
- You must be accompanied by an adult and have transportation home by car or taxi. Please bring a translator if you have difficulty with English.

- You will be asked to arrive early. Your surgery will take approximately 15 to 30 minutes and you will be required to stay for about 30 to 45 minutes after surgery.
- Please start the eyedrops received in your surgical package 1.5 hours before your surgery.
- If you are wearing an eyepatch after surgery, it remains on the eye until the first postoperative visit with the doctor. The drops will start after the patch is removed. Many patients do not have a patch and drops can start on the day of surgery.
- All patients *must* see the doctor for a follow-up visit 1 or 2 days after surgery.

fed to the public is boiled down in the interests of simplicity so that the patient often has a naive concept of the function and mechanics of ocular surgery or, even worse, a totally distorted view of it. The ophthalmic assistant should be able to intelligently handle many of the general questions regarding ophthalmic surgery and be able to relate to the patient a simple but accurate account of what is to be expected during the procedure.

Some questions and misconceptions commonly asked by patients regarding ophthalmic surgery are discussed next.

Can an eye be transplanted?

Only the cornea can be transplanted; the entire eye cannot. In the evolution of modern surgery the cornea was one of the first structures of the body to be replaced with tissues from another body. The body was found to be able to accept a transplanted cornea because of the lack of blood vessels in this structure and the inability of the immune mechanisms of the body to reach the transplanted tissue and reject it. Every ophthalmologist experiences the necessity of having to tell a blind patient, with perhaps absolute glaucoma or retinitis pigmentosa, that the patient's blindness cannot be cured by one of the "new transplant procedures." Not every eye is suitable for a transplant.

Is the eye taken out for surgery?

Some patients think that the ophthalmologist takes the eye out, places it in some kind of vise on a workbench, completes the surgery and then merely pops the eye back into place. The eye is never removed from its socket unless, of course, an enucleation was actually intended.

Will there be any unsightly scars on the eye after surgery?

Ophthalmic surgeons are very much aware of the cosmetic importance of the eyes and usually leave no trace of their incisions visible to the naked eye. This is particularly true of cataract and strabismus procedures. After fistulization procedures for the treatment of glaucoma the patient may develop a soft bulge above the cornea, but it usually is well hidden by the upper eyelid.

Will both eyes be patched after surgery?

With the exception perhaps of retinal detachment surgery, both eyes are not patched after surgery. Even after bilateral strabismus surgery, one patch usually is removed shortly after so that the patient will not feel blinded after the operation.

Is there a great deal of pain after ocular surgery?

The pain is minimal. It is controlled by medications freely available to the patient in the immediate postoperative period so that the patient's discomfort is comparatively insignificant.

Must the head be placed between heavy sandbags after surgery?

In the early days of ophthalmic surgery, before the development of good sutures, needles, and instruments, the wound was not apposed with sutures. Later, sutures for large incisions were required. The patient's head then had to be held rigid and the eyes immobilized until healing took place. Today, with microincision surgery almost all patients, with only few exceptions, are allowed up and around with minimal restrictions on the day after surgery. For most patients, cataract surgery is an outpatient procedure.

Can both eyes be operated on at the same time?

Because safety has greatly increased with small incision cataract surgery, some surgeons are operating on both eyes at the same time so the patient can return to work early. However, most are still concerned that if an infection breaks out in an operating room, there could be an irreparable loss to both eyes.

TYPES OF ANESTHESIA

General anesthesia is used for all children's surgery, most strabismus procedures, retinal detachments, enucleations, and removal of orbital tumors. Local anesthesia is often preferred for adults undergoing other types of eye surgery, such as for cataracts or glaucoma. Most cataract procedures are performed without any general anesthesia. Local anesthesia can be achieved by a combination of topical anesthetic drops instilled in the eye and infiltration anesthesia. There are four main methods of infiltration anesthesia: nerve block, direct subcutaneous infiltration, retrobulbar anesthesia, and peribulbar anesthesia.

In a nerve block the anesthetic is directed at the site of the emerging nerve and the area supplied by that nerve is affected.

Direct subcutaneous infiltration facilitates surface anesthesia of the skin and paralyzes the underlying musculature. In Figure 30.3 the purpose of the subcutaneous infiltration of the local anesthetic is to inactivate the orbicularis oculi muscle, which closes the eye. This muscle always is inactivated before intraocular surgery.

Retrobulbar anesthesia provides complete anesthesia of the globe and temporary paralysis to the muscles attached to the globe so that unwanted eye movements cannot occur during the procedure. The site of the penetration can be

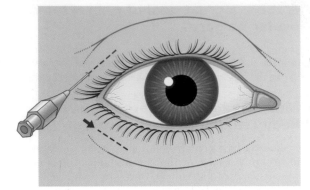

Figure 30.3 Subcutaneous infiltration anesthesia. The needle is pointed under the skin along the lower eyelid and the upper eyelid to anesthetize the skin and inactivate the orbicularis oculi muscle.
(Adapted from Berens C, King JH. An atlas of ophthalmic surgery. Philadelphia: JB Lippincott; 1961.)

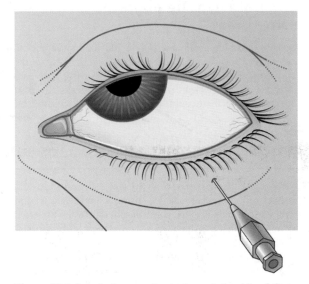

Figure 30.4 Retrobulbar anesthesia through the skin of the lower eyelid. The patient is asked to look up and away from the site of penetration of the needle. The needle penetrates the muscle cone behind the eye to paralyze the intraocular and extraocular muscles.
(Adapted from Berens C, King JH. An atlas of ophthalmic surgery. Philadelphia: JB Lippincott; 1961.)

either through the skin (Figure 30.4) or the conjunctiva (Figure 30.5), the needle coursing under the globe itself and the point of the needle emerging in the muscle cone of the eye (Figure 30.6).

Peribulbar anesthesia has become increasingly popular as a result of occasional compression damage to the optic nerve caused by retrobulbar injections. In peribulbar anesthesia a needle is directed down to the floor of the socket (or to the roof of the orbit) so that the anesthetic surrounds

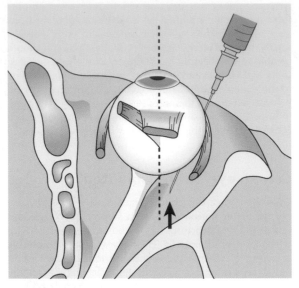

Figure 30.5 Advancement of needle in retrobulbar block.
(From Allman, KG. In: Yanoff M, Duker J, editors. Ophthalmology. 4th ed. Philadelphia: Elsevier Inc; 2014. All rights reserved.)

the soft tissue of the globe rather than being placed in the muscle cone itself.

Infiltration anesthesia may not be necessary with the new small incision and corneal incision surgery for cataracts. In intraocular (intracameral) anesthesia, developed by Dr. James Gills, an injection may be given into the anterior chamber at the start of cataract surgery to enhance patient comfort under topical anesthesia. The injection of 0.5 mL of preservative-free 1% lidocaine (Xylocaine) has resulted in a dramatic improvement in patient comfort, with a decrease in light sensitivity. This advance has led to essentially painless cataract surgery without the use of retrobulbar or peribulbar injections. Vancomycin and other antibiotics may be used. In addition, unpreserved antibiotics may be injected in the anterior chamber or behind the previously placed implant. In cataract surgery, it may be injected in the vitreous for endophthalmitis.

Questions for review and thought

1. Outline a routine to be followed in booking a patient for surgery.
2. Discuss the psychologic handling of a child who has to enter the hospital for strabismus surgery.
3. What forewarnings should be given to the adult patient before admission for major ocular surgery?
4. Discuss various types of anesthesia for cataract surgery.
5. What are the advantages of a local anesthetic over general anesthesia for cataract surgery?
6. What is the cataract-suturing technique in your center?

Figure 30.6 Point of destination of the retrobulbar injection. Note the needle point is in the muscle cone and amid the delicate nerves extending toward the eye. Injection of the anesthetic at this point paralyzes the muscles of the eye.

(Adapted from Berens C, King JH. An atlas of ophthalmic surgery. Philadelphia: JB Lippincott; 1961.)

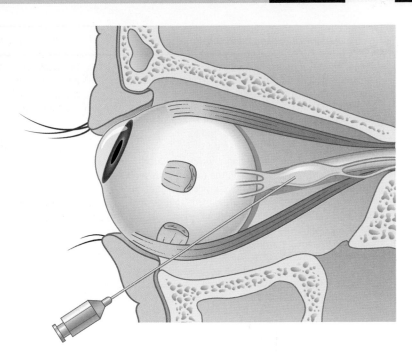

Q Self-evaluation questions

True–false statements

Directions: Indicate whether the statement is true **(T)** or false **(F).**

1. An important factor in scheduling patients for surgery is the length of the surgical procedure. **T** or **F**
2. An individual requests a certain date for surgery because of a forthcoming wedding in the family. This is considered an urgent booking. **T** or **F**
3. In advanced glaucoma, corneal transplantation may offer some hope in restoring vision. **T** or **F**

Missing words

Directions: Write in the missing word in the following sentences:

4. A lacerated globe is considered an _____ operation.
5. Children's surgery most often is performed under _____ anesthesia.
6. Anesthetic drops instilled in the eye are called _____ anesthesia.

Choice-completion questions

Directions: Select the one best answer in each case.

7. Retrobulbar anesthesia consists of placing an anesthetic agent in the:
   a. lower fornix.
   b. muscle cone behind the eye.
   c. peribulbar space.
   d. preauricular space.
   e. subcutaneous space.
8. Which of the following methods is not considered local anesthesia?
   a. Infiltration
   b. Intubation
   c. Retrobulbar
   d. Peribulbar
   e. Systemic
9. Which of the following is not required in scheduling major surgery?
   a. Phoning the patient
   b. Confirming the letter
   c. Assisting at surgery
   d. Identifying the date of surgery
   e. Determining the time required for the operation.

A Answers, notes, and explanations

1. **True.** Individual ophthalmic surgeons vary in the time they require for different procedures. A dacryocystorhinostomy by one surgeon may take only 1 hour, whereas another surgeon may take 3 hours. The same thing can occur in cataract surgery. This is an important variable in determining the overall time required for the operating room.

2. **False.** An urgent booking is one in which the nature of the ocular problem requires getting the patient in as soon as possible. Social reasons are not considered urgent. However, accommodation is often made to provide convenient times to the individual.

3. **False.** In advanced glaucoma corneal transplantation is not indicated. Corneal transplantation is indicated only for diseases and disorders affecting the cornea. In this procedure a hazy cornea can be replaced with a clear transparent cornea from donor tissue. Because of the avascular nature of the cornea, there is a minimal amount of antibody response. This permits the donor cornea to survive.

4. **Emergency.** Any laceration of the globe, eyelid, or adjacent area that requires surgical repair is considered an emergency admission. Although the patient may not necessarily have to stay overnight in the hospital or surgical center, he or she is admitted with proper documentation of the details of the injury. This detailed admission has medical and legal implications in case a lawsuit arises at a later date.

5. **General.** Almost all children's surgery is performed with the child under general anesthesia. The psychologic trauma of instruments appearing close to the eye can be devastating to children. Consequently they should be completely asleep and their eye movements controlled.

6. **Topical.** Applying drops directly to the eye is considered topical anesthesia. This can be highly effective and is used primarily in adults in combination with infiltration anesthesia.

7. **b. The muscle cone behind the eye.** Effective anesthesia of the ciliary ganglion is achieved by directly penetrating the muscle cone. There has in recent years, however, been some concern about the compression of the optic nerve or the possible perforation of the globe itself.

8. **b. Intubation.** In intubation anesthesia a tube is inserted into the trachea and the patient's complete anesthesia is controlled through gaseous vapors absorbed in the lung.

9. **c. Assisting at surgery.** Although this is an important act, it is not part of the routine in scheduling surgery. In the scheduling of surgery, it is very important that all the details are fully understood by the patient and that there is accuracy in both time and place for the surgery.

Chapter | 31 |

Highlights of ocular surgery

Many surgical procedures are performed to cure eye disorders, restore vision, prevent blindness, correct congenital abnormalities, or cosmetically improve the area in and around the eye. For each eye condition various surgical procedures, sometimes ingenious, have been devised.

To familiarize the ophthalmic assistant with some of the highlights of ocular surgery, the most commonly performed ocular procedures are outlined in this chapter.

STRABISMUS SURGERY

Preparation

When having strabismus surgery, children may be admitted to the hospital the afternoon before or on the day of surgery. Nowadays surgery is often performed on an outpatient basis because the child is more comfortable at home with his or her parents at night. Unless there is some adverse medical problem such as asthma, this seems to be a safe outpatient procedure. Parents are often encouraged to remain with the child to alleviate fears and relieve the child's feeling of abandonment. Older children are told that they may expect a bandage on one or both eyes after surgery, but that at least one bandage will be removed before they are sent home.

Surgery

Muscle surgery involves weakening or strengthening of the rectus muscles to improve alignment of the eyes.

The four rectus muscles insert close to the limbus, the medial rectus muscle being the closest (approximately 5.5 mm, whereas the lateral rectus muscle is 7 mm from it). The rectus muscles would be easily visible if they were not covered with the conjunctiva and subconjunctival tissue. To isolate these muscles, the surgeon must cut through the conjunctiva and place a muscle hook under the muscle. The oblique muscles insert at the back of the globe, so surgery on these muscles is not performed at their insertions.

The following procedures *weaken* the extraocular muscles:

1. *Recession* (Figure 31.1). The muscle is removed from its original insertion and repositioned farther back on the sclera. This loosens the grip the muscle has on the globe.
2. *Transverse margin myotomy*. Overlapping cuts are made on each side of the muscle to lengthen it. No change is made in the insertion.
3. *Complete tenotomy*. The muscle or tendon is severed completely and allowed to retract. Rare today but needed occasionally.

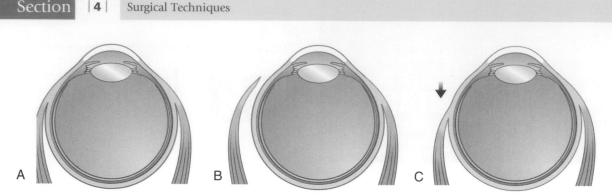

Figure 31.1 Recession operation. (A) Preoperative position of muscles. (B) Muscle detached from globe. (C) Muscle reattachment to sclera at a point farther back from its original insertion.
(From Stein HA, Slatt BJ, Stein RM. Ophthalmic terminology: speller and vocabulary builder. 3rd ed. St Louis: Mosby; 1992.)

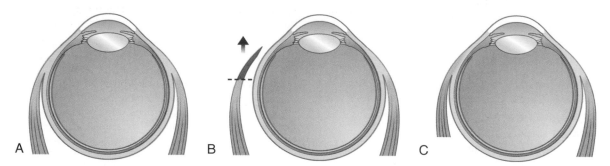

Figure 31.2 Resection operation. (A) Preoperative position of muscles. (B) Muscle detached from globe and an anterior portion of muscle cut away. (C) Muscle resutured to sclera at original insertion point.
(From Stein HA, Slatt BJ, Stein RM. Ophthalmic terminology: speller and vocabulary builder. 3rd ed. St Louis: Mosby; 1992.)

The following procedures *strengthen* an extraocular muscle:

1. *Resection* (Figure 31.2). A section of the muscle is removed from its insertion and the muscle is reattached to its original position. A resection shortens a muscle, thereby increasing its effective tension and pull.
2. *Advancement.* This procedure is usually combined with a resection. After the resection has been completed, the muscle is repositioned ahead of, or anterior to, its original insertion. Advancement increases the arc of contact of the muscle with the globe, thereby enhancing its effective pull.

Although there are six extraocular muscles, occasionally one may require surgery on the superior oblique and the inferior oblique muscle when overaction of these muscles occurs. For a full discussion of muscle function see Chapter 2.

Postoperative routine

After strabismus surgery, children are usually allowed up as soon as the effects of the anesthetic have disappeared. Normally the child is able to resume school activities almost immediately and sports within 2 weeks. The parents are informed that the operated eye may be red in the immediate postoperative period, but that this will gradually fade until the eye looks normal again. In some cases the eyes are not straight in the immediate postoperative period because of swelling, hemorrhage, and trauma to the muscles, all of which check eye movements. The parents are told of these postoperative variations so that they do not become upset if the eyes are not straight on removal of the bandages.

Occasionally a child will show an allergic response to the sutures used. This is likely to occur 2 or even 3 weeks after surgery, during a period when recovery is virtually complete. The lids suddenly swell, the conjunctiva balloons out, and the child's eyes generally look dreadful. This is a rather innocuous event, which subsides within 3 or 4 days without causing any complications. Occasionally, however, a suture granuloma may develop.

Questions often asked about muscle surgery include the following:

1. *Can vision be lost because of muscle surgery?* No. Because the muscles are attached on the surface of the globe, the eye itself is never opened.
2. *Are the eyes usually straight after one procedure?* Yes, in most cases. However, undercorrections and overcorrections do occur and no ophthalmic surgeon can say with certainty which patient will require further surgery. Therefore, parents are generally informed that two procedures may be necessary to straighten the eyes. With this approach, parents are not disappointed or

bitter if reoperation becomes necessary and they are extremely happy if surgery results in a complete success after the first procedure.

3. *Can muscle surgery improve the vision of an adult who has a turned eye that is amblyopic?* No. Strabismus surgery on an adult is strictly cosmetic. The turn can be corrected so that the position of the eyes appears normal, but the vision is not affected for better or worse.

4. *Can the eyes of an adult with strabismus be straightened?* Yes. Age is no barrier to a cosmetic strabismus procedure.

5. *Can the eyes be straightened with orthoptic exercises to avoid surgery?* Usually orthoptics is an adjunct to ophthalmic surgery and not a substitute for it. Strabismus may be corrected with the use of glasses, eyedrops, or orthoptic exercises in some patients. When possible, nonsurgical methods are used first and, in small degrees of strabismus, may result in a correction.

CATARACT SURGERY

Phacoemulsification (phaco) has evolved to be the state-of-the-art cataract surgical procedure. Patient satisfaction is extremely high with the development of a painless procedure and a rapid return of vision. The widespread use of phacoemulsification is related to improvements in surgical techniques, including incision construction, advances in machine technology, developments in intraocular lenses, and the ability to perform surgery without injections under topical anesthesia. These advancements, along with the potential complications, are discussed in this section. However, femtosecond laser may fast surpass phacoemulsification.

A cataract is opacity of the lens of the eye (Figure 31.3). The opacity may be minimal in size and faint in density so that the transmission of light is not appreciably affected, or it may be large and opaque so that light cannot gain entry to the eye's interior. When the cataract is pronounced, the examiner cannot see the interior of the patient's eye with any clarity and conversely the patient cannot see the examiner very clearly.

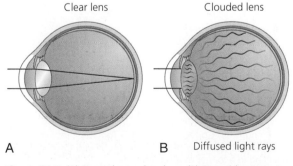

Clear lens   Clouded lens

A   B   Diffused light rays

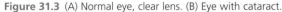

Figure 31.3 (A) Normal eye, clear lens. (B) Eye with cataract.

A cataract is removed if it endangers the health of the eye or interferes with the patient's ability to function. No visual level can be identified on the Snellen chart because contrast sensitivity, glare, pupillary constriction, and ambient lighting may significantly affect a person's functioning ability, even with an early cataract. The visual demands of patients can vary depending on occupation, stage of life, or whether they are driving, and so on.

Preoperative evaluation

The cataract, when it becomes mature, obscures all details of the fundus. When this occurs, efforts should be made to evaluate the health of the interior of the eye before cataract surgery. This evaluation has important prognostic importance. It can be performed by the following methods:

1. *Two-point light discrimination test.* Two lights are held a measured distance (60 cm) from the affected eye—the fellow eye being firmly covered—and are gradually separated until they can be identified as two lights. These measurements are recorded. The normal separable amount that two lights can be identified varies with the preoperative acuity. For visions reduced to hand movements, the lights should be identified about 12.5 cm apart. For visions better than 20/400, they should be identified about 5 cm apart.

2. *Light projection in all quadrants.* An assessment of active sensory retina in all quadrants should be performed by asking the patient to determine the position of a small transilluminator light.

3. *Ultrasound.* Ultrasound (or high-frequency waves) passes through the dense cataract and identifies any interference between the lens and the retina by rebounding off any firm obstruction. Abnormalities in the ultrasonogram can confirm the presence of a tumor mass, hemorrhage, or detached retina behind the lens. The B-scan is the main method of evaluating the area behind the lens. However, A-scan measurements (see following text) may detect defects in the central pathway.

4. *Blue-field entoptoscope.* This device permits the patient to observe his or her own white blood cells flowing in the retinal capillaries in the macular area. This flow is visible even with a dense cataract. This entoptic phenomenon is created by an intense blue light that the patient views. With normal retinal function the patient will describe "flying corpuscles" moving in the entire field. If the macula is not functioning, no flying corpuscles will be seen.

   This phenomenon occurs because the blue light is strongly absorbed by the hemoglobin and red blood cells, which results in the photoreceptors behind the capillaries becoming relatively dark-adapted. When a white blood cell moves through the capillary, the blue light passes through it and excites the photoreceptors behind it. Thus the passage of a leukocyte is perceived as a moving bright dot or a flying corpuscle. The intensity of the blue light can be adjusted so that sufficient light reaches the retina in cases of media opacities. This entoptoscopic effect can also be seen by looking at a clear blue sky on a bright day. Abnormalities in perception of the corpuscles are the result of changes in the perifoveal circulation or functional impairment of the neural elements in the retina, or both. Differentiation between the two is possible in conjunction with other tests such as those based on fluorescein angiography and electrophysiology. Abnormal entoptoscopic findings include one or more of the following:

- Total or partial absence of corpuscle perception in one or both eyes
- Absence of pulsatile motion
- Fewer corpuscles in one eye
- Lower corpuscle speed in one eye

Clinical experience with cataract patients has shown that a positive response to the blue-field entoptic test indicates a 98% probability of good postoperative macular function (visual acuity 20/40 or better). The test is especially useful when a direct view of the fundus is obscured in cases of corneal edema or scarring, hyphema, cataract and vitreous hemorrhage, membranes, or exudates.

5. *Brightness acuity tester (BAT)*. This instrument, devised by Dr. Jack Holladay, can determine a significant visual loss attributed to a bright light creating a small pupil and glare (see Figure 8.15). The excess light is the normal light that a person may experience when outdoors in bright sunshine. An individual with a small central cataract may be seriously affected in driving and participating in sports when the pupil contracts.

6. *Prediction of potential acuities.* Interferometers and potential acuity meters (PAMs) are used in office tests to predict potential acuities in patients with cataracts and those with hazy posterior capsules after cataract extractions. This allows realistic expectations on the part of the surgeon and patient before cataract surgery or a neodymium YAG posterior capsulotomy. The interferometers pass two beams of laser light through the pupil, producing a three-dimensional interference pattern within the retina. This allows the ophthalmologist to bypass problems with most opacities of the media, as well as refractive errors. If the patient can see the interference pattern, which will appear as bands in a specific direction, this is evidence of macular function. The narrower the bands that are projected and seen, the higher is the degree of macular function.

The PAM (Figure 31.4) is basically a pinpoint light source, a transilluminated visual acuity chart, and a lens. It projects a brightly illuminated Snellen acuity chart through an area approximately 0.15 mm in diameter. It

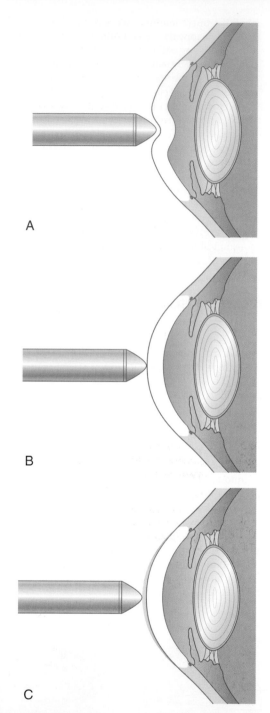

A

B

C

Figure 31.4 Errors in A-scan measurements. (A) Too much pressure with the probe indents the cornea and may cause excessive shallowness of the anterior chamber and a shorter axial length. (B) Correct pressure. (C) Too little pressure may leave a thick tear layer between the probe and the cornea, resulting in a longer axial length.

can be used to test approximate acuities through mildly dense media because of the brightness of the stimulus and the tiny diameter of the beam used for the examination.

In the clinical application of these tests, the following guidelines should be used:

- Do not shine lights into the patient's eyes before testing because this may decrease the acuity readings.
- Have the pupil well dilated.
- PAM testing: drop the chinrest to enable the patient to talk without moving the head so that the acuity chart will remain visible to the patient.
- Interferometer testing: stress that background noise will be seen (swirls of light, dots, wavy lines, half lines), but that the patient should ignore these and indicate only the direction of the lines of light seen.
- Focus the beam in the center of the pupil at the plane of the iris, then scan the pupil until best responses are obtained.
- With the interferometers, first use horizontal and vertical bands until the best acuity has been reached and then use oblique lines to verify this.
- With the PAM, start with large letters and ask the patient to read only the first two or three letters in each line. If at any time two or more letters are identified in a given line, that line, if it is the smallest read, is the endpoint even though the patient may not be able to detect that line again.
- Never tell patients they should see letters or lines, because this tends to upset them. Simply ask, "What do you see?" If they see letters, they will say so. With the interferometer, ask, "What do you see?" If they begin to see something, ask if there are any lines as you make them larger and larger until they see them.

7. *Endothelial cell function.* Although specular microscopic examination is the standard method of evaluating the morphology and cell count of the endothelial cells, the use of slit-lamp biomicroscopy can aid the clinical observation (see Figure 31.5). With the use of an objective lens in the slit lamp and careful positioning of the slit light, the endothelial mosaic may be viewed. By use of the Endo lens designed by Tomey Corporation, the image may be enhanced. The image may be compared with a grid that can be placed in the objective lens assembly. Pachymetry can be performed to measure the central thickness of the cornea. Thicker corneas, especially greater than 600 μm, increase the likelihood of a compromised endothelium. The findings of one or more of the following signs suggest an increased risk of corneal edema or decompensation following any cataract surgery: thick cornea, reduced endothelial cells, or corneal guttata.

8. *Partial coherence interferometry or A-scan.* Another important aspect of evaluation is to determine the required dioptric power of the intraocular lens to be chosen. Coherence interferometry is a noncontact method that allows determination of the axial length of the eye as well as keratometric values of the cornea. With these two values, as well as specific constants for the different implants, the ideal power of the intraocular lens can be determined. The older method of calculation of the axial length of the eye is by A-scan ultrasound, which uses a probe that makes contact with the cornea (see Figure 31.4). Special concerns that require an adjustment of intraocular lens formulas include patients with previous refractive surgery (e.g., LASIK, PRK, RK [radial keratectomy]), high myopia, or high hyperopia.

Preparation

Patients are often seen by the family physician or internist at least 1 week before cataract surgery to ensure that medical conditions such as diabetes and hypertension are under control. Also the ophthalmic surgeon should be provided with the names and dosages of the medications the patient may be taking.

Patients should be instructed to wash their hair before entering the hospital because hair washing is avoided

Figure 31.5 The slit lamp may be used for evaluation of cell density.

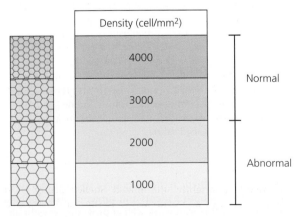

Using an objective lens of 1.6 ×

during the first few postoperative days to prevent contamination of the wound by dirty rinse water. Smoking, of course, should be discouraged because a heavy cough can easily disrupt a fresh wound or initiate bleeding. With clear corneal microincisions performed under topical anesthesia, it is not necessary to discontinue aspirin or warfarin (Coumadin). If a peribulbar or retrobulbar block is given or a scleral incision is made, it is usually best to discontinue medication that could result in bleeding.

Surgery

The object of cataract surgery is to remove the crystalline lens of the eye that has become cloudy. This is performed under an operating microscope that permits magnification. The technique of phacoemulsification is the preferred method of removing cataracts today. An ultrasonic probe that vibrates rapidly can liquefy a lens through a microincision. This small-incision surgery has resulted in an incision size that has been reduced from 10 mm for extracapsular surgery to 1.8 to 2.2 mm for phacoemulsification. Special incision construction generally eliminates the need for sutures. This leads to minimal induced astigmatism and a rapid recovery. Most surgeons today perform cataract surgery in freestanding surgical centers on an outpatient basis (see Chapter 35).

Phacoemulsification

In 1963 Dr. Charles Kelman commenced research to ascertain the possibility of removing a cataract through a small incision. After attempting many preliminary techniques, including crushing, cutting, and drilling the lens, he finally perfected an apparatus and tip that he used to apply an oscillating and ultrasonic frequency to emulsify the cataract. He was attempting to improve on the system of cataract surgery that, in that era, consisted of freezing with a cryoprobe or by using a capsule forceps. With the phacoemulsifier, a microincision of less than 3 mm is required. This means less tissue destruction, less wound reaction, a quicker operation, less chance of wound disruption and its attendant complications, less astigmatism, and earlier ambulation and visual recovery (Box 31.1). In most cases the patient is able to resume normal activities immediately after the operation.

Skin and eye preparation

Before surgery the skin around the eyelids is prepared with an antiseptic, most commonly povidone-iodine (Betadine) preparation. The eye is irrigated with a dilute solution of Betadine and balanced saline.

Anesthesia

Advances in anesthetic techniques have resulted in a dramatic change for both patients and surgeons. Retrobulbar injections into the orbit work well at providing anesthesia

---

> ### Box 31.1 Phacoemulsification
>
> **Advantages**
> Small incision
> Fewer wound problems
> Less astigmatism
> More rapid physical rehabilitation
> Less risk of expulsive hemorrhage
> Faster surgery
> Quicker visual recovery
>
> **Disadvantages**
> Machine dependent
> Longer learning period
> Complications while learning
> Expensive equipment
> Difficult with hard nucleus
> Need good pupil dilation
> Difficult with small pupils

---

and akinesia. Unfortunately the injections may be associated with complications that can include retrobulbar hemorrhage, intraocular penetration, and optic nerve penetration. The development of peribulbar injections decreases the chance of intraocular or optic nerve problems, but still can result in an orbital hemorrhage and discomfort. The use of topical anesthesia combined with intraocular lidocaine has revolutionized the way that surgery can be successfully performed.

After the superficial ocular structure is anesthetized with a topical anesthetic (e.g., tetracaine), a paracentesis is performed into the anterior chamber and 0.25 to 0.50 mL of 1% preservative-free lidocaine is injected into the anterior chamber. This results in dramatic anesthesia and has eliminated essentially all discomfort for the patient. The advantages of topical anesthesia are that it avoids all complications from orbital injections, provides increased safety for patients on anticoagulants, and results in an immediate recovery of vision because the optic nerve is not affected by this form of anesthesia.

Incision construction

Incision size has reduced with changes in techniques. The incision size for intracapsular cataract extraction was approximately 12 mm, with extracapsular cataract extraction 10 mm, and with phacoemulsification of around 2.5 mm. The advantages of a smaller incision are primarily less trauma to the eye, less astigmatic effect, and a quicker return to the former lifestyle. A self-sealing incision can be created in which there is an internal corneal lip of tissue that is closed off by the normal intraocular pressure. Sutures may not be required. The induced astigmatism is minimal.

Continuous curvilinear capsulorrhexis

The technique involves making a small opening in the limbus or in the clear cornea and introducing a cystotome to cut an opening in the anterior capsule of the lens (Figure 31.6). Previously the opening into the anterior capsule was made with a capsulotomy needle by a series of jagged punctures that converted the central capsule into a series of postage-stamp cuttings. Currently, a continuous tear opening, often called *continuous curvilinear capsulorrhexis (CCC)*, is made by tearing the capsule so that the edges remain sharp, well demarcated, and very strong. This prevents extension into the periphery of tears of the capsule and permits the capsule to hold the lens implant securely (Figure 31.7). This can be performed with better centration and circularity with the femtosecond laser. The capsulotomy with a laser can be done on the line of sight, which allows the implant to be centered in the capsular bag.

Hydrodissection and hydrodelineation

Balanced saline can be injected into the lens to separate either the cortical material from the capsule (*hydrodissection*) or the nucleus from the epinucleus (*hydrodelineation*). This allows the nucleus to be rotated freely within the capsular bag during the phaco technique. Separation of the nucleus from the epinucleus allows removal of the nucleus with phacoemulsification, leaving an underlying cushion of epinuclear tissue to protect against inadvertent rupture of the posterior capsule.

Figure 31.6 Phacoemulsification. (A) Cataract. (B) Continuous curve capsulotomy. (C) Removal of nucleus. (D) Cortex aspiration and enlargement of incision. (E) Insertion of intraocular lens. (F) Wound closure.

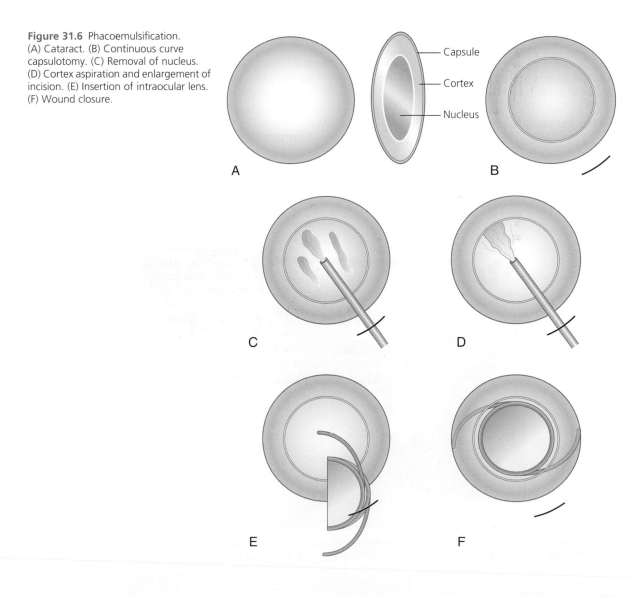

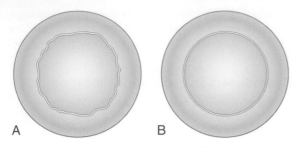

Figure 31.7 (A) Can-opener capsulotomy. (B) Continuous curve capsulorrhexis.

Machine design

Phaco equipment consists of a phaco tip that is inserted into the eye, a phaco handpiece that allows rapid vibration of the tip to liquefy the nucleus, and the machine that allows adjustments of a variety of parameters. The parameters that can be varied during each case include the amount of fluid infused into the eye, a vacuum level that allows suction of lens material, and the phaco energy that controls vibration frequency of the tip.

Phaco technique

There are a variety of techniques to emulsify and remove the nucleus, which may vary depending on the density of the cataract. A chopping technique utilizes a "chopper"

to divide a nucleus into small segments before being emulsified. The phaco tip with high vacuum impales the nucleus and the chopper is used to divide the lens into fragments. A "divide and conquer" approach may be used in which a deep trench is created in the nucleus, and instruments are used to crack the nucleus into multiple pieces that can be safely removed from the eye. A "flip" technique involves lifting or floating the nucleus above the capsule before emulsification is performed.

Sutures

The sutureless closure has resulted in more rapid rehabilitation after cataract surgery. The basic principle of sutureless incision is the creation of a valve-like self-sealing wound that is relatively small. The valve permits the incision to withstand unusual stress or intermittent raised intraocular pressure, which may follow in the postoperative period. The most common incision is made into clear cornea. If a scleral incision is made, various shapes of design have been advocated that lessen the degree of induced astigmatism. These include variations of straight incisions or a curvilinear incision, which is sometimes labeled the "frown and smile" incision.

Femtosecond laser

Advancements in technology have resulted in the development of laser cataract surgery (Figure 31.8). Combining a

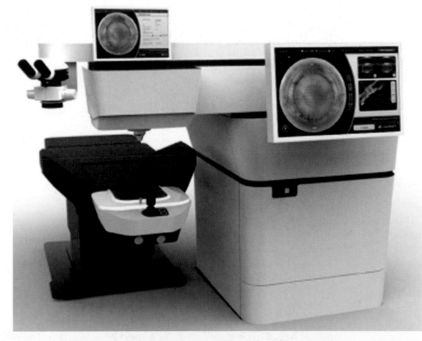

Figure 31.8 Laser cataract unit for wound construction, limbal relaxing incisions, capsulorrhexis, and fragmentation of the nucleus. *(Courtesy of Optimedica, Santa Clara, CA.)*

femtosecond (FS) laser (see following text) with a sophisticated imaging technique such as optical coherence tomography (OCT) has allowed the laser to perform corneal wound construction (main incision and side-port incision); limbal relaxing incisions to reduce astigmatism; capsulorrhexis of an exact size, shape, and centration (Figure 31.9); and fragmentation of the nucleus. The laser procedure is typically performed outside of the surgical operating room. After this procedure the patient is taken to the surgical suite, where the eye is prepped and draped in the usual manner. A dull instrument is used to open the corneal wound incisions, and a viscoelastic substance is placed in the anterior chamber. A forceps is then used to grab the central capsule and pull this out from the

eye. Hydrodissection and hydrodelineation are performed. A phaco tip is then placed into the eye, and the nucleus, which was previously dismantled by the laser, is removed from the eye. The amount of phaco energy to remove the nucleus is significantly lower than with standard phacoemulsification. In fact, a high percentage of cases can be performed without any phaco energy. The remaining cortical material is aspirated from the capsular bag. The implant is then inserted through the small phaco incision, typically around 2.2 mm.

The main advantages of laser cataract surgery include less dexterity required on the part of the surgeon, an easier learning curve for beginner surgeons, more accurate and consistent corneal incisions, limbal relaxing incisions,

Figure 31.9 Comparison of capsulorrhexis done manually (A), versus with a laser (B).
(Courtesy of Optimedica, Santa Clara, CA.)

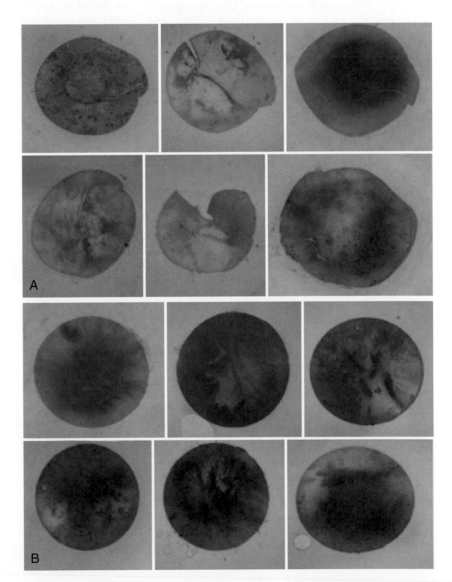

and a capsulorrhexis, which allows a more accurate effective lens position. With a more accurate lens position in the eye there is a greater chance of a more predictable refractive outcome. In addition because there is less energy used to liquefy the cataract, there should be less intraocular turbulence, which results in clearer postoperative corneas and a safer procedure.

Intraocular lenses

Historically, one of the major problems after cataract surgery was the use of aphakic spectacles. Older adult patients had to bear the attendant magnifications and distortions by spectacles following cataract surgery. Contact lenses were developed, especially those that can be worn overnight or for extended wear, to avoid the handling difficulties of insertion and removal that are a constant hazard to the insecure older adult aphakic patient. The solution today has been in the direction of intraocular lens implants, which Ridley introduced in 1949. Through the pioneering efforts of Cornelium Binkhorst of Holland, Peter Choyce of England, Edward Epstein of South Africa, and Fyderov of Russia, the intraocular lens has become the major form of visual rehabilitation after cataract surgery. With the use of sodium hyaluronate (Healon) and other viscoelastic substances, endothelial damage is minimized during implant surgery. Magnification induced by spectacles and contact lenses has been reduced to zero with intraocular lenses through the positioning of the implant within the eye (Figure 31.10).

The present-day success of intraocular lenses is a result of more skillful microsurgery, as well as better design, finish, and fixation of the lenses. In addition, a better understanding of positioning of the lenses within the capsular bag, the use of the yttrium aluminum garnet (YAG) laser for capsular opacification, and the better management and minimization of complications have led to significant success with intraocular lenses. Their use is indicated in virtually all patients undergoing cataract surgery.

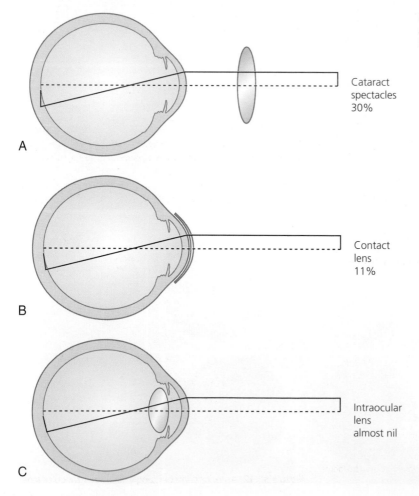

Figure 31.10 Magnification induced by aphakic spectacles, contact lenses, and intraocular lenses.

Cataract spectacles 30%

A

Contact lens 11%

B

Intraocular lens almost nil

C

Lens materials and design

Intraocular lenses are composed of an optical portion, called the "optics" of the lens, and the "haptics" (Figure 31.11). The optics portion has a dioptric power that permits focusing light from afar onto the retina. The "size" of the optics varies from 5 to 7 mm in diameter. The term *haptics* is from the Greek word *haptesthai* meaning "to lay hold of." The haptics refer to the method of holding the optical portion in place in the human eye, which consists of loops that are made of either polymethyl methacrylate or Prolene. Polymethyl methacrylate is noteworthy as a hard, firm, inert material that has been singled out for the manufacture of quality intraocular lens optics and is inert in the human body. Loops made of this material are commonly used instead of Prolene. Prolene is a suture material that is also relatively inert in the human body and provides a softness and pliability that permit its support of the optical portion of the lens. Acrylic and silicone lenses have been developed, which are also inert inside the eye and can be folded so as to be inserted through a microincision. Titanium and metal loops have disappeared in the manufacture of intraocular lenses because of the adverse reaction they produce on the human retina. Loop designs are more flexible so as to permit greater adjustments within the structure of the eye itself to variations of the ocular changes that occur with each blink and contraction of the rectus muscles. This in itself has been a major step forward in the design of intraocular lenses.

The shape of the optical portion may be *planoconvex*, in which case the anterior portion of the lens is *convex*, whereas the back surface is flat. It may have reverse optics, in which the back surface of the lens is convex and the front surface is flat. It may alternatively be *biconvex*, in which both sides of the optical portion are convex. Some lenses are made *aspheric*, in which there is an alteration in power from the center of the lens to the periphery. Because of microincision surgery, foldable lenses have become popular.

Designs have incorporated an ultraviolet filter into the optical portion of the lens. This eliminates wavelengths in the ultraviolet spectrum less than 400 nm. The health of the cornea can be determined by specular microscopy on corneal cell density (see Chapter 41) or by a guestimate using a ×1.6 objective lens with a slit lamp (see Figure 31.5).

The power of the intraocular lenses varies from eye to eye. The use of A-scan ultrasound or optical biometry with ultrasound allows the examiner to measure the axial length of the human eye and to determine exactly the required power of the implant. The more common powers are about +18.00 to +22.00 diopters, but lenses are available for any power, including minus power and very high plus power.

Intraocular lenses also may be classified according to their position and their method of fixation. Anterior chamber lenses (Figure 31.12) include lenses that lie in the anterior chamber of the eye. These may be angle-supported, in which case they are supported in the angle of the anterior chamber, or they may be iris-supported, in which case they may be attached with or without sutures to the iris. These lenses have almost become obsolete and are used only for special purposes. Lenses are usually positioned in the posterior chamber and they may be supported by capsular support, in which case they may be called *in-the-bag lenses* (see Figure 31.14C) because they are fitted directly into the capsular bag that contained the former crystalline lens, or they may be sulcus-supported (Figure 31.13), in which case they lie in front of the remainder of the anterior capsule and are supported in the sulcus of the eye (Figure 31.14B).

New developments in soft implants composed of silicone, hydrogels, and acrylic have heralded a new generation of implants, which may be folded and inserted through a much smaller incision. The development of *endocapsular* surgery with lens placement into the capsular bag has become state of the art.

Multifocal lenses *(bifocal intraocular lenses)* are another attempt to replace the human crystalline lens with an exact duplicate in function. Bifocal intraocular lenses, which are

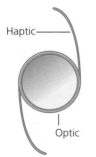

Figure 31.11 Intraocular lenses.
(From Stein HA, Slatt BJ, Stein RM. A primer in ophthalmology: a textbook for students. St Louis: Mosby; 1992.)

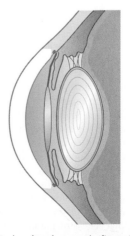

Figure 31.12 Anterior chamber, angle-fixated intraocular lens.

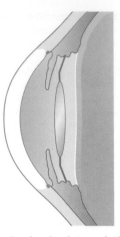

Figure 31.13 Posterior chamber intraocular lens placed in the ciliary sulcus.

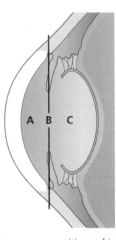

Figure 31.14 Most common positions of intraocular lenses. (A) Anterior chamber. (B) Ciliary sulcus. (C) Capsular bag.
(From Stein HA, Slatt BJ, Stein RM. A primer in ophthalmology: a textbook for students. St Louis: Mosby; 1992.)

sometimes referred to as *multifocal intraocular* lenses because they focus at many distances, have been introduced to try to eliminate spectacles entirely for the patient who has had a cataract removed. The advantage of multifocal lenses is simply that the patient does not require spectacles for most activities. Multifocal lenses separate rays of light to allow distance, intermediate, and near vision. Lens designs can include a diffractive optic, in which there are a series of rings with different step heights. Another design is a lens with different refractive zones. Because there is a separation of light rays with multifocal implants, there is an increased risk of glare and halos as well as reduced contrast sensitivity. In many patients the symptoms improve over 6 to 12 months. However, some patients can find night driving difficult.

Patient selection and expectations are critical to the acceptance of multifocal lenses. Generally the individual with type A personality is not a good candidate, nor are those who do a significant amount of night driving. In addition, patients with a limited visual potential are not good candidates, such as those with a diseased cornea (e.g., keratoconus or epithelial basement membrane dystrophy) or macular problems (e.g., age-related macular degeneration, macular hole, or epiretinal membrane). To achieve the best outcome it is important to obtain exact biometric readings and to have the lens positioned in the capsular bag. Low postoperative astigmatism is also critical; this means correction of astigmatism at the time of surgery by limbal relaxing incisions or the insertion of a multifocal-toric implant.

Accommodating intraocular implants

An ideal implant would provide excellent vision at all focal distances. There is a great deal of research into the development of such a lens. The first lens approved in the United States was the crystal lens. This is a plate design with hinges that makes it capable of flexing. The proposed mechanism of action is that ciliary muscle contraction results in increased vitreous pressure that pushes the lens forward, with a resultant improvement in near vision. A YAG capsulotomy does not diminish the effectiveness of the lens.

The Restor implant and TECNIS multifocal implant use diffractive optics to provide distance, intermediate, and near vision. It is not uncommon for patients to experience some glare and halos, especially at night. These symptoms tend to decrease over time because of the mechanism of neuroadaptation. The TECNIS Symfony is the newest multifocal implant that is designed with an elongated focal point that results in an increased depth of focus. This allows patients to have a broad range of vision and has been shown to have a lower risk of glare and halos.

It was hoped that the Synchrony or dual-optic implant would provide a full range of vision and improved quality. This lens design consists of two components: a 32.00 diopter anterior optic and a minus-powered posterior optic that varies according to the biometry of the patient. The lenses are joined by a unique spring system. With distance focus the two lenses are close together. With accommodation the anterior lens moves forward, changing the focus to intermediate or near vision. Unfortunately the promise of the Synchrony implant was never achieved and it has been abandoned from further trials.

A few new accommodative implants are under development. The FluidVision lens relies on liquid to make accommodative changes. By virtue of the natural human physiologic contraction and relaxation of the ciliary muscle, the fluid internal to the implant allows changes in shape like a pliable crystalline lens before the onset of presbyopia. The implant is acrylic and is filled with silicone oil. As the ciliary body muscle contracts and relaxes, forces are conveyed through the zonules and the capsule to the implant and the fluid in the haptics is pushed into the optic, causing the anterior curvature of the optic to increase. A nonfoldable prototype of the lens was implanted in 14 sighted eyes in 2010, and an average of 5.00 diopters of accommodative amplitude was documented.

Another prototype implant, the electroactive Sapphire AutoFocal, is an electromechanical lens equipped with a microscopic battery that stimulates shape change in the optic when sensing accommodation. As the pupil changes size and becomes smaller, the liquid crystals inside the lens are stimulated by electromechanical impulses, resulting in a change in the refractive lens to provide 3.00 diopters of reading. This implant does not rely on the muscles in the eye functioning and capsular bag contraction or hardening to be effective.

Corneal inlays for reading vision

An exciting new procedure for vision correction surgery is corneal inlays. These are small inserts placed under a LASIK flap or in a corneal pocket to enhance reading vision. The procedure is typically performed for presbyopic patients who have clear crystalline lenses and are interested in LASIK. However, pseudophakic patients, such as those following cataract surgery with a monofocal intraocular lens implant, may benefit from a corneal inlay to improve reading vision.

The Kamra corneal inlay is designed to increase the depth of field in the implanted eye. The inlay can enhance near and intermediate vision without a significant effect on distance acuity. Implantation can be combined with an excimer ablation to simultaneously address a refractive error and presbyopia. The inlay is implanted over the line of sight under a corneal flap or in a pocket. Seyeddain et al found that 96.9% of patients (n = 32 eyes) could read J3 or better in implanted eyes after 24 months. Yilmaz et al determined that the mean uncorrected near visual acuity (UNVA) improved from J6 preoperatively to J1 + 12 months postimplant in 39 presbyopic patients (12 were naturally ametropic and 27 had ametropia from previous hyperopic LASIK). There was no significant change in mean uncorrected distance VA (UDVA) in inlaid eyes. At 4 years, 20 all patients retained a 2-line improvement in near vision with no significant loss in distance vision.

The Raindrop corneal inlay is intended to improve near and intermediate vision by changing the curvature of the cornea. The inlay steepens the central cornea for near vision and leaves the curvature of the more peripheral cornea unchanged for intermediate and distance vision. The material has a refractive index and water content similar to that of the human cornea. Distance acuity is minimally affected as light rays paracentral to the 2-mm inlay remain primarily focused on the retina, particularly with a middilated or dilated pupil. Pupil constriction creates a pseudoaccommodative effect using the steep and central cornea to focus light rays for near. Six-month data in 30 emmetropic presbyopes showed that mean uncorrected near vision of the treated eye was 20/25 and J1, corresponding to 4 lines of improvement. Uncorrected intermediate visual acuity in the treated eye improved to 20/25; that is, 2 lines of improvement. No patient lost greater than 2 lines of corrected near or distance VA. In a previous animal study, the implanted eyes remained clear and free from reaction to the corneal inlay. Corneas were clear on slit-lamp examination at 1 year and histology data suggested that the inlay appeared to be inert.

Historical methods

Intracapsular cataract surgery

The intracapsular operation is rarely used today. If a lens is dislocated or has extremely poor zonular support it is generally best to remove the entire lens through a large limbal incision. Because the capsule is completely removed with this technique, an anterior chamber lens or a sutured posterior chamber lens must be inserted. A cataract with weak zonules can undergo phacoemulsification with caution and with the insertion of a capsular tension ring that is placed into the capsular bag to expand its diameter before the insertion of an implant.

Extracapsular cataract surgery

This is becoming a historic procedure in North America, but in underdeveloped countries without the advantage of new technology it continues to be a common procedure. A retrobulbar anesthetic or peribulbar injection is used to anesthetize the globe. Facial nerve paralysis may be produced by an O'Brien, Van Lint, or Nadbath anesthetic, but such anesthesia may not be necessary. The Honan intraocular pressure reducer or the superpinky ball, championed by Dr. James Gills, significantly lowers the intraocular pressure before surgery. Hand massage also may be used, but one should guard against excessive massage because of the possibility of central retinal artery or vein obstruction.

An incision is made at the superior limbus and a small opening is made into the anterior chamber. A viscoelastic substance is introduced. A small bent needle or cystotome is introduced and a cut is made into the anterior capsule in a circular can-opener, triangular, or D-shaped fashion (anterior capsulotomy) (Figure 31.15). The wound is enlarged in extracapsular surgery to a chord diameter of 10 to 11 mm (approximately a 150-degree arc or smaller) to allow removal of the cataractous nucleus.

The nucleus is then expressed from the eye. Sutures are inserted to maintain the anterior chamber so that the remaining cortex can be removed. The cortex may be

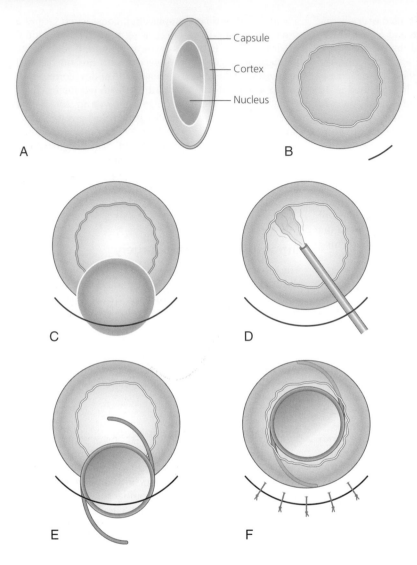

Capsule

Cortex

Nucleus

A

B

C

D

E

F

Figure 31.15 Extracapsular cataract extraction. (A) Cataract. (B) Small incision and capsulorrhexis. (C) Phacoemulsification of lens. (D) Cortex aspiration. (E) Insertion of folded lens. (F) Rotation of lens in capsule.

removed by a manual method (e.g., Simcoe or McIntyre needle) or by an automated system. These are sometimes referred to as *I/A units* (irrigating/aspirating units). These instruments irrigate balanced salt into the eye in proportion to the amount of aspiration occurring. The automated systems are foot-controlled.

Once all of the cortex is removed from the capsular bag, the posterior capsule may be "polished" to remove any residual plaques. An intraocular lens is then inserted into the posterior chamber. This lens may be positioned either into the capsular bag (Figure 31.16A) or into the sulcus (Figure 31.16B). The capsular bag is preferred.

Sutures are then placed in the cornea or the corneoscleral wound. These may be radial interrupted sutures, a continuous suture, or a combination of the two. At the end of the

procedure, an antibiotic (e.g., vancomycin) may be given intraocularly in the anterior chamber, or an antibiotic-steroid combination injection may be given subconjunctivally (Box 31.2).

The essential difference between intracapsular surgery and extracapsular surgery is that in the former the entire lens and capsule are removed from the eye, whereas in the latter the posterior capsule remains intact, permitting a pocket for an intraocular lens.

The large incision and sutures with extracapsular surgery usually result in induced astigmatism of a significantly greater degree than with phacoemulsification. Sutures may be removed at 4 to 6 weeks to reduce astigmatism. In general, the visual recovery may be more prolonged than with phacoemulsification.

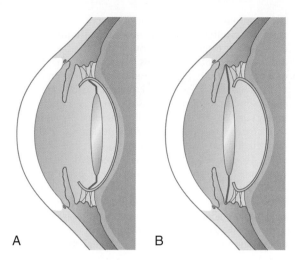

A   B

Figure 31.16 Posterior chamber intraocular lens. (A) Capsular bag insertion. (B) Sulcus insertion.

Box 31.2 Extracapsular surgery step by step

1. Draping and speculum insertion
2. Bridle suture for superior rectus
3. Conjunctival incision
4. Cauterization of bleeders
5. Scleral or corneoscleral incision
6. Viscoelastic substance introduced
7. Capsulotomy or capsulorrhexis
8. Nucleus expression
9. Cortical clean-up
10. Intraocular lens (IOL) insertion
11. Suture placement
12. Conjunctival reapproximation
13. Injections: subconjunctival or intraocular
14. Instilling medication and patching the eye

Femtosecond laser cataract surgery

FS cataract surgery is considered to be one of the most significant advances in cataract surgery in 50 years. Laser cataract surgery has shown excellent results for accurate self-sealing corneal incisions; arcuate incisions to reduce astigmatism; highly circular, strong, and well-positioned capsulorrhexis; and safer and less technically difficult removal of the cataract with almost complete elimination of phacoemulsification. Laser technology may allow ophthalmologists to meet the demands of cataract patients to the same level that has been accomplished with laser vision correction

The technology today recognizes clear corneal incisions. The benefits of clear corneal incisions are that they are well

tolerated by patients, provide a rapid recovery of vision, preserve the subconjunctival space for future filtering procedures, and allow improved visibility during phacoemulsification as a result of the shorter tunnel. There are reports of an increased incidence of endophthalmitis that may be related to the use of clear corneal incisions. Although the incidence of endophthalmitis is only 0.13%, this remains the most feared complication of cataract surgery with a potential devastating effect. Endophthalmitis after cataract surgery with a permanent decrease in vision can affect an individual's quality of life, including productivity.

Manually created incisions have potential for leakage because of difficulty in controlling the ideal length and architecture of the incision. Surgeons tend to vary their angle of incision depending on the ergonomics of the situation. Other potential causes of leakage include thickening of the incision site and detachment of Descemet's membrane. Masket et al were able to demonstrate in cadaver eyes the advantages of a clear corneal incision using an FS laser with a more reproducible square incision and a multiplanar configuration of the corneal wound.

A clear corneal incision that is poorly constructed may result in leakage, hypotony, iris prolapse, or endophthalmitis. Cataract incisions created with a blade typically have a simple uniplanar configuration, with a suboptimal construction, and fluids may leak in and out of the eye. This increases the risk of endophthalmitis because bacteria from the tear film may enter the anterior chamber of the eye. Future studies will address the ideal architecture of the corneal incision to prevent leakage and minimize astigmatism induction. The FS laser has the potential to create a more square architecture using complex multiplanar incisions (Figure 1) such as a tongue-and-groove or interlocking zigzag design, which could provide a more stable wound configuration that is more resistant to leakage.

If astigmatism management is required, the FS laser provides customized control of depth, location, and angle of entry.

An anterior capsulotomy or capsulorrhexis is required in every cataract surgery. The preciseness of this procedure with the FS laser is much superior to the manual approach for both positioning and centralization of the anterior capsulotomy, and minimization of capsular tears.

Femtosecond lasers: mechanism of action

The FS laser used in ophthalmic applications is in the near-infrared wavelength of light (1030 nm) similar to the neodymium:yttrium aluminum garnet (Nd:YAG) laser, with the exception that it has significantly shorter pulse duration. This enables a different way of laser–tissue interaction called laser-induced optical breakdown, which means that the laser produces smaller shockwaves and cavitation bubbles affecting tissue volumes. Ultrashort laser pulses used in FS lasers can ablate a very small fraction of tissue. No heat is generated during the ablation process. The FS laser can be focused with precise accuracy at different depths, using a guidance system to create the corneal incisions, astigmatic keratotomy, capsulotomy, and nuclear fragmentation. The focused laser energy increases to a level where plasma is generated. The plasma expands and causes a shockwave, cavitation, and bubble formation. The bubble then expands and collapses, leading to separation of the tissue.

Because FS lasers function at nearly an infrared wavelength, they are not absorbed by optically clear tissues. This allows the FS laser to be used to the anterior segment of the eye as the anterior chamber provides an optically clear tissue pathway. This wavelength of light is not absorbed by the cornea. The shockwaves generated by FS photodisruption dissipate within approximately 30 µm of the targeted tissue, thus protecting the posterior capsule and corneal endothelium. The surgical effect is achieved by delivering thousands of individual laser pulses per second to produce tissue separation or continuous incisions.

Education and training

Surgeons are concerned about the transition from the more familiar standard phacoemulsification to laser cataract surgery. The learning curve with laser cataract surgery will make the procedure, at least initially, slower and more difficult. Although the surgeon will spend time using the FS laser, this will result in saving time in the operating room, having already performed many of the critical steps with the laser. Surgeons who have adopted this technology have made the transition because of the potential for greater safety, reproducibility, and precision in creating the corneal incisions, capsulotomy, and nuclear removal.

In the future, ophthalmologists will still need to learn manual techniques to deal with challenging cases such as white intumescent cataracts, zonular dehiscence, perforated globes with cataracts following trauma, and ectopic lenses.

Corneal endothelial cell loss, which occurs with standard phacoemulsification, can occasionally lead to bullous keratopathy. A reduction in ultrasound energy with laser cataract surgery can lead to clearer corneas postoperatively and potentially a reduction in endothelial cell loss. Knorz reported a 25% decrease in endothelial cell loss in laser cases compared with manual cases at 1 month postoperatively.

Posterior capsular rupture and vitreous loss range from 2% to 6% of all standard phacoemulsification cases. FS cataract surgery performed with a precise capsulotomy, a reduction in phaco energy, and a decrease in intraocular maneuvers, especially when dealing with a dense nucleus, may reduce the incidence of posterior capsule rupture and vitreous loss.

In summary, we are at the beginning of a new era in cataract surgery that may be similar to the transition from extracapsular cataract extraction (ECCE) to phacoemulsification in the 1980s and 1990s. It is probable that FS lasers will revolutionize the technique of cataract surgery. The method has shown excellent results for accurate self-sealing corneal incisions; arcuate incisions to reduce astigmatism; highly circular, strong, and well-positioned capsulorrhexis; and safer and less technically difficult removal of the cataract with almost complete elimination of phacoemulsification. An improvement in the predicted final resting position of the intraocular lens can significantly enhance the refractive outcome. A precise capsulotomy can reduce implant tilt or decentration and as a consequence reduce higher-order aberrations. The laser technology may allow ophthalmologists to meet the demands of cataract patients to the same level that has been accomplished with laser vision correction.

The surgery should be more reproducible from patient to patient and surgeon to surgeon. It is likely that future new procedures, techniques, and intraocular implants will be developed as a consequence of the capabilities of the FS laser. It is also possible that a combined machine may be built that includes an FS laser and phacoemulsification.

There is a surgical learning curve with laser cataract surgery, and initially it will be more technically demanding and a longer procedure. Despite these factors, the benefits to patients are significant. Although the procedure is more expensive for an individual patient, it may turn out to be cost-effective for society. The implementation of laser cataract surgery into clinical practice should not be viewed as a step toward "robotic" cataract surgery, but rather an effort to raise our surgery standards to a new higher level of safety and clinical results. The technology is continuing to evolve but in its current state is offering patients clinical advantages.

Cataract postoperative care

The patient, who is usually ambulatory right away, may be warned to avoid bending, stooping, heavy lifting, straining, or sleeping on the side of the operated eye. If the patient lives alone or has no assistance, arrangements may be made for someone to help with any strenuous household activities.

While convalescing, the patient is more comfortable wearing dark glasses with ultraviolet protection. Protection, in the form of a metal or plastic eyeshield, only need be worn to shield the eye from the patient's own hands during periods of sleep for a few nights, to allow adequate wound healing. Reading, watching television, and walking are not restricted. There are no dietary limitations.

Usually it is safe for a patient to return to work soon after surgery, depending on occupational requirements and the need to use the operated eye for visual function.

The ophthalmic assistant should always keep in mind the patient's dependency after cataract surgery. Such a patient is handicapped because of a cataract in one eye and a fresh wound in the other. Fears increase in the postoperative period, and the person is frightened of doing anything that might jar the eye. However, the inability to see prevents the person from taking precautions to avoid bumping into things. The postoperative patient should be given every consideration. In the ophthalmologist's office, the patient should be helped off and on with his or her coat, assisted in and out of the examining chair, and given explicit verbal and written instructions about repeat visits and the timing and methods of instilling medication in the eye.

Medications that are frequently used in the postoperative period, which may last from 2 to 4 weeks, include antibiotics (e.g., Vigamox, Zymar, etc.), steroids (e.g., Pred Forte [prednisolone acetate], Maxidex [dexamethasone], Flarex [fluorometholone], etc.) and nonsteroidal preparations (e.g., Acular, Voltaren [diclofenac]). The antibiotic drops are used to decrease the risk of endophthalmitis. The steroid drops decrease ocular inflammation. The nonsteroidal drops decrease the risk of cystoid macular edema.

Early complications after cataract surgery

Subconjunctival hemorrhage

This has no effect on the visual outcome. The hemorrhage usually resolves within a few weeks without adverse sequelae. Patients need reassurance, but no specific treatment is required.

Hyphema

Blood in the anterior chamber may be from a tear of the iris or the wound. It usually resolves with time.

Raised intraocular pressure

This may occur within the first 24 to 48 hours as a result of the blockage of outflow chambers by the viscoelastic substance used at surgery. Pressure also may rise because of inflammation in the anterior chamber. Pain and corneal edema are common features of raised intraocular pressure.

Corneal edema (Figure 31.17)

This appears as a central clouding of the cornea. It may result from trauma at surgery, from intraocular injections, or from high postoperative pressure in the eye. The denser the cataract, the greater is the chance of corneal edema.

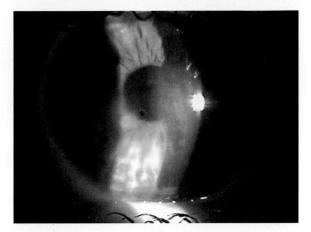

Figure 31.17 Corneal edema.

The endothelial cells (innermost layer of the cornea) function to keep the cornea transparent by maintaining it in a state of relative dehydration by means of turgescence, that is, pumping water constantly out of it. The risk of endothelial cell damage by a nuclear fragment or touch by an intraocular lens can be reduced by the use of a viscoelastic substance during phacoemulsification and before lens insertion.

Shallow anterior chamber

This temporary condition may be a result of inhibition of aqueous production by acetazolamide (Diamox) or beta-blocker drops. It must be differentiated from pupillary block glaucoma or a wound leak.

Flat anterior chamber

If corneal–endothelial touch is allowed to occur it can result in permanent corneal decompensation (see earlier text). The postoperative loss of the anterior chamber may result from any of the following events:

1. Leaking wound diagnosed by Seidel test, that is, observing the escaping aqueous wash away fluorescein from the leak in the wound; the wound requires suturing
2. Inhibition of aqueous secretion in the treatment of glaucoma by acetazolamide and beta-blocker drops
3. Postoperative ocular trauma; patients should wear protective shields while asleep
4. Pupillary block (raised intraocular pressure); treat by immediate dilation or peripheral iridectomy

Iritis

In its mildest form, iritis may manifest as broad, thin, gray, or brown deposits on the intraocular lens precipitates, sometimes with cells in the anterior chamber or aqueous flare. The goal of treatment of iritis is to prevent synechiae (adhesions of the iris) implanting because they may be the precursors of retrolenticular membrane formation and glaucoma.

It is advisable to use mydriatic agents to promote gentle dilation and pupillary motion. Therapy depends on topical steroids to control the inflammation.

Retinal detachment

This occurs more frequently after cataract surgery and YAG laser treatment, especially in patients with a history of a high degree of myopia. This risk is increased if surgery is complicated by rupture of the posterior capsule with vitreous loss. A sudden loss of full or half vision is an important symptom.

Cystoid macular edema (Figure 31.18)

This condition can be defined as an extracellular, intraretinal edema at the macula, which may be demonstrated by fluorescein angiography or with an OCT. Clinically the patient manifests a reduction in visual acuity that may disappear over a period of time with restoration of vision. A transient hyperopic shift in the refractive error usually occurs. The etiology of cystoid macular edema is unknown, but it may be precipitated by rupture of the posterior capsule and vitreous loss. In the majority of cases the macular edema occurs in an otherwise uncomplicated procedure.

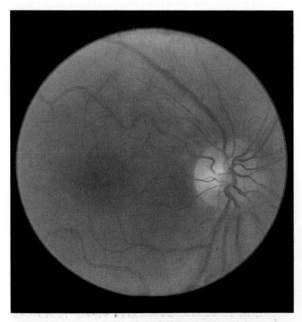

Figure 31.18 Cystoid macular edema.
(Reproduced from Spalton D, Hitchings R, Hunter P. Atlas of clinical ophthalmology. 3rd ed. St Louis: Mosby; 2004, with permission.)

The edema can occur in the early postoperative period, within 6 weeks, or later. The use of topical steroid and non-steroidal drops promotes resolution of the edema. Rarely the cystoid macular edema may be chronic, resulting in a permanent loss of vision.

Intraocular lens decentration

The implant occasionally can be noted to be decentered in a downward direction *(sunset syndrome)* or resting superiorly *(sunrise syndrome)*. If the decentration is associated with symptoms (e.g., glare, halos, or decreased vision), then surgical reposition or exchange of the implant is required.

Incorrect intraocular lens power

If the refractive error is significantly off from that intended and produces anisometropia, the implant can be exchanged. Other options include a secondary implant in the sulcus to correct the residual refractive error, or refractive surgery such as LASIK or PRK.

Retained lens material (Figure 31.19)

Occasionally cortical material, recognized as fluffy white in appearance, can be noted in the anterior chamber. This usually resolves through absorption with time. Nuclear material, characterized as yellow or brown in appearance, also may be noted. If this is minimal in size it will usually absorb with time. However, if there is more significant nuclear material, especially if a secondary uveitis occurs, surgical removal of the fragments is necessary.

Endophthalmitis (Figure 31.20)

This is a true ocular emergency. Symptoms may consist of any or all of pain, redness, and decreased vision occurring in the first week postoperatively. The overall incidence is 0.01%, often associated with pain. Patients are often admitted to the hospital and treated with topical, intravitreal, and

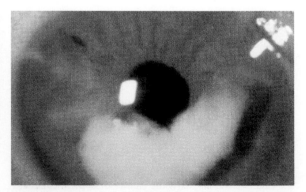

Figure 31.19 Retained lens material.

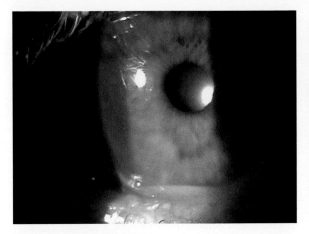

Figure 31.20 Endophthalmitis.

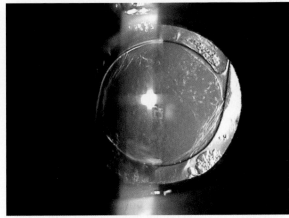

Figure 31.21 Capsular opacification.

even intravenous antibiotics after specimens are taken from the anterior chamber and vitreous. If there is significant inflammation on initial presentation, a vitrectomy is often performed to improve the prognosis.

Final visual acuity is guarded unless the infection is recognized early and treated aggressively. The use of preoperative prophylactic broad-spectrum antibiotics, attention to surgical sterility, and the use of intraocular antibiotics into the anterior chamber at the conclusion of the procedure have further decreased the incidence of this complication in recent years.

Astigmatism

Significantly induced astigmatism with small incision and no-stitch phacoemulsification is uncommon. There is usually no induced astigmatism with an incision around 2.2 mm. There is typically a 0.50 diopter change in the astigmatism with a 3-mm incision. The larger the incision, the greater is the induced astigmatism. Temporal incisions also tend to induce less astigmatism than superior incisions. If significant preoperative astigmatism exists, limbal relaxing incisions or an astigmatic keratotomy can be performed at the time of surgery. Toric implants can be inserted and aligned in the eye to decrease astigmatism. If there is induced astigmatism and the patient is unable to tolerate this in a glass or contact lens, then incisional corneal surgery or laser vision correction can be performed.

Capsular opacification (Figure 31.21)

If this is associated with diminished vision or symptoms of glare, then a YAG capsulotomy can be performed. Advances in intraocular lens designs with a square-edged optic have dramatically decreased the incidence of capsular haze. If a foldable silicone plate lens has been inserted, it is best to wait until at least 4 months postop to decrease the chance of dislocation of the implant into the vitreous following a

YAG capsulotomy. Patients should be aware that there is an increased risk of a retinal detachment or cystoid macular edema following a YAG capsulotomy.

Pseudophakic bullous keratopathy (Figure 31.22)

Corneal decompensation may occur following cataract surgery, and this may be noted in the early postoperative period or typically months to years after the procedure. Preoperative risk factors include the presence of corneal guttata, Fuch's corneal dystrophy (guttata with edema), or a low endothelial cell count. Surgical risk factors include the insertion of an anterior chamber lens, prolonged phaco procedure time, or rupture of the posterior capsule. A penetrating keratoplasty can be offered to improve both comfort and vision. An extended-wear bandage soft contact lens can improve the comfort if a patient is not interested in surgical repair or while waiting for keratoplasty. Hypertonic drops and ointment (ketorolac [Muro 128] 5%) will decrease epithelial edema and enhance comfort.

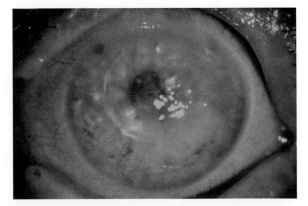

Figure 31.22 Pseudophakic bullous keratopathy.

Questions often asked about cataract surgery

1. *Is a cataract a film that grows over the eye?* No. It is not a growth of any kind. It is a haziness that occurs in the lens of the eye and interferes with sight.
2. *Can cataracts grow back once removed?* No. However, secondary membranes may form from opacities on the posterior capsule or from Elschnig's pearls that appear.
3. *If the cataract is removed completely, does this guarantee sight?* No. The recovery of vision depends on two factors: the provision of clear optic media and the integrity of the retina and macula. Because the surgeon often cannot see the fundus preoperatively, recovery of vision cannot be guaranteed despite a superb surgical result. If the patient's macula has been damaged, a successful cataract extraction will improve only the peripheral vision and not central vision.
4. *Does a cataract have to be "ripe" before it is removed?* No. In the early days of cataract surgery a completely opaque, or mature, lens was easier to deliver and therefore surgery was often delayed until the lens became mature. The patient often thought of the cataract as a fruit that had to ripen before it could be picked. In addition, physicians were reluctant to operate on one eye in cataract patients because of the troublesome double vision that could develop if the other eye is normal.

   With the surgical techniques available today, any cataracts can be removed. The disability of the patient, rather than the maturity of the lens, has become the prime consideration regarding a decision for lens extraction.
5. *How important is ultraviolet (UV) light?* Ultraviolet light can be classified as follows:
   - UVA contains wavelengths from 400 to 320 nm.
   - UVB contains wavelengths from 320 to 280 nm.
   - UVC contains wavelengths less than 280 nm.

   The ozone layer of the atmosphere absorbs all UVC from the sun. However, other sources of UVC include welding arcs and germicidal lamps. Of the total solar radiation that reaches Earth, about 90% is UVA and 10% is UVB.

   Ultraviolet light varies with the season, being greatest in summer and near the equator. It is also more intense at high noon and in high mountains. Fresh snow reflects about 68% of the incident light, whereas sandy beaches reflect about 15% and water reflects about 5%. Some laboratory experiments have shown that UV light can damage human tissues. The details may take many years to unfold and are often difficult to prove. UV light has been implicated in both cataract production and macular degeneration. Study results are inconclusive at present.

   UV filters can be incorporated into intraocular lenses. When a cataract is removed, the UV filtering mechanism is removed; thus a UV filter in the intraocular lens is valuable.

Summary

Cataract surgery has undergone significant advances since the pioneering work of Dr. Charles Kelman, who developed phacoemulsification. FS laser now brings in a new era of surgery in which many of the critical steps of the operation can be automated to enhance outcomes and safety. The adoption of laser cataract surgery by ophthalmologists is growing worldwide. Although laser cataract surgery is already at an advanced stage, further refinements are being made to optimize surgical outcomes. Innovations have also been made in lens implants to improve quality of vision and provide patients with a broader range of vision.

GLAUCOMA SURGERY

The glaucoma procedure most often performed is called an *iridectomy*. In this operation a small incision is made either directly through the cornea at the upper limbus or under a flap of conjunctival tissue. The iris is grasped with a small forceps, pulled out of the eye and partially excised. The excision of the iris may involve a sector down to the pupillary area *(sector iridectomy)* or only a peripheral area near the root of the iris *(peripheral iridectomy)*. The cornea is then sutured and the eye bandaged.

At this time, a *trabeculectomy* is the most popular glaucoma operation. In this procedure a small portion of the trabecular meshwork is surgically removed, permitting the aqueous to filter out of the anterior chamber and form a conjunctival bleb (Figure 31.23).

Laser trabeculoplasty has become a principal strategy to reduce intraocular pressure on a permanent basis. This is a procedure in which an *argon laser* is used to produce mild burns in the trabecular meshwork, causing mild shrinkage of the trabeculum, which in turn opens up the interspaces in the meshwork. This permits an increased outflow of aqueous from the anterior chamber. It is useful for mild rises of pressure in open-angle glaucoma in which peripheral synechiae are absent or minimal, with a good exposure of the trabecular meshwork. The *holmium laser* is also rapidly becoming of interest in the management of glaucoma. This technique produces subconjunctival filtration and offers great hope in the management of the condition. (See also the Laser surgery section that follows.)

In some cases a *sclerectomy* may be performed. This procedure is similar to an iridectomy except that an additional small button of the sclera is removed, usually at the superior junction of the cornea and the sclera. The scleral button may be removed with scissors or by a small punch. The sclerectomy provides for a permanent drainage of aqueous

Figure 31.23 Filtering procedure. Aqueous fluid flows from the anterior chamber through an opening in the sclera (trabeculectomy site) to the subconjunctival space where a filtering bleb is formed.

(From Stein HA, Slatt BJ, Stein RM. Ophthalmic terminology: speller and vocabulary builder. 3rd ed. St Louis: Mosby; 1992.)

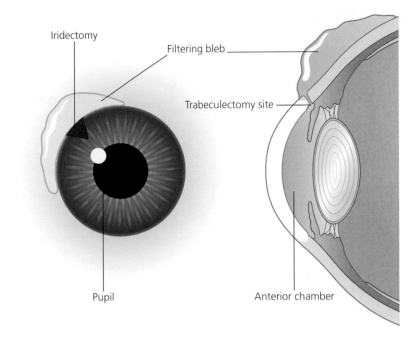

Iridectomy

Filtering bleb

Trabeculectomy site

Pupil

Anterior chamber

fluid from the anterior chamber of the eye to an area underlying the conjunctiva.

Another glaucoma operation, called an *iridencleisis,* is a filtration procedure. In this operation a flap of conjunctiva is elevated and the anterior chamber is entered with a superblade knife. The iris is then grasped with forceps and a segment is cut with scissors. One portion of the cut iris is allowed to fall back into the eye, while the other portion is drawn into the incision and left there to act as a wick to maintain permanent filtration from the anterior chamber to an area under the conjunctiva.

Occasionally glaucoma is seen at birth or in infancy *(congenital glaucoma).* A procedure that requires a small gonioknife has been devised for this condition. The gonioknife is passed across the limbus of one eye to the opposite area and a sweep is made to open the angle of the opposite portion of the eye *(goniotomy).* In some cases the knife is passed under the opposing conjunctiva as well, which allows fluid to pass through this channel *(goniopuncture).*

Selective laser trabeculoplasty (SLT) is a new form of laser treatment of the trabecular meshwork. This uses a switched 530-nm laser that delivers a 200 μm spot to the meshwork to create fine bubbles in the anterior chamber. It takes 6 to 8 weeks to be effective. See Chapter 25 for more details.

RETINAL DETACHMENT SURGERY

When looking into the normal eye with an ophthalmoscope, the examiner can see the retina lying against the choroidal layer, from which it receives part of its blood supply and nourishment. Normally the retina is loosely attached to the choroids, but when it becomes separated from the choroid it flaps loosely within the vitreous fluid of the eye (Figure 31.24). Naturally, retinal detachment leads to poor nutrition and function of the retina and eventually to loss of vision. Many things predispose to retinal detachments, such as injury, myopia, and previous surgery. Often there is a tear or hole present that permits fluid to collect under the retina. This is called a *rhegmatogenous retinal detachment* (Figure 31.25).

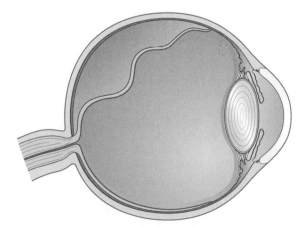

Figure 31.24 Retinal detachment superiorly. Defect in field below.

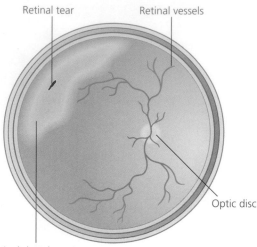

Retinal tear   Retinal vessels

Optic disc

Retinal detachment

Figure 31.25 Rhegmatogenous retinal detachment with associated retinal tear.
(From Stein HA, Slatt BJ, Stein RM. A primer in ophthalmology: a textbook for students. St Louis: Mosby; 1992.)

Correction of a retinal detachment is accomplished either by bringing the retina back to the choroid or by pushing the choroid up to the retina. To bring the retina back to the choroid, scleral punctures are made in attempts to surgically drain some of the fluid that lies between the retina and the choroid. If the retina is lying against the choroid at this stage, either electrocoagulation or cryotherapy with a cold probe against the sclera will bond the retina to the choroid. The choroid and retina are brought together by placing a buckling band of silicone on the overlying sclera and choroid, which exerts inward pressure. If the retina is not attached at this stage, then air, special gases, or oil may be injected into the vitreous to push the retina back against the choroid.

In retinal detachment surgery, cryotherapy is useful because it can create firm adhesion of the tissues so that retinal breaks and holes can be sealed. Before the development of cryotherapy, retinal surgeons used diathermy, which created a firm bond in the retinal tissues by heat coagulation. Cold treatment was found to be superior to heat treatment because it did not damage large blood vessels, with the attendant risk of thrombosis or hemorrhage in these vessels. Also the cold seal was effected without damaging other tissues such as the sclera. (With diathermy the sclera had to be moved aside surgically before the diathermy current could be applied.) In many instances cryotherapy has reduced the need for implants and buckles, which may give rise to infection and may even extrude at a late postoperative date. Cryotherapy has not rendered obsolete other methods of treatment for retinal disease, but has merely added to the surgeon's versatility in approaching the general problem. Retinal surgery has

always been difficult, but now the ophthalmic surgeon has a number of tools for handling this problem.

Today, with modern techniques, the outlook for reattachment of the retina and restoration of sight is excellent.

Summary of retinal surgery and postop care

- Surgery may last 1 to 2 hours.
- The operated eye is patched after surgery until the patient is seen the next day by the surgeon.
- If a gas bubble is introduced, the patient may be instructed to keep his or her head in a face-down position as much as possible, and to avoid exertion, heavy lifting, and going more than 2000 feet (600 m) in elevation until the surgeon says otherwise.
- Patients will have specific drops and instructions to follow for a few weeks.
- Patients are allowed to return to work after 1 to 2 weeks.
- Patients should call the doctor's office if they experience nausea or vomiting, severe eye pain, huge loss of vision, a noticeable increase in floaters, and flashes of light or pus-like discharge.

Additional information for patients having retinal surgery

- Preoperative assessment is scheduled before surgery to assess if the patient is healthy enough for neuroleptic anesthetic and the procedure.
- Aspirin or other blood thinners must be stopped 1 week before surgery if possible.
- Only the eye having surgery will be patched.

VITREOUS SURGERY

The *vitreous infusion suction cutter (VISC)* represents a major milestone in ophthalmology. This instrument can be used to treat disorders of the vitreous that were considered inoperable until its development in the early 1970s. It performs three major functions within the vitreous cavity of the eye: it is able to cut the vitreous, remove the debris from the eye by suction, and replace the aspirate with an infusion of Ringer's solution.

The VISC is introduced into the vitreous cavity anywhere over the pars plana 4 to 7 mm from the corneal limbus. In this position it is possible to avoid both hitting the lens of the eye and stripping the retina itself. In some cases in which a cataract obscures the view of the vitreous, this instrument with its cutting action can be used to remove the cataractous lens material itself.

The results of vitrectomy surgery have in many instances been astonishing. When it is effective, visual acuity can be improved from hand movements to 20/30. Despite preselection of cases, not all results are successful and the visual improvement in some instances is not so dramatic; however, when we remember that these cases were previously thought to be hopeless, any improvement is gratifying.

The most common indication for a vitrectomy is a non-clearing vitreous hemorrhage in a patient with diabetes. With removal of the blood-filled vitreous, light is able to reach the retina and therefore improve the level of visual acuity (Figure 31.26).

Vitrectomy also has been used to handle cases of retinal detachment to eliminate the traction on the retina. In such instances there are usually strong vitreous bands contracting and pulling on the retina and preventing it from being returned mechanically. In cataract extraction there sometimes is vitreous loss, and with the loss of vitreous the retina can become detached. Detachment is largely the result of shrinkage of the trapped vitreous, which is attached at the wound site of the cataract extraction. Again, the vitrectomy instrument has been effective in cutting and eliminating these traction bands, which can produce complications such as retinal detachment, macular cysts, macular holes, macular edema, and retinal holes.

The vitrectomy instrument also has been used in patients with heavy intraocular connective tissue formation after foreign body injuries. Vitrectomy is the only way of removing severe scar formation in the vitreous cavity. It also has been useful in cases of severe inflammatory reaction in the vitreous.

In some instances, though, vitrectomy is not effective. It has had poor results in eyes with massive preretinal retraction. At times vitreous hemorrhage may occur, which leads to a poor result.

LASER SURGERY

The principle of lasers was predicted by Albert Einstein in 1917. During the 1950s, Townes and Schawlow at Columbia University and Vasov and Prokhorov at the Lebedev Institute, working independently in the field of microwave physics, demonstrated that stimulated emission of radiation could be made available for practical use. The researchers received a Nobel Prize for this work in 1964.

Lasers are used in a growing number of medical procedures that permit surgeons to perform noninvasive surgery. Diseased tissue can be cut away or vaporized by lasers with less damage or trauma to neighboring healthy tissues. Surgery also can be accomplished in inaccessible parts of the body by transmitting laser beams to those parts through fiberoptics, transmission cables, and other innovative delivery systems. In ophthalmology, the delivery system is usually a slit-lamp microscope, but new laser cutting instruments are being studied.

In ophthalmology, the *argon laser* can alter the trabecular meshwork and increase outflow of aqueous (see Glaucoma section earlier). It can be used for gonioplasty and for iridotomy because it can coagulate, retard, or destroy new vessel growth in the anterior and posterior segments of the eye. The nd:YAG laser also has a wide variety of uses in ophthalmology, but its most popular use has been that of opening the posterior capsule when it has become opacified.

The YAG laser is widely used today. Contrary to popular belief, this laser does not remove cataracts. Within months or years after a cataract has been removed, eye surgeons frequently use the YAG laser to clear cloudy secondary membranes. This results in restoration of vision by a noninvasive method of opening these membranes. The procedure is not painful and requires no hospitalization. The YAG laser is a "cold" type of laser and uses quick pulses of laser energy on clear tissues within the eye. It also is used for performing an iris iridotomy in cases of narrow-angle glaucoma.

CORNEAL TRANSPLANTATION

The cornea is the clear portion in the front part of the eye that is similar to the transparent covering on a watch. When injury, degeneration, or infection occurs that causes the cornea to become cloudy, vision is disrupted. Only by replacing a portion of the cornea with a clear window taken from a donor eye can vision be restored.

Not everyone with a corneal disease can be helped by corneal transplantation.

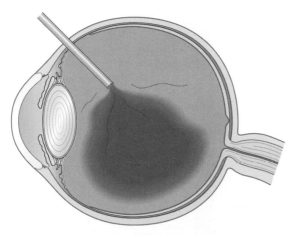

Figure 31.26 Vitrectomy performed to remove vitreous that is mixed with blood.

(From Stein HA, Slatt BJ, Stein RM. A primer in ophthalmology: a textbook for students. St Louis: Mosby; 1992.)

The cornea, because it is devoid of blood vessels, is one of the few tissues in the human body that may be transplanted from one human being to another with a large degree of success. The absence of blood vessels in both the donor and the host cornea reduces the allergic reaction, in which reactive immunoglobulins are carried through blood flow, and permits the body to retain and not reject the foreign cornea. Thus only those conditions in which the cornea is free of blood vessels are suitable for transplantation.

Two basic types of corneal transplantation are performed. One is the *lamellar* or *partial penetrating procedure,* in which a half thickness of cornea is transferred from the eye of a donor to that of the host (Figure 31.27A). In this procedure the anterior chamber of the eye is not entered and only the outer half or two-thirds of the cornea is transplanted. Union is made of the donor cornea with the host cornea by means of several interrupted fine sutures or a continuous suture around the periphery of the donor button. The donor button varies anywhere from 6 to 10 mm in diameter, depending on the extent of the disease involved. The second type of transplant operation is the *penetrating* or

full-thickness corneal transplant (Figure 31.27B). In this operation the full thickness of the cornea is removed from the donor eye and replaces the full thickness of the central portion of the host cornea. The surgery involves entering the anterior chamber, inserting the donor cornea, and establishing a tight fit by direct suture closure or a continuous suture (Figure 31.28). Healon often is used to minimize endothelial damage.

In the postoperative period the most common complications include a wound leak, suture breakage and wound dehiscence, infection, and graft rejection. If detected early and managed appropriately, these complications can be controlled or eliminated, enabling a high level of success for the operation. Thus careful monitoring by the doctor, nurse, or ophthalmic assistant is required.

In both the lamellar and full-thickness corneal transplant, the donor and the host buttons are trephined with a round cutting trephine, which cleanly and sharply removes the affected part. The cornea taken from a recently deceased person is then carefully sutured in place (Figure 31.29).

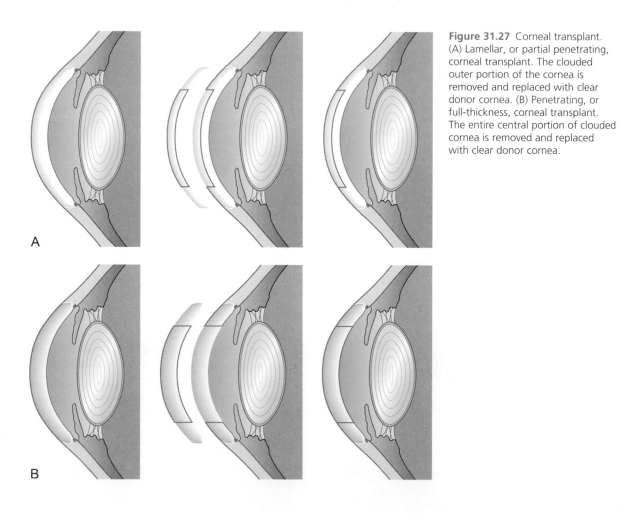

A

B

Figure 31.27 Corneal transplant. (A) Lamellar, or partial penetrating, corneal transplant. The clouded outer portion of the cornea is removed and replaced with clear donor cornea. (B) Penetrating, or full-thickness, corneal transplant. The entire central portion of clouded cornea is removed and replaced with clear donor cornea.

Figure 31.28 Penetrating keratoplasty.
(A) Preoperative corneal scar. (B) Trephine
used to cut donor cornea. (C) Trephine
used to cut patient's cornea. (D) Cut cornea
of patient is removed. (E) Donor cornea is
placed in opening of patient's cornea.
(F) Donor cornea is sutured into position.
*(From Stein HA, Slatt BJ, Stein RM. Ophthalmic
terminology: speller and vocabulary builder.
3rd ed. St Louis: Mosby; 1992.)*

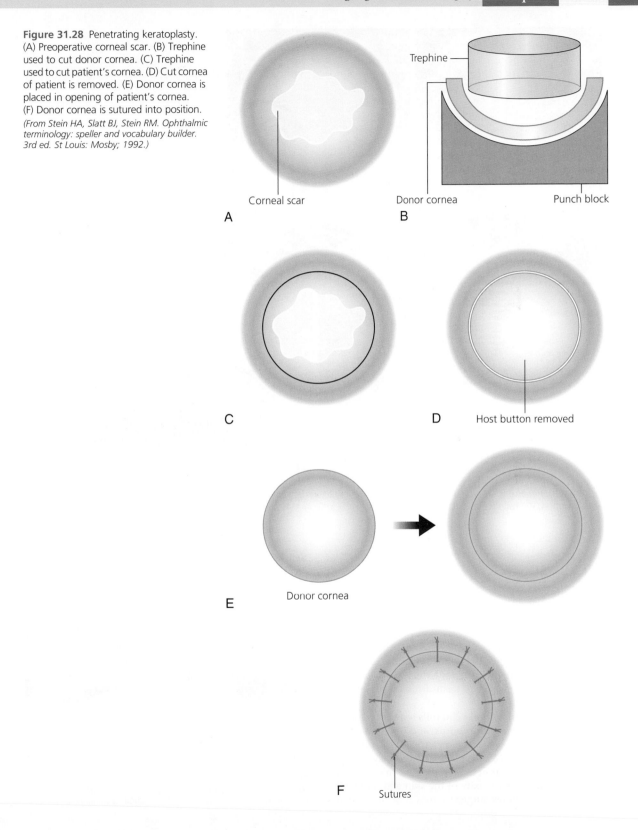

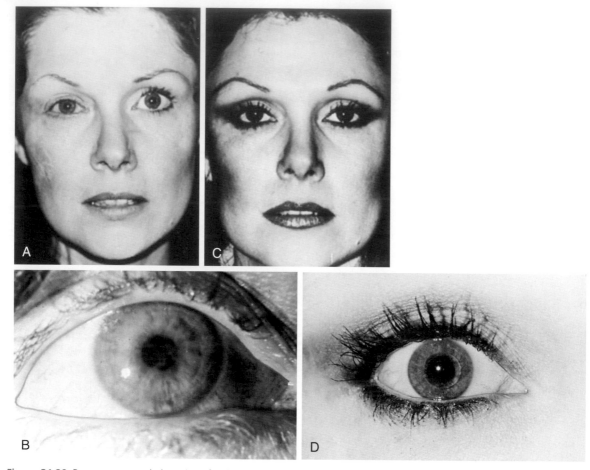

Figure 31.29 Recurrent corneal ulceration after herpes simplex virus with visual loss. (A) Full face and (B) cornea. After corneal transplantation, (C) full face and (D) cornea.

EYELID SURGERY

Entropion is a condition in which the eyelashes roll in and rub against the cornea. Numerous types of eyelid operations are performed for the correction of this condition. One of the simplest is Ziegler cautery, in which the cautery is applied to the area just below the eyelashes. Other procedures include tightening the underlying muscles of the eyelid or removing a wedge of tarsus from the inner aspect of the eyelid.

Ectropion occurs when the eyelid rolls outward. This may be the result of scarring from burns, and insertion of skin grafts taken elsewhere is required to reduce the pull from the scar tissue. Grafts of skin for the eyelids may be taken from upper eyelids or from behind the ears. In some cases, ectropion results from a laxity of the skin and underlying structures. This requires surgical removal of these tissues to properly evert the lid so that the lid margin lies in its correct position against the globe.

Ptosis occurs when the eyelid droops to cover the upper portion of the pupil (Figure 31.30). Investigation in the

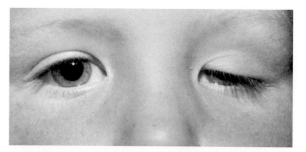

Figure 31.30 Congenital ptosis, left eye.

(Reproduced from Spalton D, Hitchings R, Hunter P. Atlas of clinical ophthalmology. 3rd ed. St Louis: Mosby; 2004, with permission.)

adult should rule out medical causes before surgery is undertaken. If the levator muscle still functions, a resection of this muscle will be performed, either from the undersurface of the eyelid or through the eyelid skin. In this procedure the muscle is identified and shortened by a measured amount of millimeters. When the levator muscle is completely paralyzed, the eyelid may be suspended from the brow muscles to the tarsal plate by use of fascia lata taken from the thigh or from cadavers, by collagen tapes, or by white silk sutures.

PTERYGIUM REMOVAL

Pterygium is a fibrovascular growth of the actinally damaged conjunctiva that invades a portion of the cornea from the limbus (Figure 31.31). It occurs in up to 7% of the population in North America and a higher proportion in warmer climates. It is usually vascular when active. A pterygium may encroach on the visual axis and interfere with vision. There are several techniques for surgical removal including the bare scleral method, transplantation of the head, and conjunctival grafting. The recurrence rate is high and can vary from 5% to 40%. In the past few years mitomycin has been applied to minimize recurrences.

DACRYOCYSTORHINOSTOMY

Blockage of the tear canal may result from obstructions arising anywhere, beginning at the small punctum on the eyelid margin and extending to the nasolacrimal duct. Obstructions involving the lacrimal sac and nasolacrimal duct require correction by dacryocystorhinostomy.

In this procedure a large opening, approximately 8 to 10 mm in size, is made in the wall of the nose and a union

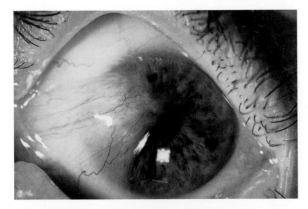

Figure 31.31 Advanced pterygium of left cornea.
(Reproduced from Spalton D, Hitchings R, Hunter P. Atlas of clinical ophthalmology. 3rd ed. St Louis: Mosby; 2004, with permission.)

is created between the mucosal lining of the nose in this area and the lacrimal sac. Thus the lacrimal sac opens directly into the nose through this large opening. The operation usually ensures relatively good success in curing both tearing and infection problems that arise from stagnation in the lacrimal sac.

ENUCLEATION AND EVISCERATION

An eye may be removed because of tumor, injury, or severe pain combined with dysfunction. Enucleation usually is performed with the patient under general anesthesia because of the psychologic effect of removing an eye.

The conjunctiva is opened around the limbus and the four rectus muscles are identified and severed from the globe. Enucleation scissors are passed behind the globe and the optic nerve is severed. The oblique muscles are then severed from the globe and the globe is removed from the socket. Pressure is applied until bleeding has stopped. An implant of glass, plastic, or silicone is placed in the socket to fill the defect. The muscles or tissues are sewn over the implant in a way that permits movement of the implant. When healing has occurred, the patient is directed to an artificial-eye maker *(ocularist)*, who fashions a cosmetic shell with a built-in painted iris and pupil to match the fellow eye. Sometimes only the contents of the globe are removed, leaving the outer shell with muscle attachments. This procedure is called an *evisceration*.

EYE DRESSINGS

Eyepatches are usually used postoperatively to prevent infection and absorb discharge. They also immobilize the eyes and protect them from accidental trauma. Most eye pads have a cotton center and a fine mesh surface to prevent the cotton from being absorbed into the discharge and wound.

An eye pad is secured in place with the application of three or four strips of adhesive or cellophane tape. The strips are directed on an angle from the cheek to the forehead, away from the margins of the mouth so that eating will not be hampered. A shield of metal or plastic is commonly applied over the eye pad to protect the eye from undue external pressure or injury.

SUMMARY

The ophthalmic assistant should maintain routines that can be adapted for every surgical patient. The management of a surgical patient involves attention to the mechanical details of surgery, as well as to education of the patient regarding the nature of the hospital stay.

Questions for review and thought

1. Outline an operative technique for strabismus surgery, cataract surgery, and glaucoma surgery.
2. What are the principles behind:
   a. cataract surgery?
   b. corneal transplant surgery?
   c. muscle surgery?
3. What is the role of laser therapy after cataract surgery?
4. What is the most common major ocular surgical procedure performed?

5. Name some complications that can occur after cataract surgery.
6. How can a patient's general health affect the outcome of surgery?
7. Identify the use of drugs during cataract surgery.
8. Identify the difference between phacoemulsification and extracapsular cataract surgery.
9. Describe the steps of the cataract phacoemulsification procedure.

 Self-evaluation questions

True–false statements

Directions: Indicate whether the statement is true **(T)** or false **(F).**

1. In muscle surgery, recession of a muscle involves moving it from its attachment and placing it at a point closer to the cornea. **T** or **F**
2. Cryosurgery refers to any surgical procedure involving cold temperatures during surgery. **T** or **F**
3. Phacoemulsification is removal of a cataract through the use of ultrasound. **T** or **F**

Missing words

Directions: Write in the missing word in the following sentences:

4. Removal of an eye is called _____.
5. Removal of a portion of the trabeculum for glaucoma is called _____.
6. An out-turning of the eyelid is called _____.

Choice-completion questions

Directions: Select the one best answer in each case.

7. In strabismus surgery, which procedure is not considered a normal surgical practice?

   a. Uncovering the eye the day after surgery
   b. Patching the unoperated eye preoperatively
   c. Giving systemic antibiotics
   d. Letting the patient go home the day after surgery
   e. Using orthoptic exercises soon after surgery

8. Which of the following is not a surgical procedure for glaucoma?

   a. Laser iridotomy
   b. Trabeculectomy
   c. Sclerectomy
   d. Cryotherapy
   e. Ziegler cautery

9. Corneal transplantation is utilized as a surgical procedure for which of the following conditions?

   a. Cataracts
   b. Advanced glaucoma
   c. Toxic keratitis
   d. Keratoconus
   e. Keratoconjunctivitis sicca

A Answers, notes, and explanations

1. **False.** In recession of a muscle, the reattachment is made at a point toward the posterior portion of the eye and away from the cornea. This in effect weakens the pull of the muscle so that it has a less effective contraction. In convergent strabismus the medial rectus may be recessed, whereas in divergent strabismus the lateral rectus is recessed.

2. **True.** Cryosurgery involves the use of a probe cooled by liquid nitrogen, carbon dioxide, or Freon, so that the temperature ranges anywhere from −20° to −70° C. By so lowering the temperature, a small probe can be applied to the lens of the eye to create an iceball formation and adhesion of the lens to the probe. This forms a bond that is useful in extracting the cataract. Cryotherapy is also used to destroy lashes and hair follicles. It is used in retinal detachment repair to create adhesions of the tissues themselves. It may be used in glaucoma to shrink the vascular coat of the eye.

3. **True.** In this procedure, which has gained widespread acceptance throughout the world, ultrasound is used in a small probe that enters the eye. By means of high-frequency sound waves, the cutting edge impinges on the cataractous lens and emulsifies it so it can be easily removed by aspiration.

4. **Enucleation.** Enucleation is performed whenever an eye is diseased and painful, or a malignant tumor is present. During enucleation all muscles are severed from the globe and then the optic nerve is severed and the globe removed. An implant of plastic, glass, or silicone is placed in the socket to fill the defect left by removal of the eye. An artificial eye is then fashioned that moves with the implant and simulates the appearance of a normal eyeball.

5. **Trabeculectomy.** Trabeculectomy is the removal of a portion of the trabeculum to improve the outflow of fluid from the eye. It thereby reduces the devastating destructive effect that the elevated intraocular pressure of glaucoma creates.

6. **Ectropion.** An eyelid that turns out is called an *ectropion,* from *ec-* meaning "out." This may occur as the result of scarring of the overlying eyelid tissue (cicatricial ectropion) or from the laxity of the muscles (senile ectropion) as occurs in older adults. Surgical correction is the only means to repair an ectropion.

7. **c. Giving systemic antibiotics.** An operation such as strabismus surgery performed in a sterile environment requires no systemic antibiotics. Topical antibiotics may be given at the time of surgery and may even be given by some ophthalmologists in the postoperative period. This is usually satisfactory to overcome any invading organism. The rich blood supply of both the vascular coat and the muscles of the eye is usually sufficient to take care of any inflammation that may arise. This situation, however, may not be true for intraocular surgery when there is an absence of blood vessels and thus an absence of the vascular response to an invading microbacterial organism. In these intraocular cases, antibiotics may be preferred to raise the intraocular level of the antibiotics to prevent infection.

8. **e. Ziegler cautery.** All the procedures except Ziegler cautery are used for either narrow-angle or wide-angle glaucoma. Ziegler cautery is used to correct a spastic entropion of the eyelid.

9. **d. Keratoconus.** Keratoconus is a progressive out-pouching and thinning of the cornea with rupturing and scar formation. A corneal transplant is required when the cone has reached the point at which contact lenses or spectacles can no longer satisfactorily correct vision. The cornea eventually may become extremely thin, in which case a penetrating corneal transplant is required.

Chapter 32

Surgical correction of presbyopia

Raymond M. Stein, Rebecca L. Stein

Surgical correction of presbyopia is an area of intense research and development. Although it would be ideal to prevent or reverse hardening of the crystalline lens, this is not a viable therapeutic option. In recent years, many different surgical procedures have been developed to allow near vision. These procedures include surgery on the sclera, the cornea, or the crystalline lens. The most common surgical options include monovision laser-assisted in situ keratomileusis (LASIK), monovision lens exchange, corneal inlays, presbyLASIK, and multifocal or accommodative lens implants. All refractive and cataract patients should understand the advantages and disadvantages of the various presbyopic procedures. Although technology will continue to advance, there are real clinical benefits to the presbyopic options that are offered today.

INTRODUCTION

Advances in refractive surgery have brought significant changes in the treatment of myopia, hyperopia, and astigmatism. Surgical correction of presbyopia is considered the final frontier in the field of refractive surgery.

Presbyopia is the gradual reduction in the amplitude of accommodation with aging that has already started by the early teenage years and ends sometime in the sixth decade of life with the complete loss of the ability to change the power of the eye. It is only when an individual's near point has receded to an inconvenient distance that any remedial action becomes necessary.

The first known reference to presbyopia is probably by Aristotle (384–322 BC), who referred to the individual suffering from it as presbytes, from which the relatively modern term *presbyopia* is derived. *Presbyopia*, literally meaning "old eye," is the most common ocular condition in the world. The basic pathophysiology involved in its development has been a matter of controversy for centuries.

The treatment of presbyopia has consisted primarily of reading glasses or contact lenses. The problem with reading glasses has been the fact that they only allow sharp vision at a given distance. Benjamin Franklin in 1760 invented bifocal glasses to allow both near and distance vision. However, bifocals can be difficult to use because the patient has to rotate the eyes downward instead of rotating the head. Eye care professionals and patients are searching for a safe, effective procedure to replace accommodation thus restoring the full range of vision typically enjoyed before age 40.

Currently all presbyopic nonsurgical and surgical approaches are considered compromises because there is no causative treatment, which would result in restoring the flexibility of the crystalline lens. A compromise means that the surgical procedure has benefits but also side effects, which must be differentiated from the inherent surgical risk to any procedure. For example, a reduction in contrast sensitivity or halos at night as a result of a multifocal implant are unwanted side effects, but endophthalmitis or cystoid macular edema is a surgical risk of the same procedure.

In addition to the goal of enhanced distance and near vision, it is important to provide functional intermediate vision. Computers, dashboards, mirrors, deskwork, and everyday facial encounters bring out the value of clear uncorrected intermediate vision.

There is a wide choice of surgical approaches to help the presbyope. Some of these, such as monovision LASIK or the creation of monovision with an intraocular lens (IOL) implant, are mature technologies. Others, including photo-disruption of the crystalline lens and capsular refilling, are at an early stage of development. Refractive surgeons now have a number of different surgical modalities to choose from including corneal inlays, presbyLASIK, intrastromal correction with femtosecond technology, multifocal implants, accommodative implants, monovision, and scleral procedures.

Surgical correction of presbyopia has been one of the most intense areas of research in ophthalmology. The purpose of this chapter is to provide an overview of the procedures and related devices currently in use or in development for treating presbyopia. This is an exciting time for those involved in vision correction for the presbyope and for presbyopic patients.

THE UNDERLYING PROBLEM

Modern physiologic studies confirm Helmholtz's theory that progressive hardening of the crystalline lens is at the root of age-related loss of accommodation. In 1855 Helmholtz observed that the center of the human lens thickened during accommodation. He theorized that when the eye accommodates, the ciliary muscle contracts, reducing the tension on the zonules that span the circumlental space extending between the ciliary body and the lens equator. This releases the outward-directed equatorial tension on the lens capsule and allows this elastic capsule to contract, causing an increase in the anteroposterior diameter of the lens and resulting in an increase in its optical power.

Many studies based on Helmholtz's theory have attempted to explain the loss of accommodation in the aging eye. Some suggest a loss of zonules or capsule elasticity with aging; thus, when the zonules are relaxed, the lens is not able to change its shape. There are some conflicting reports on whether the ciliary muscle atrophies with age. The major factor in the loss of accommodation appears to be the increased stiffness of the aging lens with inability to respond to accommodative stimuli.

The ideal treatment of the crystalline lens's loss of functionality would be either prevention or reversal of the hardening. Unfortunately we are short of realizing either therapeutic option. Surgical procedures to treat presbyopia have been developed to deal with the sclera, cornea, or lens.

SURGICAL CORRECTIVE PROCEDURES

Scleral procedures

Scleral procedures performed with a blade, laser, and/or insertion of scleral implants have had limited success. The procedures are based on expanding the distance between the lens equator and the ciliary muscle, thereby increasing zonular tension. The mechanisms underlying this concept have yet to be proven. In Schachar's view, it is growth of the lens without concomitant growth of other ocular structures, which physically inhibits the movement necessary for accommodation. A sclerotomy, which can be performed with a blade or laser, would give the lens more room for accommodation. Physiologic studies have shown, however, that the lens does not have increased space to move and, additionally, does not move equatorially. Some of the early positive results with the scleral expansion procedure may be secondary to induced multifocality, which provided some enhanced near vision. Clinical outcomes with scleral expansion bands have been neither long-lasting nor predictable. In addition, there are potential risks of scleral procedures, which include the danger of perforation, retinal detachment, choroidal or retinal hemorrhage, and ischemia. In addition, scleral implants increase the risk of infection and may migrate and extrude.

Despite disappointing results in the past, there is one new laser procedure that aims to correct presbyopia by modification of the scleral–ciliary complex. The LaserACE (Ace Vision Group, Inc., Silver Lake, Ohio) procedure uses an erbium yttrium-aluminum-garnet (YAG) laser to ablate at a depth of 90% of the sclera and a width of 600 μm, with the goal to free the ciliary muscle to contract normally. The spots are delivered in a matrix pattern of nine laser spots into each oblique quadrant. After completion of the microexcisions, a collagen biomatrix filler is applied to fill the excisions to prevent fibrosis and maintain patency of the ablations. Hipsley and colleagues presented data in 2011 on 135 eyes with a reported restoration of accommodation of 1.25 to 1.50 diopters, which remained stable through 18 months. They also reported that 89% of patients had near uncorrected visual acuity of J3 or better, postoperatively, and no significant loss of distance visual acuity. Broader clinical trials are under way to corroborate these early results. If similar results are achieved, this scleral procedure will be an option for the early presbyope to delay the need for reading glasses.

Corneal procedures

PresbyLASIK

There are two main approaches to creating corneal multifocality with LASIK: central presbyLASIK and peripheral presbyLASIK. Peripheral presbyLASIK is dependent on increasing the range of pseudoaccommodation, whereas central presbyLASIK essentially creates a bifocal. Although higher-order aberrations are responsible for decreasing the quality of vision, they can increase the depth of focus to enhance near vision. The amount of aberration that is beneficial appears to vary from patient to patient.

In peripheral presbyLASIK, the depth of focus is increased by the ablation of the peripheral cornea inducing negative peripheral asphericity. In this procedure the center of the cornea is left for distance, whereas the peripheral cornea is for near. The presbyopic correction achieved with this ablation profile is significantly influenced by the pupil diameter. If the pupil dilates, as under night conditions, more of the area of the pupil is covered by near correction, and distance vision may be compromised. Conversely, if the pupil becomes miotic, the near-vision performance is reduced.

Central presbyLASIK involves the creation of a hyperpositive area for near vision in the central cornea, resulting in a surface that functions similar to a defractive multifocal IOL. This type of ablation profile is dependent on pupil size for the presbyopic correction. If the pupil constricts, then near vision is enhanced at the expense of distance vision. One of the main advantages of this technique is that less tissue has to be removed compared with the peripheral presbyLASIK technique.

Clinical outcomes for both peripheral as well as central presbyLASIK have demonstrated a high percentage of patients achieving 20/25 distance acuity and J2. Further studies are necessary to determine the long-term success of these techniques and to further evaluate the quality of vision under low-light and low-contrast conditions.

Corneal inlays (Table 32.1)

There have been many challenges over the years in the development of corneal inlays. A clinically successful corneal inlay must be thin, have a small diameter, provide adequate nutritional and fluid permeability, and be inserted relatively deep in the cornea under a flap or in a pocket. Impermeable intrastromal inlays can interfere with corneal metabolism and lead to overlying thinning. An adequate supply of glucose from the aqueous humor, anterior to the inlay, is critical to prevent anterior stromal necrosis. Superficial implantation can lead to abrupt surface curvature changes. Inlays also have the potential to be implanted in monofocal pseudophakic patients and postlaser vision correction patients who have become presbyopic.

The benefits of intrastromal corneal inlays for the treatment of presbyopia include potential reversibility, ease of implantation, and the potential advantage to combine them with other refractive procedures to allow the simultaneous correction of distance acuity. Early intrastromal corneal inlays had been complicated by corneal opacification, vascularization, keratolysis, and decentration. Advancements in corneal inlay technology have been secondary to materials with enhanced biocompatibility, femtosecond lasers that facilitate the creation of intrastromal pockets, and a better understanding of wound healing responses. The success of this technology depends on long-term studies that can demonstrate biocompatibility and excellent refractive outcomes.

KAMRA inlay (Acufocus)

The KAMRA corneal inlay (Figure 32.1) is designed to increase the depth of field in the implanted eye. The inlay can enhance near and intermediate vision without a significant effect on distance acuity. The current inlay design is 5 μm thick, has 8400 microperforations, a central aperture of 1.6 mm, and an overall diameter of 3.8 mm. Implantation can be combined with an excimer ablation to simultaneously address a refractive error and presbyopia. The inlay is implanted in the nondominant eye, either under a lamellar flap or in a pocket at a depth of 200 μm. The inlay is positioned over the line of sight or in cases in which there

Table 32.1 Summary of corneal inlays for presbyopia				
	KAMRA	**Raindrop**	**FlexiVue**	**ICOLENS**
Procedure	Modified monovision	Modified monovision	Modified monovision	Modified monovision
Principle of action	Increases depth of focus	Steepens anterior corneal curvature	Refractive index	Multifocal effect
Surgery	Pocket or flap	Flap	Pocket	Pocket
Stromal depth	200 μm	120 μm	280–300 μm	280–300 μm
Inlay thickness	5 μm	25 μm	15–20 μm	15 μm
Diameter	3.8 mm	2 mm	3.2 mm	3 mm
Transparency	No	Yes	Yes	Yes

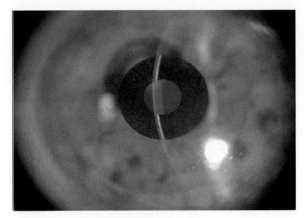

Figure 32.1 KAMRA corneal inlay.

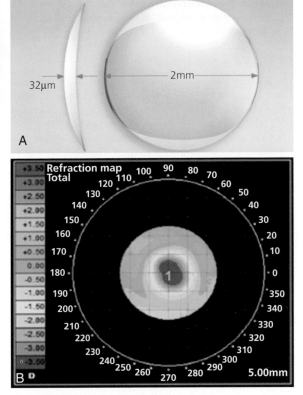

Figure 32.2 Raindrop corneal inlay. (A) Inlay size and profile. (B) Refractive map showing a central increase in corneal power.

is a significant deviation between the line of sight and the center of the pupil, an intermediate position is defined.

Seyeddain et al reported 2-year results with the KAMRA inlay in 32 eyes and found that 96.9% of patients could read J3 or better in the implanted eyes after 24 months. Yilmaz and colleagues reported 1-year data on 39 presbyopic patients in whom 12 were naturally ametropic and 27 had ametropia from previous hyperopic LASIK. Of the 39 inlays implanted, 3 were explanted during the study. At 1 year the mean uncorrected near visual acuity improved from J6 preoperatively to J1[+]. The mean uncorrected distance visual acuity in eyes with the inlay did not change significantly from preoperatively and remained 20/20 throughout the study period. All three eyes that had the inlay explanted returned to ±1.00 diopter of their preoperative refractive state for both near and distance visual acuity, with no loss of best-corrected distance visual acuity. Yilmaz et al reported 4-year results, and that all patients retained an improvement in near vision of two or more lines with no significant loss in distance vision.

Raindrop corneal inlay (revision optics)

The Raindrop inlay (Figure 32.2A) is intended to improve near and intermediate vision by changing the curvature of the cornea. The inlay steepens the central cornea for near vision and leaves the curvature of the more peripheral cornea unchanged for intermediate and distance vision (Figure 32.2B). The inlay has a diameter of 2 mm, a thickness of 25 μm, and is made of hydrogel plastic similar to that used for soft contact lenses. The Raindrop material has a refractive index and water content similar to that of the human cornea.

The inlay is inserted under either a LASIK flap or into a corneal pocket at a depth of approximately 130 to 150 μm in the nondominant eye. Distance acuity is minimally affected as light rays paracentral to the 2-mm inlay remain primarily focused on the retina, particularly with a middilated or dilated pupil. Pupil constriction creates a pseudoaccommodative effect using the steep and central cornea to focus light rays for near.

In 2010, Slade presented the visual performance of 30 emmetropic presbyopes. At 6 months, mean uncorrected near visual acuity of the treated eye was 20/25 and J1, corresponding to four lines of improvement. Uncorrected intermediate visual acuity in the treated eye improved to 20/25, corresponding to two lines of improvement. No patient lost two or more lines of corrected near or distance visual acuity. In a previous animal study, the implanted eyes remained clear without any reaction to the corneal inlay. Slit-lamp examination at 1 year revealed clear corneas, suggesting the inlay appeared to be inert.

FlexiVue microlens (Presbia)

The FlexiVue microlens is the only inlay using a refractive add power. The lens is made of a hydrophilic polymer, and has a diameter of 3.2 mm, and a thickness in the periphery of 15 μm. It is available in +1.5 to +3.5 diopter refractive powers. The inlay is inserted in the nondominant eye into a corneal pocket at a depth of 280 to 300 μm. In a study of 43 patients (average age 52 years) with a mean preoperative uncorrected distance acuity of 20/20 and mean uncorrected near acuity of 20/50, all patients had an increase in uncorrected near visual acuity after 1 week. By 1 year 93% of patients had an uncorrected near acuity of J2 or better.

ICOLENS inlay (Neoptics)

The ICOLENS is the newest corneal inlay in development and is designed to create a multifocal effect using a hydrophilic acrylic hydrogel. The lens combines a neutral central zone with a peripheral optical zone of 3.00 diopters. Similar to a multifocal IOL, this bifocal inlay delivers two simultaneous images onto the retina. The peripheral positive refractive power of the inlay provides near vision.

The ICOLENS has a diameter of 3 mm, an edge thickness of less than 15 μm, and a central hole of 0.15 mm to facilitate nutrient flow. It is made of a hydrophilic copolymer categorized as "hydrogel." The lens is a bifocal design, with a central zone for distance vision and a peripheral positive refractive zone for near vision. It is implanted in the nondominant eye with a pocket procedure.

In a study by Kohnen et al, 52 implants were performed and clinical results showed that 60% of patients gained two or more lines in near visual acuity and 34% gained three or more lines. A total of 52% of patients had no change in uncorrected distance visual acuity; 30% lost one or two lines; and no patient lost more than two lines. No corneal complications or adverse events occurred. Further clinical results will be documented to determine the long-term patient satisfaction and safety level.

Corneal intrastromal femtosecond laser treatment (INTRACOR procedure)

The INTRACOR procedure uses the femtosecond laser (VICTUS femtosecond laser platform) to create five concentric rings within the stroma to induce central corneal steepening in the correction of presbyopia. There are no incisions in the epithelium or Bowman's layer. The procedure takes approximately 15 to 20 seconds and starts in the center with a ring diameter of 1.8 mm with subsequent rings moving toward the periphery. The formation of these intrastromal rings produces a localized biomechanical change that reshapes the cornea to enhance near vision. The procedure is typically performed in the nondominant eye. Immediately following the procedure the intrastromal rings are clearly visible with slit-lamp examination, secondary to the cavitation gas bubbles from photodisruption. These gas bubbles disappear after a few hours, and within a few weeks the rings are barely visible.

This intrastromal femtosecond laser treatment was first described in 2009 by Ruiz and colleagues. By producing a series of intrastromal corneal ring incisions a multifocal cornea can be created. The hyperprolate central cornea can allow an improvement in near vision. Ruiz et al reported that at 6 months postoperatively all 83 (100%) eyes had improved uncorrected near visual acuity with

minimal or no change in uncorrected distance visual acuity. At 12 months, 22 eyes had an uncorrected near visual acuity, which had improved to J1. In addition, 2.4% of eyes lost two lines of corrected distance visual acuity at 6 months, but this did not occur in the 22 eyes seen at 1 year.

One-year data on 58 patients found that uncorrected near visual acuity improved by a mean of four lines. Further long-term study of a group of 25 patients, at 18 months' follow-up, showed the median gain of five lines of near vision and that corneal steepening remained stable during the follow-up period.

Although the majority of patients have shown distance refractive stability, the intrastromal femtosecond laser treatment has also showed significant side effects. Holzer et al, showed at 12 months, that 7.1% lost two or more lines of best corrected distance visual acuity, 11.5% lost two or more lines of best corrected near visual acuity, and 19.6% were not satisfied with the result.

The loss of best-corrected distance visual acuity is of significant concern with the INTRACOR procedure. Treatments should be used with extreme caution because the unwanted side effects may not be reversible. There is concern of a potential biomechanical disaster resulting in irregular astigmatism as a result of corneal instability, which occurred in the past with procedures like hexagonal keratotomy, automated lamellar keratoplasty, and radial keratotomy. Long-term data on the INTRACOR procedure are required to identify the risk of refractive instability, as well as the potential reduction in contrast sensitivity and increased night vision disturbances.

Monovision

Classic monovision

Monovision is a well-established procedure in refractive surgery. The limitations include loss of fusion as a result of anisometropia between the two eyes, poor intermediate vision, reduced binocular contrast sensitivity, and reduced stereoacuity. However, studies have demonstrated that many of these limitations can be avoided by limiting the anisometropia to 1.25 or 1.5 diopters. It is of interest that monovision induced by refractive surgery can be tolerated by a higher portion of patients (92%) than monovision induced by contact lenses (60%). It is unclear whether this may be related to problems with contact lens wear and tolerance.

The technique of monovision, in which the dominant eye is corrected for far vision and the nondominant eye is corrected for near vision, represents the earliest surgical attempt to deal with presbyopia. Monovision can be achieved by either corneal refractive surgery (LASIK or photorefractive keratotomy [PRK] monovision) or by a monofocal implant. Before monovision surgery, a preoperative spectacle or contact lens trial should be implemented to ensure that anisometropia could be tolerated. The success rate in pseudophakic patients is relatively high, varying from 64% to 100%. The main difficulties with the monovision technique are related to reduce stereopsis as a result of anisometropia, and blurred vision during night driving. A pair of glasses for night driving is helpful to allow improved visual function.

Laser-blended vision

Laser-blended vision is a technique that combines elements of monovision with increasing the depth of field. By increasing spherical aberration, the depth of field can be increased. A sophisticated excimer laser ablation profile is used to induce spherical aberration within a certain range to mitigate adversely affecting contrast sensitivity and quality of vision. Laser-blended vision is essentially a micromonovision technique that is performed monocularly. The technique has demonstrated satisfactory binocular fusion and functional stereoacuity compared with classic or traditional monovision. Reinstein et al demonstrated that 94% of myopes, 80% of hyperopes, and 92% of emmetropes see 20/25 and J2.

Intraocular procedures

IOL technology continues to advance with the development of multifocal and accommodating IOLs. Each IOL design has clear advantages and disadvantages. Preoperative assessment of the patient's personality and needs is critical to determine the success with IOL technology for presbyopia.

Multifocal IOLs

The goal of a multifocal presbyopia-correcting IOL is to provide spectacle independence with satisfactory distance, intermediate, and near vision. Multifocal IOLs have demonstrated a number of advantages including spectacle independence, good near and improved intermediate acuity, depth of field, easy implantation, and long-term capsular bag stability; also with neuroadaptation, the symptoms of glare and halos tend to improve. The potential disadvantages of multifocal IOLs include limited intermediate vision, reduced contract sensitivity compared with accommodating and monofocal lenses, pupil size and centration dependency, and glare and halos; unhappy patients may require explanation of the IOL. In several studies, more than 90% of patients would choose to have the same IOL implanted again. For dissatisfied patients, the cause could typically be identified and effective treatment taken in most cases. Compared with accommodative IOLs, reduced contrast sensitivity may limit multifocal IOLs in some patients who perform low-light activities. Glare and halos may be less prevalent with the newer aspheric designs.

Multifocal IOLs are designed to have multiple focal points that create multiple images at different focal lengths. Patients tend to perceive only the focused image of interest. Multifocal IOLs can be divided into refractive and defractive lenses.

Patient selection is critical to achieve success because multifocal implants typically result in reduced contrast sensitivity and may cause dysphotopic phenomena, such as glare, halos, and problems with night vision. Patients who have epithelial basement membrane dystrophy and any macular disease, such as age-related macular degeneration or epiretinal membrane, should be discouraged from having a multifocal implant. High hyperopes might face difficulties because of the large positive angle kappa that can result in multifocal intolerance. Patients who receive multifocal implants must be aware that neuroadaptation to the newly created vision might take up to 6 months.

Defractive multifocal IOLs

Defractive multifocal IOLs use defractive zones, or microscopic steps across the lens surface. As light encounters these steps, it is directed toward near and distance focal points. The amount of light directed to the near focal point is directly related to the step height, as a proportion of wavelength. At a step height of one wavelength, all light is directed to the near focal point. Similarly, a step height that is a smaller proportion of the wavelength directs more light particles to the distance focal point. These underlying principles are important in understanding the design differences of the two types of defractive multifocal IOLs, apodized or nonapodized.

Apodized defractive multifocal IOLs

An apodized lens has a gradual reduction in defractive step heights from the center to the periphery. As a consequence, as pupil size increases, more defractive zones with smaller step heights are exposed and direct a larger portion of light rays to the distant focal points. In theory, this design allows enhanced distance vision in low-light situations, such as driving at night. The Restor implant has an apodized defractive optic zone centrally and a refractive peripheral zone (Figure 32.3). This regional zone difference favors distance vision under mesopic conditions. The Restor lens is available in a +3.0 model, which provides +2.25 to +2.50 diopters at the spectacle plane, and a +2.5 model, which provides +1.75 to +2.25 diopters at the spectacle plane. The Restor +2.5 distributes more light for distance vision, has fewer diffractive zones, a larger central refractive zone, and a focal point that is about 0.50 diopter farther out than the Restor +3.0. Because visual function is dependent on pupil size for both Restor implants, satisfactory reading requires sufficient light to produce a relatively small pupil.

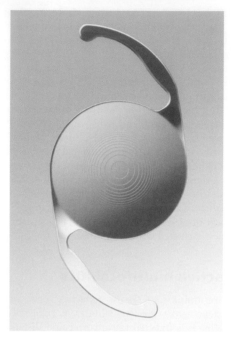

Figure 32.3 Restor implant, an apodized defractive multifocal intraocular lens (IOL).
(Courtesy of Alcon, Canada.)

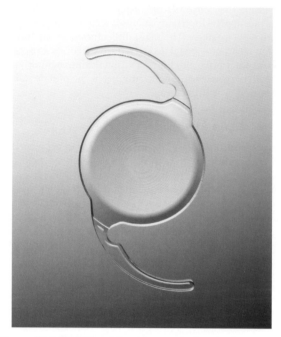

Figure 32.4 TECNIS multifocal intraocular lens (IOL), a nonapodized multifocal IOL.
(Courtesy of AMO, Canada.)

Nonapodized defractive multifocal IOLs

Nonapodized defractive IOLs are designed with defractive steps that have a uniform height from the periphery to the center, which results in an equal amount of light to near and distance foci for all pupil diameters. The two examples of the nonapodized multifocal IOLs are the TECNIS multifocal IOL (AMO, Figure 32.4) and the AT LISA 809 IOL (Carl Zeiss Meditec, Germany). Unlike the Restor implant, the TECNIS multifocal features nonapodized defractive steps on the posterior surface of the lens. The AT LISA 809 IOL, although nonapodized, does direct light asymmetrically to the two focal points, in favor of distance vision.

Rotationally asymmetric multifocal IOLs

Unlike the refractive and defractive IOLs, which are designed with rotational symmetry, a new category of IOLs uses the concept of rotational asymmetry. One such lens—the LENTIS Mplus (Oculentis, Figure 32.5)—consists of a near section add that makes the IOL independent of pupil sizes greater than 2 mm. It is a single-piece, square-edge implant composed of a hydrophilic material and is available with a +3.0 or +1.5 diopter add.

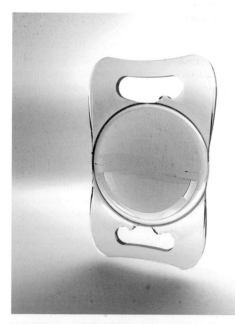

Figure 32.5 LENTIS Mplus intraocular lens (IOL), a rotationally asymmetric multifocal IOL.
(Courtesy of Clarion, Canada.)

Table 32.2 Multifocal and accommodating IOLs in Canada

	Type	Regulatory status in Canada	Contrast sensitivity
Restor +3 diopters (D)	Multifocal	Approved	Decreased
Restor +2.5 D	Multifocal	Approved	Slight decrease
TECNIS Multifocal	Multifocal	Approved	Decreased
AT LISA	Multifocal	Special access	Decreased
Mplus 3.0 D	Asymmetric multifocal	Approved	Not significantly affected
Mplus 1.5 D	Asymmetric multifocal	Approved	Not affected
FineVision	Asymmetric multifocal	Special access	Slight decrease
Crystalens	Accommodating	Approved	Not affected
Synchrony	Accommodating	Special access	Not affected
FluidVision	Accommodating	Research stage	Not affected
AutoFocal	Accommodating	Research stage	Not affected

Accommodating IOLs (Table 32.2)

There are two designs of accommodating IOLs: one with a single-optic and the other with a dual-optic system. Single-optic accommodative IOLs are designed to alter the focal length of the IOL eye optical system, based on the anterior movement of the lens and changes in lens architecture. The dual-optic accommodating IOL is designed based on the concept of not only axial movement, but also changing the power of the implant, which changes in position.

The Crystalens accommodating IOL (Bausch & Lomb) is a single-optic lens that features flexible hinges at the plate style haptic to facilitate anterior movement of the lens. Clinical trials have reported approximately one diopter of accommodation, although the mechanism has been controversial. Clinical outcomes have demonstrated that 88% of patients have achieved 20/40 vision or better for their distance, intermediate, and near vision, compared with 36% using the standard IOL. It has been suggested that one mechanism to account for the observed accommodation or pseudoaccommodation is flexing of the optic itself, as is seen during accommodation of the natural crystalline lens.

A dual-optic accommodating IOL uses two lenses, one of high power and one of negative power, typically with a higher-power lens anterior and the negative power lens posterior. An example is the Synchrony IOL, which is designed with a +32.0 diopter front optic connected by spring haptics to a posterior optic of variable negative power. Clinical trials have demonstrated a mean accommodative range of 3.22 ± 0.88 diopters. Synchrony requires a 3.7-mm incision that can induce postoperative astigmatism.

A few new accommodative implants are under development. The FluidVision lens (PowerVision) relies on liquid to make accommodative changes. By virtue of the natural human physiologic contraction and relaxation of the ciliary muscle, the fluid internal to the implant allows changes in shape like our pliable crystalline lens, before the onset of presbyopia. The implant is acrylic, filled with silicone oil. As the ciliary body muscle contracts and relaxes, forces are conveyed through the zonules and the capsule to the implant, and the fluid in the haptics is pushed into the optic, causing the anterior curvature of the optic to increase. As the ciliary body relaxes, the zonules are put on stretch and fluid goes back out to the haptic. In 2010 a nonfoldable prototype of the lens was implanted in 14 sighted eyes in South Africa. An average of 5.00 diopters of accommodative amplitude was documented. In April 2013, a foldable version of the lens was implanted in four eyes but data are not currently available.

Another prototype implant is the electro-active Sapphire AutoFocal IOL, which may offer patients the full range of vision. This implant is an electromechanical lens with a microscopic battery inside that stimulates the optic to change shape when it senses accommodation. As the pupil changes size and becomes smaller, the liquid crystals inside the lens stimulated by electromechanical impulses result in a change in the refractive lens to provide 3.00 diopters of reading. This implant does not rely on the muscles in the eye functioning and capsular bag contraction or hardening to be effective. This technology is in early development and will be undergoing an animal study in the near future.

Femtosecond laser photodisruption of the crystalline lens

Femtosecond laser technology is revolutionizing ophthalmic surgery by its capability of providing ultrashort laser pulses to a focal point without interacting with the

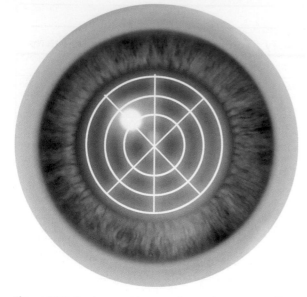

Figure 32.6 Femtosecond laser can be used to cut crystalline lens fibers in the midperiphery to restore accommodation.

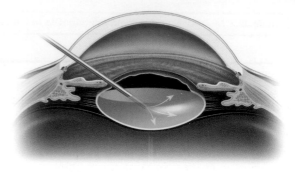

Figure 32.7 Extraction of lens followed by refilling of capsular bag with an injectable substance.

surrounding transparent ocular tissues or causing collateral damage. This laser has the potential to precisely treat the crystalline lens in a noninvasive procedure that could restore elasticity to the lens (Figure 32.6). The idea of enhancing accommodation with a femtosecond laser to soften a hard nucleus was first introduced in 1998. The cutting inside the lens could be achieved by the effect of photodisruption, whereby localized laser-induced plasma is formed, followed by a shockwave and a cavitation bubble. The idea was to increase the flexibility of the lens and hence restore accommodative amplitude. After initial experiments in vitro and safety studies in vivo, a clinical study was initiated to demonstrate the safety and effectiveness of the procedure. A clinical study performed in the Philippines in 2011, with a 2-year follow-up, showed less than 1.00 diopter of accommodation. This minimal average change suggests that the early treatments had femtosecond spot patterns that were ineffective and require further investigation to determine the ideal laser pattern. The safety of the procedure was documented, showing no progressive cataract formation. The lack of clinical efficacy in the first living human eyes treated with an ultrashort pulse laser suggests that the proper geometric pattern of laser pulses and total energy have not yet been determined. Further clinical studies have been initiated with refined algorithms, and outcomes will be reported in the near future.

Lens refilling

An ideal option to restore accommodation would be a lens-refilling procedure (Figure 32.7). An injectable material would replace the nucleus and cortex of the crystalline lens

in the presence of a functioning ciliary muscle and capsular and zonular integrity. An ideal lens-refilling procedure would create an ametropic eye, result in increasing accommodative amplitude, and be viable for several decades. The concept was mentioned in 1964 by Kessler, who suggested that after the removal of a relatively rigid presbyopic crystalline lens that the lens capsule might be refilled. The refilled capsule would have the potential to restore accommodation by mimicking the mechanical properties of the youthful natural lens. Exploratory studies have shown that the accommodative amplitude decreases significantly with capsule fibrosis, suggesting that capsule elasticity is critical in the accommodative mechanism. It also has been demonstrated that the volume of the injected material is important to determine the postoperative refraction in vivo animal lens-refilling studies. The development of capsular fibrosis was seen as a major obstacle in achieving a successful lens-refilling procedure. Attempts to eradicate regeneration of equatorial lens epithelial cells during surgery have not yet been fully successful; therefore, lens-refilling techniques are unproven to date for the long-term restoration of accommodation.

SUMMARY

The prevention or reversal of hardening of the crystalline lens would be an ideal approach to maintain or restore accommodation. Unfortunately, this is not a viable therapeutic option. Many different surgical procedures have been developed in recent years to allow near vision. These procedures include surgery on the sclera, the cornea, or the crystalline lens. The most common surgical options include monovision LASIK, monovision lens exchange, corneal inlays, presbyLASIK, and multifocal or accommodative lens implants. All refractive and cataract patients should understand the advantages and disadvantages of the various presbyopic procedures. Although technology will continue to advance, there are real clinical benefits to the presbyopic options that can be offered today.

REFERENCES

1. Aristotle. Problems. Cambridge, Mass: Harvard University Press; 1957.

2. Smyth AH. The writings of Benjamin Franklin. New York: Macmillan; 1905.

3. Mathews S. Scleral expansion surgery does not restore accommodation in human presbyopia. Ophthalmology 1999;106(5):873–7.

4. Malecaze FJ, Gazagne CS, Tarroux MC, Gorrand JM. Scleral expansion bands for presbyopia. Ophthalmology 2001;108 (12):2165–71.

5. Pepose JS, Mujtaba AQ, Shuster JJ. Implantation of sclera expansion band segments for the treatment of presbyopia. Am J Ophthalmol 2002;134:808–15.

6. Hipsley AM. Laser ACE procedure for presbyopia, In: Paper presented at ASCRS annual meeting, Symposium on Cataract, IOL and Refractive Surgery; March 27, 2011 San Diego, CA.

7. El Danasoury AM, Gamaly TO, Hantera M. Multizone LASIK with peripheral near zone for correction of presbyopia in myopic and hyperopic eyes: 1-year results. J Refract Surg 2009;25:296–305.

8. Telandro A. The pseudoaccommodative cornea multifocal ablation with a center-distance pattern: a review. J Refract Surg 2009;25:S156–9.

9. Pinelli R, Ortiz D, Simonetto A, Bacchi C, Sala E, Alio JL. Correction of presbyopia in hyperopia with a center-distance, paracentral-near technique using the Technolas 217z platform. J Refract Surg 2008;24:494–500.

10. Jackson WB, Tuan KM, Mintsioulis G. Aspheric wavefront-guided LASIK to treat hyperopic presbyopia: 12-month results with the VISX platform. J Refract Surg 2011;27:519–29.

11. Seyeddain O, Riha W, Hohensinn M, et al. Refractive surgical correction of presbyopia with the AcuFocus small aperture corneal inlay: two-year follow-up. J Refract Surg 2010;26:707–15.

12. Slade ST. Early results using the PresbyLens corneal inlay to improve near and intermediate vision in emmetropic presbyopes, In: Paper presented at European Society of Cataract & Refractive Surgery annual meeting; September 2010 Paris, France.

13. Pallikaris IG, Bouzoukis DI, Kymionis GD, et al. Visual outcomes and safety of a small diameter intrastromal refractive inlay for the corneal compensation of presbyopia. J Refract Surg 2012;28:168–73.

14. Guedj T, Danan A, Lebuisson DA. In-vivo architectural analysis of intrastromal incisions after INTRACOR surgery using Fourier-domain OCT and Scheimpflug imaging. J Emmetropia 2011;2:85–91.

15. Holzer MP, Menassa N, Fitting A, et al. Visual outcomes and corneal changes after intrastromal femtosecond laser correction of presbyopia. J Cataract Refract Surg 2012;38:765–73.

16. JCox C, Krueger R. Monovision with laser correction. Ophthalmol Clin North Am 2006;19:71–5.

17. Reinstein DZ, Archer TJ, Gobbe M. LASIK for myopic astigmatism and presbyopia using non-linear aspheric micro-monovision with the Carl Zeiss Meditec MEL 80 platform. J Refract Surg 2011;27(1):23–37.

18. Reinstein DZ, Archer TJ, Gobbe M. Aspheric ablation profile for presbyopic corneal treatment using the MEL 80 and CRS-Master laser blended vision module. J Emmetropia 2011;2:161–75.

19. Gooi P, Ahmed IK. Review of presbyopic IOLs: multifocal and accommodating IOLs. Int Ophthalmol Clin 2012;52:41–50.

20. Gooi P, Ahmed IK. Review of presbyopic IOLs: multifocal and accommodating IOLs. Int Ophthalmol Clin 2012;52:41–50.

21. Davison JA, Simpson MJ. History and development of the apodized diffractive intraocular lens. J Cataract Refract Surg 2006;32:849–58.

22. McAlinden C, Moore JE. Multifocal intraocular lens with a surface-embedded near section: short-term clinical outcomes. J Cataract Refract Surg 2011;37:441–5.

23. Gatinel D, Pagnoulle C, Houbrechts Y, et al. Design and qualification of a diffractive trifocal optical profile for intraocular lenses. J Cataract Refract Surg 2011;37:2060–7.

24. Cumming JS, Colvard DM, Dell SJ, et al. Clinical evaluation of the Crystalens AT-45 accommodating intraocular lens: results of the US Food and Drug Administration clinical trial. J Cataract Refract Surg 2006;32:812–25.

25. McLeod SD, Vargas LG, Portney V, et al. Synchrony dual-optic accommodating intraocular lens. Part 1: optical and biomechanical principles and design considerations. J Cataract Refract Surg 2007;33:37–46.

26. Donnenfeld E. An "autofocal" accommodating IOL. Cataract and Refractive Surgery Today 2013;13:73–6.

27. Myers RL, Krueger RR. Novel approaches to correction of presbyopia with laser modification of the crystalline lens. J Refract Surg 1998;14(2):136–9.

28. Nishi Y, Mireskandari K, Khaw P, Findl O. Lens refilling to restore accommodation. J Cataract Refract Surg 2009;35:374–82.

Chapter | 33 |

Assisting the surgeon

Most surgical procedures for the eye are performed on an outpatient basis. However, some procedures (e.g., retinal surgery, high-risk patients, cardiac surgery) are still performed in the hospital. This chapter highlights those patients who are admitted. Chapter 35 covers ambulatory or outpatient surgery.

BEDSIDE OPHTHALMIC ASSISTANT

One of our most important senses is that of sight. A blind or partially sighted individual is considerably impaired in the ability to move about freely, perform work, and function effectively. Daily living is seriously jeopardized. Consequently, any threat of loss or impairment of these abilities is a threat to an individual's independence.

Without sight, no longer can drivers drive their cars, pilots fly their planes, or surgeons perform their work. Because of the consequences of blindness and the fear associated with this threat, the nursing care of patients with eye disorders demands extraordinary skill.

The background for ophthalmic nursing requires a good understanding of people and their management. Psychologic problems induced by the emotional havoc created by the threat of losing one's vision must be dealt with effectively. Ophthalmic assistants interested in eye nursing will become involved in these emotional reactions.

General nurses are expected to increase their knowledge of the eye and eye disorders. They must become familiar with the terminology and acquainted with various diagnostic tests and surgical procedures. They also must become aware of the relationship between disease of the eye and disease of the body. A gentle touch and fine dexterity are prerequisites in caring for patients, particularly when administering eye medications and treating eyes that have undergone recent surgery. Nurses must move about quietly in the rooms of such patients, not dash into the room, bump into beds or chairs, or in any way startle patients who could become alarmed because they cannot see anyone's movements. Ophthalmic nursing is essentially "quiet" nursing. The successful restoration or, indeed, improvement in eyesight often provides a stimulating and rewarding experience for ophthalmic nurses.

Visually impaired patient

Blindness is considered to be a total lack of vision or vision insufficient to conduct the ordinary activities of life. It is defined as a central visual acuity of 20/200 or less in the better eye with corrective glasses or a field defect in which the peripheral field is contracted to such an extent that the widest diameter of the visual field subtends an angle not greater than 20 degrees.

With both these limitations, a person is *economically* blind. A vast majority of the blind are in the group just below this threshold. Some are able to read newspaper headlines and some can identify distant objects. They may see light in various directions – in the corridors and the windows and in the streets. Only in the most severe form is the blind person completely devoid of any light sensation.

Some blind patients live in false hope of a possible cure and refuse to adjust to their decrease in vision. Others withdraw from society and lean heavily on their visual defect. They no longer face the normal problems of daily living and become dependent on others to relieve them of their responsibilities. These blind individuals may find comfort because they do not encounter failures and disappointments and are freed from judgment and condemnation by others. Others again recognize that their visual impairment imposes limitations on their way of life. They have difficulty in accepting their disability and become aggressive and angry in their behavior, and this anger is often reflected toward others. Some adjust realistically; they measure what assets they have and use their resources positively, thereby maintaining a degree of independence. They constantly work toward making life worthwhile for themselves and those with whom they are in contact.

When a patient with poor vision arrives in the hospital, the nurse must evaluate the patient's degree of acceptance of visual impairment in terms of physical ability and psychologic dependence. The patient who denies existence of the disability and withdraws from society needs to be brought back to reality and to develop meaningful relationships with others. Gradual motivation can be instilled so that the patient eventually will assume a degree of responsibility for self-care. When confronting a patient who is aggressive and hostile because of the impairment, the nurse should establish communication so that the patient feels free to voice negative feelings about his or her limitations.

Patient orientation

When a partially sighted or blind patient has to be admitted to a hospital or surgicenter, there should be a structured system of orienting the patient to the environment. The nurse should greet the patient warmly, addressing the person by name, and rapidly clarify the nurse's position in the hospital setting. It is important that patients know to whom they are talking, who will take care of them, and what hospital personnel will do for them. Often shaking the patient's hand and touching an arm provide a feeling of welcome. The ophthalmic nurse should observe the patient's movements to decide what type of help the individual requires. Patients who walk slowly and hesitantly, with body bent forward and arms extended to find certain guiding objects, may require a great deal of assistance and orientation.

Patients with normal vision in one eye but impaired vision in the other eye have little difficulty adjusting to the hospital environment and need little orientation. Partially sighted people with impaired vision are usually aided by bright lights, such as corridor and window lights. Consequently, rooms and corridors should be kept well lit before eye surgery, and hospital design should allow for this level of increased illumination.

The partially sighted individual who is being escorted should be permitted to take the assistant's arm lightly above the elbow. This automatically places the patient a step behind the guide, which provides protection and the ability to feel slight movements and to anticipate directional changes. An individual should never be pushed or steered. Any stairs, ramps, or surface changes should be indicated and described so that footing adjustments can be made. While walking with the patient, the assistant should engage in conversation and give a description of the surroundings. The assistant should also orientate a blind person to the room and the bathroom by having the person move about, touch the furniture and equipment, and become familiar with his or her location. These objects should be kept in a fixed location so that the patient may use them as landmarks.

Many patients and parents of children undergoing surgery will ask the hospital assistant questions they have been hesitant to ask the ophthalmologist. The assistant must be sure to say the right thing with tact and diplomacy and in a quiet authoritative manner, speaking in lay terms that are readily understandable and not shocking. For example, the parents should not be told that their child is crosseyed and requires sight-saving surgery. It is more tactful to state that the child requires the surgery to correct the eyes' tendency to turn and that surgery offers the best treatment for a permanent correction. It even helps to reassure the parents by telling them that the procedure is simple and painless and requires only a short recuperation period.

Children, in particular, enter the hospital with a fair degree of apprehension. Basically they want to like and trust the people they meet, but they are afraid of the unknown, the atmosphere, the strange uniforms, the instruments, and the worry about needles. Usually a sincere smile, a soft voice, and a warm greeting will break the ice.

The ophthalmic assistant

The ophthalmic assistant can play a greater role in helping patients understand the disorder and what should be expected during both minor and major surgery.

Assistants may choose to review pictures or videos. Certification of the assistant becomes of value, not only for professional reasons but also developing greater communication and trust with the patient and a stronger understanding of ocular diseases and disorders.

The assistant can be invaluable in handling calls from pharmacists and opticians on prescriptions. They can provide indigent patients with samples and direct others to more inexpensive quality opticians and pharmacists.

Preoperative preparation

Before surgery the ophthalmic nurse should review with the patient the type of surgery that is about to be performed and what is expected of the patient to promote the success of the operation. This approach considerably lessens the patient's anxieties and elicits postoperative cooperation. Even though basic information has been given to the patient by the ophthalmologist, securing the patient's confidence helps the development of a good nurse–patient relationship, which promotes the patient's recovery.

For those procedures performed under local anesthesia, the patient should be instructed in deep breathing and movement of the limbs to encourage circulation. Older adults tend to lie rigidly in the same position for prolonged periods, fearful of movement. The voluntary movement of limbs and chest muscles greatly lessens respiratory difficulties postoperatively.

Patients also should be instructed that coughing, sneezing, and squeezing the eyelids may have a detrimental effect on the operation. Bowel evacuants are often used the night before surgery so that abdominal discomfort is relieved and harmful straining after surgery is eliminated.

If the patient has never had eyedrops instilled, it is appropriate for the ophthalmic nurse to provide instructions regarding the procedure and the purpose of medication before surgery so that undue squeezing of the eyes after medication is avoided. Ophthalmic nurses will probably be responsible for administering eye ointments and solutions and it is important that they take extreme care in administering these medications. The eyes are especially sensitive after surgery, and any abrupt manipulation will cause discomfort and squeezing, which endangers the eye. Hands should be washed before instilling drops. The dropper tip should not touch the eyelashes. The head should be tilted back, the patient asked to look up and the lower eyelid pulled down. The drop is then instilled in the lower fornix (see Figure 4.3). Topical anesthetic drops, however, are placed in the eye with the patient looking down and the solution directed to the 12 o'clock area of the sclera near the limbus. This permits the drop to run down over the cornea, where it produces maximal anesthesia.

Patients should be advised that whether they have local or general anesthesia, they will feel little discomfort during or after surgery. Some patients are very concerned that they will see everything during the operation and must be reassured that this is not so.

Postoperative care

When the patient has returned from the operating room to the bed or chair, gentleness is of the utmost importance. After intraocular procedures the patient should exercise caution and avoid rapid head movements. To prevent dislodging the eye dressing or pressing the eye bandage into the pillow and thereby injuring the eye, the patient should avoid lying on the side that has had surgery. The patient must be reminded to refrain from touching or disturbing the eye dressings so as to prevent any self-inflicted injury or infection. With older adults, during sleep, the assistant may put loose restraints on the wrists as a reminder for the sleeping patient not to touch the eye dressing.

After retinal detachment operations, the head of the bed often is placed in the position that is most beneficial for securing the reattachment. For some of these patients a considerable amount of encouragement is necessary, and every effort should be made to ensure that the patient avoids exertion or strain in the immediate postoperative period. For surgery that is not intraocular, such as for strabismus or eyelid repair, limitations seldom are placed on the patient's activity. For small-incision intraocular surgery, many of these safeguards are being abandoned.

The hospital atmosphere should be quiet and subdued. We recommend blackout drapes in each room so that the drapes may be drawn if the patient is photosensitive, as so often occurs after an eye operation. This often is caused by a low-grade iritis or a dilated pupil. The nurse should be on guard for signs of restlessness or confusion in the patient. Some patients undergo behavioral changes and may even have hallucinations. We are all dependent on sensory input from exposure to the world about us. The patient who suddenly loses the sense of sight because of a bandage often feels isolated from the environment and becomes disoriented. This creates a state of confusion, and disturbing illusions may occur. Any changes of this sort require a watchful nurse who constantly communicates with the patient and tries to effect relaxation and a return to reality. Radios may help in giving the patient this contact with reality through the auditory sense.

If nausea or vomiting occurs in the immediate postoperative period, adequate medication must be given immediately for relief. Often a light, often liquid, diet is ordered for the day of surgery as prevention. Foods should be sufficiently low in residue so that they require only a minimum amount of chewing and are not constipating. The physician's orders must be carefully followed and order abbreviations must be well known (Table 33.1).

Sometime before the first eye dressing, the patient should be made aware that removal of the bandage does not immediately result in clear vision. No matter what the surgery, it takes time for the process of healing to occur and for the final vision to be obtained.

Alarming postoperative signs and symptoms

The ophthalmic nurse undertaking the immediate postoperative treatments for eye patients should be on the watch for unusual ocular signs that indicate untoward complications. Any hemorrhage in the anterior chamber should be noted and the attending physician informed. Unusual pain may be accompanied by a prolapse of the iris, in which a knuckle of iris protrudes from the wound incision; this is an alarming sign and requires immediate attention. However, this is rare today with smaller incisions. The presence of a flat anterior chamber that has not re-formed, or one that has suddenly occurred, should be noted.

Table 33.1 Hospital chart abbreviations

Abbreviation	Meaning	Abbreviation	Meaning
aa	of each	mg	milligram
ac	before meals	non rep	do not repeat
ad lib	as desired	ocul	eye
amp	ampule	od	right eye
bid	twice a day	os	left eye
c or cum	with	ou	each eye
caps	capsule	pc	after meals
cc	cubic centimeter	po	by mouth
collyr	eyewash	prn	as needed
dr	dram	qh	every hour
g	gram	qid	four times a day
gr	grain	qs	sufficient quantity
gt	drop	s	without
hs	at bedtime	ss	half
ic	between meals	stat	immediately
IM	intramuscular	tab	tablet
IV	intravenous	tid	three times a day
lot	lotion	ung	ointment

Any evidence of small amounts of whitish material in the lower portion of the anterior chamber is an ominous sign and should be brought to the attention of the ophthalmologist immediately. It indicates a developing hypopyon, which may arise from an intraocular infection. If accompanied by severe pain, it is even more ominous and should be brought to the immediate attention of the surgeon or doctor on call.

Marked swelling of the eyelids combined with excoriation of the skin should be noted. This is a common sign of allergy to the medication that is being introduced or of an infection that may be starting. Unusual complaints of pain in the immediate postoperative period should be quickly brought to the attention of the ophthalmologist because occasionally wound rupture or infection does occur, which is marked by severe pain. Evidence of a purulent discharge postoperatively is a warning sign.

Instructions to patient on discharge

When the patient is discharged from the hospital, or even if an outpatient, he or she should be given instructions that will ensure the continuing success of the eye surgery. Eyes that have had surgery require cautious care for the first few weeks after operation (Box 33.1).

Each ophthalmologist has specific individual methods of dealing with patients. The physician's input is most important in giving directions to patients. Typed discharge instructions similar to those in Box 33.1 are helpful.

OPERATING ROOM ASSISTANT

Many ophthalmic assistants working in offices and clinics have the privilege of accompanying the ophthalmologist to the operating room. Here a new challenge awaits.

The drama of the operating room, the exactness, care, and detail required in eye surgery and the satisfaction resulting from a successful procedure instill a sense of accomplishment in the assistant at the end of each operating period. Here the operating room assistant is expected to fulfill his or her role with the utmost gentleness, care, and attention.

The ophthalmic nurse probably will be responsible for the selection, care, handling, and sterilization of the many ophthalmic instruments required. A meticulous scrub and gown routine must be followed. One should be exceptionally careful that the exact sterile technique in scrubbing, gowning, and draping in the operating room is not broken

---

Box 33.1 Directions for patients leaving the hospital after cataract surgery

Your wound is healing, but it will not be firm enough to stand much pressure. You may feel that something is in your eye. This is because of the stitches or the incision. This feeling will go away.

1. Continue to be careful.
2. Avoid closing the eyes tightly. One often closes the eyes tightly when laughing, talking, sneezing, coughing or yawning, or if irritated. At these times you should be particularly careful not to close your eyes tightly. Never rub or touch the eye.
3. Avoid stooping, straining, lifting, and bending over.
4. If there is much secretion then wipe off the lids with cotton, but avoid exerting pressure on the eye, particularly the upper lid.
5. You will be given drops to use in your eye. Please follow these directions carefully. When the drops are gone, fill your prescription and use those drops.

How to instill drops

a. Wash your hands thoroughly before and after putting in eyedrops and ointments.
b. Clean the edges of your eyelids, using a clean cotton ball or washcloth that has been moistened with tap water. Do not press on the upper lid.
c. Pull your lower lid down with one hand, forming a pouch. Look up.
d. Put one drop of medicine in the pouch. Do not touch the tip of the bottle to your lid, eyelashes, or any other place.
e. Close your eye for 1 full minute after each drop.
f. If you find the preceding difficult, lie on the bed and repeat the instructions while looking up at the dropper.
g. Never use eyedrops that are more than 2 months old. Discard them.

6. You may watch television and read.
7. You may go outdoors for a walk or drive. It is not necessary to cover the eye, but it is preferable to shield it from bright sunlight by wearing sunglasses with ultraviolet protection.
8. You may wash your hair 1 week after surgery, but do not get soapy water in your eye.
9. Mild pain and discomfort may be relieved by aspirin. If there is more severe pain, please contact us.
10. You may have the feeling of something in the eye because of the incision, but do not close it tightly. This feeling may persist for a few weeks.
11. Glasses or contact lens may be prescribed when the eye is fully healed and the prescription is stable.

---

by any member of the team, lest an infection develop that not only may cause irreparable damage but also result in blindness and even removal of the eye itself (Figure 33.1).

The use of powderless gloves has been a major help in reducing airborne particles.

The operating room must be quiet except for background music; CD players or tapes are helpful. Sudden loud noises might make the patient move unexpectedly and endanger the eye. All those who assist the ophthalmologist must ensure that the environment is pleasant and quiet from the time the patient is brought into the room until he or she leaves. Personal talk such as politics, vacation, sports, and other patients should be avoided.

Aseptic technique in the operating room

Although surgery has been practiced since ancient times, the practice of asepsis is recent. As long ago as 3000 BCE, Egyptians bored holes in skulls to let evil spirits out. Even in 700 BCE, the Hindus performed cataract and eyelid surgery. Those who performed the surgery learned to keep their fingernails short, take daily baths, and wear white clothing. It was only in the 19th century that Joseph Lister introduced modern surgical aseptic techniques. Lister recognized that results of surgery improved

tenfold if microorganisms could be kept out of the wound. Thus many methods of sterilization of instruments and preparations for cleansing and disinfecting the skin came into being, until today's modern methods were attained. Aseptic technique is discussed in Chapter 29. Strict adherence to the principles of instrument sterilization, skin disinfection, and eye preparation is essential to eliminate ocular infections, which can be visually devastating (Box 33.2).

Routine procedure for the operating room assistant

Before scrubbing

Assistants must know the operative procedure well, even if it requires additional reading for them to become familiar with the technique. There should be a regularly updated card or page listing the surgeon's preferences in instruments, sutures, and preparation of the patient. Assistants should question other operating room personnel who have worked with the surgeon to understand his or her special variations. If all are unfamiliar with the procedure, assistants should not hesitate to contact the surgeon a day or two before surgery to ensure that all necessary equipment is available.

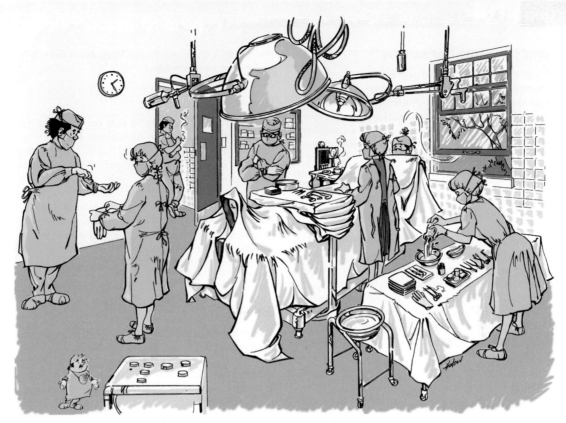

Figure 33.1 Errors in aseptic techniques. Identify all errors of aseptic technique.

Box 33.2 **Some common errors in aseptic surgical techniques (see Figure 33.1)**

Masks and caps

1. Mask covering only the mouth and not the nose
2. Mask tied too loosely
3. Hair permitted to protrude from the cap

Scrub

1. Fingernails too long (should not exceed 1 mm)
2. Allowing the runoff to drip from the hands, thus contaminating them (runoff should be from the elbow)
3. Too short a scrub time
4. Failing to develop a systematic scrub routine and thus leaving bare spots
5. Splashing the clothes, thus contaminating sterile gown later

Drying

1. Using wet section of towel to dry upper arms, thus contaminating dry fingers
2. Allowing towel to touch unsterile clothing

Gowning

1. Allowing gown to become contaminated by the hands or other unsterile objects
2. Allowing gown to touch unsterile objects by walking about the room

Powdering hands

1. Dispensing powder from the hands into the air
2. Not carefully cleansing powder from outside of gloves

Gloves

1. Touching outer portion of glove
2. Failing to detect perforations or breaks in the glove
3. Holding hands against the body while waiting

Skin preparation

1. Believing the manufacturer's claim for the product; check it out
2. Relying on aqueous antiseptics
3. Failing to realize that quaternary ammonium compounds (Zephiran) may be neutralized by even small traces of soap
4. In applying antiseptics, going back and forth from clean to contaminated areas and back to the clean area again (instead, ever-widening circles should be made, starting from the eyelid margin)
5. Forgetting to prepare the eyelashes, the eyelid margin, or the eyebrows

Bringing the patient to surgery

The patient should be as relaxed as possible. A cheerful but quiet manner will provide an atmosphere of relaxation. Assistants should try to instill optimism and confidence in patients and should be particular to point out that everything will go well. They should always express confidence in the skill of the surgeon. It has been our habit to play soft music in the operating room throughout the procedure to ensure relaxation. Coming to the operating room for surgery is a unique and often terrifying experience for the patient. Each patient should be treated as if he or she were the only one and not one of many who pass through each day.

Cutting the eyelashes is not routinely performed for all procedures and may be abandoned by many surgeons since the advent of newer draping techniques. However, when it is necessary, the eyelashes should be cut before skin preparation. A thin film of ointment is placed on the cutting edge of an eyelash scissors so that the free lashes will adhere to the blades and be prevented from falling into the eye. The patient should be reassured that the lashes will rapidly regrow.

Scrubbing

Assistants should carefully clean the area under their nails with a nail file or orangewood stick before scrubbing. The water should be at a comfortable temperature. Many sinks have elbow, knee, or foot controls so that adjustments can be made during the scrub technique. Assistants should adhere to the required time and the antiseptics used in any given hospital. They must be sure to follow a definite scrub routine so that no bare areas or blind spots occur on the sides of fingers, back of hands, or back of arms (Figure 33.2). There should be at least 20 to 30 brush strokes for every portion of skin. The water and the debris should always be allowed to run down from the elbows

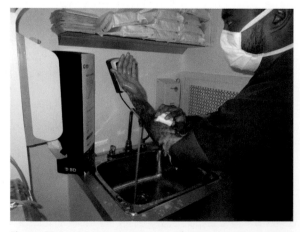

Figure 33.2 ABC steps in proper sterile gowning.

into the sink and never to run back down over the hands, which have been scrubbed first.

Gowning

The gown must be folded so that the scrub assistant can unfold and put the gown on without touching the outer side with the bare hands. A towel placed on top of the gown should be used for careful drying of the hands before taking up the gown.

Gowns should be of sufficient thickness to provide protection from contamination by underclothing. Each sleeve should have a fitting wristlet. Many gowns now have wraparound backs to prevent the back area from contaminating instrument tables. Many doctors use disposable paper gowns that require no laundering and have no lint particles.

Gloving

Several techniques are available for putting on gloves under sterile operating room conditions. The *closed gloving technique* represents perhaps the best method available for the scrub assistant. Some advantages of the closed gloving technique are reduction of possible contamination of the gloves from the hands and free glove powder, which scatters in an operating room.

In the closed gloving technique (see Figure 33.3), the scrub assistant puts on the gown but slides his or her hands into the sleeves only until the sleeve cuff seams can be grasped between the fingers and thumbs. The hands do not protrude beyond the seam of the gown. The gloves are then laid out with the gown-covered hand. The glove is placed in the sleeve thumb down, with the fingers pointing toward the shoulder, and the wrist edge of the glove is level with the sleeve cuff seam. The cuff of the glove is then grasped against the sleeve with the thumb and forefinger, which are inside the sleeve. The upper edge of the glove cuff is grasped with the sleeve-covered fingers of the opposite hand and the glove opening is pulled down completely over the gown cuff of the hand being gloved. If the glove is being placed on the left hand, the glove cuff and the stockinette cuff are grasped with the right hand and both the cuff and the glove are pulled on at the same time. With the gloved hand the other glove is now picked up and the same procedure is followed for gloving the other hand. Using this technique, the gloves are never touched with the bare hands.

Arranging the preparation table

A small table should be arranged to provide all the necessary solutions and supplies for preparing the skin and giving local anesthetic. These include antiseptic solutions, irrigation solutions, applicators, gauze, and local anesthetic solutions, as well as suitable syringes and needles. It is

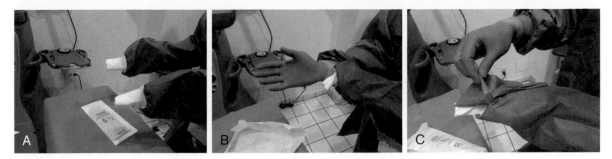

Figure 33.3 Closed gloving technique.

desirable that the sterile table be kept separate from the main instrument table and be removed once the eye and eyelid have been prepared.

Arranging the back table

The back table should be laid out in a definite order of use to provide necessary towels, gowns, and gloves for the surgeons, as well as drapes for the patient. Supplies such as gauze and applicators should be placed here. The back table should include basins for solutions and basins for waste, in addition to required syringes for mixing and drawing up special solutions. Care must always be taken that solutions are never mixed or confused. Instruments are placed on the back of the table, leaving work space in front. Additional instruments that are seldom used but occasionally required may remain on the back table and not be transferred to the instrument, or Mayo, stand.

Arranging the instrument stand (Figure 33.4)

The instrument, or Mayo, stand should be arranged according to a consistent pattern. Forceps are placed in one area, scissors in another, and needle drivers in another. Irrigating solutions, applicators, gauze, and so on have their own place on the instrument stand.

Most ophthalmic surgical procedures can be classified in two main sections:

- Intraocular, which includes cataract extractions, corneal transplants, and corneal or scleral laceration repair
- Extraocular, which includes correction of strabismus and eyelid surgery

Each surgeon uses different instruments that he or she is comfortable with.

Example of a set of instruments for basic intraocular procedures

1 right and 1 left corneal section scissors
1 pair Stevens scissors, curved
1 pair spring scissors

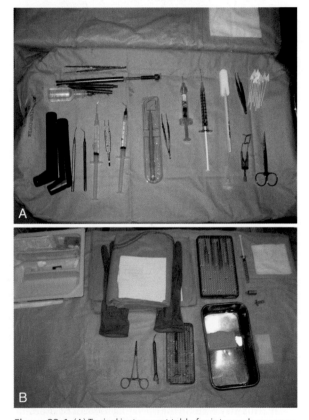

Figure 33.4 (A) Typical instrument table for intraocular surgery. (B) Back-up table for additional instruments.

1 superblade or diamond blade
1 pair iris scissors
1 pair Vannas scissors
1 straight and 1 angled fixation forceps (0.12 teeth)
2 fine-tying forceps
1 anterior chamber irrigating cannula
1 Sinskey hook
1 eye speculum
2 straight and 2 curved fine hemostats

1 muscle hook
1 iris spatula
1 synechia spatula or cyclodialysis spatula
1 lens loupe
2 needle drivers, finely curved
3 anterior chamber irrigating tips (19, 27, and 30 gauge)
1 irrigating cannula
Series of irrigating aspiration probes
Series of phacoemulsification tips and handpieces
Series of special keratomes, scleral blades for phaco incisions
Cautery cord and tip
1 Hershman spatula
1 intraocular lens-holding forceps

Instruments for extraocular procedures

1 no. 3 Bard-Parker knife handle (e.g., strabismus)
1 pair Stevens scissors
1 pair spring scissors
1 straight and 1 angled fixation forceps
1 double-pronged scleral forceps
2 muscle hooks
1 caliper
1 right and 1 left muscle clamp
2 straight and 2 curved fine hemostats
2 towel clips
2 skin hooks, fine
1 anterior chamber irrigating tip, 19 gauge
1 speculum

Special instruments for procedures such as intraocular lens implants, corneal transplants, and enucleation may be sterilized in separate packages and dispensed as necessary in addition to the basic instrument tray. This method avoids unnecessary handling and sterilization of instruments not needed for routine surgery. It applies specifically to the delicate and expensive microsurgical instruments.

Demagnetization

Poor and frustrating surgical technique may be brought about by magnetization of microsurgical instruments, which in turn magnetizes the fine needles commonly used today. This may occur in the operating room or by exposure to larger surgical instruments while being sterilized with ethylene oxide. It is most frustrating to have to dislodge a fine needle from a needle driver during a critical point in a delicate eye operation.

A number of inexpensive methods are available for demagnetization of instruments and needles (Figure 33.5). A tape head demagnetizer also can be used.

Diamond knives

The diamond blade is made from a gem-quality diamond, which is the hardest element known. Diamond knives are

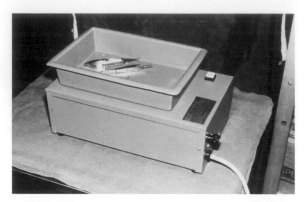

Figure 33.5 Demagnetizing tray for microsurgical instruments and needles.

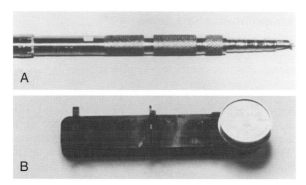

Figure 33.6 (A) Diamond knife with guarded handle. (B) Coin gauge used to check calibration of the diamond knife.

used in ocular surgery because of their extreme sharpness and ability to make a corneal or corneoscleral incision with ease and without tissue destruction. They are far superior to steel blades (Figure 33.6A). This extension of the knife may be measured by the caliper on the handle, but should also be checked against a coin gauge (Figure 33.6B), a ruler, or a microscope. Diamond knives used for cataract surgery are usually unguarded.

To care for the diamond knife, one should use the following procedure:

1. Immediately after surgery, advance the knife blade sufficiently to be exposed, but not beyond the feet, and rinse thoroughly with sterile distilled water squirted with force through a syringe.
2. Visually examine the blade under a microscope for possible dirt or residue, which can be removed by extending the diamond beyond the feet and lightly plunging the blade into Styrofoam. Caution: Cleaning should always be done by making fresh insertions into Styrofoam. Never apply excessive side motion to the diamond. Rinse thoroughly.

3. Visually examine the blade under a microscope for any remaining dirt or residue. If there is residue, repeat steps 1 and 2.
4. Retract the diamond blade.
5. Proceed with any method of sterilization normally used; 275 °F (135 °C) as maximum temperature for 3 to 5 minutes is an acceptable sterilization method for diamond knives and coin gauges. Try not to let blood, tissue, or saline solution dry on the blade, which causes susceptibility to cracking and edge chipping when the blade is autoclaved. After extended use, if a film is noted, clean the diamond blade by immersing it in a pan of distilled water with one tablet of an enzyme cleaner used for contact lenses. This proteolytic enzyme cleaner removes the protein that adheres to the surface of the diamond. Then rinse with distilled water and repeat the cleaning procedure.

Sapphire blade

The sapphire blade is made of crystal sapphire and is extremely sharp and delicate. Like the diamond blade, it is subject to chipping. The same requirements apply for cleaning with distilled water and use of an enzyme film. Before the film develops it may be appropriate to insert both the diamond blade and the sapphire blade into a wet sponge or fiberglass packing material. One should not expose the sapphire blade to ultrasound cleaning. It may be sterilized by means of steam autoclave, ethylene oxide gas, or dry heat (see following text).

Ruby blade

The ruby blade should be stored in a retracted position until it is used. Any wiping motion against the blade will dull the cutting edge. The blade should be flushed with distilled water squirted with force through a syringe. Blood, saline, or tissue should not be allowed to dry on the blade. The blade may be cleaned with contact lens enzyme cleaner. It also may be cleaned in an ultrasonic cleaner.

Special care of gem blades

The following procedure should be used to care for gem blades:

1. Always protect the tip of the blade and store it in a retracted position.
2. Use a rest when laying an extended blade on a Mayo stand.
3. Observe the blade for cleanliness and chips under high magnification with retroillumination.
4. Immediately after use, flush the blade with a steady stream of distilled water with a syringe and needle.
5. The surgeon may gently wipe the side of the blade with a wet Merocel sponge.

6. Diamond and ruby blades can be cleaned after each use by ultrasound with hydrogen peroxide. Rinse thoroughly.
7. Clean baked-on protein as follows:
   a. Expose blades as far as possible
   b. Use a soft wet Styrofoam packing peanut; stab the blade and work it through incisions for 20 to 30 seconds in the direction it is designed to cut
   c. Rinse thoroughly with distilled water.
8. Inspect with a calibration scope.
9. Dry the instrument immediately with a hot air blower. Blow drying removes excess moisture from hard-to-dry areas that are most susceptible to rust. It is a method preferred over towel drying because it prevents lint, keeps edges and tips sharp, and prevents accidental breakage or bending of delicate tips. Drying is not necessary if it is immediately followed by steam sterilization.
10. Avoid sudden hot or cold changes. Always allow the knife from the autoclave to cool in the air. Do not put it in a basin of water if in a hurry because blade damage can result.

Sutures

Sutures are available from the manufacturer in packets consisting of two parts: a primary packet enclosing the suture and a peel-apart overwrap enclosing the inner sterile packet. The inside packet is sterile as long as the overwrap remains intact and undamaged. The circulating nurse must deliver the sterile inner packet to the sterile field without touching it or permitting the inner packet to touch unsterile surfaces. The nurse may use one of three methods to accomplish this:

1. The two flaps of the overwrap may be grasped between the thumbs and forefingers and peeled back to offer the packet to the scrub assistant, who may remove it with a sterile instrument (Figure 33.7).

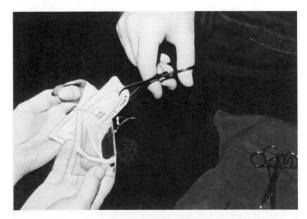

Figure 33.7 Removing suture from sterile packet.

2. The inner packet may be flipped out onto the sterile table.

3. After the outer packet is opened, a transfer forceps may be used to place the inner packet on the instrument table.

The scrub assistant will then take the suture packet and open it. Many absorbable sutures contain a preservative, which must be carefully rinsed before the suture can be used. The suture should then be laid out on the tray in preparation for use.

Types of ophthalmic sutures

Ophthalmic sutures are made of a variety of materials, each material having specific advantages that can be tailored to the individual surgeon's likes (Table 33.2). The broad categories include the following:

1. *Plain surgical gut.* This is commonly referred to as *plain catgut*, a term believed to have originated from the Arabic word *kitgut* or *kitstring* signifying a fiddle string. The Arabian dancing masters used a three-string violin called a *kit* and ancient instrument makers created these strings from the intestines of a variety of animals. This material is absorbable. It eliminates the need for suture removal, which is of prime importance in children and uncooperative individuals. The disadvantages are, in time, variability or loss of tensile strength and absorption, an increased tendency to neovascularization, and some reaction to the material with granuloma formation.

2. *Chromic surgical gut.* This is gut that is chromicized to retard the tensile strength loss and lengthen the time of absorption permitting the suture to last longer. The disadvantage is that, like any natural suture, it causes some moderate tissue reaction.

3. *Vicryl or Dexon.* This is a synthetic absorbable suture that has strong tensile strength, elicits less tissue reaction than gut, and provides excellent knot security. Because of the hydrolytic absorption process, it is more predictable in terms of tensile strength retention and absorption than are the natural absorbable sutures. There is significant absorption in 30 days and maximum absorption in 60 to 90 days. These synthetic absorbable sutures, in sizes 4-0 through 8-0, are of a braided construction to maximize the handling properties. To further improve the passage through tissue and the knot-tying characteristics, an absorbable coating has been added to Vicryl sutures. The coating affects neither the absorption nor the degree of tissue reactivity elicited by the suture.

4. *Nylon.* This is a synthetic monofilament suture commonly used in anterior segment ophthalmic surgery. It maintains its tensile strength and does not irritate the tissues or support bacterial growth. The suture degrades, however, losing approximately 10% to 15% of its strength yearly and it is more difficult to tie than silk. It is available in a variety of sizes for ophthalmic use.

5. *Silk.* This is a natural protein material derived from the silkworm but treated with resins and waxes. This handles the best of all sutures and has excellent knot-tying security. It evokes a slight tissue reaction.

6. *Polypropylene* (Prolene). This is a strong, inert suture that ties well and does not degrade with time. This suture causes minimal inflammatory reaction, is not absorbed, and is not subject to biodegradation or weakening by the actions of tissue enzyme. Because of its relative biologic inertness, there are no known contraindications. This suture is pigmented with copper phthalocyanine blue. It has more elongation than nylon and because of its hydrophobic nature and inertness in the eye, it has become increasingly useful in suturing intraocular lenses, in iris repair surgery, and in anterior segment wound closure.

7. *PDS* (polydioxanone) suture. This is a monofilament absorbable suture for corneoscleral closure. Wound-holding tensile strength is 56 days. The monofilament nature of this suture allows for easy passage through ocular tissue. Available in size 9-0, it is attached to a wide range of fine ophthalmic needles.

8. *Mersilene* polyester fiber suture. This is a monofilament polyester suture for corneoscleral closure. This suture is nonbiodegradable and has 50% more tensile strength than nylon. Mersilene is 20% less elastic than nylon; therefore, it is said to create less suture-induced astigmatism. Available in size 10-0, it is attached to a wide range of fine ophthalmic needles.

Suture evaluation

Uniform standards are required in sutures for microsurgery. The *needles* should be sharp and should not dull easily with repeated passage. They must be securely swaged onto the suture. The *appearance* is important because colored sutures are more easily seen. The suture should be

Table 33.2 Origin of suture materials used in ophthalmology	
Suture	**Raw materials**
Surgical silk	Raw silk spun by silkworm
Catgut (plain or chromic)	Submucosa of sheep intestine or serosa of cow intestine
Collagen (plain or chromic)	Flexor tendon of beef
Nylon	Polymeric amide derived from chemical synthesis
Mersilene (polyester fiber)	Polymer of terephthalic acid and polyethylene

reasonably *pliable* to permit ease of handling. The tensile strength should be adequate for the area and should not crack or break with normal handling. The *pull-through* effect should be smooth and should not drag tissue. *Tying* should be performed simply. The knots should remain secure and the suture should not *fray*.

The knots should remain secure postoperatively. There should be no marked reaction to the suture, although a minimal reaction may accelerate wound healing. With absorbable sutures the absorption time should be sufficient to maintain closure until wound healing is secure.

Ophthalmic needles

Needles have a variety of shapes, points, and curvature, each designed to perform a special task and each related to the type of material that the suture will be required to track through. The needles are attached directly to the suture

Preparing the patient's eyelids

In ophthalmic surgery skin antiseptic agents should be carefully applied, beginning at the lash margin and carefully including the lashes. Ophthalmic personnel should avoid having any of the solution enter the eye. A dry applicator is preferred for skin preparation. Beginning in increasing circles from the eyelid margin, the assistant prepares a large area above the eye. Special care must be taken that the eyebrow and underlying skin are adequately prepared with the antiseptic solution. The eye should then be flushed with saline, diluted povidone-iodine (Betadine) solution, or self-sterilizing aqueous antiseptic solution by use of an irrigating bulb or an asepto syringe.

Draping the patient

A large folded sheet is used to cover the patient's body. The head is commonly draped with a double-thickness sheet or double towels. An eye sheet, preferably with a small opening, or a disposable eye sheet is then placed over the operative site.

AMORIC ENVIRONMENT

The room for operating must be amoric (Greek *a* means "no"; *morion* means "particle"). This term was coined by Dr. José Barraquer to indicate that particulate matter can be as devastating to the visual performance of an eye as infected material. To obtain this amoric environment, it is ideal if the operating room is limited to eye surgery only and has positive pressure. The number of personnel in the operating room should be minimized, as well as movements in and out. All talcum powder should be eliminated by using powderless gloves. All cotton balls should be eliminated. All syringes, cannulas, needles, and Petri dishes should be washed at least five times. Ideally, Millipore filters should be used for any solution irrigated into the anterior chamber. A lint-free type of drape, such as plastic or paper, should be used. Instrument tips must be examined under the microscope and, if particulate matter is present, cleaned with a lint-free wipe. After any instrument has been used, it should be rinsed in saline and wiped well.

CARE AND HANDLING OF SURGICAL INSTRUMENTS

Manufacturers of quality stainless steel instruments (both in the United States and in Germany) have always done their best to produce surgical instruments that are extremely resistant to rust or corrosion. The stainless alloys used in the manufacturing are subject to strict industry and government standards. Their composition may vary to enhance certain desired qualities in the final product. For instance, to guarantee an extra hard cutting edge in scissors, the manufacturer will select a type of stainless steel that contains a higher percentage of carbon molecules, thus making the steel extra hard after hardening and tempering. For some eye instruments that need to be nonmagnetic and in which hardness is not of prime importance, the stainless steel selected will contain little carbon and more chromium and nickel. As a general rule, the greater the carbon content, the harder the steel can be made by the instrument maker. However, it is exactly the carbon content of the stainless steel that can later present a corrosion or rusting problem if the instrument was not properly manufactured or is incorrectly used by the consumer.

To increase its corrosion resistance, a properly manufactured surgical instrument will have passed through two special processing steps. The first is called *passivation*. In this process the instrument is treated with an electrochemical process to thoroughly clean its surfaces, thereby reducing its tendency to corrode. The same process can be achieved through immersing it in a bath containing a heated aqueous solution of 30% nitric acid.

The second special processing step is *polishing*. This creates an extremely smooth surface that removes areas of possible corrosive action. It actually builds a fine layer of chromium oxide on the instrument. This layer is highly resistant to corrosion and will actually continue to build up with regular handling and sterilizing of the item. Naturally, incorrect cleaning and handling may cause this layer to become damaged or disappear, thus increasing the possibility of corrosion problems.

Surfaces that cannot be effectively polished, such as knurled or serrated handles and glare-reducing satin finishes, are more prone to corrosive attack. Because this corrosion does not penetrate deeply, it may be removed by scrubbing with a brush or detergent. As an alternative, the instrument can be returned to as-new condition by passivation and repolishing by the manufacturer or a professional instrument repair service.

Use of shortcuts in instrument care can lead to rust, corrosion, stains, and spotting. Corrosion, the gradual wearing away of material, eventually impairs an instrument's function. The most common causes are:

- Inadequate cleaning and drying after use
- Corrosive chemicals or sterilizing solutions
- Use of ordinary tap water rather than distilled or softened water in the cleaning process
- Laundry detergent residue remaining in operating room linens
- Harsh detergents
- A malfunctioning autoclave

Cleanliness, lubrication, and correct handling and storage procedures ensure an instrument's proper performance. In addition, inspection, troubleshooting, and a professional instrument maintenance program can actually lengthen the serviceable life of surgical instruments. To that end, the following instrument care habits are recommended:

Rust

If the problem is one of real rust (which is rare), it is necessary to determine whether the rust originated from the instrument itself or whether it was transferred from another source. To check whether the item itself is rusting, a pencil eraser is used to remove the rust, then the surface beneath the rust is checked to see if it is pitted. A pitted and rusting instrument must be taken out of a set of instruments immediately because it can cause a rust problem for the entire set. The item is returned to the manufacturer (provided it is not too old), who, in many cases, will replace it at no charge.

If the instrument is not actually rusting but shows some rust deposits, it must be refinished by the manufacturer or a competent repair facility. An attempt should then be made to find the source of the rust. There are several possibilities, the most common one being that one or more instruments in the set are rusting because they are old and of the chrome or nickel-plated type. When this plating wears off through use or sharpening, the carbon steel below it becomes exposed and is subject to immediate corrosion during autoclaving or immersing in cold sterilization solutions.

Inexpensive instruments sometimes rust because they have not undergone the passivation process; thus the surfaces contain carbon molecules. High-quality stainless steel instruments will pass certain tests (boiling, copper sulfate), whereas some of the lesser-grade instruments will not. It is the latter that can cause a problem. The fact that these instruments were stamped "stainless" does not always guarantee that they were made corrosion-resistant by the manufacturer. The buyer must be aware of this.

Another source of rust can be the water used in the autoclave. It is recommended that distilled deionized water be used because this has been stripped of all minerals and metals. Distilled water alone may not be pure enough, because many marketed distilled waters still contain many essential minerals for plant growth or human consumption. These minerals sometimes tend to stain the instrument. Thus deionized distilled water is best.

How to avoid a stained appearance

Stains are deposited onto the instrument's surface, plated on, or, in the case of rusting, develop from the instrument itself. The most common discoloration is a result of deposit stains that commonly occur during autoclaving. Instrument stains appear in a variety of colors, and in most cases the colors suggest the origin of the stain.

Brown or orange stain

The most common stain is also the one most often mistaken for rust. After removing the stain with an eraser, which usually is not difficult, the ophthalmic assistant should check the surface of the instrument for porous signs (pits). If none is found under the stained area (usually the instrument surface is smooth), proceed to locate the cause of the staining.

With the brown or orange stain, the problem is most often a phosphate layer (brown to light orange) on the instrument, which develops as a result of the following causes:

1. *Detergents used to wash and clean instruments.* Many of the detergents sold are highly alkaline and contain polyphosphates that aid in breaking down fats and blood. Hands are also left softer after prolonged use of these detergents. However, this high alkaline content produces the brown or orange stain during the autoclave cycle. The best detergents for instrument washing are those that are neutral pH 7 (on a pH scale of 0–14). These are available from hospitals and surgical suppliers and do not cost much more than regular detergents. Also, often the instruments are not rinsed long enough to neutralize the detergents. A thorough rinsing ensures that the detergent is no longer on the instrument.
2. *Water source.* Traces of minerals or metals (or both) may be contained in the tap water in a particular geographic area. The best way to check whether the water is the cause of the staining is to take a clean (or new) instrument that has no staining on it, wash it thoroughly in distilled deionized water with neutral pH detergent, rinse it thoroughly in distilled deionized water, and put it through a sterilization cycle.

Follow the same procedure with another clean instrument, but this time wash and rinse with tap water. If the second instrument shows staining, it could reasonably be assumed that the tap water contains elements that stain the instrument. If both instruments still show stains, then a check of the autoclave is necessary. In this case clean the autoclave according to the manufacturer's instructions and run one or two cleaning cycles with a recommended cleaner.

3. *Dried blood.* This usually results in a dark brown stain that can be rubbed off. Blood should be removed from the instrument surface as soon as possible because it will break down the surface by chemical reaction.

4. *Surgical wrappings.* If the laundry uses too much detergent, or detergents that contain a lot of phosphates (which are the less expensive ones available), surgical wrappings may contain enough remaining detergents to cause a reaction during autoclaving. A telltale sign is the brown stain on the towel (the outline of the instrument in an orange stain on the towel may even be visible). This type of stain is difficult to remove and on many occasions the instrument will have to be refinished by the manufacturer.

5. *Cold sterilization solutions.* Many times, these are high in pH (like detergents) and need to be rinsed off thoroughly before storing instruments or before autoclaving.

6. *Foreign matter inside steam pipes.* Rust-colored film is particularly prevalent in new hospitals as a result of foreign matter inside steam pipes during installation. Unfortunately nothing can be done, but the situation is only temporary.

Light and dark spots

Light and dark spots are caused by the slow evaporation of condensation on instruments. Traced to mineral residue, such spots can be prevented by following the autoclave manufacturer's directions carefully and using distilled or demineralized water for all cleaning procedures and solution preparation.

Purplish black stains

Purplish black stains indicate exposure to ammonia. Thorough rinsing after use and cleaning in the usual manner should eliminate this stain.

Bluish black stains

These are usually a result of plating and are extremely hard to remove from the instrument's surface. The surface beneath the stain is always smooth, but the instrument may have to be refinished by the manufacturer to obtain good results. The cause of this staining is mixing of dissimilar metals in ultrasonic cleaners and during autoclaving.

Multicolor stains

These are caused mostly by excessive heat (chromium oxide stains) and actually show rainbow colors with a blue or brown overtone. When the instrument shows these heat stains, it may have lost part of the original hardness and may not perform as well (especially scissors, which need the extra hardness on their edges for cutting performance). Such instruments usually can be refinished by the manufacturer and the hardness can be tested. The stain can be polished off.

Black stains

The most common black stains are caused by an acid reaction. The eraser minimizes the stain, but the surface beneath remains slightly rougher than that of a normal instrument. Black stains may result from the detergents used. Similar to the brown stain caused by high pH in detergents, the black acid-type stain can be caused by low pH (<6) during autoclaving. The autoclaving temperature and pressure magnify the chemical effects of acid on steel many times, so the neutrality of the pH in the autoclave environment is of great importance.

Bluish gray stains

Bluish gray stains are indicative of cold sterilizing solutions. Following a manufacturer's directions explicitly will remedy the solution.

As described, stains are deposited onto the instrument surface, plated onto it or, in the case of rusting, develop from the instrument itself.

The most common discoloration results from deposit stains that commonly occur during autoclaving. To minimize such staining, it is important that the autoclave run perfectly and that it has a well-functioning drying cycle. The instruments should come out bone dry, whether in wrappers or loose on a tray. If any moisture is left in the pack or on the instruments, it will result in tiny water droplets that leave a circular stain on the instrument surface after drying.

An interesting fact in regard to plating stains or the stains that are a result of metal deposits is that the area of staining is always near the most magnetic parts of the instrument. New instruments are often highly magnetic in the locks, serrations, and ratchets because the carbon steel tools used to work on the instruments during production are highly magnetic themselves. This magnetism wears off gradually during handling and sterilization. This is why newer instruments tend to stain more visibly, causing the complaint that new instruments are showing stains but the old ones are not.

If there is any suspicion as to what might cause a staining problem, one clean instrument should be processed in the manner suspected of causing the problem and then autoclaved. A clean control instrument should then be processed by washing and rinsing it in distilled and deionized water only. This instrument should process without problems, whereas the first instrument will show the stain. All types of stains can be tested for in this manner, including water, detergent, wrapping, and cold sterilization solution left on the instrument.

Meticulous care during surgery will prolong the life of surgical instruments. Although blood and saline are the most common causes of corrosion and pitting, instrument contact with the following solutions should also be avoided if possible:

Aluminum chloride
Barium chloride
Carbolic acid
Chlorinated lime
Dakin's solution
Ferrous chloride
Lysol
Mercury bichloride
Mercury salts
Phenol
Potassium permanganate
Potassium thiocyanate
Sodium hypochlorite
Stannous chloride
Tartaric acid

Exposure to the following solutions is extremely detrimental:

Aqua regia (a mixture of nitric and hydrochloric acids)
Ferric chloride
Diluted sulfuric acid
Hydrochloric acid
Iodine (not to exceed 1 hour)

Steps in cleaning and sterilization

Cleaning

All instruments should be thoroughly cleaned immediately after use. Using a toothbrush is helpful. Blood or debris should never be allowed to dry on the instruments. Baked-on blood in a box lock or crevice can result in corrosion and subsequent cracking under stress. Therefore box locks should be opened and instruments with removable parts should be disassembled.

Cleaning solutions with a neutral pH level (7–8.5) are recommended. An extremely alkaline detergent (>9) may stain and might cause breaks and an extremely acid detergent (<6) may cause an instrument to pit.

After cleaning, the instruments should be dried quickly to avoid water stains. Of course, if they are to be autoclaved immediately, it is not necessary to dry them first.

Washer-sterilizers are ideally suited for washing and terminally sterilizing soiled instruments. However, it is imperative that the sterilizer itself be clean and functioning properly. Hospitals in hard-water areas should implement a water-softening or demineralizing system. Surgical wrappings must be free of any laundry detergent residue.

A helpful machine is the ultrasonic cleaner. For most offices the medium-sized unit, 10 inches (25 cm) by 4 inches (10 cm) (6–8 inches [15–20 cm] deep) is usually adequate. Ultrasound is a form of acoustic vibration occurring at frequencies too high to be perceived by the human ear, usually greater than 20,000 Hz (i.e., 20,000 cycles per second). Ultrasonic cleaning uses acoustic vibration at high frequencies through a liquid medium. The vibration of the fluid is so rapid that it forms bubbles. This process is known as *cavitation*. The bubbles adhere to and collapse on the surfaces of instruments, causing the foreign matter on the surface to be dislodged gently but totally. Millions of microscopic bubbles or "vacuum cleaners" dislodge the foreign matter from the surfaces, blind holes, pores, tight joints, and places that cannot be reached by lengthy soaking and scrubbing. Ultrasonic cleaning accomplishes this in minutes and is so gentle it will not etch glass. The instruments are thoroughly cleaned and ready for sterilization, eliminating the possibility of "disinfected dirt." The minivacuum created by the exploding bubbles removes up to 90% of all foreign matter from the instrument, particularly in the hard-to-reach areas such as the box locks, scissor locks, and other crevice-like areas.

Although an ultrasonic cleaner removes up to 90% of the soil, it does not preempt the need for sterilization. *Caution: Microsurgical instruments must not come into contact with one another during ultrasonic cleaning.* The unit's vibrations may cause premature wear on their precision tips.

Lubrication

Ultrasonic cleaners remove all lubrication from instruments; therefore, all clean instruments should be bathed in instrument milk or a similar product after ultrasonic cleaning. Instruments should be lubricated after every five procedures. It is also recommended that they be lubricated after every cleaning process to guard against mineral deposits and other water-system impurities that can lead to stains, rust, and corrosion. Previous vigorous cleaning removes all lubrication and may result in "frozen" lock boxes. To impede the growth of bacteria in the lubricant wash, only antimicrobial water-soluble lubricants are recommended. The manufacturer's instructions should be followed carefully.

Inspection

In addition to being completely clean and free-moving to ensure proper function and sterilization, instruments must be inspected before packaging for reuse.

Hinged instruments should be inspected for alignment of jaws, meshing of teeth, and stiff or cracked joints. Ratchets should close easily and firmly. To test ratchets, clamp the instrument on the first tooth. Holding the instrument at the box, tap the ratchet end against a solid object. Repair is required if the instrument springs open. Close the instrument to test its tension; when jaws touch, a space of $\frac{1}{18}$ to $\frac{1}{16}$ inch (1.6–1.4 mm) should exist between the ratchet teeth of each shank.

Ring-handled instruments can be tested by holding one handle in each hand. Open the instrument and try to wiggle it. If the box lock is loose, jaw misalignment will occur.

Large scissors should cut four layers of gauze at the tip of the blade. Smaller scissors (less than 4 inches [10 cm] in overall length) should cut at least two gauze layers. Blades should be inspected for burs.

If a needle that is clamped in the jaws of a needle holder locked on the second ratchet tooth can be turned easily by hand, the instrument should be tagged for repair or replaced.

Finally, elevated heat temperatures weaken stress points and can actually change molecular structures of the metal. This change weakens and dulls instruments, resulting in their continual diminished performance. Be on the lookout for weakened stress points.

Preparing a set of instruments

Instruments made from differing alloys should be sterilized separately. Place all sharps (such as scissors, knives, skin hooks) individually so that they do not touch each other at the sharp areas during autoclaving. The tips of sharps can be protected with small corks. Cotton or gauze also can be used to protect some of the smaller instruments. Special trays are available to keep small instruments and microinstruments in place so that they cannot move during autoclaving or storage. An extra towel can be folded to a strip and wound around the critical areas of several cutting instruments in a set.

Make sure that all instruments are in an open position. Instruments autoclaved in a closed position (especially those with ratchet locking devices) may spring the box lock because of the increased tension during the heat and pressure in the autoclave. In cases of metal-to-metal contact in a closed instrument, such as near the tips and the ratchets, make sure that the steam reaches all these areas. Otherwise, the instruments may not be sterile.

Do not overload trays. Try to standardize with as few instruments as are commonly used in the particular procedure and keep all other instruments set up separately to be available as required. Overloading causes unnecessary handling and sterilization, which not only creates extra work but also shortens the life of the instrument.

Sterilization

Sterilization is the complete destruction of all microorganisms within or about an object. Articles are either *sterile* or *unsterile*; there is no middle ground. Essentially, sterilization is accomplished by subjecting all material to either physical or chemical treatment to destroy all microorganisms. Careful sterilization must be carried out not only to avoid infection of wounds but also prevent the transmission of organisms from patient to patient. The bacterial spore is the most stubborn of all living organisms in its capacity to withstand destruction. Therefore, standards of effectiveness of sterilization are based on the destruction of these bacterial spores.

The following methods are most commonly used in ophthalmology for sterilizing instruments and material:

1. Boiling
2. Dry heat (hot oven)
3. Moist heat (autoclave)
4. Chemical disinfectants (germicides, acetone, alcohol)
5. Gas
6. Radiation (ultraviolet, electron beam)

Boiling

Most microorganisms are destroyed by subjecting instruments to boiling water for 20 minutes. However, it may take several hours of boiling to kill some resistant spores and encapsulated bacteria. A timer should be available so that ineffective sterilization does not result from removing the instruments too early. Instruments with sharp points or blades are rarely boiled because this dulls the cutting edges. Some instruments rust after sterilization in boiling water if they are not properly dried, or if they are allowed to remain in the water. It is important to use distilled water because this prevents minerals from precipitating on the instruments and the walls of the sterilizer. It is recommended that the water sterilizer be emptied, washed, rinsed well, and dried thoroughly at the end of each day.

Dry heat (oven)

Several types of dry heat ovens are available for sterilizing instruments. Run by electricity, these ovens provide a constant and controlled amount of heat to instruments, drapes, gowns, and gloves for a given time. Temperature should be maintained at 320 °F (160 °C) for 60 minutes. The disadvantage of this method is the long time required for the sterilization of instruments and packs (Figure 33.8).

Moist heat (autoclave)

The most common and practical form of sterilizing instruments is steam sterilization. The autoclave is designed to use steam under pressure to destroy microorganisms. Moist heat has a greater destructive effect on bacteria than heat alone (Figure 33.9).

In autoclaving, the higher the temperature or pressure obtained, the shorter is the time required to sterilize. For instance, instruments under 15 pounds (6.8 kg) of pressure at 250 °F (121 °C) are effectively sterilized in 15 minutes. Under the same pressure at 270 °F (132 °C), they are effectively sterilized in 3 minutes.

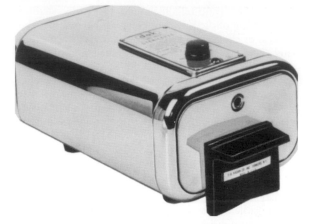

Figure 33.8 Dry heat oven.

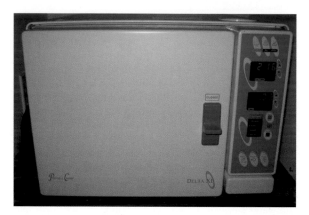

Figure 33.9 Small autoclave.

The time of effective sterilization varies with the type of material being autoclaved. For example, cloth (gauze) takes longer to sterilize than steel (instruments). Autoclaving may be used for a wide range of items of different materials, such as towels, sponges, rubber gloves, and masks. These items may be wrapped in special packages and they will remain sterile for some time after removal from the autoclave.

When ovens and autoclaves are loaded, it is important to prepare all the packs and to arrange the instruments in a way that will permit proper permeation of the materials by the moisture and heat. Crowding must be avoided. All oil and grease must be removed from instruments before autoclaving because steam does not penetrate through oil.

The autoclave has to be in good working order and operating perfectly in both steam and drying cycles. Commercially available autoclave tapes and chemical indicators may serve as controls to show that the autoclave is functioning properly.

Instruments loaded into the autoclave chamber should not be too cold because they can cause steam condensation

and staining. In some instances it may be advisable to heat the load (by using the drying cycle) to warm up the instruments before sterilization. This should be tried first whenever water stains are encountered after sterilization. Also it is important not to open the chamber immediately after sterilization, but rather to crack the door for a few minutes (7–10 minutes, as per manufacturers' recommendations) while the drying cycle is on. In any case, the instruments should come out bone dry, without any condensation moisture anywhere in the packs. To minimize steam staining, only distilled deionized water should be used in the autoclave. Also, all autoclaves should be flushed according to manufacturers' time schedules and recommendations. Iron, sodium, calcium, magnesium, or copper in hard water can cause spotting, staining, or corrosion.

Chemical

Chemicals should be used when heat would dull the sharp cutting edges or would destroy the object to be sterilized (such as plastic). The chemicals that are used on instruments and plastics are called *germicides*. (Chemicals that are used on living tissues are called *antiseptics*.) The process of chemical sterilization with germicides is commonly referred to as *cold sterilization* (Figure 33.10).

Each autoclave has its own set of instructions. All instruments should be cleaned, and when lubricating instruments, be sure to wipe off excess lubricants. Check that

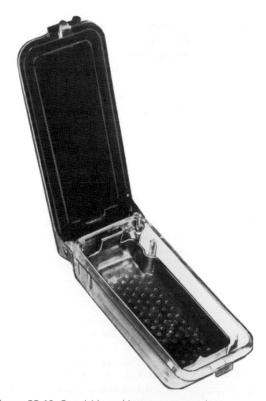

Figure 33.10 Germicide and instrument container.

all materials can be autoclaved. Examples of autoclavable organic materials are: nylon, polycarbonate, polypropylene, Teflon, acetal, polysulfone, polyetherimide, silicone rubber, and polyester. Examples of materials that cannot be autoclaved include polyethylene, styrene, cellulosics, polyvinyl chloride (PVC), acrylic (Plexiglas), latex, and neoprene.

Cold sterilization (germicidal solution bath)

Contrary to popular opinion, cold sterilization is not better for instruments than steam sterilization. With cold sterilization, most professional offices leave the instrument in germicide for hours and even days at a time. Even though the germicides are only slightly corrosive, this extralong immersion takes its toll on the instrument surface. A short (20–30 minutes) steam exposure is much less corrosive and less dulling to sharp edges of scissors and knives than is long exposure to cold sterilization. Also some of the cold sterilization solutions are either highly alkaline (high pH, >7) or highly caustic (low pH, <7) and can cause staining and corrosion when autoclaved after a germicidal bath. Make sure to rinse the instruments thoroughly after taking them out of the germicidal bath. Do not leave instruments in the following solutions for extended periods, because corrosion can result: aluminum, barium, calcium, ferrous or stannous chloride; phenol, Lysol or iodine; benzalkonium chloride (Zephiran); and any acid, mercury, or potassium solution.

The minimum time for chemical sterilization is 20 minutes. The pan in which the instruments are placed for sterilization should be padded with soft material to prevent the tips of the instruments from becoming damaged. Rust inhibitors are often added to some of the commercial germicides. The following germicides are commonly used: ethyl alcohol 70%, benzalkonium chloride (Zephiran), mercury cyanide solution (1:1000), formaldehyde germicides (Bard-Parker solution), cetrimonium bromide (Cetavlon), carbolic acid, aqueous nitromersol solution (Metaphen), phenol derivatives, alkaline glutaraldehyde, hydrochloride solution (sodium or calcium), benzyl ammonium chloride (Germiphene), and acetone (Table 33.3).

Acetone sterilization

Concentrated acetone is used by some practitioners for its rapid bactericidal effect. It has a track record of more than 50 years, is inexpensive and readily available, and evaporates rapidly at room temperature, thus eliminating residual activity. It is rapidly effective against bacteria, but it is only sporistatic (inhibits spores) rather than sporicidal (kills spores) against spores.

Acetone in 100% concentration may be used to disinfect instruments that have become contaminated in surgery. A 1-minute dip is sufficient for disinfection of minor surgical instruments for chalazia, foreign bodies, and eyelids. However, acetone does not kill some spores and may not be effective against the virus of serum hepatitis; it is not

Table 33.3 Advantages and disadvantages of germicides		
Germicide	**Advantages**	**Disadvantages**
Ethyl alcohol	Good bactericidal and virucidal activity in the presence of protein; reduced toxicity; not harmful to instruments, lenses, or plastics; inexpensive	No sporicidal activity
Benzalkonium chloride (Zephiran)	Controversial bactericidal activity; low toxicity	Reduced bactericidal activity against *Proteus* and *Pseudomonas* organisms; no sporicidal activity
Phenol derivatives (Staphene)	Good bactericidal activity	Poor sporicidal activity; toxic
Alkaline glutaraldehyde (Cidex)	Good sporicidal and bactericidal activity in presence of protein; rapidly effective but instruments should be soaked 3–10 hours and rinsed well; low toxicity; not harmful to lensed instruments	Three hours required to kill some spores; before product is effective, it must be activated with sodium bicarbonate
Benzyl ammonium chloride (Germiphene)	Rapid bactericidal activity with 30 seconds; no toxicity; not harmful to plastic, instruments, or rubber	Poor sporicidal activity

nearly as reliable as autoclaving. Acetone neither corrodes instruments nor damages sharp edges. It does not pass biologic tests for sterility, but it is a practical effective solution for minor nonintraocular surgical procedures.

Alcohol disinfection

Like acetone, alcohol is rapidly effective against vegetative bacteria and mycobacteria. Its action against fungi (30–60 minutes) is slower and virucidal activity is highly erratic. An ophthalmologist has to decide whether an item should be sterile or simply clean. If the item need only be clean, then the disinfection process of alcohol should destroy most microorganisms known to cause disease in that situation.

Gas and radiation

Ethylene oxide is an effective gas for sterilizing instruments and materials. It is useful in sterilizing articles that would be damaged by heat or by exposure to strong liquid disinfectants. It is the method of choice in sterilizing intraocular lens implants. Some of the advantages of gas sterilization are that it can be used on most materials, can sterilize materials that cannot be sterilized by other means, is effective against all organisms, and achieves good penetration. The disadvantages of gas are that it is slow, costly, flammable, and toxic and it requires special equipment.

Electron beam irradiation may be applied to completely sealed articles, such as sutures.

Effectiveness

To test the efficacy of sterilization methods, one may attempt to culture organisms from the instruments after obtaining what is considered proper sterilization. If any organisms are cultured, the method and solution used must be reevaluated. In standard tests, specific organisms may be placed in the sterilizing apparatus and cultures analyzed to test effectiveness.

Sterile packs

Many microsurgical instruments and supplies are provided as disposables in sterile packs. Single-use instruments such as blades, injection needles, trephines, and suture needles should conform to standards established and described in the manufacturer's promotional material.

A potential problem in shipping, storage, and use of sterile packs is the possibility of contamination or loss of sterility, or both. A sterile pack should contain an indicator to confirm maintained sterility and freedom from exposure to ambient air and possible contamination through cracks, tears, or perforations in packs sterilized by heat, ethylene oxide, or radiation.

OPERATING ROOM MICROSCOPE

Ophthalmic surgery has become microsurgery. The operating room microscope is the most important piece of equipment in ophthalmic surgery. Zeiss designed the first microscope so well that Zeiss operating microscope equipment is the kind most commonly used in operating rooms. Other brands such as Mueller, Olympus, Weck, and Wild are also available throughout North America, with minor improvements over the more common Zeiss equipment.

An advantage of Zeiss microscopes is that they are interchangeable with existing components and accessories.

The modern operating room microscope supplies the surgeon with illumination, magnification, and controlled positioning. Equipment is designed to minimize clutter and to be placed in the most accessible part of the operating room. Because of the magnification involved, a minimal amount of vibration is tolerated, and therefore heavy bases or ceiling mounts are required. A lightweight microscope beside the table stand is inconvenient and commonly causes troublesome vibration for the operating surgeon.

The first Zeiss microscope was the Omni One, developed in 1956. It has been improved and updated several times. Its microscope provides motorized zoom and focus capability in a short body, in addition to zoom capability that allows greater magnification and fine focusing adjustments. Also available is a movement attachment in two planes called the XY movement, which provides smooth, controlled movement in repositioning the microscope. The oculars of the microscopes are usually × 12.5 and may be increased to × 16. The objective lens of the microscope, found under the microscope, should be suitable for a definite working distance compatible with the surgeon's requirements. The focal length of the objective can be interchangeable. Most surgeons use a 200- or 175-mm objective lens depending on their arm length.

A number of accessories can be obtained for most microscopes. These include observer systems, accessory lights, ultraviolet filter, occluder filter, photo or video adapters, XY coupling to include alignment and self-centering devices, pupillary distance adjustment, foot-control switch, hand-control switch, voice activation, and Retrolux fit that will move the fixation beam so it is coaxial with the microscope light.

A *beam splitter* is required to provide accessories such as the observer system and the photo or video adapter. Additional lights may provide slit-view or diffuse side lighting.

The microscope may be covered by a microscope drape, knob covers, or light plastic sterile drapes. Adjustment knob covers that can be readily sterilized between procedures and applied at the beginning of the surgery are available from Zeiss and other manufacturers.

Troubleshooting

Lamp failure

If the microscope lamp fails to go on at the outset or goes off during the procedure, it may not always be the bulb. The main power to the operating room may fail, of course. On the other hand, microscopes have fuses in a variety of locations. Replacement fuses should always be available. Microscope lamps may fail and additional lamps must be available. Newer microscopes have a double system of lamps so that easy interchange into another box unit is possible. The personnel in the operating room should be familiar with the method of reinstituting the light in cases of failure.

Failure of the zoom operation

The zoom operation is powered by a small motor. This motor may become wet, in which case it may not function properly. As the microscope ages, it also may fail. Professional maintenance may be required.

Power focus

The most common failure of microscopes is jamming of the power focus in the down position. If this should occur, jiggling the up focus switch while tapping on the microscope body may cause the clutch to engage. Again, professional maintenance is required.

Failure of foot switch

The foot switch may be dampened by balance salt that flows from the incision into the mechanisms of the foot control. Corrosion may reach the electrical contacts, causing the foot switch to become unreliable and perform intermittently. This requires professional servicing. Covering the foot controls in a light plastic bag often prevents this problem.

Blurred image

Blurred images may occur if breath fogs the surface of the oculars. It may require skin taping of the mask to prevent the surgeon's breath from appearing from the upper portion of the mask. Blurring also may occur if eyelashes smear skin oil on the glass surface. Periodically, outer surfaces and the objective lens should be cleaned carefully with lens cleaner to prevent fogging. In humid rooms, moisture condensation may occur on the optical surface of the microscope.

Filters

Ultraviolet filters can be placed within the system of the microscope to impede ultraviolet light from entering the eye. This is important because ultraviolet rays may have an injurious effect on the macular area. This is more important if there has been a break in the capsule. A central eclipse filter is available that can be added to the microscope by turning a knob to bring it into position. This feature may be valuable in occluding light rays from entering the eye while suturing is occurring.

Back-up generators

Back-up generators are available to attach to phaco machines. They provide 4 to 6 hours of extra power to continue and finish the operation in case of power failure.

ETHICAL BEHAVIOR OF THE OPHTHALMIC ASSISTANT

1. Never betray a patient's confidence. During this trying period, patients may take you into their confidence and tell you details about their personal lives that they do not wish communicated to others.
2. You may learn things from observations or from coworkers that are highly private, for example, that someone wears a wig or a person's real age. These must be kept private.
3. People in public life or well-known personalities may come under your care and wish to remain anonymous.
4. Do not discuss any surgical case or complication of a patient with anyone outside the hospital environment.
5. Respect the confidence of your coworkers. If you cannot respect their abilities, do not gossip about them. Some of your coworkers may have personal problems that should not be relayed to others.
6. Develop a sense of loyalty to your coworkers.
7. Do not overstep the limits of your legal responsibility. There will be restrictions placed on you in many areas, and these are for your own protection. The minute you overstep these limitations, you are placing yourself in legal jeopardy.

For further information see Chapter 52.

MEDICOLEGAL TIPS

1. Ensure the identification of the correct patient and the correct side for any surgical procedure. Often these are X-marked on the forehead.
2. Establish good rapport with the patient. The patient who likes the physician and the environment in which surgery is performed is less likely to sue. Some lawsuits evolve from a patient's vindictiveness even if the physician is not at fault. A practitioner whom the patient views as compassionate and understanding has already acquired some protection against legal actions.
3. Operative notes should be made soon after surgery, not weeks or months later.
4. Be sure there is a good consent form that is well outlined to the patient. Effective personnel communication with the patient concerning risks, benefits, and alternatives is extremely valuable.
5. Maintain good records in the office and the hospital. The quality and legibility of one's records affect the quality of one's practice. It is important to attach to the records a log of telephone advice. Cursory, sloppy, or nonexistent notes call the practitioner's credibility and standards of practice into question. The physician should initial all laboratory and x-ray reports before they are filed.

For further information see Chapter 52.

Questions for review and thought

1. In a 5-minute period, identify as many errors as you can in Figure 33.1.
2. What are some possible fears of a patient admitted to the hospital for eye surgery?
3. What are some of the problems facing the almost-blind patient?
4. How should you go about orienting a partially blind patient who is admitted to the hospital?
5. Delicate handling of eye patients after intraocular surgery is important. Outline the measures you would take to ensure a smooth postoperative course.
6. What significant postoperative signs and symptoms should be brought to the attention of the ophthalmologist after eye surgery?
7. Outline a routine for postoperative care that a retinal detachment patient could follow after discharge from the hospital.
8. How would you prepare a child for strabismus surgery?
9. When should skin sutures be removed after a blepharoplasty?
10. What instructions should be given to a patient for a retinal detachment?
11. Describe the function and care of cataract instruments.
12. Describe the rationale for proper technique of scrubbing, gowning, gloving, preparation, and draping.
13. Outline the components of the operating microscope.

 Self-evaluation questions

True–false statements

Directions: Indicate whether the statement is true (**T**) or false (**F**).

1. The ophthalmic assistant in a hospital setting is commonly a nurse. **T** or **F**
2. Blind or partially sighted individuals should take the assistant's arm, and follow. **T** or **F**
3. Preoperative orientation is not a function of the hospital ophthalmic assistant. **T** or **F**

Missing words

Directions: Write in the missing word in the following sentences:

4. An environment that is free of particles is called _____.
5. Sterilization of the operator's skin is called _____.
6. A technique of putting on gloves by not hand touching the cuffs of the gloves is called the _____ glove technique.

Choice-completion questions

Directions: Select the one best answer in each case.

7. Which is not an alarming immediate postoperative sign after cataract surgery?
   a. Blood in the anterior chamber
   b. Severe pain
   c. Photophobia
   d. Pus in the anterior chamber
   e. Prolapse of the iris
8. Which is an incorrect postoperative instruction?
   a. Avoid heavy lifting.
   b. Avoid straining at bowel movement.
   c. Keep hands and face clean.
   d. Avoid car rides.
   e. Wear sunglasses outdoors.
9. Which is not an error in surgical technique?
   a. Splashing the surgical gown
   b. Permitting hair to protrude from cap
   c. Cleaning nails in scrub sink before scrubbing
   d. Mask not covering the nose
   e. Leaving skip spots while scrubbing

A   Answers, notes, and explanations

1. **True.** Most often the nurse, when employed by a hospital or by an ophthalmologist, is the individual who assists in the care of eye patients. A nurse is usually the individual in the operating room who, by training and experience, can quickly learn the skills of assisting, aseptic technique, and microsurgery. At the bedside, the nurse can follow the progress of a patient, identify abnormal signs and symptoms, and report progress to the ophthalmologist. However, in many states someone who is not a nurse, but who is well trained in these functions, may accompany the ophthalmologist and assist with preoperative, operative, and postoperative care of the patients. In surgicenters, a trained layperson is taking on increasing importance in this role.

2. **True.** By taking the assistant's arm just below the elbow, the partially sighted individual will be protected from interfering objects in the pathway and will be able to anticipate directional changes. In this way the person will feel more secure when walking. A blind person should never be steered. The assistant should engage in conversation and provide information on the patient's surroundings.

3. **False.** No matter how well the patient has been oriented to any particular surgery by the office personnel of the ophthalmologist, he or she is still apprehensive on the night before surgery. The evening before, the hospital ophthalmic assistant should review the routines that will occur before the surgery and the convalescent care that may be required. The patient should be given necessary cautions that are routine at the hospital. The patient should be forewarned as to what to expect from the type of anesthetic to be given, be it local, intravenous, or general.

4. **Amoric.** Creating an amoric or particle-free environment is as important as creating a sterile environment for ocular surgery. Fine particles of dust, debris, or powder can be devastating if they enter the eye.

5. **Scrubbing.** The operator's skin may be rendered safe temporarily by vigorous scrubbing with a scrub brush soaked in antiseptic solution, although bacterial flora return to the skin rapidly (within minutes) and so the skin does not remain sterile. However, pathogenic microorganisms will be permanently destroyed. Thus although scrubbing does not produce sterility, it does produce a considerably decreased risk of transferring pathogenic organisms.

6. **Closed.** This is the most sterile way of putting on gloves. Here the hands enter the sleeves of the gown only down to the cuffs and then the gloves are grasped with the sterile gown cuffs until the hands enter the gloves. The purpose of this technique is to minimize bacterial recovery on the scrubbed hands from the outside of the glove.

7. **c. Photophobia.** Generally, because of a traumatic iritis with cells on the anterior chamber, most eyes are light-sensitive after cataract surgery. A darkened room or sunglasses may be comforting for the first few days. A dilated pupil often contributes to the photophobia.

8. **d. Avoid car rides.** As long as the driver is careful to avoid bumps and jars, there is no reason why an individual cannot ride in a car, go for walks, or lead a reasonably normal life during the postoperative period. Today's modern suturing techniques avoid the one major complication of wound rupturing with iris prolapse that was seen in the past. However, excessive straining can raise thoracic pressure and, secondarily, the venous return. This may give rise to intraocular hemorrhage on relatively fragile vessels.

9. **c. Cleaning nails in scrub sink before scrubbing.** This is a correct and important part of achieving cleanliness before scrubbing. All of the other activities are serious breaks in surgical technique. For sterility and cleanliness, attention must be paid to three participants in the operation: (1) the operator and assistants, (2) the patient, and (3) the instruments, drapes, and surgical accessories that are used. All must be carefully cleaned and sterilized or disinfected.

Chapter | 34 |

Lasers in ophthalmology

Ernest R. Simpson

Perhaps more than any other recent advance in medical science, the advent of laser technology has produced a major effect on clinical ophthalmology. The effect of solar radiation was well known in ancient times; the first description of a central scotoma after a solar burn of the retina was reported in the mid-17th century. Although Albert Einstein described the concept of stimulated emission of light in 1917, a doctoral student Gordon Gould in 1957 figured out a way to make light waves march in unison, and Bell Labs produced the first useable laser in 1960.

Medical applications of this new energy were explored at an early stage, but the first experiments were poorly controlled and commonly produced unsatisfactory results. Some of these early investigators used effects of the sun or the carbon arc to produce a lesion in the retina. In 1927 Maggiore focused sunlight on two eyes that were later enucleated. These eyes showed a significant reaction in the retina as a result of this focused energy. In 1949 Dr. Meyer-Schwickerath focused light from the sun through a rudimentary optical instrument and successfully photocoagulated the human retina with a retinal hole.

In 1960, the first optical laser (*light amplification by stimulated emission of radiation*), as it was eventually called, was produced, which provided the ophthalmologist with an intense, pure beam of light that could produce extremely small burns of varying intensities. The use of the argon ion laser in treating various retinal vascular diseases was first considered in 1965, and in 1971 clinical trials concerning the photocoagulation potential of the krypton laser, as well as the neodymium:yttrium-aluminum-garnet (Nd:YAG) laser, were begun, and shortly thereafter this equipment became available commercially.

Several external ocular growths were removed by a carbon dioxide laser in 1971. Various glaucoma conditions became treatable in 1973 with high-powered laser. Since then the Nd:YAG laser has been used extensively to cut membranes and persistent capsular material in the human eye after cataract extraction. As an investigative tool, laser light is being used to treat sensitized malignant ocular tumors and to produce highly accurate incisions in corneal tissue to correct refractive errors.

LASER THEORY

A laser is a source of extremely intense monochromatic coherent light. The electromagnetic spectrum is composed of radiant energy that ranges from short cosmic waves (10 nm) (nanometers; a nanometer is 1 millionth of a meter) to the longest radio waves (1000 m). Laser light is basically the same as light from the sun or a household light bulb. It is formed by photons and, like any other form of light, is propagated in an electromagnetic wave form. In the visible portion of the electromagnetic spectrum, the radiation with the shortest wavelength is in the violet region. These wavelengths are in the region of 400 nm. The visible radiation with the longest wavelength is red light. Red light waves may be up to 700 nm.

Lasers can produce light energy with wavelengths shorter than the visible spectrum (ultraviolet) or longer than the

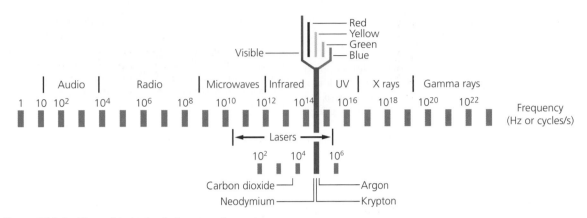

Figure 34.1 Positions of lasers in electromagnetic spectrum.
(From L'Esperance FA Jr. Ophthalmic lasers: photocoagulation, photoradiation and surgery. 3rd ed. St Louis: Mosby; 1989.)

Figure 34.2 Elementary laser scheme illustrating active medium within optical resonant cavity formed by mirrors and pump, which creates population inversion in active medium.
(From Steinert RF, Puliafito CA. The Nd-YAG laser in ophthalmology: principles and clinical applications of photodisruption. Philadelphia: Saunders; 1985.)

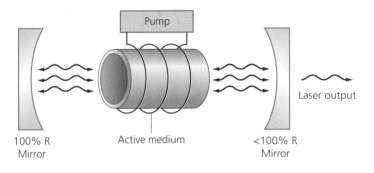

visible spectrum (infrared), each one causing different forms of tissue destruction in the eye (Figure 34.1).

Three basic conditions must be met for most lasers to operate (Figure 34.2):

1. There must be an active medium, that is, a material such as a gas or solid in which the atoms, molecules, or ions emit optical radiation when properly stimulated.
2. There must be a suitable energy source that can pump the atoms, molecules, or ions in the active medium, producing the emission of photons of radiation.
3. There must be some form of optical feedback or gain, which usually is provided by mirrors or other reflecting surfaces in the laser's optical cavity.

Argon, krypton, carbon dioxide, helium-neon, various liquids (dyes) and solids, such as neodymium supported by YAG, as well as many other types of semiconductors, are all in use as lasing media. The active medium in the Nd:YAG laser, for instance, consists of an insulating crystal fabricated from yttrium, aluminum, and garnet and doped with the rare earth neodymium (Nd) ion. The energy source used to pump or excite the neodymium ions is typically a quartz body or flashlamp for pulsed applications or a direct current arc lamp when continuous laser output is

desired. Optical gain is provided by placing mirrors at each end of the Nd:YAG rod in this type of laser to reflect the light back and forth through the crystal. Alternatively, the ends of the laser rod can be coated with reflective material and thereby serve as the laser mirrors.

PUMPING AND SPONTANEOUS EMISSION

When photons of light from the pumping lamp collide with the active lasing medium, they often impart enough energy to raise some of their orbiting electrons to higher-than-usual energy levels. This is referred to as *optical pumping*. These electrons remain at the higher energy levels for varying periods of time, dropping back to lower energy levels randomly and spontaneously. When they drop from a higher to a lower level, they in turn emit energy in the form of photons of radiation. This phenomenon is called *spontaneous emission*. The wavelength of the radiation emitted depends on the difference in the potential energy of the two levels.

STIMULATED EMISSION

If a photon strikes an electron that is in a high (or pumped) energy level, the electron instantaneously drops back to a lower energy level only if the triggering photon is of the same wavelength or frequency as the one that is emitted when the electron falls to the lower energy level. When an electron is stimulated to give off a photon of radiation, the photon emitted travels in exactly the same direction as the photon that triggered it. Therefore, the laser light is reflected back and forth along the axis. In a short period, many identical photons form in a standing wave (all of them in phase), producing coherent radiation. This standing wave, which has now become a beam of laser radiation, continues to be amplified as it passes back and forth through the laser rod cavity between the two mirrors. This process is referred to as *stimulated emission.*

Spontaneous emission therefore occurs randomly without any need for external intervention, whereas stimulated emission occurs when an ion, in its excited state, interacts with a photon of the proper wavelength. To achieve release of the stimulated emission, one of the mirrors is made fully reflective and the other only partially reflective. The portion of the light wave striking the second mirror leaves the cavity as the emitted laser beam, and the reflectivity of the mirror is selected to satisfy the requirements for efficient application in a particular system of reflecting mirrors, which are then fitted to either a slit lamp or another delivery system.

TYPES OF LASERS AND THEIR CLINICAL USE

Each lasing medium produces a different wavelength with a selective absorption effect in tissue. Tunable dye lasers are capable of providing a broad range of wavelengths and a wide range of tissue responses. The most powerful lasers are generally used in industrial applications. Although such lasers may generate many kilowatts of energy, those used in medicine require much less, generally no more than 100 watts.

Many factors other than power levels determine a laser's effectiveness as a medical instrument. The characteristics of both the target tissue and the laser source determine the biologic consequences of laser radiation. This fit between the laser light and its target is what allows for selective damage or alteration of ocular tissue. For example, red objects strongly absorb green or blue light, but reflect most red light. Thus the argon laser, with its blue-green light, is used for many procedures that involve coagulating blood or sealing off blood vessels. In general, longer wavelengths penetrate tissue more deeply than do shorter wavelengths; that is why krypton laser red light produces damage at a deeper level in tissue than argon laser green light. Carbon dioxide laser light, at 10,600 nm, is absorbed completely by water in tissue and is therefore effective in cutting tissue with a high water content. Medical lasers produce tissue damage by three basic mechanisms: thermal, photodisruptive (ionizing), and photochemical.

Thermal mechanism

The human eye transmits light between wavelengths of 380 and 1400 nm. In principle, light throughout this range may be used to treat intraocular structures by delivery through the pupil. At wavelengths shorter than 380 nm, the ultraviolet-absorbing properties of the lens and cornea limit the exposure to the retina. At wavelengths longer than 1400 nm, water absorption sharply limits this transmission. Because laser light is monochromatic, highly columnated and intense, and because the eye is an optically open system, laser irradiation is well suited to produce thermal effects resulting in photocoagulation. When absorbed by tissue, laser light is transformed to heat energy, causing a thermal response.

Absorption of laser light is related to wavelength and absorption characteristics of the tissue. When light strikes a tissue surface, part of this light is reflected, part is absorbed by various cells or cell layers, and part is transmitted inward until the energy is depleted. The absorption of laser light depends on the chromophore content of the tissues. Tissue chromophores include hemoglobin (present in blood vessels), melanin (present in the retinal pigment epithelium, iris pigment, epithelium, uvea, and trabecular meshwork), and xanthophyll (present in the inner and outer plexiform layers of the retina in the macula) (Figure 34.3). When these tissues absorb light, the light is transformed into heat energy, a thermal reaction occurs, and photocoagulation results with surrounding tissue destruction. Argon blue-green (composed primarily of the 488 and 514.5 nm emission lines), argon monochromatic green (514.5 nm), and krypton red (647 nm) are commonly used in ocular photocoagulation to induce thermal effects. Krypton yellow (568 nm) and continuous wave and long-pulsed Nd:YAG (1064 nm) sources also have been used for thermal photocoagulation.

Thermal photocoagulation (Figure 34.4) is used extensively in treating diabetic retinopathy, branch or central retinal venous occlusion, retinal telangiectasia, closure of retinal holes, and certain varieties of localized retinal detachment without traction. Choroidal neovascular membranes (200–2500 nm from the center of the foveal avascular zone) also may be treated with thermal photocoagulation. The target ocular chromophores for producing the desired effects in this type of treatment are melanin in the retinal pigment epithelium and hemoglobin in the retinal and choroidal vessels. Central venous retinopathy with active leakage also can benefit from thermal photocoagulation.

Figure 34.3 Light wavelength absorption in certain tissue chromophores.

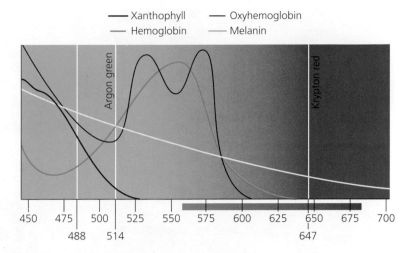

Figure 34.4 (A) Moderately severe nest of papillovitreal neovascularization *(arrows)* extending from the optic nerve before photocoagulation. (B) Appearance of the posterior retinal region after panretinal photocoagulation. (C) Complete disappearance of neovascularization 3 months after completion of panretinal photocoagulation.
(From L'Esperance FA Jr. Ophthalmic lasers: photocoagulation, photoradiation and surgery. 3rd ed. St Louis: Mosby; 1989.)

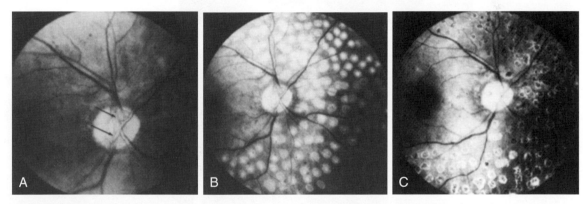

Tunable dye laser systems (Figure 34.5)

Although there is an advantage to a laser system that offers a wide selection of wavelengths to interact with different tissue chromophores in the eye, the absorption characteristics of melanin are the single most important consideration in applying laser energy to melanin-containing ocular tissue to produce a thermal effect.

Dye lasers, which have become important in treating vasculopathy in tissue of low melanin content, have permitted new approaches in treatment through photosensitization. In the anterior segment of the eye, thermal photocoagulation can be used to produce an iridotomy in the treatment of angle-closure glaucoma, improve trabecular meshwork function in the treatment of open-angle glaucoma (trabeculoplasty), and produce alterations in pupil size and shape (iridoplasty).

Most of these procedures take just several minutes to perform under local anesthesia and usually require a contact lens to focus the energy in the desired location. Patients are usually seated during the procedure and most require only topical anesthetic. In some instances, when extensive procedures are required, retrobulbar anesthesia is accomplished so that the procedure is relatively pain-free.

Laser light from a carbon dioxide source is absorbed by water. Because a high percentage of cellular content is water, this laser is effective in cutting tissue because it can be focused to vaporize cells in a very fine line. Its use in ophthalmology is reserved primarily for removing skin lesions and producing fine skin incisions for various forms of lid surgery (Figure 34.6). The Nd:YAG laser in a continuous waveform is only partially absorbed by hemoglobin or water and penetrates much more deeply than does the

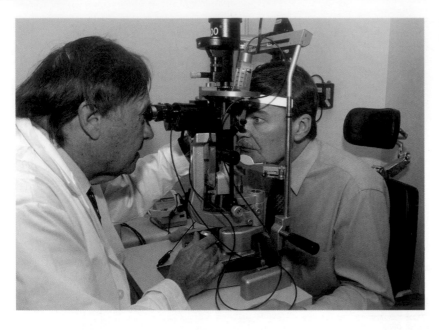

Figure 34.5 Tunable dye laser in clinical use.

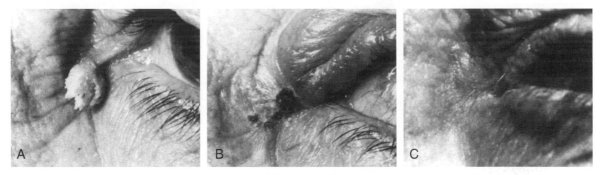

Figure 34.6 (A) Keratitic growth near inner canthus before CO_2 laser photovaporization. (B) Appearance of keratitic area immediately after CO_2 laser photovaporization. (C) Appearance of area of photovaporization of keratitic growth 3 weeks after CO_2 laser photovaporization.
(From L'Esperance FA Jr. Ophthalmic lasers: photocoagulation, photoradiation and surgery. 3rd ed. St Louis: Mosby; 1989.)

argon laser. Although the Nd:YAG laser can be used for thermal photocoagulation, its main function uses the principle of photodisruption.

Diode lasers

Diode lasers that use gallium-arsenide plates to induce rapid electron transfer induce thermal photocoagulation. These systems are efficient and cost-effective but lack wavelength flexibility. These systems are compact and frequently portable, permitting a wide range of clinical applications requiring absorption in the 600- to 800-nm range.

Photodisruptive (ionizing) mechanism

If the power of laser energy is released over an extremely short time (1 billionth or 1 quadrillionth of a second), tissue ionization or complete ablation results, giving rise to local intense heating and generation of mechanical and acoustic shock waves in tissue. This form of laser tissue destruction is known as *photodisruption* and can be accomplished by the Nd:YAG laser. The laser beam itself is invisible, having a wavelength of 1064 nm, and focusing is therefore accomplished by placing a red helium-neon laser in the beam path. The laser energy is "q switched" (quality switched) or "mode locked" and is delivered in a single pulse or train of pulses over an extremely short time interval of nanoseconds (q switched) or picoseconds (mode locked). The energy is supplied to the tissue so quickly that damage is produced by a microexplosion rather than by a heating effect, as in thermal photocoagulation.

It is critical that this laser be focused with extreme accuracy, with the minimum power and the minimum number of shots to achieve the desired effect. An appropriate contact lens is usually used because it forms part of the optical focusing system in the laser beam path. This improves accuracy and allows a higher power density, thus minimizing the total energy required to accomplish a given task such as opening a posterior capsule after cataract surgery (Figure 34.7). Vision can be improved immediately, as soon as the small opening is produced.

Patients with thick capsules or secondary cataracts occasionally may be treated with this form of laser surgery. Cyclitic membranes that form after trauma to the eye, surgery, or uveitis sometimes can be treated in this manner. High laser energies are usually required and generally it is safer to use multiple treatment sessions. Iridotomies for the treatment of angle-closure glaucoma are accomplished with this form of laser application. Infrared laser systems that use short pulses are being evaluated in a number of clinical settings including the production of

a fistula as a filtering mechanism in the treatment of glaucoma. Most of these procedures can be carried out with use of a topical anesthetic, as in the case of thermal photocoagulation. Occasionally, however, local anesthesia is required.

Photochemical mechanism

When certain wavelengths of laser light interact with a photosensitizing agent, the absorbed light energy is converted into a highly reactive oxidative process that can bring about cell death. The therapeutic use of laser-induced photochemical damage in ophthalmology has been limited. Attempts have been made to treat cancer in the eye by shining red laser light at a photosensitizing agent known as *hematoporphyrin derivative*, which is preferentially localized in cancerous eye tissue. Cancer cell death has been achieved by this form of therapy, although results remain preliminary. Efforts to control age-related macular degeneration with photodynamic therapy using newer, more specific sensitizers hold promise for this disabling and common condition of the aging eye.

Photorefractive and phototherapeutic keratotomy

The development of short-wavelength lasers, called *excimer* (*exci*ted di*mer*) lasers, which can efficiently generate high-power ultraviolet light, has prompted the use of short-pulsed ultraviolet radiation for tissue destruction. Surgical modification of corneal refractive power occurs because this tissue possesses about two-thirds of the total refractive power of the phakic eye and is the only refractive surface once the lens is removed.

Pulsed 193-nm light is used to ablate a small amount of corneal stroma (30–100 µg) to induce corneal flattening in a spherical or cylindric manner. Early results indicate that the procedure is safe and generally stable. Predictability for correction of myopia varies with the degree of refractive error correction required.

First-generation excimer lasers have large beams (6–7 mm) and very large diaphragms that expand or contract relatively slowly. Smoother ablations resulted with second-generation lasers by incorporating wobbling beams and less energy. Third-generation lasers are equipped with small scanning and tracking beams to assist patient fixation. These lasers also use less gas and require less optical maintenance but take longer to produce ablations because of smaller beam technology. Photorefractive keratotomy (PRK) using removal of the corneal epithelium has been safely applied for lower myopic corrections; laser-assisted in situ keratomileusis (LASIK) may prove of greater benefit for higher refractive

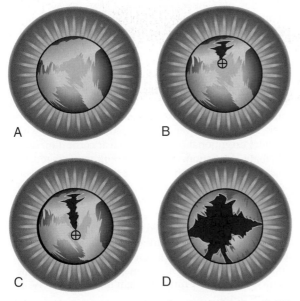

Figure 34.7 Progressive opening of posterior capsule with Nd: YAG laser photodisruption.
(From Steinert RF, Puliafito CA. The Nd-YAG laser in ophthalmology: principles and clinical applications of photodisruption. Philadelphia: Saunders; 1985.)

errors, particularly as microkeratome technology improves. Details of the excimer laser are found in Chapter 37.

SAFETY IN THE LASER CLINIC

Everyday supermarket product-marking lasers, CD lasers (5 milliwatts [mW]), DVD players (10 mW), and DVD burners (100 mW) can produce vision damage if improperly used. Lasers used in surgical techniques (30,000–100,000 mW) have significant damage potential from direct or indirect exposure. Even low-mW class 2 lasers, such as those that used as fixation or target devices, can damage vision. Variables such as eye health, duration of exposure, and fixation time must be monitored carefully to avoid direct and indirect macular injury.

Safety features that protect the operator and patient from accidental laser exposure have been incorporated into most laser systems. Each product should be carefully scrutinized with these features in mind. It is difficult to formulate mandatory safety rules for an ophthalmic laser clinic because of lack of extensive clinical experience. It is possible, however, to suggest a list of precautions to be followed in the use of such an instrument:

1. Insist that all onlookers wear appropriate laser eye protection.
2. Keep all delivery optical equipment, including contact lenses, clean.
3. After extensive maintenance or unusual jolting of the instrumentation, check the laser beam alignment by firing the beam at a sample target; a sudden change in laser output for the same setting can indicate problems with the laser energy monitor.
4. Always use the lowest energy to accomplish the task.
5. In the case of Nd:YAG lasers, avoid procedures close to the retina and cease laser use if the plasma formation becomes sporadic, which implies malfunction or lowered energy output.
6. Position the patient to avoid accidental exposure, either directly or indirectly, to laser light.
7. Use appropriate signs or indicators to prevent direct viewing of the operating laser by a person entering the room.

FUTURE APPLICATIONS OF LASER TECHNOLOGY

As experience with laser energy increases in the field of ophthalmology, existing forms of therapy are undergoing revision and new treatments are emerging. Noninvasive ciliary body ablative procedures for glaucoma using frequency-doubled Nd:YAG and diode sources are being evaluated. Nd:YAG laser photodisruption of vitreous opacities and traction bands has been accomplished. Cataract degradation laser procedures may offer an alternative to ultrasound phacoemulsification in the quest for small-wound, low-energy cataract surgery. Photochemical interaction between laser light and specific sensitizers continues to show promise in producing selective tissue damage in the treatment of age-related macular disease, certain retinal hemangiomas, and other choroidal neovascular membranes. Excimer laser modification of corneal tissue continues to evolve as an effective method to modify refractive errors safely and consistently.

Finally, the introduction of a variety of laser-based imaging techniques used in optical coherence tomography (OCT), macular assessment devices, and wavelength technology is improving the clinician's diagnostic capabilities in managing a number of ocular conditions. Micropulse modification, which is available in certain solid-state diode lasers, can maximize desired laser effects while reducing unwanted collateral laser damage to surrounding tissue. With micropulse variation, the continuous wave emission is chopped into a train of short laser pulses that can be adjusted by the surgeon, thus providing an advantage to disease control. A longer pulse interval between pulses allows cooling of tissue to take place before the next pulse is delivered. Also, the advance of automatic or preplanned laser delivery can minimize laser exposure time for patients and reduce operator treatment times.

Femtosecond laser technology has advanced the accuracy and refinement of tissue ablation in the anterior segment of the eye. The femtosecond laser used in ophthalmology uses near-infrared light applied with shorter pulses than Nd:YAG laser interaction. These ultrashort laser pulses disrupt very small fractions of tissue, which provides exceptional accuracy for clear corneal incisions, astigmatic correction, anterior capsulotomies, and lens fragmentation. With these laser systems, corneal dissection for flap formation in refractive procedures can be applied with greater safety, more consistency, and greater precision over shorter time intervals. Femtosecond laser technology also has advanced the potential for intraocular lens disruption in the continuing quest for minimally invasive cataract surgery. Technologies using laser applications such as photoacoustic image capture are in their infancy, but promise further insight into more precise disease description.

As the future unfolds we can look forward to further advances in laser applications in the field of ophthalmology that will bring novel diagnostic and treatment options to the management of ocular disease.

Questions for review and thought

1. What are the different types of lasers used in ophthalmology?
2. What are the indications for laser use?
3. What anatomic structures must the argon laser light pass through before being absorbed by the pigment epithelium of the retina?
4. What safety precautions should be in place when lasers are used?

Q Self-evaluation questions

True–false statements

Directions: Indicate whether the statement is true **(T)** or false **(F).**

1. Laser application to the eye requires the patient to undergo general anesthesia. **T** or **F**
2. The argon and krypton lasers work on the principle of thermal photocoagulation. **T** or **F**
3. The Nd:YAG laser works via the mechanism of photodisruption. **T** or **F**

Missing words

Directions: Write in the missing word(s) in the following sentences:

4. The letters of the word *laser* stand for _____.
5. The lasers that use ultraviolet radiation for tissue destruction are referred to as _____.
6. The letters of the word YAG stand for _____.

Choice-completion questions

Directions: Select the one best answer in each case.

7. Laser light is consistent with which of the following?
   a. Monochromatism
   b. Coherence
   c. Low divergence
   d. Brightness
   e. All of the above

8. Of the lasers, which has the shortest wavelength?
   a. Argon
   b. Krypton
   c. Nd:YAG
   d. Carbon dioxide
   e. Excimer

9. The argon laser is not used to:
   a. ablate ischemic retina in proliferative diabetic retinopathy.
   b. produce a full-thickness iris hole (iridotomy) in angle-closure glaucoma.
   c. create burns of the trabecular meshwork in patients with open-angle glaucoma.
   d. create a central opening in an opacified posterior capsule after cataract surgery.
   e. ablate ischemic retina in central vein occlusions.

A Answers, notes, and explanations

1. **False.** Laser surgery can be performed under local anesthesia. If a specialized contact lens is used to focus the laser light, topical anesthesia is used. If the surgery involves coagulating the retina, for example panphotocoagulation, then a retrobulbar block in addition to topical anesthesia will often make the patient more comfortable.
2. **True.** The light from argon and krypton lasers is absorbed by tissues, resulting in sufficient heat energy for the surrounding tissue to be coagulated.
3. **True.** Unlike the argon and krypton lasers, the Nd:YAG laser uses high energy and an extremely short period of light exposure, which results in vaporization of tissue.
4. *Light amplification by stimulated emission of radiation.*
5. **Excimer lasers.** Because the laser light has a wavelength less than 380 nm, this light will not penetrate to the back of the eye; it will be completely absorbed by the cornea and lens. For this reason, the laser can be used to produce fine cuts in the cornea to change the refractive error of the eye.
6. **Yttrium, aluminum, garnet.** These are the components (in addition to neodymium ions, an energy source that can excite the molecules and an optical feedback mechanism) that comprise the Nd:YAG laser.
7. **e. All of the above.** Lasers are composed of monochromatic light in that one or more specific wavelengths are characteristic of each type of laser medium. Coherence refers to the light waves traveling in perfect step. The low divergence means that as light rays leave the laser cavity they are nearly parallel. The brightness of laser light exceeds all known artificial and natural light sources.
8. **e. Excimer.** The excimer laser has the shortest wavelength (193 nm). The other lasers in increasing order of wavelength are argon (488 and 514.5 nm), krypton (568 and 647 nm), Nd:YAG (1064 nm), and carbon dioxide (10,600 nm).
9. **d. Create a central opening in an opacified posterior capsule after cataract surgery.** The Nd:YAG laser, unlike the argon, acts to vaporize tissue. For this reason an opening in an opacified posterior capsule can be made. All the other answers are appropriate indications for use of the argon laser, which acts by photocoagulation.

Chapter | 35 |

Ambulatory surgery

Ambulatory—often called outpatient—surgery has been one of the most dramatic changes in an ophthalmic practice. In contrast to the previous patterns of hospitalization and restricted activity, most types of ophthalmic surgery, including cataract, glaucoma, and intraocular surgery, are now performed on an ambulatory, outpatient basis. For example, whereas 85% of cataract surgery used to be performed on an inpatient basis, now more than 85% of cataract surgery is performed on an outpatient basis in one of three specially designed ophthalmic surgery areas: hospital-based facilities, free-standing surgical centers, and office surgical suites. The patient goes home soon after the surgery.

Several factors have influenced this dramatic change. The shift from intracapsular surgery to extracapsular ophthalmic surgery and now small-incision phaco and femtosecond laser has contributed to the safety of cataract surgery performed on an ambulatory basis. Wounds have become smaller and the capsule has remained in place to prevent vitreous herniation. Suture material has improved, with increased tensile strength and elasticity; there is also a greater knowledge about better wound closure. Valve-like wound architecture is now possible.

However, a hospital admission may be required in cases of cardiovascular risks, older adults, the uncontrollable patient, and the infant and young child in whom general anesthesia may be required.

AMBULATORY SURGERY CENTERS

The development of ambulatory surgical centers (ASCs; surgicenters) throughout North America has contributed significantly to the changes in ophthalmic surgery. The overall emphasis of surgery is now placed on keeping hospital inpatient beds reserved for ill patients who require acute or prolonged care and attention. By avoiding hospitalization, significant financial savings can be realized by the public, the insuring agent, and governments.

Economics, however, was not the primary motivating factor for the directional change toward ambulatory surgery. Progressive ophthalmologists have long questioned the medical necessity of keeping patients immobilized for 24 hours after surgery, with gradual ambulation over several days. Dr. Norval Christie was a pioneer in this area, having operated on thousands of cataract patients annually in Pakistan on an outpatient basis. Other leading surgeons in the world followed with ambulatory surgery and immediate ambulation for their patients. Phacoemulsification surgery, with its small wound opening, gave impetus to this approach to surgery. Thus ambulatory surgery was ushered in and the Outpatient Ophthalmic Surgery Society (OOSS) was created to form a union of those who have free-standing eye centers.

One major value of an office-based or a free-standing surgical facility is that there is continuity of patient care. The same people are involved from the initial workup to the final discharge. This continuity with familiar faces, combined with trained personnel who care, eases the patient's anxiety.

The American Society of Cataract and Refractive Surgery (ASCRS) and OOSS have established standards for surgical ophthalmic centers that address the areas of construction, asepsis, and record keeping. These standards provide for the safety of patients, as well as the legal responsibility of the surgicenter for monitoring and maintaining continual self-assessment programs for quality control. Periodic site reviews are carried out. Equipment standards also are required.

To be eligible to receive Medicare payments, ASCs must be inspected by state Medicare agencies and certified that they meet federal standards. These standards require the ASC to:

1. Comply with state licensure requirements
2. Name a governing board that assumes full legal responsibility for the ASC's policies
3. Have an effective procedure for the immediate transfer to a hospital for emergencies, as well as a written transfer agreement with the hospital; all of the ASC's physicians must have privileges at the hospital
4. Have policies relating to surgical procedures and ASC privileges for qualified physicians, including examination of the patient by the physician before and after anesthesia
5. Have policies on the discharge of patients, including who should be discharged in the company of a responsible adult
6. Have procedures for ongoing, comprehensive self-assessment of the quality and necessity of care
7. Have a safe and sanitary environment
8. Be accountable to the ASC governing board; policies must be established for granting clinical privileges, periodic reappraisal, and supervision of the nonphysician staff
9. Have direct and staff nursing services to ensure that the nursing needs of all patients are met
10. Maintain complete, comprehensive, and accurate medical records to ensure adequate care
11. Provide drugs and biologic agents in a safe and effective manner, according to accepted professional practice and under the direction of a responsible designated individual
12. Have arrangements for obtaining routine and emergency laboratory and radiologic services from approved facilities.

The advantages of a surgical outpatient facility have been pointed out by Dr. Sanford Severin of Albany, California. These advantages include the following:

1. Patient acceptance. A more pleasant and comforting environment is provided, with ready access to familiar faces.
2. Cost-effectiveness. There is a major saving for the patient and the government or insurance company. The government can save more than $1 billion per year if the 1 million cataract extractions in the United States are charged a small facility fee.
3. Complete control of the operating room. Personnel can be chosen who work well together and are effective, not only in knowing the surgeon's routines and the purchasing and replacement of equipment and supplies but also in maintaining good public relations with the patients and answering questions in a meaningful way, allaying patients' fears. Thus a surgical team is evolved that relates to both the surgeon's and the patient's wishes.
4. Scheduling. Scheduling is at the convenience of the surgeon. There is no waiting for surgical time or being "bumped" for emergencies of other surgeons. One can schedule late in the day and on weekends.
5. True effectiveness. There is a better efficiency of time for the surgeon and the patient. There is less travel time for the surgeon, less waiting time for surgery for the patient, and a reduction in the wait between cases for maximum use of the operating room and the staff's time.
6. There are commercially available sterile and disposable drapes, gowns, and medical supplies.

The disadvantages of a free-standing ophthalmic surgical center or an office surgical center include the following:

1. The surgeon and staff must assume more responsibility in maintaining adequate stock, equipment, and sterility
2. Medicolegal responsibilities increase; if a patient should become seriously ill during surgery, the ASC staff is responsible for the care of the patient and the transfer to a general hospital
3. The need for ongoing interaction with agencies for payment reimbursement and peer review for certification standards
4. Expenses can be greater than the reimbursement rate unless a large number of procedures are being performed; the center may not be cost-effective for small numbers
5. The ambulatory center as a major financial commitment is threatened in the case of sickness of the primary surgeon or key staff members or a reduction in surgical volume
6. There may be a lack of patient compliance with the postoperative regimen after the patient is discharged from the surgical center.

TIPS ON MEDICAL/LEGAL PROTECTION

About 1 in 10 physicians will be sued at some time during their average medical career. Approximately 75% of these claims result from surgical procedures. Ophthalmologists, fortunately, have the lowest rate of malpractice and litigation in the medical profession. Only about 2.5% of

Box 35.1 **Ways to avoid a lawsuit**

1. Ensure that you identify the correct patient and the correct side for any surgical procedure. Mark the procedure site preop and double-check before proceeding.
2. Establish good rapport with the patient. The patient who likes the physician and the environment where surgery is performed is less likely to sue. Some lawsuits are started because of the patient's vindictiveness, even if the physician is fault-free. A doctor whom the patient views as compassionate and understanding has already acquired some protection against legal actions.
3. Discharge the patient into the care of a competent adult, one who will take care of the patient at home. The name of this individual should be recorded on the chart.
4. Provide written, easy-to-understand directions for the follow-up care and return visits. These should be read and explained to the patient or relative and all questions answered.
5. Include in the list problems or symptoms that may arise at home and what to do if they occur.
6. Provide in the instructions some directions for obtaining an appropriate physician for medical problems. Telephone numbers of the physician, ophthalmologist, and a nearby hospital emergency room should be given.
7. Arrange for a nurse or assistant to telephone that evening or the next day to check on the patient's condition if the situation warrants it, and record this on the chart.
8. Make operative notes immediately after surgery, not weeks or months later.
9. Instruct patients to leave valuables at home or arrange some system for safekeeping of the patient's valuables during surgery. Often lockers are provided.
10. Make sure that life-sustaining equipment is available and in good working order.
11. Be sure there is an adequate consent form that is well outlined to the patient. Good personal communication with the patient as to risks, benefits, and alternatives is highly valuable. An informed consent for major surgery is mandatory. These consent forms can range from a simple page or two to an elaborate 12-page document with video viewing and the patient's response questionnaire. Each physician determines his or her own comfort level. Appendix 3 contains the principles of informed consent.
12. Maintain good records in the office and the hospital. The quality and legibility of your records affect the quality of your practice. It is important to attach to the records a log of telephone advice. Cursory, sloppy, or nonexistent notes call the physician's credibility and standards of practice into question. The practitioner should initial all laboratory and x-ray reports before they are filed.

practicing ophthalmologists claim to have been sued. The most common suits are negligent performance of cataract surgery, negligent treatment of ophthalmic conditions, failure to diagnose ophthalmic conditions, postoperative vision loss, and complications as a result of negligent surgery or follow-up (Box 35.1).

All surgical patients should be given extensive education concerning their problem. Videotapes may be shown and visual aid instructions may be given. Every effort should be made to have the family present at the teaching session. Providing written handouts also can be of some value (Box 35.4).

PREPARATION FOR ADMISSION

In preparation for admission to an ambulatory surgery center, each patient should have a careful medical evaluation by the family physician or internist. A checklist should be made of such events as routine laboratory tests and electrocardiograms (Box 35.2). A complete eye workup should be performed. A-scan measurements should be determined. If the power of the intraocular lens is beyond the range of stock maintained, then a correct dioptric power intraocular lens should be obtained from the manufacturer. An additional visit may be required for the patient to consult with the anesthesiologist, who can review the laboratory results and the workup of the family physician (Box 35.3).

ADMISSION FOR SURGERY

Each surgicenter has its own specific requirements for admission for cataract surgery. We arrange to have our patients report 1½ hours before surgery to ensure adequate dilation of the pupil before the procedure. We apply name tags with the site of operation on each patient to avoid mistakes.

Vital signs are recorded. The patient is free to move around and sit with relatives. Preoperative intramuscular sedation may be given to the nervous patient. Local anesthesia is administered by way of topical drops. Peribulbar or retrobulbar injection may be given. Some surgeons prefer to give an injection of intravenous methohexital (methohexitone, Brevital) or sodium thiopental (thiopental,

Box 35.2 **Surgical checklist**

*Type of surgery; e.g., secondary IOL
  *Site of surgery; e.g., rt eye (or OD)
  CAT/IOL
  SECONDARY IOL
  OTHER _____
  OD/OS
  _____

DATE OF SURGERY _____
**SPECIAL REQUESTS, E.G., TYPE OF IOL, e.g. toric, bifocal
  manufacture, power
PREOPERATIVE VISIT
_____ Preoperative booklet given
_____ Operative instructions given
_____ History and physical form given
_____ Laboratory tests arranged
_____ Appointment scheduled with Dr. _____
for _____
_____ A-scan scheduled for _____
_____ A-scan result: Lens style _____
Diameter _____

_____ Endothelial studies
_____ Financial planning
_____ Insurance
_____ Surgery scheduled: Date _____
PATIENT _____
ADDRESS _____
PHONE NO. _____
RELATIVE'S NAME _____
PHONE NO. _____
SURGERY DAY
_____ Operative consent reviewed and signed
_____ Premedication given
_____ Postoperative instructions given
_____ Postoperative appointment made for_____
_____ Responsible home person: _____
_____ Medication given
_____ Ultraviolet glasses given or ordered

Box 35.3 **Anesthetic questions**

The following questions have been designed for use by the Department of Anesthesiology. They are to be completed before your operation. Please answer each question carefully. Bring the completed form to the preadmittance laboratory.

Name _____
Address_____
Phone_____ Age_____ Sex_____
Health Card No._____

Answer ☑	Yes	No	Do not know
1. What is your approximate weight? _____ (pounds/kg)?			
2. Did you ever have trouble with your heart?	☐	☐	☐
3. Did you ever take any medicine or pills for your heart?	☐	☐	☐
4. Did you ever take any medicine or pills for your blood pressure?	☐	☐	☐
5. Did you ever have high or low blood pressure?	☐	☐	☐
6. Did you ever take any medicine or pills for your breathing?	☐	☐	☐
7. Did you ever have any trouble with your breathing?	☐	☐	☐
8. Did a doctor ever tell you had asthma?	☐	☐	☐
9. Do you take any medicine, pills, or injections of any type regularly while you are not in the hospital? If so, see Question 27	☐	☐	☐
10. Within the past year, have you taken any medicine for rheumatism, arthritis, or allergies?	☐	☐	☐
11. Have you taken a drug called cortisone or prednisone within the past year?	☐	☐	☐
12. Have you taken any tranquilizers or nerve pills within the past 2 weeks?	☐	☐	☐
13. Have you been pregnant within the past 3 months?	☐	☐	☐
14. Do you have any bleeding or bruising tendencies?	☐	☐	☐
15. Do you take pills for thinning your blood?	☐	☐	☐
16. Have you had a general anesthetic within the past 3 months?	☐	☐	☐

Continued

Box 35.3 Anesthetic questions—cont'd

17. Were you ever been told that you were unusually sick after a previous general anesthetic? ☐ ☐ ☐
18. Have you ever been jaundiced or had liver trouble? ☐ ☐ ☐
19. Do you have a family history of problems with anesthesia or of malignant hyperthermia? ☐ ☐ ☐
20. Do you have loose, false, or capped teeth? ☐ ☐ ☐
21. Do you wear contact lenses? ☐ ☐ ☐
22. Do you have glaucoma or use eyedrops regularly? ☐ ☐ ☐
23. To the best of your knowledge, are you allergic to anything? ☐ ☐ ☐
24. If so, to what are you allergic? _____
25. Please list below the operations you have had during your life:

_____
_____
_____
_____

26. Please list below the illnesses you have had during your life:

_____
_____
_____
_____

27. Please list below the names of the medicines you have taken regularly and the reasons for taking them:

_____
_____
_____
_____

Anesthetist's comments:

_____
_____
_____
_____

Date: _____ Signature of patient: _____

Box 35.4 Patient instructions for ambulatory surgery

Your procedure is scheduled for: _____
  (Date to be inserted by surgeon's office)
1. Come to the admitting office at: _____
  (Time to be inserted by surgeon's office)
2. Bring this form with you.
3. You must not eat or drink anything after 11.30 p.m. on the evening before your procedure.
4. Leave valuables at home. Your stay will be short. You will not be staying overnight.
5. Remove makeup before coming to hospital.
6. If you have a cough or cold, whether taking medication or not, please call your surgeon as soon as possible, because your operation may have to be rescheduled.
7. You must not drive a motor vehicle for 24 hours after surgery. You must arrange for a responsible person to pick you up and accompany you from the hospital as soon as you are able to go home. Please arrange to have this person call _____ approximately 3 hours after you arrive to establish the time of pickup.
8. Male and female patients will be prepared for procedures in the Ambulatory Procedure Unit. After surgery you will be taken from the operating room to the recovery room and then be discharged to go home.
9. It is expected that a parent will stay with children younger than 10 years of age until time of discharge.
10. You must not take any drugs or alcohol 24 hours after surgery unless prescribed by a physician.

thiopental sodium, Sodium Pentothal, Trapanal) during this latter procedure to reduce any awareness of this injection. Either the Honan balloon or the super pinky may be used for compression. Some patients are given intravenous medication such as Valium or Innovar for sedation.

The patient is then brought into the operating room and helped onto the operating table and made comfortable. The electrocardiograph leads and blood pressure cuffs are put in place. The eye is prepared with antiseptic solution. The nurse explains these procedures as they are being performed. The specialized ophthalmic assistant often participates actively in the surgery in an outpatient facility where a medical assistant may not be available (Figures 35.1 to 35.3).

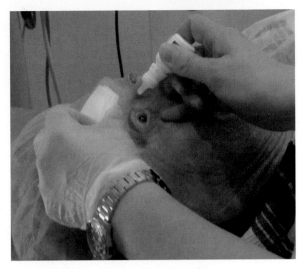

Figure 35.3 Instilling medication after surgery.

The most important factors in success are meticulous surgery, good wound closure, cleanliness and sterility of the operating facility, and friendliness and competency of the staff.

POSTOPERATIVE RECOVERY

The patient's family is invited to remain in the waiting room during surgery. After surgery they are invited to be with the patient in the recovery area. Here, vital signs are checked regularly. The patient may sit up and be served juice, coffee, tea, or light refreshments. The patient is given counseling in postoperative care. The patient is discharged shortly after surgery and an appointment is arranged for the following day for examination. The only restriction is to avoid excessive exertion. The total time spent in the surgical center is minimal. The patch is removed the following day, eyedrops are prescribed, printed instructions are given, and a pair of dark glasses are often provided.

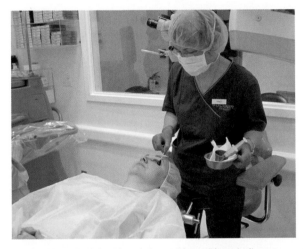

Figure 35.1 Prepping the patient with povidone-iodine (Betadine) before cataract surgery.

SUMMARY

In ASCs, the operation is performed in a friendly environment that is familiar to the patient and relatives. Each step from check-in before surgery to check-out after surgery is designed to allay fears and make the patient as relaxed as possible. It is important that the center has caring dedicated personnel, with compassion and a real willingness to cater to the needs of elderly persons, who are the typical eye

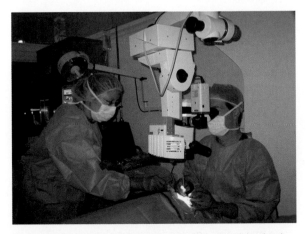

Figure 35.2 Specialized ophthalmic assistant participating in ophthalmic surgery.

patients. In addition, staff must be well trained and competent.

Outpatient ambulatory surgery is based on the fact that, with currently available techniques, complications are no greater than with inpatient cataract surgery in hospitals.

The patient's acceptance is, however, much greater with ambulatory surgery. Everywhere in the world, outpatient cataract surgery has become the rule rather than the exception. Certified ASCs are as high in quality as major hospital operating rooms.

Questions for review and thought

1. List the significant advantages of ambulatory surgery.
2. List the possible disadvantages of ambulatory surgery.
3. Outline safety standards in a free-standing surgical facility.
4. What are the operative routines followed in your practice?
5. What are the preoperative testing routines before major surgery?
6. What medication, both ocular and systemic, is given before a cataract operation by your ophthalmologist?
7. What is the role of the ophthalmic medical assistant in the care of patients before and after cataract surgery?
8. What is the medicolegal responsibility of the ophthalmic assistant?

Q Self-evaluation questions

True–false statements

Directions: Indicate whether the statement is true **(T)** or false **(F).**

1. Operative notes must be detailed in a free-standing surgical facility. **T** or **F**
2. A consent form is required only in some major eye operations. **T** or **F**
3. Drugs and biologic agents can be administered only by a physician. **T** or **F**

Missing words

Directions: Write in the missing word(s) in the following sentences:

4. A _____ is used to record that all necessary preoperative and postoperative evaluations have been ordered.
5. The abbreviated form for medication given by injection in the muscle is called _____.
6. _____ is the Latin term for medication taken by mouth.

Choice-completion questions

Directions: Select the one best answer in each case.

7. Which is not true? Ambulatory cataract surgery may be performed in:
   a. a hospital-based facility.
   b. office treatment rooms.
   c. free-standing surgical centers.
   d. office surgical suites.
   e. hospital emergency operating rooms.
8. Which condition is least likely to be treated with ambulatory surgery?
   a. Cataract with intraocular lens (IOL)
   b. Orbital tumor
   c. Strabismus surgery
   d. Glaucoma surgery
   e. Pterygium surgery
9. Standards for an ambulatory surgical center involve a number of requirements. Which of the following is not required?
   a. A governing body responsible for policies
   b. A mechanism for transfer to a hospital for emergencies
   c. A mechanism for ongoing care
   d. An attending nurse at all times
   e. Maintenance of complete records

A   Answers, notes, and explanations

1. **True.** The requirements for an ambulatory surgical center are as rigid as those of major hospital operating rooms. The details of the surgical procedure must be outlined in a standard operative report attached to the records.

2. **False.** All major surgery requires an informed consent form.

3. **False.** Drugs and biologic agents can be given orally or by eyedrops by allied health personnel who have been trained to do this. Intramuscular or subcutaneous injections must be given either by a physician or by someone licensed in the state to invade tissue. This may be a registered nurse.

4. **Surgical checklist.** Checklists are important to jog one's memory that all items necessary for preoperative and postoperative evaluations are available and the results tabulated. Such information as A-scan measurements may be critical when the time comes for surgery. A checklist is vital.

5. **IM.** The injection is given into the muscle mass.

6. **Per os.** When medication is given orally, it is often written per os, meaning through the mouth.

7. **b. Office treatment rooms.** Office treatment rooms usually do not have the sterility required for major surgery. They also are not adequately equipped for respiratory or cardiovascular emergencies that could occur.

8. **b. Orbital tumor.** Orbital tumors may result in bleeding postoperatively, which may require blood transfusions. There also is a danger that there could be an invasion of adjacent tissue or some unusual tumor found that requires more extensive dissection.

9. **d. An attending nurse at all times.** An attending nurse is not required at all times. Often the physician may supervise a great deal of the ambulatory surgery personally. The ophthalmic medical assistant can be trained to be responsible for a great deal of the patient's care.

Chapter | **36** |

Refractive surgery

Raymond M. Stein, Rebecca L. Stein

BASIC PRINCIPLES OF REFRACTIVE SURGERY

The cornea's function is to maintain the integrity of the eye and the transparency of the anterior surface of the globe so that light can pass through to the retina. Most important, this anterior surface is responsible for 70% of the refraction of light entering the eye. In myopia, either the cornea may be too convex or the axial length of the eye may be too long, causing light to converge at a focal point anterior to the retina. Corneal reshaping is an important concept in refractive surgery and is the procedure most commonly used. The surgery aims to flatten the center of the cornea so that light will focus more posteriorly (Figure 36.1).

Laser-assisted in situ keratomileusis (LASIK) and photorefractive keratectomy (PRK) are the dominant refractive procedures. These laser correction procedures tend to remove less than two-tenths of the full thickness of the cornea (about 50–100 μm). The procedures can correct nearsightedness, far-sightedness, and astigmatism. LASIK and PRK have replaced the technique of radial keratotomy (RK) in which a diamond blade is used to make radial corneal incisions. This procedure weakened the midperipheral cornea, resulting in central flattening to correct nearsightedness. Laser vision correction has been shown to be more predictable and stable than RK.

PHOTOREFRACTIVE KERATECTOMY, PHOTOTHERAPEUTIC KERATECTOMY, AND LASER IN SITU KERATOMILEUSIS

Excimer laser corneal surgery may be divided into phototherapeutic keratectomy (PTK), PRK, LASIK, and LASEK (laser-assisted subepithelial keratectomy or laser-assisted epithelial keratomileusis). PTK is the removal of tissue from the cornea to correct a medical problem with the eye; PRK, LASIK, or LASEK, is the removal of tissue from the cornea to correct a refractive problem of the eye (near-sightedness, far-sightedness, or astigmatism). These procedures are performed with an excimer laser beam.

The word excimer is a contraction of "'excited"' and "'dimer."' The laser is a product of a reaction between a rare gas (argon) and a halogen (fluorine) in the presence of a strong electrical discharge. This reaction creates short-lived molecules (excited dimers) that emit strong pulses of light in the form of ultraviolet radiation at 193 nm. When precisely focused on the cornea, this pulse of light can remove tissue from the cornea in a manner that is cleaner and more controlled than any diamond knife. It can remove tissue to within a fraction of a micrometer (Figure 36.2). The excimer laser energy is almost totally absorbed by the epithelial cells, Bowman's layer, and the stroma as the energy is pulsed onto the cornea at a 0.25-μm depth per pulse. Ablation of the corneal layers results in flattening and reduction of the myopic error.

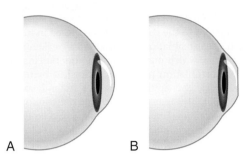

Figure 36.1 (A) Normal, smoothly contoured cornea. (B) Flattened, central cornea after radial keratotomy (RK) or laser surgery.

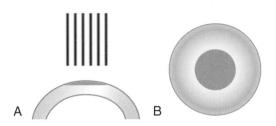

Figure 36.2 Excimer laser vaporizes a thin layer from the surface of the cornea. (A) Cross-section of the cornea. (B) Direct view of the cornea.

History

The excimer laser was first developed by IBM in 1975 for etching microchips. In 1981 Toboada and Archibald investigated the clinical aspects of the excimer. Stephen Trokel and Charles Mulleryn saw its clinical application to the cornea and became involved. Trokel, Pulofito, Hanna, MacDonald, and others began the process of scientifically studying the procedure, first in the laboratory and later in blind human eyes. Clinical trials around the world have documented the predictability, stability, and safety of PRK for low and moderate degrees of myopia, astigmatism, and hyperopia.

Photorefractive keratectomy

The PRK procedure, which is performed using a topical anesthetic such as proparacaine 0.5% or tetracaine drops, takes anywhere from 2 seconds to 45 seconds depending on the degree of myopia, astigmatism, and hyperopia. Most excimer lasers use flying spot technology in which a small laser beam is emitted that is computer-controlled. The rapid firing of the laser beam to the cornea systematically ablates tissue to correct refractive errors. All lasers use a tracking system to increase the chance that the laser pulses will be delivered to the intended area. This decreases the

chance of a decentered ablation. The epithelium is removed by mechanical means (spatula or brush) or by using the laser to reveal Bowman's layer. The laser beam is activated by a foot control, and the ablation process typically removes less than 100 μm of tissue. The higher the correction, the more tissue is removed. A bandage soft contact lens is inserted for 4 to 5 days and medication is given.

In refractive surgery to treat myopia, more tissue is removed from the center than from the periphery, so that flattening of the cornea occurs. In treatment of hyperopia, more tissue is removed from the midperiphery than from the center, which results in steepening of the cornea and a decrease in hyperopia.

Results

The results of excimer laser surgery have been excellent in recent years. A majority of patients (95%) achieve a level of uncorrected vision of 20/25 or better and within 0.50 diopter of correction. Clinical data have shown that with proper patient selection, laser vision correction has been an effective and safe procedure, and a viable alternative to glasses or contact lenses. However, a number of side effects can occur.

1. *Delayed epithelial healing.* With PRK, the outer layer of the cornea is removed before excimer laser surgery. Normally this layer replaces itself within 4 or 5 days.
2. *Light sensitivity.* Because of temporary disturbance of tissues, sunglasses probably should be worn in sunlight for at least the first week. This is not a major factor.
3. *Corneal haze.* This occurs in some cases. However, it usually does not interfere significantly with vision. The patient may notice some glare. The haze is a result of keratocytes that enter the cornea after the ablation procedure and begin the healing process. Eventually they disappear, but they may persist and cause impaired vision. The use of dilute sterile mitomycin solution as an intraoperative application for 12 to 60 seconds has reduced the incidence of haze by acting directly on the keratocytes to reduce new collagen synthesis.
4. *Overcorrection.* Overcorrection of myopia, hyperopia, and/or astigmatism can occur during the healing process. If there is no resolution after 6 months and the amount of overcorrection is visually significant to the patient, an enhancement can be performed.
5. *Undercorrection.* Undercorrection can occur with the treatment of myopia, hyperopia, or astigmatism. If there is no significant improvement after 6 months and the patient is not satisfied with the level of vision, an enhancement can be performed.

How does it work?

The excimer laser uses a mixture of argon and fluorine gases in a mirrored tube to produce a cold, ultraviolet beam of light that vaporizes tissue by breaking molecular bonds a few molecular layers at a time. This process allows for vaporization or ablation of tissue without burning or disturbing the underlying tissue. Ultraviolet laser beams break up tissue by excitation of the atomic links, a photochemical process. The result is a precise cut with very straight edges and no discoloration or dehydration of surrounding tissue. The excimer laser is so precise that it can remove tissue 0.25 µm at a time (1 µm = $\frac{1}{1000}$ millimeter). The treated area of the cornea is so smooth and the ablation amount is so accurate that very precise modification of the corneal curvature is possible.

Before excimer laser surgery was performed on sighted humans, a wealth of information on the procedure was gathered from testing first on animal eyes and later on blind human eyes.

In addition to its use in eye surgery, the excimer laser is being tested by heart specialists as a way of clearing out clogged coronary arteries.

Advantages and disadvantages

The advantage of excimer laser surgery is that it is computer-driven and is more reproducible than a handheld surgical knife. Excimer laser removes tissue by ablation. Usually neither deformation of the cornea nor induced astigmatism occurs. The sculpting is computer-programmed, leaving less room for human-generated variables. In addition, the procedure is quick.

With PRK, incision problems are avoided because the surgery ablates only a very thin layer of the cornea. Anatomically the eye is almost unaffected because laser surgery does not cause detectable weakening of the cornea, and susceptibility to injury is prevented.

Other advantages of excimer laser surgery are as follows:

- Surgery with the excimer laser is more reproducible than a handheld surgical knife.
- The speed with which the laser sculpts minimizes the variability as a result of corneal dehydration during the course of surgery; hence accuracy is much more complete.
- The laser is capable of creating a variety of patterns currently not practical with the handheld knife.
- With the excimer laser there are no incision healing problems because the surgery removes a very thin layer of the cornea, less than ($\frac{1}{10}$) of its thickness. In RK, the cornea is permanently weakened because the cuts have to be more than ($\frac{9}{10}$) of its thickness to achieve the flattening effect required.
- Because a very small amount of the cornea is affected (microscopic layers on the surface of the cornea), the eye is almost unaffected anatomically.

The disadvantage of PRK is that the procedure carries some risks because the ablation process is performed in the central 5.5 to 6.5 mm of the cornea. The depth is usually not more than 50 to 100 µm of the cornea. However, software has been designed to provide a sculpting of the borders and a blending of the curves to reduce the greater ablation process and depth in the cornea that is required in high myopia. Too deep an ablation may result in a weakening of the entire cornea, which may lead to a central bulging or ectasia. After the ablation process is performed by use of the excimer laser, the epithelium slides in and covers the denuded area. This may take 4 to 5 days. Discomfort during the healing process has been greatly reduced by the fitting of a bandage soft contact lens, nonsteroidal antiinflammatory drops, ice packs, and systemic pain relief medication.

Therapeutic corneal surgery (phototherapeutic keratectomy)

The excimer laser for therapeutic use (PTK) offers tremendous potential for improving sight to literally millions of persons affected by corneal scars or corneal dystrophy. Superficial ablation of the stroma up to 150 µm in depth can remove scars and permit normal regularly aligned stromal fibers to be covered by regenerated epithelial cells. Astigmatism that may follow cataract or corneal transplant surgery can be corrected by the excimer laser with the astigmatic module.

The use of the excimer laser in corneal surgery enables physicians to treat a number of corneal injuries, scars, and diseases without having to go to the extreme of a corneal transplant.

Therapeutic areas in which the excimer laser has been very useful are removal or reduction of superficial corneal scars, dystrophies, or deposits. These conditions may include scars from trauma or superficial infections, superficial corneal dystrophies such as granular dystrophy, or calcium deposits referred to as band keratopathy. The excimer also can be used to smooth the corneal surface in cases of scars or dystrophies that create irregular astigmatism. Another therapeutic application is the treatment of recurrent corneal erosions by removing 5 to 10 µm of Bowman's layer. By roughening Bowman's layer the newly regenerated epithelium sticks down better, thus decreasing the risk of erosions.

Laser-assisted in situ keratomileusis

LASIK is a laser vision correction procedure in which a thin flap of corneal tissue with a hinge is created, the flap is then retracted, the excimer laser is used to ablate tissue beneath the flap, and then the flap is repositioned. The LASIK flap can be created with a femtosecond laser or a mechanical microkeratome that uses a blade. Femtosecond laser technology is gradually capturing the market share because of accuracy, ease of use, and safety. The LASIK flap is typically 90 to 110 µm thick. As with PRK, the excimer laser is used to ablate tissue of the corneal bed to correct nearsightedness, far-sightedness, and astigmatism.

Advantages and disadvantages

LASIK has a number of advantages over PRK:

1. Minimal or no discomfort postoperatively
2. Rapid return of vision because it is not dependent on epithelial migration
3. Earlier refractive stability than with PRK, usually by 2 months
4. Ease of enhancement or retreatments, in which the flap can be lifted generally without cutting and further treatment with the excimer laser applied
5. Minimal healing response, so that corneal haze is generally not a problem

The disadvantages of LASIK compared with PRK are related to problems in creating the corneal flap. These include an incomplete flap, a free flap, a buttonhole flap, a dislocated flap, and wrinkles in the flap. Fortunately the incidence of flap-related complications is decreasing with surgical experience, improvements in the microkeratomes, and especially with femtosecond lasers. Another potential complication is interface debris that is not irrigated out at the time of surgery.

As in PRK, complications of LASIK can be secondary to the excimer laser. These problems include decentration, central island (i.e., focal central steep area), irregular astigmatism, undercorrection, or overcorrection.

Follow-up

Follow-up after LASIK is relatively simple and straightforward. Patients recover quickly, have little pain, and are usually extremely pleased with their new vision, which they begin to enjoy almost immediately after surgery. Good guidelines and a clear idea of what to look for make the LASIK follow-up process fit easily into a comprehensive ophthalmology practice.

Initial follow-up

The surgeon performs the initial follow-up within an hour after surgery. The surgeon checks for the following four primary items:

- Flap position. Incorrect positioning of the flap should be rectified (Figure 36.3).
- Significant wrinkles (or folds) in the flap. If these are found, the flap has to be refloated and repositioned (Figure 36.4).
- Significant debris beneath the flap. If there is enough debris to compromise vision, the flap must be lifted and the debris irrigated out.
- Epithelial defects close to the cut edge of the flap (other than the cut edge itself). Because defects increase the chance of epithelial ingrowth, a bandage soft contact lens may be required until the epithelium heals.

Before leaving, the patient is provided with a broad-spectrum antibiotic moxifloxacin ophthalmic solution

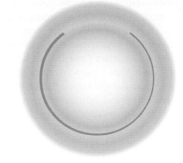

Figure 36.3 Poorly positioned flap after LASIK. The gutter is wider on one side than the other.

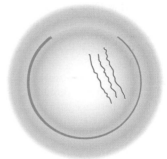

Figure 36.4 Significant wrinkles in the flap after LASIK.

(Vigamox) and gatifloxacin ophthalmic solution (Zymar) and a steroid. Both are typically taken five times a day for 5 days. Unlike PRK, there is no need to prescribe either an anesthetic or a nonsteroidal antiinflammatory drug (NSAID) after LASIK. However, we do use a few drops of NSAID at the conclusion of the LASIK procedure.

Although routine in PRK, a bandage lens is rarely used after LASIK. Instead, the patient should be provided with a protective shield or safety glasses to be put on at bedtime for the next few nights. The shield is designed to prevent eye rubbing during sleep. Although use of this shield or safety glasses can be discontinued after these few nights, we recommend that patients not rub the operated eye(s) for an entire month. They can take showers at any time, but they should be careful to keep water out of their eyes for a few days. The use of makeup and all other normal activities can resume after the fifth to seventh postoperative day.

When to use a bandage lens

Epithelial defects (other than the normal cut from the microkeratome) found after the LASIK procedure usually indicate an underlying anterior basement membrane dystrophy. These patients are better treated with PRK than with LASIK; however, the diagnosis is not always made before surgery.

If the anterior basement dystrophy goes undetected and LASIK is performed, the epithelium can come off in sheets. In these cases, a bandage soft contact lens may be necessary. The lens should remain in place for a few days after the epithelium is shown to be intact (usually 3–4 days), at which time the bandage lens can be gently removed.

Remove the lens at the slit lamp. Rather than pinching the lens between two fingers, lubricate the eye liberally with artificial tears and, using a curved forceps, gently slide the lens off the eye.

Postoperative pain

Significant, long-lasting pain is very rarely a complaint in LASIK. Most patients experience ocular irritation and are somewhat light-sensitive in the hours immediately following their procedure, but close to 100% of them are comfortable by the next morning. If the patient is still uncomfortable after a night's rest, the doctor who sees the patients on postoperative day 1 should look carefully for a dislocated flap or an epithelial defect that was either missed or created after the patient left the laser center.

Pain in the first postoperative week may also signal an inflammation. LASIK patients should be advised to call immediately if they experience pain.

Follow-up schedule

The follow-up for the comanaging eye doctor can begin on postoperative day 1, and it progresses through three phases. In the first phase, flap integrity and epithelial healing are the main concerns. In the next, attention shifts to the quality and precision of the correction, and, in a few cases, there is a third phase in which the patient is referred for enhancement.

We recommend follow-up visits at 1 day, 1 week, 1 month, 3 months, 6 months, and 1 year.

Infection

The signs of infection in the immediate postoperative period include a white infiltrate in the stroma, increased redness of the eye, and an increased anterior chamber reaction. The patient will likely experience pain, which is otherwise unusual following LASIK.

If there is suspicion of infection or inflammation, a culture should be considered. The broad-spectrum antibiotic should be stopped and the infection treated with fortified antibiotics such as tobramycin (15 mg/mL) and cefazolin (50 mg/mL).

EpiLASIK

EpiLASIK is a variant of surface ablation or PRK in which an epiLASIK microkeratome is used to create a flap of epithelium away from Bowman's layer. The epithelial flap is lifted, and the excimer layer is used to remove tissue from the stroma. The flap can then be repositioned. Recent studies have not shown any significant advantages of this technique over standard PRK.

ADDITIONAL PROCEDURES

Small-incision intrastromal lenticule extraction (SMILE)

A procedure has been developed that uses a femtosecond laser to cut a lenticule of tissue within the stroma. This tissue is then extracted through a small superior incision. Clinical outcomes have shown equivalent long-term outcomes to LASIK. The potential advantages of SMILE are the elimination of a flap and possible fewer dry eye symptoms. It was hoped that the incidence of ectasia would be lower by preserving some of the anterior corneal lamellae, but at the time of this writing there have been a number of reported ectasia cases. Another issue is the slower visual recovery, which typically takes a few days to a week compared with the rapid return of vision with LASIK in 24 hours. Other issues are that one is unable to correct hyperopia or mixed astigmatism, and that enhancement must be performed using PRK.

Intracorneal ring

An intracorneal ring can be inserted into the eyes of patients with low degrees of myopia (1.00–4.50 diopters) and 0.75 diopter of astigmatism or less. This is a permanent, but reversible, procedure in which a PMMA ring of variable thickness is inserted into the midperipheral cornea. The increase in thickness of the peripheral cornea induces central flattening and correction of low degrees of myopia. If the refractive correction is not satisfactory, the ring can be removed. This procedure is appealing to the successful contact lens wearer who is anxious about laser vision correction, or who believes there may be better procedures or better technology in the future.

The advantages of the intracorneal ring include no risk of losing best corrected vision because the central cornea is spared, reversibility, exchangeability, and maintenance of normal asphericity of the cornea (steeper in the center and flatter in the periphery), which results in excellent night vision.

The intracorneal ring is most commonly used in eyes with keratoconus or ectasia after LASIK to flatten the cornea or area of ectasia. The use of LASIK or PRK has generally replaced the intracorneal ring for the correction of myopia. Laser vision correction has been shown to be more accurate and predictable.

Keratomileusis

José Barraquer first described the procedure of keratomileusis in the early 1960s. In this procedure, lamellae of the patient's own cornea are removed and lathed on a cryolathe in a frozen state and resutured back to the cornea in a flattened condition centrally. The cornea can be either steepened or flattened. This procedure requires a sophisticated cryolathe and a well-trained cryolathe technician. It can be used after cataract operations and can correct up to 12.00 diopters of hyperopia. Complications may include induced irregular astigmatism, interface debris, undercorrection, and overcorrection. It is a sophisticated procedure that requires an experienced surgeon and an experienced technician for precise measurement. It is not user-friendly.

Automated lamellar keratoplasty

A slightly more user-friendly, nonfreeze method is automated lamellar keratoplasty (ALK). The patient's own cornea is removed with a microkeratome, the cornea is reshaped in a flattened state, and the anterior layer is simply placed on the eye. New modifications of reshaping the stroma with excimer laser have been developed using the technique of LASIK.

Epikeratoplasty

Epikeratoplasty comes from the Greek *epi* ("on top of") and *kerato* ("cornea") (Figure 36.5). Epikeratoplasty was developed at Louisiana State University by Herbert Kaufman, Marguerite MacDonald, and Theodore Werblin. This procedure is most useful for pediatric aphakia and keratoconus. When performed after cataract surgery, it is called epikeratophakia. In this procedure a precarved corneal donor button is rehydrated at the time of surgery when the surgeon sews it into a recipient bed after the epithelium has been mended.

Phakic implant

A phakic lens or implant can be used to correct myopia, hyperopia, and astigmatism. Typically very high corrections are treated with this technology. The implant is custom-ordered for power and sometimes size, and inserted through a microcorneal incision. A variety of

different models are available including those that attach to the iris, anterior chamber angle lenses, or sulcus lenses. Patients must have an anterior chamber depth of greater than 2.8 mm (distance between the back of the cornea and the crystalline lens). Potential complications include pupillary block glaucoma, corneal endothelial cell loss leading to edema, and a focal or diffuse cataract.

Refractive lens exchange

Refractive lens exchange involves removal of the crystalline lens and the insertion of an intraocular lens implant to correct refractive errors. The operation is similar to a cataract operation except for the fact that surgery is performed on a clear lens. The procedure is typically used to treat presbyopia with the insertion of a multifocal or accommodating implant, or the correction of high refractive errors that are outside the normal range for LASIK or PRK. As with any intraocular procedure, complications may occur that are similar to those after cataract surgery, which include intraocular infection (endophthalmitis) and retinal detachment (see Chapter 31).

Corneal inlays

Corneal inlays are being evaluated as another option to correct presbyopia. The inlay is inserted under a LASIK flap or through a pocket. A number of inlays have been developed, each with a different design. One inlay is the Kamra and works on the principle of a small aperture increasing the depth of focus. Another is the Raindrop, which creates a small area of elevation over the pupil to enhance reading. LASIK can be performed at the same time to enhance distance vision (Figure 36.6).

A major concern with corneal inlays has been the body's reaction to foreign material, with resultant fibrosis around the structure or corneal melting leading to diminished vision. The inlays have undergone significant modifications in design, which have resulted in improved outcomes.

Holmium laser for hyperopia

The holmium laser has been used to correct hyperopia by shrinking the periphery of the cornea, permitting the central part of the cornea to steepen and thus reduce hyperopia. This procedure has generally been abandoned

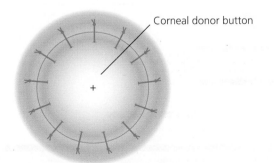

Corneal donor button

Figure 36.5 Epikeratoplasty. A lamellar graft is sutured in place.

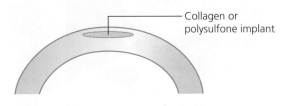

Collagen or polysulfone implant

Figure 36.6 Corneal implant.

because of problems of instability and regression. Most surgeons use LASIK or PRK for the correction of mild to moderate degrees of hyperopia.

Thermokeratoplasty (thermal collagen shrinkage)

Fyodorov, a Russian ophthalmologist, developed the technique of thermokeratoplasty, which applies radial heat in the periphery to shrink the collagen of the cornea and produce central steepening. This results in a reduction of hyperopia. Regression is common and at this time its effect is not predictable. This evolved to the procedure of conductive keratoplasty (CK), with the use of radio waves to shrink the collagen fibers. As with the holmium laser, the outcomes have been disappointing because of regression.

SURGERY: PATIENT SELECTION, COUNSELING, AND EXAMINATION

Refractive surgery patients must be seen as different from the typical patient who comes to an eye care professional's office. The people who come for refractive surgery are healthy, active, working people who don't have the time or inclination to sit in a waiting room. This is important because laser vision correction (Figure 36.7), phakic intraocular lenses (IOLs), and refractive lens exchange are elective procedures, and patients are selective about where they go.

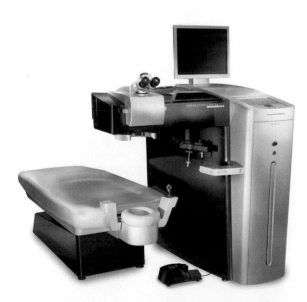

Figure 36.7 Laser room suite. Laser vision correction gives patients the option of decreasing their dependence on glasses or contact lenses. *(Used with permission from Alcon.)*

Respect for patients' time and their anxieties about a refractive procedure are vital to the success of an eye care professional. How well the office manages the patient's experience, from the first phone call to the last follow-up visit, determines how rewarding refractive surgery will be for the practice.

This section explores the role from the standpoint of both the ophthalmologist and comanaging eye doctor in preoperative and postoperative care. Comanagement is very different from a simple referral in which the patient, along with some basic information, is sent to the refractive surgeon. The comanaging doctor plays a central role in patient selection and counseling and has a responsibility for both pre- and postoperative care.

Indications

Patients selected for refractive surgery should be 18 years of age or older, with a stable refractive error. One exception to this rule is that if the patient wants refractive surgery to qualify for an occupation (e.g., firefighter, police officer), it does not matter if the refraction changes slightly from year to year. Patients will not be dismissed from an occupation just because, several years after qualifying, they refract at −1.00 diopter.

The refractive indications for LASIK, advanced surface ablation (PRK), phakic IOLs, and refractive lens exchange are listed in Figures 36.8 and 36.9.

Laser vision correction

Although each refractive surgeon has his or her own upper and lower limits, the range of correction for LASIK and PRK is approximately +5.00 diopters to −10.00 diopters. Astigmatism between −0.25 and −6.00 diopters may also be laser-corrected. For borderline cases, the comanaging eye doctor may wish to consult with the refractive surgeon.

Options in laser vision correction for both LASIK and eye doctor include standard ablation; prolate or aspheric ablation; custom wavefront-guided ablation (see Chapter 38),

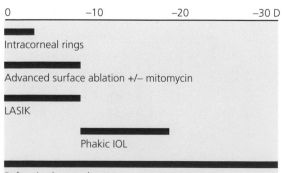

Figure 36.8 Refractive indications for myopic refractive surgery. *IOL*, Intraocular lens.

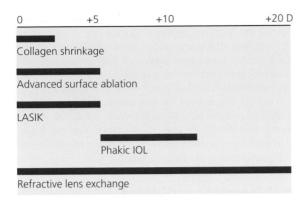

0 +5 +10   +20 D

Collagen shrinkage

Advanced surface ablation

LASIK

Phakic IOL

Refractive lens exchange

Figure 36.9 Refractive indications for hyperopic refractive surgery. *IOL*, Intraocular lens.

and topography-guided ablations. Our clinical experience has taught us that the best quality of day and night vision is obtained by either a prolate wavefront-guided ablation, or topography-guided ablation. Our determination of which procedure is best for an eye is based on either wavefront analysis that measures higher-order aberrations or topography that can measure irregular astigmatism. These measurements are performed on all laser vision correction patients. Patients with a low incidence of higher-order aberrations do extremely well with a prolate ablation. Patients with a high incidence of higher-order aberrations should have a wavefront-guided ablation or with irregular astigmatism should have a topography-guided ablation.

Patients following cataract extraction or corneal transplantation who have a significant refractive error (myopia, hyperopia, and astigmatism) can be treated with refractive surgery. Most patients are satisfied with glasses or contact lenses following major eye surgery; however, if they desire clarity without correction, then laser vision correction is a reasonable option. Following a corneal transplant, it is best to wait at least 1 year postoperatively until all the sutures have been removed and the wound is strong. In such cases, PRK with mitomycin can be offered or a phakic implant. If there is irregular astigmatism, a customized topography-guided ablation should be performed to decrease the surface irregularity.

Following radial keratotomy, if patients are overcorrected or have residual myopia or astigmatism, laser vision correction can be offered by PRK. It is important for the patient to understand that any glare, starbursts, fluctuation in vision, or loss of best corrected visual acuity (BCVA) as a result of the radial keratotomy will generally not improve following laser vision correction.

Phakic intraocular lens and refractive lens exchange

For higher degrees of myopia (>−10.00 diopters) or hyperopia (>+5.00 diopters), an intraocular procedure should be considered such as a phakic IOL or refractive lens

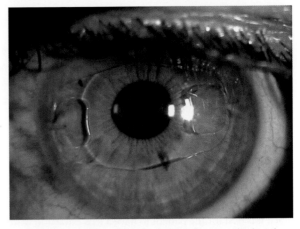

Figure 36.10 Artisan phakic intraocular lens attached to the midperipheral iris.

exchange. The phakic IOL is a lens that can be inserted into the anterior chamber, attached to the iris (e.g., Artisan lens, Figure 36.10) or behind the iris and in front of the crystalline lens (e.g., implantable contact lens, Figure 36.11). The advantages of a phakic IOL are reversibility and retention of accommodation. Contraindications are large pupils greater than 8 mm and an anterior chamber depth of less than

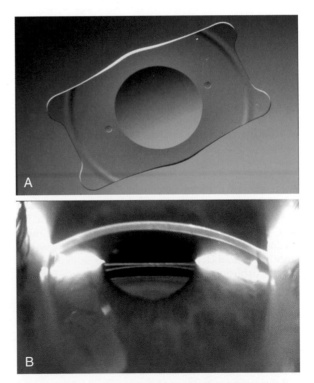

Figure 36.11 (A) The implantable contact lens. (B) The implantable contact lens positioned between the crystalline lens and the iris.

611

3 mm. Many high hyperopes do not qualify for a phakic IOL because of a shallow anterior chamber. The refractive center orders the phakic implant (power and diameter) based on manifest and cycloplegic refraction, anterior chamber depth, and the horizontal corneal diameter (white-to-white measurement).

A refractive lens exchange is simply a lens extraction with insertion of a foldable posterior chamber implant. The procedure is performed under topical anesthesia with a clear corneal incision. Neither sutures nor a patch are required. Astigmatism can be treated by the insertion of a toric implant or astigmatic keratotomy. In addition to the correction of high myopia or hyperopia, another case to consider is the patient more than 60 years of age who has lost most accommodative ability. If there are signs of early cataract, it is best for the patient to have a lens extraction with an implant rather than laser vision correction.

Intraocular procedures are typically associated with a minimal healing response and a rapid return of vision. The main risk is infection or endophthalmitis. Fortunately, this is extremely rare, occurring in less than 1 in 10,000 eyes. The quality of vision is generally excellent with a phakic IOL or refractive lens exchange. If there is a residual refractive error, then laser vision correction can be used to optimize uncorrected visual acuity (UCVA). This is usually performed at least 2 to 4 months following the intraocular procedure. The combination of procedures is termed *bioptics*.

Monovision

Patients must be counseled that reading correction is necessary after the onset of presbyopia following laser vision correction or phakic IOL. For all practical purposes, only patients older than the age of 40 will be interested in monovision. However, discussing it with younger patients is part of the process of helping them understand the limitations of refractive surgery. Patients who have a refractive lens exchange will require reading glasses unless either a multifocal implant is used or monovision is achieved.

Ideal monovision candidates for refractive surgery are those who have already adapted to monovision, that is, those who are successfully wearing two different contact lenses, one correcting distance vision, the other correcting near vision. Particularly apt for consideration are those occupations that require intermittent focusing between distance and near, such as sales representatives, schoolteachers, lawyers, or business individuals who are frequently involved with meetings.

For monovision, it is typically the dominant eye that is treated to correct for distance. A number of different tests can be used to determine ocular dominance. A simple one is to hand the patient a camera and ask him or her to pretend to take a photograph of some distant object. The eye he uses to look through the viewfinder is the dominant eye.

If the patient expresses an interest in monovision, a trial with contact lenses may be in order. This trial will determine the patient's suitability for monovision and indicate the appropriate power for each eye. A satisfactory, well-tolerated trial is a good indicator of probable success of surgically created monovision. If the contact lens trial is not well tolerated and the trial has been adequately long (approximately 2 weeks), avoid using this approach.

In the eye that is used for near vision, the typical degree of residual or induced myopia for successful monovision is usually between 0.75 and 1.5 diopters. Leaving higher degrees of myopia often results in too much anisometropia and interference with distance vision.

Problematic candidates

Box 36.1 lists some of the attitudes and ocular conditions that make a patient a poor candidate for refractive surgery. Recognition of these clinical factors is essential to decrease the risk of postoperative problems.

In many situations, a patient may be a candidate for PRK or LASEK but not for LASIK. Surface ablation is the procedure of choice among patients with:

- Epithelial basement membrane dystrophy (EBMD) because there is an increased risk of epithelial ingrowth with LASIK
- Relatively thin central corneas (such that less than 300 μm of tissue would be left in the bed after ablation)
- Narrow palpebral fissures and/or deep-set eyes (which make work with a femtosecond laser or microkeratome difficult)
- Keratoconus or forme fruste keratoconus (as there is an increased risk of corneal ectasia with LASIK)
- Extremely steep corneas (>48.00 diopters) with an increased risk of a buttonhole flap with LASIK when utilizing a microkeratome. This risk is eliminated with a femtosecond laser.

The quality of vision can deteriorate with a postoperative cornea that is either too steep (>50.00 diopters) or too flat

---

Box 36.1 Poor candidates for refractive surgery

- Less than 18 years old
- Unstable refraction or progressive myopia
- Irregular astigmatism with loss of best corrected visual acuity (BCVA)
- Dry eyes, with punctate keratopathy or filaments
- Cataract
- Herpes simplex (eye must have been quiet for at least a year)
- Vision-threatening macular disease (e.g., diabetic retinopathy)
- Pregnancy
- Unrealistic expectations
- Unwilling to commit to follow-up

(<36.00 diopters). The postoperative curvature should be predicted; if this is outside an acceptable range, it is best to recommend either a phakic IOL or refractive lens exchange.

Medicolegal issues

Some patient situations are problematic for medicolegal reasons. For example, if a patient with an underlying disease (e.g., diabetic retinopathy, myopic macular degeneration, age-related macular degeneration) suffers a loss of vision in the year or two after refractive surgery, he or she may hold the surgery rather than the disease accountable. One should exercise extreme caution here. Because patients' vision is almost always correctable by spectacles or contact lenses, avoiding surgery may be wise in these circumstances.

Pregnancy can affect refraction and wound healing. In addition, any untoward event in pregnancy may be blamed on the procedure or related medications. Hence it is wise to put off refractive surgery during pregnancy.

Patient selection

Serious complications of refractive surgery are, fortunately, extremely rare. Disappointment is much more common and may cause more problems for the refractive surgeon and comanaging optometrist than serious vision loss. Two actions on the part of the eye care team can minimize disappointment: patient selection that weeds out inappropriate personality types and careful presentation of facts to the patient, so that nothing said or done will impart unrealistic expectations.

Patient selection is more than a matter of meeting objective criteria. Perfectionists, individuals who cannot tolerate small disappointments, and others who are likely to be grossly upset if they don't achieve 6/6 (20/20) or better vision from their surgery should be avoided. With limited exposure to the patient, it is very hard for the refractive surgeon to spot these personality traits. This is one great advantage of comanagement: often the comanaging doctor has known the patient for years and may have greater insight into the patient's personality.

The best candidates for refractive surgery are those who are strongly motivated to be rid of corrective lenses, but who recognize that their postoperative uncorrected vision may not be quite what it was with correction before surgery.

Good candidates are relatively easygoing and able to tolerate mild disappointments. Some of the traits common to good candidates for refractive surgery are noted in Box 36.2.

Managing patient expectations

It is all too easy to create unrealistic expectations. Patients want a great outcome and this may make them selective in their hearing. Therefore, nothing that the doctor or staff

---

Box 36.2 **Traits desired in candidates for refractive surgery**

- Very unhappy with their dependence on corrective lenses
- Think they are poor candidates for contact lenses
- Believe wearing corrective lenses restricts them in sports and similar activities
- Think they look better without glasses
- Worry about what would happen to them if they lost or broke their glasses or contact lenses
- Would prefer merely functional vision without correction to excellent vision with corrective lenses
- Would be happy if their uncorrected vision could be much improved, even if corrective lenses were still necessary
- Adjust well to change
- Are easygoing; can tolerate disappointment
- Are not perfectionists

---

says or does should support unrealistic expectations. Any mention of '6/5' ('20/15') or 'perfect vision' can lead to an expectation of that outcome.

One should avoid making promises. Instead, '"greatly improved vision"' or '"reduced dependence on glasses and contact lenses"' should be used to create realistic expectations. Marketing materials and staff interactions must also follow this pattern of refusing to overpromise.

For patients having PRK, one should not understate the possibility of some postoperative discomfort and delay in achieving optimum acuity. It is better to overstate the possibility of postprocedural pain and a slow return of vision than for the patient to be surprised by it. This is much less of an issue with LASIK, in which patients tend both to be comfortable postoperatively and experience an early return of BCVA.

The preoperative examination

Candidates for refractive surgery require a complete preoperative eye examination. Important history includes:

- Good general health
- No allergies or sensitivities to the medications used, especially in PRK; this is less important with LASIK, for which medication is used for much shorter time
- No systemic lupus or collagen vascular disease that requires treatment with systemic immunosuppressive medication.

Contact lens wearers must cease lens wear before the procedure and refrain from it long enough for their corneas to stabilize (as shown by refraction and topography). For rigid gas-permeable contact lens wearers, this may require cessation for a month or longer (Figure 36.12). The corneas

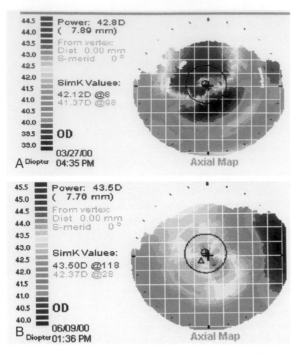

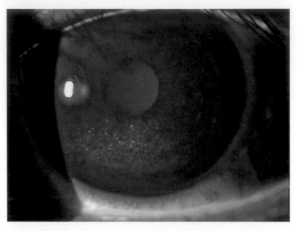

Figure 36.13 Inferior superficial punctate keratopathy secondary to exposure from incomplete lid closure. This can lead to poor wound healing after refractive surgery.

Figure 36.12 (A) Irregular astigmatism seen after a rigid gas-permeable (RGP) lens has been removed. History of lens wear for over 20 years. (B) Irregular astigmatism has resolved after discontinuing contact lens wear for 3 months. The patient is now a satisfactory candidate for laser vision correction.

of soft lens wearers stabilize very quickly, sometimes within hours; however, 1 week's wait is recommended to be certain that the cornea is stable.

The examination should include the following:

1. External eye examination. This may uncover lid abnormalities that result in exposure keratopathy (Figure 36.13) and lead to poor wound healing after refractive surgery. The detection of a significant chalazion can result in induced astigmatism.

2. Pupils. Although best checked with infrared light (Colvard pupillometry) (Figure 36.14), an estimate can be made with a narrow slit-beam with all the room lights off and the patient fixating on a point in the distance. Glare and halos are less common today with laser vision correction using large optical and transition zones. In general, there are no contraindications to advanced laser eye surgery based on pupil size. However, with phakic implants the pupil size should be less than 8 mm.

3. Slit-lamp. Findings may include the following:
   a. Blepharitis, though not a contraindication, should be cleared up to the greatest degree possible before surgery to decrease the chance of infection (Figure 36.15). Treatment may include the use of warm compresses to the lids, an antibiotic ointment

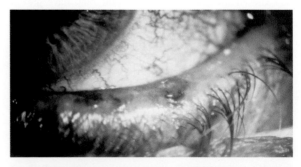

Figure 36.14 Measuring the pupil with the Colvard pupillometer.

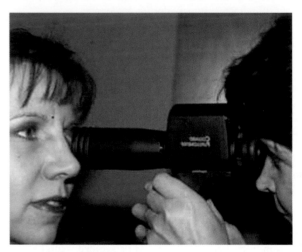

Figure 36.15 Blepharitis. Patients with blepharitis should be treated with appropriate lid hygiene before refractive surgery to decrease the chance of infection.

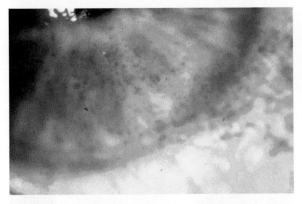

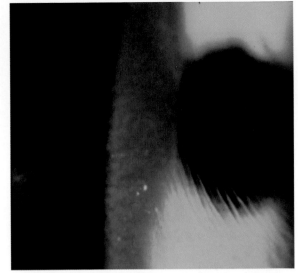

Figure 36.16 Advanced keratitis sicca with diffuse punctate keratopathy. Laser vision correction is contraindicated unless the cornea becomes clear with appropriate dry measure (e.g., artificial tears, ointments, punctual occlusions, etc.).

at bedtime (e.g., erythromycin), and oral medication (e.g., doxycycline [Vibramycin] pills 100 mg by mouth every day or twice a day for 2 to 4 months).

b. Significant dry eye with punctate keratopathy should be aggressively treated (Figure 36.16), with lubricating drops, gels, ointments, or silicone plugs. If symptoms or corneal findings cannot be resolved, the patient is a poor candidate for laser vision correction.

c. Corneal scarring is not a contraindication; advanced surface ablation is the procedure of choice when there is a superficial scar encroaching or overlying the pupil. However, if the scar is secondary to herpes simplex there is a risk of recurrence following surgery (Figure 36.17). The eye should be quiet (with no herpes simplex flare-ups) for at least 1 year before considering laser vision correction. Oral antivirals (e.g., acyclovir) should be prescribed for 1

Figure 36.18 Epithelial basement membrane dystrophy with map-like changes within the epithelium. LASIK is contraindicated because of the increased risk of epithelial ingrowth. Photorefractive keratectomy (PRK) may be of value.

to 2 weeks preoperatively and 1 month postoperatively to decrease the risk of virus reactivation.

d. Neovascularization is not a contraindication unless blood vessels extend into the central 6- or 7-mm zone. (Bleeding can occur after creating the flap in LASIK or with PRK, but this is rarely a problem.)

e. Epithelial basement membrane dystrophy (Figure 36.18) is a relative contraindication to LASIK, but not PRK. Sloughing of the epithelium during the microkeratome pass increases the risk of epithelial ingrowth. Although the results with PRK can be excellent, there is a greater degree of under- or overcorrection because of variable epithelial thickness.

f. Cataract is a contraindication. If present, consider a cataract extraction with an intraocular lens. Opacities that are not visually significant and have been stable for years are not a contraindication.

4. Tonometry. Rule out glaucoma. Patients with glaucoma are more susceptible to elevated pressures when topical steroids are used. In addition, a baseline disc evaluation and, if indicated, a visual field may be of value because postoperative intraocular pressures may be artificially low following myopic laser vision correction, secondary to significant corneal flattening. Corneal thickness is important in evaluating intraocular pressure.

5. Fundus examination. Look for any vision-threatening disorder such as myopic macular degeneration (Figure 36.19), age-related macular degeneration,

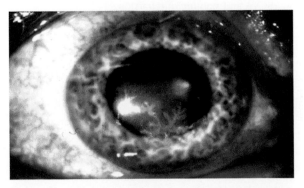

Figure 36.17 Herpes simplex keratitis with a corneal dendrite. The eye should be quiet, with no recurrence for at least a year before refractive surgery.

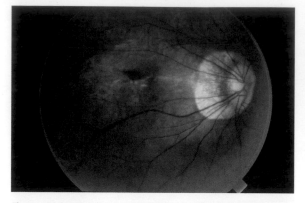

Figure 36.19 Fundus examination.

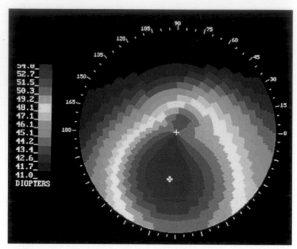

Figure 36.21 Computerized videokeratography with significant inferior steepening, which confirms the diagnosis of keratoconus.

diabetic retinopathy, and so on. These patients are at risk for vision loss in the future and are not considered good candidates for refractive surgery.

6. Refraction. Do both a manifest and cycloplegic refraction. Accurate refraction is the key to success in refractive surgery. Correct cylinder axis measurement is particularly critical. If the cylinder axis is off by 15 degrees, one can have a decreased effect of up to 50% following laser vision correction. An inaccurate refraction will lead to a laser correction procedure that removes either too much or not enough tissue. With the ultrahigh expectations and the demand for perfection that exist today, unpleasant surprises are most unwelcome. Suboptimal outcomes result in an increase in the number of postoperative visits, excessive time demands for patient counseling, and, sometimes, the need for an enhancement procedure.

7. Keratometry. Look for irregular astigmatism (Figure 36.20). Computerized videokeratography is performed to rule out keratoconus (Figure 36.21) or forme fruste keratoconus.

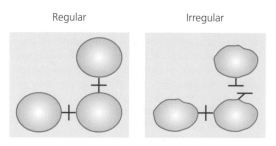

| Regular | Irregular |

Figure 36.20 Keratometric astigmatism.

Interaction with the refractive surgeon

In our comanagement system, the comanaging doctor can call the refractive surgeon to discuss patient issues; however, in the majority of cases the information is exchanged by means of fax or email. Most calls to the refractive surgeon pertain to the choice between refractive procedures (PRK, LASIK, phakic intraocular lens, or refractive lens exchange), when there is something unusual and whether a particular patient is an appropriate candidate. Good staff training and carefully crafted guidelines make the patient's transition from comanaging doctor to refractive surgeon and back again routine and uneventful.

The information that the comanaging doctor sends ahead of the patient includes:

- Manifest and cycloplegic refractions
- BCVA and stability of refraction
- Intraocular pressure and keratometry
- Fundus and slit-lamp examination results
- Pupil diameter
- Topography, if available
- A recommendation for LASIK, PRK, EpiLASIK, phakic IOL, or refractive lens exchange. Also, decide whether monovision is desired.

In the case of laser vision correction, it can be arranged for the patient to have a consultation and full workup with the surgeon or refractive counselor if the comanaging doctor so desires. On the day of either the consultation or surgery, a variety of tests are performed including pachymetry, computerized videokeratography, and wavefront imaging. These tests may indicate a preference for PRK over LASIK or a preference for a wavefront-guided ablation over a prolate ablation.

All patients referred for phakic IOL or refractive lens exchange require a consultation with the surgeon before scheduling surgery. Preoperative measurements are performed at the surgical center to determine the appropriate implant (spherical power plus or minus toric implant). Yttrium Aluminium Garnet (YAG) iridotomies are required for some of the phakic IOLs to prevent pupillary block glaucoma.

Informed consent

The comanaging doctor should discuss the potential complications with the patient. The refractive surgeon will discuss the consent form and answer patient questions. The comanaging doctor will prepare the patient, and the ophthalmologist doing the surgery can provide details of the procedure and answer any questions the patient may have before or on the day of surgery.

Postoperative care

Postoperative examinations allow for listening to and counseling of the patient. They also permit the evaluation of UCVA, BCVA with a manifest refraction, and the detection of any complications. If there is a loss of BCVA (Boxes 36.3–36.5) the cause must be identified.

Laser vision correction

The loss of acuity in laser vision correction may be secondary to irregular astigmatism from an ablation problem (decentered or irregular ablation, central island), flap complication (e.g., striae or buttonhole), diffuse lamellar keratitis, superficial keratitis, corneal haze, or an intraocular problem. In the absence of slit-lamp evidence of corneal

---

Box 36.4 Loss of best corrected visual acuity in phakic intraocular lens

Early (<1 month)
Transient corneal edema
Pupillary block glaucoma
Endophthalmitis

Late (>1 month)
Cataract
Pigmentary glaucoma
Corneal edema

Box 36.5 Loss of best corrected visual acuity in refractive lens exchange

Early (<1 month)
Transient corneal edema
Endophthalmitis
Macular edema

Late (>1 month)
Macular edema
Capsular opacification
Retinal detachment
Pseudophakic bullous keratopathy

---

abnormalities or intraocular problems, computerized videokeratography should be used to rule out an ablation problem as the cause of the irregular astigmatism and loss of acuity. Additional laser treatment may be needed if BCVA does not improve, or if any symptoms do not resolve.

Best corrected vision and refractive stability occur earlier with LASIK than with advanced surface ablation. In the LASIK patient, BCVA is typically achieved in 24 hours and refractive stability occurs between 1 and 3 months. The lower the refractive error, the earlier is the refractive stability. With surface ablation, BCVA is usually achieved by 1 month and refractive stability by 4 to 6 months. Fluctuation in vision is uncommon after 3 months with LASIK and after 6 months with PRK. Most of the early fluctuation in vision is secondary to an induced dry eye condition. If so, the use of lubricating drops, gels, ointments, or punctal plugs may be helpful.

For those patients with an under- or overcorrection, an enhancement procedure can be considered, but it is suggested that you wait at least 4 months following LASIK or 6 months following surface ablation. These delays are only approximate; the key is to wait until the refraction

---

Box 36.3 Loss of best corrected visual acuity in laser vision correction

	LASIK	PRK
Infection	+	+
Decentered ablation	+	+
Irregular ablation	+	+
Central island	+	+
Corneal haze	+	+
Superficial keratitis	+	+
Diffuse lamellar keratitis	+	−
Flap striae	+	−
Flap buttonhole	+	−
Epithelial ingrowth	+	−

LASIK, Laser-assisted in situ keratomileusis; *PRK*, photorefractive keratectomy.

is stable, with less than 0.5 diopter change from the previous month's examination. If a patient has residual or consecutive myopia and is presbyopic or early prepresbyopic, consider a trial to determine the acceptability of monovision before you undertake any surgical enhancement.

A patient who is surgically treated to intentionally create monovision and who experiences difficulty, especially with night driving, can be given a prescription for glasses that correct distance vision in both eyes. If the patient experiences problems with binocular vision and sporting activities, try fitting a contact lens for the reading eye to improve distance vision.

Postoperatively, if a patient complains of glare, halos, monocular diplopia, or poor quality of vision that does not resolve after a few months, it is important to identify the cause. Any residual uncorrected refractive error can result in significant visual complaints. Computerized videokeratography can be used to identify an abnormal ablation pattern. If no abnormality is found on topography, consider wavefront analysis to determine whether any significant higher-order aberrations have been induced. If so, a customized or wavefront-guided ablation can be performed, with the goal of resolving the patient's symptoms and improving the overall quality of vision.

Refractive lens exchange

Complications are uncommon but may occur. The risks are similar to a cataract operation with insertion of an intraocular implant. The most serious complication is endophthalmitis. This usually presents in the first week postoperatively with diminished vision, redness, and pain. Fortunately, the incidence is less than 1 in 10,000 eyes. Cells in the anterior chamber and vitreous are usually present. Stat referral to a refractive surgeon is mandatory. Other complications that can occur include corneal edema (transient or permanent), subluxation of implant, cystoid macular edema, toxic keratopathy from eyedrops, capsular opacification, and retinal detachment. Detection of these complications and communication with the refractive surgeon are critical in the early rehabilitation of the patient. A residual refractive error can be treated by a secondary implant in the sulcus to correct hyperopia or myopia, astigmatic keratotomy to reduce astigmatism, or laser vision correction.

Phakic intraocular lens

As with all intraocular procedures, there is a small risk of endophthalmitis. A more common complication with a phakic IOL is pupillary block glaucoma. The patient presents with pain, elevated intraocular pressure, and a shallow anterior chamber. The previous laser iridotomies may be closed, requiring emergency retreatment. In general, the complications vary depending on the phakic IOL and include subluxation of the implant (Artisan > ICL),

transient corneal edema (Artisan > ICL), cataract (Artisan < ICL), pigmentary glaucoma (Artisan < ICL), and pupillary block glaucoma (Artisan < ICL). A residual refractive error, if unsatisfactory to the patient, can be treated with laser vision correction.

The bottom line

Refractive surgery patients require a high level of attention from the practice, beginning with the first phone call and continuing through the last follow-up visit. Determining a patient's suitability for refractive surgery is based on both objective criteria and evaluation of the patient's motivation and personality. Patients who cannot tolerate less than a 6/5 (20/15) result, as well as pregnant patients and patients with vision-threatening retinal disease, should be discouraged. The examination of candidates for refractive surgery includes an external eye examination, slit-lamp findings, fundus examination, manifest and cycloplegic refractions, keratometry, and pupil size. The patient's general health and sensitivity to medications are important parts of the history. Monovision should be discussed with all presbyopic and early prepresbyopic patients. The surgeon must help the patient to make an informed decision as to the best procedure: laser vision correction, refractive lens exchange, or phakic IOL. The doctors and staff must take great care to say nothing that will give the patient unrealistic expectations or create alarm. Clear guidelines and a well-run system can make refractive surgery rewarding for the refractive surgeon, comanaging doctor, and the patient.

SUMMARY

Refractive surgery is an elective procedure performed for relief of myopia, hyperopia, and astigmatism, with the goal of eliminating the need for glasses and contact lenses. It also has been found to be effective in correcting surgically induced refractive errors after cataract surgery and corneal transplantation. Because refractive surgery, with a track record of more than 25 years, has had few complications and a level of predictability that rivals that of intraocular lens implantation, many ophthalmologists are adding it to their routine surgical practice. The lay press also has awakened the general public's interest in refractive surgery.

A large segment (20%–25%) of the world's population is myopic. In the United States alone, more than 75 million people require some form of refractive correction. For many occupations, good vision unencumbered by spectacles or contact lenses is important for safety reasons. In addition, many performers and professional athletes want to be free of spectacles and contact lenses. For some spectacle and contact lens wearers, it may be a lifestyle change.

The cornea is the most refractive component of the eye, accounting for more than 70% of the eye's refractive ability.

In addition, more than 70% of the outside world is introduced to us from the visual senses. Therefore, most of the procedures in refractive surgery involve the cornea. The development of equipment for corneal topography has significantly improved our understanding of the cornea before and after surgery. Corneal topography equipment (see Chapter 40) provides a colored picture of corneal curvature taken from several thousand points from the center of the cornea.

Certain traits are desirable in candidates for refractive surgery. The best candidates are those who are strongly motivated to be rid of corrective lenses, but recognize that their postoperative uncorrected vision may not be quite what it was with correction before surgery. Good candidates are relatively easygoing and able to tolerate mild disappointments.

Patients who want to have refractive surgery should be aware of all the inherent risks of these procedures. As with any new procedure in medicine, there are positive and negative comments from within the medical profession. Reputable ophthalmologists and optometrists may disagree concerning the safety and efficacy of laser vision correction, RK, or other procedures for near-sightedness, far-sightedness, or astigmatism. Their skepticism is probably based on the concept of operating on an essentially healthy eye and putting it at risk. It is important to know that refractive surgery procedures, whether excimer laser or other procedures, have been developed to correct myopia, hyperopia, and astigmatism. Refractive surgery does not treat glaucoma, cataracts, or other disorders that affect and damage vision. It cannot make a blind eye see.

A person who is happy with his or her present method of correction (glasses or contact lenses) should by all means continue with it and not have surgery. Before refractive surgery is performed, a clinical evaluation is necessary to determine the patient's suitability. Corneal topography has proved most valuable in this evaluation to screen out keratoconus or any irregularity of the cornea. It is important that the proper information be given to the patient. An informed consent means that the physician has outlined the risks and complications of the procedures so that the person can make an informed decision as to whether to proceed.

Chapter 37

Corneal collagen crosslinking in the management of ectatic diseases

Raymond M. Stein, Rebecca L. Stein

Corneal crosslinking (CXL) is recognized as a major therapeutic advance in the management of ectatic diseases. There is increasing evidence from review of the literature that CXL is an effective means of halting progressive corneal thinning and steepening in patients with keratoconus, pellucid marginal degeneration, and ectasia after laser-assisted in situ keratomileusis (LASIK). Other potential applications include treatment of corneal edema in bullous keratopathy, infectious corneal ulcers, enhancing corneal flattening after the insertion of intrastromal corneal rings, strengthening the cornea before PRK treatment in high myopia or mild or forme fruste patients with keratoconus, and reducing the fluctuation in vision and hyperopic shift following radial keratotomy. More than 100 peer-reviewed articles support its efficacy in halting the progression of keratoconus and numerous reports support its use for other potential indications.

CXL treatment involves the use of riboflavin drops (vitamin B_2) and ultraviolet A (UVA) light. The main goal of CXL is to stabilize the corneal curvature and prevent the need for corneal transplantation. The treatment is being rapidly adopted by ophthalmologists around the globe as the standard of care for progressive ectasia.

KERATOCONUS

Keratoconus is a degenerative disorder of the cornea with an incidence of approximately 1 in 1000. Structural changes of the cornea cause it to thin and become conical. The disease usually presents in adolescence and tends to peak in severity in the 20s or 30s; 10% to 25% of patients with keratoconus may require a corneal transplant. CXL offers hope to prevent the need for a transplant.

Clinical signs of keratoconus

The diagnosis of keratoconus is made based on a number of clinical signs and topographic imaging (Figure 37.1). One of the earliest signs on routine examination is an irregular scissors reflex on retinoscopy. With further ectatic disease Vogt's striae or stress lines appear as vertical lines in the deep stroma. The striae temporarily disappear if slight pressure is applied to the cornea. A ring of yellow-brown pigmentation known as a Fleischer ring can be observed in around half of keratoconic eyes. This ring is caused by

Diagnosis of keratoconus

Late

- Corneal hydrops
- Munson's sign
- Apical scarring
- Vogt's striae
- Irregular keratometry mires
- Abdominal computerized topography
- High coma
- Epithelial thickness abnormalities

Early

- Posterior corneal curvature

Figure 37.1 Clinical signs of keratoconus may be early or late in the disease process.

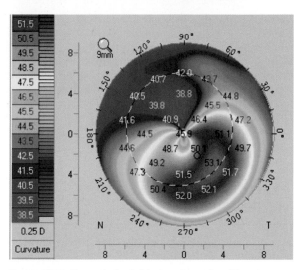

Figure 37.2 Computerized videokeratography of keratoconus with inferior steepening.

deposition of the iron oxide hemosiderin within the corneal epithelium. Further progression can lead to breaks in Bowman's membrane, resulting in apical scarring. A break in Descemet's membrane results in rapid stromal and often epithelial edema, referred to as corneal hydrops. An advanced cone can create a V-shaped indentation in the lower eyelid when the patient's gaze is directed downward, known as Munson's sign. This finding, though a classic sign of the disease, tends not to be of primary diagnostic importance because it occurs late in the disease process.

Computerized topography

Sophisticated imaging today allows for an early diagnosis of keratoconus. Computerized corneal topography can take the form of curvature analysis or elevation topography. Asymmetric astigmatism with inferior steepening is a typical topographic pattern (Figure 37.2). Elevation topography allows for the comparison of the anterior surface or posterior surface with a best-fit sphere. Changes to the posterior corneal curvature may represent the earliest clinical sign of keratoconus (Figure 37.3). Corneas are typically thinner in keratoconus, and the finding of the thinnest spot on the cornea in the steepest region associated with posterior corneal elevation is characteristic for keratoconus. Clinical studies on the measurement of the thickness of the epithelium indicate that eyes with keratoconus typically have thinner epithelium overlying the cone and thicker at the base of the cone.

Etiology of keratoconus

The etiology of keratoconus remains unknown. Keratoconus likely arises from a number of factors: genetic, environmental, or cellular, any of which may form the trigger for

Figure 37.3 (A) Computerized topography shows a relatively normal bowtie pattern of astigmatism. (B) However, posterior corneal elevation shows a focal area of bulging, characteristic of keratoconus.

Keratoconus

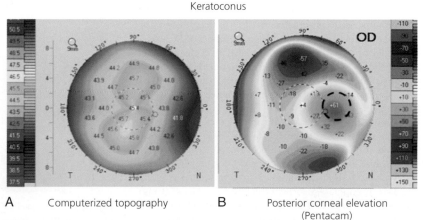

A   Computerized topography   B   Posterior corneal elevation (Pentacam)

the onset of the disease. A genetic predisposition to keratoconus has been observed, with the disease running in certain families, and incidences reported of concordance in identical twins. Most genetic studies agree on an autosomal dominant mode of inheritance. The condition is seen at a higher frequency in those with Down syndrome. Keratoconus also has been associated with atopic diseases, which include asthma, allergies, and eczema. There is support for the finding that excess eye rubbing contributes to the progression of keratoconus.

PELLUCID MARGINAL DEGENERATION

Pellucid marginal degeneration (PMD) is a degenerative corneal ectatic disease that is often confused with keratoconus. It is characterized by thinning in the periphery of the cornea. The corneas typically have a normal thickness in the center. The inferior cornea exhibits a peripheral band of thinning. There is usually high against-the-rule astigmatism. Computerized topography shows a classic butterfly appearance. No known cause for the disease has been found. Like keratoconus, PMD represents a contraindication to LASIK.

CORNEAL ECTASIA FOLLOWING LASIK

Corneal ectasia is a rare, potentially devastating complication following LASIK. Ectatic changes may occur as early as 1 week, but are usually delayed by many years after LASIK. The actual incidence of ectasia is undetermined, although incidence rates of 0.04%, 0.2%, and 0.6% have been reported.

Risk factors for corneal ectasia include:

1. Abnormal preoperative topography as seen with keratoconus, pellucid marginal degeneration, or forme fruste keratoconus.
2. Low residual stromal bed (RSB) thickness is an important factor after LASIK because tensile strength analysis indicates greater strength in the anterior 40% relative to the posterior 60% of stroma. LASIK reduces anterior corneal structural integrity; it is clear that a cutoff of 250 μm of the corneal bed does not absolutely discriminate development of ectasia; however, the risk of ectasia increases reciprocally relative to RSB thickness.
3. Young age may be a significant risk factor for ectasia in patients without other risk factors. One hypothesis is that some of these individuals would have developed delayed-onset forme fruste or keratoconus even without LASIK procedure.
4. Low preoperative corneal thickness is a factor along with the degree of myopia and RSB. RSB thickness is the most significant predictor of ectasia among them.

5. High myopia, especially greater than 12.00 diopters, is associated with a higher risk of ectasia. Despite this finding, post-LASIK ectasia has been reported in numerous patients with low myopia and even hyperopia.

Other risk factors include eye rubbing, family history of keratoconus, refractive instability, and best corrected visual acuity (BCVA) of less than 20/20 preoperatively.

DEVELOPMENT OF CORNEAL CROSSLINKING

The derivation of the concept of CXL came from the recognition that diabetic individuals tend not to develop keratoconus because of natural crosslinking from high blood glucose levels and exposure to UV light. The basic research on corneal crosslinking was conducted from 1993 to 1997 by Doctors Theo Seiler and Eberhard Spoerl in Germany. Research has shown that CXL increases corneal rigidity by 328%. New bonds are formed across adjacent collagen fibers to enhance the cornea's mechanical strength. The procedure has been effective in treating keratoconus, pellucid marginal degeneration, and ectasia following laser vision correction.

The idea of crosslinking is not new. The practice has been used since around 1940 in the field of material science in the conversion of silicone oil to rubber. Dentists have been using crosslinking for more than 25 years (Figure 37.4). Natural crosslinking occurs as a normal aging change in connective tissues of the body. This may explain why the progression of keratoconus tends to slow down with age.

BASIC RESEARCH ON SAFETY OF CXL

CXL with riboflavin solution and UVA light at 370 nm has been shown to be safe when using an irradiance of 3 mW/cm² with a minimum corneal thickness of 400 μm.

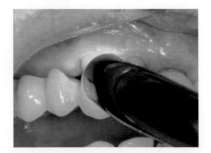

Figure 37.4 Crosslinking has been used in the field of dentistry for more than 25 years.

With a thickness of 400 μm or greater, minimal energy gets delivered to the corneal endothelium, and this level is below the threshold for any damage. The damage thresholds for keratocytes and endothelial cells are 0.45 and 0.35 mW/cm², respectively. In a 400-mm thick cornea saturated with riboflavin, the irradiance at the endothelial level was 0.18 mW/cm² (Figure 37.5), which is a factor of 2 smaller than the damage threshold. Studies have looked at the amount of radiant energy that gets into the eye that could affect the iris, the lens, and the retina, and this also has been shown to be below the damage threshold (Figure 37.6). For the development of cataract, various dose values have been discussed in the literature with wavelengths between 290 and 365 nm. The retina is damaged by thermal or blue light-induced photochemical damage in the wavelength range of 400 to 1400 nm. Studies with confocal microscopy have shown that keratocytes are depleted to a depth of 300 μm, with repopulation of new keratocytes taking up to 6 months (Figure 37.7).

CXL results in the creation of additional chemical bonds inside the corneal stroma by means of photopolymerization. Because UV light causes an effect only where it is absorbed, it is desirable that the treatment be designed so that as much as possible of the irradiation be absorbed in the corneal stroma. This is achieved by the selection of a wavelength of UV light at 370 nm, a wavelength that corresponds to one of the absorption maxima of the riboflavin chromophore. Riboflavin acts as a photomediator, creating free radicals to induce new chemical bonds. CXL has been a major breakthrough in the mechanical and biochemical stability of ectatic diseases.

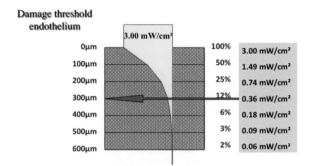

Figure 37.5 Radiant energy exposure from ultraviolet A (UVA) light versus damage threshold of structures in the eye.

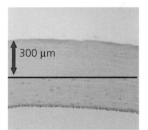

Figure 37.7 Depletion of keratocytes to a depth of 300 μm following collagen crosslinking (CXL). Minimum thickness of 400 μm, the corneal endothelium will not experience damage, nor will deeper structures such as lens and retina.

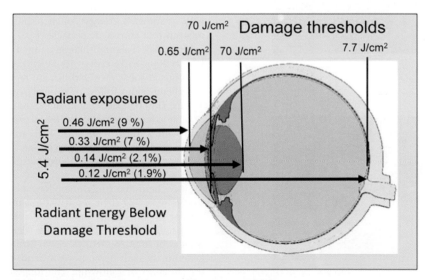

Figure 37.6 Amount of energy that enters into the eye with respect to depth.

TECHNIQUE OF CXL

The standard crosslinking technique involves removal of the central corneal epithelium of 8 to 9 mm in diameter, the application of riboflavin 0.1% drops every 2 minutes for 30 minutes (Figure 37.8), and exposure to UVA light of 370 nm (+ or − 5 nm) applied for 30 minutes (Figure 37.9). During the irradiation the cornea is rinsed with riboflavin drops every 5 minutes. The cropped light beam has a diameter of 9 mm. The energy of the crosslinking device is measured preoperatively and should be around 3 mW/cm^2 and should deliver a homogeneous illumination. Removal of the epithelium can be accomplished by a variety of techniques including the use of a rotary brush, a dilute concentration of alcohol, or mechanical debridement. Riboflavin drops are applied for 30 minutes. After the UVA light exposure for 30 minutes, antibiotic, nonsteroidal, and steroid drops are inserted along with a bandage contact lens, typically for 5 days or until the epithelium becomes intact.

Techniques have been developed that are being evaluated and compared with standard techniques. These techniques include higher energy levels and an epithelium-on approach referred to as a transepithelial technique. Instead of using the standard energy level of 3 mW/cm^2, the energy can be increased up to 45 mW/cm^2. The higher energy level decreases the time for UVA exposure, and shortens the procedure, which makes it easier for the patient. Another technique, the transepithelial approach, is gaining support as an effective CXL technique with a quicker return of vision. This approach involves a specialized formulation of riboflavin to allow this large molecular substance to pass through the corneal epithelium into the stroma. The UVA light exposure is then performed in a standard manner or with an increased energy level. Clinical studies on the higher energy level and the epithelium-on approach will eventually provide answers as to whether these technique are effective long term in preventing progressive ectasia.

CONTRAINDICATION TO CXL

Corneas thinner than 400 μm represent a contraindication to corneal crosslinking. However, the use of a hypotonic riboflavin solution to induce corneal swelling allows satisfactory transient stromal edema to permit safe crosslinking. At the Bochner Eye Institute we found that there is a 95% chance of inducing satisfactory swelling for corneas between 300 and 399 μm with hypotonic drops.

CLINICAL OUTCOMES OF CXL

The first CXL treatments were performed in Europe in 1998. This is a relatively new treatment in North America since 2007. The success of CXL is based on the lack of progressive ectasia. In addition, often some corneal flattening occurs, with asymmetric changes often resulting in an improvement in best corrected spectacle visual acuity (BCSVA).

Wollensak et al published their initial outcomes report on CXL in 2003, in 16 eyes of 15 patients with progressive keratoconus. A subsequent publication reported on 22 eyes of 24 patients with a follow-up time of between 3 months and 4 years. They reported that in all treated eyes the progression of keratoconus was halted. In 70% of eyes, there was a regression with a mean reduction of the maximal keratometry readings by about 2.00 diopters and refractive error of approximately 1.00 diopter. Visual acuity improved slightly in 65% of eyes.

Since the initial study, there have been numerous other studies reporting their results, summarized in Table 37.1. The methodologies are variable and as such are not directly comparable; however, all reports demonstrated varying degrees of improvement in visual acuity and reduction in keratometry with a progressive trend of improvement in the duration of follow-up. The longest study to date by Raiskup-Wolf et al reported their 7-year results in Germany.

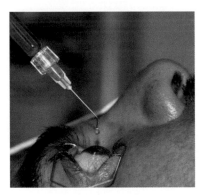

Figure 37.8 Riboflavin drops are instilled after removal of 8 to 9 mm of corneal epithelium.

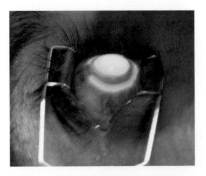

Figure 37.9 Ultraviolet A (UVA) light treatment.

Table 37.1 Summary of characteristics of efficacy studies performed to date

Author	Year	Type of study	No. of eyes	Follow-up
Caporros	2006	Prospective, nonrandomized	10 eyes	6 months
Hoyer	2008	Retrospective	153 eyes	12 months
Wittig-Silva	2008	Prospective, randomized	66 eyes	Up to 12 months
Raiskup-Wolf	2008	Retrospective	241 eyes	Min. 6 months
Jankov	2008	Prospective, nonrandomized	25 eyes	4–7 months
Vinciguerra	2009	Prospective, nonrandomized	28 eyes	12 months
Agrawal	2009	Retrospective	37 eyes	12 months
Grewal	2009	Prospective, nonrandomized	102 patients	12 months

Adapted from Ashwin PT, McDonnell PJ. Collagen cross-linkage: a comprehensive review and directions for future research. Br J Ophthalmol 2010;94:965–970.

They reported a decrease in maximum keratometry of 2.7 diopters in year 1, 2.2 diopters at 2 years, and 4.8 diopters at 3 years. BCSVA improved by one line per year in 54% of patients in the first 3 years. Two patients had continued progression and had to undergo repeat crosslinking procedures.

In the only randomized prospective controlled clinical trial of collagen crosslinking in progressive keratoconus published to date, Wittig-Silva et al reported on 66 eyes of 49 patients with documented progression of keratoconus. Interim analysis of treated eyes showed a flattening of the steepest simulated keratometry (*K*-max) by an average of 0.74 diopter at 3 months, 0.92 diopter at 6 months, and 1.45 diopters at 12 months. A trend toward improvement of BCSVA was also observed. In the control eyes, mean *K*-max steepened by 0.60 diopter after 3 months, 0.60 diopter after 6 months, and by 1.28 diopters after 12 months. BCSVA decreased by a logmar of 0.003 over 3 months, 0.056 over 6 months, and 0.12 over 12 months.

Complications following CXL are uncommon, but a few have been reported: herpes simplex virus (HSV) keratitis, sterile infiltrate, and a corneal ulcer, secondary to *Escherichia coli*.

At the Bochner Eye Institute we reported on 12-month data of 30 consecutive eyes of 19 patients who had an average age of 34.4 years with a range of 17 to 44. There were 12 right eyes and 18 left eyes. All corneas were clear preoperatively. The minimum corneal thickness was 400 μm. Pachymetry data showed an average minimum corneal thickness of 461 μm (range 401–548 μm) and at the 3-month level the average thickness had gone down to 431 μm (range 337–514 μm). By 6 months the average thickness increased to 441 μm and then at 9 to 12 months to 442 μm (Figure 37.10). When we looked at the percentage of corneal thinning from preoperative average measurements, at 3 months there was a decrease in corneal thickness by 6.5%, at 6 months 4.3%, and at 9 to

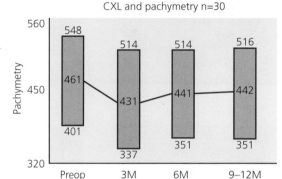

Figure 37.10 Pachymetry decreases post-collagen crosslinking (CXL) as the collagen fibers become more compact (n = 30). *M*, Months.

CXL and pachymetry n=30

	% Corneal thinning from Preop
3M	6.5%
6M	4.3%
9-12M	4.1%

Figure 37.11 Pachymetry changes over time post-collagen crosslinking (CXL): percentage thinning from preoperative measurement (n = 30).

12 months 4.1% (Figure 37.11). There is significant variability in the degree of corneal thinning from patient to patient, and even in the same patient between the right and left eyes (Figures 37.12 and 37.13). The average

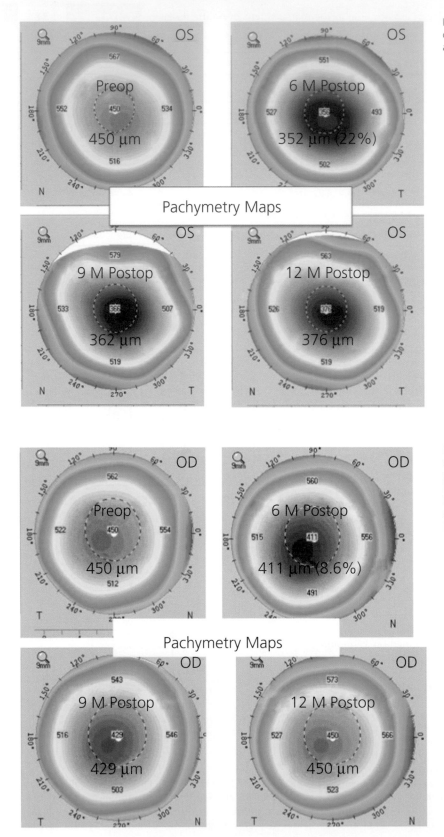

Figure 37.12 Pachymetry post-collagen crosslinking (CXL) changes at 6, 9, and 12 months (M).

Figure 37.13 Pachymetry post-collagen crosslinking (CXL) of the patient's other eye depicted in Figure 37.12. Note variable reaction between eyes as these maps show a return to preoperative levels by 12 months (M).

Figure 37.14 Computerized topography with a difference map post-collagen crosslinking (CXL). Significant changes noted with an area of 7.7 diopter (D) flattening. *M*, Months.
(Courtesy of Bochner Eye Institute, Toronto.)

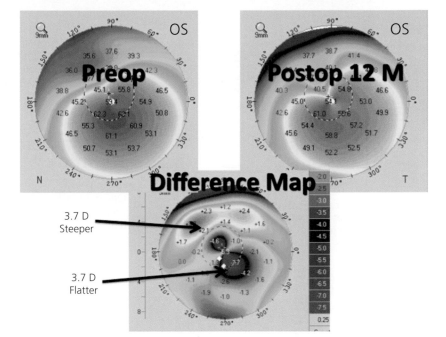

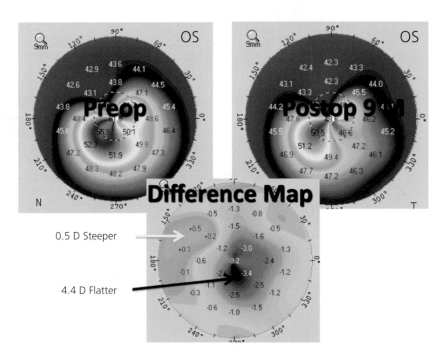

Figure 37.15 Computerized topography with a difference map post-collagen crosslinking (CXL). Significant changes noted with an area of 4.4 diopter (D) flattening. *M*, Months.
(Courtesy of Bochner Eye Institute, Toronto.)

decrease in corneal curvature looking at the steepest diopter region of the cornea was 1.00 diopter at 12 months.

The change in the steepest power or average *K* does not provide all the important information when analyzing the effects from CXL. It is important to look at difference maps to appreciate the change in curvature (Figures 37.14 and 37.15). There is some mild postoperative corneal haze that peaks at 6 months and gradually decreases over time

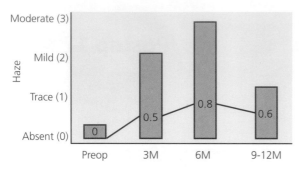

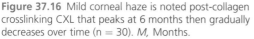

Figure 37.16 Mild corneal haze is noted post-collagen crosslinking CXL that peaks at 6 months then gradually decreases over time (n = 30). *M,* Months.

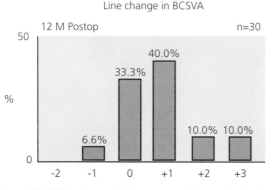

Figure 37.17 Line change in best corrected spectacle visual acuity (BCSVA) post-collagen crosslinking (CXL). *M,* Months.

(Figure 37.16). One of the most important clinical signs is the change in BCSVA (Figure 37.17). In our series of 30 eyes, at 12 months postoperatively 60% of eyes gained one or more lines of vision, 33.3% were the same, and 6.6% showed a one line decrease in BCSVA.

Following CXL the epithelium becomes intact usually by 4 to 6 days. A pseudodendrite is typically seen, which is a normal healing response to any corneal abrasion. BCSVA may be worse during the first 1 to 2 months, as the epithelium undergoes remodeling that results in a thinner layer of cells over the cone and thicker over the base to reduce irregular astigmatism.

Post-LASIK ectasia and CXL

Post-LASIK ectasia is a serious complication that rarely follows laser vision correction. Patients typically do well in terms of uncorrected visual acuity and best corrected visual acuity for years until ectasia develops. The topographic findings are similar to that of keratoconus. The biomechanical properties of the cornea have been weakened and this may be secondary to preoperative keratoconus, or minimal residual bed depth from the correction of high myopia, thin preoperative pachymetry, or a thicker flap than intended. The success rate of using CXL in ectasia cases has been reported and is the only current procedure to prevent progressive thinning and bulging (Figure 37.18).

TOPOGRAPHICALLY LINKED ABLATION

One approach to improving the visual rehabilitation of keratoconus eyes is the use of a topography-guided photorefractive keratectomy (PRK) to reduce irregular astigmatism (Figure 37.19). In this scenario the epithelium is removed either by a laser or rotary brush, alcohol, or debridement. This is followed by a topography-guided PRK in which the steep portion of the cornea is flattened and the flat area is steepened. Following laser ablation, riboflavin eyedrops are applied, and the UVA light source is then used for the CXL treatment. In addition to the asymmetric laser ablation to reduce the irregular astigmatism, a portion of the prescription can be treated. Because the CXL procedure induces flattening, typically less than 50% of the prescription is treated in this way. To preserve the biomechanical properties of the cornea usually less than 50 μm of tissue are removed.

INTRASTROMAL CORNEAL RINGS

If patients continue to have significant irregular astigmatism following CXL, and possibly despite the adjunctive use of a topography-guided PRK, the use of intrastromal corneal rings may be of further benefit to reduce irregular astigmatism. One or two intrastromal corneal rings can be inserted. This procedure was developed initially for the correction of low degrees of myopia. Dr. Colin from France began using intrastromal corneal rings for the correction of keratoconus, and this is the most common indication today. The corneal channels may be constructed by a mechanical dissector or with a femtosecond laser. The channel can be made easily with enhanced depth accuracy with the laser. Depending on the topographic pattern one or two rings are inserted. After the rings are inserted, one suture is used to close the small corneal wound. The suture is typically removed in 6 to 8 weeks. The ring procedure offers the benefit of being reversible and potentially exchangeable because it involves no removal of tissue. Early studies on intrastromal corneal rings involved use of two segments to cause general flattening of the cornea. A later study reported that better results could be obtained for those cones located more to the periphery of the cornea

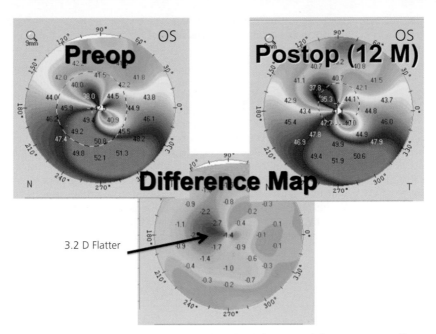

Figure 37.18 Computerized topography post-collagen crosslinking (CXL) for ectasia following LASIK. Difference map shows 3.2 diopter (D) of flattening. *M,* Months.
(Courtesy of Bochner Eye Institute, Toronto.)

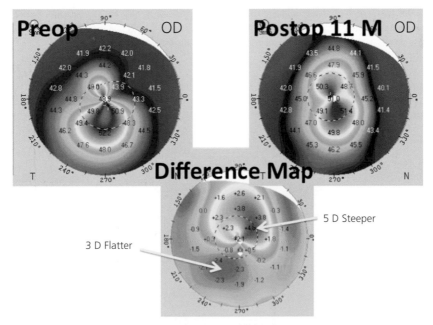

Figure 37.19 Computerized topography post-collagen crosslinking (CXL) and topographically linked ablation. Significant improvement in irregular astigmatism achieved by steepening superiorly and flattening inferiorly.
(Courtesy of Bochner Eye Institute, Toronto.)

by using a single ring segment. This leads to preferential flattening of the cone below, but also to steepening of the overflat upper part of the cornea.

POTENTIAL FUTURE ADVANCES IN CXL

CXL is one of the most significant advances in the therapeutic treatment of keratoconus, pellucid marginal degeneration, and ectasia following LASIK. A great deal of research and clinical studies are ongoing to enhance outcomes. Can we direct the UVA light to specific areas of an abnormal cornea to improve outcomes? Although patients want their disease process to be halted by CXL, they want their quality of vision to be enhanced. Further research will provide more answers.

SUMMARY

Because CXL can prevent progressive disease, the earlier the disease stage when CXL is performed, the better is the final visual result. It is important for clinicians to make an early diagnosis of keratoconus and this is greatly aided by the use of computerized topography. If there is a family history of keratoconus then topography would be helpful at an early age. If there is no family history of keratoconus then, if there is a scissors reflex on retinoscopy, a decrease in best corrected spectacle visual acuity, or increasing astigmatism, then keratoconus should be suspected and a topographic evaluation be performed. Today the CXL procedure has been approved in 65 countries and is becoming the standard of care for keratoconus, pellucid marginal degeneration, and ectasia following LASIK to halt progression.

FURTHER READING

Caporossi A, Mazzotta C, Baiocchi S, et al. Long-term results of riboflavin ultraviolet a corneal collagen cross-linking for keratoconus in Italy: the Siena eye cross study. Am J Ophthalmol 2010 Apr;149(4):585–93. Epub 2010 Feb 6.

Kanellopoulos AJ, Binder PS. Collagen cross-linking (CCL) with sequential topography-guided PRK: a temporizing alternative for keratoconus to penetrating keratoplasty. Cornea 2007;26(7):891–5.

Nawaz S, et al. Trans-epithelial versus conventional corneal collagen cross-linking: A randomized trial in keratoconus. Oman J Ophthalmol 2015;8.1:9.

Raiskup F, et al. Corneal collagen cross-linking with riboflavin and ultraviolet-A light in progressive keratoconus: ten-year results. J Cataract Refract Surg 2015;41(1):41–6.

Randleman JB, Russell B, Ward MA, et al. Risk factors and prognosis for corneal ectasia after LASIK. Ophthalmology 2003;110:267–75.

Spoerl E, Seiler T. Techniques for stiffening the cornea. J Refract Surg 1999;15:711–3.

Spoerl E, Mrochen M, Sliney D, et al. Safety of UVA–riboflavin cross-linking of the cornea, safety of UVA–riboflavin cross-linking of the cornea. Cornea 1 2007;26(4):385–9.

Chapter | 38 |

Wavefront aberrations and custom ablation

Daniel Epstein

In clinical practice, myopia, hyperopia, and astigmatism have long been the familiar refractive errors (i.e., lower-order optical aberrations) for which patients have received corrective glasses and contact lenses. However, the optical system of the eye displays many other imperfections, referred to as higher-order aberrations. They include such errors as spherical aberration and coma. These have not been addressed in routine office work because they could not be measured in clinical practice and there were no means to correct them optically. Also in the normal eye, these aberrations do not degrade the image quality below 20/20 vision.

With the advent of laser refractive surgery, higher-order aberrations have come into focus both because the laser procedures induced unwanted aberrations into the eye and because improvements in the lasers and the software that runs them now make it possible to correct some of the eye's higher-order aberrations.

Laser refractive surgery induces various amounts of spherical aberration and coma in treated eyes. For example, the procedure may correct myopia perfectly but at the same time introduce an increase in spherical aberration. These aberrations are generally not significant when the pupil is small, but they become important at low light levels when the pupil dilates. As a result, driving at night may become a problem because induced spherical aberration can cause glare, halos, and ghosting. The optical problems caused by spherical aberration in dim illumination cannot be corrected with glasses and, although a laser retreatment may be attempted, there is no guarantee that a second operation will eliminate the patient's complaints.

With the growing realization of the importance of higher-order aberrations in laser refractive patients, new measuring devices have been introduced to help the surgeon plan the procedure more accurately. These devices are based on well-known systems used for many years in optical engineering and physics. Referred to as wavefront sensors or aberrometers, they can measure the aberrations of the entire system of the eye. By documenting the aberrations preoperatively, the surgeon can theoretically aim at correcting not only the spherocylindric errors of the eye but also some of the higher-order aberrations. Also, by obtaining a more accurate picture of the preoperative optical system of a given eye, the laser ablation can be tailored to that eye ("custom ablation"), reducing the amount of aberrations induced, possibly avoiding the induction of such aberrations altogether, and even eliminating some of the preoperative higher-order aberrations.

Such a scenario sounds enticing, but is difficult to accomplish because it calls for micrometer precision and a fairly perfect conversion of the aberrometer data into an ideal ablation pattern. Imperfections in the laser beam and unpredictable individual healing responses add to the problems of designing a custom ablation.

The current intense research and development activity in the field of custom ablation has produced some systems (laser + aberrometer) that are precise enough to correct an impressive part of the eye's higher-order aberrations. However, this precision does not always translate into highly accurate outcomes because the response of the treated eyes is variable. For example, during the laser procedure the hydration of the cornea may vary, thus limiting the accuracy of tissue removal even when an extremely precise system is used. The cornea's healing response after laser surgery is a further confounding factor; postlaser epithelial thickness may vary from patient to patient (epithelial thickness changes occur not only after surface ablation but also, surprisingly, after laser-assisted in situ keratomileusis [LASIK]) and can thereby influence the refractive outcome of a procedure. Stromal remodeling after laser ablation and postoperative biomechanical changes of the cornea do not follow standard patterns and may derail the most meticulously planned custom ablation. Also, aside from the difficulties in predicting the individual eye's healing response, aging changes—especially those of the lens—may degrade the effect of the aberration correction over time.

There are further stumbling blocks when considering the discrepancy between an ideal custom ablation scenario and realistic expectations. Studies of the aberrations of normal human eyes (eyes without disease and with minor or no refractive errors) show that there appears to be a certain ratio between the magnitudes of different higher-order aberrations in normal eyes and that this ratio seems to shift for different pupil diameters. This implies that changing such a ratio (for example, by reducing spherical aberration without a proportional reduction of other higher-order aberrations) could in fact increase an eye's total aberrations.

A further observation made was that even a normal eye displays a substantial increase in spherical aberration as the pupil dilates from 5 to 7 mm (as it does in low luminance). In view of that, it may be unrealistic to expect that custom ablation can improve on nature by substantially decreasing spherical aberration for 7-mm pupils in excimer-treated eyes.

Aberrometers work on the principle that light can be defined as an electromagnetic wave and that the propagation of such a wave can be described as a wavefront (Figure 38.1). If the eye were optically perfect (i.e., aberration-free) and focused at infinity, a wavefront entering the eye would exit unchanged as a flat plane. In the presence of aberrations (as is the case in the normal eye), a deviation from the ideal wavefront is registered. In other words, the exit wavefront deviates from that of the plane wave. A wavefront aberration of the eye is thus defined as the deviation of the actual wavefront from an ideal reference wavefront.

The custom ablation laser systems currently on the market use one of a variety of aberrometers or wavefront sensors to document the eye's optical imperfections (Figure 38.2). Aberrometers can be based on a number of different optical principles. One common aberrometer is referred to as the Hartmann-Schack wavefront sensor. It works by focusing a laser beam to a point on the retina. The emerging beam from this point source is projected onto an array of lenslets (i.e., small lenses). The lenslet array forms a point pattern that is captured by a video camera. The obtained pattern is compared with that of an aberration-free beam. The wavefront is then computed from the displacement of the points from the unaberrated pattern.

For customized corneal ablation, the ablation profile produced by the laser is derived from the wavefront aberration at the corneal plane. For an object to achieve perfect focus in an aberrated eye, laser ablation of the cornea is performed, in a sense etching a lens onto the cornea.

There is, however, some disagreement as to whether the laser correction of aberrations should take account of the wavefront aberration of the whole eye or of the cornea only. Because the cornea is considered to be responsible for 80% to 85% of the aberrations of the entire eye and because the cornea is the part of the eye that is actually altered by the laser, proponents of the cornea school maintain that custom ablation should be planned on the basis of

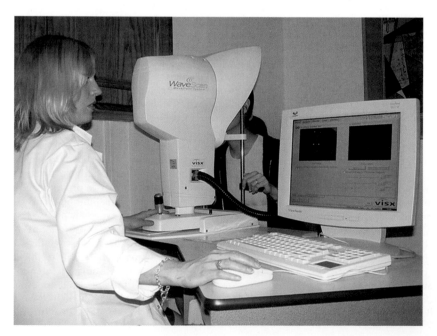

Figure 38.1 Taking a wavefront scan of the eye to detect higher-order aberrations.

Figure 38.2 The Allegretto Wave Analyzer provides the required wavefront data for treating higher-order aberrations.

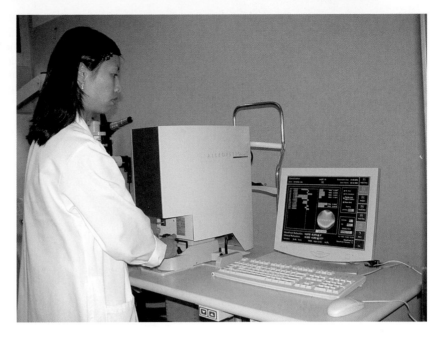

corneal aberrations only. They also point out that corneal aberrations can be calculated via topography maps, which provide a much higher resolution (and thus higher accuracy) than the aberrometers now on the market.

Others call the corneal approach nonsensical, emphasizing that the internal aberrations of the eye cannot be ignored because they are in balance with those of the cornea. By correcting only corneal aberrations, they argue, that balance is disturbed, leaving the eye with internal aberrations in disharmony with the altered cornea. It will take well-planned prospective studies to resolve this issue, but the two schools agree on one point: when treating pathologic corneas with irregular surfaces (either after corneal refractive surgery or after corneal disease), custom ablation should be based on a combination of corneal aberrations and corneal topography.

US Food and Drug Administration (FDA) data (published and unpublished) previously indicated that wavefront-guided LASIK increased the proportion of patients with a postoperative uncorrected visual acuity (UCVA) of 20/20 or better, but differences in preoperative refraction made interpretation difficult. In a more recent prospective, randomized contralateral study, comparing custom and conventional photorefractive keratotomy (PRK), investigators found that there were no differences in the outcomes between the two surgical approaches. Specifically, there were no statistically significant differences with respect to postoperative uncorrected distance visual acuity, corrected distance visual acuity, contrast sensitivity, or higher-order aberrations. Such findings inject some confusion into the whole issue of wavefront-guided

ablation, and some surgeons use the technique mainly when the preoperative higher-order aberrations are high (RMS >0.3 μm)

Wavefront aberrations can be represented by a series of terms called Zernike polynomials. These are a mathematical tool for describing the optical aberrations of the eye, and they make it possible to distinguish the spherocylindric aberrations (those that are corrected with glasses or contact lenses in routine office practice) from higher-order aberrations.

To provide a treated eye with the best possible visual acuity coupled with the highest possible optical quality, the laser system must be able to sculpt the cornea with sufficient precision. Such modern lasers need to have small spot scanning and extremely accurate eye tracking. Also the wavefront sensors that feed the data used by the laser to plan the ablation profile have to be extremely accurate.

Because the object of customized corneal ablation is to improve the optical quality of the eye, moving beyond standard laser surgery, which in fact generally increases corneal and total eye aberrations, traditional tests for measuring visual performance do not suffice to assess the outcome of custom ablation. Acuity charts (like the Snellen chart) test high-contrast visual acuity by using high-contrast letters. However, high-contrast visual acuity measurements (the time-tested golden standard of office practice) are fairly insensitive to the kind of more subtle visual complaints expressed by refractive surgery patients. The postoperative lamentation of a patient who achieves an uncorrected visual acuity of 20/20 but maintains that the vision is not as good as preoperatively cannot be comprehended if a high-contrast chart is used as the only visual performance test. Low-contrast charts, by lowering letter contrast, increase the sensitivity of the visual acuity test, making it possible to detect more subtle changes in optical quality. Several studies have shown that low-contrast acuity is a more sensitive measure of changes in visual function after refractive surgery than is high-contrast acuity.

A further examination that improves the assessment of the postrefractive surgery eye is the contrast sensitivity test. If a custom ablation succeeds in reducing an eye's higher-order optical aberrations (in addition to eliminating the spherocylindric error), the outcome is likely to result in higher-contrast images, making it easier for the patient to drive at night or to perform other tasks in dim illumination.

Chapter | 39 |

Optical coherence tomography

Raymond M. Stein, Rebecca L. Stein

Optical coherence tomography (OCT) is a revolutionary diagnostic technique that performs high-resolution cross-sectional imaging of the internal structures of the eye (Figure 39.1). It enables imaging in real time with resolutions of 1 to 15 μm. This high-resolution imaging is 1 to 2 orders finer than with the use of ultrasound, magnetic resonance imaging (MRI), or computed tomography (CT). The OCT, which was developed in 1991, has become a major advance in the field of ophthalmology, allowing for the imaging of the anterior segment and retina at resolutions that allow for a proper diagnosis.

An anterior segment OCT can image the anterior structures of the cornea, measure the corneal thickness, and allow visualization of the anterior chamber angle and related internal structures. Imaging of the retina can evaluate the optic disc, nerve fiber layer, vitreoretinal relationship, and macula. The high-resolution images allow for a diagnosis of glaucoma, an epiretinal membrane, cystoid macular edema, macular hole, macular degeneration, macular complications of diabetic retinopathy, and other conditions.

The OCT device is a noncontact method that allows for detailed cross-sectional imaging of the anterior eye and retina. The cross-sectional information obtained is complementary to the conventional testing of fundus photography and fluorescein angiography. In addition to its diagnostic ability, the monitoring of diseases such as macular edema and glaucoma can provide helpful information as to disease progression. A measurement of the thickness of the nerve fiber layer is a diagnostic indicator for early glaucoma and disease progression. OCT imaging is useful in determining the effectiveness or adequacy of treatment in disease conditions like glaucoma, macular edema, central serous retinopathy, macular holes, and exudative age-related macular degeneration.

OCT performs cross-sectional imaging by measuring the time delay and intensity of back-scattered or back-reflected light from structures inside tissue. Unlike with the use of light, ultrasound imaging depends on the reflection of sound waves from intraocular structures; it requires a direct contact of the ultrasound probe with the cornea or immersion of the eye in a liquid bath in order to transmit sound waves into the eye. It is the frequency or wavelength of the ultrasound waves that determines resolution of the images. Although typical ultrasound systems yield a resolution of 150 μm, high-resolution imaging devices using higher-frequency sound waves can achieve resolutions of 20 on the 20 μm scale. At these high-frequency sound waves the ultrasound signal is greatly attenuated in tissue and is limited to a depth of only 4 to 5 mm, which means that high-resolution imaging of the retina is not possible.

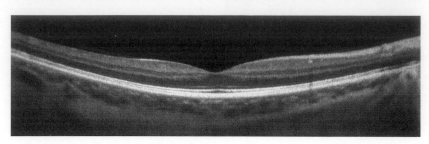

Figure 39.1 Optical coherence tomography (OCT) image of normal retina.

OCT is an optical imaging technique that uses light instead of sound, so the optical imaging is limited to tissues that are optically assessable. In addition to its use in ophthalmology, it can be incorporated into devices such as endoscopes or catheters. Patients are more comfortable with OCT imaging than ultrasound because the former is a noncontact testing device. OCT imaging devices have continued to improve in terms of resolution. The initial OCT units had resolutions of 10 μm. Current-generation units are in the 5 to 7 μm range, with a potential in the future for even finer resolution of 2 to 3 μm. The high-resolution devices today allow visualization of individual retinal layers, thus allowing for the diagnosis of a wide range of retinal conditions.

Histologic evaluation of the retina allows for the distinction of 10 layers, including 4 cell layers and 2 layers of neuronal interconnections. High-resolution OCT imaging allows for the detection of these internal retinal structures. These distinct layers, from the inner retina to the outer retina, are the inner limiting membrane, the nerve fiber layer, the ganglion cell layer, the inner plexiform layer, the inner nuclear layer, the outer plexiform layer, the outer nerve layer, the external limiting membrane, the photoreceptor inner segment and outer segment of the photoreceptor layer, and the retinal pigment epithelium. The choriocapillaris and choroid are immediately posterior to the retinal pigment epithelium. Ultrahigh resolution allows for excellent visualization of the retinal microstructure.

THE TECHNICIAN'S ROLE

Many OCT devices have come to market in recent years. The software and hardware of these devices can vary, but the basic principles are similar. If it is a new device for a practice, proper training should come from the distributor. If the device has been in the practice for some time, then training may come from a knowledgeable in-house technician. A grounded power supply is a requirement; in areas where the power supply is unstable, it is advisable to install an uninterrupted power supply. The OCT unit should be placed in a room in which there is a satisfactory area for both the operator and the patient to maneuver. The room

should generally be void of sunlight and the lighting condition should be adjustable with a dimmer switch. The room should have a solid floor to minimize vibration. The unit must be kept in a fairly stable temperature environment because extreme fluctuations in temperatures can have an adverse effect on the internal settings. The practice should decide on which scan protocols are used for evaluation of the cornea, anterior chamber angle, optic nerve head, nerve fiber layer, and macula. In addition to onsite training sessions, some companies offer online sessions (called webinars).

The patient should be seated in front of the OCT device in a sturdy chair with a back, and locking or no wheels. Make sure that the patient is comfortable by adjusting the table height and chin rest. Basic information needs to be entered into the computer system, including the first and last names. The technician then activates the required testing to be performed. On the first evaluation the patient's data are compared with those of normal patients with similar characteristics. On a follow-up visit, in addition to the normative database one also has the patient's previous records. Whereas the normative database can determine whether the patient is relatively normal, the progression reports allow the determination of any deterioration.

NORMATIVE DATABASES

Macular thickness data can be used for comparison with a normative database. The thickness values are compared with a normative database and a color scale is used to indicate which percentile each given thickness value falls into compared with normal thicknesses: red indicates greater than 99% of normal, yellow indicates greater than 95%, green is between % and 95%, light blue is less than 5%, and purple is less than 1% of normal thickness.

PROGRESSION ANALYSIS

When patients return for a repeat OCT, image thickness calculations can be compared from visit to visit using this software. These important values can be used to monitor disease progression or response to treatment.

NONEXUDATIVE AGE-RELATED MACULAR DEGENERATION

Age-related macular degeneration (AMD) is a common cause of central vision loss among individuals ages 70 years and more. The nonexudative form of macular degeneration accounts for close to 90% of all diagnosed cases. AMD can be classified into early, intermediate, and advanced stages based on clinical findings of the amount of drusen and retinal pigment epithelial atrophy. OCT evaluation can recognize findings of AMD with hard and soft drusen, pigmentary abnormalities, and geographic atrophy with dropout of photoreceptors (Figure 39.2).

EXUDATIVE AGE-RELATED MACULAR DEGENERATION

Although only 10% of AMD patients have the neovascular form of the disease, more than 80% of individuals that are legally blind (20/200 or worse) as a result of AMD have the exudative form. The exudative form of AMD, also called neovascular AMD or wet AMD, is characterized by neovascularization within the macula, detachment or tears of the retinal pigment epithelium (RPE), fibrovascular scarring, and vitreous hemorrhage. OCT is a complement to fluorescein angiography. Small changes in the structure of the retinal layers and subretinal space may signal progression or regression of the neovascular lesions. Choroidal neovascular lesions can appear with OCT imaging as an enlargement of the RPE-Bruch's membrane-choriocapillaris. A pigment epithelial detachment can be precisely imaged using OCT (Figure 39.3), which appears as a localized prominence. OCT imaging can identify an increase in foveal thickness, cystoid macular edema, subretinal fluid, RPE tears, and subretinal fibrosis or disciform scarring. One of the most valuable aspects of the OCT is in following up patients after treatment in which the central retinal thickness, as well as subretinal fluid volume, can be evaluated accurately.

OTHER MACULAR ABNORMALITIES

An OCT can be very useful in diagnosing a macular hole (Figure 39.4) and in following up eyes after treatment, to observe closure of the hole. Patients who are highly myopic are at greater risk of a choroidal neovascular membrane. An OCT is valuable in detecting early disease. Central serous chorioretinopathy is characterized by a

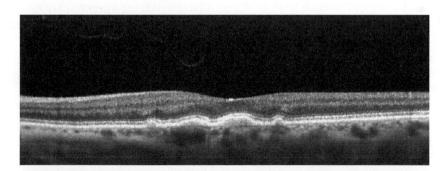

Figure 39.2 Optical coherence tomography (OCT) image of age-related macular degeneration.

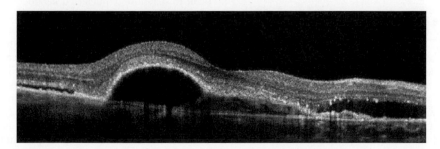

Figure 39.3 Optical coherence tomography (OCT) image of a pigment epithelial detachment.

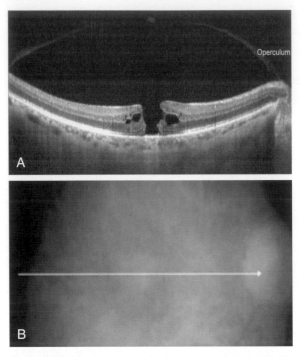

Operculum

A

B

Figure 39.4 (A) and (B) Optical coherence tomography (OCT) image of a full-thickness macular hole.

serous detachment of the retina in the area of the macula (Figure 39.5). An OCT is useful in making the diagnosis and following the course of the disease, either with or without treatment. An OCT can visualize an epiretinal membrane as a hyperreflective line on the retinal surface (Figure 39.6). As the thickness of the epiretinal membrane increases, its visibility with the OCT is more clearly defined. Contracture of the epiretinal membrane results in stretching of the retinal layers, which can be visualized. Cystoid macular edema (Figure 39.7) can be seen as a complication following intraocular surgery, a retinal vein occlusion, uveitis, and an epiretinal membrane. An OCT is useful in making the diagnosis and determining the stage of resolution with treatment.

VITREOMACULAR TRACTION

With age, liquefaction of the vitreous occurs with a resulting vitreous detachment. Usually the vitreous is most adherent out in the periphery, which is referred to as the vitreous base that overlies the ora serrata. Occasionally, there are significant vitreomacular adhesions that can result in traction and a variety of disease entities. These disease states include partial- or full-thickness macular holes, and subretinal fluid and/or macular edema. Using the

OCT this vitreomacular traction syndrome can be identified (Figure 39.8).

GLAUCOMA

OCT evaluation of the optic disc and nerve fiber layer is useful in the diagnosis of glaucoma and in follow-up to identify stability or progression (Figure 39.9). As an initial measurement the thickness of the nerve fiber layer is determined and compared with a normative database. Follow-up OCT evaluations can determine whether the nerve fiber layer is stable or there is progressive fiber loss, which indicates that the glaucoma treatment is unsatisfactory. An OCT can also provide three-dimensional images of the optic disc (Figure 39.10) and surrounding area, which can be valuable in follow-up examinations.

The OCT is also useful in identifying whether an angle is open or narrow, thus assisting the clinician to determine whether a prophylactic iridotomy is required (Figure 39.11). High-resolution OCT allows for the measurement of the anterior chamber angle with detailed imaging of Schwalbe's line, Schlemm's canal, and the trabecular meshwork. Measurement of the distance between Schwalbe's line and the anterior surface of the iris is a method of quantifying the angle width. Patients with a narrow angle are at higher risk for acute angle-closure glaucoma. The use of a prophylactic laser iridotomy can prevent the acute attack of glaucoma. An OCT evaluation is also useful in evaluating the anterior segment in the presence of diffuse corneal edema or scarring. This information can be helpful in preoperative planning for the surgeon.

KERATOCONUS SCREENING

Keratoconus is characterized by progressive thinning and bulging of the cornea. In moderate to advanced states, the diagnosis is relatively easy to make based on a variety of clinical signs and tests including computerized corneal topography (see Chapter 40). However, the early form of the disease, referred to as *forme fruste keratoconus*, can be difficult to diagnose. Undetected keratoconic eyes that have laser vision correction can lead to progressive ectasia and a poor visual outcome. OCT testing can accurately measure the corneal thickness of the cornea. The finding of eccentric focal corneal thinning is a characteristic feature of keratoconus. Parameters that have been identified to be suggestive of keratoconus include a superonasal-less-inferotemporal pachymetry reading greater than 51, a minimum corneal thickness measurement less than 472 μm, and a minimum-less-maximum pachymetry reading of less than 62 μm. If any of these readings are present then it is highly likely that the cornea is keratoconic (Figure 39.12).

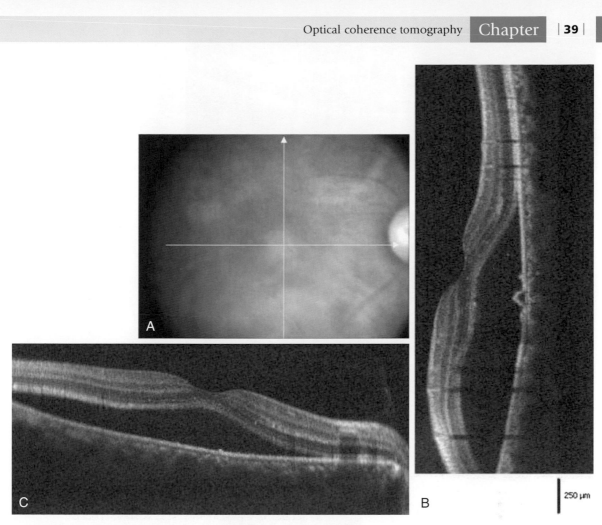

250 µm

Figure 39.5 (A)–(C) Optical coherence tomography (OCT) image of central serous retinopathy with elevation of the retina.

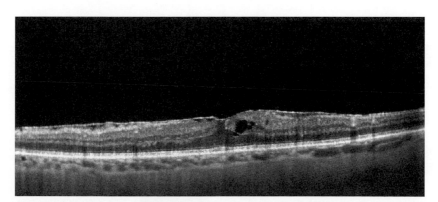

Figure 39.6 Optical coherence tomography (OCT) image of epiretinal membrane and diabetic retinopathy.

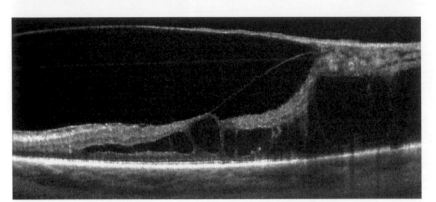

Figure 39.7 Optical coherence tomography (OCT) image of cystoid macular edema.

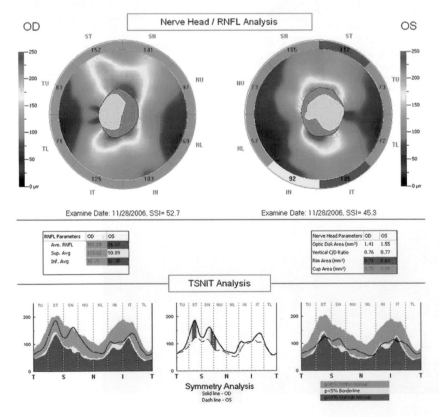

Figure 39.8 Optical coherence tomography (OCT) image of vitreomacular traction and cystoid macular edema.

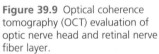

Figure 39.9 Optical coherence tomography (OCT) evaluation of optic nerve head and retinal nerve fiber layer.

Figure 39.10 (A)–(D) Optical coherence tomography (OCT) image of the optic disc in glaucoma.

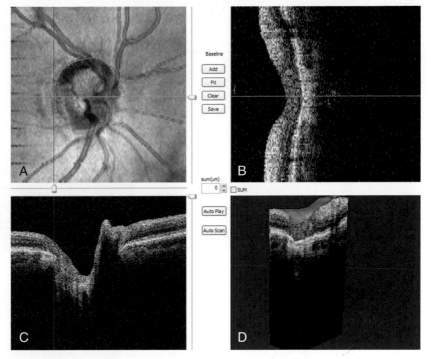

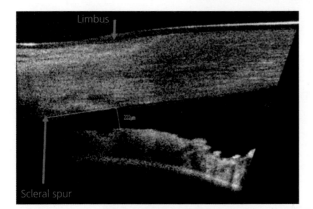

Figure 39.11 Optical coherence tomography (OCT) documenting a narrow angle (angle opening distance 200 μm anterior to scleral spur [AOD 500]; occludable angle AOD 500 < 190 μm).

(From Radhakrishnan S, Goldsmith J, Huang D, et al. Comparison of optical coherence tomography and ultrasound biomicroscopy for detection of narrow anterior chamber angles. Arch Ophthalmol. 2005 Aug;123(8):1053–9.)

REFRACTIVE SURGERY

An OCT anterior segment evaluation can accurately measure the thickness of the flap and the residual corneal bed after laser-assisted in situ keratomileusis (LASIK) (Figure 39.13). The earlier that the measurement is performed postoperatively, the easier it is to visualize the flap–bed interface. It is essential to routinely monitor LASIK flap thickness because the actual versus the intended thickness may vary. The use of femtosecond technology has significantly improved the accuracy and reproducibility of the LASIK flap compared with a mechanical microkeratome that uses a blade. Evaluation of eyes that have undergone ectasia following LASIK typically shows a flap thickness that was thicker than intended and a residual stromal bed of less than 250 μm.

An OCT evaluation can be useful in measuring the epithelial thickness following photorefractive keratectomy. Central thickening of the epithelium, referred to as *epithelial hyperplasia*, is a common response after laser vision correction, especially photorefractive keratotomy (PRK), and this may explain an unexpected outcome with significant regression.

A variety of phakic implants is available, including iris clip, anterior chamber, and posterior chamber or sulcus implants. The Visian lens, referred to as the *implantable contact lens*, is a sulcus lens, which vaults the crystalline lens. An OCT evaluation can document the position of the implantable contact lens and the distance of clearance over the crystalline lens. If the lens does not have satisfactory clearance, then there is an increased risk of cataract formation.

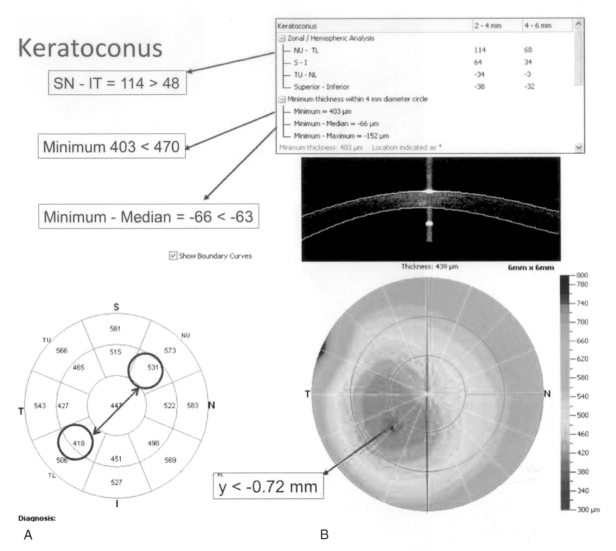

Figure 39.12 (A) and (B) Optical coherence tomography (OCT) imaging of the cornea to identify keratoconus.

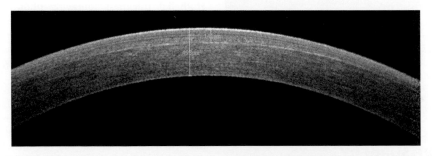

Figure 39.13 Optical coherence tomography (OCT) image of cornea with measurement of laser-assisted in situ keratomileusis (LASIK) flap.

Intracorneal rings are used primarily in the treatment of keratoconus, pellucid marginal degeneration, and ectasia following laser vision correction. The corneal rings are placed in a channel that is typically made 400 μm below the surface. OCT evaluation can confirm the exact depth of the rings. This information is of help to the corneal surgeon, so as to refine the technique of depth-related problems.

New corneal inlays are being developed for the correction of presbyopia. One such device is the Kamra inlay, which consists of a biocompatible polymer that increases depth of focus through a pinhole effect. The corneal implant is inserted into a corneal pocket that is made either with a femtosecond laser or with a microkeratome. OCT evaluation can demonstrate the exact depth of the implant.

CORNEAL PATHOLOGIES

The exact depth of corneal opacities can be measured with the OCT (Figure 39.14). Using this information the surgeon can then decide which surgical procedure would be best to enhance the patient's vision. With superficial opacities, a phototherapeutic keratectomy can be performed. With deeper opacities, a lamellar graft is usually the treatment of choice. OCT evaluation of corneas following surgical procedures such as a corneal transplant (Figure 39.15) can provide the surgeon with valuable information as to technique or complications.

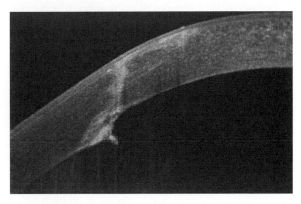

Figure 39.15 Optical coherence tomography (OCT) image of a penetrating keratoplasty.

Figure 39.14 Optical coherence tomography (OCT) image showing significant scarring at the level of Bowman's membrane in Reis-Buckler's corneal dystrophy.
(A) Reis-Buckler's corneal dystrophy with superficial corneal scarring.
(B) Optical coherence tomography (OCT) image showing significant scarring at the level of Bowman's membrane.

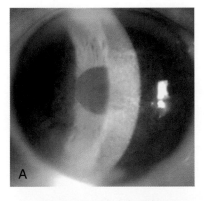

A

Dramatic epithelial masking

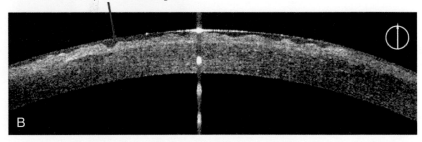

B

Femtosecond laser cataract surgery

The majority of femtosecond lasers use OCT imaging of the anterior segment to guide surgical planning of many of the critical steps of the cataract operation. Detailed images are obtained of the cornea, iris, lens, and anterior vitreous. This information allows for surgical planning of the corneal wound incisions, arcuate relaxing incisions in the cornea for astigmatism, anterior capsulotomy, and fragmentation of the nucleus. OCT imaging allows the laser to be directed to the exact location and depth of the cornea and lens to enhance outcomes.

SUMMARY

OCT is a sophisticated cross-sectional imaging device that allows the clinician to make an accurate diagnosis of a variety of conditions of the anterior segment, retina, and optic disc. It also provides a great tool with repeat imaging to determine stability, improvement, or deterioration of an eye condition. This information allows the clinician to determine the success of treatment. If there is progressive disease, then further clinical steps need to be taken.

Chapter 40

Computerized corneal topography

A. Ghani Salim

INTRODUCTION AND BASICS

Computerized corneal topography analysis is the measurement of the curvature of the corneal surface. This tool is based on the principles of keratometry and photokeratoscopy developed in 1880 by Placido. He placed a planar target with concentric alternating black-and-white rings in front of a patient's eye and then observed the shape of the rings in the virtual image of that target created from the reflection of the patient's anterior corneal surface. If the cornea is spherical, the rings appear circular and concentric. Deviations of the corneal shape appear as either distortions in shape or eccentricity of the rings.

Photokeratoscopy provides the user with only qualitative information about the curvature of the cornea, changes that accompany surgery, and progressive corneal abnormalities. The keratometer yields quantitative data, but only at four points. These points are located at approximately the 3-mm optical zone along two perpendicular meridians. One pair of points is aligned along the steepest axis of the corneal surface, with the second pair 90 degrees away. The keratometry has fundamental limitations in that it is able only to measure points along the annulus of the 3-mm optical zone.

With the capability of modern computers and software technology to qualify the data obtained from reflected Placido disc images, it has become feasible and practical to precisely analyze the radius of curvature (mm) and corresponding refractive power (diopter) on the corneal surface from inside the 1-mm optical zone to outside the 9- to 11-mm optical zone. This information is then translated into a complete color-coded map. The map is interpreted much like other topographic maps. These topographic maps provide the ability to monitor corneal curvature changes from the apex to the periphery.

There are a variety of corneal topographer systems available. Some use a back-lit conical dish as its Placido target; other systems use a cylindric light cone as the Placido target. With either a conical dish or a cylindric light cone, a Placido ring image is produced on the cornea.

The Orbscan IIz, Galilei G2, and Oculus Pentacam (Figure 40.1) are the latest in the state-of-the art technologies for mapping the surfaces of the cornea and for anterior segment analysis. The Orbscan takes multiple cross-sectional scans of the cornea with an advanced Placido disc system and is able to analyze elevation and curvature measurements on both the anterior and posterior surfaces of the cornea, white-to-white measurement, anterior chamber depth, angle kappa, and corneal pachymetry values. Galilei G2 merges two technologies, the rotating Scheimpflug and Placido technology, into one measurement, leading to accurate values of the posterior and anterior surfaces. The dual Scheimpflug approach offers accurate pachymetry readings and needs only to rotate 180 degrees. Pentacam is a rotating Scheimpflug camera that generates Scheimpflug images in

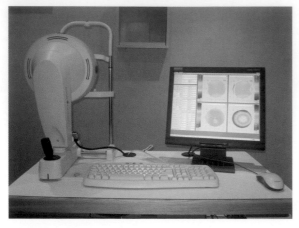

Figure 40.1 Oculus Pentacam.

the entire anterior and posterior surfaces of the cornea from limbus to limbus are calculated and depicted in Figure 40.2. The analysis of the anterior eye segment includes calculation of the chamber angle, chamber volume, and height. Images of the iris and anterior and posterior surfaces of the lens also are generated. The densitometry of the lens is automatically qualified. This chapter's focus is on the cornea.

Most corneal topography systems available today can generate various map displays. When performing computerized corneal topography for prerefractive surgery screening, diagnosis of a corneal pathology, or contact lens fitting, the most commonly used maps include the following:

Axial map or sagittal map

This is the most widely used and simplest of all topographic displays. It shows the curvature of the anterior surface of the cornea as a topographic map in diopteric values and measures it in axial direction relative to the center.

Every map has a color scale. Cool colors such as blue and green represent flatter areas of the cornea, whereas the warmer colors of orange and red represent steeper areas of the cornea. The analysis should include the keratometric values and should not be interpreted based on the colors alone.

three dimensions, with the dot matrix fine-meshed in the center as a result of the rotation. It takes a maximum of 2 seconds to generate a complete image of the anterior segment. Any eye movement is detected by a second camera and corrected in the process. The pachymetry and topography of

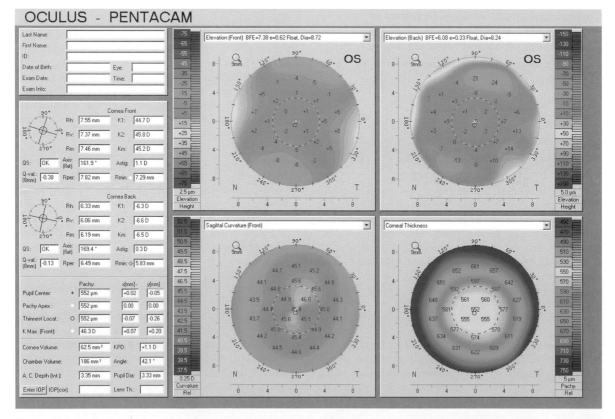

Figure 40.2 Oculus Pentacam, normal four-map selectable showing *(top two images)* anterior and posterior elevation, *(lower left image)* corneal surface power, and *(lower right)* corneal thickness representation map.

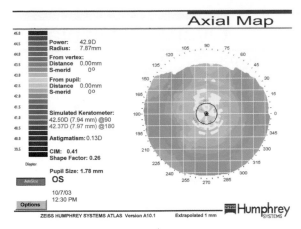

Figure 40.3 Normal aspheric axial corneal map.

Corneal irregularity measurement (CIM) and shape factor measurements are statistical indices that some topography units such as Humphrey Atlas provide on their axial map printout. The increase or decrease of these two over time indicates a change in the progress or healing of a condition. CIM values less than 0.5 indicate a normal-shaped cornea, and 1.0 or higher indicates corneal surface irregularities. Shape factor 0 to 0.3 is normal. Shape factor more than 1.0 indicates high irregularities (Figure 40.3).

Elevation map

This is the difference in height between the measurements of the cornea and a reference shape called best fit. This value can be negative if the measurement is less than the reference and positive if it is greater than the reference. The reference shape could be a best fit sphere, best fit ellipsoid, or a toric reference shape (Figure 40.4).

Corneal thickness map

This describes corneal thickness measurements distributed across the cornea

Other types of topography displays include tangential map, true net power, refractive map, keratometry map, multivue map (Figure 40.5), differential map, photokeratoscopic view, profile view, and so on.

CLINICAL USES

Of all currently available technology, the corneal topography is the best to provide specific and detailed information about the curvature of the cornea. It offers an exact evaluation of the profile of the cornea and a better interpretation and control of some of the pathologic conditions that can occur and affect the cornea.

Variations that occur in corneal topography can be the result of the changes of the corneal stroma and epithelium. Tissue loss and scars cause a flattening of the area and increase the curvature of the cornea around the lesion. With thinning processes such as keratoconus and pellucid marginal degeneration, thin tissues actually protrude and therefore the curvature of the cornea becomes greater.

The most commonly performed laser eye surgeries such as photorefractive keratectomy (PRK) and laser-assisted

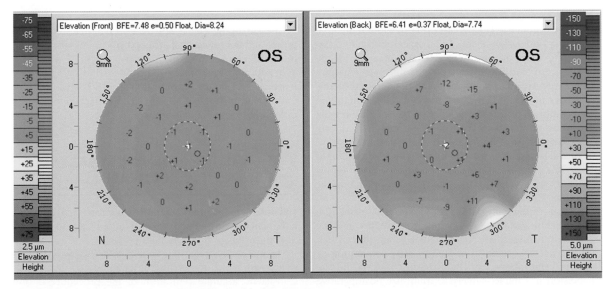

Figure 40.4 Oculus Pentacam anterior and posterior elevation maps.

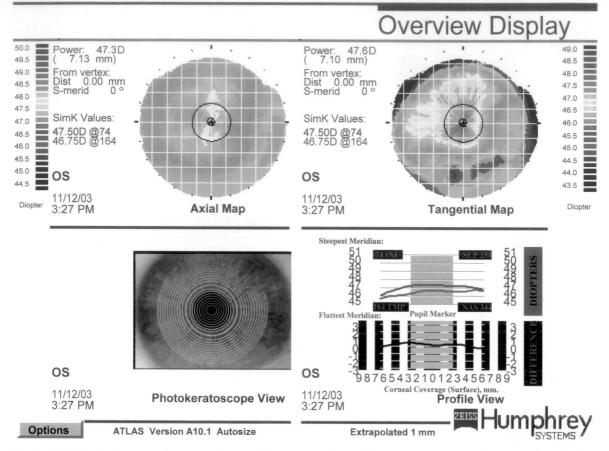

Figure 40.5 Multiple view maps: *(top left)* axial, *(top right)* tangential, *(lower left)* photokeratoscope, and *(lower right)* profile view.

in situ keratomileusis (LASIK) for the correction of myopia, hyperopia and astigmatism, and corneal collagen cross-linking (CXL) for the treatment of keratoconus, can greatly benefit from corneal topography. Corneal topography can identify irregular astigmatism and potential problems, as well as early forms of keratoconus and pellucid marginal degeneration. Corneal topography precisely measures the alterations produced in corneal shape and follows any regression or remodeling that may occur over time.

Corneal topography is useful for the correct evaluation of high corneal astigmatism. These cases often pose significant challenges when performing retinoscopy, automatic refraction, and standard keratometry.

Corneal topography is very helpful in assessing the quality of the surface of the cornea, the stability and the effect of the surgery after CXL, radial keratectomy (RK), and the selective removal of sutures after penetrating or lamellar keratoplasty. Also it assists in choosing the site of incision in cataract surgery to minimize postoperative astigmatism.

Corneal topography is very beneficial in determining the power and axis of corneal astigmatism in implanting toric intraocular lenses in cataract surgery.

In addition, corneal topography is used in fitting contact lenses, especially gas-permeable lenses. It is also useful in monitoring and evaluating contact lens effect on the cornea in long-term contact lens wearers.

CORNEAL TOPOGRAPHY ANALYSIS IN REFRACTIVE SURGERY

The development and evaluation of keratorefractive surgery have benefited from the parallel advances made in the field of corneal topography analysis.

The major advantage of laser refractive surgery is the precision with which the excimer laser ablates corneal tissue. Consistent, accurate centration of the procedure is one component of the technique that is critical to its success.

From the topographic map of a cornea it is possible to determine the amount of spherocylindric aberration before surgery and objective measurement of surgical results, as well as the precise location of the ablation zone in laser refractive surgery.

Preoperative analysis

The normal cornea is aspheric (see Figure 40.3), being steepest centrally with progressive flattening toward the periphery.

A commonly encountered corneal topographic finding is that of regular and symmetric astigmatism with a bowtie shape. A with-the-rule regular corneal cylinder is vertically aligned (Figure 40.6, lower left), whereas against-the-rule corneal astigmatism takes the form of a horizontally aligned bowtie pattern (Figure 40.7).

The steepest axis of the cornea may not be symmetric. Asymmetrically distributed astigmatism has potentially important implications in surgical correction. For patients who have asymmetric astigmatism, it is very important to ask about contact lens wear, and whether there is a family history of keratoconus.

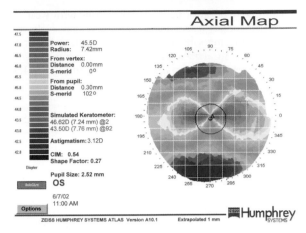

Figure 40.7 Axial map of normal against-the-rule astigmatism.

Although topography is important in achieving good visual outcomes, it is essential to ensure that the cornea is stable before performing any refractive procedure. Operating on an unstable cornea usually leads to disappointing visual outcomes.

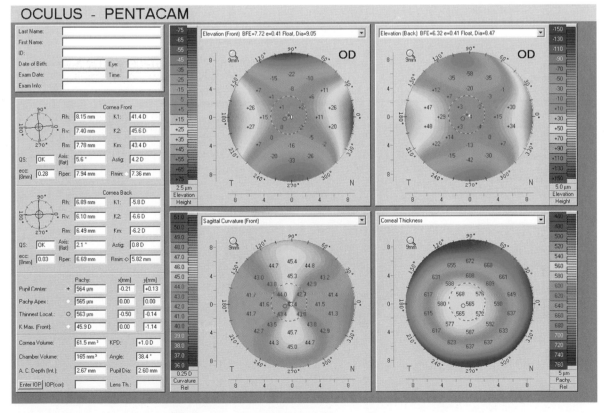

Figure 40.6 Normal bowtie type with the rule astigmatism *(lower left)*.

Chronic hypoxia of the cornea and long-term wear of poorly fit contact lenses, particularly if the lens is decentered, cause changes in the contour of the cornea with resultant change in refraction. This reversible condition is referred to as corneal warpage (Figures 40.8 and 40.9). This condition is not as prevalent today with rigid gaspermeable lenses as it was in the era of polymethyl methacrylate (PMMA) lenses. Therefore, corneal topography is very useful in monitoring and evaluating the contact lens effect on the cornea for patients wearing contacts for a long

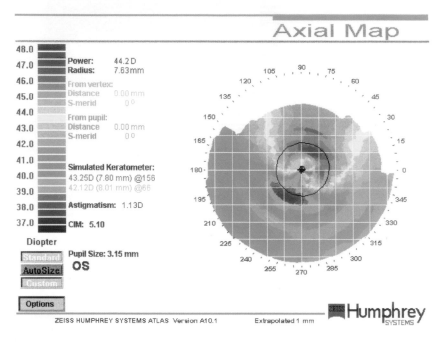

Figure 40.8 Axial map of corneal warpage from rigid gas-permeable contact lenses.

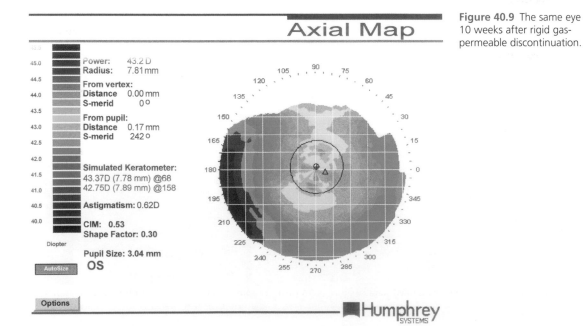

Figure 40.9 The same eye 10 weeks after rigid gas-permeable discontinuation.

time. Corneal refractive surgery is contraindicated until the warped area has reversed and refraction has become stable.

It is important to distinguish between corneal warpage induced by contact lenses and true keratoconus. Keratoconus is a red flag in refractive surgery, especially LASIK. Patients suspected of keratoconus are at greater risk of ectasia after LASIK. Even with advanced diagnostic tools and careful screening, the incidence of ectasia after LASIK could be as high as 1 in 2500 cases.

Corneal warpage is a reversible condition. It is important to distinguish between real corneal alterations and irregularities induced by contact lenses. A corneal pachymetry map shows no thinning at the warped area. Because differentiation may be difficult, the patient must abstain from wearing contact lenses until refraction and corneal topography are stable. Significant changes suggest that corneal warpage from contact lenses has not yet resolved. If contact lens wear is discontinued only a few days before the preoperative evaluation, the final refractive result may be unpredictable because the time for reestablishment of corneal stability after contact lens warpage may take days to months to occur. Stability can vary with soft lenses from minutes to 1 week or longer. One month is the minimum for discontinuation of rigid gas-permeable lenses, although it may take up to 6 months or longer before the cornea is stable. On a practical note, if serial refractions performed every 2 weeks show no change in refraction (<0.50 diopter) and computerized corneal topography is stable and appears normal, it is probably safe to proceed with laser surgery.

Topography is helpful in predicting outcomes. For example, patients achieve better visual results if their refractive astigmatic axis approximates their topographic axis. Theoretically, in these cases, PRK and LASIK that treat astigmatism can create a spherical cornea. These patients may achieve outstanding acuity levels as a result of the creation of a spherical cornea.

The preoperative identification of early or mild keratoconus is very important because lamellar refractive surgery is generally not indicated in these patients. Up until recently, irregular astigmatism could not be satisfactorily treated with the standard excimer laser treatments. Even if the myopia were reduced, any residual irregular astigmatism would require a rigid contact lens for correction. In addition, the correction of asymmetric astigmatism was difficult to treat with the older laser technologies because more laser pulses were required at the steeper quadrant compared with the meridian 180 away. Although keratoconus is still a contraindication for lamellar laser refractive surgery such as LASIK, limited topography-guided and wavefront-guided customized PRK ablation has shown promise in reducing the irregular astigmatism and improving best corrected vision. The concern of treating unrecognized keratoconus patients is the potential for litigation if keratoconus is detected postoperatively and is thought to be caused by the laser procedure.

The newer topography systems such as Orbscan IIz, Galilei G2, and Oculus Pentacam provide true elevation and depression maps, as well as a map of pachymetry values. The measurement of the corneal thickness has important diagnostic and clinical implications in the planning of refractive surgeries such LASIK and PRK and monitoring the progression of conditions such as keratoconus or corneal edema. When the apex has been displaced inferiorly and is associated with the most prominent area of thinning, the surgeon can be confident of a keratoconus diagnosis.

Postoperative assessment of the cornea

In corneal laser refractive surgery, the excimer laser is used to reshape the cornea to correct myopia, hyperopia, and astigmatism. In cases of myopia the center of the cornea is flattened (Figure 40.10), and in hyperopia it is steepened (Figure 40.11). In cases of astigmatism the steep axis is flattened and the flat axis is steepened. Corneal topography, along with other tests, qualifies and quantifies the changes induced by refractive surgery. It evaluates the centration of the ablated area and monitors the stability of the changes.

Ablation decentration (Figure 40.12) relative to the entrance of pupil may produce increased glare and distortion from the edge of the ablation zone encountering the edge of the pupil. Patients with small pupils may be asymptomatic yet still have a slight or moderate decentration. Eccentric ablation zones always result in manifest refractive astigmatism.

Postoperative topography is helpful in assessing both symptomatic and asymptomatic patients. It provides feedback to the surgeon on the quality of the ablation and determines the changes such as regression.

CORNEAL TOPOGRAPHY AND CATARACT SURGERY

Clinical studies have demonstrated that posterior corneal astigmatism could be a factor in generating unexpected postoperative outcomes after cataract or refractive lens exchange surgeries. One of the new devices that measures total corneal astigmatism is the Cassini Corneal Shape Analyzer (Figure 40.13). Reliable Purkinje imaging and precision ray tracing technologies are used to determine corneal shape and optical aberrations. Posterior and anterior data are calculated to provide surgeons with the total corneal power, as well as steep axis and magnitude of astigmatism (Figure 40.14). Understanding the relationship between the anterior and posterior of the cornea should help to provide a more customized planning approach to correcting astigmatism at the time of cataract surgery.

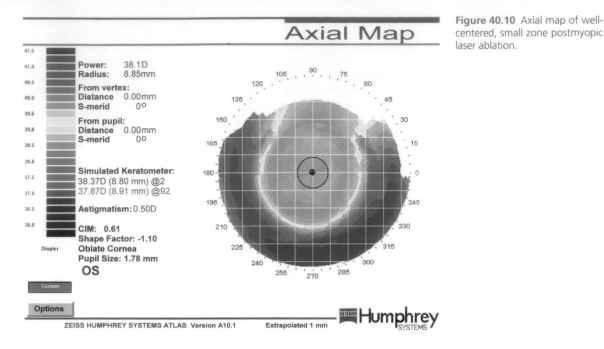

Power: 38.1D
Radius: 8.85mm

From vertex:
Distance 0.00mm
S-merid 0°

From pupil:
Distance 0.00mm
S-merid 0°

Simulated Keratometer:
38.37D (8.80 mm) @2
37.87D (8.91 mm) @92

Astigmatism: 0.50D

CIM: 0.61
Shape Factor: -1.10
Oblate Cornea
Pupil Size: 1.78 mm

OS

Custom

Options

ZEISS HUMPHREY SYSTEMS ATLAS Version A10.1   Extrapolated 1 mm

Figure 40.10 Axial map of well-centered, small zone postmyopic laser ablation.

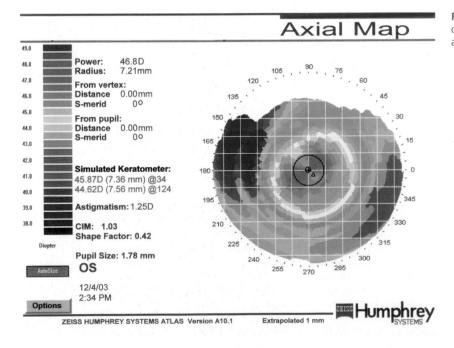

Power: 46.8D
Radius: 7.21mm

From vertex:
Distance 0.00mm
S-merid 0°

From pupil:
Distance 0.00mm
S-merid 0°

Simulated Keratometer:
45.87D (7.36 mm) @34
44.62D (7.56 mm) @124

Astigmatism: 1.25D

CIM: 1.03
Shape Factor: 0.42

Pupil Size: 1.78 mm

AutoSize OS

12/4/03
2:34 PM

Options

ZEISS HUMPHREY SYSTEMS ATLAS Version A10.1   Extrapolated 1 mm

Figure 40.11 Axial map of normal cornea posthyperopic laser ablation.

Figure 40.12 Anterior sagittal curvature map of ablation decentration postmyopic laser vision correction.

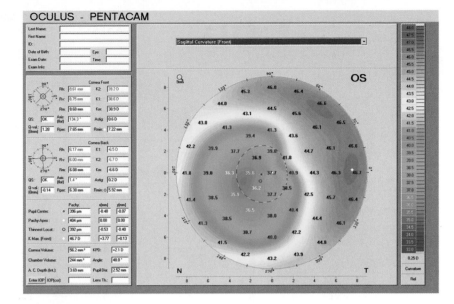

Color-coded maps have now become a universally accepted method of displaying corneal topography. Since the early 1990s the instruments have been promoted as one of the better tools to aid in the fitting of rigid gas-permeable lenses, especially in patients with abnormal corneal topographies. Most of the current corneal topographers have software that has been installed to help in the contact lens fitting.

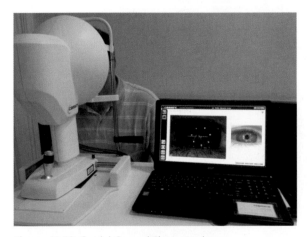

Figure 40.13 Cassini Corneal Shape Analyzer.

CORNEAL TOPOGRAPHY AND CONTACT LENS FITTING

Much of the success of a rigid contact lens fit is predicated on the delicate balance that exists between the anterior corneal surface and the posterior contact lens design. This interaction creates a number of bearing and clearance points that must be of appropriate location and pressure to maintain optimum lens dynamics and ocular health.

Of the more recent technologies to emerge, computerized corneal topography, has had the greatest commercial success and worldwide clinical acceptance.

Today, computerized corneal topographies have demonstrated their usefulness in quantifying the maps of normal eyes as well as those involving corneal injuries, surgery, or disease.

KERATOCONUS

Keratoconus is a bilateral, progressive disease of the cornea in which the cornea becomes conical and protrudes. The protruded area is usually the thinnest part of the cornea (Figure 40.15). In the majority of cases the cone is located in the inferior part of the cornea, but it can be found nasally, temporally, and even centrally. The ectatic part is about 3 to 6 mm in diameter.

Patients with advanced keratoconus (Figure 40.16) showing clinical signs such as an iron ring, corneal Descemet's folds, corneal scarring, or corneal hydrops do not require corneal topography to make the diagnosis. It is the patients who present with a clear cornea on slit lamp and less than 20/20 best corrected visual acuity that need corneal mapping.

The keratometry is helpful if corneal mires are irregular or distorted, and the cornea is relatively steep (>49.00 diopters). Also helpful in the diagnosis is the finding of scissoring of the retinoscopic reflex, less than 20/20 best corrected visual acuity, careful biomicroscopy to see an iron ring, and the changes in Descemet's membrane.

Today corneal topography is the gold standard for diagnosing all types of keratoconus including early and

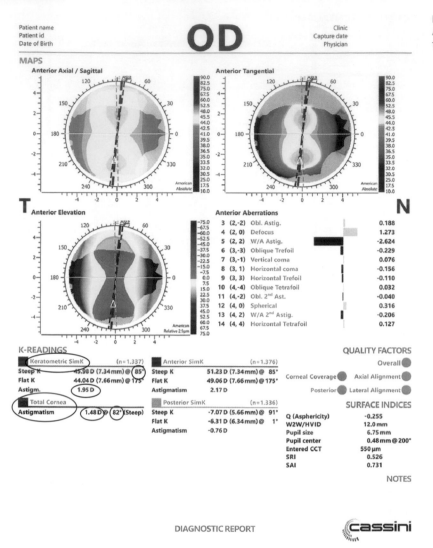

Figure 40.14 Cassini Corneal Shape Analyzer shows 0.47 diopter less total corneal astigmatism.

asymptomatic (forme fruste keratoconus). Asymptomatic forme fruste keratoconus (Figure 40.17) without affecting best corrected visual acuity can remain undiagnosed unless corneal topography is performed.

Corneal topography provides information on the location, size, and curvature of the cone apex and helps follow the progress of the disease. The typical findings of keratoconic corneal topography are irregular steepening of the cornea, decentered thinning (Figure 40.18), inferior steepening of greater than two diopters compared with superior cornea (Figure 40.19), elevation of the anterior surface of the cornea greater than 15 microns, and elevation of the posterior of the cornea greater than 20 microns (Figure 40.20).

The most difficult keratoconus to diagnose are the apical ones because of regularity and symmetry (Figure 40.21). In these cases one should look for keratometry readings and corneal pachymetry. Unexplained increased myopia and astigmatism, K higher than 49.00 diopters and corneal pachymetry less than 500 microns is suggestive of apical cone.

A new treatment for keratoconus that has shown great success is corneal CXL, a onetime application of riboflavin eyedrops to the eye. The riboflavin, when activated by illumination of ultraviolet A (UVA) light, augments the collagen crosslinking within the stroma and recovers some of the mechanical strength of the cornea. CXL has been shown to slow or arrest and in some cases slightly

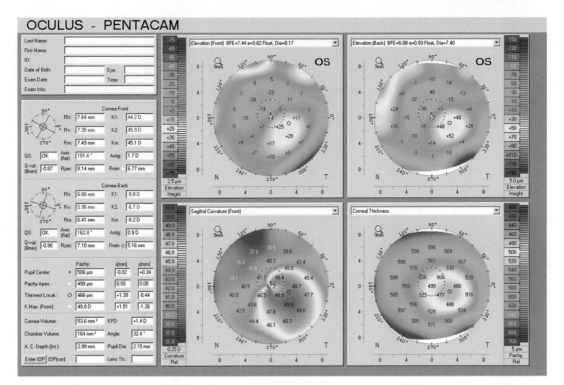

Figure 40.15 Midkeratoconus extending from the center of the cornea. Note that the cornea is greater than 49.00 diopters steep at the apex of the cone.

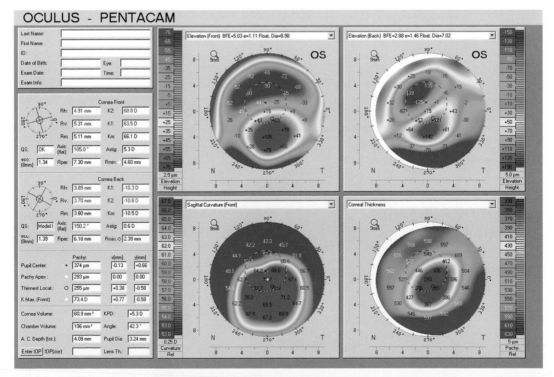

Figure 40.16 Advanced keratoconus with the anterior elevation more than 100 microns, posterior elevation more than 140 microns, steepest *K* greater than 72.00 diopters, and the lowest corneal thickness less than 260 microns.

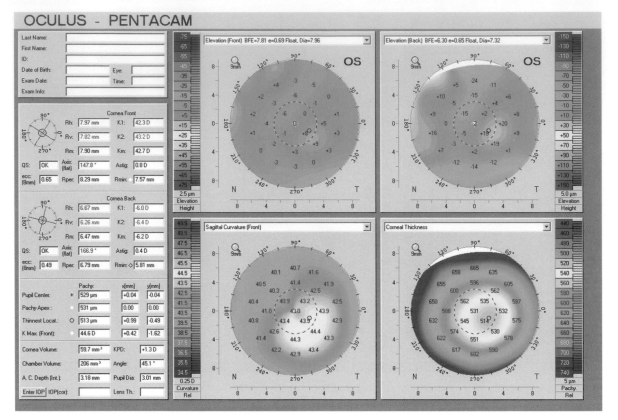

Figure 40.17 Forme fruste keratoconus. This patient's spectacle best corrected visual acuity is 20/20.

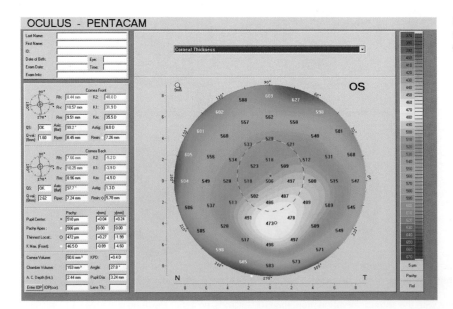

Figure 40.18 Corneal thickness map in keratoconus. Note decentered thinning of the cornea.

Figure 40.19 Anterior sagittal map in keratoconus suspect. Note that the cornea is more than 2.00 diopters steeper inferiorly compared with the superior cornea.

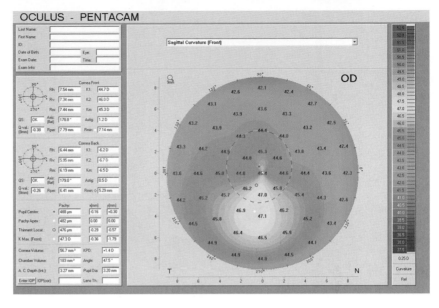

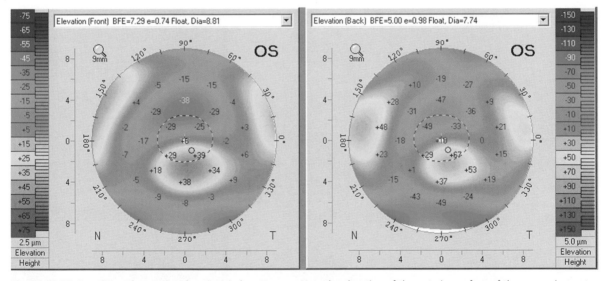

Figure 40.20 Anterior and posterior elevations in keratoconus. Note the elevation of the anterior surface of the cornea is greater than 35 microns and elevation of the posterior of the cornea is greater than 60 microns.

reverse the progression of keratoconus (Figure 40.22). After CXL the patient can be fitted with contact lenses, or with limited customized topography-guided or wavefront-guided advanced surface laser ablation (LASIK is still a contraindication for diagnosed or suspected keratoconus). The goal of the treatment is to partially correct the refractive error and astigmatism as well as to create a regular spherical surface on the cornea. This can be achieved by soft or rigid gas-permeable contact lenses in mild to moderate keratoconus and with rigid lenses or piggyback lenses in cases of advanced keratoconus. Sometimes surface ablation can help to flatten the cornea to fit with the contact lenses. When all attempts fail, corneal transplant is advised.

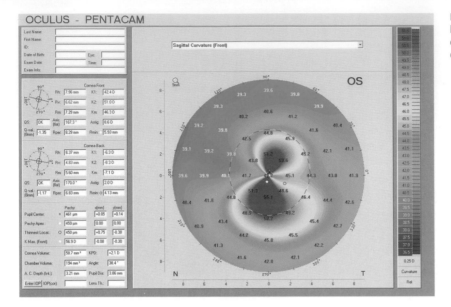

Figure 40.21 Central apical keratoconus. Note that the center of the cornea is more than 50.00 diopters steep.

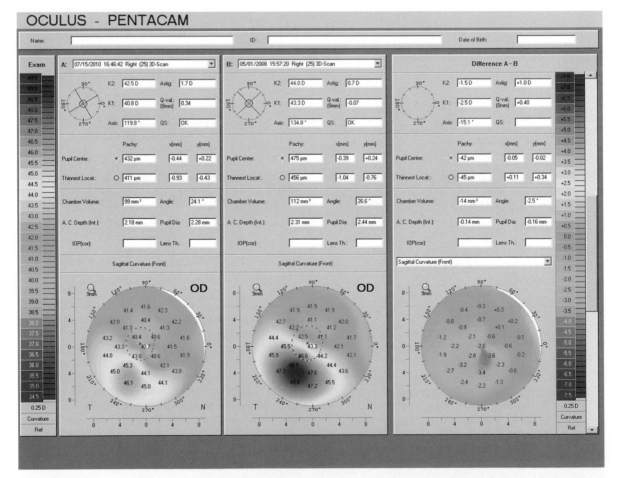

Figure 40.22 Anterior sagittal curvature maps in keratoconus: *(left)* 2 years following corneal collagen crosslinking (CXL), *(center)* pretreatment, and *(right)* difference map. Note that the cornea has flattened by more than 3.00 diopters in the difference map.

SUMMARY

Computerized topography is an important tool for the anterior segment surgeon and contact lens fitter. It is an integral part of the pre- and postoperative evaluation of the cornea. The slit lamp and keratometry are not of great clinical value in assessing patients preoperatively for diagnosis of corneal warpage, keratoconus, and irregular astigmatism and postoperatively for those who complain of halos, glare, or monocular diplopia. Computerized corneal topography, however, often enables the clinician to make the correct diagnosis. It not only evaluates subjective complaints but also gives positive feedback to the surgeon about the size of the ablation, centration, regularity of the surface, development of ectasia, and progression of keratoconus. Some of these instruments directly input data into the laser computer (topography-guided customized laser ablation) so that laser pulses can be distributed to produce a more natural prolate cornea.

Corneal topography plays an important role in design and parameter calculation of contact lenses. Manufacturers are trying to design custom contact lenses that directly use corneal topography information. This would have exciting clinical implications for those patients who have been unable to wear contact lenses with comfort and substantially reduce the number of required visits to achieve adequate fitting in difficult cases.

Chapter | 41 |

Specular microscopy

Harold A. Stein, Raymond M. Stein, Melvin I. Freeman

SPECULAR MICROSCOPE

The specular microscope is used to examine the endothelium of the cornea, which is the layer of the cornea in contact with the aqueous humor transfer (Figure 41.1). The specular microscope permits visualization and photography of the endothelium. Analysis by computer can quantitatively and qualitatively identify the cell loss of the endothelium from contact lenses and intraocular surgery. Without a viable endothelium the cornea would swell, lose its transparency, and become a painful debilitating organ, such as occurs in bullous keratopathy.

The specular microscope is an instrument in which light passes through a slit aperture into a system of mirrors with a direct light, moves out through an objective lens, and is attached to a "dipping cone." This cone lens is a flat surface extension of the $\times 20$ water immersion objective. Specular microscopes can be contact or noncontact regarding the cornea. A focusing knob adjusts the movement of the cone lens to focus the image on a cornea for different thicknesses. This process is used for an objective measurement of the corneal thickness. The light that is reflected from the endothelium and back through the objected eyepiece at $\times 200$ magnification can be observed through an eyepiece or directed into a single-lens reflex camera. The xenon flashcube permits clear photographs despite continuous small eye movement (Figure 41.2).

Endothelium counts are expressed as cells per millimeter squared. The average central endothelium cell count rate is from 1800 to 4000 cells/mm^2, with an average of 2800 cells/mm^2. A significant decrease in cell density occurs with age, indicating a continuous cell loss throughout life. The endothelial cell has no capacity for cell division and reproduction so that when loss occurs there is no replacement. The endothelial cell population of the human cornea decreases from approximately 1 million cells from the first year of life to one-third of that number by the eighth decade of life.

The greatest effect of specular microscopy has been in the area of cataract extraction, particularly with regard to intraocular lens insertion. It has been shown that patients with routine cataract extraction have endothelial cell losses ranging up to 8%. With some anterior chamber intraocular lenses, cell losses can range from 24% to 62%. It has been established that such endothelial cell loss is a result of the intraocular lens touching the endothelium. This has caused a change in our thinking to have posterior chamber lenses inserted in the capsular bag. The introduction of sodium hyaluronate (Healon) and other viscoelastics has significantly minimized the endothelial trauma during the surgery. The use of the specular microscope has made the practitioner aware of factors that encourage a concerted effort to minimize irreparable endothelial damage.

The clinical specular microscope has become an important clinical aid in helping the surgeon operating on the anterior segment to plan a more rational presurgical approach. In those practices in which a great deal of surgery is being performed and a specular microscope is used, it is important for the ophthalmic technician to learn how to use this instrument, to understand its significance, and to know how to use it for taking pictures of endothelium for the surgeon to examine (see Figure 41.4).

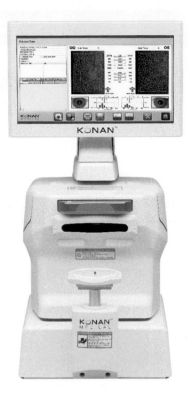

Figure 41.1 The specular microscope is used to determine the cell count (cells/mm^2) and morphology (shape and size) of the corneal endothelium to evaluate the health of this important cell layer.

(Courtesy of Konan Medical USA, Inc., Irvine, CA, USA)

Of equal importance is its role in establishing oxygen deprivation in long-standing contact lens wearers. The corneal endothelium can undergo changes to the shape and size of cells as a result of hypoxia.

ENDOTHELIAL SPECULAR PHOTOMICROGRAPHY

As its name implies, specular photomicrography is based on a system of projecting a light onto the endothelial surface and photographing the information contained within the specular reflection of that light source. Specular, from the Latin *specularis*, means "mirror-like." A specular reflection can be obtained from any relatively smooth surface. To be visible, however, it must be viewed at an angle from the perpendicular directly proportionate to the angle of incidence. The glossy surface of the endothelial cells reflects a considerable amount of light, whereas their borders, not being smooth and flat, absorb the light, thus providing a discrete "negative" outline of the cells (Figure 41.3).

Although endothelial cells play a critical role in maintaining corneal clarity, they are of a finite number and do not regenerate. Several conditions, including age, can contribute to their compromise; an assessment of their density and general health can therefore be of significant value when considering procedures such as cataract extraction or intraocular lens implantation (Figure 41.4).

Two types of endothelial microscopes, contact and noncontact, are available. The former requires direct contact with the patient's cornea. Before use of the contact microscope, the patient's cornea must be anesthetized and extreme care taken during the procedure to avoid inadvertent, excessive pressure on the eye. To this end the patient

Figure 41.2 CellChek cellular analysis detail.

(Courtesy of Konan Medical USA, Inc., Irvine, CA, USA)

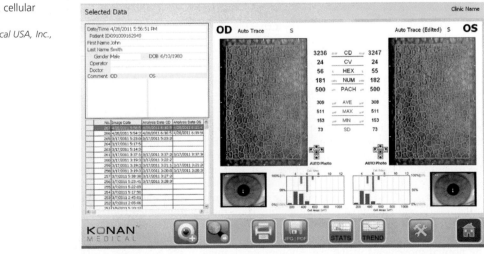

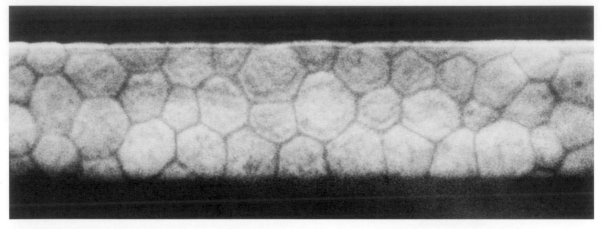

Figure 41.3 Mosaic pattern of corneal endothelial cells.

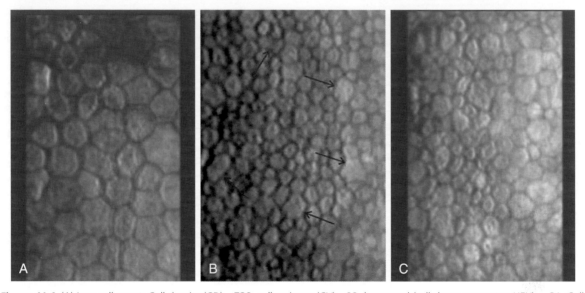

Figure 41.4 (A) Low cell count: Cell density (CD)=739, cell variance (CV)=22, hexagonal (cell shape geometry; HEX) = 31. Cell density is low (CD = 739) and shows abnormal shape (HEX=31%), but fairly equally enlarged (cell volume [CV]=22). Therefore, the endothelium is fairly stable and the cornea still clear. (B) Cell coalescence. This image shows several cells going through the process of coalescence *(arrows)*, one mechanism of the wound-healing process. (C) Another example of high cell volume: CD=2169, CV=51, HEX=48. To avoid a sampling error, one must count all visible cells. More the better by Center Method (Semi manual). *(Courtesy of Konan Medical USA, Inc., Irvine, CA, USA)*

must be positioned in the headrest assembly so as to be able to maintain steady, gentle pressure against the chin rest and, most important, the forehead-stabilizing bar. If the patient's forehead is allowed to move away from the camera, there is the risk of the patient moving abruptly forward and applying excessive pressure to the eye. The slight amount of pressure required for photography is no more than that needed to slightly flatten the cornea against the applanator surface. Contact microscopes help minimize the normal movements of the eye. Appropriate cleaning and disinfecting procedures should be followed between patients.

Noncontact microscopes may be extremely useful when direct contact with the patient's cornea is contraindicated.

The newer digital endothelial microscopes are of the noncontact type, and are easier to use than the older film-based contact models, which required touching the cornea. A digital display shows a sample image of the cells, from which the count can be made to determine cell density (see Figure 41.2).

Diagnostic ultrasound

Ultrasound is an indispensable tool in medical imaging
and plays an important role in ophthalmologic diagnoses.
It is the most important imaging technique in eyes with
anterior segment opacities. This chapter discusses the basic
techniques of ultrasound examination and the technique
of ultrasound biomicroscopy, which uses higher-frequency
ultrasound to produce images of much higher resolution.

GENERAL CONSIDERATIONS AND CONVENTIONAL ULTRASOUND DIAGNOSES

Theoretic considerations

Mechanical waves and vibrations occur over a wide range of
frequencies called the acoustic spectrum. This spectrum
extends from the audible range (10–20,000 Hz), with
which we are all familiar, to the range of phonons
(>1012 Hz) that comprise the vibrational states of matter.

The frequency most commonly used in ocular imaging is
10 MHz. Higher-frequency ultrasound provides higher resolution of the order of 20 to 40 μm, but the penalty to be
paid is loss of penetration. All human tissues exhibit
ultrasound attenuation coefficients that increase with frequency. The maximum penetration that can be achieved

for a 10 MHz system is approximately 50 mm. For a
60 MHz system, penetration is only 5 mm.

Electrical impulses are converted to sound by a vibrating
crystal (transducer). These sound waves are propagated
through tissue at various speeds and are reflected or scattered from interfaces between tissues of different acoustic
impedance (a property related to the density of the tissue
and the speed at which sound passes through it). After
emitting a pulse, the transducer "waits" for the reflected
waves to return, strike the quartz crystal, and initiate the
reverse process. The electrical impulses thus produced are
electronically amplified and modified to produce the
familiar A-scan and B-scan displays.

Two common types of ultrasound displays are used: the
A-scan and the B-scan. The A-scan is a single linear image.
The longer an impulse takes to return, the farther it is
placed on the display. This time can be converted to distance if one knows the speed of sound in the tissue through
which the sound is traveling. Each tissue has a characteristic
speed at which the sound travels through it. The longer it
takes to return, the farther away is the structure that
reflected the sound. Figure 42.1 shows a typical A-scan of
the globe. The height of the spike on the graph relates to
the intensity of the returned echo.

A B-scan is produced by a moving transducer. At each
point along the path of transducer movement, a pulse is
sent out and received. The intensity of the returning sound
is represented on the screen as brightness instead of height
on a graph. This series of lines produces a two-dimensional
cross-sectional representation of the object being imaged
(Figure 42.2). This type of display is easier to interpret than
an A-scan and is used for most diagnostic work, such as
determining the state of the retina behind an opaque cataract or imaging intraocular tumors.

between the lens echo and the echo from the retina. Artifacts can occur, but the presence of any persistent echo in this region should alert the operator to the need for further assessment before surgery. A B-scan examination is indicated in any eye in which the posterior pole cannot be visualized.

Intraocular disease

Some typical ocular problems that can be diagnosed on B-scan examination are discussed in the following text. It is important to remember that ultrasound is a nonspecific examination technique and can be used on any problem within the penetration range of the instrument.

Retinal detachment

Frequently a major diagnostic question in an eye that we cannot see into is whether the retina is detached. The typical B-scan appearance of retinal detachment is that of a funnel-shaped, highly reflective membrane that inserts into the optic nerve. Figure 42.5 shows the V-shaped membrane inserting into the low reflective optic nerve. Detachments can be incomplete, but they always insert into the nerve.

Choroidal detachment

Choroidal detachments have a different appearance on ultrasound. Because the choroid is tethered to the sclera at the exit of the vortex veins, choroidal detachments appear as smooth elevations that insert into the globe at a short distance from the optic nerve (Figure 42.6).

Intraocular tumors

Ultrasound is an indispensable tool for the diagnosis and follow-up of intraocular tumors. Differential diagnosis is performed by reference to the shape of the tumor and the pattern of intratumor reflectivity, which can vary

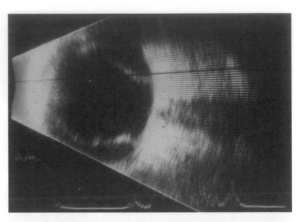

Figure 42.6 Choroidal detachment. The detached choroid inserts into the posterior pole some distance away from the optic nerve.

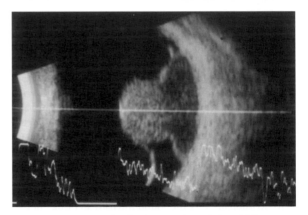

Figure 42.7 B-scan of collar button-shaped choroidal melanoma.

depending on the internal structure of the tumor. Melanomas are the most common primary intraocular tumors. They are generally dome-shaped or collar button (mushroom)-shaped (Figure 42.7) and have a medium to low internal reflectivity. The collar button shape occurs when the tumor breaks through Bruch's membrane, a dense barrier at the surface of the choroid.

Treatment of melanomas is based on the height obtained on ultrasound, and follow-up to determine growth is very important. Measurement is generally done by imaging the greatest height of the tumor with B-scan, freezing the image, and using the vector A-scan to do the actual measurement (Figure 42.8).

Anterior segment tumors

Anterior segment problems are best imaged using a mini water bath technique with a biometry eyecup filled with

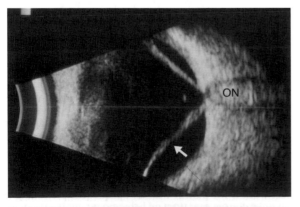

Figure 42.5 A complete retinal detachment. B-scan shows a V-shaped membrane inserting into the optic nerve (ON).

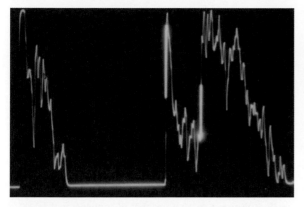

Figure 42.8 An A-scan of a melanoma showing medium to low reflectivity. The electronic gates are used to measure the height of the tumor.

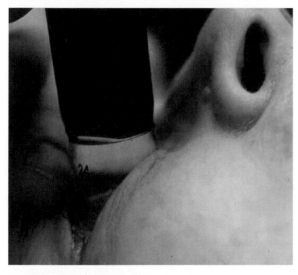

Figure 42.9 A mini water bath using a biometry eyecup to examine the anterior segment.

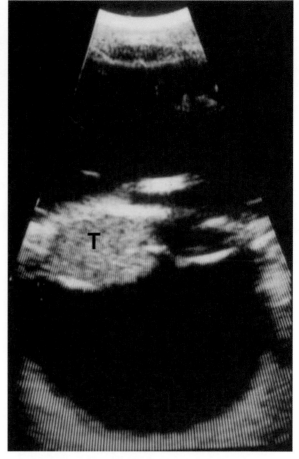

Figure 42.10 A ciliary body tumor (T) examined in a water bath.

ULTRASOUND BIOMICROSCOPY

There are limitations to conventional ultrasound, particularly in terms of resolution. In our attempts to gain a greater understanding of the mechanisms of ocular disease, we have a never-ending need for higher resolution. In the same way that optical microscopy has allowed improved understanding of basic processes, improved imaging resolution allows us to see and understand that which has not been seen before. The basic physics and techniques of using higher-frequency ultrasound to image living structures were developed at the University of Toronto in the laboratories of Stuart Foster. We subsequently applied these techniques to ocular imaging and named this process ultrasound biomicroscopy (UBM), that is, the imaging of living structures at microscopic resolution. The ability to see below the surface at microscopic resolution has allowed improved diagnoses and clarified mechanisms of ocular disease that had previously only been speculated upon.

methylcellulose (Figure 42.9). An anterior segment tumor such as a ciliary body melanoma can then be imaged (Figure 42.10) and measurement performed in the reverse direction, from the sclera in.

Orbital ultrasound

Ultrasound can penetrate most of the orbit and image problems such as tumors behind the eye. There are limitations, because ultrasound cannot penetrate the bony walls of the orbit and imaging is difficult at the orbital apex. Computed tomography (CT) scans and magnetic resonance imaging (MRI) are generally more commonly used for orbital imaging.

The method uses very-high-frequency ultrasound in the range 20 to 100 MHz. Resolution exceeds that of conventional ultrasound by a factor of up to 10. The price to be paid is penetration; this is limited to 5 to 6 mm depending on the tissue one is examining. In the laboratory we use instruments with frequencies between 40 and 100 MHz. The commercial instrument we most commonly use has a 50 MHz transducer, which is a good compromise between resolution and penetration. Various instruments are available with frequencies between 20 and 50 MHz.

Technique

The technique of eye examination using UBM is similar to conventional B-scan examination of the anterior segment. A fluid immersion technique is required to provide an adequate stand-off from the structures being examined. This is necessary to avoid distortion of the image close to the transducer and to prevent contact of the transducer and the eye. We have designed eyecups that hold the eyelids open and allow more rapid patient preparation (Figure 42.11). These eyecups resemble those used in conventional ultrasound biometry, with a lip that slides under the eyelids and holds the cup in place. They differ from biometry eyecups in being shallower and having a distinct flare that allows a good view of precisely where the scanning head is being placed; 1% methylcellulose is used as a coupling medium.

Unlike a conventional 10 MHz B-scan, high-frequency transducers are generally not covered by a membrane, which would provide excessive sound attenuation and defeat the purpose of doing examinations at this frequency.

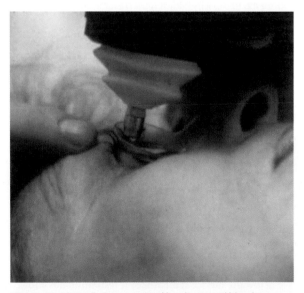

Figure 42.11 Eye being examined by ultrasound biomicroscopy (UBM) using a flared cup filled with methylcellulose.

Because the transducer is moving, contact with the eye and resulting corneal abrasion must be carefully avoided.

Any part of the eye that can be approached directly over the surface can be examined. The cornea and anterior segment structures are easily examined in any meridian. The conjunctiva, underlying sclera, and peripheral retina can be examined by rotating the eye as far as possible away from the region being examined. Any adnexal structures that can have their surfaces exposed can be examined.

Measuring ocular structures

Measurement accuracy is improved by UBM, which has an axial resolution 5 to 10 times that of conventional 10 MHz ultrasound. Measuring a structure accurately with ultrasound requires knowledge of the speed of sound in the structure being examined. We have used a speed of sound of 1540 m/s to make the majority of measurements. This speed is used in conventional ultrasound scanning to measure distances in most tissue.

Ultrasound biomicroscopy in ocular disease

Because UBM is a nonspecific imaging tool, it is suitable for examination of a large range of diseases that fall within the penetration limits of this technique. It is particularly useful in those conditions in which structural abnormalities are present, that is, those conditions that produce rearrangement of normal anatomy.

Glaucoma

Several types of glaucoma are caused by structural abnormalities of the anterior segment of the globe. This is particularly true of angle-closure glaucoma and infantile glaucoma. The ability of UBM to image structural abnormalities on a much finer scale than previously provides us with a quantitative new tool for research and clinical assessment of glaucomatous disease.

Pupillary block

In pupillary block the iris assumes a convex profile as a result of the pressure differential between the posterior and anterior chambers (Figure 42.12). Following iridotomy the profile changes to a much straighter configuration. Of interest is the fact that the degree of iris–lens contact is relatively small in pupillary block, as the iris is lifted off the lens. The block is thus not related to the area of contact. The area of iris–lens contact becomes even smaller when the pupil dilates. Anatomic angle closure in the dark in pupillary block occurs rapidly and relates to increased iris thickness and increased anterior bowing as the iris tip moves toward the iris root. A dark room provocative test

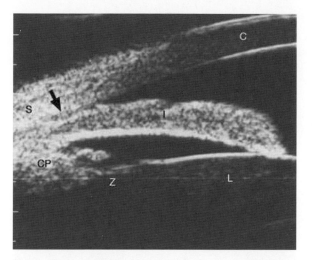

Figure 42.12 In pupillary block the iris shows anterior bowing narrowing the angle *(arrow)* and a small iris lens contact. *C,* Cornea; *CP,* ciliary processes; *I,* iris; *L,* lens; *S,* sclera; *Z,* zonule.

can be done using UBM, which detects whether appositional angle closure occurs in the dark.

A very common case for referral for UBM is the patient in whom the angle does not open completely after iridotomy. The usual cause for this is an imperforate iridotomy, anterior synechiae, or plateau iris.

Anterior synechiae

Angle closure by synechiae is illustrated in Figure 42.13. Here the iris takes an angular form as opposed to the smooth curve of pupillary block. The state of the angle behind synechiae can be defined by UBM.

Plateau iris syndrome

UBM has been used to elucidate the etiology of *plateau iris syndrome.* In this syndrome the ciliary processes are anatomically anteriorly located, closing the ciliary sulcus and providing structural support behind the peripheral iris (Figure 42.14). This prevents this portion of the iris from falling away from the trabecular meshwork following iridotomy. In studies of plateau iris in the dark and after pilocarpine administration, we demonstrated that the distance between the ciliary processes and trabecular meshwork remained constant, the only variable contributing to angle narrowing being iris thickness. We have shown that the axial anterior chamber is shallower in plateau iris than in pupillary block. The false sense of a deeper chamber likely relates to the deeper peripheral chamber that occurs when the iris flattens following iridotomy. Pupillary block and plateau iris frequently coexist.

Supraciliary effusions and malignant glaucoma

Supraciliary effusions that cannot be detected by conventional ultrasound can be imaged by UBM. These effusions occur in a variety of conditions including inflammatory disease, vein occlusions, and following retinal detachment surgery. Supraciliary effusions produce rotation of the ciliary processes and iris around the scleral spur. This can result in angle closure, particularly if the angle is narrow to begin with. We have found that most cases of malignant glaucoma have supraciliary effusions and anteriorly rotated ciliary processes (Figure 42.15). It is likely that effusions play a major role in the clinical manifestation of this condition.

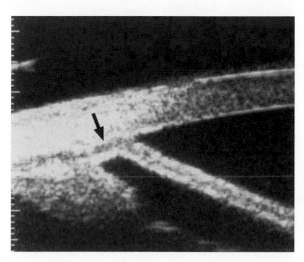

Figure 42.13 Anterior synechiae show an angled appearance of the iris with attachment to the trabecular meshwork *(arrow).*

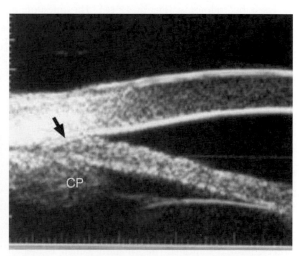

Figure 42.14 In plateau iris the ciliary processes *(CP)* are forward, supporting the peripheral iris and producing peripheral angle narrowing *(arrow).*

669

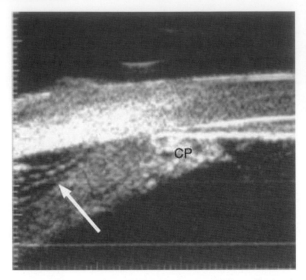

Figure 42.15 In malignant glaucoma, a supraciliary effusion is present *(arrow)* with anterior rotation of the ciliary processes *(CP)* and iris.

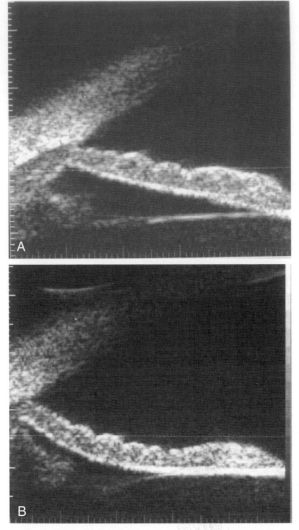

Figure 42.16 Pigment dispersion. (A) The iris profile is straight on distance fixation. (B) The iris bows backward on near fixation.

Pigmentary dispersion

Pigmentary dispersion syndrome is characterized by loss of pigment from the pigment epithelial layer of the iris and subsequent pigment deposition in the trabecular meshwork leading to glaucoma. The concept of reverse pupillary block implies temporary reversal of the pressure differential in the anterior and posterior chambers, producing posterior bowing of the iris, which leads to iris–zonule contact with mechanical pigment loss. UBM has shown that accommodation produces posterior iris bowing, which is reversed by iridotomy (Figure 42.16). The question of whether an iridotomy is indicated in this condition has not been answered clearly, but it is probably not indicated in older patients with diminished accommodation.

Anterior segment tumors

Iris and ciliary body tumors

UBM is a very useful adjunct in the management of anterior segment tumors. It provides a clear image of even the smallest anterior segment lesions (Figure 42.17). The ability to measure these lesions accurately adds the dimension of depth to our criteria for demonstrating growth. The ability to determine the underlying structure of the tumor allows improved classification and the ability to determine ciliary body involvement. When observation is elected, lesions may be followed with greater precision. Where surgical intervention is indicated, information gained is helpful in planning the approach.

It is difficult to be too specific as to histologic diagnosis with ultrasound, even with the added detail presented by UBM. Resolution is not at the level that can differentiate individual cells.

Cysts

Cysts are clearly imaged by UBM. The usual clinical presentation of an iridociliary cyst is an elevation of the peripheral iris without iris involvement. The typical ultrasound biomicroscopic appearance of a thin-walled cyst with no internal reflectivity (Figure 42.18) is diagnostic and essentially eliminates any question over whether a lesion is a cyst or a solid tumor. Small cysts also are found occasionally, either as an isolated finding on examination for some other clinical indication or in association with solid lesions of the iris or ciliary body.

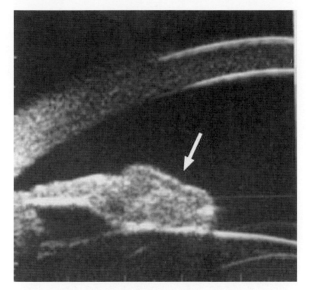

Figure 42.17 Tumor of the iris *(arrow)* in radial section. Tumor thickness can be measured and followed.

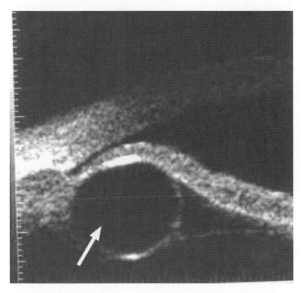

Figure 42.18 Iridociliary cyst *(arrow)* produces peripheral iris elevation.

The zonule

The anterior zonule can be imaged clearly with UBM. We are frequently asked to determine the state of the zonule in various disease and traumatic conditions before cataract surgery. The absence or irregularity of the zonule can generally be determined and the clock hours involved reported.

Corneal and scleral disease

UBM can be helpful in patients with opaque corneas before transplantation. Anterior segment details such as the depth of the anterior chamber, state of the angle, presence of anterior synechiae, and intraocular lens positioning can be determined preoperatively. Intracorneal abnormalities also can be imaged. Corneal edema can be assessed and measured. An arc scanner has been developed that uses a transducer path that follows the corneal curvature, allowing imaging of the entire cornea in one sweep. This instrumentation has allowed construction of three-dimensional depth maps of corneal thickness, epithelial thickness, and depth of intracorneal incisions in refractive surgery. UBM is also useful in scleritis, allowing both differentiation between extrascleral and intrascleral disease and assessment of the degree of scleral thinning.

Intraocular lens complications

UBM can easily assess the position of intraocular lens haptics (Figure 42.19). This is very useful in assessing malpositioned lenses, assessing the source of intraocular bleeding, and determining haptic freedom if removal or repositioning is required.

Hypotony and trauma

UBM can image cyclodialysis clefts even when the anterior chamber is shallow and the cyclodialysis cleft is not obvious with gonioscopy. There are always 360 degrees of supraciliary fluid present in these cases. The region of the cleft is usually obvious from the displacement of the iris root from the scleral spur. Other causes of hypotony in which UBM can provide useful information include occult wound leaks and ciliary body membranes. In other

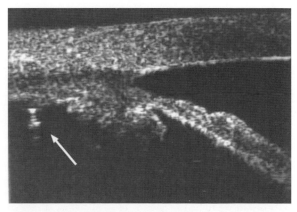

Figure 42.19 IOL haptic *(arrow)* over the pars plana.

trauma problems, UBM can image the state of the anterior chamber under traumatic opacities and detect small foreign bodies that are difficult to image using conventional techniques.

Conjunctival and adnexal disease

UBM can be used with any lesion that can be approached over the surface. It can provide valuable information in the differential diagnoses of tumors, aid in judging the depth of conjunctival and limbal lesions, and allow imaging of intracanalicular conditions. Recently we have imaged malpositioned punctal plugs in the canaliculus.

Future directions

UBM presents us with a new method of imaging the anterior segment of the eye at high resolution. Its strengths lie in its ability to produce cross-sections of the living eye at microscopic resolution without violating the integrity of the globe. Although histologic assessment of various disease types is sometimes available from pathology specimens, this usually occurs at a late stage in the disease and is susceptible to the inevitable distortions of the preparation process. UBM, though lacking the resolution of optical microscopy, gives us images in living eyes without affecting the internal relationships of the structures imaged. This method has proven valuable in both clinical practice and ophthalmic research. New methods of using high-frequency ultrasound are in development, including three-dimensional imaging, Doppler, and the use of contrast agents. These developments should extend the use of this technique to new areas.

ACKNOWLEDGMENT

The editors would like to acknowledge the contribution to the chapter in previous editions from Charles J. Pavlin (now deceased).

FURTHER READING

Pavlin CJ, Foster FS. Plateau iris syndrome: changes in angle opening associated with dark, light and pilocarpine administration. Am J Ophthalmol 1999;128:288–91.

Pavlin CJ, Harasiewicz K, Foster FS. An ultrasound biomicroscopic dark-room provocative test. Ophthalmic Surg 1995;26:253–5.

Pavlin CJ, Macken P, Trope GE, et al. Accommodation and iridotomy in the pigment dispersion syndrome. Ophthalmic Surg Lasers 1996;27:113–20.

Pavlin CJ, Rutnin SS, Devenyi R, et al. Supraciliary effusions and ciliary body thickening after scleral buckling procedures. Ophthalmology 1997;104:433–8.

Chapter 43

Ocular motility, binocular vision, and strabismus

Ocular motility refers to the movements of the eye in all directions of gaze and to its relationship in movement with its fellow eye. Strabismus is failure of the eyes to spontaneously direct their gaze at the same object because of muscular imbalance (such as crossed eyes). Orthoptics is a paramedical specialty that investigates the motor and sensory adaptations to strabismus and deals with nonsurgical treatments to help patients regain the ability to use both eyes together normally to obtain comfortable, binocular single vision. Orthoptics originates from the Greek words *orthos* (meaning "straight") and *ops* (meaning "eye").

In the investigation of strabismus, the orthoptist is required to assess the vision or fixation of each eye, the alignment of both eyes in all directions of gaze, and the ability of the two eyes to work together binocularly. Orthoptic therapy is directed toward the elimination of suppression and amblyopia and toward the correction of anomalies in binocular vision. Therapy includes prescription glasses, optical correction with prisms, eye exercises, patching, and sometimes the use of drugs that modify the focusing power of the eye. The work of the orthoptist is an adjunct to that of the ophthalmologist, not a substitute for it.

Because the brain controls visual sensation and ocular muscle coordination, orthoptic practice must involve a process of mental retraining. In terms of vision, the eye is not strengthened by the amblyopia therapy; rather, the brain becomes readapted so that it can accept, receive, and store all the visual imagery received by the eye. Because therapy is directed toward the higher centers of the brain controlling all visual responses, the child receiving orthoptic therapy must be alert, cooperative, and properly motivated. The age of the patient controls the approach the orthoptist takes and largely determines the success of the entire program. Younger children have visual patterns that are not well established. Therefore, abnormal patterns can be restored to normal by vigorous retraining. After the age of 6 or 7 years, the vision and ocular motor control and the reflexes governing these areas become more difficult to change. The older patient, being more mature, may be easier to work with, but established visual patterns are much more difficult to disrupt.

Ultimate responsibility for every stage in the treatment of all patients with strabismus rests with the ophthalmic surgeon. Orthoptic assessment and treatment are carried out by a well-trained orthoptist. An understanding of the techniques available is important to the ophthalmic assistant. Thus a brief outline of some of these tests is presented to familiarize the assistant with the more commonly used orthoptic instruments and methods.

EVALUATION OF STRABISMUS

History

When the history of a child with strabismus is documented, the following points should be noted:

- Age at onset and type of onset (rapid or slow)
- Whether the turn is intermittent or constant

- Whether one eye turns at all times, or whether either eye alternately turns
- Whether it is more apparent with close work or when looking in the distance
- Precipitating causes before onset of squint (illness, trauma, and so forth)
- Previous family history of strabismus
- Previous therapy for treatment of strabismus
- Birth history
- General health and past health

Vision testing

Vision is tested by using the conventional Snellen chart, the illiterate E chart, Landolt's broken-ring chart, the picture chart, the Allen cards, 'Sjögren's hands, and, more recently and effectively, the Sheridan-Gardiner (see Chapter 8). If the child is too young to be tested, some statement should be made of the child's fixation. This can be accomplished by means of the central, steady, and maintained classification. Central indicates that the corneal reflex is the same in both eyes; steady means that fixation is not wandering (common with amblyopia) and nystagmus is not present; and maintained denotes that fixation is sustained by a given eye either through a blink or through an induced smooth pursuit movement. This method for testing a young child can be accomplished by holding an interesting toy nearby.

The visual acuity of an infant is much poorer than that of an older child. The orderly improvement of visual acuity is greatest in the first few months of life. Normal adult vision (20/20) is achieved somewhere after 6 months of age, depending on the method of vision assessment. Vision tests based on preferential looking techniques, such as Teller acuity cards, are helpful in assessing vision in a clinical setting.

Hirschberg's test

Hirschberg's test is a rather gross method of determining the presence or absence of strabismus and its magnitude. The examiner shines a light in the child's eyes and notes the position of the reflex of light, which normally falls centrally on the cornea or on a slightly nasal spot off the center of the pupil of each eye. If this reflex is temporally placed in one eye and is normal in the other eye, the child obviously has an esotropia (Figure 43.1). Each millimeter of deviation from the normal position of the light reflex represents 7 degrees. To be displaced 3 mm from its normal position on the temporal side, the magnitude of the esotropia would be grossly judged at approximately 20 degrees. The corneal reflection test is not sensitive enough for the detection of small-angled strabismus. However, Hirschberg's test is commonly used as a preliminary assessment to determine the magnitude of deviation in an older child and may be the easiest method of assessing the amount of strabismus in an infant.

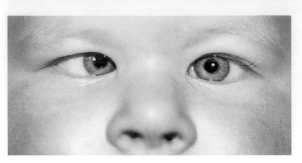

Figure 43.1 Essential infantile esotropia. Note the decentered position of the corneal reflex
(Reproduced from Kanski J. Clinical ophthalmology: a systematic approach. 5th ed. Burlington, MA: Butterworth-Heinemann; 2003.)

Krimsky's test

Another method for measuring angle of strabismus that is more accurate than Hirschberg's test is named after Krimsky, who first described it. This test is used on infants or those with deep amblyopia. Prisms are placed in front of the fixating eye to force it to move over. This draws the fellow (deviated) eye to a straighter position so that its corneal reflex is centered. The strength of the prism required to center the corneal reflection in the strabismic eye is equal to the amount of deviation present.

Cover test

The cover test is perhaps the one most widely used by ophthalmologists to detect and measure a strabismus angle. It is reliable, easy to perform, and requires no particular equipment. This test is conventionally performed at both distance and near, with and without glasses, the eyes being examined in the primary position. To ensure fixation in very young children, the fixation object should be an interesting and detailed article, such as a brightly colored toy or a toy with a squeaker. A flashing clown or dog in the distance is useful for fixation. A strabismus misalignment is called heterotropia or tropia.

Once the examiner is sure that the child is looking at the fixation object, an occluder is interposed in front of one eye. If the child has a strabismus of the right eye and the left eye is occluded, the following possibilities may ensue:

1. The right eye, which is deviating, may move horizontally (esotropia: moves from an inward position to take up fixation; exotropia: moves from an outward position to take up fixation) or vertically (hypertropia: moves from an upward position to pick up fixation; hypotropia: moves from a downward position to pick up fixation), indicating that the child has a manifest strabismus.
2. The right eye may wander, indicating that the fixation of the eye is defective or absent, as may occur with gross amblyopia.

3. There may be no movement of the right eye, indicating that this eye is straight. The procedure is then repeated, this time covering the right eye, without allowing the patient to become binocular during testing.

A manifest strabismus tropia is revealed by observation of any eye movements of the uncovered eye to take up fixation when the cover is placed before the fellow eye. In addition to the primary straight-ahead position of gaze, the cover test may be executed in each of the eight diagnostic positions of gaze.

On occasion, a child is referred who appears to have an ocular deviation but has no detectable strabismus. This condition is called pseudostrabismus. In most instances the appearance of a strabismus is caused by the presence of prominent epicanthal folds that extend from the upper lid, cover the inner canthal region, and blend into the medial aspect of the lower lid. The child's eyes commonly appear to be turned in because a minimal amount of the "'white of the eye"' shows medially and a normal amount laterally. This false impression of a turn inward (esotropia) is augmented when the child looks to either side. The adducting eye commonly slips under the epicanthal fold that bridges the corner of the eye. Parents, when commenting on this phenomenon, commonly state that the turn is so severe when the child is looking to the side that the eye almost disappears from view.

Pseudostrabismus can be differentiated from true strabismus by means of the cover test. With pseudostrabismus, neither eye has to move to pick up fixation with alternate occlusion if the eyes are straight. Once pseudostrabismus has been detected, the parents can be reassured that even the appearance of a turn will disappear with growth. This occurs because the growth of the root of the nose displaces these epicanthal folds medially and eventually eliminates them so that the amount of white of the eye visible on the medial aspect is in proportion to that found on the lateral aspect.

The measurement of the magnitude of a true strabismus is carried out by means of a prism (Figure 43.2) and an alternating cover test, whereby the cover is shifted back and forth between the two eyes. The apex of a prism is placed in the direction of the eye turn. The purpose of the prism is to displace the image of the object of regard onto the fovea of the turned eye so that, on alternating cover, there is no movement of either eye to take up fixation. Prisms of gradually increasing magnitude are introduced before one eye, the other being occluded. The magnitude of deviation with use of prisms is indicated by the prism that, when placed before a deviated eye, allows no movement of either eye with the alternating cover test. The patient must maintain fixation on a suitable accommodative target, such as a letter or number for an older child or an interesting toy for a young child. If the patient is too young to cooperate, the examiner must exercise ingenuity to attract the patient's attention and to maintain his or her interest on a particular fixation target.

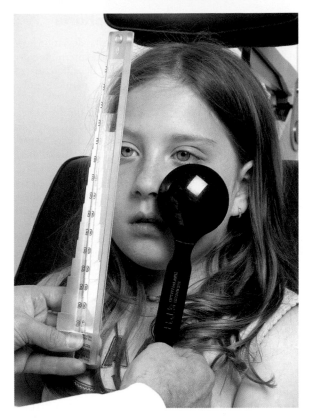

Figure 43.2 Measurement of degree of strabismus by a prism bar.

Eye rotations (versions)

Weakness of an extraocular muscle is detected by simple observation of the two eyes as they track together in the different directions of gaze. One looks for defects in ocular movement in one or both eyes. The positions of gaze that should be tested are along the horizontal and vertical meridians and the oblique positions between them. Versions are commonly designated dextroversion (right gaze), levoversion (left gaze), supraversion (straight-up gaze), and infraversion (straight-down gaze). The eyes also should be examined in the four oblique positions. Versions are binocular eye movements in which both eyes move in the same direction, such as both eyes moving into left gaze (levoversion) or both eyes into right gaze (dextroversion).

Vergence movements are also binocular movements in which both eyes move in opposite directions in an effort to attain and maintain fusion, such as convergence and divergence that are required when changing fixation distance.

Electrooculography assists in the understanding of the function of the eye muscles in normal and pathologic states. It can detect various types of nystagmus and can determine velocities of eye movements.

Measurement of a heterophoria

A heterophoria (or phoria) is a latent ocular deviation kept in check by the power of fusion and made intermittent by disrupting fusion. A heterophoria must be differentiated from a heterotropia, which is a constant manifest ocular deviation.

Heterophorias are classified in a fashion similar to heterotropias: esophoria is the tendency of the eyes to turn in; exophoria is the tendency of the eyes to turn out; hyperphoria is the tendency of one eye to turn up. Any of these conditions may occur normally when fusion is disrupted.

The prism and alternating cover test is the most useful test for measuring a phoria (as with a tropia). The Maddox rod (see following text) is sometimes used; however, it is not as accurate.

During cover–uncover testing, the clinician pays attention to movement of the fellow eye and, on alternate cover testing, to the movement of the eye at the moment it is being uncovered.

The cover disrupts fusion, and any latent tendency of the eye to turn is revealed by the deviation of the eye under cover. For example, if the eye moves from an inturned position outward to fixate when the cover is removed, then esophoria is present. The alternate cover test, combined with prisms, provides a measurement of the deviation.

The Maddox rod has a series of red cylinders that distort a point of light into a fine red band, thereby changing the size, shape, and color of an image before one eye. Thus, as the patient views a fixation light, one eye sees the light and the other sees a fine red line. Because these images cannot be fused, the eyes take up the fusion-free position.

The direction of the red line is perpendicular to the direction of the red cylinders. If the Maddox rod is held horizontally before one eye, the red line will appear either through the light (orthophoria) or to one side of the light (esophoria or exophoria). Measurement of the magnitude of the phoria is determined by the amount of prism required to displace the red line so that the patient sees it running through the muscle light. If the Maddox rod is held so that the red cylinders are running vertically, the red line will appear as a horizontal band either through the light (orthophoria), above it (hypophoria), or below it (hyperphoria). Again, prisms are used to measure the magnitude of the deviation.

The Maddox rod test can be used to measure the magnitude of both vertical and horizontal phorias at either distance or near.

Hess screen test, Lees screen test, and Lancaster screen test

The Hess, Lees, and Lancaster screen tests are similar in principle and purpose. The difference is in the type of screen used and the method of charting.

For the Hess and Lancaster screen tests, the patient wears red-and-green goggles. The patient is given a flashlight that projects a green light and the examiner holds a flashlight that projects a red light. In the Hess test, the examiner places his or her light at the indicated dots on the chart and the patient tries to place his or her light over that of the examiner. The patient fixates on the examiner's red light with the eye covered by the red lens and projects the green light in the direction toward which the eye under the green lens is pointing. If the eyes are not straight, the displacement of the green light in relation to the red light is a measure of the deviation (Figure 43.3).

The Lees screen test is plotted in the same way as the Hess; however, it is not as dissociating a test because the patient does not wear red-and-green glasses. The patient sits approximately 3 feet (1 m) away from two screens that are at right angles to one another. A two-sided mirror with an attached chin rest bisects the junction of the two screens. The patient is shown targets on one screen and asked to point with his or her light to localize the points on the second screen while looking into the mirror. The displacements of the patient's perceived points from their true locations are proportionate to the muscle imbalances.

The Lancaster screen test is similar to the Hess test except that the examiner usually begins at the zero position and then moves his or her light to the cardinal positions of gaze.

These tests are useful in the detection of paretic ocular muscle palsies and strabismus. They are based on the fact

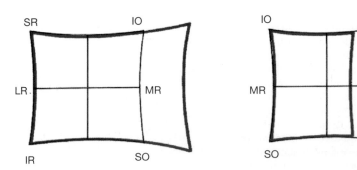

Figure 43.3 Hess chart of a recent right lateral rectus palsy. *IR, inferior rectus; IO, inferior oblique; LR, lateral rectus; MR, medial rectus; SO, superior oblique; SR, superior rectus.*

(Reproduced from Kanski J, Bowling B. Clinical ophthalmology. 7th ed. Philadelphia: Saunders; 2011.)

that foveae of straight eyes project to the same point in space. In patients with strabismus, the foveae do not project to the same point in space. The measurement of this difference is a measure of the deviation.

RETINAL CORRESPONDENCE

Normally, images from the foveae of the two eyes project in the same visual direction. This is known as normal retinal correspondence (NRC). Anomalous retinal correspondence (ARC) is another faulty sensory adaptation to a strabismus in which the fovea of one eye projects to the same point in space as an extrafoveal point on the retina of the other eye. Conversely, the definition may be stated as a condition in which the foveae of both eyes do not point in the same visual direction.

Anomalous retinal correspondence develops most commonly in relatively long-standing monocular strabismus. It is a sensory adjustment on the part of the turned eye. The fovea of the turned eye is suppressed to avoid confusion of images and diplopia, but a nonfoveal point on the retina takes up the function of the fovea so that its projection comes in line with the projection of the fovea of the other eye. In a sense, the patient does develop binocular vision, but of a gross form.

Worth four-dot test

The Worth four-dot test is a gross test to detect the presence of fusion or the suppression of one eye. It consists of an illuminated panel of lights in diamond formation. It is housed in a flashlight for near-vision testing and in a panel for distance testing. In this apparatus the two lateral lights are green, the upper one is red, and the lower one is white (Figure 43.4). The patient wears red-and-green glasses and is merely asked to note the number and color of the lights. The white light is usually described either as a combination of red and green in the presence of fusion or as changing from red to green. When one eye is definitely dominant, the light is either red or green, depending on the dominant eye. If the patient has single binocular vision, four lights will be seen: the red above, the two greens at the side, and a pale pink or green below, depending on which eye is dominant. If the patient has diplopia, five lights will be noted: three green and two red. If the patient is suppressing, only the colored lights observed by one eye will be seen, that is, either two red lights or three green lights. The patient may have one response for distance and an entirely different response for near.

Bagolini striated-glasses test

The Bagolini striated-glasses test is the least dissociative of the three most common tests for determining the presence of anomalous retinal correspondence. In this test, patients wear two lenses (one over each eye) with striations placed at 90-degree angles to each other. The responses are interpreted as follows.

Normal retinal correspondence exists if the patient has no manifest deviation on the cover test and sees a perfect cross.

Abnormal (anomalous) retinal correspondence exists if the patient has a manifest deviation on the cover test and sees a perfect cross. A streak with a gap indicates suppression with abnormal retinal correspondence. Two separate streaks (not in the form of a cross) indicate diplopia with normal retinal correspondence (see below).

Afterimage test (Figure 43.5)

In the afterimage test the patient fixates, with one eye occluded, for 10 seconds on a dot on a bulb containing an electrical filament. During this time the electrical

Figure 43.4 Worth four-dot test used to detect suppression and diplopia. *ARC*, abnormal retinal correspondence; *NRC*, normal retinal correspondence.

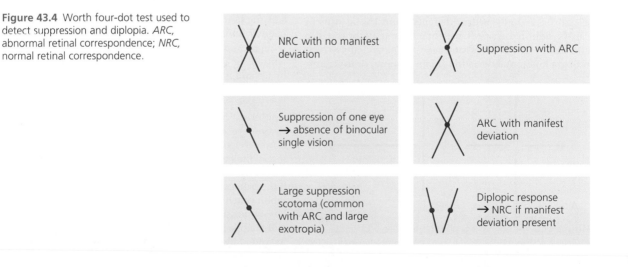

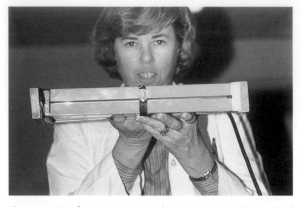

Figure 43.5 Afterimage test used to detect anomalous retinal correspondence.
(Reproduced from Kanski J. Clinical ophthalmology: a systematic approach. 5th ed. Oxford: Butterworth-Heinemann; 2003, with permission.)

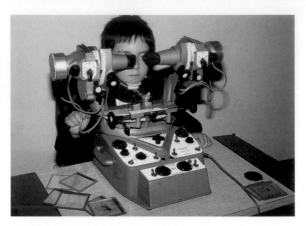

Figure 43.7 Using the major amblyoscope.
(Reproduced from Spalton D, Hitchings R, Hunter P. Atlas of clinical ophthalmology. 3rd ed. St Louis: Mosby; 2004, with permission.)

filament is held vertically and flashed. This imprints a vertical afterimage across the macula of the fixating eye. Then the eye is covered and a horizontal flash of light is presented to the fovea of the other eye. If the patient has normal retinal correspondence, the afterimages are seen as a perfect cross. If the patient has anomalous retinal correspondence, the position of the two bars will be displaced. For example, if the patient has a right esotropia and if the vertical bar is presented to the right eye and the horizontal bar to the left eye, the afterimage would consist of a vertical line to the left of the horizontal line (Figure 43.6).

Major amblyoscope

The major amblyoscope is a device for the measurement of strabismus and the assessment of binocular vision. In the past it was additionally used as a treatment for suppression and amblyopia (Figure 43.7).

The instrument itself has two viewing tubes so that each eye can be presented with a different picture. The instrument can be adjusted to each patient's interpupillary distance and chin level. The tubes can be moved horizontally to neutralize a horizontal deviation (main purpose) or to create a demand for convergence or divergence. They also can be moved vertically to neutralize a vertical deviation or to create a demand for a vertical vergence movement, or they can be displaced vertically. In addition, cyclotorsion can be measured subjectively. Each optical tube contains a slide carrier, a low-intensity light source for the illumination of the slides, and a high-intensity light source for creating afterimages. Some of the amblyoscopes also contain a device called Haidinger's brushes, which is used to test macular function and projection. A 6.50 diopter lens is placed in front of each tube to eliminate the accommodation required for viewing through a short tube that is only about 6 inches in length.

To assess the grades of binocular vision, disparate targets are presented to the eye.

Grade 1 binocular vision requires simultaneous perception (parafoveal, foveal, or macular slides may be used; this choice depends on visual acuity). Dissimilar targets, such as a lion and a cage, are presented to each eye. The patient who sees the lion in the cage is seeing with each eye simultaneously and has grade 1 binocular vision (Figure 43.8). If suppression is present, one image disappears intermittently. The "'jump'" is caused by the disappearance of an image and is therefore repetitious.

Grade 2 binocular vision requires fusional ability. Similar targets presented to each eye must be fused before a complete picture is identified. A grade 2 target may present to one eye a picture of a rabbit with no tail, clutching flowers (Figure 43.9); the other eye is presented with a picture of the same rabbit but it has a tail and held in its paw is a stem without flowers. Grade 2 binocular vision is present if the patient fuses these images and reports seeing a tailed rabbit clutching a group of flowers by a stem. If the patient has suppression, one of the controls (the tail or the flowers) will disappear. With grade 2 targets, fusional reserves can be measured by moving the arms of the instrument in or out

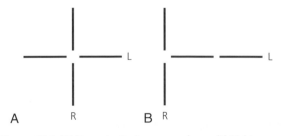

Figure 43.6 (A) Normal retinal correspondence. (B) Right esotropia with abnormal retinal correspondence (crossed images).

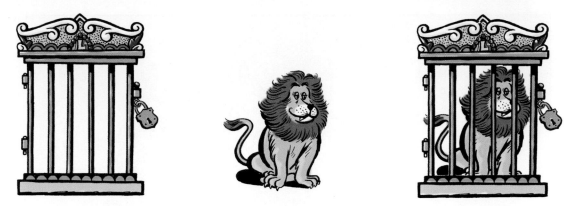

Figure 43.8 Grade 1 targets used for determining simultaneous macular perception. The targets are dissimilar and cannot be fused but the brain superimposes the images when the slides are brought together.

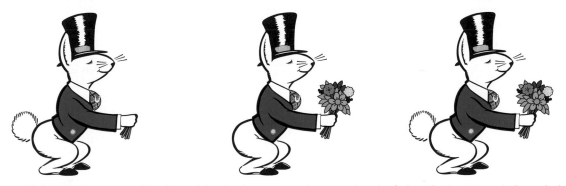

Figure 43.9 Grade 2 targets used for determining simultaneous macular perception plus fusion. The targets are similar and when fused present a complete picture.

(fusional convergence and divergence) until a point is reached where the patient complains of diplopia (sees two rabbits) or suppression (flowers or tail disappear) at the break point.

Grade 3 binocular vision requires the coordinated use of the two eyes together to yield the sensation of stereopsis (depth perception). Grade 3 slides present to the viewer pictures that are not quite superimposable. The fusion of these slightly disparate images by the brain creates the sensation of depth or stereopsis. If fused correctly, one of the seahorses will appear distinctly in front of the others (Figure 43.10).

Clinical measurements of strabismus using the major amblyoscope

The patient is placed before the amblyoscope, chin on the chin rest, which has been adjusted so that each eye looks straight through the lenses. All the readings on the amblyoscope are set at zero.

Consider a patient with a left esotropia. Grade 1 targets are placed in the tube; the patient is looking with one eye through the right tube and the left eye is turned in. The targets are presented alternately, first to one eye and then to the other. To take up fixation, the turned eye moves. The arms of the tube on the left side are moved in the direction of the deviation until no movement occurs on flashing. This measurement is called the objective measurement and corresponds to the amount of manifest deviation.

If the patient fuses images when the angle of strabismus is corrected, then the patient is said to have normal retinal correspondence. When abnormal retinal correspondence is present, the patient fuses even if the angle is only partially corrected (subjective angle). A difference between the two angles is referred to as the angle of anomaly. If this angle is the same as the objective measurement of the deviation, the abnormal retinal correspondence is called harmonious. If the angle is less than the objective measurement of the deviation, the retinal correspondence is called unharmonious.

Detection and treatment of suppression

Theoretically any child whose eyes are crossed and whose foveae are not pointed to the same position in space is expected to see double. The reason that children do not

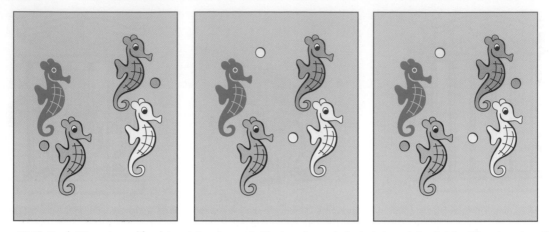

Figure 43.10 Grade 3 targets used for determining stereopsis. The targets are similar but viewed at a slightly different angle so that a sensation of depth occurs.
(Courtesy of M. Blair, American Orthoptic Council.)

see double or have diplopia awareness is that they are capable of suppressing an area of the retina to avoid double vision and confusion of images. It is the constant habit of continuous suppression that eventually leads to loss of binocular visual function and to strabismic amblyopia. In the past, antisuppression devices were used to make the patient aware of diplopia and to try to overcome suppression. Some examples of these devices (which no longer are in active use) are the stereoscope, the Tibbs binocular trainer, the amblyoscope, red-and-green glasses, and the reading bar.

AMBLYOPIA

Amblyopia is a term for loss of vision in one or both eyes in which no organic pathologic condition is seen in the eyes or optic nerves. The incidence is approximately 2.5% of the population. Vision is reduced in the affected eye to 6/12 (20/40) or worse.

Unilateral amblyopia is caused by conditions that affect vision in one eye only. The most common cause is a manifest strabismus of one eye, and suppression is often associated with it. Other causes include a significant refractive error of one eye and conditions of stimulus deprivation that block or blur images to the retina, such as ptosis, cataract, or corneal opacities. Thus unilateral amblyopia can occur in conditions other than strabismus, in which the eyes may be straight.

Bilateral amblyopia is caused by symmetric abnormalities of the two eyes, causing blurring of retinal images. These conditions include bilateral significant refractive errors and bilateral stimulus deprivation, such as in bilateral cataracts or corneal scars.

Amblyopia caused by refractive errors or strabismus usually responds well to treatment in children younger than the age of 6 or 7, after which the success rate declines with age. This interval of reversibility is known as the critical period. Although the critical period for reversing amblyopia caused by refractive error or strabismus is the first few years of life, such is not the case for stimulus-deprivation amblyopia caused by congenital cataracts or corneal scars. These disorders must be treated within the first few weeks of life or the visual deficits may be permanent and irreversible. Thus early detection and therapy are fundamental to the treatment of amblyopia.

The treatment of amblyopia depends on the cause. Any causes of stimulus deprivation such as cataracts must be removed and appropriate refractive correction instituted. Significant refractive errors in one or both eyes are corrected by glasses or contact lenses. A unilateral amblyopia caused by strabismus is treated by patching the sound eye to force the amblyopic eye to work harder for most of the child's waking hours.

The most common amblyopia therapy is occlusion of the good eye and use of the amblyopic, or lazy, eye. Occlusion, to be effective, needs to be maintained constantly during all waking hours until visual acuity is equal and voluntary alternation is attained.

Many types of occluders are available. The Elastoplast occluder is an extremely effective one that seals off the eye and prevents peeking in any direction (Figure 43.11). However, this type is uncomfortable in hot weather, often tends to slip off, and may cause contact dermatitis with prolonged wear. An alternative patch is Micropore tape and tissue. This tape is hypoallergenic, fully adhesive, and nonirritating to the skin during removal. The tissue is cut into the appropriate shape and size and is placed in the center of the tape and positioned over the eye. The Opticlude is

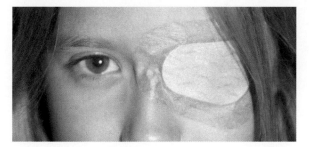

Figure 43.11 Elastoplast occluder.
(Reproduced from Spalton D, Hitchings R, Hunter P. Atlas of clinical ophthalmology. 3rd ed. St Louis: Mosby 2004; with permission.)

a hypoallergenic type of occluder patch. Another type is the rubber suction-cup occluder, which is applied to the posterior lens surface and totally occludes the eye because of a temporal extension that prevents peeking. Frosted lenses and clip-on occluders are not satisfactory because the patient tends to peek over, under, or around the occluder.

If the child is uncooperative and tears off patch after patch, occlusion can be provided by placing atropine ointment in the fixating eye. Atropine has the outstanding merit that, once instilled in the eye, the child cannot remove it. It can be extremely effective in a child who is hyperopic because the atropine paralyzes the child's ability to compensate for the hyperopia by eliminating accommodation. The atropine ointment is preferred because it is less apt to produce systemic reactions (fever and flushing) and is easier to instill.

Once the child has accepted the occlusion therapy and the performance of the amblyopic eye has improved to 20/25 or 20/30, occlusion of the dominant eye can be maintained by painting the front and back surfaces of the lens with two or three coats of clear nail polish. The only advantage of this method of occlusion is that it is less noticeable and psychologically easier for the patient to accept.

Children between the ages of 1 and 3 years respond quickly to occlusion therapy and are seen weekly to avoid occlusion amblyopia. Because conventional visual acuity tests cannot be performed on this age group, the child's response to occlusion therapy is estimated by his or her fixation pattern. With a successful result, the child should be able to maintain fixation on a target steadily and centrally with the affected eye. If no improvement occurs after 3 months, occlusion therapy is usually discontinued.

The older child, between the ages of 4 and 7 years, usually requires a much longer period of therapy to produce improvement in visual acuity. Although older children are more resistant to therapy, they are easier to work with because conventional vision tests can be used. If improvement in vision does not occur after 3 months of constant effort, amblyopia therapy is usually discontinued. Occlusion is maintained until the vision in the affected eye is brought up to 20/25 or 20/20 or until vision no longer improves. Then the daily hours of patching are tapered over several weeks as long as visual improvement is maintained.

The success of occlusion therapy often depends on the child's cooperation and enforcement of the regimen. Some parents become terrified at the thought of a patch on their child's good eye, believing that the child will become accident prone and be in physical danger. Parents should be reassured about such fears, because patching the good eye does not produce a blind child and accidents in the home as a result of patching are rare. Also some parents regard the patch as a stigma of weakness in their child and remove it when the child is playing with friends at school or is seen by adults. It is vital that the parents be informed about the principles of amblyopia therapy and the necessity for total occlusion. It should be impressed on them that neglect of total occlusion only prolongs the duration of amblyopia therapy and that failure to achieve significant gains in visual acuity by the age of 6 or 7 years usually results in a defective eye and an absence of stereopsis for the rest of the child's life.

With older children, amblyopia therapy can be enhanced by encouraging the child to engage in activities involving eye–hand coordination. Such home activities include tracing, coloring, cutting out patterns, threading beads, watching television, and putting models together. All these activities are performed, of course, with the use of the amblyopic eye. Visual games can be played in the automobile or while out walking by having the child attempt to read street signs, billboards, license plates, and so forth.

Before one discontinues any amblyopia program as a total failure, it is important to reassess, first, the method of occlusion (ensuring that the occluder completely covered the eye and prevented the dominant eye from being used) and, second, the duration of occlusion (ensuring that the supervision of the child was close and that occlusion was maintained fully). Finally, any child with amblyopia should be given the opportunity for a patching trial, even one who is older than 7 years of age. Some children will respond well beyond the age of 7 into the teenage years.

ECCENTRIC FIXATION

Eccentric fixation is the culmination of damaging sensory habits in strabismus, primarily suppression and amblyopia. With this condition, the vision loss in the affected eye is usually profound because an area other than the fovea is used for fixation. Visual acuity is often less than 20/200 and the patient is unable to gaze directly at an object when the sound eye is covered.

Eccentric fixation may be detected by the visuscope, combined with a reduction in visual acuity. An abnormal position on the corneal reflex may be a clue to eccentric fixation.

TREATMENT OF STRABISMUS

The first concern in treating strabismus is the elimination of any coexisting amblyopia. Some forms of strabismus can be corrected by improving the vision in the amblyopic eye inasmuch as the eye muscle control may improve at the same time. In addition, the eyes may straighten in some patients with strabismus who require glasses to correct vision or amblyopia.

Patients with well-controlled heterophorias or small heterotropias may need no treatment at all. Some forms of strabismus, such as nerve palsies, are temporary and will subside with time. Other forms, such as convergence problems that cause reading difficulties, will respond to orthoptic exercises.

Patients who have diplopia may experience relief of the double vision and regain fusion through the use of prisms. Both permanent and temporary types of prisms are available. Sometimes eyedrops that constrict the pupil (miotics) aid in straightening eyes with certain forms of esotropia.

If none of these treatments is indicated or is successful in straightening the eyes, then two options are available. One is eye muscle surgery, which involves the strengthening of weak eye muscles and weakening of overactive or tight muscles. In adults this can be performed by means of an adjustable suture technique whereby the alignment of the eye can be altered on the same day as the surgery while the patient is awake. The techniques of eye muscle surgery of young children are described in more detail in Chapter 31. The other option is the injection of botulinum toxin into eye muscles, which paralyzes them and straightens the eyes with certain forms of strabismus.

SUMMARY

The main function of an orthoptist is to evaluate muscle imbalances and to promote binocular cooperation between the patient's two eyes by a reeducation process. Orthoptics is not a cure for strabismus, but is an excellent adjunct in the preoperative and postoperative management of patients who can cooperate for the required procedures. Orthoptic training attempts to improve the quality of fusion and to break down faulty adaptive sensory habits of strabismus, such as suppression and abnormal retinal correspondences.

The role of the ophthalmic assistant is to assist either the ophthalmologist or the orthoptist in the practical diagnosis and therapy of strabismus. Participation by the ophthalmic assistant in orthoptics depends on the enthusiasm and knowledge of the assistant and the facilities available in a given office or clinic.

Questions for review and thought

1. Many patients, particularly infants, have facial features that make them appear to have strabismus although their eyes are orthophoric. What is this condition called?

2. When an eye truly deviates outward, what is it called?

3. If the eye has a tendency to turn in, the condition is called esophoria. What is it called when there is a tendency to turn up?

4. Vision is depressed in one eye and the eye obviously appears to turn in. However, when the fellow eye is covered, the eye does not take up fixation on a muscle light. What type of fixation is said to exist?

5. How does amblyopia come about? What are some of its causes?

6. The light reflex demonstrated by the Hirschberg test is centered on one pupil but falls to the outer portion of the cornea on the fellow eye in a given patient. What condition exists?

7. A patient complains of double vision. Outline a method of detecting which muscle or muscles are at fault.

8. Outline a method of measuring the amount of strabismus present in a patient.

9. The Worth four-dot test is used to detect suppression of one eye, the presence of fusion, or diplopia. How is this test performed?

10. Discuss the treatment of amblyopia.

Q   Self-evaluation questions

True–false statements

Directions: Indicate whether the statement is true **(T)** or false **(F)**.

1. The primary difference between the alternate cover test and the cover–uncover test is the use of prisms. **T** or **F**

2. Abnormal retinal correspondence is a monocular adaptation to strabismus. **T** or **F**

3. To neutralize an exodeviation with prisms, the base of the prism is held toward the nose. **T** or **F**

Q Continued

Missing words

Directions: Write in the missing word in the following sentences:

4. A term synonymous with binocular single vision is

_____.

5. An alternating deviation is usually indicative of _____ visual acuity.

6. _____ are conjugate eye movements and _____ are disconjugate eye movements.

Choice-completion questions

Directions: Select the one best answer in each case.

7. When performing the alternate cover test:
   a. use a light for fixation.
   b. allow the patient to be binocular.
   c. observe the occluded eye only.
   d. never have the patient wear his or her glasses.
   e. never allow the patient to be binocular.

8. When a constant monocular deviation is present, the patient:
   a. may have anisometropia.
   b. may have fusion ability.
   c. has a deviation that cannot be neutralized.
   d. never demonstrates suppression.
   e. has an esodeviation.

9. Strabismus:
   a. is only monocular in nature.
   b. has motor and sensory adaptations.
   c. is always present when the corneal reflexes are not properly positioned.
   d. indicates that visual acuity is always lower in both eyes.
   e. requires surgical correction.

10. The Worth four-dot test:
    a. is used to quantitate a deviation.
    b. is a test for color blindness.
    c. detects the presence and type of diplopia.
    d. detects the presence of amblyopia.
    e. is used to evaluate fusional amplitudes.

A Answers, notes, and explanations

1. **False.** The primary difference between the alternate cover test and the cover–uncover test is binocularity. During the alternate cover test, the patient is never allowed to become binocular. While the cover–uncover test is performed, the patient must be allowed to become binocular between the occlusion of each eye.

2. **False.** Abnormal retinal correspondence is a binocular adaptation to strabismus. By definition, it is an abnormal relationship that develops between retinal elements in each eye.

3. **True.** To neutralize an exodeviation with prisms, the base of the prism is held toward the nose. In an exodeviation the object of fixation stimulates the temporal retina and is therefore projected nasally. A prism displaces an image toward its apex. Therefore, when a prism is held base-in in front of an eye, the object of fixation appears to the temporal side and thus the deviation can be neutralized.

4. **Fusion.** Fusion is the unification of visual impressions by the brain into a single visual image, received as the result of stimulation of corresponding retinal elements.

5. **Equal.** An alternating deviation is a condition in which first one eye and then the other fixates. Both eyes are used, which assists in providing good visual acuity in both eyes. Monocular fixators develop amblyopia.

6. **Versions, vergences.** Versions are binocular eye movements in which both eyes move in the same direction, such as moving into left gaze (levoversion) or into right gaze (dextroversion).

   Vergence movements are also binocular movements in which both eyes move in opposite directions in an effort to attain and maintain fusion, such as convergence and divergence that are required when changing fixation distance.

7. **e. Never allow the patient to be binocular.** The alternate cover test is performed to provide an accurate determination of the amount of deviation present. One essential factor to eliminate is motor fusion. The motor fusion mechanism is sufficient to keep the eyes aligned. Therefore, the patient is constantly dissociated by occlusion and is never allowed to become binocular to eliminate any attempt to fuse.

8. **a. May have anisometropia.** Anisometropia is a condition in which the refractive error is unequal in the two eyes. Therefore, one eye perceives an image that is much clearer than the other eye, an obstacle to fusion. Anisometropia may be a precipitating factor in amblyopia and strabismus.

The imaging sensor and film

The digital imaging sensor has replaced film as the light-gathering component in digital photography. It comes in different sizes and types, but whereas the choice of film and developing combinations was vast and had to be established before the photograph was made, once a digital camera with a certain sensor is purchased the choices for photography are made using settings available on the camera. Choice of color balance, black-and-white imaging, and light sensitivity can be made at the camera. This is wildly different from the days of film that required stocking different film types to accommodate different lighting situations. Once a roll of film was placed in the camera, all the pictures taken on that roll of film had to be taken based on the characteristics of that film type. Now, with digital, each image taken can be set to entirely different settings, frame by frame if desired.

Focal length

The focal length of a lens is the distance between the lens and the film plane in the camera (measured from the principal plane of the lens when focused at infinity). The focal length, expressed in millimeters, is engraved on most lens systems along with the serial number and trade name. The normal, or standard, camera lens is that which will produce an image of a scene in the same perspective as that seen by the unaided eye. The normal focal length for a camera is roughly equivalent to the diagonal measurement of the image sensor. Different-sized cameras often have different-sized digital sensors, and consequently the lenses used have different magnification settings.

Most modern digital cameras still refer to their focal length in comparison to 35 mm film. For a 35 mm film camera (with a film image area measuring 24 × 36 mm), the standard lens is 50 mm in focal length and has approximately a 45- to 55-degree angle of view. A wide-angle lens, such as a 24 mm, has a short focal length and an angle of view of about 74 degrees. A telephoto lens, such as a 135 mm, has a long focal length and is restricted to an angle of 18 degrees. Digital cameras often refer to their image magnification size in relation to the 35 mm standard. For example, the typical digital SLR camera has an image sensor that is two-thirds the size of a 35 mm frame of film. Consequently, a 40 mm lens on a digital SLR is equivalent to a 60 mm lens on a film camera.

Lens speed

Lens "speed," or a lens's widest aperture, refers to the maximum light-gathering power of the lens. It is expressed in the form of an "f" number, which represents the ratio of the diameter of the lens to the focal length. Engraved on the lens system, it may appear as f2.5 or f1:2.5 (or merely 1:2.5) (Figure 44.1). The diameter of an f1 lens is equal to

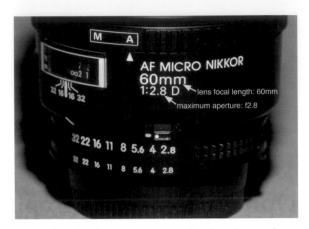

Figure 44.1 Autofocus Nikon lens, with a focal length of 60 mm and a maximum aperture of f2.8.

its focal length and it is termed a fast lens because it permits a great amount of light to reach the film. Such a lens is well suited for photography in available light. Most lenses have adjustable f-stops, operated by a diaphragm between lens elements.

Depth of field

The distance between the nearest and farthest objects from a camera that are acceptably sharp is called the depth of field. Depth of field is a function of focal length and lens aperture (or f-stop). It increases with the use of larger f-stops (smaller apertures) and decreases with smaller f-stops (larger apertures) (Figure 44.2). Depth of field is also greater for a wide-angle lens (short focal length) and less for a telephoto lens (long focal length) when both are set at the same f-stop. Depth of field is further affected by the camera-to-subject distance. The effective distance covered by the depth of field when a lens is focused at or near infinity is far greater than that of the same lens focused on a very near object. The closer a lens is focused, the more 'shallow' becomes the depth of field.

Because most photography in ophthalmology is done at high magnifications with a short distance between the camera and the subject, natural limitations in depth of field must be compensated for by using the highest possible f number (referred to as stopping down) and by using a light source that is sufficiently bright to provide the necessary exposure. The fundus camera, by design, has a single maximum aperture. Consequently, retinal photographs have a very shallow depth of field, and good focus can be difficult to achieve.

Resolution

Resolution, or resolving power, is the ability of a lens, film, digital imaging chip, or the eye to distinguish fine detail.

Figure 44.2 (A) The shallow depth of field with a lens set to its maximum aperture of f3.5. (B) The smaller aperture of f22 results in greater depth of field.

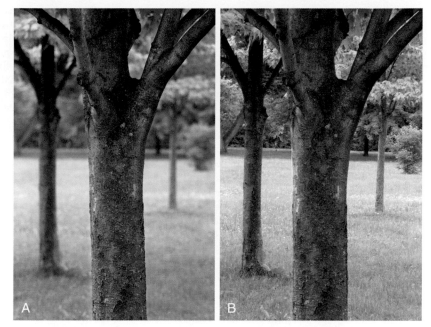

This resolving ability is measured by the highest number of line pairs per millimeter that are definable without blurring together.

Shutter speed

Shutter speed is measured by fractions of a second, indicated by numbers such as 30, 60, and 125, which stand for $1/30$, $1/60$, and $1/125$ of a second. These numbers represent the length of time the shutter is open when the shutter release is activated; the interval during which the light passing through the lens strikes the film. A slow shutter speed allows more light to pass to the image sensor than a faster shutter speed.

Setting

A specific area should be set aside for ophthalmic photography if possible. The photographic environment, including background and room lighting, can thus be better controlled, providing more consistent results. A degree of privacy, an important courtesy to the patient, also will be ensured.

Sensor sensitivity

The sensitivity of an imaging sensor refers to its sensitivity to light, expressed as ISO numbers, established by the International Organization Standards. A higher number indicates that the sensor is more sensitive or 'faster.' The sensitivity of a digital chip is established during its manufacture, and usually has a base sensitivity of 100 to 200 ISO. This number can be adjusted higher to optimize results in low light situations. Set to a low ISO number, an image sensor will produce less image noise and higher resolution than when it is set to a higher ISO number. The sharp detail offered by low ISO settings makes these valuable to scientific or diagnostic study, particularly when large prints are to be made. Color fundus photographs are normally taken with the camera set to 100 ISO. Because the exciter and barrier filters used in fluorescein angiography absorb a lot of light, the fundus camera software is set to a higher ISO setting (400–800 ISO) to compensate.

DIGITAL IMAGING

Digital imaging chips

The charged coupled device (CCD), complementary metal oxide semiconductor (CMOS), and Foveon chips are the three currently competing technologies within digital imaging. The CCD used in still photography was adopted from video technology and, with the benefit of considerable fine-tuning since the mid 1980's, has evolved into a high-quality imaging standard. CMOS is a more recent challenger. Although far less expensive to produce than a CCD, it initially suffered from poor contrast and image noise. These problems have been resolved and the CMOS chip is now used in most cameras. The Foveon chip promises even more resolution and detail, but has been slow to enter the market.

Whichever chip is used, it is located in the camera at the same plane normally occupied by the film emulsion, known as the "film plane." Working in conjunction with the chip's ISO sensitivity, the shutter speed and lens aperture are adjusted according to the prevailing light levels.

Much like the variety in film formats, the digital chip comes in many sizes. Because the chips are expensive to produce, the manufacturers have tried to reduce cost by keeping the chip size small. Most digital SLR cameras are currently equipped with chips that are two-thirds the size of 35 mm film. Consequently, images produced on these digital cameras appear magnified compared with the same image on film. Because most fundus cameras are designed for 35 mm film, either a reducing lens is placed between the fundus camera and the digital camera back or a more expensive, larger chip is used.

Color balance

Unlike film, which needs to be matched for correct color temperature (daylight or tungsten), digital cameras correct for proper color balance by adjusting what is known as 'white balance.' Although this white balance can be set to automatically correct itself, it is sometimes preferable to set it to match the specific type of lighting environment.

All lighting sources have a color temperature, which is expressed in degrees Kelvin (K). Normal daylight, around midday, has a color temperature of approximately 5400K. The light produced by an electronic flash has the same color temperature. Standard household lighting is often much warmer in color, and tungsten bulbs are approximately 3000K. Fluorescent lighting and halogens all have their own color temperature, some cooler, some warmer. Whereas the human eye and brain constantly adapt to correct for these color imbalances, the camera must be told to adjust. Otherwise, a color balance setting for outdoor lighting will have a blue cast if that setting is used with indoor tungsten lights. A tungsten color balance setting used outdoors will look orange. Fortunately, most digital cameras can automatically adjust for color balance changes by constantly monitoring lighting conditions and self-adjusting using the "auto white balance" (AWB) setting. However, it is sometimes good to manually make this setting, especially if complex lighting conditions cannot be established with AWB.

Digital imaging software

The image on a 35 mm slide may be viewed by just placing it in front of a light source, such as a light box. To observe a digital image the process is not as direct. Without a computer running compatible software, the image bits are meaningless. Imaging software is just as important as the hardware used to make it. With just basic software, one can look at a few images, but to manage thousands of images of hundreds of patients, a more sophisticated software program not only allows a more efficient review of these images, but also provides a system of image management that far exceeds the capabilities of film. There are a number of professional ophthalmic image and management programs available, and they all do a good job of taking, storing, and retrieving photographs.

Resolution

Among many other factors, the quality of a digital image is dependent on pixel resolution. The term *"pixels per inch"* (ppi) refers to the density of pixels in an image. *"Dots per inch"* (dpi) refers to the number of dots used by a printer to make a print based on the ppi of the image. Generally, the higher the dpi, the finer is the detail in a print. However, how the dots are managed is just as important. A dye sublimation printer may have a low dpi rating, such as 300, but it uses heat to increase the tonal range of a print. Inkjet and laser printers use various algorithms to enhance performance beyond their dpi rating.

Image resolution is affected by many factors, including lens quality and exposure setting. Whereas different films have different resolving powers, digital imaging resolution is largely determined by the density of pixels. High resolution begins with a large number of pixels on an imaging chip. However, the amount of resolution actually needed is relative to how the image is used. Smaller images require fewer pixels than larger ones. Images displayed on a computer monitor require fewer pixels per inch than those displayed as a print.

File formats

Numerous imaging file formats accommodate different uses of images. The two main categories are uncompressed and compressed. An uncompressed file saves one pixel for every pixel. A commonly used uncompressed format is tagged image file format (TIFF). Image compression can be either lossless or lossy. *Lossless* compression reduces the file size by generalizing areas of common data. For instance, a large area of 100% black is stored with a more efficient description than repeating every pixel as black. *Lossy* compression takes more liberties with describing the data, but also enables a more efficient storage and transporting of that data. Joint Photographic Experts Group (JPEG) is a common compression format that can be adjusted to various levels of compression. It is also widely recognized by most imaging programs and across Macintosh and Windows platforms, making it a format of choice when maximum versatility is required. Because there is some level of quality loss in JPEG, although slight to negligible at its "best" setting, it is best practice to work with an image in a lossless format until all corrections are made. As the final step, the image can be saved as a JPEG file.

Readjusting already JPEG'd images may introduce undesirable image artifact.

Many other file format types are available and are used by different camera manufacturers. It is important to know what these formats are to use these images outside that particular operating system.

Exposure

Exposure is the total volume of light that strikes the image sensor. It is the sum of light intensity and duration of exposure. Correct exposure is achieved through the balanced interaction of sensor, sensitivity, brightness of illumination, f-stop, and shutter speed.

With the use of available light, the shutter speed is used to control the duration of the exposure and the f-stop is used to regulate the intensity of the light striking the film. Each full f-stop setting (f8, f11, f16, and so on) and each shutter speed setting ($\frac{1}{30}$, $\frac{1}{60}$, $\frac{1}{125}$, and so forth) affects the total exposure by a factor of two. For example, if the camera were set at a correct exposure of $\frac{1}{60}$ of a second at f11 and then the lens were opened to f8, twice as much light would reach the sensor and the image would be overexposed. Conversely, if the lens aperture were closed down to f16, only half the needed light would reach the sensor, and the image would be underexposed. Likewise, if the f-stop remained constant and the shutter speed varied, the same alteration in total exposure would result. By decreasing the shutter speed from $\frac{1}{60}$ to $\frac{1}{30}$ of a second, the exposure is doubled; by increasing the shutter speed from $\frac{1}{60}$ of a second to $\frac{1}{125}$ of a second, the exposure is halved. Correct settings, therefore, are vital to correct exposure. If either f-stop or shutter speed is off by just one setting, a serious overexposure or underexposure may result on the sensor.

Exposure meters

Whenever a light source other than a flash is used, the correct exposure can be determined with the light meter, which is built in to most consumer digital cameras. For the best exposures, it is good to be familiar with how your camera's light meter reads the light in the viewfinder. If the light meter is allowed to respond to an area that is either much brighter or much darker than average, a proportionate underexposure or overexposure will result.

Flash illumination

With the use of electronic flash, the duration of the exposure is usually determined by the duration of the flash. Because most modern electronic flash units have a duration of approximately $\frac{1}{1000}$ of a second, the length of the exposure is $\frac{1}{1000}$ of a second. This very short, motion-stopping duration makes the electronic flash ideally suited for eye photography. Because the duration of the exposure is now essentially beyond our control, correct exposure is achieved by regulating the intensity of the light, either at its source or when it passes through the lens, or both. In most cases, the intensity of the flash source itself need not be altered. In fact, it is desirable to have ample light to guarantee a good exposure at very high f-stops, thereby ensuring the greatest possible depth of field at close working distances.

Electronic flash sources have different amounts of light output, and exposure is greatly determined by the flash's distance from the subject. The farther the flash is away from the subject, the darker it gets, so either the camera's lens aperture must be adjusted or its ISO must be set higher.

The camera's shutter speed also must be set at the speed prescribed by the manufacturer to provide proper synchronization (maximum light output coincident with a fully open shutter). Shutter speeds that are too slow may allow extraneous ambient light to affect the exposure. Shutter speeds that are set faster than the shutter's synchronization result in partial or no pictures (Figure 44.3).

EXTERNAL PHOTOGRAPHY

A digital single-lens reflex (D-SLR) camera with interchangeable lenses is recommended for external eye photography. The D-SLR feature permits viewing and photography through the same lens system. Composition and sharp focus are thus made much simpler because the image being photographed is seen in the viewfinder exactly as it will appear on the sensor.

To achieve the necessary magnification, a macro lens (specially designed to permit focusing on very near objects) is recommended. Macro lenses for D-SLR cameras are available from approximately 50 to 200 mm in focal length. The advantage of a longer (100 mm and greater) focal length macro lens is that it permits a greater working distance between camera and subject and produces less perspective distortion. A good, practical magnification-to-working distance ratio can be achieved with the use of a 100 mm lens. Photography of an intraoperative procedure may dictate the use of a longer focal length lens to provide a greater working distance-to-magnification ratio.

Using a D-SLR with interchangeable lenses, a good choice is a 100 mm macro lens. The longer focal length provides the close focusing capability and comfortable working distance away from the patient that is needed in ophthalmology.

A fixed (noninterchangeable) lens camera may provide adequate working distance and magnification, but not all cameras have this capability. Before purchasing a new digital camera with a fixed lens, determine that it can focus closely on a single eye and that the flash functions at close distances.

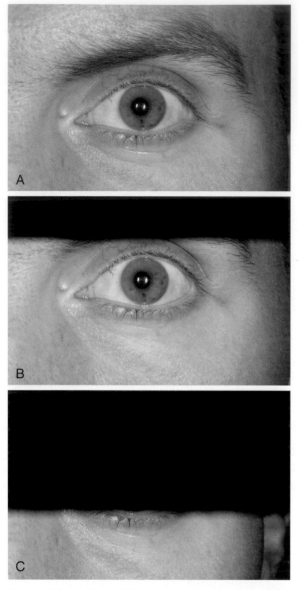

Figure 44.3 The Nikon D100 camera can synchronize with an electronic flash up to a shutter speed of $^1/_{80}$ second (A). Increasing the speed to $^1/_{250}$ second results in partial exposure (B) and even less at the faster speed of $^1/_{500}$ (C).

Illumination

For illuminating external photographs, an electronic flash device is recommended. Problems created by rapid eye movements or blinking are eliminated by the extremely short duration of the flash. Many inexpensive flash units with automatic exposure control are available, eliminating the need to change f-stops while providing the ability to alter the distance between camera and subject over a given

range. If such a flash is being contemplated, its ability to function in the automatic mode at such close distances must be ensured. Not all have that capability.

A flash source should always be positioned to provide even, diffuse illumination over the area being photographed. The bridge of the nose and prominent brows should not be allowed to cast a shadow onto the area of interest. When taking photographs of a single eye area, the light should be positioned on the patient's temporal side. For taking a two-eye view or full-face photograph, the light should be positioned directly above the lens. In some types of portrait photography, a ring flash is used to provide soft and even illumination. However, for close-ups of corneal pathology, the large ring of light reflex created by these flash units often obscures what is meant to be documented. The Nikon SB-29s (Figure 44.4) is a convenient lens-mounted flash that uses two smaller flash tubes rather than a single large ring of light. The unit is mounted directly to the front of the lens and can be rotated and variously controlled for satisfactory illumination. The resulting photograph will show uniform illumination over the subject area, with shadows falling directly behind and below the patient. The use of a lens of a 100 mm focal length considerably lessens the problems arising with the use of sharply oblique illumination, which results from working at too close a range to the subject.

A suitable background should be provided. A simple solution is to obtain several large (30×40 inches [0.75×1 m]) matte boards available in a variety of colors. In general, a medium blue works well for most subjects.

PHOTO SLIT-LAMP BIOMICROGRAPHY

Many conditions affecting the anterior segment of the eye—especially the transparent cornea, anterior chamber, and lens—are of such a subtle nature that they defy detection by any means other than slit-lamp biomicroscopy. Because the adverse conditions occurring in these transparent or translucent structures are themselves commonly transparent, conventional, diffuse illumination is unsuitable for their visualization. Only the specialized capabilities of the slit-beam illuminator and high magnification of the slit-lamp biomicroscope provide an adequate view of subtle changes of interest to the ophthalmologist.

Fundamental to producing consistently useful photo slit-lamp documentation is a thorough knowledge of the structures of the eye, the location and general appearance of the diverse conditions affecting the eye, and the basic forms of illumination and their application to these conditions. Basic illumination techniques include direct focal, tangential, direct, and indirect retroillumination from the iris; retroillumination from the fundus; transillumination; sclerotic scatter; proximal illumination; and Tyndall's phenomenon for aqueous cells and flare.

Figure 44.4 The Nikon SB-29s flash unit mounts directly onto the front of a camera lens. It has two flash units on either side of the lens that can be controlled independently, as well as rotated. The flash is well situated for good illumination at close working distances, and the unavoidable specular reflection from the cornea is much smaller than with a ringlight flash.

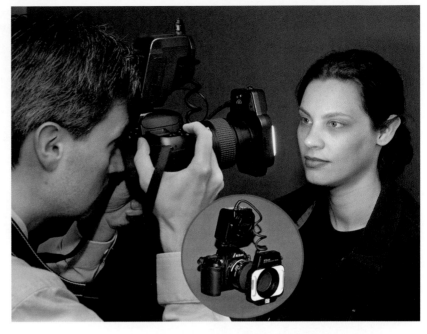

A slit-lamp biomicroscopic examination is a dynamic process. With the use of a narrow slit beam to provide optic sectioning, transparent structures, such as those in the cornea, can be examined in minute detail a small section at a time. The result is, in essence, a composite, mental image of the entire cornea. In slit-lamp photography, however, each photograph is restricted to a single moment of that examination. To overcome this limitation, some slit lamps are equipped with an additional diffuse illuminator. When used in conjunction with the slit illuminator, the result can be a pleasingly illuminated image of the overall eye with a superimposed narrow slit beam to provide specific information about that section of the structure that it isolates (Figure 44.5).

Whereas diffuse illumination causes some fine detail to become obscured through the scattering of light, it is useful to provide general, introductory photographs. With these as a basis, additional photographs can illuminate areas of more precise interest, further isolated through increased magnification. The result then is a series of images that leads the viewer through a logical progression from an overview to the subtlest detail. Figure 44.6 shows some of the forms of illumination, along with recommended exposures as used on the Zeiss Standard photo slit lamp. For other photo slit lamps, exposures should be established by exposing test films based on the manufacturer's recommendations.

Photo slit lamps may be film-based or digital. Desirable features include coaxial viewing (viewing and photography through the same lens system) and a flash source for both the slit and diffuse illuminators. Slit lamps not designed for

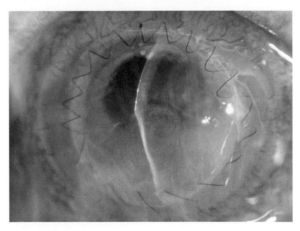

Figure 44.5 Slit-lamp photograph of a corneal ulcer shown in diffuse, overall illumination with a superimposed narrow slit beam to demonstrate inferior corneal thinning.
(From Mártonyi CL, Bahn CF, Meyer RF. Clinical slit lamp biomicroscopy and photo slit lamp biomicrography. Ann Arbor, MI: Time One Ink; 1985.)

photography may, on occasion, produce satisfactory photographs with the appropriate attachments. Of these attachments, electronic flash illumination is the most essential to provide the short exposures necessary to "freeze" eye movements. Additionally, when camera backs with auto exposure are used on slit lamps not equipped with electronic flash within the slit illuminator, the metering system responds to the lightest portion of the image and

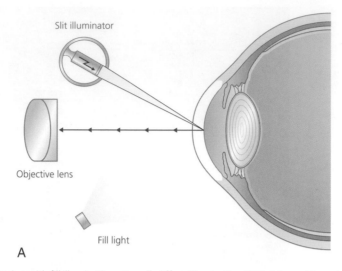

Slit illuminator

Objective lens

Fill light

A

Figure 44.6 (A) Optic sectioning with fill illumination. Overall, diffuse illumination (fill light) provides a view of the entire eye, and the superimposed direct focal illumination of the narrow slit beam provides specific information about the area that it isolates. Direct focal illumination in the form of a very narrow slit beam, without overall diffuse illumination, is the most selective, direct method of examining the structures of the eye.

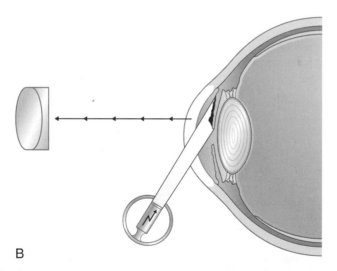

B

Figure 44.6 (B) Tangential illumination. A moderate to wide slit beam is projected onto the area of interest at a sharply oblique angle to produce clearly defined highlights and shadow areas, greatly enhancing topographic detail.

underexposes most areas of interest illuminated by indirect methods. Electronic flash also provides the correct color temperature of light for daylight film. (Most tungsten bulbs used in slit-lamp biomicroscopes do not produce the exact color temperature required by available films.) With a digital camera back, this limitation can be minimized by using the white balance control. Another important attachment for a nonphotographic slit lamp is a diffuse illuminator to provide the overviews mentioned earlier.

Beyond the mastery of the mechanics of a photo slit lamp, the diligent practice of slit-lamp biomicroscopy is important to gain experience in disease entity recognition and light source manipulation to achieve maximum detail enhancement.

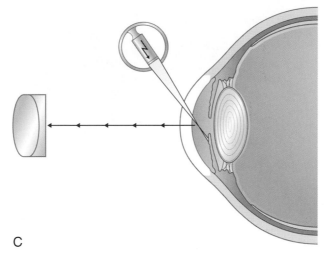

C

Figure 44.6 (C) Pinpoint illumination. Pinpoint illumination, based on Tyndall's phenomenon, is used to visualize and photograph aqueous cells and flare. The smallest circle beam is directed through the anterior chamber at an oblique angle. If the aqueous is turbid with cells and protein, the small cone of light will be visible to a variable degree depending on the amount of abnormal material it contains, demonstrating anywhere from "one" to "four plus" aqueous cells or flare.

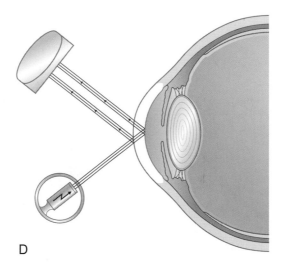

D

Figure 44.6 (D) Specular reflection. A moderate slit beam is projected onto the surface of interest (the corneal endothelial surface in this example) and viewed at an angle from the perpendicular that is equal to the angle of incidence. An area of nonreflectance from normally flat, reflective surfaces indicates an abnormality.

GONIOGRAPHY

Certain important structures of the anterior segment of the eye, such as the filtration angle, cannot be seen directly. To obtain a view of the angle, a gonioscope (contact lens, some types containing mirrors) is placed on the eye. With use of a moderate beam from the slit-lamp illuminator and the standard exposure for that slit width, excellent photographs are obtainable (Figure 44.7). Diffuse illumination is not used in goniography because of the increase in light scatter within the gonioscope.

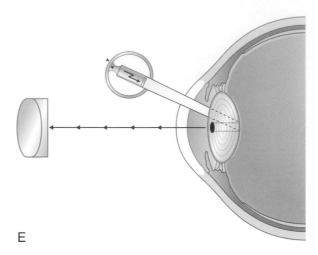

E

Figure 44.6 (E) Proximal illumination. A moderately narrow slit of light is directed to strike an area just adjacent to the area of interest. The light is absorbed by the surrounding tissue and scattered behind the abnormality, outlining it in relief against a now lighter background. This is an especially useful technique for delineating the general size and shape of an opaque object obscured by overlying soft tissue (such as an imbedded foreign body).

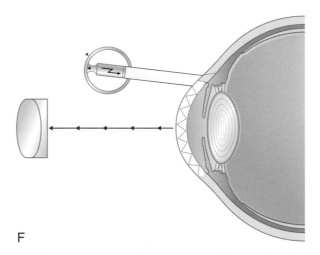

F

Figure 44.6 (F) Sclerotic scatter. A wide slit beam is directed to strike the limbal area where the light is absorbed and "piped" throughout the cornea. When corneal changes are present, they become visible by reflecting a small portion of the light passing through the cornea.

Before the placement of the lens on the eye, a topical application of proparacaine hydrochloride 0.5% is used to anesthetize the corneal surface. The concave, contact end of the lens is filled with a viscous solution of methylcellulose to provide the necessary optical medium and a cushion between the lens and the eye.

Once on the eye, the lens is rotated to place the desired mirror opposite the area to be viewed and photographed (see Figure 44.6K). (Goldmann and Haag-Streit lenses are available with three mirrors set at varying angles to facilitate a view of the angle, anterior vitreous, and retina.) Care should be taken to position the lens to eliminate reflections from its flat, anterior surface. A three-mirror Haag-Streit lens with a special antireflection coating (similar to coatings on photographic lenses) is available from Ocular Instruments Inc., Redmond, Washington.

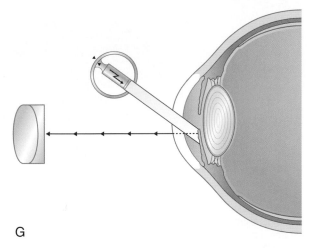

G

Figure 44.6 (G) Direct retroillumination from the iris. A moderate slit beam is directed onto the iris surface behind the corneal abnormality. (The slit beam must not strike the corneal changes directly.) The corneal abnormality is then examined or photographed in silhouette against the light background of the illuminated iris. The slit illuminator is rotated from its normally isocentric position to permit centration of the principal subject area in the final photograph.

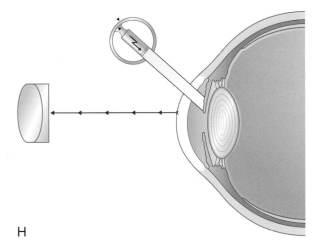

H

Figure 44.6 (H) Indirect retroillumination from the iris. A moderate slit beam is directed to strike the iris just adjacent to the area that lies directly behind the corneal abnormality. The light striking the iris is reflected in all directions and the subtle corneal changes can be seen, diffusely retroilluminated, against the dark background of the unilluminated iris and even darker pupil. The most useful zone of information is often at the interface of light and dark backgrounds at the pupillary margin. The slit illuminator is rotated from its normally isocentric position to permit centration of the principal subject area.

This coating, as on photographic lenses, permits a more efficient passage of light and contributes to the quality of the photographs.

Another type of goniolens, the Koeppe, not containing mirrors, is ideal for examining or photographing patients in the supine position, or children under anesthesia. In this case a handheld fundus camera, such as a Kowa, is used instead of the slit lamp and produces excellent results.

When desired, slit-lamp photographs of the fundus can be obtained through the center of the Goldmann type of contact lenses (Figures 44.8 and 44.9). The slit-lamp illuminator must be placed in a fairly coaxial position with the

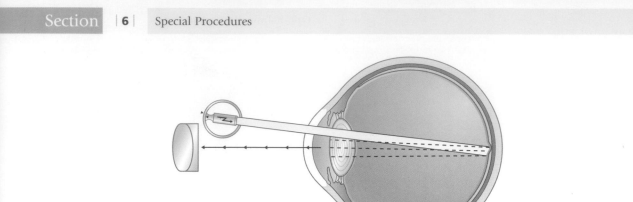

I

Figure 44.6 (I) Retroillumination from the fundus. A moderate slit beam is projected through the dilated pupil to strike the fundus in an area behind the abnormality to be examined or photographed. The slit illuminator must be brought into a nearly coaxial position with the biomicroscope and the slit beam decentered to enter at the pupillary margin. Through careful positioning of the slit illuminator and the slit beam in the pupillary area, the red reflex can be seen, against which subtle corneal and lenticular changes are outlined. Considerably greater levels of illumination may be achieved by rotating the subject eye to position the optic nerve head to provide a much brighter background. This is an especially useful technique in photographing patients with dark fundi.

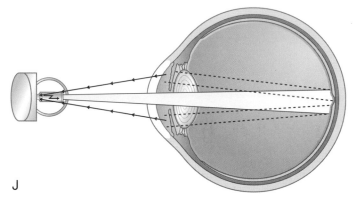

J

Figure 44.6 (J) Iris transillumination. Photographs should be taken with the pupil only partly dilated (3–4 mm when light-stimulated). With the slit illuminator in a coaxial position with the biomicroscope, a small, full circle beam of light is projected through the pupil into the eye. Defects in the iris are visible by transmission of the orange light reflected from the fundus.

microscope to provide adequate illumination through the relatively small aperture of the pupil.

All contact lenses, especially those used for photography, must be carefully maintained. By rinsing with running warm water immediately after each use, the methylcellulose is easily removed, which prevents the formation of a crusty residue that can easily scratch the surface of the lens if one attempts to wipe it away. Following standard procedures for decontamination, the lens should again be rinsed,

carefully dried with a soft cloth or tissue to remove droplets (which may leave precipitates behind), and stored in a sturdy, dust-free container.

To ensure the quality of goniographs, new lenses should be purchased and their use restricted to photographic purposes only.

Gonioscopy, like all slit-lamp biomicroscopy, should be practiced as often as possible under the direction of the ophthalmologist.

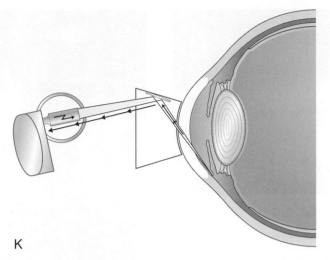

K

Figure 44.6 (K) Goniography. After placement on the eye, the goniolens is rotated to bring the desired mirror into position opposite the area to be examined or photographed. A slit beam of moderate width, made parallel with the angle, is usually used. The same basic technique is used for the study and documentation of peripheral vitreal and retinal conditions, through a well-dilated pupil.

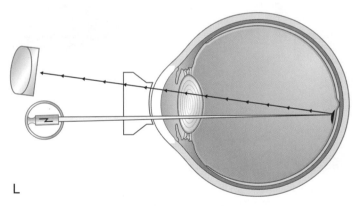

L

Figure 44.6 (L) Photography of the posterior pole through a fundus lens. A contact lens is placed on the eye, which permits a view of the fundus with the biomicroscope. With a narrow or moderate slit beam, the structures of the posterior fundus can be examined in minute detail. The slit illuminator must be placed in a relatively coaxial position with the biomicroscope; the larger the pupil, the better is the opportunity for oblique sectioning.

(From Mártonyi CL, Bahn CF, Meyer RF. Clinical slit lamp biomicroscopy and photo slit lamp biomicrography. Ann Arbor, MI: Time One Ink; 1985.)

ENDOTHELIAL SPECULAR PHOTOMICROGRAPHY

Specular micrography is a method of photographing and evaluating the endothelial surface of the cornea (see Chapter 37).

FUNDUS PHOTOGRAPHY

Fundus cameras are used to document the posterior segment of the eye. Viewing and photography are done through a single-lens system and correct exposures are ensured by predetermined flash intensity settings. With a

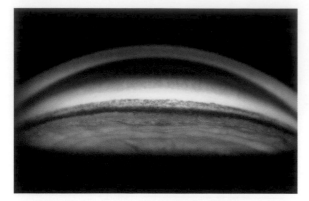

Figure 44.7 Goniograph demonstrating pigment dispersion syndrome.
(From Mártonyi CL, Bahn CF, Meyer RF. Clinical slit lamp biomicroscopy and photo slit lamp biomicrography. Ann Arbor, MI: Time One Ink; 1985.)

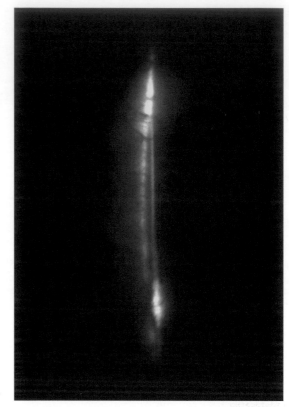

Figure 44.9 Double slit indicates shallow detachment of neurosensory retina.
(From Mártonyi CL, Bahn CF, Meyer RF. Clinical slit lamp biomicroscopy and photo slit lamp biomicrography. Ann Arbor, MI: Time One Ink; 1985.)

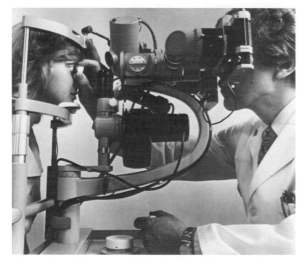

Figure 44.8 Zeiss photo slit lamp in use with contact lens to obtain slit fundus photograph shown in Figure 37.10.

little practice, even the novice can produce consistently acceptable photographs of the posterior pole.

The fundus camera system consists of a camera mounted on a specially designed instrument table equipped with a chin rest assembly to provide a comfortable and steady support for the patient's head (Figure 44.10). A power supply provides viewing illumination and rapid recycling flash illumination (up to three flashes per second). A digital sensor camera records the image, and this is connected to image capture software that processes and stores the images.

The fundus camera, like the slit-lamp biomicroscope, uses an aerial image system of focusing. Unlike the single-lens reflex camera in which the image is projected onto a ground-glass surface, the aerial image is projected into space. This space is, in fact, a well-defined plane designated by a "crosshair" reticule. With this system the only means of ensuring a sharp image at the film plane is to maintain the crosshair reticule and the fundus detail in sharp focus simultaneously. Because accommodation on the part of the photographer can result in a dramatic shift of the aerial image away from its intended plane, neglect of the crosshair reticule can result in unsharp photographs.

The eyepiece of the fundus camera has an adjustable diopter range to correct for the photographer's refractive error. To establish the correct eyepiece setting, the eyepiece must be turned to its maximum up, or "plus," position. Then, while the examiner looks through the camera at some distant object with both eyes open, he or she slowly rotates the eyepiece downward toward the "minus" side, until the crosshair reticule is sharply seen (Figure 44.11). The examiner should stop at this point. This procedure should be repeated several times or until the photographer's accommodation is relaxed and the same setting is consistently arrived at. Accommodation can be more easily

Figure 44.10 Zeiss Fundus Flash IV fundus camera.

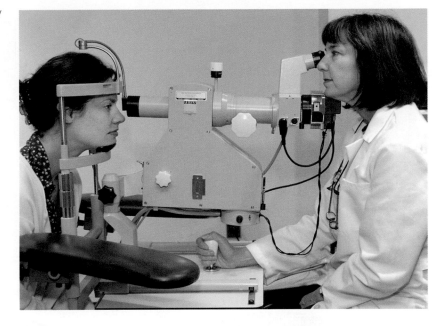

controlled if the examiner works in a darkened room with both eyes open while viewing through the fundus camera.

Before fundus photography is performed, the patient's pupils must be dilated. The minimum pupil size through which acceptable photographs are achievable varies from one fundus camera to another. Wide-angle cameras (45–60 degrees) generally require a proportionately larger pupil for acceptable results. The larger the pupil, the easier it is to obtain good photographs. In the presence of opacity, such as a central cataract, a poor image of the fundus results when the camera is properly centered. If the pupil is large enough, however, the camera can be placed off center, resulting in a much clearer photograph. The use of a cycloplegic is also recommended to minimize the patient's accommodation. As the optical components of the eye— the lens and cornea—become part of the total optical system of the fundus camera, continued, active accommodation by the patient results in an image that drifts in and out of focus.

Before the patient is seated in front of the camera, it is good practice to enter the patient's demographics into the imaging software database.

After seating the patient comfortably, the examiner should position the camera to produce a well-delineated, circular image of the viewing bulb filament on the cornea or, if not well visualized there, on the closed eyelid (Figure 44.12). With the camera aligned at this distance on the center of the pupil, a good view of the fundus should be attained. Without alteration of the camera position, the image should be sharply focused, after which final adjustments in camera position can be made.

Correct saturation, or maximum intensity of the correct color of the fundus, is achieved by moving the camera toward or away from the eye. When the camera is too far from the eye, a blue-gray halo forms around the image. As the camera moves forward, the color becomes more saturated.

When the camera is placed slightly off center and moved closer to the eye, an orange to bright yellow crescent appears on one side. This crescent signals maximum saturation beyond which the examiner should not go. By moving the camera laterally away from the crescent it will disappear but, by moving too far in that direction, the crescent will reappear on the opposite side. A crescent appearing on the top of the picture is eliminated by moving the camera down; moving the camera up eliminates an inferior crescent.

In attempting photography through a small pupil or other media opacity, it may be impossible to avoid the bluish haze or crescent, but both should be minimized as much as possible. When a view of the fundus is so dark that it requires an increase in the viewing illumination intensity, a proportionate increase in the flash intensity must be made to ensure correct exposure. Conversely, for extremely light fundi, both viewing and flash intensities may be proportionately reduced.

The photographic sequence should begin with the posterior pole of the right eye and should include the disc and macula for positive identification of the eye being photographed. Stereo photographs of the macula and disc can be taken at the same time. When a fundus "map" is required, following a routine sequence will aid in

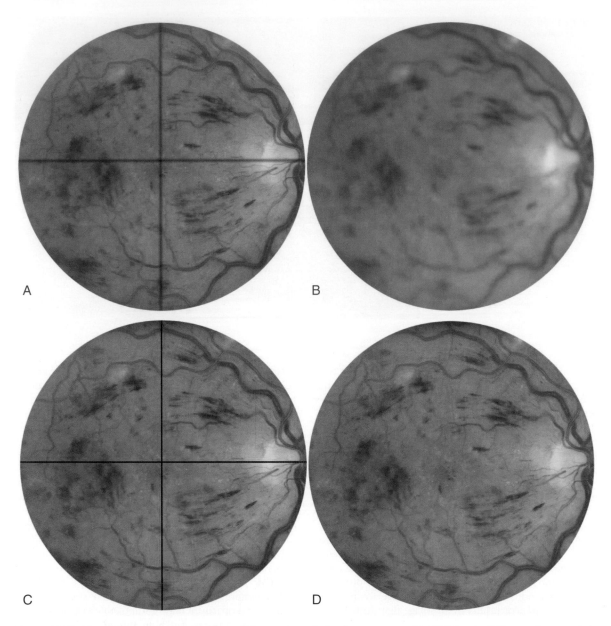

Figure 44.11 A fundus image when viewed through the eyepiece of a fundus camera may look in focus, but if the eyepiece crosshairs are not in focus at the same time (A), the photographic results will be out of focus (B). Both the fundus image and the crosshair image must be in focus at the same time (C) to obtain a well-focused fundus photograph (D).

reconstruction of the photographic map after processing (Figure 44.13). To achieve a view of other areas of the fundus, the patient's eye can be rotated by moving the fixation target and moving the camera to stay lined up on the center of the dilated pupil.

When fundus photography is attempted for the first time, or when a new camera is being tried, careful documentation of exposures and procedures provides a baseline from which appropriate adjustments can be made.

Stereo fundus photography

Sequential stereo fundus photography is achieved by aligning the camera initially as described, then moving it laterally from one side of the dilated pupil to the other, taking a photograph in each position to provide the three-dimensional (3-D) effect. When crescents are encountered, the camera should continue in the direction of the crescent, which should cause it to disappear. If a crescent persists, the camera should be moved slightly back from the eye. By previewing the area to be photographed in stereo while moving the camera briskly between the two laterally displaced positions, the examiner can get an excellent appreciation for the elevation or depression of the structure or lesion being viewed. Optimum camera position for each side of the stereo pair can thus be appraised before making the actual exposures. The greater the stereo base (distance between the two camera positions), the greater is the 3-D effect. Because stereo photography requires using the camera in a drastically off-center position, it may not be possible to eliminate all artifacts. At times, especially when the patient's pupil size is relatively small, stereo photography may involve a compromise to the quality of the individual frames. However, the two frames reinforce each other considerably in addition to providing the 3-D effect so vital to the evaluation of many disease entities. Whereas some cameras offer the option of a mechanical locking device to help establish a degree of stereo separation, its use is

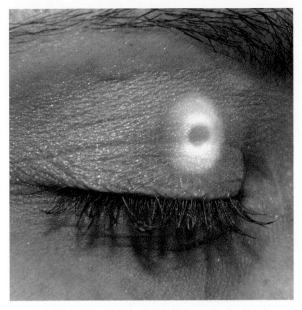

Figure 44.12 Appearance of correctly focused image of viewing lamp filament on closed eyelid.

Figure 44.13 Suggested format of successive fields to provide a composite of posterior fundus. Proceed counterclockwise in the right eye and clockwise in the left.
(Courtesy of Hackel R, Saine P. In: Saine P, Tyler, ME, editors. Ophthalmic photography. Burlington, MA: Butterworth-Heinemann; 2003.)

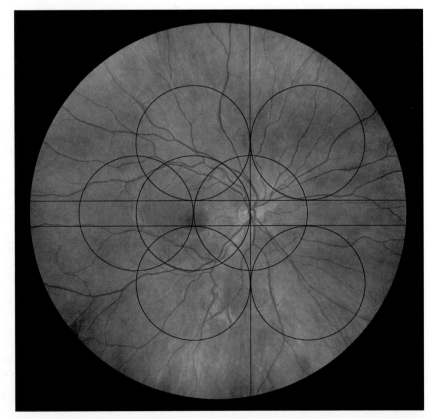

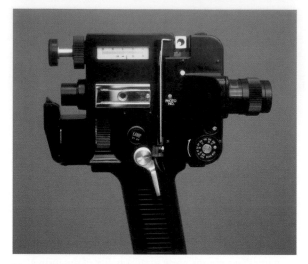

Figure 44.14 Kowa handheld fundus camera.

discouraged. Not only is it unreliable, given the wide disparity in pupil sizes, but it is also limiting when stereo photographs are required in the presence of ocular opacities. Under such circumstances, an unrestricted manual displacement technique will provide better results.

A wide range of fundus cameras is available: most are table-mounted and a few are handheld. Most systems offer two or three angles of view, usually from 20 to 50 degrees. Some older models have only one angle of view. Some specialized cameras using a contact lens arrangement are capable of photographing 180 degrees of the fundus in a single image. Handheld fundus cameras (Figure 44.14) are useful for photographing children under anesthesia or other patients who are unable to sit at a table-mounted system. The handheld fundus camera also can also serve as a helpful external camera.

FLUORESCEIN ANGIOGRAPHY

For fluorescein angiography, a fundus camera must be equipped with a rapid-recycling, high-output power supply and an exciter and barrier filter combination. The exciter filter is placed in the path of the light and allows only a specific wavelength of blue light (approximately 490 nm) to strike the fundus. When fluorescein is introduced into the circulation of the eye, the blue light excites the fluorescein molecules to a higher state of activity, causing them to emit a greenish yellow light of a higher wavelength (approximately 520 nm), creating the fluorescence that we record. The barrier filter is positioned to filter out the blue exciter light and allow only the excited yellow-green light of actual fluorescence to strike the image sensor.

Modern filter combinations are so efficient that they permit the recording of true fluorescence only. Older filter combinations were less efficient and commonly produced a dim but discernible image of light structures within the eye (such as the optic nerve head) even without the injection of fluorescein. This level of exposure of light objects without fluorescein is generally referred to as *pseudofluorescence*. As a means of dealing with pseudofluorescence, a "control" photograph of the area to be documented should be taken. The exposure is made before the injection of fluorescein, with the exciter and barrier filters in place and the flash intensity set at the level for fluorescein angiography. When this procedure produces an image, it is generally indicative of filter failure, perhaps requiring filter replacement.

Before fluorescein angiography is undertaken, the patient is informed of the procedure and its implications, and consent is obtained. (Laws and regulations for obtaining consent vary among states and institutions.)

To produce an angiogram (Figure 44.15) the following steps are recommended:

1. Set the image capture software to record for fluorescein angiography. This sets the camera and computer to process the image in black and white, and it raises the ISO setting because the fluorescein filters absorb a lot of light.
2. Set the flash intensity to the level used for color photography.
3. Introduce the green or "red-free" filter into the light path.
4. Position the patient at the camera and take a stereo photograph of the area to be studied with the green filter in place.
5. Set the image capture software and the camera to its fluorescein angiography settings. This may automatically increase the flash output to the level required for fluorescein angiography, or you may have to change these settings manually.
6. When the needle is correctly inserted into the patient's vein, check the patient's head position and viewing through the camera's viewfinder, to again ensure proper alignment and focus.
7. Initiate the rapid injection of the fluorescein and simultaneously activate the timer.
8. At 5 to 7 seconds following the start of the injection, the exposure sequence should commence. The average arm-to-eye circulation time in an adult is between 8 and 15 seconds. In a child, it can occur within 4 to 7 seconds and requires earlier initiation.
9. After the rapid-sequence documentation of the initial circulation of fluorescein through the full arteriovenous phase, the frequency of exposures may be reduced considerably because further development in the angiographic pattern occurs much more slowly beyond this point. (An understanding of the

interval can also be used to monitor the patient for any signs of adverse effects from the fluorescein angiographic procedure. Stereo fluorescein photography can be incorporated at any stage of the angiogram by using the procedure described for stereo photography.

Indocyanine green chorioangiography

Advances in digital imaging technology facilitated the practical use of indocyanine green (ICG) dye for the study of choroidal vessels. As ICG dye is excited in the near-infrared range, effective penetration of the retinal pigment epithelium is achieved, with a correspondingly improved view of the choroidal vasculature. It is most often used to identify occult neovascularization of the choroid. Although its applicability is limited, for certain patients it can result in the treatment of conditions that might not otherwise be adequately outlined.

A conventional fundus camera design must be enhanced to function in the near-infrared range (Figure 44.16). The procedure for ICG angiography is essentially the same as for fluorescein angiography. With some retinal diseases, the earliest frames are all that is necessary to identify a feeder vessel. In other cases, it is the very late phase, at 30 minutes postinjection, that is more important (Figure 44.17). Because ICG is more completely plasma-bound, it takes longer to leak from abnormal blood vessels in sufficient quantities to be visible. Unlike the fluorescein procedure, the late phase for ICG pictures is taken at 30 minutes postinjection.

Digital systems can be equipped to capture fluorescein and ICG angiograms electronically. Resultant images can be adjusted for contrast and density and subjected to various subroutines for maximizing their usefulness in determining the treatability of certain conditions.

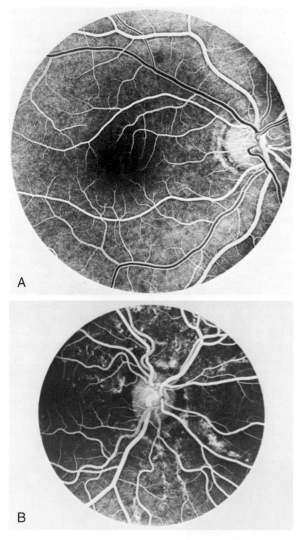

Figure 44.15 (A) Normal angiogram showing early venous "laminar" or "lamellar" stage of circulation. (B) Angiogram in full arteriovenous stage of circulation in eye affected with angioid streaks.

hemodynamics of the choroidal and retinal circulation, as well as the appearance of fluorescein angiographic characteristics of the various lesions studied, improves judgment.)

10. Intermediate or recirculation phase: photographs should be taken at approximately 1 to 3 minutes after injection.

11. A late photograph, approximately 8 minutes after injection, is also recommended. Certain conditions are not delineated until this point, and the time

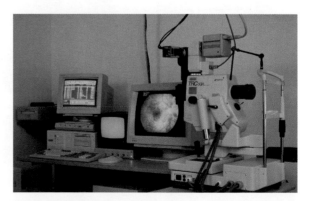

Figure 44.16 Topcon ImageNet system for digital fluorescein and indocyanine green (ICG) angiography.

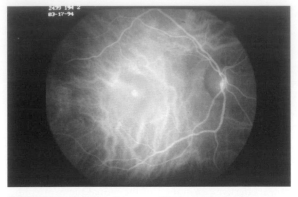

Figure 44.17 Indocyanine green (ICG) angiogram showing large choroidal vessels and a "hot spot" near the fovea, indicating possible choroidal neovascularization.

VIDEO RECORDING

Requests for motion recording may be made for patient eye motility studies and intraoperative procedures. Technologic advances in video recording have made it easier to obtain quality results. Whereas analog tape formats such as VHS were once adequate, they were difficult to edit and suffered from quality loss because the tape had to be copied with each successive edit. The newer digital formats, such as compact digital and MPEG, combined with basic computer editing software, offer a useful way to capture, edit, and distribute motion picture documentation of patients. Because the signal is digital, progressive copies of the file do not degrade the image quality.

When video is used to document a patient's eye movements, instructions to the patient can be recorded simultaneously with the video to positively identify the direction of gaze being attempted. If desired, the sound portion can be eliminated or recorded over at another time. With many of the newer compact digital cameras, short motility studies can be effectively recorded onto compact flash media. Not only does this allow for easier access and cataloging than videotape, but it also allows for direct importation into a PowerPoint type of presentation.

For much of the intraoperative recording of surgical procedures, such as vitrectomies, a video camera is mounted on the operating microscope and is coaxial with the surgeon's view. The video system is generally left on for an entire procedure. Even if the case is not recorded onto videotape or digital media, the progress of the procedure can be effectively monitored by other members of the surgical team. It also allows a number of observers to benefit from the view normally seen only through the microscope oculars (Figure 44.18).

For documenting procedures not requiring an operating microscope, a system as described for ocular motility may

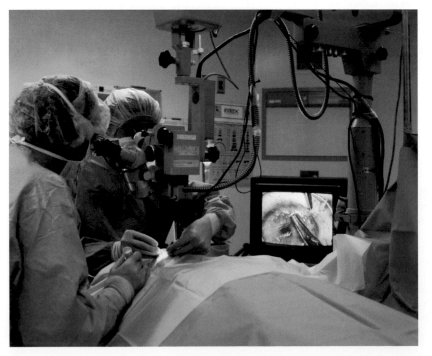

Figure 44.18 A surgical procedure displayed on closed-circuit television.

be used. A long-focal-length macro lens is recommended to provide a suitable magnification-to-working-distance ratio. Especially for long video sequences, the camera should be placed on a sturdy tripod of sufficient height to provide the desired angle of view. The photographer may have to stand on a short stepladder to provide an optimal view.

IMAGE PRESENTATION

Images from a digital system can be imported directly into Microsoft PowerPoint, Apple Keynote, or other presentation software, along with video files and other scanned material. Printed materials can be scanned using a flatbed scanner. With the addition of a transparency adapter, 35 mm slides, film-based x-rays, computed tomography (CT) images, and magnetic resonance images (MRIs) can be easily integrated into the digital presentation.

The file size requirements are much less for an on-screen display than for prints. Whereas an 8×10 color print will usually require a 300 ppi, 20 megabyte (MB) file to print on an inkjet printer, the same image projected on-screen with PowerPoint requires only a 96 ppi, 2 MB file. Using a larger file size in PowerPoint has no effect on the image quality; it only makes the file size of the presentation larger.

Video clips can be imported directly into PowerPoint, but care should be taken as to file compatibility. There are many competing formats on the market, such as MPEG, QuickTime, AVI, and many others. Because some formats do not work on all systems, it is important to learn which ones work with the current version of software you are using.

Up until the most recent version of PowerPoint, the way image files were handled (using the older .ppt format) was different for photographs and videos. When photographs are imported into any PowerPoint version, they are embedded into the presentation and become part of the file. When copying or moving PowerPoint file, it is not necessary to also include copies of the image files. Videos, however, when imported into the older .ppt PowerPoint version, were "linked," not embedded. Therefore, it was important to keep the video file in the same folder as the PowerPoint presentation. This entire folder had to be copied whenever the file was moved.

The good news is that the current versions of PowerPoint, for both Macintosh and Windows, which use the .pptx file format, do embed the videos, so the linking concerns are no longer a problem.

SUMMARY

In ophthalmology, a picture can truly be "worth a thousand words" and ophthalmic photography has indeed become an indispensable adjunct to the eye care profession.

To provide this vital service the ophthalmic photographer must learn proven methods and stay abreast of new developments in technique and instrumentation. The success of each individual hinges primarily on the person's interest in photography and ophthalmology, along with a keen desire to excel in this challenging specialty.

Questions for review and thought

1. The aperture of a camera refers to the size of opening that permits light to enter the camera. Is an f16 opening a large or small opening?
2. The depth of field indicates how much of the picture will come into sharp focus. Does an f2.6 opening have a large or small depth of field?
3. A fast image sensor setting is used when there is insufficient light available. Name an image sensor speed that is relatively fast.
4. What are the chief sources of lighting for external photographs of the eyelid and cornea?
5. How can you obtain steadiness of the patient and the camera during photography?
6. Fundus photographs may be taken with special cameras designed for this purpose. Name the camera type that you are familiar with and outline a routine of photographing the fundus.
7. Outline a method of performing fluorescein angiography and photography.
8. What is color balance, and how is it managed with digital cameras?

Q Self-evaluation questions

True–false statements

Directions: Indicate whether the statement is true **(T)** or false **(F)**.

1. A longer than normal focal length lens tends to reduce perspective distortion. **T** or **F**
2. Fluorescein angiography should be recorded on a low ISO setting. **T** or **F**
3. The normal average arm-to-retina circulation time is in the range of 8 to 15 seconds. **T** or **F**

Q Continued

4. A digital image saved as a JPEG file is always the same size as a TIFF file. **T** or **F**

Missing words

Directions: Write in the missing word(s) in the following sentences:

5. The sensitivity, or "speed," of an image sensor is expressed in _____ numbers.

6. Normal daylight has a color temperature of _____ Kelvin.

7. Before performing gonio slit-lamp photography, a drop of _____ must be instilled into the eye.

Choice-completion questions

Directions: Select the one best answer in each case.

8. The ability of a lens to discriminate fine detail is called:

a. speed.
b. angle of acceptance.
c. focal length.
d. resolution.
e. depth of field.

9. When an exposure is adjusted from $^1/_{30}$ of a second at f16 to $^1/_{60}$ of a second at f5.6, the total volume of light striking the film:

a. becomes one-half as much.
b. remains the same.
c. becomes twice as much.
d. becomes four times as much.
e. becomes one-third as much.

A Answers, notes, and explanations

1. **True.** A lens of a wide angle of acceptance must be used close to the subject with a resultant overemphasis of things nearest the camera. With a long-focus lens, the camera is used farther from the subject, resulting in more normal-appearing perspective.

2. **False.** Fundus cameras require the use of a high-speed setting such as 400 ISO for adequate exposures. The slow speed of 100 ISO makes it unusable for angiography in normal situations.

3. **True.** Arm-to-retina circulation time for the average adult is approximately 12 seconds. A child's is from 5 to 8 seconds and in individuals with certain problems the dye circulates much more slowly. It is important to be prepared for this factor to ensure correct sequencing during the initial phase of the angiogram.

4. **False.** A JPEG file is a compression format that helps to reduce file size. A TIFF file has every pixel represented as a discrete bit.

5. **ISO. International Standards Organization.** The sensitivity setting for an image sensor is designated by a numeric value, its ISO number, which must be calculated into the exposure. A higher ISO number requires less light, so in a dark environment, faster shutter speeds or smaller apertures can be set on the camera.

6. **5400K.** The color temperature of fluorescent lights is approximately 3700K, photofloods are 3400K, and

ordinary household light bulbs are approximately 2700K. Care must be taken to set the white balance correctly on the camera.

7. **Proparacaine hydrochloride 0.5%.** The surface of the cornea must be anesthetized before placing the gonio lens into contact with it.

8. **d. Resolution.** The resolution of a lens is measured by its ability to discriminate the maximum number of lines per millimeter. In other words, if a lens can produce a negative of a 1 mm area containing 200 line pairs so that those lines can be counted on the negative but in an attempt to record 200 line pairs the lines become blurred together and cannot be counted, that lens has a resolving capability of 200 line pairs per millimeter.

9. **d. Becomes four times as much.** The basic exposure is $^1/_{30}$ of a second at f16. Each setting of either shutter speed or f-stop influences the total exposure by a factor of two. Changing the shutter speed from $^1/_{30}$ to $^1/_{60}$ of a second cuts the exposure in half. By 'opening up' from f16 to f11, that half is again increased by two to the original total exposure of 'one.' One-sixtieth of a second at f11 equals $^1/_{30}$ of a second at f16. By opening up to f8, the exposure is doubled and is then doubled again, or increased to four times, at f5.6.

Chapter | 45 |

Visual aids for the partially sighted

Harold A. Stein, Gwen K. Sterns, Eleanor E. Faye

The partially sighted comprise that group of individuals whose vision is not sufficient for ordinary reading or ambulation despite correction with conventional glasses. Normally a person's visual function is not considered impaired until the vision in the better eye has deteriorated to at least 20/50 or worse. Included in the classification of the partially sighted are people deemed legally blind, who have either a visual acuity of 20/200 or worse in the better eye or field restriction of 20 degrees or less. In a special category are individuals with nuclear sclerosis or severe myopia whose uncorrected near or reading vision remains normal, or near normal, although distance vision may have worsened.

Most people with subnormal vision can be assisted by properly selected optical aids. The assistance does not mean restoring vision, but rather facilitating the use of available vision to restore the person's functional capacity, including the potential for employment. In industries in which partially sighted individuals have been employed, their work output has been on a par with that of fellow workers and their safety record is usually superior. Children can be given the opportunity to obtain an education using modern computer technology. For the older adult, visual assistance may provide a new lease on life, enabling the person to continue working, reading, writing, and pursuing hobbies.

Vision rehabilitation is an essential part of comprehensive eye care. Many patients have been told that their vision cannot be improved, which has caused them to believe that they will be forced to abandon their enjoyment in work or their special interests, or both. Witnessing a visually impaired individual reading after being convinced that nothing can be done is a more dramatic event than seeing a postoperative cataract patient read the 20/20 line.

FACTOR OF AGE

An appreciation of the etiology of a patient's vision loss helps us to better prescribe low-vision aids. Most patients with subnormal vision can be assisted by properly selected optical aids that can restore the person's functional loss and sense of self-sufficiency. To an adult this may mean the opportunity for resuming or gaining employment. Children can be given the opportunity to be mainstreamed in their classrooms to allow them to participate with their sighted peers. For the older adult, visual assistance may provide a new lease on life, preventing depression because of inability to read, write, or maintain hobbies. The rehabilitation of the partially sighted is extremely gratifying, for both the patient and the provider.

Management of the partially sighted varies with the patient's age. Affected children comprise a small but important group because if they are not helped to deal with their vision problem they may fail to achieve a level of education that will allow them to live an independent life. They have the longest period in which they have to live with their disability and therefore must acquire the necessary skills from their earliest years when their motivation, a necessary factor in learning to use an optical aid, is likely to be high. Also, children have an excellent range of accommodation, which enables them to perform visual tasks at near despite poor distance vision.

Many children with distance vision of 20/200 have excellent reading vision. In this group are those who have congenital nystagmus, high myopia, albinism, or congenital retinal conditions. In the early grades children often require no special optical aids because they have sufficient accommodation to compensate for the disability by holding printed material close. Also, children's books are printed in large type in the first four grades; for children ages 7 to 8 years the size of the print is about 18 points (requiring 20/100 vision), whereas for ages 9 to 12 years it is 12 points (requiring 20/80 vision). As the child progresses into the higher grades, the textbook print invariably becomes smaller. It is usually between the fifth and seventh grades that the child who had been able to get along previously may need assistance from visual aids and from the special education teaching staff. At this point optical aids become important because they may enable these children to continue on a level with their sighted peers.

Young adults actually constitute the smallest group of those becoming partially sighted because the adult usually experiences the onset of loss of vision because of injury or disease. The situation of young adults is often critical, however, because their livelihood depends on successful rehabilitation. Young adults are understandably depressed and anxious about their recently acquired visual disability. They need support in their vocational restructuring from the private and state rehabilitation programs that specialize in visual retraining using sophisticated computer technology.

Older adults constitute the largest group of the visually handicapped because of the increase in age-related eye conditions, as well as other physical infirmities such as poor hearing, difficulty in walking, or tremor. However, many older people, in spite of other infirmities, are motivated to continue their interests and their occupations, even if in a somewhat modified form. The current aging generation that is computer-literate is able to make the transition into both optical and computer-generated visual aids with help from private and state programs for older individuals.

Assistance for patients with subnormal vision is provided through a careful eye examination, a good history from the patient, including an assessment of the reaction to vision loss, the degree of adjustment made, and a survey of the patient's educational background, interests, and visual needs, and the provision of optical and nonoptical aids. Many enterprising patients have discovered magnifying lenses on their own and welcome the introduction of more sophisticated or technically superior devices.

It is important in the eye examination to test visual acuity accurately. The partially sighted patient should therefore be tested at 10 feet (3 m) rather than at 20 feet (6 m). Most projectors have no test print between 20/100 and 20/200

or beyond 20/200. If a patient is tested at 10 feet with Snellen charts or specially designed early treatment diabetic retinopathy study (ETDRS) test charts, this deficiency is remedied.

To convert to standard notations, the results are multiplied by 2; for example, $10/70 = 20/140$. If the acuity is less than 10/200, the chart is brought closer to the patient until the 200 letter is identified (5/200, 3/200). Counting fingers should not be used as a visual acuity test. A careful refraction is important because correction of a basic refractive error may not only improve the impaired vision but also serve as a baseline acuity for the prescription of other optical magnifying devices.

The history provides many essential details about the patient's response to loss of vision. Adjustment to a recent vision loss may require counseling and introduction of a change in lifestyle. Not everyone accepts such a loss immediately, but with vision rehabilitation and introduction of new skills, most people eventually learn to modify their customary activities with the use of optical and nonoptical aids. Some individuals are content to be able to read hockey scores and manage their shopping and personal mail, whereas for others reading may play a much larger part in their daily life, whether for personal pleasure or for earning a living.

It is the role of the ophthalmologist and ophthalmic assistant to make sure that all of these patients receive low-vision care either onsite or by referral to a low-vision specialist. We need to treat the vision loss as a medical problem and relate the diagnosis to a functional vision loss. Our history should include a functional history as well as the goals and expectations of the patient and family.

LOW-VISION OPTICAL DEVICES

Refraction

Refraction is one of the most important parts of the low-vision examination. Refraction and an understanding of the needs of your patient are the first step in providing low-vision care. Often refractive errors are overlooked in patients who have been followed for macular degeneration or glaucoma. A good refraction gives the baseline visual acuity of the patient, corrects astigmatic errors, and corrects both for a myopic shift from a progressive cataract and for aphakia. Many doctors overlook refracting an amblyopic eye, which, with progressive disease in the opposite eye, may become the eye that provides the best acuity for the patient. A good refraction and an increase in a bifocal add is often the best solution for a patient with early vision loss. A patient with high myopia may be able to read without glasses, but need a new prescription for distance. Once a good refraction is obtained, the reading add is determined.

Refracting a low-vision patient may require more patience than with other patients, but the principles are the same. It is important for the patient to see the chart and more than one letter or number. By placing a printed low-vision chart on an intravenous (IV) pole, you can move the chart closer to the patient to enable more than one letter and line to be visualized. When checking between two lenses, give the patient more time to see and answer than a patient with normal vision; patients with nystagmus need extra time to focus before establishing the preferred choice.

Spectacles

Spectacles allow the patient to function hands-free, that is, the patient does not need to hold a magnifier.

It is important to understand the needs of the patient when prescribing a reading aid. Often the patient may want to have a more effective intermediate distance for the computer or for meal preparation. It may be necessary to increase the bifocal strength to enable reading fine print. The patient must be told that it may be necessary to hold the reading material at a closer working distance. Spectacles allow the incorporation of tints to reduce glare and improve contrast. We can incorporate prisms in the spectacles to assist the patient in finding an area of the retina that offers improved vision. In a patient with a visual impairment, every small improvement in vision offers the opportunity for improved function.

Spectacles also can provide the incorporation of high adds to be used for magnification. These lenses may require base-in prism to reduce the demand on convergence. They also provide a large reading field, but with a close and fixed working distance. The degree of magnification required depends on the patient's visual acuity, age, and the work for which the optical aid is being used.

OPTICAL AIDS

Optical aids are divided into conventional corrective lenses (strong minus lenses for high myopes, corneal contact lenses for those with corneal scars, keratoconus, and so forth) and magnifying or convex lenses.

The patient often can see details only if they are magnified. Magnification devices are available for both distance and near vision. The degree of magnification required of course depends on the patient's visual acuity and age and the work for which the patient wishes to use the optical aid.

In terms of visual acuity alone, the Kestenbaum rule is a good starting point. When the numerator of the patient's distance visual acuity is divided into the denominator, the result should approximately equal the magnification required for seeing Jaeger's test type 5 (J5) or 1-meter print on the near-vision chart. This figure is doubled to achieve J1, for example:

20/100 = +5.00 for J5, 10.00 for J1
20/200 = +10.00 for J5, 20.00 for J1
20/400 = +20.00 for J5, 40.00 for J1

An adult patient with 10/100 would require a +5.00 lens in addition to the ordinary spectacle correction for seeing print of this size. This may be used as a rule of thumb, with further refinement for a patient's specific task requirement. A young person, especially a child, would need less than a +5.00 lens because of accommodation, and usually the addition to the ordinary spectacle correction would be the weakest lens that enables reading of J5 on the near-vision chart. In addition, word and text charts are available that assist in assessing magnification requirements of partially sighted patients.

For viewing distant objects, telescopes or binoculars can be useful. Although Kestenbaum's rule is helpful, the patient usually will have to try two or three aids before matching an aid to the desired activity or task.

All magnifying devices function by effectively enlarging the size of the retinal image (Figure 45.1). A similar effect can be produced by bringing the object closer to the eye because an object viewed at 10 inches has a retinal image twice the size of the same object viewed at 20 inches. However, only in children is the range of accommodation sufficient to provide exceptionally close viewing. The clarity

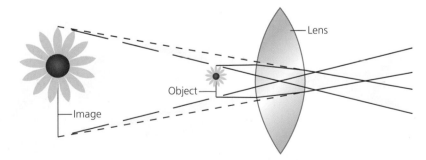

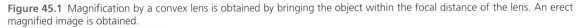

Figure 45.1 Magnification by a convex lens is obtained by bringing the object within the focal distance of the lens. An erect magnified image is obtained.

of distant objects often can be improved by walking or sitting closer to them. This is useful, for example, when watching television or reading a sign.

TYPES OF MAGNIFYING DEVICES (FIGURES 45.2–45.5)

Hand readers

The dioptric strength of most hand magnifiers already owned by most patients can be checked on a lensmeter. Some hand magnifiers are of a power greater than the range of a lensmeter. One has the option to hand-neutralize the lens with a lens of the opposite power so that no movement of the image occurs when the lens is moved back and forth.

Another option is the test described here to determine the magnification power of any hand magnifier.

1. Focus a magnifying lens to form a clear image of some print. Measure the distance from the paper to the lens

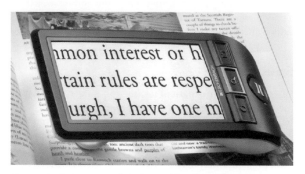

Figure 45.3 SmartLux digital portable video magnifier.
(Courtesy of Eschenbach Optik; http://www.eschenbach.com.)

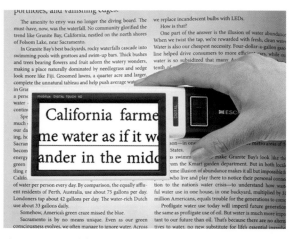

Figure 45.4 Mobilux Digital Touch HD portable video magnifier.
(Courtesy of Eschenbach Optik; http://www.eschenbach.com.)

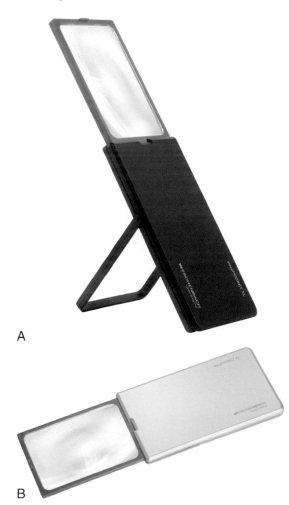

A

B

Figure 45.2 EasyPocket XL LED stand (A) and handheld (B) magnifiers.
(Courtesy of Eschenbach Optik; http://www.eschenbach.com.)

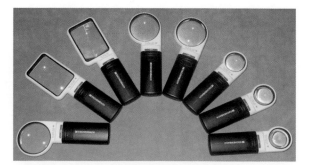

Figure 45.5 Mobilux LED handheld magnifiers.
(Courtesy of Eschenbach Optik; http://www.eschenbach.com.)

in inches and divide this distance into 10. This gives the magnifying power of the lens (e.g., a lens that focuses at 2 inches is a $10/2 = \times 5$ magnifier). Note: Those who prefer to work in centimeters will arrive at the same answer by dividing the measurement in centimeters into 25: $25/5 = \times 5$.

2. The magnification of the lens in $\times$power multiplied by 4 equals the approximate dioptric power of the lens. A $\times 5$ lens $\times 4 = +20.00$ diopters.

The advantage of a hand magnifier is that it is small and relatively inexpensive and easy to carry in a pocket or purse. The strength of hand magnifiers ranges from $\times 1$ (4.00 diopters) to $\times 20$ (80.00 diopters). The aspheric lens has been developed for many spectacles, hand and stand readers and is a considerable improvement over the older lenses because it effectively reduces the distortion ordinarily found at the edge of the field.

Most patients, when buying magnifiers, believe that the larger the lens area, the greater is the magnification; exactly the reverse is true. A large plus lens cannot be a strong plus lens or, conversely, the higher the plus power of the lens, the smaller the lens must be to reduce distortion. Most patients relate large devices with high power and must be shown how the optics of magnifiers affects the size of the lens. Patients may be shown how holding a strong lens close to their eye increases the viewing area.

Stand magnifiers

Stand magnifiers provide a prefocused mounting, allowing stability for patients with tremors to rest the magnifier directly on the material to be seen. The power of these magnifiers can be as great as 60.00 diopters, and some have illumination incorporated within their design. A reading stand used with a stand magnifier can reduce postural fatigue. Some patients using a stand magnifier may need a reading aid to maximize the effect of the magnifier and make it easier to use. Some patients use the stand magnifier to assist in writing by placing the pen or pencil under the magnifier between the legs of the stand. For older adults with tremors, and for younger children trying to maintain their place while reading, a stand magnifier may be the best device.

Telescopes

Telescopes allow magnification of an object in the distance by increasing the retinal image size. Telescopes can be handheld or spectacle-framed. They come as binocular or monocular and most can be focused. Telescopes allow the spotting of street signs, classroom materials, bus signs, shows and movies and speakers in a classroom or church. The field of view is small and illumination may be poor. There is a limited depth of focus. Patients with nystagmus have limited success as do patients with tremors. These patients may need telescopes that are mounted in a spectacle carrier.

For many other patients, though, they provide invaluable support for distance viewing, giving the user greater flexibility.

Desktop projection devices

Video desktop magnifiers are a useful aid, with the camera scanning the reading material and projecting the image onto a monitor (Figure 45.6). The benefits include magnification available to $\times 60$, adjustable contrast and brightness levels, and now text-to-speech functionality. In addition, a negative image can be projected onto the television screen to convert black letters printed on a white background to white letters on a black background. Desktop projection devices provide the best contrast and most normal reading posture of any visual aid.

A number of companies have introduced several models of video desktop magnifiers to see text such as a book or newspaper. These instruments are also available as portable battery units that can increase the magnification and yet view a line of text with practice. The text can be viewed at the reader's desired speed.

Strong convex lenses

The use of strong convex lenses (i.e., +4.00–60.00 diopters) is one method of providing magnification. The strong convex lens has a short focal distance so that reading material must be brought close to the eye. For example, with spectacles of +5.00 diopters, print is held about 9 inches (22.5 cm) away, whereas with a +20.00 diopter lens, the reading distance is only about 2 inches (5 cm) from the spectacles. Cosmetically, they are no more unsightly than cataract lenses. Anything greater than +12.00 diopters ($\times 3$), however, cannot be fitted binocularly. These high-plus

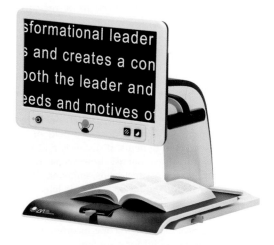

Figure 45.6 MagniLink Vision desktop video magnifier. *(Courtesy of Eschenbach Optik; http://www.eschenbach.com.)*

lenses may be made up in lenticular form to reduce weight, or in bifocal form.

Important considerations in the spectacle reading aid are freedom from aberrations, light weight, and a relatively wide field of view. Spectacles also allow both hands to be used for holding the reading material so that reading often is faster than with a magnifying glass.

A major disadvantage of spectacle lenses is that the reading material must be held still in the hand at the critical focal point. With older adults, early fatigue may occur when maintaining this fixed posture. Also, their hands may be tremulous, making reading at a fixed distance impossible. At higher-power corrections, the reading material is so close to the face that it often cuts out the light that normally would fall onto the type. Despite these disadvantages, the high-powered spectacle lens remains a widely used and popular aid.

In addition to the Kestenbaum rule as a method of determining how much magnification a patient needs to read, there is a Keeler low-visual-acuity word chart. The patient should be wearing correction spectacles to focus on print held at 10 inches (25 cm) in good light. The chart then indicates the magnification required to read small print. The patient should be prevented from moving the chart closer than 10 inches. Devices with the indicated magnification are then tried. Children (or adults who have not read for many years) are asked to spell the letters or read them out, whichever is most comfortable.

If a patient is a high myope, merely removing the glasses and reading without them may produce sufficient magnification. If the patient with low visual acuity has had a cataract operation with an intraocular lens implant, standard convex low-vision aids may be used as with any person. Finally, children have ample accommodation and can achieve excellent reading ability by holding their reading material in focus close to their eyes. This is not harmful and parents and teachers may need to be reassured on this point.

Distance magnifiers

Distance magnifiers are seldom worn permanently by the partially sighted. For the partially sighted to travel alone safely and efficiently, a wide field of vision is more important than good central visual acuity. Telescopes that magnify distant objects seriously reduce the field of vision, interfere with correct judgments of distance, and magnify lateral motions. For occasional use, however, such as identifying bus numbers and street signs, enjoying films and stage plays, or recognizing faces, telescopic lenses can be useful. These devices include binocular and monocular telescopes. For sustained reading at a distance, such as from a blackboard, a monocular telescope incorporated into a spectacle lens can be useful for a student.

Monocular telescopes can be held to the better-seeing eye and may be preferable to binoculars. A variety of

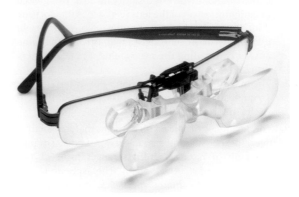

Figure 45.7 MaxTV clip telescope.
(Courtesy of Eschenbach Optik; http://www.eschenbach.com.)

lightweight, small monocular telescopes are readily available in strengths from ×2.5 to ×10.

For most patients, a telescope serves for occasional use out of doors and for watching a stationary scene such as a television screen or theater.

Some telescopes are constructed so that in addition to viewing distant objects they can be focused to reading distances. Some telescopes designed for distances accept reading caps of various strengths. Finally, some telescopes are designed for reading only and are mounted in an eyeglass frame (Figure 45.7). The advantage of a reading telescope is that the reading distance is increased. The small field of view, the increased motion of print as the head is moved in reading, and the limited depth of field are disadvantages for some patients, but with persistence these can be overcome.

LIGHTING

Good lighting is an important visual aid for everyone, but it is particularly important for partially sighted patients. What is good light for normal vision may be inadequate for the partially sighted. Lighting increases contrast between print and the background, thereby making details more legible. The best contrast is achieved by good type with black print on a white or near-white background.

Valuable improvement in lighting often can be achieved by having the patient simply alter the position of existing lamps or their shades, or even by altering the strength of the bulbs used. The patient will soon realize the benefits. Even those who may have mild photophobia can usually obtain some benefit.

A valuable lamp is one that uses a 60- or 75-watt bulb, with a metal reflecting shade and adjustable metal spring-mounted extendible arms, which can bring light efficiently onto such things as reading material, writing, financial accounts, sewing, and playing cards. This type of light is readily available in lighting stores in a variety of mountings. Chromolux bulbs offer lighting without glare and can help a patient achieve success with a visual aid.

Halogen reading lamps are not recommended for patients with retinal or corneal problems. The light is very bright and fatiguing and the bulb may be dangerously hot. Ambient halogen room lighting is safe.

The failure of an optical or nonoptical visual aid to work in the patient's home when success was indicated in office testing often means that the home setting has inadequate lighting.

NONOPTICAL VISUAL AIDS

Several accessory, nonoptical visual aids are commonly helpful to the patient with subnormal vision. These devices operate mainly by achieving magnification through the use of large print and special lighting effects. Another device includes the reading rectangle (typoscope), filters, check-writing guides, and marking pens.

Reading rectangle (typoscope)

The reading rectangle is a black matte plastic device in which a rectangular opening shows only a few lines of type (Figure 45.8). Reducing the glare from the surrounding page can often produce improvement in the vision of patients with incipient cataracts or corneal opacities by cutting off the reflected light from the page. It also is a useful means of finding the beginning of the next line of print to be read. This feature is particularly helpful with high-magnification aids, through which only a few words or even a few letters of print are discernible.

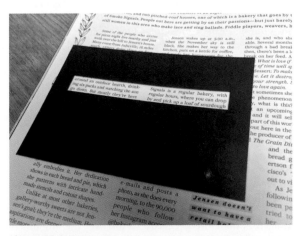

Figure 45.8 Typoscope.

Large type

Large-type visual aids include magazines, newspapers, and books printed in 18-point type as well as telephone dials or keypads with large numbers, playing cards with large figures, and school textbooks from grades one to four. The variety of large-print reading material can be somewhat limited if the patient's reading activity is restricted to material available only in large format. Most patients prefer using an optical device to provide the magnification so that the range of reading, both for pleasure and for work, is unrestricted. However, copy machines that enlarge type to any size are convenient to enlarge personal reading material. Computers have adaptable font sizes and special programs that use large print, such as job access with speech (JAWS).

Yellow filter

In some cases in which a patient reports fuzzy vision, yellow light will improve the contrast between the dark letters and the white paper. Yellow light can be provided by dark yellow clip-ons, coating of the lenses with dark yellow, use of a dark yellow light bulb in the reading lamp, or a yellow plastic sheet laid on the page.

Writing guides

Often the partially sighted patient cannot use an ordinary magnifier to write because the field of vision is not large enough to encompass a line. The writing guide gives direction, which could not be accomplished otherwise and so may be useful for this purpose. Patients who write a great deal prefer using a closed-circuit television (CCTV) to other more cumbersome methods.

Marking pens

Marking pens are nylon or felt-tipped with which one can write or print in dark and bold print so that a partially sighted person can not only receive messages from others but also keep lists and telephone numbers or even do personal bookkeeping. The partially sighted person writes or prints as large as is needed to be able to read the writing. These pens are readily available in all stationery and hardware stores.

Additional aids and devices

Large-print magazines, books on tape, and, in many areas, a radio reading service may be available for the visually impaired. Signature guides and check guides help to ease these tasks and are readily available. Broad-tipped markers are invaluable for notes and phone numbers and many patients appreciate large-dial thermostats, clocks, and telephone dials. Those who play cards may enjoy large-print playing cards. A reading stand is invaluable for the patient with arthritis or stroke who needs the reading material supported.

Many ingenious devices have been designed to assist the blind person to cope with everyday living. Among these devices are Braille or talking watches and clocks. Talking watches announce the time aloud at the press of a button and many also include auditory alarms. These watches are available in various designs, including both pocket and wrist types.

Many computer-based technologic aids are available that provide audible access to information or Braille displays. Small portable devices such as the Braille 'N Speak, which has a Braille input keyboard and speech output, allow the user to access a note taker, calculator, and appointment book, all in a device that weighs less than 2 pounds (0.9 kg). There is a programmable device that will speak the name of a medication and frequency of use.

Kitchen aids available for the homemaker include microwave ovens with Braille or large timers and controls, liquid level indicators, and triangular pie cutters. There are self-threading needles that include a groove at the back of the needle before the actual eye of the needle. The thread is positioned into this groove and a small tug pulls the thread into the eye of the needle. Measurements can be made with a tape measure with inches or centimeters marked off in elevated markings. There are check-writing guides and large checks with raised lines to guide the patient where to write. Talking thermometers announce the temperature aloud and talking scales are available. For the blind diabetic patient, insulin needle guides enable the person to locate the center of the rubber cap over the insulin bottle. There are also tactile raised markings on the syringe itself to measure the amount of insulin drawn up.

Tactile games have been developed by adapting standard games such as bingo, chess, Scrabble, Monopoly, dominoes, and playing cards.

Selection of low-vision aids

No single visual aid is best because each patient must be considered in terms of functional loss, age, interests, motivation, and the type of activity for which the aid is intended. For example, an older adult with a tremor might prefer a standard magnifier or spectacles. High-tech devices might be essential for someone at work to maintain employment. Children, especially those in the early grades, should be exposed to visual stimuli in the world around them. Simple magnifiers are valuable at early ages to allow the child to explore his or her environment.

Patients who have recently lost vision may need time to accept this. A multidisciplinary approach to the care of these patients is very helpful. Low-vision rehabilitation includes training for mobility, learning how to work in the kitchen safely, and how to navigate the home. The important thing to keep in mind is that even a small visual improvement can often enable patients to accept further

intervention, allowing a greater chance of their agreeing to more extensive visual rehabilitation.

THE PARTIALLY SIGHTED CHILD

A question commonly posed to the ophthalmologist is, should the child with partial sight be allowed to continue in regular grade school? There are no hard and fast rules because so many factors are involved besides those attributable to loss of sight. Of great importance are the child's intelligence, motivation, and ability to cope emotionally with the disability among regular schoolchildren. If a particular child is bright, social, alert, competitive, and capable of maintaining grades at a level commensurate with his or her age, then attending a regular school is to be encouraged. In effect, a child who can carry on such a program despite the disability must have superior ability and a supportive family. Certainly the early experience of competing with sighted children will prepare the child better for future life.

Every attempt should be made in the normal school system to provide special help from a teacher of the visually impaired. However, if the child experiences nothing but frustration and defeat in the environment of the better-sighted, it might be preferable in the long run to acquire basic educational skills at a school where children can proceed at their own pace and obtain the individual attention needed. Nevertheless, even in this setting it is best for the child to learn from regular and large-print textbooks and materials as long as possible, rather than resort to Braille. The trend has been to mainstream all disabled children, with special classes as needed.

If the child with a visual disability is excluded from ordinary children's games, such as basketball, football, throwing a ball and catching it, and baseball, the loss of peer support can be just as discouraging as failure at school. Such a child requires guidance even in choice of play. This youngster can be encouraged to participate in team activities in the capacity of manager or coach, to feel included in the group, or can be encouraged to develop skills in sports not requiring visual accuracy, such as track and field events, wrestling, and weightlifting.

SELECTION OF A VISUAL AID

No single visual aid is best because each patient must be considered in terms of age, interests, motivation, and the type of activity for which the aid is intended. For example, an older adult with a shaky hand is better off with a stand magnifier; a handheld magnifier is almost useless. Other patients have to see to make their living and they have to read. It is therefore necessary to discover the amount of reading required for a given patient and to consider the distance at which work must be carried out. In this context, the general rule is to give patients the weakest magnification that will enable them to function, because as the magnification is increased so too is the difficulty in working and reading. Children, especially those in the early grades, because they have a large range of accommodation and because their texts usually are printed in rather large type often require no visual aids until they reach grade five or six. It is recommended that children be examined after the beginning of each school year, bringing workbooks and textbooks with them. The evaluation is ongoing throughout their education.

Patients who have recently lost vision may need special counseling before they can use visual aids. With the new treatments available, they secretly harbor a notion that their vision may be restored. Also, the emotional upheaval in reaction to sensory deprivation may be so great that the factor of motivation is difficult to introduce in the early period of visual loss. A period of adjustment and adaptation—which varies, of course, with each patient—must usually pass before the patient accepts the fact that the disability is permanent. Providing supportive counseling and vision rehabilitation is the first step in guiding a person to establishing a new life.

Some older adults who have had poor vision for many years without a remedial education program may have accepted their disability and be uninterested in trying to learn to read again. In addition, they may have been unable to read for such a long period that they have forgotten how and, in the meantime, have learned other adaptive skills to replace visual activity.

The important thing to keep in mind is that even a small visual improvement can ease many people's problems, allowing a greater chance for education and employment or simply enabling them to enjoy activities of daily living again.

Questions for review and thought

1. Most people with reduced vision can be assisted by proper optical devices. What are the simplest devices that they can use?

2. Although a patient with subnormal vision has difficulty seeing at both distance and near, which of these two is the most important for most patients? Which is easier to correct optically?

3. Why can children with subnormal vision in the early grades of school manage in the regular classroom, but as they progress in school they often require optical aids?

4. Often partially sighted patients will have tried some optical aid on their own. What types of optical aids are readily available? Discuss different types of these optical aids as to the value of size and shape.

5. Discuss the effect of lighting on the activities of the visually impaired person.

6. Jewelers and other specialized workers require magnification for their work. Discuss how you would incorporate magnification for their work and how you would evaluate their magnifying devices.

7. The magnification of a lens is stated as ×3.5. What is the approximate dioptric power?

8. A lens has a back focal length of 25 mm. How much magnification would this give?

9. Why do large-diameter hand magnifiers fail as an aid for the patient with low visual acuity?

Q Self-evaluation questions

True–false statements

Directions: Indicate whether the statement is true **(T)** or false **(F).**

1. Many people who are legally blind are able to see well enough to work for a living and read normal-sized print. **T** or **F**

2. Patients should be given the weakest aid in terms of magnification. **T** or **F**

3. Children require the same magnification as adults. **T** or **F**

Missing words

Directions: Write in the missing word in the following sentences:

4. Equally important to the power of the lens is _____.

5. The best form of 'eye exercise' for a partially sighted person is _____.

Choice-completion questions

Directions: Select the one best answer in each case.

6. Magnification power of a lens is determined by:
   a. the reading of a lensmeter.
   b. the neutralization by another lens.
   c. taking the focal distance in inches and dividing this number into 10.
   d. the lighting present.
   e. all of the above.

Q Continued

7. The use of strong convex lenses creates which of the following?
   a. Aberrations similar to those of highly myopic spectacles
   b. An exceptionally close near point; for example, 20.00 diopters has a focal point of 2 inches
   c. Distortions that are best controlled with a single-cut lens
   d. Headaches if the correction is not bilateral
   e. All of the above

A Answers, notes, and explanations

1. **True.** One of the greatest handicaps of being legally blind is the common notion that such people are sightless and no longer can render a service to society. This is simply not true. Being legally blind with vision of 20/200 or less is a disability but not a total handicap. Blind people have prospered through ingenuity, determination, and selected visual aids.

2. **True.** As the magnification of a device increases, so too does its weight, distortion, and the critical nature of its focal point. Rather than depend on magnification alone, the patient may be better served by increasing illumination, which aids contrast. Also with high-power magnification devices, a patient cannot read by scanning but must labor like a child, going from word to word.

3. **False.** Children who are partially sighted can achieve better magnification by simply holding the book or paper a little closer to their eyes. Adults, especially those older than 45, have virtually depleted their accommodation ability and cannot naturally hold things close. A child may have an accommodative reserve of 14.00 diopters, whereas an adult counterpart may not have more than 2.00 diopters.

4. **Illumination.** Good lighting can make the difference between comfortable reading and labored reading. Tensor lamps, yellow light, and focal lighting all have their advocates. It is important to remember that the best light is that of the sun.

5. **Reading.** Many partially sighted people feel that their eyes are like tires: that if they are used too much they will wear out. This is a myth. Although reading is not an ocular exercise per se, it should be encouraged. It gives the person more contact with his or her world and helps destroy that psychologic feeling of being different and handicapped. If a person can read, most of the visual handicap is gone.

6. **c. Taking the focal distance in inches and dividing this number into 10.** A lens that focuses at 2 inches has a magnification of 10/2 or 5. In centimeters, the correct answer is found by dividing the measurement in centimeters into 25. On the other hand, magnification times 4 equals the dioptric power of the lens. Aspheric magnifiers for lenses +10.00 or greater (magnification of ×25) should be ordered because of the enlargement and the relative lack of distortion of the peripheral field.

7. **b. An exceptionally close near point; for example, 20.00 diopters has a focal point of 2 inches.** A magnifying lens is always convex: +10.00 to 20.00 diopter lenses are used the most. Lenticular lenses were popular to reduce weight and distortion.

Chapter 46

Blind persons in the modern world

Harold A. Stein, Gwen K. Sterns, Eleanor E. Faye

BLINDNESS DEFINED

The most widely accepted definition of blindness considers an individual to be blind whose central visual acuity does not exceed 20/200 in the better eye with a correcting lens, or whose visual acuity if better than 20/200 has a limit to the central field of vision to such a degree that its widest diameter subtends an angle no greater than 20 degrees.

Almost 1% of the US population is blind and almost 2% of individuals have low vision. The leading cause among White Americans is age-related macular degeneration (54%), whereas cataracts and glaucoma lead the way among African Americans (60%). Two-thirds of legally blind people have sight of various degrees. Some can distinguish only the difference between light and darkness, whereas others see vague shapes and patterns as if a thick fog were always in front of their eyes. Still others have peripheral sight and see the world around the edges of a blank or distorted area in the center of their vision (macula); they do not see the whole shape of anything if they look directly at it, but by shifting their eyes slightly to one side or up and down they see an image, although not with the detail of the normal macula. Others have no peripheral vision, but normal central vision.

In the visually impaired population the degrees and different types of vision loss are almost as varied as the people themselves. It is estimated that among blind individuals in the United States and Canada, less than 10% are totally blind (with no light perception). Nonlegally blind but visually impaired individuals outnumber those who are legally blind. The Eye Diseases Prevalence Research Group concluded that approximately 1 in 28 Americans more than the age of 40 years is affected by low vision or blindness, and that by 2020 the number of blind and low-vision persons in the United States will increase by 70% to 1.6 million. This study used data on blindness as defined by the World Health Organization (WHO) (<6/120 [<20/400]) and by the United States (<6/60 [<20/200]) and, for low vision, defined as vision in the better-seeing eye of less than 20/40.

A resolution adopted by the International Council of Ophthalmology, held in Sydney, Australia, April 2002, recommended to the world vision community the use of the following terminology to describe visual loss:

- Blindness. To be used only for total vision loss and for conditions in which individuals have to rely predominantly on vision substitution skills
- Low vision. To be used for lesser degrees of vision loss, so individuals can be helped significantly by vision enhancement aids and devices
- Visual impairment. To be used when the condition of vision loss is characterized by a loss of visual functions (such as visual acuity, visual field, etc.) at the organ level; many of these functions can be measured quantitatively
- Functional vision. To be used to describe a person's ability to use vision in activities of daily living (ADL);

presently, many of these activities can be described only qualitatively

- Vision loss. To be used as a general term, including both total loss (blindness) and partial loss (low vision), characterized either on the basis of visual impairment or by a loss of functional vision

Vision impairment and blindness are feared by most people throughout the world. Seventy percent of Americans older than age 45 fear blindness more than losing a limb, needing a wheelchair, or deafness. When patients or families of affected patients hear the word "blindness" they think of loss of all vision, darkness, and gloom. Telling a patient or a parent of a child that he or she is losing vision should therefore be handled with sensitivity, knowledge, and hope. Options for rehabilitation for the patient must be introduced. The patient and family should be expected to grieve for their loss and we as professionals need to understand the grieving process and accept and support it. These families and patients must be given the opportunity to see there is hope for their independence and for attaining and maintaining meaningful lives, education, and jobs.

PARTIAL SIGHT AND BLINDNESS

When patients are classified as legally blind, they have not always lost all of their visual function. In the United States blindness is defined as reduction of central visual acuity to no more than 20/200 in the better eye with a correcting lens or limitation of the central field of vision to less than 20 degrees at its widest diameter. The WHO defines blindness as visual acuity less than 20/400. The definitions of blindness used by the WHO and the United States are intended as legal classifications and they do not necessarily convey important functional information. Most patients classified as legally blind can still distinguish between objects, can read with low-vision aids, and maintain their independence with visual aids and training; a smaller number can distinguish only the difference between light and darkness. Low vision is an impairment that cannot be corrected by medicine, surgery, or conventional aids and interferes with functional vision. Many people who are not legally blind are visually impaired and need low-vision rehabilitation.

Most people who are legally classified as blind have some sight. However, it is inaccurate to label a visually impaired person as blind. An individual with sight can learn to use that residual vision in many ways, using a variety of optical devices and computerized reading machines. No one with sight is blind in the sense of having to use alternative nonvisual methods exclusively as the primary mode of functioning. For this reason, no one should be advised to learn to read Braille if he or she can read type, even though classified as legally blind. More than 90% of the legally

blind children between 7 and 17 years of age attend regular school. Low-vision aids and computers make this possible.

Braille is probably useful when a person has profound loss of vision (5/200 or less) and cannot read type, or read fast enough, with a closed-circuit television (CCTV) or strong magnifier. If possible, children with profound vision loss should be taught print letters and numerals to aid visualization of text, even if they eventually have to switch to Braille.

RECENT VISION LOSS

In most instances it is the ophthalmologist who is responsible for telling a person that he or she has a permanent loss of vision. Most authorities in the field of rehabilitation believe the person should be informed as early as possible once the diagnosis has been made. The sooner the disability is faced and accepted, the sooner the reality of vision rehabilitation can be accepted. The practice of prolonging hope of vision restoration not only impedes effective rehabilitation, but also delays facing reality.

Although it is important for the ophthalmologist to present the diagnosis in a candid and factual manner, it is just as essential for the practitioner to appreciate the emotional effect of such information. The doctor should provide a supportive environment in which the person is allowed time to ask questions, as well as be given information about community rehabilitation resources.

For most individuals, any loss of vision arouses an emotional response, usually fear of blindness. Depression is a normal response to becoming dependent and having to rely on others for help in basic living activities. Young adults fear loss of a job; older adults fear financial dependence, isolation, and loss of their friends and community.

TOTAL BLINDNESS

Myriad repeated frustrations occur in the daily lives of the totally blind that accentuate the dependency of the condition. Maintaining a job and personal life becomes a feat in itself. The routines that the sighted do automatically and without thought must be deliberately learned, step by step, by the blind. For example, the blind person must learn how to eat all over again. If the portions on a plate are not placed in a certain location, the blind person must explore the plate with a fork to discover where the food is placed.

Simple tasks can arouse feelings of insecurity, fear, and anxiety, especially when they have to be performed in public. Blind people may be afraid of making mistakes and of being clumsy and awkward for fear that they will become an object of attention. It is these little things—such as eating out in public, combing the hair or shaving, putting on makeup, or setting down a glass of water without knocking it over—that the blind must be able to learn to do with confidence. One of the first decisions to be made is whether the person would be safer learning long-cane travel or whether a guide dog would be more compatible with the individual's temperament. Each method has its adherents, advantages, and disadvantages; it is a highly personal choice.

Totally blind people may choose to withdraw into a familiar and unchanging environment that can be controlled with their visual incapacity. If they withdraw, they will be safe from physical harm and public ridicule, but limited in thoughts and actions. The other extreme is to tackle the problem head on, that is, to ignore the disability and continue with life despite the inconveniences, dangers, and hardships, learning in a specialized agency or organization for the blind how best to adapt to life without sight. The most desirable reaction is one that balances the disability with new ability and redirects interests, skills, and strengths so that the visual need in selected activities is minimized. The physician can be supportive of this reorientation by referring the blind person to trained rehabilitation personnel who can transmit the new skills to help the individual move toward physical and psychologic adjustment.

Ophthalmic assistant's role

The ophthalmic assistant will encounter in his or her daily work individuals who have a variety of different vision impairments, including blindness. The assistant should be familiar with the methods used to provide orientation to those with visual disabilities and to facilitate their mobility.

On first meeting a blind person, one should introduce oneself. The assistant should always offer his or her arm to the blind person. With a hand lightly on the assistant's arm, the patient feels the body movement and, because the assistant is slightly in front, the patient will have a feeling of confidence with each step. To be propelled from behind can be most awkward and unnerving. The assistant should be sure to ask a blind person if he or she needs help because the need for assistance should not be assumed without question. When you reach the examination chair, tell the patient where the chair is and place his hand on the chair so that he can position himself properly. Naturalness, kindness, and inherent human respect result in the most successful relationships and avoid an overdose of assistance, which makes a handicap more noticeable and damages the value of the assistant's role.

The assistant should realize that he or she should go to the patient to escort the latter to the examination room, rather than expecting the patient to navigate the office alone. Also any paperwork to be completed by the patient should be handled by either the assistant or office personnel in a private setting. If a blind person has been guided to a place and is to be left alone, he or she should first be

informed about the surroundings. It is also desirable, under such circumstances, to establish some position of safety and orientation, such as a table, chair, or wall, and to let the patient know if the door will be left open, so the person can call out for assistance if needed and be assured that someone will return shortly to check on the patient.

Because most patients with visual loss have normal hearing, medical personnel should avoid talking loudly to them. A patient with a visual impairment doesn't want to have his history discussed out loud in a waiting room any more than a sighted person would. You should not assume that the person accompanying the visually impaired patient is the one to whom questions of a sensitive nature should be directed. It is possible that this person is a neighbor or taxi driver and not someone with whom the patient wants to discuss private information. Visually impaired patients deserve the same courtesy as sighted patients.

The ophthalmic assistant should be aware of the thin line between giving someone assistance and making him or her feel helpless. Many blind people are quite proud of the many functions they can perform for themselves. They do not like having their disability emphasized and their dependency magnified. The assistant can ask the patient, in a quiet voice, if he or she can help him with this or that and let the patient make the decision about the degree of assistance wanted.

The ophthalmic assistant should avoid discussing with patients the status of their eyes, the state or federal assistance they can expect, or the details of the facilities available for them. Each of these areas should be handled by professionals trained in their fields. The assistant should also avoid giving false hope to patients by casually mentioning the miracles being achieved every day in the fight for sight.

Blind people should not be regarded as unimportant or incompetent. Patients should be asked questions directly, not through a second party. Conversation should never be allowed to flow around or through them as though they did not exist. They should be treated as individuals without sight, not as ones without insight.

THE BLIND CHILD

Congenitally blind children, unlike some of their adult counterparts, have no recollection of the visual world to assist them. Without this visual memory, blind children must learn about the world by being exposed to the environment and provided with the opportunity to explore it through other senses. Although parents know their child best, early intervention by child development specialists who have training in visual impairment can offer additional support to parents and assist them with encouraging their child's normal development. Other professionals who can offer support with the habilitation needs of blind children include orientation and mobility specialists and life skills instructors. These personnel are trained to assist blind children and their families with the development of daily living skills and the attainment of safe independent travel skills.

The young child who does not have a visual memory may have to be physically shown and encouraged to develop skills such as creeping, walking, holding a spoon, and drinking from a cup. The blind child who has never seen these activities cannot rely on visual modeling as a learning tool. Parents of blind children must be patient and firm, allowing their child the opportunity to succeed by independently doing a task, as well as permitting the child to fail at times and learn from his or her mistakes.

It is important that some routine be established in the home to assist the blind child with understanding his or her environment. For example, it is easy for a totally blind child to confuse day with night; thus the routine of going to bed is important. Because bedtime is not accompanied by a change of light, a preliminary quiet period can be substituted. The blind child's language and concept development can be facilitated by bringing the child into direct association with the object or action while the appropriate words are being used. This helps the child to acquire a meaningful conceptual base.

Many congenitally blind children develop mannerisms such as rocking, touching and rubbing their eyes, or waving their hands. These and other repetitive motions are known as blindisms. Early intervention with blind children focuses on trying to help the child prevent these blindisms from developing. Once blindisms are established, diminishing them may require persistent effort on the part of the blind person to correct them.

It is estimated that up to 60% of young blind infants and preschool children in North America have additional motor and cognitive disabilities. One reason for this is the greater ability of modern medicine to save low-birthweight infants. Although many of these infants may be perfectly normal, premature infants with very low birthweights (<750 g) tend to have a greater incidence of disability. Blind children with additional disabilities require either a transdisciplinary team approach or a special school to effectively meet their diverse and unique habilitation needs.

Although most blind children receive their education through local schools in an integrated educational setting, the totally blind child requires some form of educational support services to assist with meaningful learning in the integrated classroom. Residential schools for blind children still exist in some areas, thus allowing families and school placement personnel choices and options to best meet the educational needs of the individual child.

Braille

One form of written communication the blind child may use is Braille, a system of raised dots on paper read by touching them with the ends of the fingers (Figure 46.1).

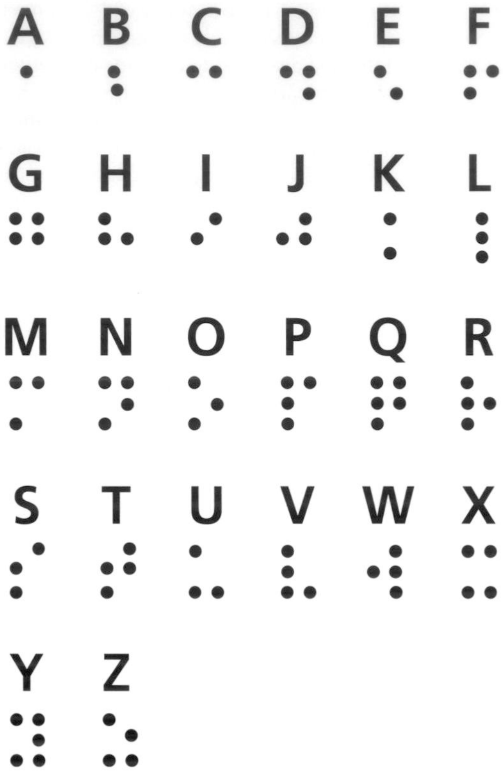

Figure 46.1 Braille alphabet based on six-dot system.

Although modern technology presents blind children with more communication options, the importance of Braille has not diminished as a tool for literacy.

The Braille system was developed by Louis Braille, a blind student who in 1824 developed a six-dot raised code. The Braille alphabet consists of combinations of one or more raised dots in a six-dot square known as the Braille cell, which is three dots high and two dots wide. There are 63 possible combinations of dots; after the letters of the alphabet are arranged, the remaining signs are used for punctuation, music, codes, and mathematics. Braille can be written through the aid of a slate, a Braille writer, or a computer system using a Braille printer. To facilitate the development of later Braille skills, young children are introduced early to activities to assist with the development of tactile sensitivity, manual dexterity, and fine motor development. Later, the preschool blind child receives training and materials that focus on pre-Braille readiness skills. The reading and writing of Braille are taught to blind children in the early years, and Braille is still useful in spite of the advanced computer technology available for many simple labeling and writing tasks (Figure 46.2). Some skilled Braille readers enjoy reading at night in the dark.

Braille libraries are available from which the blind student can obtain books. To supply textbooks for blind

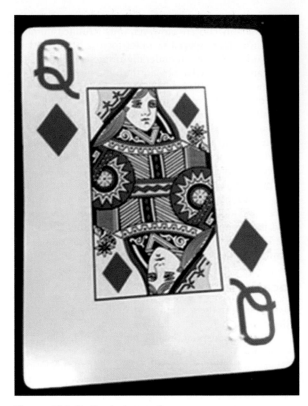

Figure 46.2 Braille playing card.

students in higher education in Canada, the Canadian National Institute for the Blind has developed a large group of volunteers who have learned to write the Braille system and spend many hours each week transferring printed pages into Braille. In other countries, similar organizations provide this service. Many popular magazines, trade journals, and periodicals are available in Braille. There is still a place for Braille for blind people, although it is less prevalent than in the past century.

Blind children now have access to the latest development in written communication. The proliferation of communication technology has made it possible for blind students to gain access to print information by computer through synthesized speech, large print, or Braille access modes. The combined use of these devices makes possible a scenario in which blind students can access a print exercise through synthesized speech or Braille modes, respond to the exercise in their chosen medium of Braille, and then make a print copy of their answers for the sighted teacher and a Braille copy of the answers for their own files. The Americans with Disabilities Act makes it possible for visually disabled children to receive a good education.

Some blind people may find it difficult to read Braille in an efficient manner with their fingers. To help these individuals, the talking book was developed. Books are recorded on a cassette. The blind person places the tape cassette into a device similar to a tape recorder, which is called a talking book machine. Some blind people do not like to be read to and do not enjoy talking books. They often say that the radio is their chief source of information and that they "listen" to television.

With the right support and appropriate early intervention for families, the capabilities of the blind child are limitless. Blind individuals today are independently employed successfully in an astounding variety of work roles. If society does not limit its expectations of the blind child, these children are capable of living fulfilling lives.

Ophthalmic assistant's role

The orientation of the blind child in an office or any situation is similar to that of an adult in that the assistant first introduces himself or herself to the child and family. With small children, the ophthalmic assistant can take their hand. With older children, the assistant can offer an arm, as for an adult. Children should be told in advance about the general geography of a room and the location of steps as they come to them. In the ophthalmologist's office, the assistant should lead the child to a chair, gently turn him or her, and, placing the child's hand on the arm of the chair, tell the child to sit on the chair at the side where the hand is placed. Again, the right and left sides should always be designated with reference to the position of the blind person. A blind child should be spoken to in a natural manner; these children are skilled in assessing people by the tone of their voice, just as a sighted child would assess a stranger by the person's facial expression.

REHABILITATION

Rehabilitation assists a totally blind person to acquire the practical skills to minimize the effects of disability and lead to independence and social competence.

Rehabilitation programs are often essential for working-age blind people to regain basic independent living skills that make possible further educational training or gainful employment. However, more than 70% of blind and visually impaired individuals are more than 65 years of age. For these individuals, prescribing low-vision aids and offering a rehabilitation program in daily living skills can contribute substantially to their quality of life and assist them with continuing to live in as independent an environment as possible.

Rehabilitation programs are usually staffed by a multidisciplinary team of professionals. The rehabilitation team assesses specific learning needs, develops a training program to meet these needs, and evaluates the blind person's progress in achieving established goals. Services include counseling, daily living skills instruction, orientation and mobility training, Braille and tape library services, sight enhancement services, and concept and sensory development, as well as the provision of consultation and educational information to caregivers, family members, and the general public.

Career development and employment

The goal of rehabilitation for working-age blind persons is competitive employment. Barriers faced by blind individuals seeking employment are related to educational background, skills, and attitudes.

In making an occupational choice, blind people must have information to make meaningful decisions. They need information about their own skills and interests, various occupations that they might find suitable, the technologic knowledge that would qualify them for the job, and how other blind persons have adapted various job tasks.

Occupations pursued by blind and visually impaired people cover the whole range of occupational categories, so there need be very few limits placed on their career aspirations. Obtaining the necessary information is still a problem for many blind and visually impaired persons. Expertise related to the disability and employment opportunities is often hard to find as mainstream employment services possess little knowledge of blindness and visual impairment. The specialized employment services for blind people are available from private organizations and from every state commission for the blind.

Prevailing public perceptions of the potential of blind people tend to influence employers' hiring practices. For this reason, the public education function of agencies for the blind is of critical importance. So too is the outreach function of specialized employment services for blind and visually impaired job seekers, in which employment counselors perform a marketing function on behalf of their clients.

The greatest single factor in increasing employment of blind individuals has been the emergence of information technology. Blindness is handicapping in terms of availability of information; thus access to information is of the utmost importance. Today, the prevocational education component of blind and visually impaired people, whether they are children or newly blinded adults, is in the field of electronic communications.

Vocations

Most rehabilitation programs place blind persons in a job within the sighted community. Job placements require, of course, that special safeguards be made available for the blind worker. It has been shown conclusively that the output of the blind worker in assembly work may be equal in both quantity and quality to that of sighted colleagues if the work is suitably chosen. However, only a limited number of industries have special facilities for the blind worker. Many workshops are run under the auspices of blind institutions and are geared to obviate the blind person's disability. Some blind people actually prefer working under these conditions because of the protections afforded them both physically and psychologically.

The active rehabilitation of blind people depends on many individual factors, such as aptitudes, skills, and training. The advancement of information technology has enabled the blind person access to the Internet and the ability to participate in many of the same things as their sighted peers. Blind people have gone on to attain advanced degrees and hold positions of management, law, social work, and economics. Many musicians are blind, and some have achieved a great measure of fame; pianist George Shearing is an excellent example.

Vocational teaching

The key figure in the rehabilitation of the blind is the rehabilitation teacher. These teachers, some who are blind themselves, are inspirational figures to an individual who has recently lost his or her sight and feels life is over. Such teachers understand very well the many small frustrations that accumulate daily and reduce the morale of the blind trainee. Their understanding of these frustrations and their own unwillingness to be defeated by such problems serve as an excellent example to individuals who have recently lost their sight. Rehabilitation teachers may teach Braille reading and computer skills. The function of the teacher is to show the newly blind person that skills still can be learned and acquired despite a handicap. The teacher is fundamentally a builder of confidence and self-esteem and one to open the minds of the blind person to the opportunities available.

AVAILABLE AIDS

Many ingenious devices have been designed to assist the blind person to cope with everyday living. Among these devices are Braille or talking watches and clocks (Figure 46.3). Braille watches typically have a spring catch that when pressed causes the watch glass to open, allowing the user to read the location of the raised hands on the Braille face of the watch. Talking watches announce the time aloud at the press of a button and many include auditory alarms. These watches are available in various designs, including both pocket and wrist types.

In addition, many computer-based technologic aids are available that provide audible access to information or Braille displays. Small portable devices such as the Braille 'n Speak, which has a Braille input keyboard and speech

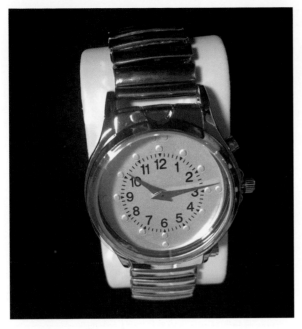

Figure 46.3 Braille watch.

output, allow the user to access a note taker, calculator, and appointment book, all in a device that weighs less than 2 pounds (0.9 kg).

Kitchen aids available for the blind homemaker include microwave ovens with Braille timers and controls, liquid level indicators, and triangular pie cutters. There are self-threading needles that consist of a groove at the back of the needle before the actual eye of the needle. The thread is positioned into this groove and a small tug pulls the thread into the eye of the needle. Measurements can be made with a tape measure with inches or centimeters marked off in elevated markings.

Among the medical aids are talking thermometers that announce the temperature. For the blind diabetic patient, insulin needle guides enable the person to locate the center of the rubber cap over the insulin bottle. There are also tactile raised markings on the syringe itself to measure the amount of insulin drawn up.

Recreation is a vital part of everyone's life in today's modern world. Tactile games have been developed by the adaptation of standard games such as bingo, chess, Scrabble, Monopoly, dominoes, and playing cards. For more vigorous exercise and recreation, blind individuals participate in all sports, including swimming, track, bowling, horseback riding, golf, hiking, and wrestling.

Questions for review and thought

1. In your area, what level of vision qualifies an individual to be considered as legally blind?
2. Imagine yourself having both eyes bandaged for 24 hours. Outline the inconvenience and problems you may be confronted with in your normal living.
3. Cover both eyes during a meal and try to cope with the problems of finding your silverware and eating.
4. What is the basis of the Braille system?
5. Name the agency or agencies in your area that help blind people.
6. What aids are available to help blind people?
7. Spend half a day touring your nearest agency for the blind and visually impaired. Outline your impressions and the facilities available.

Q Self-evaluation questions

True–false statements

Directions: Indicate whether the statement is true **(T)** or false **(F)**.

1. A legally blind person cannot read. **T** or **F**
2. The Braille system was developed by Louis Braille, a blind student who in 1824 developed a six-dot raised code. **T** or **F**
3. There is an association between blindness and mental retardation in the adult. **T** or **F**

Missing words

Directions: Write in the missing word(s) in the following sentences:

4. The mannerisms of blind children, such as rocking and rubbing their hands, are called _____.
5. Blindness is defined in the United States and Canada as vision of _____ or less in the best eye and a peripheral field no greater than _____.

Q Continued

Choice-completion questions

Directions: Select the one best answer in each case.

6. The blind person can:
   a. ski.
   b. go to university and become a doctor.
   c. be employed, with better records for safety, productivity, and punctuality than for sighted counterparts.
   d. play golf.
   e. all of the above.

7. Braille should be taught:
   a. to every blind person.
   b. only to the young blind person.
   c. to a person recently blinded.
   d. only to those who cannot possibly read with visual aids.
   e. to people going blind.

8. In North America the leading cause(s) of blindness is (are):
   a. cataracts.
   b. corneal disease.
   c. retinal disease.
   d. diseases of the vitreous.
   e. diseases relating to dryness of the eyes.

A Answers, notes, and explanations

1. **False.** A legally blind person may have 20/200 vision and, with adequate visual aids and good lighting, can read normal-sized print. The ability to compensate depends on the person's drive, determination, and intelligence. The worst handicap a blind person has is acceptance of his or her blindness as a totally incapacitating event. Only 25% of blind people have no light perception and are truly blind.

2. **True.** The Braille cell is three dots high and two dots wide. Most popular books are available in Braille. Also many magazines, such as *Reader's Digest,* have a Braille edition. Textbooks in Braille are also available and blind students have graduated in medicine, law, accounting, and other demanding courses of study.

3. **False.** People who are blind may have macular degeneration, diabetes, or glaucoma, none of which is associated with mental deterioration. In developing countries trachoma can cause blindness because of corneal scarring. Simple cataracts, undetected and untreated, are a common source of blindness. Whatever the cause, the blind person is commonly treated with pity, as though he or she not only cannot see but also cannot think properly.

4. **Blindisms.** These habit spasms are difficult to eradicate, but with trained help, they can be. They should be removed because such traits are an obvious stigma of a person's blindness.

5. **20/200, 20 degrees.** Blindness is not the absence of light perception; a person is considered blind only if unable to function in the ordinary world. With this definition there are many legally blind people who neither consider themselves blind, nor are they considered blind by others. In a sense, it is a state of mind.

6. **e. All of the above.** A protected environment is not needed for an ambitious, hardworking blind person. Blind people cannot fly a plane, drive a car, or play baseball. However, they can do many things at home, at work, or in sports without special assistance.

7. **d. Only to those who cannot possibly read with visual aids.** Although Braille has served the blind well for over 150 years (through Braille watches, typewriters, and so on), it does narrow the range of options for the blind. Only a small segment of the world's literature is turned into Braille symbols. The options for learning and promotion are far greater if the blind person can stay in the sighted world, even if it means a constant struggle. It is better to have a handicap than to be handicapped.

8. **c. Retinal disease.** Fortunately, cataracts and most forms of corneal disease can be treated surgically with great success. Diseases of the vitreous are usually secondary to retinal or ciliary body disorders. Whereas great advancement has been made in retinal disease, there are no replacement parts for a sick macula or optic nerve. When the macula is injured by disease or trauma, the effects are permanent. The optic nerve, the victim of such common disorders as temporal arteritis, glaucoma, and arteriosclerosis, cannot be helped once damaged. The retina and optic nerve play a major role in creating blindness simply because there is no therapy for these problems. Years ago, the same could be said for diseases of the cornea or lens.

Chapter | **47** |

Art and the eye

Phyllis L. Rakow

Vision is defined in *Webster's College Dictionary* as "the act or power of sensing with the eyes; sight." To an artist vision is much more than simply seeing. It represents a marriage of eye and brain: an interpretation of color, light, line and form, clarity, tone, proportion, depth, and dimension. As sight diminishes we see and record the world in a different light. A look at the works of many well-known artists raises a multitude of questions in the eyes of the astute observer. Did the painter deliberately change his style as he (or she) matured? Are the changes in color or technique related to changes in the way in which the artist was seeing things? If so, what was happening to his vision? Refractive error? Presbyopia? Cataracts? Diabetic retinopathy? Macular degeneration? Other pathology? Was he actually trying to depict the world as he saw it? Art history takes us behind the scenes. It explores evidence that helps to explain the theories that have been presented and leaves us with thoughts to contemplate when we have no way of obtaining documentation or proof. Let us examine some of these theories as we look into the lives and works of artists whose vision was dimmed by disease.

EL GRECO (1541–1614)

Art historians and ophthalmologists alike have studied the paintings of El Greco, born in 1541 on the Greek island of Crete, a possession, at that time, of the Republic of Venice. Although he trained in Italy, El Greco was most noted as a Spanish painter. It was to Spain, in 1570, that he brought his style of predominantly vertically elongated, isolated figures and mystical atmospheres, a style considered shocking at the time. Why were his figures so elongated? For almost a century, art connoisseurs and physicians alike have advanced theories attributing his elongations to an astigmatic refractive error. Patrick Trevor-Roper, a British ophthalmologist, stated that "in nearly all his paintings there is a vertical elongation but on a slightly oblique axis, so that all his characters seem to be in danger of falling off the bottom right-hand corner of the picture." Astigmatism elongates along its axis and Trevor-Roper notes that the distortion can be neutralized by photographing the paintings through a cylindric lens, plano -1.00×15.

When we place his paintings in the context of their times, however, we discover that a style of painting termed *mannerism* had developed and was popular in Europe from about 1520 to 1600. Mannerist paintings displayed great emotion and were characterized by figures that were distorted and deformed, stretched and exaggerated. X-rays of El Greco's paintings show the elongations superimposed on his normally proportioned original sketches. More evidence pointing to the influence of style, rather than astigmatism, on his work can be observed in paintings such as *Saint Andrew* (Figure 47.1), in which the fingers of the right hand are held *horizontally* and elongated; the fingers of the left hand point *vertically* and

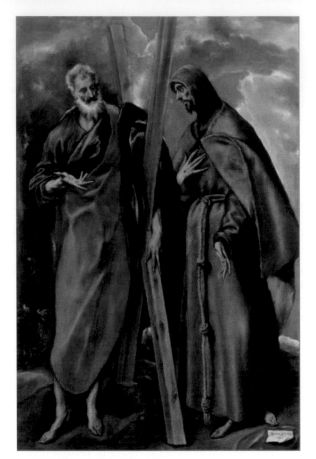

Figure 47.1 El Greco: *Saint Andrew.*
(From Marmor MF, Ravin JG. The eye of the artist. St Louis: Mosby; 1997.)

are also elongated. Could he have had one eye with hyperopic astigmatism that he used to see his subjects at a distance and the other with myopic astigmatism that he used at close range to see his canvas, one eye with with-the-rule astigmatism and one eye with against-the-rule astigmatism? As he grew older his figures became more and more elongated, an unusual occurrence if the elongations were caused by astigmatism, because astigmatism tends to remain stable in adults. The answer to our questions will forever remain an enigma.

THE EYES OF THE IMPRESSIONISTS

A fast-forward to the latter half of the 19th century brings us to the era of *Impressionism*. In their day, Impressionist paintings were considered shocking, radical, and revolutionary. Brushstrokes were quick and spontaneous, coarse,

thick, and sometimes broken; colors were often bold and daring and mixed directly on the canvas to be blended not by the painter but by the observer's eye. The artists attempted to capture a fleeting moment, an *impression*, and chose subjects from everyday life, from nature, from the rapid changes that were transforming the Western world into an industrial society: locomotives, bridges, city scenes, and factories rather than paintings that portrayed historical, religious, or mythical subjects or taught moral lessons. They attempted to portray the real world and experimented with light, color, candid groupings, off-center focal points, deep perspectives, and spontaneity. To many, their work seemed crude and unfinished, but the Impressionists felt themselves liberated from the strict formats that had ruled technique and subject matter in the past.

Many of these new works of art seemed out of focus. Had these unique techniques originated because of defects in sight? Did the rough brushstrokes portray the subjects the way the artists actually saw them, or did they represent the attempt of the artist to capture an instant in time with rapid, incomplete movements of the hand that suggested motion: trains, parades, people at work, dancers, strollers, party-goers?

Because so many of the well-known Impressionist paintings appear misty and obscure, it has been written that most Impressionist painters were myopic and preferred to view their subjects without optical correction. Paul Cézanne was reported to be myopic (as well as affected with diabetic retinopathy) and, although glasses were available to correct his refractive error, he stated: "Take those vulgar things away." His landscapes are hazy and indistinct; his still-life paintings, done at close range, show clarity and detail. Would he agree with the remark of Mr. Cross, the Vicar of Chew Magna in Somerset, England, who was purported to say, "The newly invented optick glasses are immoral because they pervert the natural sight and make things appear in an unnatural and false light" or an epitaph in the church of Santa Maria Maggiore in Florence, Italy, that reads "Here lies Salvino d'Armato, of the Armati of Florence, Inventor of spectacles: may God forgive him his sins. AD 1317." Or, by painting through his myopic eyes, was he trying to portray a softer, gentler world?

CLAUDE MONET (1840–1926)

The term *Impressionism* was coined in 1873 when Claude Monet was asked to name one of his paintings for an exhibition. He called it *Impression: Sunrise* and he and his contemporaries in the fledgling movement of innovative painters soon came to be known as *Impressionists*. Monet studied the subtleties of changing light and recorded these nuances with different versions of the same motif at different times of day and changing weather conditions, moving from one canvas to another to capture the sun and shadow as the world turned. He is said to have wished that he "had been born blind in order to experience sight suddenly: to see the world naively, as pure shape and color." He actually did experience temporary blindness at the age of 27, which was attributed to worries about his wife, Camille, who was about to give birth to his son, Jean.

As he entered his 66th year, Monet became aware of changes in his vision, although bilateral cataracts were not diagnosed until 4 years later. He consulted with several ophthalmologists, but was advised to defer surgery. Although the cataract in his right eye was almost mature and the eye virtually useless, he was deathly afraid of surgery. His close friend, the diplomat Georges Clemenceau, had been a physician and helped to provide both medical advice and a shoulder to lean on. Although Clemenceau assured Monet that his sight could be restored through surgery, Monet remained opposed to an operation. By 1918, then 78 years old, Monet reported:

"I no longer perceived colors with the same intensity. I no longer painted light with the same accuracy. Reds appeared muddy to me, pinks insipid and the intermediate or lower tones escaped me...."

"'At first I tried to be stubborn. How many times, near the little bridge where we are now, have I stayed for hours under the harshest sun, sitting on my campstool, in the shade of my parasol, forcing myself to resume my interrupted task and recapture the freshness that had disappeared from my palette! Wasted efforts. What I painted was more and more dark, more and more like an "old picture," and when the attempt was over and I compared it to former works, I would be seized by a frantic rage and slash all my canvases with a penknife.'"

Subtle differences in color became difficult to distinguish, although vivid colors were still visible against a dark background, and the bright noonday sun forced him to abandon painting at midday. Aware of his problems differentiating colors, he arranged his paints according to their labels, in a set sequence, on his palette. Acknowledging that he was unable to select colors appropriately, he destroyed a number of canvases. By now, his cataracts had become brunescent and were affecting his color perception by filtering out blue, violet, and some shades of green. His paintings reflected his vision and became increasingly hazy and more red, yellow, and brown (Figures 47.2 and 47.3).

Although Monet had agreed to produce 19 large water lily panels that the French government would place in the Orangerie Museum in Paris, he felt, by 1922, that he would be unable to complete the project. In a letter, he lamented:

"I wished to profit from what little [remained of] my vision in order to bring certain of my decorations to completion. And I was gravely mistaken. For in the end, I had to admit that I was ruining them, that I was no longer capable of making something of beauty. And I destroyed several of

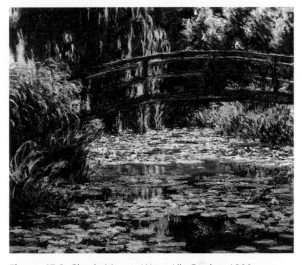

Figure 47.2 Claude Monet: *Water Lily Garden,* 1900.
(From Marmor MF, Ravin JG. The eye of the artist. St Louis: Mosby; 1997. Mr. and Mrs. Larned Coburn Memorial Collection. Reproduction, The Art Institute of Chicago.)

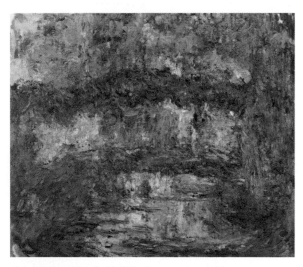

Figure 47.3 Claude Monet: *Japanese Footbridge at Giverny,* 1923.
(From Marmor MF, Ravin JG. The eye of the artist. St Louis: Mosby; 1997. Musée Marmottan, Paris. Bridgeman Art Library.)

my panels. Today I am almost blind and I have to renounce my work completely."

By September 1922, Monet's vision had decreased to light perception with projection OD and 20/200 OS. Yet he continued to resist surgery. An attempt was made to enhance the vision in his left eye by dilating the pupil with eucatropine hydrochloride, a mydriatic used at that time, so he could see around the opacity. For a brief period of time, it seemed to help. Monet wrote to his ophthalmologist:

"It is all simply marvelous. I have not seen so well for a long time.…The drops have permitted me to paint good things rather than the bad paintings which I had persisted in making when seeing nothing but fog."

Within a month, however, he realized the futility of his strategy to circumvent surgery and agonized over the inevitable procedure. He wrote to Clemenceau about his torment and nightmares. At the time, cataract surgery was a complex procedure. Monet knew of others, including the American Impressionist Mary Cassatt and the French caricaturist Honore Daumier, who had undergone unsuccessful cataract extractions and he became increasingly despondent. Finally, in January 1923, in response to the strong urging of Georges Clemenceau, who reminded him of his agreement with the French government to complete the water lily panels, Monet underwent an extracapsular cataract extraction, which had been preceded by an iridectomy the month before. The only anesthetic available was cocaine and the surgeon probably used no sutures or perhaps just one.

Monet found it difficult to adapt to the postsurgical regimen of lying in total darkness, both eyes bandaged shut, flat on his back (with no pillow), his head between sandbags to prevent movement and with no nourishment except bouillon and lime tea, for 10 days. The only time light entered his eyes during this period was when the bandages were removed from his right eye every hour or two to instill eyedrops. Monet had to be forcibly restrained from tearing off his bandages and expressed a preference for being blind rather than having his eyes covered. He was attended by a guardian at night, not only to make sure he did not move but also to engage in conversation because lack of contact with the outside world could cause delirium or psychotic behavior. Three weeks after surgery, he was given a pair of temporary cataract glasses and began his "adjustment" to the aphakic world.

As anticipated by his ophthalmologist, the posterior capsule opacified, necessitating still another surgical procedure. Severe depression set in. He wrote to his surgeon, Dr. Charles Coutela:

"'I am absolutely discouraged and as much as I read, not without effort, 15 to 20 pages per day, outdoors from a distance, I cannot see anything with or without glasses [with the right eye]. And for 2 days, black spots have bothered me.

"Remember that it has been 6 months since the first operation, 5 since I left the clinic and 4 that I have been wearing glasses. It has taken me 4 or 5 weeks to get used to my new vision. Six months that I would have been able to work if you had told me the truth.

"It is to my chagrin that I regret having had this fatal operation. Pardon me for speaking so frankly and let me tell you that it is criminal to have put me in this situation."

Dr. Coutela noted Monet's "profound discouragement and despair" and related that "Monet saw himself as blind

forever and, completely demoralized, refused to leave his bed." The secondary membrane was removed at Monet's home in Giverny in July 1923, after which he was able to achieve vision of about 20/30 in his right eye with a prescription of $+10.00 + 4.00 \times 90$. Unfortunately, because he refused to have the cataract in his left eye removed, he was unable to use his eyes together. The brunescent cataract in his left eye caused him to experience a marked difference in color perception between the two eyes. The colors seen with his left eye were muddied by the cataract; with his right eye, the lost blues and violets returned with a vengeance. He painted his house, as seen from the rose garden, through the mature cataract in his left eye (Figure 47.4) and the aphakic (probably uncorrected) vision in his right (Figure 47.5).

Monet found it difficult to adjust to aphakic spectacles. He was bothered by the abnormal curvature of objects caused by the high-plus astigmatic lens for his right eye and had difficulty walking with his glasses. He expressed his disappointment in a letter to Dr. Coutela:

"I have just received them [new glasses] today but I am absolutely desolated for, in spite of all my good will, I feel that if I take a step, I will fall on the ground. For near and far everything is deformed, doubled and it has become intolerable to see. To persist seems dangerous to me."

And to Clemenceau, he wrote:

"I'm doing exercises and can read easily but the distortion and exaggerated colors that I see are quite terrifying. As for going for a walk in these spectacles, it's out of the question for the moment anyway and if I was condemned to see nature as I see it now, I'd prefer to be blind and keep my memories of the beauties I've always seen."

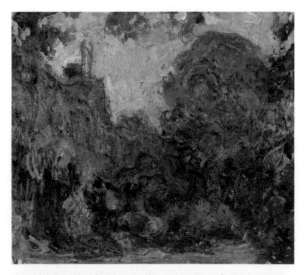

Figure 47.4 Claude Monet: *The House Seen from the Rose Garden*, 1923.
(From Marmor MF, Ravin JG. The eye of the artist. St Louis: Mosby; 1997. Musée Marmottan, Paris. Bridgeman Art Library.)

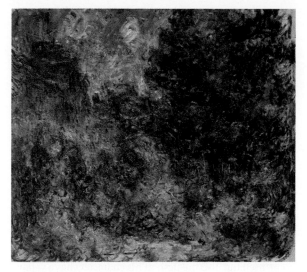

Figure 47.5 Claude Monet: *The Artist's House Seen from the Rose Garden*, 1923.
(From Marmor MF, Ravin JG: The Eye of the Artist. St Louis: Mosby, 1997. Musée Marmottan, Paris. Bridgeman Art Library.)

Clemenceau urged him to have surgery on the second eye but he responded:

"I absolutely refuse, for the moment at least, to have the operation done to my left eye. … You can have no idea of the state I'm in as regards my sight and the alteration of colors…so unless I find a painter, of whatever kind, who's had the operation and can tell me that he can see the same colors he did before, I won't allow it."

Aphakic glasses, even today with corrected curve lenses, have a great deal of aberration; they create a ring scotoma that restricts the wearer's peripheral vision and induce magnification of 1.5% to 2% per diopter of correction, making it impossible for patients who have had surgery in only one eye to use their eyes together. Monet had to block his unoperated left eye with a piece of paper or, in a later pair of glasses, what appears to be an occluder lens. He had separate glasses for near and distance rather than bifocals, and experienced far greater distortion, as well as spherical and chromatic aberration, than a wearer of contemporary aphakic spectacles would today. The high magnification and high astigmatic correction contributed to his depression and his refusal to have surgery on the contralateral eye. A pair of his aphakic spectacles on display at the Musée Marmottan in Paris reads: OD + 14.00 + 7.00 × 90; OS plano. He complained of overwhelming blue and yellow vision and expressed his desolation to Dr. Coutela:

"For months I have worked with obstinacy, without achieving anything good. I am destroying everything that is mediocre. Is it my age? Is it defective vision? Both certainly, but vision particularly. You have given me back the sight of black on white, to read and write and I cannot

be too grateful for that but I am certain that the vision of [this] painter…is lost and all is for nothing.

"I am telling you this confidentially. I hide it as much as possible but I am terribly sad and discouraged. Life is a torture for me."

Eventually Monet was fitted with a Zeiss aphakic spectacle lens, which had a wider field of vision. He continued to complain about colors:

"I see blue; I no longer see red or yellow. This annoys me terribly because I know that these colors exist, because I know that on my palette there is some red, some yellow, a special green and a certain violet….It's filthy, it's disgusting, I see nothing but blue. …"

Relief was finally achieved and a more normal perception of blue obtained with glasses that were tinted yellow-green, allowing him to better adapt to his aphakic vision. He still experienced dramatic mood swings that are evidenced in letters he wrote in the final years of his life:

"I am more certain than ever that a painter's eyesight can never be recovered. When a singer loses his voice he retires; the painter who has undergone an operation of the cataract must renounce painting and this is what I have been incapable of."

But a few months later, in a letter to Dr. Coutela, he wrote:

"I am very happy to inform you that I have recovered my true vision and that nearly at a single stroke. I am happily seeing everything again and I am working with ardor."

Monet continued to paint until his death, at age 86, from lung cancer and chronic obstructive pulmonary disease, retouching and completing his water lily series, which can be seen today at the recently restored Orangerie in Paris.

VINCENT VAN GOGH (1853–1890)

Vincent Willem van Gogh was born into a Dutch family of preachers a year to the day after his stillborn brother and given the same name as the firstborn son. Although he studied for the ministry and tried his hand at teaching, he gradually drifted into a troubled and tragic life as an artist.

Many theories have been put forth in an attempt to explain his mental illness, bizarre behavior, and artistic technique. As an adult, particularly during the last 2 years of his life, he experienced periods during which he appeared to be perfectly normal and lucid, interspersed with episodes of severe mental disturbances. His mental illness has been attributed to epilepsy, bipolar illness, schizophrenia, Méniére's disease, and chemical toxicity. More recently, the possibility of porphyria, a genetic disease caused by an enzyme deficiency and manifested by symptoms that include abdominal pain and neurologic and psychiatric disturbances, has been proposed as the cause of his bizarre behavior because others in his family also exhibited symptoms of insanity. However, dark urine is characteristic of porphyria, and scholars have found no references to this in his letters nor has any other medical documentation been uncovered.

How can we envision van Gogh's vision? Did his paintings reflect an abnormality of vision? Trevor-Roper hazards a guess that van Gogh was short-sighted, based on the fact that his paintings are best viewed within a short radius; the subjects in his paintings are placed at an unusually close range; and that he had a "childhood habit of walking with half-shut eyes, hunched shoulders, looking at his feet, and being a duffer [incompetent] at ball games." Ravin and Marmor, though, report that in May of 1890, van Gogh's vision was informally tested by Dr. Paul Ferdinand Gachet, a homeopathic physician, amateur artist, and rather eccentric individual himself. Gachet was entrusted with van Gogh's care after van Gogh left the mental institution in Provence, where he had admitted himself after cutting off part of his left ear. Van Gogh was intrigued by an eye chart hanging on the wall of Gachet's country home in Auvers-sur-Oise, north of Paris. On reading the letters on the chart and also being tested for color vision with the materials that Gachet used to test railroad workers, he was found to have excellent visual acuity and normal color vision. In spite of these findings, many questions have been raised about his style and use of color, particularly during the last 2 or 3 years of his life.

Van Gogh's halos

The colored halos and swirls in the sky in *Starry Night* (Figure 47.6), perhaps van Gogh's most well-known painting, and similar waviness and halos in some of his other works, have been the subject of much analysis. In *Starry Night* the moon and sun are superimposed, stars magnified and surrounded by halos, and the sky filled with swirling nebulae. Some think that the painting resulted from a dramatic revelation that he experienced during a vivid hallucination. Others have entertained the possibility that the colored halos were indicative of an attack of angle-closure glaucoma, although there is no reference to the nausea, intense pain, and severe clouding of vision that accompany an angle-closure glaucoma attack in any of his letters, most of which have been preserved. Perhaps, as used by previous artists symbolically in religious paintings, the aura in the sky represented his "sentimental attachment to stars from his youth…when he felt a need for religion, he went out at night and painted them."

Xanthopsia

Even more fascinating is van Gogh's preoccupation with the color yellow. In many of his paintings, not only the scene itself but also the flesh of his characters has a yellowish cast (Figures 47.7 and 47.8). Was this a result of a conscious choice of yellow pigments or was the yellow vision caused by xanthopsia? If, indeed, he was experiencing

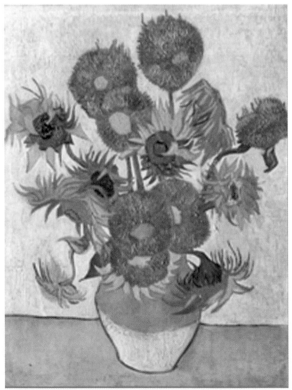

Figure 47.7 Vincent van Gogh: *Still Life With Fourteen Sunflowers*, 1889.
(From Mühlberger R: The unseen Van Gogh. Chesterfield, MA: Chameleon Books; 1998. Van Gogh Museum, Amsterdam, The Netherlands.)

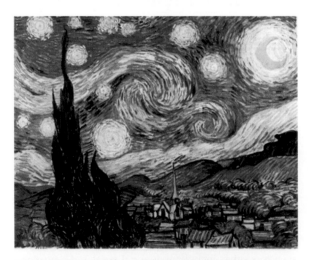

Figure 47.6 Vincent van Gogh: *Starry Night*, 1889.
(From Mühlberger R: The unseen Van Gogh. Chesterfield, MA: Chameleon Books; 1998. Museum of Modern Art, New York, NY.)

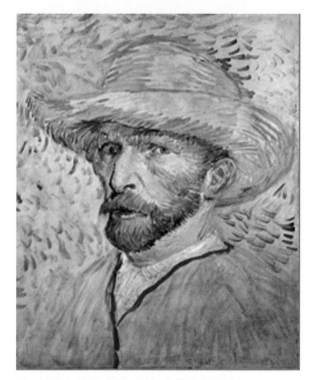

Figure 47.8 Vincent van Gogh: *Self-Portrait With Straw Hat,* 1889.

(From Mühlberger R: The unseen Van Gogh. Chesterfield, MA: Chameleon Books; 1998. Van Gogh Museum, Amsterdam, The Netherlands.)

xanthopsia, was it caused by substance abuse or chemical toxicity?

In March 1889, in a letter to his brother, art dealer Theo van Gogh, he wrote:

"M. Rey [a physician] says that instead of eating enough and at regular times, I was keeping myself going by coffee and alcohol. I admit all that but it is true all the same that to attain the high yellow note that I attained last summer, I really had to be pretty well strung up."

By July he appeared to have given up alcohol and wrote to Theo:

"I drank in the past because I did not know how to do otherwise. Anyway, I don't care in the least!!! Very deliberate sobriety—it's true—leads nevertheless to a state of being in which thought, if you have any, moves more readily. In short it is a difference like painting in grey or in colors. I am going in fact to paint more in grey."

While van Gogh was hospitalized in Arles after cutting off part of his ear, he was diagnosed by a psychiatric intern as having a seizure disorder. Today we think of digitalis as a medication used for patients with heart abnormalities. In van Gogh's day the drug was also used to treat seizure disorders, and digitalis toxicity was a known cause of yellow vision. No evidence has ever surfaced to indicate that van

Gogh's seizures were ever treated with digitalis, but some interesting theories have been put forward.

The eccentric Dr. Gachet, responsible for the care of van Gogh in Auvers, "was known as Dr. Saffron because he dyed his hair yellow." Van Gogh was much aware of Gachet's unconventional demeanor and wrote to Theo:

"I have seen Dr. Gachet, who made the impression on me of being rather eccentric but his experiences as a doctor must keep him balanced while fighting the nervous trouble from which he certainly seems to be suffering at least as seriously as I."

Digitalis was also a homeopathic remedy used, among other things, for managing "melancholic thoughts, hypochondria, mental illness, headache, nausea, vomiting, pain in the eyes, swelling of the eyelids, tearing, and inflammation of the eyes" and Gachet was a homeopathic practitioner. He has been accused of overdosing van Gogh with digitalis and mismanaging his care. Yet Gachet was said to understand the physiologic dangers of digitalis and its potential for problems. He also felt that van Gogh's mental illness, which he diagnosed as manic depression (which would explain the periods of lucidity that alternated with periods of mania and melancholy), was not treatable at that time with medication.

There are substances other than digitalis that can cause yellow vision, one of them being santonin, which was used at that time as a preventive medicine and antibacterial agent to treat intestinal parasites. Van Gogh was known to have digestive problems and may have been treated with santonin for them. He was thought to have abnormal cravings (pica) for camphor, thujone, and turpentine, which are chemically similar to santonin. He might have ingested santonin to relieve the pica. He was also an insomniac and known to use large doses of camphor as a sleep remedy, often drank absinthe, a potent alcoholic beverage that contained thujone, and was reported by the artist Paul Signac to express the desire to consume a large amount of turpentine.

Although there is much support for the hypothesis that van Gogh's xanthopsia was chemically induced, other evidence fails to substantiate the findings. Van Gogh often experimented with color. In a letter he wrote:

"Monticelli was a painter who painted the south all in yellow, orange and sulfur colors. Most painters do not see these colors because they are not really experts in color."

And in 1885, he argued:

"Suppose I have to paint an autumn landscape, trees with yellow leaves. All right—when I conceive it as a symphony in yellow, what does it matter if the fundamental color of yellow is the same as that of the leaves or not?"

And Gauguin commented:

"Oh yes, he loved yellow, this good Vincent, this painter from Holland—those glimmers of sunlight rekindled his soul that abhorred the fog, that needed the warmth."

The collection of van Gogh's letters contains numerous passages dealing with his experimentation with other colors and he studied the basic color triangle, complementary colors, color harmonies, and color contrasts. The truth remains a mystery.

Fame came to van Gogh only after his death. On July 27, 1890, at the age of 37, he could bear his loneliness and torments no longer. He shot himself with a revolver in the fields through which he had often wandered and painted, and although mortally wounded and in excruciating pain, struggled back to his room at the inn. He died 2 days later, in his brother Theo's arms. Although only one of his paintings was sold during his lifetime, he always felt that fame would be achieved after his death. He had written:

"Just as we take the train to get to Tarascon or Rouen, we take death to reach a star. One thing absolutely true in this reasoning is that we cannot get to a star while we are alive, any more than we can take a train when we are dead."

EDGAR DEGAS (1834–1917)

When we hear the name Degas we often visualize ballet dancers in motion, soft, hazy pastel renditions, smudges of flesh coloring across a featureless face, off-center focal points. Were these deliberate stylistic schemes, or were they related in some way to a disturbance in his vision? Examination of Degas' early works of art reveals finely detailed facial features and central focal points. His medium of choice in the early years was oil on canvas, and his color vision appeared to be normal.

We have learned from Degas' letters and accounts from his contemporaries that he began to experience progressive loss of vision at an early age and, by the time he was 36 years old and a member of the National Guard during the Franco-Prussian war, he was unable to see a rifle target with his right eye. He attributed this loss of vision to exposure to extreme weather conditions that he experienced during his service as a sentinel at the time of the siege of Paris. Later, he blamed it on a "cold in the eye" that he developed at the age of 19 when forced to live in a garret after his father cut off his allowance. He was bothered by bright sunlight and cold weather, blaming them for his eye weakness, and, unlike his fellow Impressionists, abandoned open-air painting for the comfort of cafés, dance studios, opera houses, offices, and other indoor venues.

During a trip to New Orleans in 1873, Degas complained of the strong Louisiana sunlight. He also became acquainted with his first cousin, Estelle, who had become his sister-in-law. By the time she was 25, little vision remained in her left eye and, within 7 years, she became blind in both eyes. Like Degas, her loss of vision was progressive, affected just one eye initially and ultimately resulted in bilateral loss of vision. The trip to New Orleans increased Degas' anxiety about his own vision and he began to realize that he, too, probably had a progressive, incurable eye condition, which at that time was simply referred to as *ophthalmia*. After his return, he wrote to fellow artist, James Tissot, that he expected to remain in the ranks of the infirm until he passed into the ranks of the blind.

As his vision deteriorated, he described a blind spot in the center of his field of vision and spoke of his difficulty in trying to see around this blind spot when he was drawing or painting. He described painting as "an exercise of circumvention." He experienced a loss of central vision in both eyes during the next two decades, which, today, would classify him as legally blind. Eventually he lost the ability to differentiate colors and needed assistance to identify them. The softness of his early works evolved into coarser compositions with more intense colors. When he became resigned to the reality that there was no hope for his eye condition to improve, he looked for solace and help from the sisters of a religious order and began exploring other media. Pastels replaced oils. Faces lost their features. Focal points moved to the periphery (Figure 47.9), with few details in the center. He turned to sculpture (Figure 47.10) because he was able to use his sense of touch, and he experimented with photography.

Degas' medical records have been lost, but his symptoms have received much attention from contemporary ophthalmologists. Some of his glasses are in the possession of the Musée d'Orsay in Paris. They include neutral gray plano pince-nez glasses, which block out 85% of incoming light; deep blue-tinted pince-nez glasses with a small correction for myopic astigmatism; deeply tinted regular spectacles with a −1.50 sphere correction OU; and an unusual pair of spectacles with an occluder lens for the right eye and a stenopeic slit at 160 degrees for his left, which aligned with

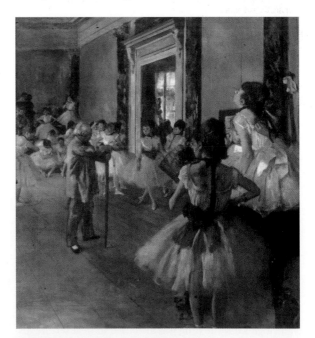

Figure 47.9 Edgar Degas: *La Classe de Danse,* vers 1873–76. Musée D'Orsay, Paris.

What Degas might have created if he had retained good vision throughout his life will never be known, but the masterworks that he did produce have not only contributed to the annals of art but also enabled the medical community to analyze and interpret the path from his eye, to his brain, to his canvas.

CAMILLE PISSARRO (1830–1903)

The French Impressionist movement was profoundly influenced by a West Indian-born Sephardic Jew of Portuguese Marrano descent, Camille Pissarro, who, with Claude Monet, is regarded as a cofounder of Impressionism. Educated in France and returning there at the age of 25 to establish a long and prolific career, his wisdom, integrity, and benevolence made his fellow artists turn to him for comfort and advice and earned him the title of "Père Pissarro."

Pissarro's early years in France were spent in the Île de France, just north of Paris, where he painted under open skies, applying Impressionist techniques to the everyday scenes around him…village streets, country meadows, landscapes with peasants, farmers, strollers, fruit gatherers, fragments of rural life. He was characterized as myopic, with scarring from corneal ulcers that dated back to childhood, making his personal world a constant Impressionist panorama.

As the sixth decade of his life drew to a close he developed a chronic inflammation of his right nasolacrimal duct. A firm believer in homeopathic medicine and one who regarded conventional medicine with mistrust ever since the death of his friend, the artist Edouard Manet, he located an ophthalmologist, Dr. Daniel Parenteau, who was an advocate of homeopathic therapy. Initially he was advised that the problem was not serious and that rest would bring recovery, but recurrent inflammation, necessitating a probing, revealed a bony obstruction. Pissarro described his visit to Dr. Parenteau:

"After having skillfully probed the lacrimal canal, he told me there was a growth of bone that was obstructing the canal's passage: generally one forces the passage but he told me that it is absolutely dangerous. The consequences are disastrous.…Here is what he advised me: To take a homeopathic medicine [Aurum] in order to reconstitute the covering of the bone, which is bare and let the tissues heal themselves; it will take at least 6 months. But precautions must be taken—avoid wind, dust, wash the eye with boric acid immediately. All that is hardly easy for a painter who has to face the elements."

The inflamed passages eventually had to be incised and drained to obtain relief. Recurrent abscesses developed and, with each episode, Pissarro was forced to protect the eye from the elements with a patch. The homeopathic medication failed to prevent abscess formation and Pissarro, unable to paint, returned to Paris for additional therapy, this time with injections of silver nitrate.

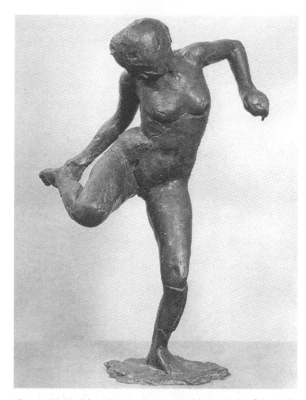

Figure 47.10 Edgar Degas: *Dancer Looking at Sole of the Right Foot.*
(From Marmor MF, Ravin JG. The eye of the artist. St Louis: Mosby; 1997. Musée Marmottan, Paris. Bridgeman Art Library.)

his astigmatic axis. This was meant to reduce dispersion of light, but Degas found the spectacles useless and embarrassing to wear. Trevor-Roper assumed that the stenopeic slit was used to improve vision that was affected by irregular astigmatism, but stenopeic slits were also used for other eye conditions, particularly for reducing glare.

Degas' condition was referred to as *chorioretinitis*, a catch-all term used in the 19th century for a broad spectrum of retinal diseases, and some analysts suggested that he might have had uveitis or corneal disease. Present knowledge points to a form of macular degeneration, certainly not age-related, and possibly familial. Retinal disease would also explain his extreme sensitivity to light and progressive loss of color perception. Because blue cone deficiencies are associated with central retinal disease, this might explain the prevalence of red and limited use of blue as his vision loss increased, as well as his use of more intense colors.

Did Degas eventually become totally blind? In photographs taken late in life his eyes appear to be orthophoric, which would indicate that he retained at least some peripheral vision and was thus able to attain peripheral fusion. It has also been pointed out that if the right eye was totally blind, he would not have needed an occluder lens in his glasses.

"Right now Parenteau [who was not averse to using conventional medical treatment when necessary] is giving me injections of silver nitrate [to close off the abnormal passageways that had been created by probing] while waiting for another abscess to form. When that happens and the eye is sufficiently inflamed, he will perform the slight operation necessary [to drain the abscess]. So the thing is only deferred. I will probably now not suffer from abscesses so constantly, thus I will be able to do a little work. Besides, I am getting used to the idea of working with just one eye, which is certainly better than none."

Pissarro consulted with other ophthalmologists and received conflicting advice that ranged from destruction of the lacrimal sac, which could cause constant tearing, to attempting to locate the passage through the bone to the nose, the only two ways of treating dacryocystitis that were available in France at the time. Complications of probing included the creation of false passages, cellulitis, and further scarring. Afraid of surgery, Pissarro decided to remain a patient of Parenteau. Large doses of quinine were prescribed as preventive medicine, but recurrences erupted from time to time. He described his treatment to his son, Lucien, in a letter dated 1897:

"I am afraid of complications for my eye. I have gone daily for a dozen days to Parenteau, who has been cauterizing me and has been putting an astringent on the veins of the eye…Parenteau gave me silver nitrate drops to put in the eye and on the lids. This is hardly easy. Every morning there is more pus in the eye, so that I dare not venture a trip. Your mother advised me not to leave [to see his son, Titi, who was dying of tuberculosis in London]."

Abandoning the woods and fields of the Île de France (Figure 47.11) for the comfort and safety of an indoor environment, Pissarro moved his paints and easel indoors and

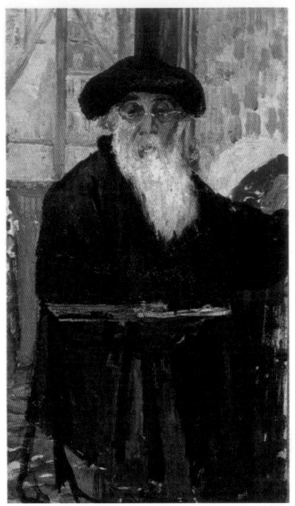

Figure 47.12 Camille Pissarro: *Self-Portrait*, 1898. *(From Marmor MF, Ravin JG. The eye of the artist. St Louis: Mosby; 1997.)*

set them up in front of windows. There, he could paint without cold, wind, and dust and, looking out, he created cityscapes that are now considered to be some of his finest works. It was not until 1904, a year after Pissarro's death, that an Italian surgeon, Toti, published a paper on his procedure, dacryocystorhinostomy, which opened the door to modern lacrimal surgery. One mystery remains: if, as Trevor-Roper claims, Pissarro was myopic, why is he wearing half-glasses, pushed slightly down on his nose, in several of his self-portraits (Figure 47.12)?

MARY CASSATT (1844–1926)

Mary Cassatt, the most well-known American Impressionist, spent most of her life in France, developing friendships with her French contemporaries and exhibiting at four of

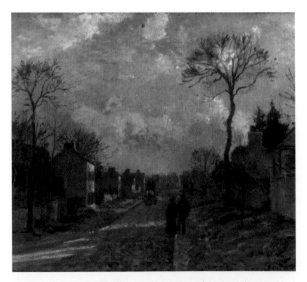

Figure 47.11 Camille Pissarro: *La Route de Louveciennes*, 1872. Musée d'Orsay, Paris.

the eight Impressionist shows. Unlike her French counterparts, she eschewed landscapes and chose predominantly indoor settings of mothers and children. Her paintings also differed from theirs in technique, her brushstrokes being smooth rather than coarse and broken (Figures 47.13 and 47.14).

Cassatt began to experience difficulty with her vision around 1900, although cataracts were not diagnosed until she was 68, in 1912. She had also been diagnosed with diabetes and, because insulin was not available until the 1920s, bizarre methods of treatment were attempted. Radium was the miracle discovery of the early 20th century and was being used to treat diabetes and even cataracts. In a letter dated December 14, 1911, while undergoing treatment for her diabetes, Cassatt wrote:

"I am at the doctor's taking inhalations of radium. This is the eighth day and I am suffering very much, which it seems would prove that it is doing me good, that it will be a success provided I can stand it."

There is no mention about Cassatt being treated with radium for her cataracts, but a 1920 article in the *American Journal of Ophthalmology*, titled "Radium for Cataract," reported that:

"Of the 31 patients under observation, 84.3% showed a change for the better. In the cases that showed a marked improvement, the opacities were definitely thinned out; one of these, a very early nuclear cataract, disappeared entirely, leaving no trace of the opacities. Radium is of proven value in the treatment of incipient cataracts."'

Another article, "The Technic of Radium Application in Cataracts," was published in 1920 in the *American Journal of Roentgenology* and concluded that "the application of radium is harmless to the normal tissues of the eye." The dangers of radium were yet to be discovered. In fact, Marie Curie, the discoverer of radium, developed cataracts herself and had to undergo surgery in both eyes.

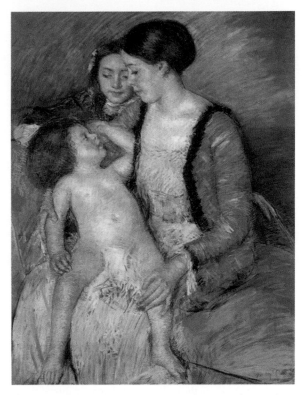

Figure 47.14 Mary Cassatt: *Young Mother, Daughter and Baby.*
(From Marmor MF, Ravin JG. The eye of the artist. St Louis: Mosby; 1997. Memorial Art Gallery of the University of Rochester. Marion Stratton Gould, Fund.)

As Cassatt's cataracts progressed, her brushstrokes became coarser and thicker, her colors harsher, her paintings less delicate. By 1913, she wrote:

"My eyes, which have always been my strong point, are troubling me. If I only was sure of a good oculist but Dr. Whitman is again away. I don't know for how long."

And, later that year:

"My oculist has turned out terribly. I have conjunctivitis, an inflammation of the eyelids. He said it was nothing, that I had good sight, one eye very good, the other not so good but not very bad. Then when I saw him again, change of front. Wants to keep me here 2 months and try experiments on the poorer eye, trained nurse to assist at the operation twice a week! Dr. Whitman was horrified. He told me plainly it was to make money…one goes for a little simple advice and to be tested for glasses and they see a chance of making money and do not hesitate to rush making you blind! My theory is that they get so hardened with vivisection that human suffering is nothing to them."

Cassatt underwent cataract surgery in her right eye in 1917. On December 28, 1917, she wrote:

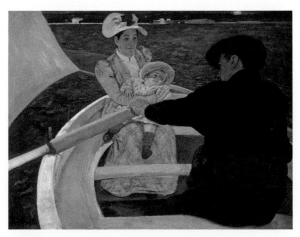

Figure 47.13 Mary Cassatt: *The Boating Party.*
(From Marmor MF, Ravin JG. The eye of the artist. St Louis: Mosby; 1997.)

"Operating on my right eye before the cataract was ripe is the last drop. …The sight of that eye is inferior but I still saw a good deal in spite of the cataract. Now I see scarcely at all."

Following the extracapsular extraction, the capsule opacified, necessitating additional surgery the following year. Cassatt wrote:

"The secondary cataract is covering the right eye which was operated on in October and no doubt it can be removed in the fall. The operation, which was made in October and followed by so long a treatment, was a complete failure and ought not to have been attempted, if only it has not injured what there was of sight in that eye! The cataract over the left eye, which is the eye in which depends my hope of future sight, is not nearly ripe or I could not write this to you.…'"

A month later, she wrote:

"My sight is getting dimmer every day. I find writing tires my eyes. I look forward with horror to utter darkness and then an operation which may end in as great a failure as the last one."

The cataract in her left eye was removed in October of 1919 and was probably an intracapsular extraction. Afterward, Cassatt wrote:

"The operation was a very daring one as the cataract was not ripe but he [Dr. Louis Borsch, an American ophthalmologist married to a French woman] staked his reputation on the result. He is the only man in Paris capable of doing such an operation and I am told few anywhere in the US.…"

Results were poor and she wrote:

"I am old and so blind that I don't feel up to much…I see less with the eye that was operated in October than I did with the one with the secondary cataract in it! …I think the state of my eyes will, I hope, shorten my life."

And a 1921 letter reads:

"Last May I had an operation upon my best eye. The operation was very successful and the oculist promised me I should paint again but a hidden abscess in an apparently sound tooth caused a violent inflammation and I have not yet recovered from it. Nor has the sight of the eye returned."

And, finally:

"I have had a very serious operation for cataract several weeks ago and have my eye still bandaged and can see very indifferently with the other eye which is my poor eye. I shall not be able to use my eyes, nor be allowed glasses for several months to come, after that my oculist promises great results. I do not allow myself such sanguine hopes."

As Cassatt's vision diminished, she turned from oils to pastels, using broad strokes on large sheets of paper. The delicacy of her earlier works and her careful color choices disappeared with her dimming sight. By 1915, her days as an artist had ended and by 1918, she could no longer read. Though she lived until 1926, the same year Monet died, her diabetes and cataracts cut short her career and deprived her of the work she loved.

SUMMARY

The artists we have discussed represent only the tip of the iceberg. Other artists showed signs of color deficiencies or presbyopia; some had symptoms indicative of syphilis and various genetic and neurologic diseases. Unfortunately, the absence of medical records or other documentation precludes us from accurately diagnosing their eye disorders and they remain only conjecture. The works of many artists were profoundly influenced by their eye conditions, a great many of which are treatable today.

The eye diseases of the Impressionists were managed with treatments that seem primitive and even barbaric. Today, three of the four major causes of visual loss in older adults are treatable: simple outpatient, minimally invasive surgery with the implantation of intraocular lenses enables us to quickly restore normal vision to patients with cataracts. They no longer have to wait until their vision is severely impaired before undergoing the procedure. Lens implants enable them to maintain binocular vision when only one eye is involved. They no longer have to endure prolonged recuperation periods and adapt to a highly magnified, distorted world. If their postoperative vision becomes hazy owing to opacification of the lens capsule, a painless YAG laser capsulotomy can restore clarity in a few minutes. Insulin and oral medications have helped those with diabetes control their blood sugar and prolong their lives. Diabetic retinopathy can be treated with argon lasers and vitrectomy. Glaucoma can be treated medically and/or surgically. Macular degeneration, though, still remains a challenge and we are currently unable to restore normal color perception to those with color deficiencies or cure a number of retinal problems and genetic eye conditions.

Many patients suffering from mental illnesses respond well to modern psychotherapy and treatment with psychotropic drugs. Seizure disorders can be controlled. The wearing of glasses has become accepted not only as a means of vision correction, but also as a fashion accessory; contact lenses or refractive surgery can correct vision invisibly. Progressive multifocals have replaced conventional bifocals or separate glasses for near and distance. Patency of the lacrimal system can be safely established and modern antibiotics are available to treat dacryocystitis and other infections.

Would these acclaimed artists have achieved the same degree of achievement, recognition, and renown if modern medical and surgical procedures had been available to treat their pathology? If they lived in current times, would the Impressionist movement have even occurred? And if it had, would they be, as they were in the latter half of the 19th century, shunned by traditional artists and art patrons?

DEDICATION

This chapter is dedicated to Michael F. Marmor, MD, and James G. Ravin, MD, whose book *The Eye of the Artist* served as my major resource and my inspiration.

FURTHER READING

Marmor MF, Ravin JG. The eye of the artist. St Louis: Mosby; 1997.

Metzger R, Walther IF. Van Gogh. Köln, Germany: Taschen; 1998.

Ravin JG. Monet's cataracts. JAMA 1985;254(3):396.

Ravin JG, Kenyon CA. Degas' loss of vision: evidence for a diagnosis of retinal disease. Surv Ophthalmol 1994;39(1):57.

Seitz W. Monet and abstract painting. In: Stucky CF, editor. Monet: a retrospective. New York: Hugh Lauter Levin Associates; 1985.

Trevor-Roper P. The world through blunted sight. London: Souvenir Press; 1997.

Chapter | 48 |

Reading problems in children

The child with a reading problem has a disability as incapacitating as any physical infirmity. Basically, the poor reader is thwarted in the attempt to acquire knowledge. Just like children with a physical deformity, poor readers cannot effectively compete with their classmates because of a handicap. However, unlike the physically handicapped child, whose deformity is obvious, the poor reader is difficult to distinguish from others as having a special problem. This child usually passes all preschool medical examinations and is declared healthy and able to meet the challenge of early grade school. Of course, the youngster does poorly and either suffers a major failure at a young age or is carried by the current of regular promotion to higher grades, but is insecure, unprepared, and destined to become an early school dropout. It is estimated that 10% to 20% of the school population has some form of reading disability.

There are many reasons for poor achievement at school. The operative factors include immaturity, cultural deprivation, discord in the home (divorce, separation, or inadequate or hostile parents), poor health, and intellectual disability. The child with a reading problem does not necessarily have any cultural, social, or intellectual failings. In many cases the youngster does poorly in spite of being gifted with every tangible advantage both at home and at school.

WHOSE PROBLEM IS IT?

Because many children with a reading disability become juvenile delinquents, marginal unskilled laborers, or severely emotionally disturbed adults, the problem is obviously a matter of public health and welfare, with major responsibility directed toward both federal and local government bodies. Many heterogeneous groups have or should have a vested interest in this disability. These groups include departments of education and, more specifically, subdepartments of special education; the medical schools, in particular departments of ophthalmology, neurology, psychology, psychiatry, and pediatrics, and schools of social work; and the paramedical groups, such as optometrists, orthoptists, ophthalmic assistants, and technicians. Obviously, with such a large number of subsidiary groups, there is plenty of room for each to avoid or ignore its responsibility toward the entire subject. Thus instead of disciplined group responsibility, the situation has deteriorated to the point of undisciplined group evasion. For example, many poor readers are incorrectly assumed to have poor vision. The ophthalmologist, after careful examination, usually will find that vision is 20/20 in each eye and will reassure the parents that there is no ocular pathologic condition present. The ophthalmologist's responsibility toward that patient usually ends at that point. Unfortunately, the problem does not.

Many of these children develop behavioral problems. They are listless or hyperactive and cannot concentrate on their lessons at school. Their failure at school and subsequent admonishment both at school and at home lead to acts of rebelliousness, disregard of authority and, of course, further failure. Often the secondary behavior problem overshadows the primary problem and many are sent for psychiatric evaluation as emotionally disturbed children. The psychologist may be consulted to conduct a battery of tests to determine the child's IQ, verbal and nonverbal skills, and abilities. Other areas of nonperformance may become apparent. The child may have difficulty with speech and with coordination of fine motor skills (writing, tying shoelaces, throwing a ball) or may show faulty spatial orientation. Many questions are raised and a pediatric or neurologic consultation may become desirable and helpful. Some children show faulty development patterns (e.g., in crawling and walking) during the formative years, whereas others reveal clinical and electrophysiologic evidence of minimal brain dysfunction.

A brief glance at the subject of reading disabilities indicates that many different professions and groups have a stake in the diagnostic and therapeutic aspects of this disorder. A multidisciplinary approach is mandatory. Until teams of effective and interested specialists are mustered and captains of the teams chosen to coordinate their productive efforts, the problem of the poor reader will remain a conundrum tackled by anyone who shows an interest in the subject, regardless of qualification. In the partial vacuum of any treatment center, some good work has been done by interested individuals, but the need for treatment also has been exploited by quacks, charlatans, and the demigods of truth who, in effect, make a cult of their beliefs.

TERMINOLOGY

Dyslexia is the inability or reduced ability to read and *developmental dyslexia* refers to the presence of that condition from childhood and the first attempts to read. This is different from the dyslexia occurring in an adult who formerly read, but who has lost the ability because of brain damage. *Agraphia* is the inability to write. The ability to read and the ability to write are not mutually dependent because a person can have difficulty with reading but none with writing.

Inability to recognize an object or a written or auditory symbol is called *agnosia*. Inability to correlate verbal information into meaningful terms by means of sensory organs is called *aphasia*. The individual, then, who cannot recognize a spoon or fork has agnosia, but the one who can state what it is but has forgotten its function has aphasia.

Apraxia is inability to perform a previously learned task in spite of an intact sensory and motor system. In terms of reading, apraxia may be applied to the child who cannot recall what has been previously assimilated, so that errors of reading are made repeatedly.

The terms *agnosia*, *aphasia*, and *apraxia* belong to the neurologic jargon used to describe organic lesions of the parietal and temporal lobes. Because many children with general perceptual motor defects have signs and symptoms that are similar to acquired organic disturbances of the parietal and temporal lobes, the terminology used to describe their symptoms is most easily understood in the context of organic lesions.

ACT OF READING

The ability to read depends on different overlapping cerebral mechanisms, each functioning independently and yet totally dependent on the other. These overlapping processes include visual sensation, recognition, and comprehension.

Visual sensation begins with visual experience, which depends on the penetration of an adequate amount of light through the clear optical media of the eye. This stimulates the retina with the relay of visual information mediated through an intact afferent visual pathway from the optic nerve to the visual striate area of the cerebral cortex.

Vision in human beings can be either *monocular* (using one eye) or *binocular* (using both eyes). Binocular vision occurs when the images from both eyes are fused into a single mental impression. Binocularity depends, then, on strict anatomic alignment of the eyes and the ability of the eyes to project to the same point in space at a given distance. *Stereopsis*, a higher aspect of binocular vision, features the ability not only to form a single visual picture but also to perceive depth by parallax.

Adequate visual sensation per se is not defective in most children with reading problems. They can see with the uncorrected eye or with properly prescribed spectacles and they have 20/20 vision in each eye when tested with the Snellen chart. There is no dispute on this point. Contention arises on the subject of binocular vision. Some people believe that the harmonious act of binocular coordination is faulty in the perceptually handicapped child. They find difficulties in eye muscle balance, abnormal ocular movements, and faulty sensory fusion and they actively treat these disabilities. Other workers cite the lack of harmony between ocular and hand dominance as a paramount problem in the perceptually handicapped. Although many points are still unsettled, most ophthalmologists believe that disorders of ocular motility have little to do with perception or comprehension.

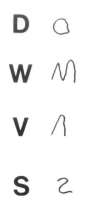

D	⊖
W	⋀
V	⋀
S	⸑

Figure 48.1 Copying of a 6-year-old dyslexic child. Note the mirror writing and reversals of letters.

Yet the child may reveal a visual imagination, excel in oral composition, and appear bright when spoken to in a casual conversation. It is this ability that parents see at home, and therefore they often blame the schools or the teachers for the child's lack of achievement.

Perceptual motor defects

Children with perceptual motor defects are commonly described as awkward and clumsy. Any skill that requires finely coordinated motor ability is performed poorly (Figure 48.2). In the early grades, when copying from the board or from visual aid posters is vital, these children are inordinately handicapped. They cannot trace a figure, copy a geometric form either from memory or directly, draw, or even print in neat fashion between two lines (Figures 48.3–48.5). This gross failure to complete the simplest tasks in the classroom is augmented outside the classroom. Success eludes them in this setting as well; they perform poorly in athletics because they are unable to throw or catch a ball with any degree of constancy.

The characteristics of the perceptually handicapped child are not uniform. They vary in accordance with the child's level of intelligence, disposition, cultural environment at home, and the integrity of the family unit. These modulating factors will influence the child's adaptation to the disability and to a great extent determine behavior patterns.

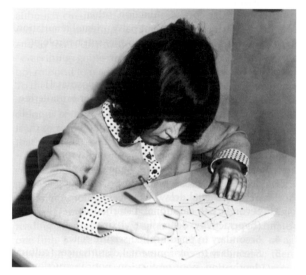

Figure 48.3 Child is asked to connect dots to improve hand–eye coordination. This is part of the Marianne Frostig test of visual perception.

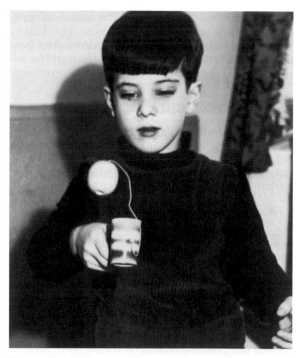

Figure 48.2 Game to test coordination.

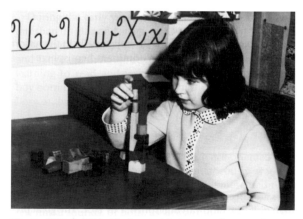

Figure 48.4 Building blocks used to improve fine muscle coordination.

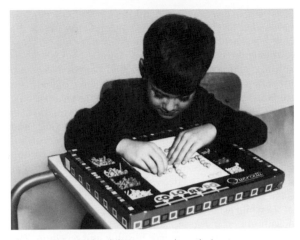

Figure 48.5 Child's ability to reproduce designs on a pegboard is tested.

The natural course of a child with a reading problem is an interruption of learning. The child falls farther and farther behind in reading ability, becomes increasingly frustrated in academic areas that require reading, and so as a rule comes to dislike school. Consequently the youngster does not rely on reading for information or pleasure. Without practice, the student actually regresses. Thus begins the vicious circle: lack of progress, frustration, dislike for reading, and avoidance of tasks, leading to further failure in related areas.

ROLE OF BRAIN AND EYE DOMINANCE

It has been estimated that 65% of patients with reading difficulty have some conflict in establishing laterality. These patients show right–left confusion and are ambidextrous; they fail to establish a cerebral dominance, often until the age of 8 or 9 years. Also these children commonly fail to show harmony between their dominant hand and dominant eye. The view that inability to establish a synchronous complex between hand and eye coordination is paramount in causing reading disabilities has many advocates in both Canada and the United States. Acting on this premise, the disciples of this belief have set up schools, training centers, and remedial reading centers with the singular objective of establishing a dominance in the perceptually handicapped child. The most vigorous of these theorists train the children to relearn every motor act acquired since birth (including reaching, creeping, and crawling) and claim success in their efforts to overcome reading problems, difficulties in motor coordination, and even strabismus. The object of these programs is to establish well-defined cerebral dominance.

In literature on the topic, little attention or credibility is placed on the role of ocular dominance. Good readers are found among children who do not have well-established motor laterality (e.g., Leonardo da Vinci wrote with his left hand and did mirror writing).

Many centers use extensive visual exercises, designed to establish harmonious eye–hand dominance, improve defects in binocularity, or help overcome faulty visual spatial projection disorders. The exercises themselves are usually simple and designed to hold the child's interest. They may include, for example, following a pendulum, copying blocks, and tracing figures and designs. The eye exercises are regarded by most ophthalmologists as of no value in terms of the major problem.

NEUROLOGIC FACTORS

Many perceptually handicapped children are regarded as having *minimal brain dysfunction*. However, this is only by definition. It has not been demonstrated neurologically that minimal clinical signs are in fact related to minimal brain abnormalities. Minimal signs may be concomitant with significant lesions of the brain. Of course, the converse also holds true. To complicate the situation further, many neurologically impaired children do not present any specific learning problem in the classroom, whereas children without brain injury but with supposedly aberrant behavior do have difficulty.

EDUCATIONAL CONSIDERATIONS

Probably the greatest problem in this area lies in the identification of the child with a specific learning disability. In most schools there are no formal screening tests to detect overt or latent perceptual inadequacies in children, and the diagnosis initially rests with the teacher. Dyslexia first becomes evident as the child reaches kindergarten and first grade, although it is often not recognized until much later and, indeed, is commonly never recognized for what it is (Figure 48.6).

Teachers of an early grade have two roles to fill. They must teach the group as a whole, a task for which the teachers are prepared by virtue of their training, and they must sort out and refer for special instruction the child who fails to progress at the expected rate. It is the second role in which teachers may fail because of the inadequacy of their training. Teachers, like general practitioners of medicine, are the first line of defense before the specialist takes over. Unlike their medical counterparts, however, their training is primarily concerned with teaching methods rather than diagnostics.

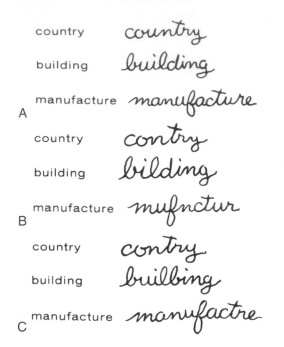

Figure 48.6 Writing of a 9-year-old boy. (A) Words dictated one syllable at a time. (B) Words dictated at normal speed. (C) Words copied from blackboard.

Ideally, the dyslexic child's learning program takes into account the handicap and tries to surmount it. The classroom should be geared physically to this child's distractibility, the main stumbling block to learning. The desk position—the child's place in the class—is designed to shut out many of the distractions that divert this youngster from the lesson. Also, the material is presented so that these children learn at their own pace, either in a special classroom or in a special place in the ordinary classroom. If they are forced to compete with their classmates, as opposed to themselves, they struggle and usually fail to make much progress.

In some areas that are equipped with special classrooms and highly specialized teachers, children with perceptual problems have been isolated for periods of 1 to 3 years and then successfully returned to their regular classes. With special training they not only make academic progress but also show remarkable changes in behavior.

PROBLEMS AT HOME

Children with a learning disability, although failing at school, often appear bright to their parents. Indeed, most of these children are alert, possess a vivid imagination, and do well on intelligence tests that avoid their particular disability. The parent is usually perplexed by the inability of the child to learn to read and may regard the whole business as a temporary aberration. Eventually, consistently poor achievement drives parents to find a rationale for it. Slightly bewildered and somewhat angry, parents may blame the child's teacher or the school system. Later, as they attempt to correct these injustices by home tutorials and fail miserably in teaching their own child to read, parents may accuse the child of laziness, lack of ambition, truancy, or just plain stupidity. Needless to say, the loss of parental regard is only the prelude to the child's own loss of self-esteem.

In the neighborhood the child's unpredictable and sometimes negative or hostile behavior leads to rejection by other children. Such children do not stay with group games very long because they do not possess the motor skills needed to play effectively and often cannot understand the basic organization of the game.

The child who finds rejection at school, rebuff in the neighborhood playgroup, and criticism at home is bound to develop feelings of intense hostility and rebellion. The child may become totally unmanageable. Being impulsive, hyperactive, and emotionally labile, the child with a severe emotional crisis augments these tendencies, and behavior problems soon eclipse the initial one.

Parental reaction can vary from frank hostility to bland indifference or indulgence. Sympathetic parents who do understand the nature of the child's problem are probably the most frustrated. Desiring of a solution, they first attempt to discover whether a physical disability is present. The investigation may trail through an array of professionals, including general practitioners, pediatricians, ophthalmologists, neurologists, and psychiatrists, only to reveal that the child has no gross physical disability.

The quest for a solution carries them to the schools. If the school has facilities for psychological testing and the waiting list for such tests is not interminably long, the child may be assessed and assigned to special classes. Most schools, however, do not have enough classrooms for the regular students, let alone facilities for special students. Even if enough physical space could be found and structured to meet the needs of the distractible child, there would be difficulty in finding a sufficient number of teachers with special training to meet the demand. In some instances, parents have reacted to this void by sending their children to private remedial reading schools, optometrists, or small centers for the learning disabled. Some of these private agencies and individuals obtain good results because of their knowledge, enthusiasm, and general integrity. Their facilities, however, are not subject to inspection by any government department and their abilities are not tested by any particular credentials committee. Thus it is found that among the available therapists, many will alleviate the problem, whereas others will exploit it.

Isolated groups of frustrated parents have formed associations for the child with a learning disability. The function of these lay bodies is to disseminate information on the subject and to encourage the professions of medicine, psychology, and pedagogy to take a more active interest in the child with a perceptual motor disorder. These groups acknowledge the isolated efforts of interested therapists, but have concentrated their efforts on bridging the gap among the various professions so that a multidisciplinary approach can be offered to each child.

CONDITIONS THAT ARE CONFUSED WITH A LEARNING DISABILITY

Hearing deficit

Many learning-disabled children have some defect in hearing. Some cannot differentiate sounds, as opposed to differentiating visual symbols, and they do not respond well to hearing tests. Hearing ability, therefore, is difficult to determine, and some children are mistakenly placed in classes for deaf children. Others may appear to hear properly, but they do not understand and are considered to be mentally retarded.

Mental retardation

In many respects learning-disabled children and mentally retarded children are very much alike. Both groups fail to progress at a rate appropriate for their age. Both may have difficulty caring for themselves and may be late in becoming toilet trained and in dressing and feeding themselves. Both fail to establish good personal relationships with other children. The retarded child commonly does not even make an effort to be part of the group, whereas the learning-disabled child may try and fail miserably. The fundamental difference between the two children is that the latter does not have a low intelligence quotient (IQ). The child's interest can be aroused, but it is difficult to sustain. Also, this child does not necessarily underachieve in all subjects and may even show brilliance in some courses of study while doing poorly in others.

Childhood schizophrenia versus autism

Autistic children live in their own world of social isolation and often behave in the same manner toward most people, be they strangers or members of their own family. Learning-disabled children do not behave as though the outside world were of little importance. They not only know the difference between people but will also adjust their behavior to individuals according to their importance. They can be diverted from undesirable social behavior when pride and interest in accomplishment are established through proper teaching; the autistic child cannot be diverted.

Emotional disturbance

There is often great difficulty in differentiating the truly emotionally disturbed child from the child whose behavior is the result of frustration caused by inability to communicate orally and to understand language. There are no easy methods of distinguishing the two groups, and this task must be left in the hands of professional psychologists and psychiatrists.

TREATMENT

The treatment of learning-disabled children has followed three general patterns, the emphasis varying with the individual therapist and the particular needs of the child.

One approach is to reorient the teaching program to suit the child's particular handicap. This program is usually devised by the department of special education of large school boards. In ideal situations, extra classrooms are built in such a manner as to aid the student to focus attention on school material. These rooms are located at the end of corridors, out of range of other children passing back and forth. The walls are built of sound-absorbing materials and the windows are made translucent to reduce distracting visual stimuli coming in from the outside. The number of children in a class is small; eight in a group usually is regarded as a high optimum number. The teachers, the focal point of the entire operation, are specially trained in both special teaching methods and psychology. It is desirable that they be warm, friendly, and patient. Some authorities even believe that such teachers also should undergo psychotherapy to understand themselves in their relationship to their students. Of utmost importance is that the teachers be given extensive opportunity to evaluate the case records and to talk with the psychiatrist, neurologist, and psychologist because the teachers are an integral part of the team.

When the learning disability is more circumscribed and behavior problems are not dominant, the child can be left in the ordinary classroom while receiving special attention. This type of child may need a more phonetic approach to reading and should not be required to compete with the other children. If the teacher is made aware of the child's problem, the little extras—extra help, extra understanding, extra tutorials, and extra inducement—may be of great value.

Another method of treatment is to approach the child as a whole and concentrate on rehabilitating the child in all aspects: visual, auditory, kinesthetic, and motor. The practical implications of this method are rather vague and broad. The Frostig method tries to encompass visuo-perceptual training and sensorimotor training concurrently with language training. The training in sensorimotor function includes four areas: general training of movement skills through a program of physical education, development of body awareness, training in eye–hand coordination and manipulation skills, and training in eye movement through tracking exercises.

Other groups have emphasized the difficulty of establishing lateral dominance as the major cause of a child's problem and have concentrated their efforts on this. The exercises are fundamental initially, and the child is retrained in hand reaching, creeping, crawling, and even sleeping posture.

A more segmental approach is taken by optometrists who deemphasize the emotional and neurologic aspects of the learning-disabled child and focus only on supposed errors of binocular function, ocular motor coordination, and ocular dominance. In regard to ocular motor coordination, the theory is that children, to complete or trace an oblique line, must be able to nimbly perform oblique movements of their eyes. Therefore, they are started on tracking exercises with pendulum-gazing devices, projection exercises, and so forth.

In most large training centers therapy is broadly approached, with several therapists working with problems of speech, motor skills, penmanship, verbal formulation, auditory and visual perception, visual memory, and directional confusion.

Regardless of the treatment initiated, it is essential that each child have a complete diagnostic evaluation to discover weaknesses as well as strengths. The workup should include a medical evaluation and a behavioral assessment. The medical evaluation is essential to prevent the development or continuation of unsuspected disease processes. The behavioral assessment provides the basis for a logical management and education program.

CLINICAL TESTS

Vision

Each child's vision should be fully evaluated to ensure that each eye is seeing normally. Refraction with a cycloplegic agent should be performed to detect any latent refractive error.

Letter reversal

When the child is given standard test letters to read at either distance or near, the examiner should be alert for letter reversals such as *b* for *d*, *d* for *p*, or *p* for *q*. The examiner also should observe whether the child reads from right to left instead of from left to right. Occasionally a child will read vertically when asked to read across.

Color vision

Commonly, defects in color vision are detected among children with a reading disability. Color vision should be tested by the colored yarn test when the child is small, or by pseudoisochromatic plates in the older child.

Dominance test

Although the relationship of the dominant eye to perceptual motor difficulties is still questionable, it may prove of interest for research projects. To identify the dominant eye, the child is asked to point to a distant object. By first covering one eye and then the other eye, the examiner can identify the dominant eye as the one that, when left uncovered, does not require a shift of the finger to the target.

Line drawings

The child should be asked to draw a clock complete with numbers. Children with normal spatial relationship usually space the numbers evenly around the circle; those who do not crowd them on one side.

Visual perception and comprehension tests

The child is asked to read a standard paragraph geared to his or her approximate grade level while the examiner notes the number and type of errors that the child makes. The examiner then asks a few pertinent questions about the paragraph just read to detect lack of comprehension.

Auditory perception test

The examiner can test auditory perception by dictating a simple sentence, preferably using words with *b*, *d*, and *p*, and asking the child to write out the sentence. The child with dyslexia will be unable to transfer the spoken word to the written word. It is important that these children have an audiogram to rule out primary hearing defects.

SUMMARY

Children with a reading disability can function efficiently and effectively in a calm emotional climate if they are allowed to compete only with students of their own caliber. These children require custom-designed educational facilities so that the sensory input or information does not come at them through a blocked system.

Children with a reading disability suffer from lack of simple identification. They do not possess a gross physical disability that can be easily pictured or publicly championed to elicit funds and facilities. Because their handicap is broad and subtle, it is poorly comprehended and it does not receive the allowance due to it. If these children were deaf or blind, they would be spared the necessity of functioning in the areas in which they were affected.

The prognosis depends on the age at which the handicap is identified, the family background, the presence or absence of severe secondary emotional reactions, and the magnitude of the disability. The earlier children with a handicap are discovered, the less apt they are to become a behavior problem. By the time they are 8 or 9 years of age, they have already developed a dislike of reading and learning that eventually spills over in hostility toward those who teach them. Before long, their hostility is directed at everyone of authority, including parents.

It has been estimated that about three out of four children with a mild reading disability will learn to read well if presented, on a group basis, with modifications of current teaching methods. Of the remainder, about two-thirds, if they are given enough time and are protected from emotional stresses, improve through remedial teaching techniques applied on an individual basis. The remaining third, who are the "hard core" of children with reading

disability, are eventually forced to join the ranks of the school dropouts and usually lead a marginal existence in the unskilled labor pool.

ACKNOWLEDGMENT

The editors would like to acknowledge the contribution to the chapter in previous editions from Bernard J. Slatt.

Questions for review and thought

1. Record the names of members in your community who can be of aid to the child with a reading problem.
2. Eye disorders play what part in learning disability?
3. What exercises are available for the slow reader?
4. Outline the characteristics of children with a reading disability.
5. What conditions are often confused with a learning disability?
6. Do eye exercises help the learning disabled?
7. Do children with reading problems usually have impaired vision?
8. Do children with perceptive difficulties have a low IQ?
9. Are children with learning disabilities likely to be (a) placid or (b) emotionally disturbed, with hostile behavior? Explain.
10. Does reading take place (a) when the eye moves or (b) when the eye pauses?
11. Are reading glasses of value in remedying learning disabilities?
12. Do some children with reading problems have minimal brain dysfunction?
13. Do children with strabismus have greater problems with reading? Explain why or why not.

Q Self-evaluation questions

True–false statements

Directions: Indicate whether the statement is true **(T)** or false **(F).**
1. The child with a reading problem is usually of normal intelligence. **T** or **F**
2. Reading problems are often the cause of abnormal ocular movements or faulty sensory function. **T** or **F**
3. Eye exercises help remedy learning disabilities. **T** or **F**

Missing words

Directions: Write the missing word(s) in the following sentences:
4. The inability or reduced ability to read is called *dyslexia*. The presence of that condition from the first attempts to read is called _____.
5. Among children with reading disabilities, there is a great preponderance of _____.
6. Reading problems are a subgroup of a more general classification called _____.

Choice-completion questions

Directions: Select the one best answer in each case.
7. The child with a learning disability often has:
   a. reading problems.
   b. visuoperceptual problems.
   c. auditory perceptual problems.
   d. a and c.
   e. a, b and c.
8. The treatment of a reading disability is primarily the work of the:
   a. optometrist.
   b. pediatrician.
   c. psychologist.
   d. special education teacher.
   e. psychiatrist.
9. One of the most serious side effects of a reading disability is:
   a. minimal brain dysfunction.
   b. right–left confusion.
   c. poor self-image.
   d. eye muscle imbalance.
   e. hyperactivity.

A Answers, notes, and explanations

1. **True.** Although reading problems in children can occur in many different kinds of populations—for example, in the learning disabled—the problem that is currently of particular interest to educators is a reading problem that occurs in children who are of normal or above-normal intelligence. The child of average intelligence with a reading problem has difficulty in reading for a variety of reasons. Some have difficulty with language generally and, because reading is a language process, they cannot comprehend what they read. Other children, however, have good oral language skills but cannot grasp the mechanics of reading. Because a child's intelligence is normal, the expectation is that with the appropriate remedial help the child can begin to read. Of course, this often depends on the severity of the learning disability. The better a child's overall language abilities, the more he or she is able to compensate for the reading problem.

2. **False.** Although some people blame reading problems on abnormal ocular movements or faulty sensory fusion, studies show that reading problems occur because of difficulties at a higher level of cortical functioning. In other words, there is nothing wrong with the peripheral ocular mechanism. The difficulty is the result of the brain's inability to integrate and deal with some of this information. Reading problems do not occur only because of visual processing difficulties. As was pointed out previously, reading problems also can occur because of difficulties with auditory processing and with general language difficulties. Examiners should avoid the mistake of interpreting the cause of reading problems as a difficulty with the external eye mechanism, because this certainly affects how they go about helping these children. Those professionals who try to correct ocular movements or faulty sensory fusion are wasting precious time that would be better spent in remedying reading problems in the more traditional ways. Traditional methods of remediation are usually best carried out by a teacher who has been well trained in special education.

3. **False.** This statement obviously follows from the incorrect premise that it is the external eye that is causing the child to be learning disabled. As mentioned, the difficulties occur at a different level of functioning, namely at the cortical level, and eye exercises certainly cannot help remedy this problem. The best kind of remedial intervention not only deals with the areas of difficulty but also helps the child to compensate by using some of his or her strengths. The magic ingredient in all of this, of course, is to build up the child's self-image and feeling of self-worth as a learner.

4. **Dyslexia and developmental dyslexia.** The term *dyslexia* has been traditionally used to describe an individual, usually an adult, who formerly could read but lost the ability to do so because of brain damage. This word also has been applied to the inability to learn to read from childhood and has often been referred to as *developmental dyslexia*. (The term has not been used as readily in the field.) People generally use the term *learning disabilities* to describe many different kinds of difficulties with learning. Learning to read is one of them. It is rare to find a child who has only an inability to learn to read and no other problems. Often these children also show difficulties with visual or auditory processing. These children are also often characterized by specific kinds of behaviors or learning styles; some have a poor attention span, are impulsive, are emotionally labile, or show a combination of all of these.

5. **Males.** Boys are affected more commonly than girls, the ratio varying from 4:1 to 10:1, although a ratio of 5:1 usually is given. It is difficult to know for certain why there is a great preponderance of males, although it has been suggested that this is related to their general physiologic maturation lag. This condition is also familial, although how it is carried from one generation to another is unknown. It is not uncommon to find that the father of a learning-disabled boy had similar problems when he was a youngster.

6. **Learning disabilities.** To understand the field it is important to think of reading problems as a subgroup of the more general classification of "learning disabilities." A learning disability has been defined as a disorder in one or more of the basic psychologic processes involved in the understanding or use of spoken or written language. It may manifest in disorders of listening, understanding, speaking, reading, writing, spelling, or computation.

   It has been variously referred to as a *perceptual handicap, minimal brain dysfunction,* and *dyslexia.* Learning disabilities do not include learning problems that primarily are a result of a visual, hearing, or motor handicap; mental retardation; emotional disturbance; or environmental disadvantage. It is sometimes beneficial to think of learning disabilities as two types: (a) developmental learning disabilities and (b) academic disabilities. The developmental disabilities include such factors as difficulties in visual processing, auditory processing, kinesthetic functions, integration of modalities, language, and attention. The academic disabilities are often the result of some of the developmental learning disabilities, and they show up as difficulties in reading, writing, spelling, mathematics, and written expression. The assumption, then, is that developmental learning disabilities are the forerunners of academic learning disabilities.

7. **e. a, b and c.** As mentioned in the explanation for question 6, the child with a learning disability often has reading problems as well as visuo- and auditory perceptual problems. All of these difficulties can exist in one child. Often the visuo- and auditory perceptual problems are the main contributors to the reading problem.

8. **d. Special education teacher.** It has been found that the treatment of a reading disability is best done by the special education teacher who uses his or her knowledge in remedying this kind of disability. Other professionals should certainly be involved in dealing with the problem of the learning-disabled child.

A | Continued

The best kind of remediation is done by the teacher who has a full and complete psychologic and educational assessment of the child. This assessment must outline the child's strengths and weaknesses and the areas in which help is needed. The pediatrician who is the child's primary care physician certainly has an involvement with the child and family and should know what is going on with the individual child. Sometimes the emotional difficulties secondary to the problem are great enough to warrant some kind of psychiatric involvement as well. Other professionals such as occupational therapists, speech and language therapists, and ophthalmologists have a role to play in dealing with the child and family and sometimes even in helping to remedy specific problems. The best kind of treatment is carried out by a multidisciplinary team that deals with all of the difficulties. There is great need for open communication among parents, teachers, and other professionals so that each individual helping the child knows what the goals are and what the other people are doing.

9. **c. Poor self-image.** There is no doubt among those who have worked with children with reading disabilities that one of the most serious side effects of a reading disability or learning disability is the child's poor self-image. Building up a child's self-image and helping the youngster to gain confidence are among the primary goals of treatment of these children. It sometimes is more difficult to deal with this aspect of the problem than it is to deal with the remediation of specific difficulties in the areas of visual processing or auditory processing, or even in teaching the child to read. Good remedial therapists will begin the remediation by attempting to build a solid and warm relationship with the child and in this way give the child confidence that is lacking. It also is important, because of the pervasiveness of this poor self-image, that a parent be involved in helping build up the child's confidence.

Chapter | 49 |

Cardiopulmonary resuscitation

Joseph D. Freeman

When a patient, family member, friend, or stranger stops breathing, his/her heart stops beating, or is found unresponsive, it can be one of the scariest situations of your career. However, this is also one of the times in which your knowledge and practice as a trained health care provider can make the difference between life and death. Basic life support (BLS) and cardiopulmonary resuscitation (CPR) is the skill set you will use to attempt to save the life of someone who otherwise would have no chance of survival. The rapid initiation and appropriate resuscitation of a person in sudden cardiac or respiratory arrest give that person the best hope of survival.

CARDIOPULMONARY RESUSCITATION

How does CPR work?

For all of us to remain alive, our brains must have a constant flow of basic nutrients to function. One of the most important of these basic nutrients is oxygen. Oxygen is taken in from the air we breathe, absorbed into our blood through our lungs, and pumped by our hearts into our brains. If there is any significant interruption in this constant cycle of oxygenated blood flow to the brain, we die.

The heart is, in essence, a large muscle that pumps blood to the brain and all other parts of the body. As it is a muscle,

the heart also needs the nutrients found in blood so that it can have energy to function. It gets these nutrients through the blood delivered by the coronary arteries, the arteries that run over the top of the heart and come directly off of the aorta, the central artery of the body.

Blood is able to store a certain amount of oxygen and other basic nutrients for a short amount of time. This is why we are able to hold our breath for short periods and do not have to be constantly eating food to remain alive.

In essence, CPR is attempting to re-create the function of the heart and lungs when they are not able to function on their own. This is why it is called cardiopulmonary resuscitation: *cardio-* (Latin/Greek: "heart"), *pulmo* (Latin/Greek: "lungs") *resuscitation* (Latin: "the act of reawakening something/someone"). By pushing down on someone's chest and breathing air into the lungs, you are re-creating the function of the heart and lungs in an attempt to get the blood's nutrients to the brain.

The first step of CPR: identify the need

How do you know if someone needs CPR? Identifying the need to start CPR can often be one of the hardest steps. A sense of shock and disbelief, in response to an event so out of the ordinary, often overwhelms the potential caregiver. However, rapid initiation of CPR leads to improved survival (the less time the brain is without the nutrients in blood, the better) and therefore is the most important step in CPR.

"Shake and shout" is the first step to establish if a person is responsive. If a person is responsive, he or she does not need CPR. If a person does not respond to attempts to be physically awoken (shaking a shoulder, pinching the arm, or doing something that would be uncomfortable for a person but would not cause harm) and shouting loudly into the ear, then you need to check if the person is breathing.

Look at the person's chest to see if it is rising and falling with breathing. Some people also find it useful to put their hand on the person's chest. Look at the person's face to see if any air is coming in or out of the mouth or nose. To determine whether someone is breathing, observe if the mouth is open slightly or nostrils are expanding. If a person is not responsive and not breathing, it is time to start CPR.

Common mistakes

Most people are able to recognize if someone is not breathing; however, distinguishing "agonal gasping" or "agonal breathing" from normal breathing can be hard. Agonal gasping is movement that mimics breathing but doesn't actually get air into the lungs. It often occurs right before a person dies. Agonal gasping can take on several forms, the most common of which is gagging and irregular chest and mouth movements. Agonal gasping is not breathing, and you must start CPR.

The second step of CPR: call for help and get an automated external defibrillator

A crucial step in starting CPR is obtaining help. If you are alone, yell for help. If someone responds, first tell him or her to call an ambulance immediately (phone 911 in the United States and Canada, 080 in Mexico, 999 in the UK, 112 in many countries in Europe), then try to find an automated external defibrillator (AED). An AED may be found in many public spaces designed for large groups of people (such as sport arenas, airports, large business offices), and is often marked by special signs (Figure 49.1). If you are alone and no one responds to your yells for help, your first priority is to call for an ambulance, even if this requires you to leave the patient temporarily. If you see an AED sign and can quickly get to it on your way back, obtain the AED. Otherwise, return immediately to the patient and check for a pulse.

The third step of CPR: check for a pulse

Use no more than 10 seconds to check for a pulse. The most reliable parts on the body to find a pulse are the neck (for the carotid pulse, Figure 49.2A), followed by the groin (for the femoral pulse, Figure 49.2B), and then the wrist (for the radial pulse, Figure 49.2C). If the patient has no pulse, begin chest compressions. If the patient does have a pulse but is not breathing or has agonal gasping, give one breath every 5 to 6 seconds for 2 minutes ("rescue breathing," see following text) and then recheck to see if the patient has a pulse. If there is a pulse but the person is still not breathing, or are having agonal gasping,

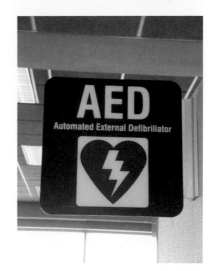

Figure 49.1 A sign alerting the provider where an automated external defibrillator (AED) can be found.

continue rescue breathing. If there is no longer a pulse, begin chest compressions.

Hints

It can often be very difficult to feel a patient's pulse because of a multitude of factors (if the patient has a large amount of fat overlying the pulse, if the patient has a weak pulse because his or her heart is not functioning well, or if the pulse is irregular or very slow). There are several techniques you can use to feel for a pulse.

The first is to make sure that you are feeling in the correct location on the body. For the carotid pulse, begin at the midline of the neck and feel the hard tubular structure, the trachea or "windpipe." Slide your fingers to either side of it and into the slight nook or soft spot between the trachea and neck muscle (the sternocleidomastoid). There are two carotids, one on either side of the trachea. For the femoral pulse, find the hip bone (the anterior superior iliac spine, which is the hard bony point on top of the hip, not on the side of the hip) and go halfway across the hip toward the groin as a starting point. Move your fingers every few seconds to the right and left if you do not feel a pulse. For the radial pulse, mentally divide the back side of the wrist in half. Using the half of the wrist that is on the thumb side, mentally divide this area in half again. Put your fingers along this imaginary line.

For all pulse checks, use two fingers (your index and middle finger) and the most sensitive area of your finger (this is the very tip of your finger just underneath your fingernail). If there are multiple people, have at least two people check for pulses simultaneously (carotid and femoral or carotid and radial if the patient is clothed).

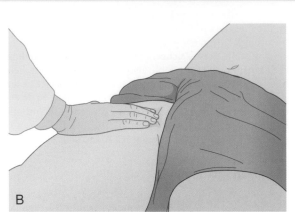
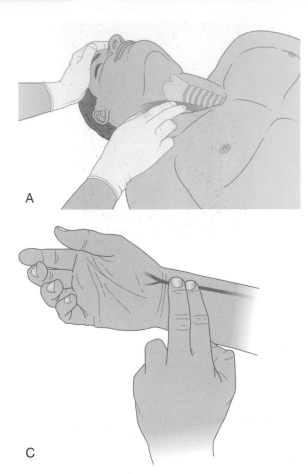

Figure 49.2 (A) Finding the carotid pulse. (B) Finding the femoral pulse. (C) Finding the radial pulse.

If you still do not feel a pulse, if you are unsure that you are checking the correct spot, or if you think the patient has a pulse but you are unable to feel it, you must start chest compressions. If the patient really does have a pulse and you are unable to feel it, chest compressions will not stop a heart from beating. If the patient does not have a pulse, then you have taken the correct step by starting chest compressions immediately.

The fourth and most important step of CPR: perform chest compressions

Of all the steps you do as part of CPR, early and correctly performed chest compressions are the most critical to saving a patient's life. These are done as a cycle: 30 chest compressions followed by two breaths, done for 2 minutes, then 10 seconds to feel for a pulse. If there is no pulse, continue the cycle of 30 chest compressions followed by two breaths, done for 2 minutes, before checking for a pulse again. If two rescuers are available, one person should do chest

compressions and the other person should perform the rescue breaths (Figure 49.3) as well as help the person doing the chest compressions to count and provide feedback when needed ("go faster," "push deeper," "let the chest recoil").

How to perform chest compressions

Performing chest compressions can be exhausting. However, fast and deep chest compressions are critical to saving a patient's life. High-quality chest compressions should have all of the following elements: between 100–120 compressions per minute, pushing down between 2–2.5 inches (5–6 cm) into the chest, letting the chest wall recoil all the way so that it comes back to its normal starting position between each chest compression, and having as few interruptions or pauses in chest compressions as possible.

Tips

Correct positioning allows for effective chest compressions as well as preventing the rescuer from getting exhausted too

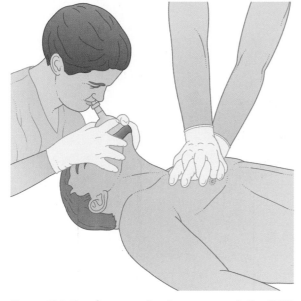

Figure 49.3 Two-rescuer cardiopulmonary resuscitation (CPR) with one person performing chest compressions and the other performing rescue breathing.

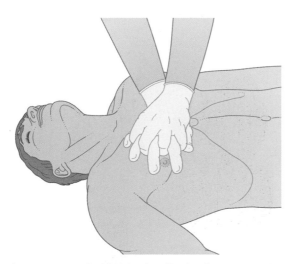

Figure 49.4 Hand positioning for effective chest compressions.

early in the resuscitation. Pushing down on the middle of the chest (above the xiphoid process, where the soft abdomen meets the hard chest wall in the middle of the body), have one hand on top of the other and use the heel of your hand to push down hard in the middle of the chest (Figure 49.4). Keep your elbows just slightly bent and your back straight. Instead of using your shoulder, back, and arm muscles to push down on the chest, have the motion start near your lower back from your waist. Performing CPR by using your waist will make you feel hot and sweaty, but allows for more muscle endurance so that you can perform

effective CPR longer. Have your chest leaning over the patient so you can use the weight of your chest pushing down on your arms. This will increase the strength of your chest compressions while decreasing the amount of energy your muscles are using to further increase your endurance (Figure 49.5).

One of the most common mistakes in performing chest compressions is going too slowly. You should be doing at least 100 chest compressions per minute, though no faster than 120 chest compressions per minute, as long as you are performing them effectively. To avoid going too slowly, either have someone count for you or frequently ask yourself if you can go faster. To be effective, however, compressions must be between 2–2.5 inches deep and allow for full chest recoil.

Sometimes, especially in the case of older adult patients, chest compressions break the ribs. When doing chest compressions, broken ribs have a crunching, clicking, or popping sensation. If you feel this, continue CPR without any interruptions or pauses. Though it is not ideal to break ribs, it is better to have broken ribs and be alive than be dead without broken ribs.

If you have multiple trained people available during CPR, use them: performing CPR is exhausting. Switch out the person performing chest compressions often. Do this with minimal amounts of pauses in chest compressions by having the next person to perform get into position with arms ready. Place yourself right next to and in parallel to the person currently performing chest compressions and count down to switch so that it happens smoothly and without pauses. One provider can check the pulse while the other performs chest compressions. Well-performed chest compressions should result in one pulse per chest compression.

How it works

The concept behind chest compressions explains why appropriate compression depth and allowing for recoil are so important. By pushing down on a patient's chest, you are creating a pressure within the chest cavity that causes the blood in the heart to go forward toward the brain. Pushing down hard enough provides the appropriate amount of pressure necessary to allow for the blood to move forward. During the temporary pause in a chest compression, the chest is able to recoil, causing a negative "sucking" pressure within the chest that allows blood to fill up the heart as well as to flow through the coronary arteries, giving the heart much needed oxygen and nutrients.

Rescue breathing

Rescue breathing becomes more important the longer CPR continues before a patient's heart starts beating and he or she begins breathing spontaneously. The oxygen that is stored in the blood is used up by the brain and other parts of the body and needs to be replenished.

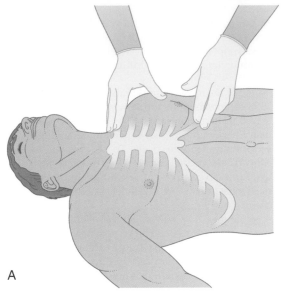

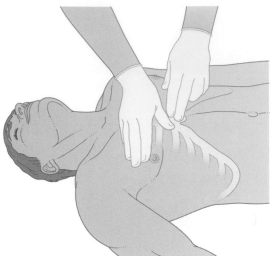

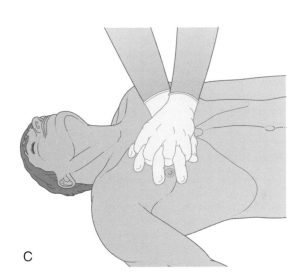

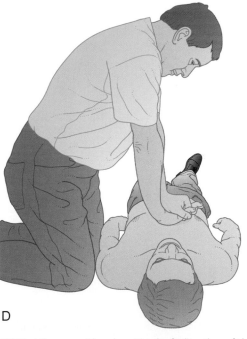

Figure 49.5 Proper body positioning for effective chest compressions. (A) Find the correct hand position by feeling the soft belly. (B) Move up the belly until you feel the hard chest wall and xiphoid process. (C) Place the heel of your hand at this spot on the chest wall, then place your other hand on top with fingers interlaced. (D) Proper body positioning.

Effective rescue breathing first requires proper positioning of the airway (the mouth, throat, and windpipe). This can be done through the head tilt–chin lift maneuver (Figure 49.6). Place one hand on the back of the head and the other hand underneath the chin. Push with both hands (down with the hand that is on the back of the head, up with the hand underneath the chin) so that the patient's head moves upward. It will seem as if he or she is trying to look up toward the forehead. This movement, called extension, straightens out the larynx and trachea and locks down the tongue into the floor of the mouth. This way air can pass smoothly from the mouth into the lungs. Using the hand that was on the back of the head to hold the head in place in extension, breathe one full breath into the patient's mouth over the course of one second (mouth-to-mouth resuscitation, Figure 49.7). Breathe enough to see the patient's chest rise. Let the air come out

Figure 49.6 (A) Airway in need of proper positioning. (B) Head tilt–chin lift for proper airway positioning.

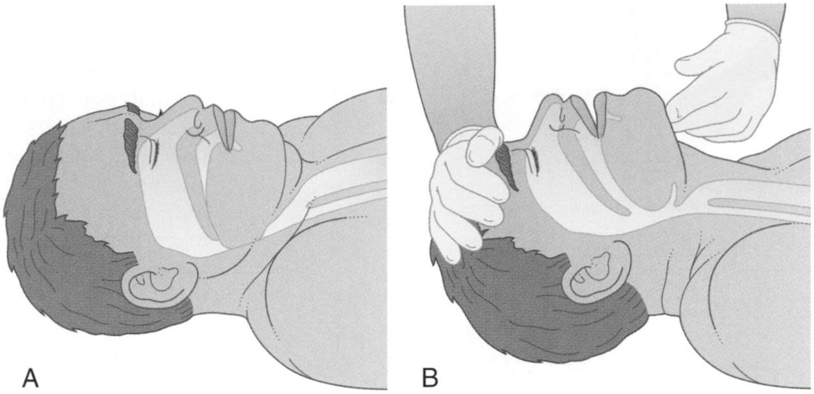

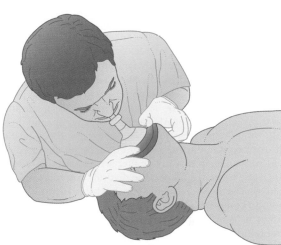

A   B

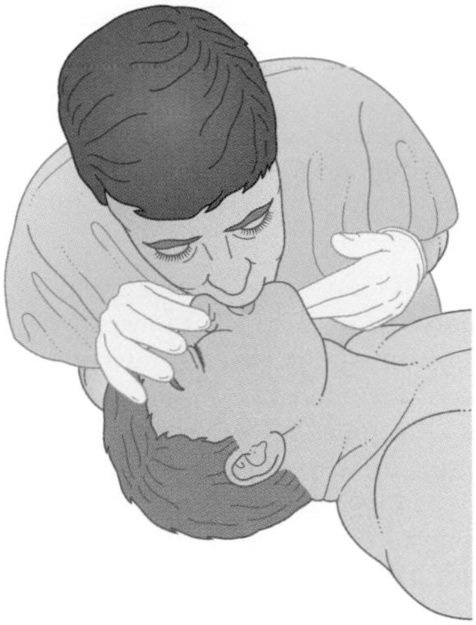

Figure 49.7 Mouth-to-mouth resuscitation.

Figure 49.8 Proper use of one type of protective mouth barrier.

of the chest fully and then repeat one more full breath: a total of two rescue breaths. Then immediately return to chest compressions. When performing rescue breathing as part of CPR, it should be done in cycles of 30 chest compressions to two rescue breaths.

Hints

When performing mouth-to-mouth resuscitation, you should first feel a small amount of resistance to your breath as the chest starts to rise. This will be followed by easier and smoother air flow. If you meet resistance (you try to blow hard but you are unable to move any air and your cheeks puff out), try to reposition the patient's head. Repeat the same technique you used to position the head the first time (one hand behind the head, the other hand underneath the chin and move the head as if the patient is looking upward).

If you try mouth-to-mouth resuscitation again and still are unable to blow air into the patient's mouth, consider the possibility that the patient has a foreign body in the airway (see following text). If when looking at the airway you see a large amount of blood or vomit in the mouth, attempt to clear it out of the airway. Put the patient on his or her side and with gloved hands, suction (if available) or scoop out the material. Do not put your hand into the patient's mouth unless you are sure he or she is unconscious and unresponsive and will not bite your hand. If at all possible, always use some form of protective mouth barrier (Figure 49.8) when performing mouth-to-mouth resuscitation, for your protection.

The AED

It is important to use the AED as soon as it arrives (Figure 49.9). There are several different companies that manufacture AEDs, and they look and work slightly differently. However, all of them work using the same basic principle and components. First, look for the directions located on top of the AED or inside the large panel, if present.

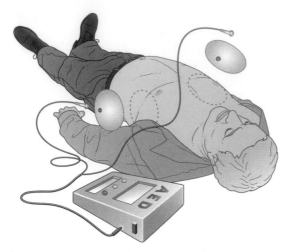

Figure 49.9 An example of an automated external defibrillator (AED).

Follow the instructions. This typically involves placing a large conducting pad on the chest and one on the back or side of the chest, connecting the wires from the pads to the AED (if they are not already connected), turning on the AED, letting the AED analyze the rhythm, and then following the prompts to initiate an electric shock to the heart or continue CPR. Some AEDs have an audio voice and some have a small computer screen with text. Some AEDs use the terms "shockable rhythm" (you need to initiate an electric shock) and "nonshockable rhythm" (you need to continue chest compressions immediately).

When using an AED, it is important to minimize the amount of time the patient is without chest compressions. If the AED tells you to initiate a shock or if it automatically initiates a shock, resume chest compressions immediately after the shock has been delivered. Use the cycle of 30 chest compressions and two rescue breaths for 2 minutes before performing a 10-second pulse check. If the AED says that no shock needs to be delivered (a nonshockable rhythm), immediately continue 30 chest compressions and two rescue breath cycles for 2 minutes before performing a 10-second pulse check.

How AEDs work

To understand how an AED works, you first need to understand how the heart coordinates itself to make a large muscle contraction to forcefully pump blood through the body. The pacemaker of the heart (the sinoatrial node) uses chemicals to create electricity that travels down electric highways in the heart. This causes the heart muscles to contract in a fast, consistent, and organized fashion. Sometimes this electric rhythm can become disrupted, either through certain chemicals that are out of proportion in the body or because of damage to the heart. Two of these types of abnormal electric rhythms—ventricular

fibrillation and pulseless ventricular tachycardia—are shockable rhythms. By causing a large external electric shock to the heart through an AED, it is possible that the external electrical shock will reset the heart's abnormal electrical rhythm back to a normal "perfusing" (the heart is now pumping blood through the body) rhythm. It should also be noted that during the delivery of a shock by the AED, people helping with the resuscitation should not touch the patient so that they will not accidentally get shocked themselves. That being said, it is extremely rare to get shocked even if touching the patient. Care should be taken to minimize all interruptions in chest compressions.

SPECIAL SITUATIONS

Children

The previous sequence and techniques for CPR are the same for a child found to be unresponsive, not breathing, or with agonal gasps except for the following seven exceptions:

1. If the child is found unresponsive and not breathing or with agonal gasps, but with a pulse, perform rescue breathing with one breath every 3 seconds (versus every 5–6 seconds in adults).

2. If during the initial pulse check the child has no pulse or if during the second pulse check (after a cycle of rescue breathing has been given) the pulse is slower than 60 beats per minute, start chest compressions (different than adults). Chest compressions are also done in cycles. If the child's pulse rate becomes greater than 60 beats per minute, go back to rescue breathing. Check the pulse every 2 minutes to determine whether it has started to go slower than 60 beats per minute and if you need to resume chest compressions.

3. If you are the only person able to perform the resuscitation, perform chest compressions in cycles of 30 compressions and two rescue breaths. If there is at least one other person who can help, perform chest compressions in cycles of 15 compressions and two rescue breaths (different than adults).

4. If you are the only person able to perform the resuscitation and do not know when the child was last seen breathing normally (an unwitnessed arrest), you should perform 2 minutes of cycles of 30 compressions and two rescue breaths immediately, then yell for help or temporarily leave the child to call an ambulance (versus immediately call for an ambulance with both adults and children in witnessed arrests).

5. The depth of chest compressions is different in infants (children less than 1 year old) versus adults. In infants, push down the chest about one-third of the way, or 1.5 inches (4 cm). In children greater than 1 year old, push

down the same amount as you would for an adult (2 inches, or 5 cm).

6. The hand position for infant or small child chest compressions is also done differently than with larger children and adults. In infants, if you are the only person available, perform chest compressions by pushing down on the chest, between the nipples, with your index and middle fingers (Figure 49.10).

7. If there is more than one person available to help with the resuscitation, perform chest compressions by encircling the infant's chest between your hands and using your thumbs to push down on the chest between the nipples (Figure 49.11). In small children you may choose to use the heel of just one hand to perform chest compressions (Figure 49.12).

Hint

A child's airway anatomy is slightly different than that of an adult (Figure 49.13). In proportion to their body, children's heads are much bigger and therefore cause the head to flex (looking down instead of looking up) when they are lying flat. Be sure to use the head tilt–chin lift technique to fully extend the head (looking upward) so the larynx and trachea become a straight tube for air to easily pass (Figure 49.14). If it is still difficult to breathe air into the child's mouth despite repositioning, look for a foreign body in the airway. Because a child's head is large, chest compressions may be difficult to perform effectively. If this occurs, try placing a small towel underneath the child's shoulders for support.

Airway foreign body

If the throat becomes blocked by a foreign body (most often a piece of food in adults, and food or a toy in children) it can stop oxygen from entering the lungs and getting into the blood. This can quickly cause the brain and heart to stop functioning from lack of oxygen, and lead to death. Suspect that the airway is blocked by a foreign

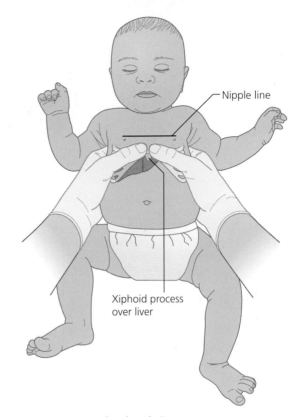

Figure 49.11 Two-thumb technique.

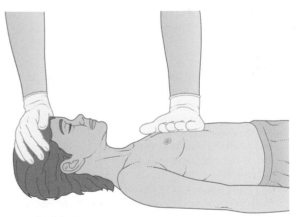

Figure 49.12 One-handed chest compressions in small children.

body if witnesses said that the patient was choking before becoming unconscious, or if despite positioning and repositioning the head and airway you are unable to blow breaths into the mouth. If the patient is unconscious and unresponsive, lay him or her on the floor, face up, put one hand on top of the other and, with the heel of the

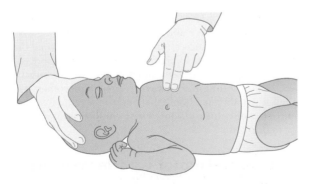

Figure 49.10 Two-fingered chest compressions for single-rescuer chest compressions in infants.

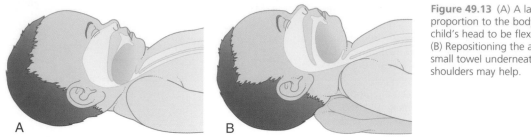

Figure 49.13 (A) A large head in proportion to the body causes a child's head to be flexed forward. (B) Repositioning the airway using a small towel underneath the child's shoulders may help.

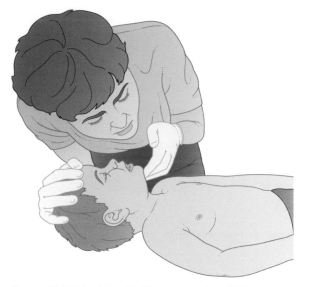

Figure 49.14 Head tilt–chin lift maneuver in a child.

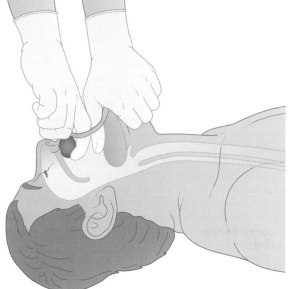

Figure 49.15 Finger sweep.

bottom hand, push hard and fast on the belly button angling toward the head several times. This is called the Heimlich maneuver (chest compressions). You will usually need to straddle the patient with your legs to get into the proper position if they are on the floor.

Next open the mouth by holding the head and pushing down on the chin, and look at the back of the throat to see if there is any foreign body. If there is, use a finger to scoop it out (Figure 49.15). Do this only if you are sure that the patient is unconscious and unresponsive or else he or she may bite down on your finger. If you are unsure, you may use any type of safe instrument to remove the foreign body. If you see no airway foreign body, reposition the head again by extending the head and attempt to breathe air into the patient's mouth. If air will still not go in, attempt several chest compressions just as you would in performing CPR. Continue this cycle of alternating abdominal thrusts and chest compressions and checking the airway for a foreign body with pauses for pulse checks, until an ambulance arrives. Begin CPR if no pulse is present.

The Heimlich maneuver is performed differently in children, infants, and pregnant women. In infants, five back blows followed by five chest thrusts should be done in sequence (Figure 49.16) and repeated as necessary. In children, five abdominal thrusts should be performed in quick succession followed by checking the airway to see if the foreign body has been dislodged. If no foreign body is seen, attempt two rescue breaths after repositioning the airway. In pregnant women, no abdominal thrusts should be performed so as not to hurt the baby. Instead, only chest compressions should be performed.

Trauma and motor vehicle accidents

Basic life support care in the setting of trauma is performed in the same manner as in nontrauma cases, with a few

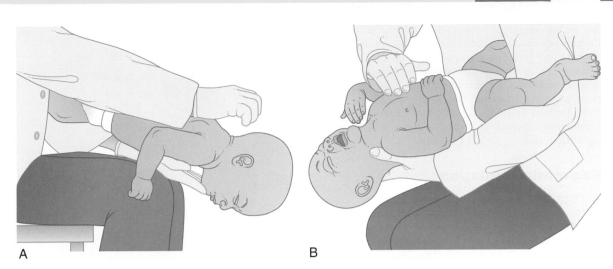

A

B

Figure 49.16 Infant airway foreign body: perform five back blows (A) followed by five chest thrusts (B).

important exceptions. A common cause of severe injury or death from trauma is in the setting of motor vehicle accidents. If you witness a motor vehicle accident in which you think people may be seriously hurt or dying, your first priority is to call an ambulance. Once this is done, your second priority is to assess for scene safety. You must be sure that you and other noninjured bystanders do not sustain injuries during the rescue and resuscitation efforts. If on a road, make sure that all traffic has stopped, especially if on a freeway with other vehicles traveling at high speeds. Rescuers have been seriously hurt and killed when hit by cars while attempting to help accident victims. If the scene is safe, approach the vehicle, telling the patient that you are there to help and ask if he or she is hurt. If possible, tell the patient to turn off the car's engine. If the patient does not talk back to you, assess as you would an unresponsive patient. Check the patient's breathing and pulse, and initiate CPR if indicated. If there is any evidence or concern that the patient may have hurt the neck or back, do all tasks, including CPR, with cervical spine precautions (see following text).

The most common cause of death from trauma is bleeding. Blood carries the necessary nutrients that the brain and heart need to survive. If through a serious injury a patient loses too much blood, there will be no way for the necessary nutrients to reach these vital organs. Thus it is important to control bleeding. This is most easily accomplished by covering the site of bleeding and pushing down hard until the blood clots and stops actively bleeding. In an emergency situation when medical supplies are not available, balled up clothing works well to stop bleeding. If the patient is awake and responsive, this step can be done immediately. If the patient is not responsive and requires CPR, begin it immediately and have another person control bleeding by covering the site and applying direct pressure.

Cervical spine injury

In the case of a serious trauma victim, it is best to assume that the patient has sustained a cervical spine injury until proven otherwise. The brain controls the function and sensation of the rest of the body through nerves. The vast majority of these nerves leave the brain through the bottom of the skull, forming the spinal cord. The spinal cord travels down the spine and branches off to innervate various parts of the body. The spine vertebrae, or backbones, protect the spinal cord from damage. If any of these bones become broken, the spinal cord is at risk of becoming injured, potentially resulting in permanent neurologic disability. In patients who have undergone trauma, the cervical spine (backbone of the neck) is the most at risk of getting broken, resulting in cervical spinal cord injury.

To prevent further injury after a trauma, precautions must be taken to minimize all neck movements such as twisting, bending, and flexing. Keep the neck in a neutral position with the head looking straight ahead and neck relaxed. This is accomplished through "in-line immobilization." If you must move a patient with a possible cervical spine or spinal cord injury, do your best to keep the neck in line (e.g., in parallel) with the rest of the body. Minimize all twisting movements by being at the patient's head, placing your hands along the patient's upper shoulders (above the shoulder blades), and using your forearms to lightly press against the patient's head. When the upper body moves, the neck and head will move in the same direction, trying to prevent further neck injury.

One important change to CPR in trauma victims is that you do not perform the head tilt–chin lift maneuver to check the airway. This moves the neck and could cause further injury. Instead use the jaw thrust method. There are two ways to perform a jaw thrust, depending on whether you are standing at the patient's head or chest. If you are at the patient's head, use both your palms to cup the side of the head and your fingers to grab the angle of the jaw and pull upward, causing just the lower jaw to move up without causing the head or neck to move. If you are at the patient's chest, use your palms and fingers to grab the side of the patient's head and your thumbs under the angle of the jaw and push upward, again causing the lower jaw to move up without moving the head or neck.

Bag-mask ventilation

You might have access to a bag-mask during CPR. Ventilations given by bag-mask are better and safer than mouth-to-mouth rescue breathing and should always be used if available. To properly use a bag-mask, the most important technique is to create a good seal between the mouthpiece of the mask and the patient's mouth. In this way no air escapes. If you are the only person who is available to help with rescue breathing, place the mask on the patient, use your thumb and index finger to create a "C" that pushes the mask firmly and evenly across the patient's mouth, and use your middle, ring, and pinky (little) fingers along the patient's jaw line, pulling the patient's lower jaw up toward the mask (Figure 49.17). Use your other hand to squeeze the ventilation bag.

If two people are able to help with rescue breathing, one person uses one hand on each side of the mask and jaw in the same way that you would hold the mask and pull up on the jaw as if you were by yourself (Figure 49.18). The other person squeezes the ventilation bag. Squeeze the ventilation bag just enough to see the chest rise each time to give the correct amount of air.

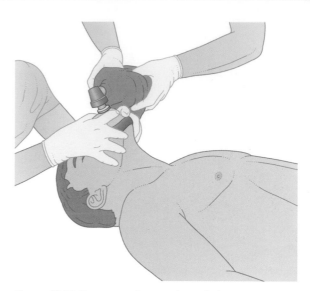

Figure 49.18 Two-person bag-mask ventilation.

Hints

If you have difficulty getting the chest to rise with bag-mask ventilation, first check to make sure that you have a good mask seal. Listen carefully: if you hear air escaping out the side of the mask, make sure that the mask fits correctly, covering only the nose and mouth. If you do have a good mask fit, then try to reposition the neck with the head tilt–chin lift or the jaw thrust technique, again pulling up on the jaw to open the throat and windpipe as much as possible.

Advanced cardiac life support/ advanced airways

If you have interest in learning more about resuscitation, consider taking a course in advanced cardiac life support (ACLS) or an advanced airway course. In ACLS you will learn further resuscitation management. Topics covered include giving the patient very strong drugs that work directly on the heart and blood vessels as well as what to do in other life-threatening situations. In an advanced airway course, you can learn how to use nasopharyngeal airways (NPAs). These are soft rubber tubes pushed down the nose that go to the back of the throat and help air reach the lungs. You will also learn about oropharyngeal airways (OPAs): hard rubber devices that go into the mouth and down the back of the throat to help air reach the lungs. Endotracheal intubation uses a special instrument called a laryngoscope to look directly into the back of the throat so as to place a tube into the windpipe to deliver air directly into the lungs. Courses are also available in pediatric advanced life support (PALS), neonatal resuscitation program (NRP), and advanced trauma life support (ATLS), among others.

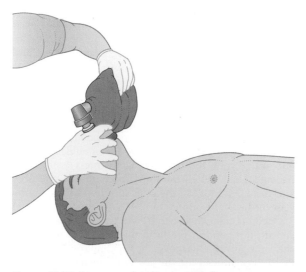

Figure 49.17 One-person bag-mask ventilation.

FINAL THOUGHTS

Seeing someone suddenly become unresponsive or finding an unresponsive person can be a frightening experience as a health care provider. Thankfully, these situations are rare. However, this can make performing CPR correctly very difficult because you will have little practice. It is important to periodically review the CPR guidelines and techniques so when the unexpected situation occurs, the skills you have practiced will come naturally. The quick initiation of CPR with minimal interruptions in fast and deep chest compressions will give someone the best chance of survival. When the situation arises, take a deep breath, try to remain calm, and trust yourself to quickly start CPR.

Questions for review and thought

1. In what cases should you start CPR?
2. Outline your procedure for performing one-person CPR.
3. What are the differences between one-person and two-person CPR?
4. What are the various procedures to deal with obstructed airways?

Q Self-evaluation questions

True–false statements

Directions: Indicate whether the statement is true **(T)** or false **(F).**

1. In an adult patient found unresponsive but with irregular gasps, you do not need to start the CPR sequence. **T** or **F**
2. The most common cause of death in trauma is as a result of spinal cord injury. **T** or **F**
3. If after an initial cycle of CPR a child remains unresponsive, is still not breathing but has a heart rate of 50 beats per minute, chest compressions should be started immediately. **T** or **F**

Missing words

Directions: write in the missing word(s) in the following sentences:

4. The _____ maneuver should be used to open the airway in a patient with a potential cervical spine injury.
5. If at all possible, use a _____ when performing mouth-to-mouth resuscitation.
6. The _____ pulse, followed by the _____ pulse and then _____ pulse are the most reliable locations to feel for a pulse.

Choice-completion questions

Directions: Select the one best answer in each case.

7. When seeing a motor vehicle injury in which you are concerned about serious injury, the most important first step is to:
   a. assess scene safety.
   b. call an ambulance.
   c. assess if the patient is responsive.
   d. perform in-line stabilization of the cervical spine.
   e. turn off the damaged car's engine.
8. If you are alone and come upon a child who had an unwitnessed arrest and is found to be unresponsive or not breathing without a pulse, the first step is to:
   a. call an ambulance.
   b. reposition the airway.
   c. perform 2 minutes of 30 chest compressions and two rescue breath cycles.
   d. search for an AED.
   e. perform the Heimlich maneuver.
9. Effective chest compressions should:
   a. be at least 100 compressions per minute.
   b. have the chest pushed down at least 2 inches (5 cm) in an adult.
   c. allow the chest wall to fully recoil after each chest compression.
   d. have all attempts made to have the minimal amount of interruptions or pauses in chest compressions.
   e. all the above.
10. The correct algorithm of adult chest compressions is:
   a. cycles of 30 chest compressions and two rescue breaths for 2 minutes, followed by a 10-second pulse check.
   b. cycles of 15 chest compressions and two rescue breaths for 2 minutes, if you have another provider to help you with the CPR.
   c. one cycle of 30 chest compressions and two rescue breaths followed by a 10-second pulse check.
   d. if an AED is available and the patient has a shockable rhythm, a 10-second pulse check should be performed after a shock and before starting cycles of 30 chest compressions and two rescue breaths for 2 minutes.
   e. if an AED is available and the patient has a shockable rhythm, continuous cycles of 30 chest compressions and two rescue breaths should be performed without any interruptions for pulse checks.

A Answers, notes, and explanations

1. **False.** If the patient is unresponsive and has irregular gasps (agonal gasping) you need to continue the CPR sequence. Call for an ambulance and perform a pulse check to see if chest compressions need to be initiated. Though agonal gasping can take on several forms, the most common is irregular, ineffective, short, loud air movements in the mouth that do not reach the lungs.

2. **False.** Though spinal cord injury is a common and potentially serious injury, bleeding is the most common cause of death from trauma. It should be addressed by trying to stop the bleeding with direct pressure early in resuscitation.

3. **True.** In children, chest compressions should be immediately started if there is no pulse or if the pulse is less than 60 beats per minute after a cycle of rescue breathing.

4. **Jaw thrust.** If near the patient's head, place both palms along the head and use your fingers to pull the jaw upward. If near the patient's chest, place your fingers along both sides of the head and use your thumbs to push the jaw upward. It is important to minimize all neck movement during this maneuver.

5. **Mouth barrier.** Unfortunately, mouth barriers are rarely available outside a hospital scenario. If available, they should always be used for your safety.

6. **Carotid, femoral, radial.** It can be hard to feel a pulse in a high-stress situation and within the required amount of time (10 seconds) before chest compressions should be started or resumed. If available, it is always best to have multiple providers feeling for a pulse simultaneously.

7. **b. Call an ambulance.** Once this is done, assess if the scene is safe. If you get injured while trying to help, there will now be one more injured person that requires care. Once these two steps are done, begin your CPR assessment by seeing if the patient is responsive.

8. **c. Perform 2 minutes of 30 chest compressions and two rescue breath cycles.** Contrary to an adult found unresponsive, not breathing, and without a pulse, a child in the same condition should immediately have 2 minutes of cycles of 30 chest compressions and two rescue breaths, if you are by yourself. Then an ambulance should be called. If there are multiple providers, one provider should call for an ambulance and look for an AED, while other providers perform cycles of 15 chest compressions and two rescue breaths for 2 minutes.

9. **e. All of the above.** Quality chest compressions will contain each one of these elements. Early initiation and minimal interruptions in chest compressions have the greatest effect when attempting to save the life of a person whose heart has stopped beating.

10. **a. Cycles of 30 chest compressions and two rescue breaths for 2 minutes, followed by a 10-second pulse check.** This is the correct CPR algorithm for an adult. The correct CPR algorithm in children, if you have another provider, is cycles of 15 chest compressions and two rescue breaths for 2 minutes. If an AED is available and the patient has a shockable rhythm, after the shock is delivered, cycles of 30 chest compressions and two rescue breaths for 2 minutes should be initiated immediately without first assessing for a pulse after the shock. However, you should assess for a pulse at the end of the 2-minute cycle of CPR.

Chapter 50

Computers in ophthalmic practice

Michael L. Gilbert, Gerald E. Meltzer

Computer technology is relatively young, the first digital computer as we know it having been built in 1937. However, the computerization of the civilized world has had an enormous effect on nearly every aspect of contemporary daily life and a major effect on the way ophthalmology is practiced. It is estimated that more than 95% of all ophthalmologic offices use computers for such tasks as insurance billing, practice management reporting, payroll, sending recall notices, or even calling patients automatically to remind them of missed appointments or to notify them that their contact lenses have arrived. Beyond the myriad practice-centered uses of desktop, laptop, and tablet or handheld computers, computerization not only controls but also aids in interpreting the results of many of the instruments commonly used in direct patient care, including the lensometer, keratometer, phoropter, perimeter, ultrasound, and optical biometry, as well as nonophthalmic but otherwise critical tools such as Internet-based telephone, digital copy machine, and the cell phone. Thus computers increasingly contribute fundamentally to better patient care as well as to increased office productivity.

The effect of computers in the field of ophthalmology is a reflection of an accelerating trend in office automation. Universal acceptance of computer technology by worldwide industries, coupled with markedly decreasing costs and widespread availability of inexpensive computer hardware and software programs, has defined a new era in computer-assisted medical care. Well-used computerization is a boon to quality patient care, staff efficiency, and practice success at all levels. This chapter is designed to expand the ophthalmic assistant's knowledge base about computers, how they work, and what they can do for an ophthalmologic office and its personnel.

COMPUTER BASICS

A computer is a device capable of accepting, storing, retrieving, and manipulating or processing information automatically at high speeds by applying a sequence of logical arithmetic or textual operations. In simpler terms, a computer is able to execute a series of instructions that allow the user to ask questions as simple as "What does Fred Smith owe on his account?" The ability to instantly and invisibly respond to sequential instructions allows computerization to aid in more sophisticated tasks such as the analysis of complex data generated by the automated lensmeter, autorefraction, retinal tomography, or corneal topography. With mounting hardware speed, complexity, and capability, computers can even make some complex decisions through the use of artificial intelligence. By comparing new patient data with stored historical databases of comparable results from normal patients, computers are able to aid in the interpretation of visual fields, corneal topography, or optic nerve analysis. This ongoing evaluation process not only aids in the initial diagnosis of disease but also helps track clinically significant changes involved in monitoring glaucoma, keratoconus, and retinal edema.

COMPUTER COMPONENTS

The physical components of a computer are referred to as the *hardware,* and the programs that instruct the computer what to do are known as *software.* Computer hardware includes four major parts: the central processing unit (CPU), input devices, output devices, and storage devices. These elements are common to all computer devices, from smartphones and tablets to the largest mainframe servers.

Central processing unit

The CPU is the brains of the computer. It performs logical and mathematic functions such as addition and subtraction, as well as comparing numbers or names. The CPU also controls the flow of information within the computer, retrieving and storing information at the same time it is processing data. The CPU is closely integrated with the temporary memory known as random access memory (RAM).

Input devices

Despite the popularity of alternative input devices such as the mouse, touch screen, character recognition, and voice recognition, the keyboard remains the most commonly used device for input of alphanumeric data into computers. Predominantly the keyboard is used as a text entry interface, although software may alter the interpretation of each key. The mouse is a popular and efficient input tool used to manipulate data on the computer screen, perform additions or deletions in word processing, and draw or alter graphics. Sophisticated mouse technology allows accurate forward and reverse scrolling, together with programmable functions for the mouse-actuating keys. Most offices now use scanners to capture images or digitize text through optical character recognition (OCR). Increasingly computer input is achieved by light pens, touch screens, barcode scanners, and various wireless devices to enter data and images as well as to control computer operation.

Networking of computers and diagnostic equipment allows the ophthalmic assistant to enter the output of devices such as an automated lensmeter, visual field machine, or corneal mapping device directly into the computer. Broadband cable and related technologies allow users to enter data *remotely* as well as review charts, images, and other vital data whether it is in the next room or a satellite office hundreds of miles away.

Voice recognition technology is used in some ophthalmic offices for medical record entry, transcription of professional correspondence, and even to control equipment such as the operating microscope. This technology allows automated translation from the spoken word to a desired action, or simply the entry of text into the intended medical record or program.

Output devices

The two main output devices of a computer are monitors and printers. Along with most technologic advances, monitors have become thinner and larger and present higher resolution while also becoming more affordable. The need for printers has rapidly evolved in the medical practice. Whereas the dot matrix printer was once important to produce multiple sequential copies of billing forms, the laser printer rapidly eclipsed it on speed, clarity, and cost. Laser printing in turn is being replaced by electronic transmission of professional correspondence, and billing is done by direct transfer of information electronically by direct upload and download of claims-related data, or by transfer over the Internet.

Storage devices (memory)

With increasing computerization throughout the ophthalmic office there is a growing explosion of data, especially from diagnostic technologies that generate large image files. The contemporary ophthalmic practice is likely to have multiple digital imaging systems, for topography, slit lamp, optic nerve, and retina. Such increasing storage needs can be met by increasingly large hard drives as well as secondary storage to optical discs or alternative drive technologies or even remote cloud storage.

Back-ups

Computers should be backed up on a regular basis to prevent loss of data. This is especially true for practices which have implemented electronic health records (EHRs). One cannot stress enough how critical multiple back-ups are to make sure that data are never lost or compromised. There are numerous protocols and technologies for backing up office data. Data are initially stored on network servers or on cloud storage. These servers are then backed up to storage media such as tape drives or remotely located disc drives. Although slower than some alternatives, tape drives can hold large amounts of data retrieved from multiple networked computers. Alternative back-up technologies include writing to CD, DVD, or flash drives as well as optical drives, or even direct off-site storage achieved by broadband transfer of data copies to contracted data storage enterprises.

Whatever the combination of technologies used to back up data, the regular and consistent commitment to creation of data copies is critical for each and every device because eventually one or more will fail. Such unexpected failure leaves the practice totally reliant on a back-up of data to avert loss or corruption of critical practice records.

COMPUTER TASKS

Applications software

Computers can perform a variety of tasks in an ophthalmic office, including billing patients, scheduling appointments, keeping medical records, sending insurance forms to Medicare and other health insurance companies, and tracking their subsequent payment. Computers aid physicians in statistical analysis of their surgical results, managing complex practice finances, modeling cost–benefit considerations of equipment purchases, coordinating projects, writing journal articles, or doing literature searches. Computerization of the ophthalmic office significantly increases practice productivity and staff efficiency by automating many of the ophthalmic assistant's routine tasks such as history taking, patient testing, and ordering contact lenses. Software packages specifically written for ophthalmic offices are becoming increasingly available. Properly designed and installed computer hardware and software should make the ophthalmic assistant's task of seeing and treating patients easier and more rewarding.

General office software

Many general office software products find powerful utility in the ophthalmic practice. Software is widely available for word processing, spreadsheets, contact management, computer presentation, website authoring, project management, and accounting. Such software tools are often integrated into powerful, successful, and familiar product packages available off the shelf that are immediately adaptable for the ophthalmic practice. However, many needs of the ophthalmic office are unique and create an opportunity for customized software applicable to the medical office in general and the ophthalmic practice in particular.

Practice management software

There is a growing array of choices for sophisticated software packages designed specifically for the ophthalmic practice. Increasingly this means resources to handle billing, accounts receivable, and appointments. The availability of the electronic medical record is an expanding option in ophthalmic practice. As the community practice of ophthalmology evolves, such dedicated software packages meet expanding practice needs through increasingly available modules to address various departments with specific and unique needs. Such modules can address the needs of the contact lens practice, inventory and laboratory management for optical departments, and even the demanding needs of running an ambulatory surgery center.

Appointment scheduling

The use of computers for scheduling is almost universal regardless of practice size. Larger practices with several offices and multiple physicians find it mandatory to use networking resources to centralize appointment scheduling. Such software makes it relatively easy to answer a quick patient question such as your next available routine appointment or to identify the exact time and date of a previously made appointment. For the computerized office it is hard to imagine having to manually search pages of appointments to find one name. The computer can also be programmed to track insurance benefits and required referrals or copay amounts; produce patient reminders; keep clinical records; track allergies, medications, and contact lenses; and flag patients who repeatedly miss appointments. Computers also can call attention to patients who are receiving critically needed drugs and fail to return for routine follow-up visits. Such software also directs general periodic recalls either by e-mail or by self-dialing computerized calling equipment.

Billing and accounting

Accounts receivable software allows an office to easily prepare bills, convert codes for services into statements, submit claims electronically or by hard copy, produce reminder letters for delinquent accounts, and analyze accounts and referral sources. This is a formidably complex task made manageable only through well-developed software and computerization.

Because most patients have some form of insurance, it is imperative to have a way to properly complete insurance documents, direct its receipt to the appropriate entity, track payments, and alert the office staff when not paid promptly and completely. Billing software has been written to automate many tasks that previously had to be performed manually, such as checking for appropriate coding, posting charges and payments, sending claims to insurance companies, and closely monitoring accounts receivable.

Many medical billing packages include software to write checks, maintain payroll, and keep the general ledger. Other software may facilitate electronic transfer of billing data offsite where accounting services may be performed remotely or otherwise outsourced. When any practice employee writes a large number of checks each month to the same people, computerization can provide precision and efficiency while saving tedious work and, in the long run, can save many dollars by automating the monthly payment and posting functions.

Management reporting

Historically the main reward of computerizing a medical office has been that of more efficient use of the data collected daily in the business office. Such data include patient names, zip codes, referral sources, diagnoses, and procedures done. Thus computers make it possible for office management to easily determine where patients are coming from, whether a marketing program is successful, and how

extending JCAHPO to associate with, and develop, regional certification standards in developing countries. Thus specialists have developed in a wide variety of technical areas, including optics, eye movements, contact lenses, surgical science, mechanics, lasers, computers, photography, and imaging (x-ray, ultrasound, nuclear magnetic resonance). These scientific fields have produced specialized groups that assist patients with clinical and laboratory procedures measuring essential data necessary to evaluate and treat eye problems.

Allied health fields in eye care have expanded outside the control of ophthalmology. These include optometry, opticians, and ophthalmic registered nurses.

CLINICAL ROLES FOR OPHTHALMIC MEDICAL PERSONNEL

Modern eye care has developed a wide range of career choices for ophthalmic medical personnel.

General ophthalmic assistant

This multitasking role usually involves administrative functions (patient appointments, greeting, chart preparation, filing, and billing) and clinical functions (history taking, visual acuity, measuring glasses, intraocular pressure, and basic eye movements) (Figure 51.1).

Specialized ophthalmic assistant

The greatest numbers of assistants work in clinical offices where, subject to training and patient needs, the ophthalmic medical personnel may undertake highly specialized

functions. In the general ophthalmologist's office, a single assistant may complete administrative and basic clinical duties to assist the ophthalmologist. Larger offices and clinics, and those that specialize in limited areas of eye care, require a variety of highly specialized, mainly technical, ophthalmic medical personnel to aid in diagnosis and management of special eye problems. Contact lenses, cataract, refractive, glaucoma, pediatric ophthalmology, and retinal surgery require specially trained ophthalmic medical personnel. In these specialized clinics it is common to have several ophthalmic medical personnel each performing their unique special function (Figures 51.2 and 51.3).

Therefore, it has developed that ophthalmic medical personnel have been directed by the needs of society, the ophthalmologist, and personal interests and skills to

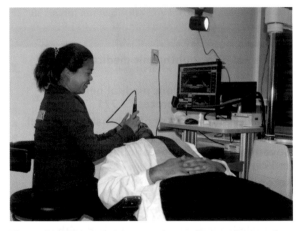

Figure 51.2 The technician completes a B-scan ultrasound.

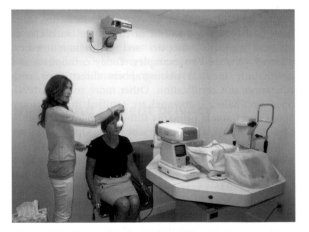

Figure 51.1 The assistant completes vision testing.

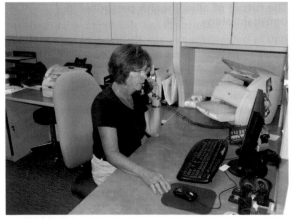

Figure 51.3 Office administrator, manager.

formally become educated and certified in highly specialized areas. These assistants provide a quality of service mandated by current medical standards, government regulations, and the needs of patients with eye problems.

EDUCATION OF OPHTHALMIC MEDICAL PERSONNEL AND THE CERTIFICATION PROCESS

Candidates generally require a high school diploma to enter training as ophthalmic medical personnel (OMP). General characteristics essential for success include enjoyment in working with people and dealing with visual health problems, a curious scientific nature, responsible and analytical thinking, multitasking ability, and a desire to solve problems.

The greatest numbers of OMP start their careers in clinical offices, but there is an increasing number attending formal training programs. Financial support for the education of OMP is available through a wide variety of sources, including the JCAHPO Education and Research Foundation.[1]

Informal training: on the job

With the support of an ophthalmologist, an interested employee can complete an approved independent home study course. Home study courses under several authorities in Canada and the American Academy of Ophthalmology in the United States provide the basic academic training required for office personnel to acquire certification. Successful completion allows the registrant to seek certification as a Certified Ophthalmic Assistant (COA). Training and coursework enable the employee to achieve the Certified Ophthalmic Technician (COT) and Certified Ophthalmic Medical Technologist (COMT) certifications. Other countries are separately, or with the support of International JCAHPO (IJCAHPO), developing their own appropriate programs.

Formal training: institutional programs[2]

Colleges, universities, and special educational institutes mainly in Canada, the United States, and other parts of the Western world offer formal training programs of 1 or more years' duration in more specialized areas of visual science. Further information can be obtained from websites documented in Table 51.1. With these diplomas or degrees, ophthalmic medical personnel are routinely certified as technicians or technologists (COT or COMT).

All certified OMP receive their education and certification under ophthalmic medical academic and clinical personnel. Senior certificants (COT and COMT) often become teachers in the family of education and policymakers by participating in the certifying bodies. Others use their skills to enter the business world.

It is estimated that about 125,000 people work as allied health personnel in ophthalmology in North America. The majority of these assistants do not have certification. They provide basic administrative and clinical needs in general ophthalmology offices. JCAHPO has approximately 22,730 COA registrants in 33 countries. There are about 700 COMT registrants. Health care standards and government regulations relating to quality-of-care and medicolegal issues are rapidly leading to necessary certification and recertification of all health care personnel.

In 2015 there were 40 CoA-level programs in Canada, the United States, Fiji, and Puerto Rico approved by the Commission on Accreditation of Ophthalmic Medical Programs (CoA-OMP).[3]

IJACHPO and the International Council of Ophthalmology, have already developed two core curricula for (1) ophthalmic assistants, and (2) refractive error, which are available in some countries. Information on IJCAHPO services is available on the JCAHPO website.

THE CERTIFICATION PROCESS OF OPHTHALMIC MEDICAL PERSONNEL

Professional specialty groups of ophthalmologists created the JCAHPO in 1969 as an educational and certifying body for OMP. As of 2015 JCAHPO is made up of 21 ophthalmic physician/surgeon and ophthalmic allied health societies/associations from Canada, the United States, and around the world (see Table 51.1). There are now 15 regular member organizations and 6 affiliate member organizations in the commission. The commission governs the JCAHPO.

Educational meetings at local, regional, and national levels have been supplemented with published JCAHPO courses. Web-based programs (EyeCare) are increasingly making education available worldwide. Many of the

---

[1]The JCAHPO Education & Research Foundation is available online at www.jcahpo.org/foundation.htm.

[2]The Committee on Accreditation for Ophthalmic Medical Personnel (CoA-OMP) is a good start when looking for institutional programs. Its website is http://www.coa-omp.org/.

[3]CoA-OMP information is available at their website, http://www.coa-omp.org/.

OPHTHALMIC MEDICAL PERSONNEL ALLIED WITH JCAHPO

Ophthalmic photographers

An ophthalmic photographer takes photographs of external or internal parts of the eye, often with specialized single-frame or movie, digital, and film-based cameras. They use drugs to evaluate functions of blood vessels in diabetes and other eye diseases. Computers and digital cameras allow telemedicine, where satellite transmission sends images to another location, for interpretation by an ophthalmologist.

The Ophthalmic Photographers' Society educates and certifies ophthalmic photographers in North America.

Orthoptists

An orthoptist measures eye movements and relates eye and brain controls of single and binocular vision. These measures lead to diagnosis and treatment of strabismus (squint), lazy eye (amblyopia), and other problems of eye movement, refraction, and sensory and motor control of eye movement within the brain. These problems are mainly seen in children, but occur throughout life as a result of trauma, cancer, and vascular and neurologic diseases.

The American Orthoptic Society in the United States, the Canadian Orthoptic Society in Canada, and equivalent societies around the world educate and are integrated in their own certifying processes.

INDEPENDENT ALLIED HEALTH PERSONNEL IN VISUAL SCIENCE

Ophthalmic operating room nurses

Ophthalmic operating room nurses (OORNs) are specially trained registered nurses. OORNs work as independent partners with surgeons under hospital and government regulatory authority. They educate and certify their own personnel.

Opticians

Opticians work in two specialty areas: as technicians making and repairing optical devices such as spectacles and contact lenses, and dispensing and fitting these optical devices to patients' needs. Contact lens manufacturing and fitting are often entirely separate from the field of spectacles, including training and certifying in some countries.

Registered nurses and opticians are trained and certified outside the control of medicine, although medicine (including ophthalmology) participates at the regulatory and management levels of these specialties.

THE FUTURE OF ALLIED HEALTH PERSONNEL IN OPHTHALMOLOGY

Medical science is advancing at a rapid rate, and new technologies are being presented to aid diagnosis and treatment in all medical fields. This has been particularly true in ophthalmology as a result of extensive advancements in microsurgery and technical testing procedures involving a wide range of wavelength energy machines that are used to analyze every part of the eye and visual system. Technical assistants use more sophisticated machines as medical science unfolds new fields of study. Genetics may introduce new opportunities in the fields of biochemistry. Qualified medical personnel are required to provide skilled services in these areas. The future will see all visual science fields working closely together as scientific knowledge, public requirements, and high costs require that assistants be trained to keep these services available at the lowest possible cost. Increasing office management requirements, especially with electronic records and increased regulation, will require highly qualified office staff. Thus there is a strong, and growing, market for ophthalmic medical personnel.

Chapter | 52 |

Ophthalmology ethics

Alex V. Levin

INTRODUCTION

Issues that challenge our ethical and moral value systems have been part of medicine throughout recorded history. As early as the 5th century BC, Hippocrates recognized the role of ethics, virtue, and moral compass in the practice of medicine in what has become known as the *Hippocratic oath*, which physicians in many countries pledge upon receiving their medical degrees. In 1241 Frederick II, the King of Naples, recognized the risks of conflict of interest when physicians engage in business relationships with apothecaries in his Law for the Regulation of the Practice of Medicine. Sir William Osler's 1906 treatise, *Equanimities*, is filled with commentary on many examples of the ethical issues that physicians face in their daily lives.

The 1960s brought an accelerated evolution of medical technology. Medicine was now able to prolong the end of life, engage in heroic surgical interventions, and save the lives of infants born at increasingly earlier ages of prematurity. With this progress also came increased attention to the ethical issues that attended such advances. The field of bioethics began to take shape and has undergone remarkable growth to the point where it has become a fundamental part of undergraduate, graduate, and continuing medical education as well as everyday practice.

In 1993 the American Academy of Ophthalmology (AAO) published its manual, *The Ethical Ophthalmologist: A Primer*. In 1995 the Royal College of Physicians and Surgeons of Canada mandated that ethics education must be part of all residency program curricula regardless of the medical or surgical specialty. Later, the Royal College would develop the Core Competencies of the CanMEDS program for physicians: Medical Expert (the central role), Communicator, Collaborator, Health Advocate, Manager, Scholar, and Professional. Each role has components that involve ethical considerations. Many training programs in ophthalmic assisting and other ophthalmic fields now include ethics in their curricula. Today most professional societies, including the AAO and the American Academy of Optometry, have published codes and guidelines for ethical behavior.

Every individual who plays a role in the ophthalmic care of patients will face ethical dilemmas. In trying to resolve these moral quandaries, each of us brings our own set of moral values and knowledge to the process. Given the almost infinite variety in our religious, family, cultural, and experiential backgrounds, it seems impossible to have a set of "right answers" that could dictate our response to ethical dilemmas when they arise. This is further complicated by the intricate details of each situation and the rich context of the lives of our patients, each with their own unique background and circumstances. The writings of philosophers and bioethicists represent many schools of thought (which are well beyond the scope of this chapter) that attempt to give us formulas or orientation of our thought processes to address our ethical challenges. Policymakers have laid out for us guidelines that prescribe acceptable and unacceptable actions and decisions as judged by peers and colleagues in the same institution or field. The law, reacting to events that question our actions within the context of our society's regulations on behavior, places further boundaries on our actions and decisions. Figures 52.1 and 52.2 offer diagrammatic approaches— one more simple and workable (see Figure 52.1) and the other perhaps more complex and attuned to the deliberations of the person with a deeper interest in bioethics (see Figure 52.2)—to how these circles of considerations

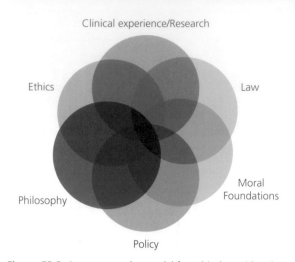

Figure 52.2 A more complex model for ethical consideration that is perhaps more applicable to a person with a deeper interest in bioethics.

in our lives might intersect to help us address ethical issues in our minds and in our practice.

Each reader of this chapter and every professional in the field of ophthalmic care will be faced with the task of resolving ethical dilemmas. The word *ethics* is indeed a plural word. There is more than one ethic depending on the specifics of the situation at hand and the background of the professional. Understanding the rich context of the patient's situation—culture, family, disease, prognosis, education level, religion, support systems, alternative health care practices, and wishes—is perhaps the first step in laying the foundation for understanding and conflict resolution. Practitioners must also understand their own orientation and bias when dealing with these issues. Each of us may make different decisions, but we must do so in a comfort zone that lies within the policy guidelines and law that govern our practice as well as the ethics boundaries beyond which most reasonable people would recognize transgression. Within those boundaries is a wide zone of possible pathways to resolution of an ethical quandary. Choosing the resolution that best suits the needs and desires of the patient is paramount, and finding a solution that is agreeable to the ophthalmic team and the individual practitioner responsible for the patient's care is most desirable.

This chapter is not intended to be a prescription of correct answers to every ethical issue that might confront eye care professionals; each issue addressed could itself become an entire chapter or book. Rather, it offers identification of issues, and a context in which they might be considered, and raises questions one might ask in trying to bring to consciousness those variables that should be addressed in trying to resolve a moral quandary. The readers of this textbook will likely come from many jurisdictions,

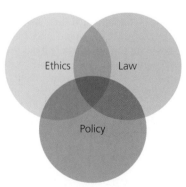

Figure 52.1 A simplified model for ethical consideration recognizing the intersection of ethics, policy, and law.

professions, and societies, so the following discussion must be interpreted within each specific context.

INFORMED CONSENT

Gone are the days when physicians simply told their patients what must be done to their bodies to treat their disease. Rather, we have developed a healthy recognition of the importance of autonomy: the right of people to make their own decisions about what they will and will not allow. Informed consent represents a partnership between medical professionals and their patients. Doctors have a fiduciary duty to ensure that each patient understands the treatment recommendations. Admittedly, this is not always entirely possible because patients rarely can achieve the same level of understanding as the doctor. In some cases patients may have such strong feelings of trust toward their physician that they make little effort to attain the knowledge level of truly informed consent and instead wish for the doctor to "do what's best for me." Yet the obligation of the physician remains to at least attempt to demonstrate that the patient does indeed have some comprehension of the medical plan.

Informed consent is more than the signed piece of paper titled "consent form." Informed consent is a process, documented in the patient's health record, wherein the physician or a trained delegate (e.g., the ophthalmic assistant) educates the patient and asks for his or her participation in the decision-making process. When the physician delegates this process, there should be an opportunity for the patient to ask questions of and speak directly to the physician if desired. Some situations require little more than the patient's action. When a patient sits at the slit lamp and puts the head forward, it is an implied consent to be examined. But when the medical encounter is to involve aspects of risk, in particular risks of bodily harm as in surgery or laser treatment, then more formal informed consent, preferably documented by the patient's signature, is required. Performing a procedure without consent may be considered as battery. Clearly there will be situations—usually those surrounding emergency medical issues—when the informed consent process must be either abbreviated or abandoned, assuming reasonable effort has been made.

The eye doctor must inform the patient of all common risks, no matter how small (including those that might result not only in changes in function but also appearance), and also all serious risks, no matter how uncommon. The disclosure of risk should be considered in the context of what a reasonable patient would want to know. Although the risks are very small, reasonable people would likely want to know about the risk of death from general anesthesia or the risk of blindness from cataract surgery.

Comprehension is another foundation of informed consent. Patients may refuse treatment, even if their decision will result in death or blindness, if they are deemed to have the capacity to do so. If the decision-making capacity of the patient is in question (e.g., in Alzheimer's disease), then a substitute decision maker must be found. In some jurisdictions this is a legal designation by power of attorney, whereas in other cultures it may be a family designation by virtue of marriage, age, or sibship. Informed consent for children is discussed in the following text.

Even when the patient is deemed capable, the ophthalmologist must ensure that the necessary information for decision making is presented in an understandable way. Risks may be described in relative terms rather than with incidence data. For example, one might say that the risk of an entirely well young adult dying from general anesthesia is less than the risk of dying in a road traffic accident. Although written information is helpful, it must be readable, preferably on a grade 6 to 8 level. Consent forms with many pages have become common, yet one can question whether they are likely to be read and understood by an average patient. No document can fully replace the conversation between physician and patient. The patient must be given the opportunity to ask questions and receive answers before making a voluntary decision without influence or coercion.

CONFIDENTIALITY

The ophthalmic health care team, like all medical professionals, has a duty to protect the confidentiality of the patient. The fulfillment of this duty enhances the trust relationship with and respects the autonomy of the patient.

Sharing of health records with other medical professionals is just one aspect of the confidentiality issue. One should remember that although the chart itself belongs to the physician or the health care institution, the information in the chart belongs to the patient. Information should not be shared with others, especially those outside the patient care team, without the patient's documented consent.

Ophthalmic professionals must also guard against accidental violations of confidentiality that can occur through the discussion of cases in public places such as elevators and registration desks or in easily overheard phone conversations. Patient charts should not be left in accessible view and computer screens with patient information should be protected by a password or screen saver. The use of email is governed by a variety of jurisdiction-specific law and policy because society is still addressing the challenge such communication imposes in our world of increasing electronic interaction. Encryption of messages may be a helpful safeguard. Portable electronic devices and hard-copy documents taken out of the patient care setting may be easily lost or stolen. Identifiable patient information should not leave the patient care setting in either form unless appropriate safeguards are in place (e.g., remote access to a secure server via a handheld device). Attention must be paid to photographs and other communications such as texts that exist on cell phones, tablets or other portable devices. Such content should be immediately transferred to the patient's chart or electronic medical record and deleted from the device. Password protection of such devices may be an insufficient safeguard. Electronic medical records, although secure, may also increase opportunities for access to patient information by curious individuals who are not directly involved in the patient's care. Without specific patient consent, such access is not allowed.

The medical professional may also be faced with situations in which there is a conflict between the patient's desire for confidentiality and the medical professional's desire to transmit information about the patient to other individuals. A patient may disclose to an ophthalmic assistant that the cause of his or her periocular ecchymosis was an assault by their spouse, but then ask that the ophthalmologist not be told. The ophthalmologist may become aware through evaluation of ophthalmic findings that a patient is infected with human immunodeficiency virus (HIV), but the patient does not wish to tell his or her sexual partner. Sometimes these situations can be anticipated and the patient forewarned that disclosure will obligate the physician to make the necessary transmittal of information either to public authorities (e.g., reportable communicable disease) or private individuals who may be at risk. Yet this obligation may hold even if the patient disclosed without being forewarned. In a landmark United States case, *Tarasoff v. Regents of the University of California,* where a psychiatrist came to know that a patient was likely to murder, the court ruled that the physician did have a duty to warn and protect by either notifying the intended victim or informing the police. The most desirable outcome in such difficult cases would be the resolution of conflict through a trusting partnership between patient and physician, perhaps with the assistance of nursing, counseling, and social work support, but if the ophthalmic professional feels that such partnership is not reasonably achievable in a satisfactory time frame, then the duty to breach confidentiality may apply.

TRUTH TELLING

Truth telling is another fundamental tenet that underlies the ethical practice of medicine. It is a foundation to the resolution of many issues discussed in this chapter (e.g., informed consent, duty to warn). Truth telling enhances trust and partnership and aids patients in understanding their disease. Sometimes, however, the ophthalmic team will receive requests to withhold the truth. The daughter of a 75-year-old man with ocular melanoma might say, "Please don't tell my father he has cancer." Although the physician may empathize with the daughter's sentiment

and truly feel that such information might do more harm than good if disclosed to the patient, it should be recognized that the courts in the Western world have found this principle of "therapeutic privilege" to be tenuous at best. Research studies have shown repeatedly that, in general, patients do want to be told the truth about their condition, and the health care team should endeavor to do so. Much has been written about patient communication and the breaking of bad news. It would benefit the members of the health care team to become skilled in these techniques. Exploring the reasons for the request of nondisclosure will likely lead to a strengthening of the doctor–family–patient relationship and easier resolution of the ethical dilemma.

BOUNDARY ISSUES

Respect for people also entails that their bodies not be violated in nonconsensual ways such as sexual advances or touching. This principle applies not only between coworkers in an ophthalmology office or clinic but also between health care professionals and their patients. Violation of boundaries may also come in the form of personal affronts without actual physical touching. Examples might include comments with inappropriate sexual content or aggressive and condescending behavior. The field of organizational ethics addresses many of these scenarios and the relationships between coworkers in various roles. In general, it is advisable for health care professionals to similarly avoid such behaviors, gestures, and advances toward their patients, including activities such as dating or sexual liaison.

MULTICULTURALISM

Many societies represent a rich blend of ethnicity, religion, and culture. With this variety in the patient population, ophthalmic professionals will likely encounter behaviors that seem foreign, if not objectionable. One must respect that there are a wide variety of behaviors to which the terms *right* and *wrong* do not apply. Rather, tolerance and understanding, often reached simply through dialog, become the basis of therapeutic success and patient compliance. For example, there are ways for a patient's appointment to be altered to a time that does not conflict with a religious holiday rather than demanding compliance with the original date.

There may be times when a cultural belief is not consistent with the laws or policies that govern the society in which the patient lives. If a mother has used her urine to treat her child's red eye and in doing so caused the child to contract gonorrhea conjunctivitis, then education to avoid this practice (in addition to bacterial culture and treatment for gonorrhea in the family as well as communicable disease reporting) is certainly indicated. To do so in a culturally sensitive way may be challenging. All medical professionals working in culturally diverse communities are encouraged to read Anne Fadiman's book, *The Spirit Catches You and You Fall Down* (Farrar, Straus and Giroux, New York, 1997).

VULNERABLE POPULATIONS

One must be particularly careful when addressing ethical dilemmas where the patient is part of a vulnerable population such as children (see following text), prisoners, minorities, and other groups who may, by virtue of their position in society, prejudice, mental incapacity, and prior unjust treatment, have impaired decision-making capacity or a lack of proper empowerment. Illness and infirmity may in themselves make the patient more vulnerable and less able to engage in capable decision making. The ophthalmic team must guard against bias and parentalism in these cases and maintain a healthy respect for the autonomy of these individuals. It is easy to become "blinded" by our beneficent parentalistic desires to benefit the patient and in so doing ignore the importance of autonomy for all patients. One might argue that extra care is required in order to ensure the rights, boundaries, privileges, and autonomy of such patients.

PEDIATRIC ETHICS

The ethical issues surrounding the care of children have enormous scope that extends well beyond the reaches of this chapter. Children are indeed a vulnerable population yet they do have a right to respect for their autonomy, which, even if they are not currently able to express it, will eventually blossom.

It is recommended that children be involved in their health care as much as possible, including discussions about their disease and proposed treatment. Infants and young children may not have the ability to participate meaningfully in the informed consent process so their parents or guardians become substitute decision makers, although the physician must ascertain that the decisions of these individuals are indeed in the best interest of the child. Although adults have the right to refuse treatment for themselves, even though such refusal could lead to death or blindness, they do not have the right to make such decisions for their children in most jurisdictions in North America. In such cases, if the health care team is unable to form a partnership with the family that would lead to a satisfactory resolution of the conflict, then the physician may be obligated to approach the child protection or legal

system for intervention on behalf of the child. Before resorting to these means, attempts to resolve conflicts with the use of social workers, clergy, mental health professionals, and other mediators can be helpful.

Likewise, parents may not harm their children and there is a firm legal obligation to report a suspicion of child abuse or neglect to child protection authorities. This is a legal as well as a moral obligation. Some health care professionals fail to report because of a lack of confidence in the system, a fear that parent and child will be separated unjustly, uncertainty over the diagnosis, a feeling that a well-known "good family" could never abuse or neglect their child, a fear of lost patient referrals, or a disinclination to have to take time to go to court to testify. In reality, the facts suggest that these fears and concerns are largely unjustified and inaccurate. In all cases, the health professional's legal obligation to report is the primary responsibility.

Older children may have some ability to participate in their own care decisions even if they are not mature enough to give full consent. In these situations one should try to obtain the child's *assent*, or agreement, to proceed with the medical plan. This can be done by involving the child in the decision-making process with the parents or guardians, asking the child directly about questions or concerns and even documenting in the chart that this process occurred, with or without the child's signature. Ascertaining when a child is able to give full consent, separate from that of the parents, may be defined by law (and varies by jurisdiction) or simply by the assessment of the ophthalmic team. In Ontario there is no legal age of consent. Older children and adolescents may have wishes that differ from those of their parents. Taking a family-centered approach to care, which attempts to find therapeutic alliance, requires time, patience, and perhaps the support of other professionals in the field. The health care team is advised to maintain a manifest respect for the child's autonomy, confidentiality, and right to know the truth about his or her care.

FUTILITY

Just as the adult patient may decide against treatments proposed by the physician, the physician may refuse to give a treatment requested by the patient if, in the best judgment of the physician, the treatment is unlikely to result in any benefit. For example, if an eye is hopelessly blinded by glaucoma and the entirely asymptomatic patient (i.e., with no pain) desires another surgery to bring the pressure down from 30, the doctor may refuse. Of course, there should be ample evidence to support the physician's position. If this difference in viewpoint leads to an irresolvable conflict between the doctor and patient, then the doctor can attempt to find an alternative care provider for the patient. Indeed, physicians may do this under any circumstance in which they feel they can no longer provide a therapeutic alliance with the patient, provided that the decision is not made on the basis of class or cultural distinction, prejudice, or malicious intent.

MEDICAL ERROR

Error is part of medicine. Much attention has been paid to error in medicine, with large studies confirming its high incidence and prevalence. Every ophthalmic team member will at some time make an error that may or may not lead to patient harm. Of course, we must always strive to reduce error and many strategies have evolved to encourage this, including the systems approach, which attempts to prevent error by adapting the environment in which we work. For example, if two eyedrop bottles are so similar that they could easily be mistaken for each other, it may be desirable to place colored tape around one bottle or move the two different medications to different locations in the office. Marking the eye to be operated before surgery and preoperative "time outs" are system interventions to avoid performing surgery on the wrong eye or patient.

Another approach to error, which has been unfortunately all too prevalent in medicine, is that of individual blame, punishment, and secrecy. The aviation industry has been a leader in the recognition that a nonpunitive approach and the encouragement of error reporting with team problem solving is the most productive path toward error reduction.

Disclosure to patients is a fundamental part of an ethical response. Research studies continue to show that patients do want to know when errors are made. Disclosure of error leads to a reduction in malpractice claims and judgments as well as an increase in the trusting partnership between doctor and patient. Disclosure may present difficult challenges. Is a rupture of the posterior capsule during cataract surgery by a skilled surgeon a complication (i.e., a known adverse event with a known frequency that accompanies any procedure) or an error? If the outcome of surgery is not influenced (i.e., intraocular lens in the bag, no vitreous loss, quiet eye), does the patient need to know? Some would argue that disclosure of such an event would be too complicated for the patient to understand even though this same patient was presumed to understand enough to give consent for surgery. Others would wish not to worry the patient unnecessarily, although the principle of such therapeutic privilege, as discussed earlier, is tenuous and runs contrary to what patient-based research would recommend. Indeed, the outcome for posterior capsule rupture may include a higher risk of retinal detachment and glaucoma. The surgeon may take special actions (e.g., dilated postoperative examination, more frequent postoperative visits) to guard against such complications. The patient may wonder why his or her care is different from other patients who were befriended in the pre- or postoperative waiting areas before surgery and are seen again at follow-up visits.

Disclosure of error is difficult for physicians and all members of the health care team. It is recommended that the health care team address error in a positive alliance designed to identify error and the factors that led to its occurrence as well as the measures that can be taken to prevent its recurrence. Patients will want to know what the expected outcome of an error might be and what measures are being taken to prevent or address those complications should they arise.

IMPAIRED PHYSICIANS AND OPHTHALMIC PROFESSIONALS

Patients have the expectation that their ophthalmic caretakers are competent. To violate this entrustment by allowing the practice of professionals who are under the influence of drugs or alcohol, or otherwise impaired by medical illness or knowledge deficiency, would be an unethical breach of our duty to do no harm (nonmaleficence). Most professional regulatory bodies have mechanisms by which such professionals can find supportive help designed to achieve reentry, when possible, into the medical care system once the individual is deemed competent to practice again.

Difficulties arise when a member of the team is unsure about the status of a colleague's competence, in particular with regards to deficiencies of knowledge, suboptimal skillsets (e.g., the surgeon with "bad hands"), or unsatisfactory decision making. Older professionals may be felt to be "not with the times." One must be careful that such determinations are made without prejudice and not by individual observations. Some practitioners, such as the retinal surgeons who are asked to retrieve dropped pieces of lens matter from the vitreous, may occasionally or even regularly see what at first appears to be the error or incompetence of another ophthalmologist. They must be careful to remind themselves that the true story of the events that led to the occurrence is not known and may have a satisfactory explanation. Assuming the incompetence of another surgeon, and in particular reporting this to the patient, is fraught with danger on many levels. Consultation with coworkers and even frank discussions with the individual about whom there is concern are advisable. If there is sufficient evidence that incompetency to practice exists, then delay in intervention will inevitably lead to patient harm. It is highly recommended that these issues be addressed before such events occur.

RESOURCE ALLOCATION

The allocation of scarce resources has become an increasingly frequent ethical challenge as the cost of ophthalmic care continues to rise as a result of remarkable technologic advances. Should only those with the means to afford it have access to multifocal intraocular lenses? Should limited operating theater time be allocated to the surgeons who do the most expensive operations with remarkable powers to restore vision on patients with uncommon diseases or to the surgeons who do much less expensive operations on larger numbers of patients with less profound effects on vision? Should we use the most expensive suture in keeping with the surgeon's preference even if there is no demonstrable benefit to the patient? Should the donor cornea go to the 1-month-old infant with unilateral Peters anomaly or to the 80-year-old person with bilateral pseudophakic bullous keratopathy?

Resolution of these issues is often difficult, complex, and far removed from the patient, yet still affecting their care. A full discussion of these issues is beyond the scope of this chapter, but perhaps the starting point is recognition of the best interest of the patient *(beneficence)*, if not most patients, in the resource allocation decision-making process. There is also an ethical duty to best represent the interests of society, which can at times compete with the interests of an individual patient. Clearly we cannot provide every possible aspect of medical care to every patient but we can use a utilitarian approach to achieve the greatest good.

RESEARCH ETHICS

In academic health science centers, and sometimes in community ophthalmic practice as well, there is a desire to achieve advancement in ophthalmic care through research. The researcher has certain ethical responsibilities toward the research subject, which include informed consent, confidentiality, disclosure, and respect for the subject's autonomy. There is also a duty to ensure that the patient is not enrolled in a frivolous project unlikely to yield meaningful results, a project in which the potential benefits are outweighed by potential harm, or a project that enhances discrimination toward the patient or the group they represent. Refusal to participate must not influence the care or the access to care that a patient receives.

Recognizing the difficulties in honoring these obligations, all research should be evaluated in advance and approved by a research ethics board (REB, also known as an institutional review board, IRB), the membership of which should be multidisciplinary, with representation of the lay public as well. REBs are available both inside and outside academic institutions. Research done in the community is not an excuse for avoidance of REB review. Most jurisdictions are now requiring even retrospective chart reviews to obtain such approval. REBs may try to streamline these processes. Although the process of REB approval may seem arduous, its objective is to facilitate good research rather than impede progress, while protecting both the researcher and the patient.

INNOVATION

Ophthalmology is a highly technologic field. It is not uncommon for ophthalmologists to find themselves "trying something new." Such presumed advances may come as the result of publications in the peer-reviewed literature, a "throw-away" publication, a presentation at a meeting, conversations with colleagues, or de novo from the creative mind of a thoughtful practitioner. The innovation may be as simple as a new way of tying a knot during surgery or as complex as a piggyback intraocular lens implanted into a neonate to deal with aphakic high hyperopia with a predicted removal of the second lens at a later date. Other examples include new intraocular lenses, new techniques for refractive surgery, and smaller instrumentation for retinal surgery. Some innovations are applications of technology and experience from one patient population to another (e.g., specialty intraocular lenses in children or anti-vascular endothelial growth factor [VEGF] injection for retinopathy of prematurity) and others are new only to that physician (e.g., switching to smaller-gauge phacoemulsification). Should innovation be allowed to proceed outside that purview of the research paradigm with involvement of a REB?

Research is designed to answer questions and improve patient care. Research studies are constructed to follow the scientific method, which allows these questions to be answered in a fashion that minimizes bias and the influence of chance. Research is also distinguished by the informed consent, which allows patients to understand the level of evidence base for the proposed intervention in the context of their care, and the REB-mandated monitoring, which protects participants from unintended harm as early as possible. Unfortunately there are many examples of innovation that proceeded without a research protocol and led to disaster; anterior chamber closed loop intraocular lenses are but one example. Some would argue that a better understanding of innovation would arise if we instead referred to it as "nonvalidated" intervention. One might doubt that patients would have much interest in being subjected to nonvalidated care. Yet patients are attracted to "sexy" innovations that they read about in the media (e.g., "bladeless" refractive surgery); they want to be cared for by ophthalmologists who are "on the cutting edge." Others would argue that innovation is part of clinical care and an intrinsic part of medicine, especially the surgical subspecialties, and therefore not a form of research.

Some innovations occur in emergency settings where REB review is not possible. When faced with an expulsive hemorrhage, the surgeon will use any reasonable means at that moment to close the eye. Other situations require somewhat urgent innovation, but perhaps with enough time to get an expedited review and compassionate approval from an REB with not much more effort than a letter to the REB chair. The majority of major practice changes are done with sufficient forethought that REB approval could indeed be sought, with the aim of ensuring the optimal outcome while protecting the best interests of patient and researcher. Some centers have tried a system parallel to the REB specifically for innovation, a system designed to be more expeditious and attuned to the unique nature of surgical practice. Institutions may adopt procedures where peer review is a minimum, perhaps in the form of approval by the departmental chief, before proceeding.

All of these considerations have in common a desire to enforce some regulation of the current freedom of ophthalmologists "to do whatever they want" and thus respect the rights of the patient to informed consent, truth telling, and protection from harm while facilitating the progress of ophthalmic care.

GENETICS ETHICS

Genetics has become an increasingly prominent part of virtually every aspect of medicine. Ophthalmic professionals, in almost every aspect of the field, must have a working knowledge of genetics, from age-related macular degeneration and cataract to steroid-induced glaucoma and congenital malformations. Advances in genetics are already bringing to ophthalmology the possibility of gene-based therapy for a variety of diseases.

Recognition of the role of genetics in eye disease brings with it some special ethical challenges. There may be confidentiality issues with the sharing of information within families and the need to obtain such information to give appropriate genetic counseling. Insurance companies may have a desire to obtain information about patient risk for diseases not yet developed and then classify the asymptomatic disorder as preexisting, and therefore uninsurable in the United States; the Genetic Information Nondiscrimination Act of 2008 prohibits insurance companies for some insurance products from using genetic information in this fashion.

Parents may ask about prenatal testing for ocular disease and consider terminating pregnancies of otherwise healthy infants. They may ask for presymptomatic predictive testing of their children for genetic disease that is unlikely to develop until the child is an adult. There is some evidence that there may be harmful psychosocial effects to both positive and negative predictive test results. Perhaps children identified as having the gene mutation for retinitis pigmentosa in the family will be steered away from certain career options only to find that when they become of age to pursue a career, there is a cure for their disease and they have missed the opportunity to prepare for the field they desire. Depression and even suicide may follow a positive predictive test. A negative test in a highly affected family with a disease-based identity may result in the child being ostracized as not one of the group.

Ultimately, ophthalmologists might even have to contend with the issue of eugenics as we become capable of eliminating gene defects from society through sperm and egg selection or gene repair. Should parents be allowed to choose the iris color of their children? There is a primate model for correction of X-linked recessive red–green color deficiency. Is this a disease? With the recent promising treatment of Leber congenital amaurosis using intraocular gene therapy we are beginning to see the power and potential of ocular gene therapy. With that must come a careful appraisal of the potential ethical implications.

It would be unreasonable to expect all ophthalmologists to be up to date with every genetics advancement, but the ophthalmic team must be cognizant of these ethical issues in genetics. When faced with such dilemmas, it is useful to call on the support and intervention of genetics professionals such as ocular geneticists, genetic counselors, or medical geneticists. They can act as consultants and partners to help address the concerns brought forward by the patient or anticipated by the team.

ADVERTISING

Physician advertising is now legal in many jurisdictions. Some ophthalmologists have rejected this as an affront to the profession that degrades our field to a business no different from auto sales. Others have embraced advertising as a means of public education at a time when informed consent has received so much attention.

The main ethical principle that applies to this and the financially related issues in the following text is that of conflict of interest. Rarely do physicians advertise solely for the altruistic benefit of disseminating information to patients. Advertising presents a conflict of interest wherein the physician's motive of financial gain, practice advancement, and perhaps ego enhancement could result in techniques that are either coercive or even untruthful. This would likely violate our duty to do no harm. Of course, physicians can choose not to advertise, at which point the ethical issue is moot. But if they do choose to advertise they should do so in a way that addresses some of these concerns.

Advertisement should be truthful and not misleading. Advertising does not replace informed consent. Some jurisdictions prohibit patient testimonials or acrimonious comparisons with other colleagues. Some professional societies review and regulate advertising to ensure that the potential patient is not influenced by style rather than content. Catchy radio jingles or print slogans may unduly influence and coerce patients into uninformed choices. Consultation with professional regulatory bodies is advised to ensure that the undesired effects of the conflict are minimized and the benefits to the patient maximized.

FEE SPLITTING

There are several forms of fee splitting. In the most typical arrangement, one caretaker (e.g., an ophthalmologist) "pays back" the referring professional (e.g., an optometrist) as a demonstration of gratitude for a referral and presumably to provide an incentive for further referral. This reward is referred to as a kickback or profit sharing and may take the form of cash or other benefits such as tickets to a sporting event, free meals, gift certificates. Another arrangement might involve a shared practice wherein members of the group all benefit from the aggregate activity of the group and therefore encourage referrals to each other. An example might be the multispecialty ophthalmology group who sends cataract patients to the retina specialist within the group for preoperative examination. Lastly, fee splitting may take the form of comanagement. The ophthalmologist delegates the postoperative care of patients to another provider, often an optometrist, and provides a payment in cash or in kind for that service. Alternatively, the optometrist may bill the patient directly for services that would otherwise fall under the care of the surgeon's postoperative care and as such may not have been billable.

Although some may perceive these arrangements as beneficial to the patient, providing continuity of care and improved access to care, others have identified the conflict of interest that may be inherent, particularly if the patient is unaware of the arrangement. Research has shown that patients are in general unhappy with these relationships. Some jurisdictions have policy or law that proscribes against these arrangements.

Health care providers should initiate and sustain referral practices based on the best interest of the patient rather than their own financial gain. The AAO's stance has been to encourage ophthalmologists to provide postoperative care for their own patients unless there are compelling reasons why this cannot be accomplished (e.g., surgeon leaving town for holiday) and only if the patient is informed in advance. When the conflict of interest persists, physicians are encouraged to disclose these relationships to the patient in a further attempt to avoid any illusion of impropriety.

One must recognize that disclosure of a conflict of interest does not remove the conflict. Patients may not be empowered, especially when made vulnerable by status, illness, or age, to act in response to such disclosures because they may feel that to do so would deny them access to the provider they want and to whom they were referred. This may leave the patient uncomfortable, suspicious, and more likely to be a dissatisfied participant in their care.

MEDICAL INDUSTRY

The medical industry provides us with our therapeutic agents, diagnostic agents, medical technology, and surgical equipment. It is a necessary and integral part of medicine. In addition to the use of these products, physicians will have direct interaction with representatives of medical industry in the form of sales representatives wanting to give information about new products, opportunities to try new products, invitations to participate or lead industry-sponsored educational events with or without social components, invitations to become a spokesperson for industry products, invitations to write papers/conduct research/write monographs sponsored by industry, offers of grants to support research activities or program development, gifts of free samples of medications or gifts ranging from items of nominal value for medical use (e.g., notepads with the drug company name on each page), to more significant gifts such as sporting event tickets, free meals, and even all-expenses-paid trips to lovely locations with or without a sometimes nominal educational component. At large meetings companies present enormous and elaborate displays, and every conference participant may be given a tote bag and a neck strap for their identification badge emblazoned with drug company logos.

As reasonable patients would likely expect that the medical decisions of their ophthalmologist are free from influence and conflict of interest, it is not difficult to see why multiple studies have shown that patients generally object to such relationships between physicians and the medical industry. Research also indicates that despite the often-heard claims of physicians to the contrary, these practices do affect our prescribing patterns. It is then not surprising to learn that the medical industry spends billions of dollars worldwide on advertising and contacts with physicians, presumably not out of purely altruistic motives but rather in recognition of the positive effect such expenditures have on company profit.

Most ophthalmic and other medical professional societies, as well as the institutions in which physicians work, now have policies regarding interaction with the medical industry. These policies grew out of the recognition of the potential for influence on the decision making of medical personnel if they stand to benefit from the largesse of industry in a personal way. Some physicians have rejected restrictions out of a feeling of entitlement, especially in times when physician fees are dropping and other restrictions on practice are increasing. Physicians may assert that their own autonomy to conduct their lives as they see fit is no less important than that of the patient. This conflict rages on.

The pharmaceutical industry also has recognized the ethical dilemmas these relationships and activities engender. As a result, some have implemented voluntary restrictions. Companies may contribute much in the way of information and financial support for medical meetings and claim that they have not influenced the scientific content (although there may be drug company-sponsored talks on exhibit floors in addition to the official scientific program). The risk of the public perception of impropriety and the potential for adverse manifestations of conflict of interest in direct patient care remain to be resolved.

COSMETIC SURGERY

As discussed, patients have the autonomous right to choose what they will and will not allow to be done to their bodies (with the exception of futile interventions; see earlier text). Cosmetic surgery acts on a patient's wish to have something normal about his or her body changed to another normal variant, often at large cost. Proponents of cosmetic surgery would argue that the patient does not perceive the condition as normal and therefore making the change, so that the patient feels more normal, is well within the helping nature of the medical profession. Analyzing the philosophic differences on this topic is beyond the scope of this chapter, but the ethical issue of conflict of interest is again worthy of consideration.

Laser and intraocular refractive surgery has proliferated worldwide. In many communities, as a procedure not covered by insurance plans, surgeons may charge sizable fees and perform the surgery exclusively in private clinics. People have flocked to have this surgery, allowing enormous numbers of patients to abandon their contact lenses and glasses. But interviews of the lay public suggest that many go for the procedure because they believe that the surgery will "fix" their bad eyes. Most of these people have normal healthy eyes, seeing 6/6 with their preoperative glasses or contact lens. Their eyes are just a different shape from the average. If the surgery were presented as a procedure that "cuts their healthy eyes" to allow them to go without glasses, would there be as much interest?

FINANCIAL ISSUES

In addition to the ethical issues discussed, many of which have financial implications for the physician (e.g., fee splitting, advertising, medical industry, cosmetic surgery), all medical practitioners are also faced with moral challenges related to charging and collecting fees for services rendered. Although altruism is an ethical principle that should pervade much of medicine, there will in almost every setting be a business component: expenses must be covered, employees must be paid, and the physician deserves an income commensurate with his or her skill, training, and success. Opportunities abound for making minor, or even major, manipulations in billing practices that will further increase income while staying within the law and out of detection by the patient.

This potential conflict of interest and the ethical issues that such practices raise, have long been troubling to the ophthalmic profession and served as the basis over the past

century for the emergence of the AAO's increasing interest in ethics with the establishment of a Code and an Ethics Committee. The potential conflict of interest was also recognized in the United States in the form of safe harbor legislation that put restrictions on potentially unethical arrangements. More subtle billing practices may also raise similar concerns that profit motives conflict with the best interest of the patient. In the past, in some Canadian provinces, ophthalmologists got paid more if the patient was referred from a physician as opposed to an optometrist even though the same service is performed. Some ophthalmologists were very creative in getting around this rule by writing consultation letters back to the patient's family doctor or refusing referrals from optometrists. The former act is a type of deception, whereas the latter causes the patient inconvenience and potential care delays in having to seek an alternative referral route. This is but one example of bending the billing rules, other forms of which range from illegal to legal but questionably ethical. In the United States an entire industry is devoted to advising physicians on how to best code for patient visits and surgery to achieve the greatest reimbursement. Although all illegal acts are not within the ethical and moral acceptability of the practice of medicine, some legal acts may also challenge our ethics boundaries. Creative billing also tends to raise the cost of health care to society, creating yet another conflict of interest and potential nonmaleficence.

TRAINEES IN PATIENT CARE

When trainees (e.g., medical students, ophthalmology residents, ophthalmic assistant students) are participating in the care of patients, there may be a reluctance to inform the patient for fear that the patient may reject this arrangement. In fact, research shows that patients do want to be told about the nature of such arrangements and, if properly informed and assured that appropriate supervision is in place, usually welcome this interaction and may even feel that they are making a positive contribution to the health care system. Some authors have argued that patients have a moral obligation to participate in the training of future professionals, particularly in a publicly funded health care system such as Canada, but this does not necessarily abrogate our truth-telling duties. The ethical principles of truth telling and disclosure play a strong role in this setting. A utilitarian approach, seeking the greatest good for both the patient and society, argues that the success of these relationships, largely through the graded allocation of responsibility to trainees and the provision of appropriate supervision, is supported by the high functioning of the training system and its lack of demonstrable negative outcome effects on patient care. In fact, the highest level of care is often delivered at the academic centers where trainees are routinely part of health care delivery.

RESOLUTION OF ETHICAL DILEMMAS

The ophthalmic team is confronted by a wide variety of ethical issues. This chapter has attempted to identify many of those issues and offer some pertinent points for reflection and consideration when attempting to resolve the dilemmas. Although there may not be a perfect right answer in each case, ophthalmic professionals should consider the relevant key ethical principles, institutional policies, and societal law. Multidisciplinary conversations with peers and colleagues can be particularly helpful. Difficult situations arise when an employee (e.g., ophthalmic assistant) has a different viewpoint on an ethical issue than his or her supervisor or employer. Open conversation can often resolve these conflicts. Consultation may be sought from bioethicists or other professionals who have had formal training in the field. Many written resources are available; ethical issues have found their way into hundreds of journal articles on virtually every topic. The University of Toronto Joint Centre for Bioethics website (www.jointcentreforbioethics.ca) is a useful resource that can link readers to a wide variety of information on bioethics and case management.

Chapter | 53 |

Ophthalmic allied health personnel: scope of practice

Lynn D. Anderson, William H. Ehlers, Craig Simms

INTRODUCTION

Ophthalmic medical personnel are classified as allied health personnel and are defined as individuals with training and responsibilities that support, supplement, and assist physicians, including ophthalmologists and other health professionals providing patient care. Ophthalmic medical personnel include ophthalmic nurses, ophthalmic assistants, ophthalmic technicians, ophthalmic medical technologists, refractionists, orthoptists, optometric assistants, opticians, contact lens technicians, and others. Other allied health occupations include medical assistants, dental assistants, radiology technicians, and sonographers. To standardize the classification of allied health care workers globally, the World Health Organization (WHO) established a classification of the eye care profession: allied ophthalmic personnel (AOP).

As vital members of the professional eye care team, AOP assist the ophthalmologist in providing quality care by gathering patient information. AOP perform tasks and testing under the direct supervision of an ophthalmologist licensed to practice medicine and surgery. Governments may require licensure or certification, or certification of AOP may be voluntary. This chapter discusses the scope of practice of AOP.

DEFINING SCOPE OF PRACTICE

Various governmental agencies regulate all physicians with regard to their scope of practice and the functions and procedures that they can delegate to others under their supervision. The range of responsibilities and functions performed by AOP, as dictated by laws and regulations and as specified by ophthalmologists, may be considered their "scope of practice." Scope of practice regulations also may determine medical reimbursement for health care services performed by ophthalmologists and their assistants.

Because there are no statutes or regulations defining the practice of nonlicensed AOP, the most important issues concern what tasks can and cannot be delegated by the physician and what can and cannot be performed by various ophthalmic assistants. Ophthalmic assistants can never diagnose disease, treat disease, or perform surgical procedures, whether using a blade, a laser, or any other instrument, technology, or modality. AOP should check local, state, or provincial laws as well as institutional and practice policies.

LICENSURE AND CERTIFICATION

Licensure and certification are two processes that govern scope of practice in the medical profession. Licensure is defined and understood as having been granted authority or legal permission to practice as regulated by federal, state, or provincial governmental agencies. Certification denotes that a person is recognized by the private sector as having achieved standards set by the profession. Certification is generally granted by an independent organization, but may also be mandated by a government regulation. In addition, registration is another term that recognizes government regulation. AOP, such as ophthalmic nurses, are licensed as well as certified.

Most AOP are not licensed by government agencies but may be voluntarily certified, based on their knowledge and skill levels, to perform delegated tasks and procedures. The Joint Commission on Allied Health Personnel in Ophthalmology (JCAHPO) certifies AOP at three levels: ophthalmic assistant, ophthalmic technician, and ophthalmic medical technologist. The JCAHPO is an internationally recognized, accredited organization by the National Commission of Certifying Agencies. Certificates of completion are also recognition that AOP have obtained specific knowledge and skill levels in particular areas. Other examples of certification programs include orthoptist and ophthalmic photographers that are certified by the Ophthalmic Photographers' Society (OPS), American Orthoptic Council (AOC), and the Canadian Orthoptic Council (COC); in addition, there is the National Contact Lens Examiners (NCLE), and the American Board of Opticianry (ABO).

Government agencies also may implement regulations requiring certification of AOP in order to perform certain ophthalmic or administrative tasks. These regulations that require only certified personnel to perform various tasks are often based on patient safety, access to care, and government reimbursement for patient services. For example, regulatory changes in the United States allowed licensed or certified personnel to enter orders in electronic medical records for reimbursement; however, the certification must be administered by an accredited national certifying organization.

DETERMINING THE SCOPE OF PRACTICE

AOP may not diagnose or treat disease or perform surgical procedures. Their primary role and responsibility is the collection of data and the performance of clinical evaluations as authorized by the supervising licensed clinician. Examples of the task of gathering patient data include patient ocular history, present illness complaint and medications, and the performance of diagnostic testing includes such tasks as muscle balance testing determination, keratometry, and tonometry. The ophthalmic assistant then provides the data and information to the ophthalmologist for interpretation and treatment. Ophthalmic assistants certified at one of JCAHPO's three different levels may perform similar duties. However, assistants with higher levels of certification are expected to perform the tasks at an advanced level of expertise and to exercise considerable technical clinical judgment as they perform those tasks.

The performance of tasks by AOP is measured by national standards that are based on statistically valid, reliable data collected in the United States and Canada. The certifying agencies conduct extensive surveys of job incumbents and their employers and ophthalmologists on tasks performed, importance of the tasks, frequency with which tasks are performed, and the task's level of difficulty. This research provides the foundation for the certification examinations, which test the knowledge and skills needed for minimal competency on the tasks performed and job descriptions used by ophthalmic practices.

Core competencies that comprise the scope of practice of ophthalmic assisting include:

- Assessment skills
- Assisting in intervention
- Corrective lenses
- Imaging
- Office responsibilities

AOP in countries other than Canada and the United States may have a scope of practice that looks very different. Some countries may combine AOP job roles and responsibilities. For example, in Africa and the South Pacific, it is common for a nurse to have job tasks that are both surgical and clinical.

INSURANCE RISK AND MALPRACTICE

Allied ophthalmic personnel should always ascertain that they are insured under the umbrella of their employer's medical malpractice policies. In addition, they should seek expressed, written indemnification from their employers for all activities performed, within the scope and capacity delineated by their supervisors and employers.

PRIVACY PRACTICES

There is a complicated balance between patient privacy and health care providers' need to use and disclose medical information. In most countries, national privacy standards regulate patient health information rights. These include the right to:

- Request restrictions on the use and disclosure of health information
- Receive confidential communication concerning the patient's medical condition and treatment
- Inspect and copy health data and information
- Amend and/or submit corrections to health information
- Receive an accounting of how and to whom health information has been disclosed
- Receive a printed copy of the privacy practice of the health care provider

AOP, as part of the health care provider team, are required to maintain the privacy of the patient's protected health information and to provide the patient with notice of the privacy practices of the provider. Notices typically address the uses and disclosure of health information.

TREATMENT

Health information may be used by staff members or disclosed to other health care professionals for the purpose of evaluating the patient's health, diagnosing medical conditions, and providing treatment. For example, results of evaluations and testing are available in the patient's medical record to all health professionals who may provide treatment or who may be consulted by staff members.

PAYMENT

Health information may be used to seek payment from the patient's health plan, from other sources of coverage such as an insurer, or from credit card companies that the patient may use to pay for services. For example, the patient's health plan may request and receive information concerning dates of service, the service provided, and the medical condition being treated.

PROVIDER INTERNAL OPERATIONS

The patient's health information may be used to support the day-to-day activities and practice management of the provider. Examples of information use include services received by the patient that are used to support budgeting and financial reporting, outcome studies, and quality improvement evaluations; sending appointment reminders to patients; and providing information about new technology relevant to patient and health-related goods and services.

LAW ENFORCEMENT

Health information may be disclosed to law enforcement agencies, without the patient's permission, to support government audits and inspections, to facilitate law enforcement investigations, and to comply with government-mandated reporting.

PUBLIC HEALTH REPORTING

Health information may be disclosed to public health agencies as required by law.

ETHICS AND SCOPE OF PRACTICE

AOP have not promulgated ethical standards as self-regulating rules of conduct. However, they perform their duties at the direction of and under the supervision of licensed employers. The hierarchy of values and the standards of conduct of the physicians, hospitals, surgical centers, and other allied health care workers become the code of conduct and ethical guidelines for ophthalmic personnel.

Today's ophthalmology practice demands that busy ophthalmologists be more efficient and delegate appropriate tasks and procedures to competent, qualified allied ophthalmic personnel. The ophthalmologist also must ensure that quality patient care is being extended when delegating responsibilities. Allied ophthalmic personnel need a good understanding of ethics in serving the best interests of the patient and the practice.

The eye care practitioner's ongoing responsibility for prevention, diagnosis, and treatment of disease must be carefully balanced when delegating tasks to make the most effective use of the eye care team in delivering quality patient care. The ophthalmologist who allows AOP to treat patients without adequate supervision compromises the licensing standards set by the government and erodes the standards of patient care. The eye care team must never neglect patient safety in the pursuit of efficiency for the practice.

SUMMARY

Major shifts in health care are driven by rapidly advancing technology, by the pressure on lawmakers for open access to medical systems, and by the desire to cut health care costs. New laws are often supported by third-party payers to save money, reduce premiums, and reimburse nonphysicians' services at a lower rate.

In this changing environment, delegation of responsibility and authority within the eye care team will progressively increase to prevent overloading the ophthalmologist, to increase the practice's efficiency, and to manage the costs of eye care to the public, third-party payers, and government. As important physician extenders, AOP are a critical part of the eye care team in providing quality patient care.

FURTHER READING

Health Insurance Portability and Accountability Act of 1996.

WHO Universal eye health: a global action plan. 2013; 2014–2019.

Chapter 54

Testing and certification of ophthalmic skills

Lynn D. Anderson, Edyie G. Miller-Ellis

INTRODUCTION

An important milestone in the career of allied ophthalmic personnel (AOP) is achieving certification. Certification demonstrates a professional commitment to ophthalmic assisting, and completing the certification process carries with it many professional and personal benefits, such as the assurance of competence in the clinical skills and knowledge required by the field of ophthalmology and increased confidence and self-esteem. The most important benefit of certification is standardization of the knowledge and skills needed in the profession, which improves the quality of patient care. This standardization occurs through identification of the profession's essential knowledge base and the skills needed to perform tasks required in an ophthalmic practice. This chapter provides an overview of the certification standards and examinations for the ophthalmic assisting profession.

KNOWLEDGE-BASED EXAMINATIONS

Certification examinations are based on several fundamental principles. One important element of certification testing is the requirement that test content be related to tasks actually performed at the level of certification sought. The Joint Commission on Allied Health Personnel in Ophthalmology (JCAHPO) conducts a national and international job task analysis every 5 years to identify the standard duties and tasks performed by an AOP at each level of certification. These data are used to develop the certification examination content with test items or questions determining the tasks actually performed by AOP. JCAHPO's certification examination content and subcontent areas are outlined in Table 54.1.

Another important element of certification examinations is objectivity. The examinations are carefully designed to test relevant core knowledge of job incumbents without subject matter bias or trick questions. The examination length is determined by the required content, which also dictates the number of test questions presented in various subject areas and the amount of time allowed to take the test.

To ensure the value of certification, the examinations require exacting security procedures at all levels. Certification examinations are administered in a proctored or monitored environment. Security measures protect the integrity of the examination, as well as the test data and the certifying agency itself. Security policies and procedures are also designed to protect test results and examinee privacy.

EXAMINATION FORMAT AND ADMINISTRATION

Certification examinations may be administered using a paper-and-pencil or computer-based format, often referred to as "written examinations." Paper–pencil examinations may be offered only a few times during the year at select locations, whereas computer-based examinations give

Table 54.1 COA, COT, COMT examination sub-content areas

Content areas	Certified ophthalmic assistant (COA)	Certified ophthalmic technician (COT)	Certified ophthalmic medical technologist (COMT)
Assessments	**42%**	**45%**	**46%**
Sub-content area			
A. History and documentation	5%	4%	3%
B. Visual assessment	6%	5%	3%
C. Visual fields testing	4%	4%	6%
D. Pupil assessment	3%	4%	3%
E. Tonometry	4%	3%	3%
F. Keratometry	2%	3%	2%
G. Ocular motility testing	4%	5%	7%
H. Lensometry	3%	4%	4%
I. Refractometry: retinoscopy & refinement	5%	5%	6%
J. Biometry	3%	4%	3%
K. Supplemental testing	3%	4%	6%
Assisting with interventions and procedures	**22%**	**17%**	**19%**
Sub-content area			
A. Microbiology	3%	2%	2%
B. Pharmacology	3%	3%	4%
C. Surgical assisting	4%	4%	4%
D. Ophthalmic patient services and education	12%	8%	9%
Corrective lenses	**4%**	**9%**	**9%**
Sub-content area			
A. Optics and spectacles	2%	3%	2%
B. Contact lenses	2%	6%	7%
Imaging	**13%**	**15%**	**14%**
Sub-content area			
A. Ophthalmic imaging	5%	7%	6%
B. Photography and videography	8%	8%	8%
Office responsibilities	**19%**	**14%**	**12%**
Sub-content area			
A. Equipment maintenance and calibration	3%	1%	2%
B. Medical ethics, legal, and regulatory issues	4%	3%	2%
C. Communication skills	3%	2%	3%
D. Administrative duties	9%	8%	5%

Note: Percentages indicate the amount of content area covered for each examination level.
COA, Certified Ophthalmic Assistant; COT, Certified Ophthalmic Technician; COMT, Certified Ophthalmic Medical Technologist.
Used with permission of the Joint Commission on Allied Health Personnel in Ophthalmology, Inc. Certification Criteria Book, 2016.

Question 2 of 5	Jane Mason Demo	Time Remaining: 14:22

The near reflex consists of:

    ○ a. accommodation, convergence
    ● b. accommodation, convergence, pupillary constriction
    ○ c. accommodation, pupillary constriction
    ○ d. convergence, pupillary constriction

Directions: Select the best answer.

⇐ Previous	Next ⇒	Mark

Figure 54.1 Sample multiple-choice items from computerized examination.

(Used with permission of the Joint Commission on Allied Health Personnel in Ophthalmology, Inc.)

examinees more options and benefits in testing. Use of the computerized format allows the certification agency to offer the examination in multiple locations (testing centers) with flexible dates and times.

JCAHPO also administers open-book certification examinations and certificates of completion through the Internet. Two open-book examinations delivered online are JCAHPO's Ophthalmic Scribe Certification and the Ophthalmic Coding Specialist examination in collaboration with the American Academy of Ophthalmology and the American Academy of Ophthalmic Executives (AAO/AAOE).

Certification examinations test specific subject matter knowledge, and the test questions (items) are most often given in multiple-choice format. Other types of items may include true/false questions, fill-in-the-blank questions, and short answer or essay questions. In addition, tests may use diagrams, photos, animations, and video.

JCAHPO's examinations primarily use multiple-choice formats, such as presented in Figure 54.1. Practice examinations give the examinee the opportunity to become familiar with computer testing and the examination. At the end of the test, many certification examinations provide immediate performance feedback and unofficial pass/fail test results with automated scoring. Box 54.1 gives some sample COA examination test items (answers are in Box 54.2).

SKILL-BASED EXAMINATIONS

In addition to knowledge-based examinations, the certification process may also include the testing of ophthalmic skills and abilities. JCAHPO, Ophthalmic Photographers' Society, American Orthoptic Council, and the Canadian Orthoptic Society conduct skill-based examinations after candidates successfully complete the written portion of certification examinations. The JCAHPO's Certified Ophthalmic Assistant (COA) test is a knowledge-based examination only. JCAHPO

Box 54.1 Sample certified ophthalmic assistant (COA) examination test items[a]

1. The specific reason a patient is being seen for an eye examination is referred to as the:
   a. patient history.
   b. chief complaint.
   c. status of the patient's visual acuity.
   d. onset of any current vision problem(s).
2. Aniscoria is described as:
   a. unequal corneal diameters.
   b. differing iris colors.
   c. different refractive errors.
   d. difference in pupil size.
3. Keratometry is the procedure for measurement of the patient's:
   a. pupil size.
   b. crystalline lens curvature.
   c. macular radius.
   d. corneal curvature.
4. Washing hands between patients is an example of which of the following?
   a. Aseptic technique
   b. Disinfection
   c. TASS control
   d. Standard precaution.
5. Strabismus is failure of both eyes to spontaneously direct their gaze at the same object as a result of:
   a. retinal dysfunction.
   b. muscular imbalance.
   c. corneal aberrations.
   d. crystalline lens atrophy.

[a]Sample Certified Ophthalmic Assistant (COA) questions used with the permission of the Joint Commission on Allied Health Care in Ophthalmology, Inc. (JCAHPO).

Box 54.2 **Answers**

1. b. Chief complaint
2. d. Difference in pupil size
3. d. Corneal curvature
4. d. Standard precaution
5. b. Muscular imbalance

advanced certifications that require skill-based testing in addition to knowledge-based testing are the JCAHPO's Certified Ophthalmic Technician (COT) and the Certified Ophthalmic Medical Technologist (COMT).

Skill tests or performance tests evaluate specific skills and abilities performed in a clinical setting. Subject matter experts have identified standardized processes for common clinical skills and have established acceptable performance measures to evaluate these skills.

Skill-based tests are traditionally conducted with the examinee performing various tasks while being observed and rated by evaluators. These are typically timed tests, conducted in a clinical setting with the examinee performing assigned tasks on patients, schematic eyes, or ophthalmic equipment.

A modern alternative to skills evaluation tests conducted with live patients is computer-based skills evaluations. The JCAHPO's COT and COMT skill evaluations use innovative computer-based simulations specially designed and developed to evaluate the knowledge and skills required for these advanced levels of competency. An examinee performs required tasks on computer-simulated ophthalmic equipment using a mouse and keyboard. The COT skill evaluation evaluates seven skills performed in a typical clinical practice: keratometry, tonometry, ocular motility, lensometry, visual fields, retinoscopy, and refinement. The COMT skill evaluation tests the candidate's abilities in pupil evaluation, advanced lensometry, motility, fundus photography, and angiography. Experts in the field of ophthalmology developed these simulations to ensure that the computer-based evaluations accurately reflect and test the skills needed to perform these tasks on actual patients.

Before taking computer-based skill evaluations, the examinee is given a tutorial and training material for use in studying and preparation for the test. The tutorial provides an opportunity to learn how the computer functions, understand how the simulated equipment works, and practice manipulating the dials and controls on simulated equipment using the computer mouse. By studying the tutorial, candidates become familiar with the examination format, which helps to ensure that they can approach the test with confidence. Figure 54.2 is a computer screen shot showing dials and controls of the lensometer from the COT skill evaluation tutorial.

The COT and COMT skill evaluation tests begin with a patient scenario based on real cases that an ophthalmic technician would encounter in a clinical practice. The examinee

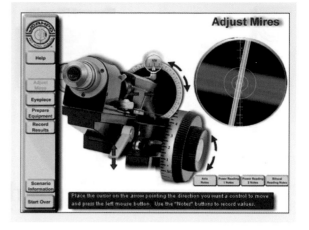

Figure 54.2 Certified ophthalmic technician (COT) skill evaluation tutorial: lensmeter.
(Used with permission of the Joint Commission on Allied Health Personnel in Ophthalmology, Inc.)

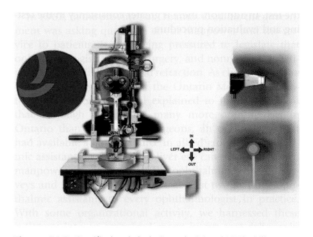

Figure 54.3 Certified ophthalmic technician (COT) skill evaluation: tonometry patient examination.
(Used with permission of the Joint Commission on Allied Health Personnel in Ophthalmology, Inc.)

must make decisions based on information given, perform the skill correctly, and obtain an accurate reading or measurement for the skill. Figure 54.3 shows the tonometer examination from the COT skill examination, and Figure 54.4 shows the retinoscopy examination from the COT skill evaluation.

In the COT and COMT skill evaluation tests, an examinee receives two scores. The examinee is first evaluated on the technique or process used to perform the skill. Secondly, the examinee must accurately record the results within a tolerance range determined by subject matter experts. The use of computer-based performance evaluations has certain advantages over evaluations performed with live patients. The tests may be scheduled conveniently

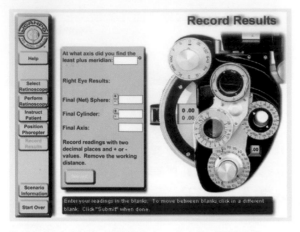

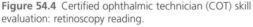

Figure 54.4 Certified ophthalmic technician (COT) skill evaluation: retinoscopy reading.
(Used with permission of the Joint Commission on Allied Health Personnel in Ophthalmology, Inc.)

at local computer testing centers, thus reducing the cost of the test. In addition, there is greater consistency in the testing and evaluation procedure.

SUMMARY

Credentialing and career ladder opportunities for the ophthalmic assistant start with JCAHPO's three core certifications. Careers can advance with specialty certifications in Ophthalmic Surgical Assisting (OSA), Registered Ophthalmic Ultrasound Biometrist (ROUB), and the Certified Diagnostic Ophthalmic Sonographer (CDOS). These career paths can lead to obtaining credentials in other eye care professions.

Certification by examination remains a primary method to assess learning and competency in many eye care professions. Advanced studying and review of resource materials that lists examination content are essential elements in reducing test anxiety and improving performance. Becoming familiar with the examination format (paper–pencil or computer-based tests) is important. The ultimate key to successfully passing the examination is adequate preparation. Certification offers greater standardization of processes, enhanced objectivity in evaluation and measurement, and improved overall quality of testing, all of which will enhance the profession of ophthalmic assisting.

Chapter | **55** |

The development of ophthalmic assistants in North America

Harold A. Stein

INTRODUCTION AND HISTORY

Until the late 1950s, ophthalmic assistants were an unorganized and uncertified group of individuals who assisted ophthalmologists in their day-to-day technical activities. No credentialing was required. Ophthalmic assistants were allied to ophthalmologists in offices and hospitals.

Skilled and specially trained assistants have been aiding ophthalmologists for many years. The most highly organized are the orthoptists, a paramedical group that originated to deal with the numerous and serious problems related to strabismus or crossed eye. The function of the ophthalmic assistant is broader than that of either the orthoptist or the visual field technician. There have been ophthalmic assistants in an informal way for as long as there have been ophthalmic offices. Training standards and efficiency have varied greatly and have depended heavily on the talents of the individual assistant and the teaching ability of the supervising ophthalmologist. Ophthalmologists have a major role as mentor to the ophthalmic assistant. Formal courses have been established in Canadian and American colleges, and official textbooks have been written that have been accepted, indeed welcomed, by both the Canadian and American ophthalmologic associations.

In 1962, in the province of Ontario, Canada, the government was asking questions about manpower and the service to patients. It was being pressured to legislate that ophthalmologists do only surgery, and nonmedical practitioners do medical work and refraction. As chairman of the Ophthalmology Section of the Ontario Medical Association, my colleagues and I explained to the government that although there were many more optometrists in Ontario than ophthalmic surgeons, an ophthalmologist had available a large resource in allied groups of ophthalmic assistants available to deliver eye care. This combined manpower was substantial. The ophthalmologists did surveys and found that there were at least two or three ophthalmic assistants to every ophthalmologist in practice. With some organizational activity, we harnessed these assistants into an organized group in eye care delivery in the province of Ontario. This was the start of the formalization of the role of ophthalmic technicians.

In the early 1960s, Dr. Slatt and I organized instructional short courses in Ontario and provided credit for examination for already existing ophthalmic personnel. Dr. William Hunter and I formed a loose association of ophthalmic assistants in the mid-1960s to provide recognition with a membership certificate and pins. This has developed into the Canadian Society of Ophthalmic Personnel, which was a forerunner of similar societies in other parts of the world.

Along with Ms. Debra Kaplan, in the late 1960s formal training courses were started at junior college level at the Centennial College of Applied Arts, Scarborough, Ontario, Canada. The course ran for 6 weeks during the day. After graduating 35 ophthalmic assistants from this intensive course, we were faced with the problem of finding them employment with ophthalmologists. This became difficult and for some impossible. Consequently we shifted the course to an evening course and took in only those ophthalmic assistants who were already employed by an ophthalmologist. This evening course, held once weekly, has continued in Toronto since 1965 and has been highly successful. We use ophthalmologists who have subspecialty interests who either volunteer their time or are paid from registration fees. There are 30 to 40 registrants per class. The training includes field trips.

In addition to this, one started a home study course from Centennial College based in Toronto and later Alberta. This was directed at assistants working for ophthalmologists from across Canada. The course updated their skills; a graduate was given a "certificate of completion" of the course with no licensing or any other academic qualification.

In 1968, the late Dr. Bernard Sakler of Cincinnati asked me to make a presentation to the American Association of Ophthalmology annual meeting, at which several thousand people were present. I gave a lecture about how we were developing the training of allied health personnel in ophthalmology in Canada. We were able to provide statistics showing that there were a large number of ophthalmologists and ophthalmic assistants in Ontario. In fact, the combined manpower numbers were sufficient to service the eye care needs of the Ontario population.

The AAO accepted this concept and began a program similar to our own. Dr. Slatt and I were asked by the AAO to start a home study course for technicians, which went out across the United States to upgrade the skills of ophthalmic assistants in offices. I eventually became the chairman of the House of Delegates of the AAO. Under the executive director, Larry Zupan, this ophthalmic assistant home study course was a landmark of success for the association. Eventually, the American Academy of Ophthalmology adopted the American Association of Ophthalmology as their council with delegates from across the United States.

Concurrently with these events, Dr. Slatt and I co-authored the first clinical textbook for allied health personnel in ophthalmology, titled *The Ophthalmic Assistant*, published by the CV Mosby Company in 1968. It is now in its tenth edition and accepted worldwide.

Following my Chicago presentation in 1968, Dr. Hugh Monahan, who was in the audience, established the Joint Commission on Allied Health Personnel in Ophthalmology (JCAHPO). This was established with three delegates from each of the major ophthalmology organizations in North America. They developed examinations and certification for a more senior level called the ophthalmic technician and later a higher level called the ophthalmic medical technologist (see Chapters 51 and 53).

There are currently 45,000 certified and noncertified ophthalmic assistants/technicians in the United States and Canada. This is approximately a 3:1 ratio of technician to physician. These serve as ancillary groups only to ophthalmology. They have no licensing arrangements. There is a technical association that holds annual scientific meetings, the Association of Technical Personnel in Ophthalmology (ATPO).

Just as the dental technician serves the dentist and the x-ray technician serves the radiologist, so the ophthalmic assistant serves the ophthalmologist in preventing blindness and restoring sight. Improvements in technology and new tests are regularly introduced that are often delegated to the ophthalmic assistant. Assessment of vision, measurement of spectacles, and recording of case histories are part of the skills required. The ophthalmologist guides, manages, and directs the assistant's work. The assistant makes no decision involving professional judgment on matters affecting the health of the patients' eyes; the ultimate responsibility for care of the patient rests with the ophthalmologist.

NATURE OF THE WORK

Probably the most important role of the ophthalmic assistant is that of public relations officer for the office, clinic, or hospital. In an increasingly technologic society, where Medicare and the influence of mass information media have placed heavy demands on the medical profession, personal relationships between doctor and patient have been somewhat shortened. An important function of the ophthalmic assistant, therefore, is to assist all patients and to reemphasize instructions in the management of their individual problem as they leave the office. This last may be a minor task, such as directing the patient to a competent optician, or it may be one of major importance, for example, instructing the patient in how to place glaucoma drops in the eyes or the importance of returning for follow-up examination.

The main role of the ophthalmic assistant is to help the ophthalmologist in patient care. The assistant can and should be responsible for taking the patient's history and conducting the preliminary examination, for maintaining sterile equipment in the office, and assisting in minor surgical duties. The position is not a secretarial role. Knowledge of computers and the operation of business machines is of secondary importance to the ability to help patients and to manage the ophthalmic office.

There are many technical tests that the ophthalmic assistant may perform in the course of the day's work. These include assessing vision, visual fields, topography, and tonometry. Because the eye is so accessible to observation, many ophthalmologists often check pathologic lesions about and within the eye by means of photography. Thus photographing the eye has become another challenging aspect of the ophthalmic assistant's role.

WORKING CONDITIONS

The ophthalmologist authorizes and directs activities at all times in his or her professional capacity. The role of the ophthalmic assistant is that of liaison between the doctor and the patient. Ophthalmic assistants are part of the eye care team.

The assistant must be discreet and invite confidence, so that a bond of trust may be established with the patient. Private and privileged information such as case histories are encountered in carrying out the role as an extension of the ophthalmologist. Naturally, such information must be kept confidential.

Today there is increasing emphasis on preventive measures in dealing with eye problems. There are also a greater number of older patients and an increased demand for and use of eye services on the part of our present highly insured general population.

In the community at large, the ophthalmic assistant is a significant help in such matters as glaucoma screening programs, understanding the blind, the rehabilitation of partially sighted adults, and cataract and refractive surgery. They may also help in developing countries.

As refractive surgery has expanded with LASIK, PRK, laser epithelial keratomileusis (LASEK), and newer intraocular lenses, more sophisticated instruments have been developed for analysis of the eye and cataract and glaucoma surgery. The technicians play a useful role in these diagnostic testing procedures including pachymetry, wavefront analysis, optical coherence tomography (OCT), specular microscopy, and topography.

Chapter 56

Ophthalmic assisting in the international community and in the prevention of blindness

Peter Y. Evans

INTRODUCTION

The purpose of this chapter is to present current efforts in line with the Global Initiative to Eliminate Avoidable Blindness, as defined by the World Health Organization (WHO) in 1997, aimed at creating alternative pathways to overcome the severe shortage of ophthalmologists in developing countries, specifically through the use of paramedical ophthalmic personnel. Because many of the leaders of these efforts abroad are increasingly looking at

In 2015 the World Health Organization in its Cambridge Declaration stated "The definition of Allied Ophthalmic Personnel may be characterized by different educational requirements, legislation and practice regulations, skills and scope of practice between countries and even within a given country. Typically, allied ophthalmic personnel comprise opticians, ophthalmic nurses, orthoptists, ophthalmic and optometric assistants, ophthalmic and optometric technicians, vision therapists, ocularists, ophthalmic photographer/imagers, and ophthalmic administrators."

the North American experience, particularly with regard to planning and organization, a short historical review appears for comparison and better understanding.

The 1960s was a turbulent decade for the United States, not only politically with presidential and other assassinations, the Vietnam War, and bloody antiwar demonstrations, but also socioeconomically with the introduction of Medicare and Medicaid. In anticipation of significant patient increases, government and academic health planners got together early to discuss challenges and explore solutions. Funds were made available to drastically enlarge medical school classes. In ophthalmology, new residency positions were to be created. Eye patients had to wait already 3 to 5 months for their appointments. The ophthalmologist's time for each patient became shorter and shorter. The doctor needed help. But to be effective and safe, that help needed also to be reliable and well trained.

In 1963, after 2 years of preparation, the first US full-time 2-year training program for ophthalmic technicians opened at Georgetown University in Washington, DC. Soon similar programs followed in university departments across the country and in Canada. And in due time it became clear that not only could more patients see their ophthalmologist in a timely fashion, but also at the same time a greater number of often time-consuming but important tests could be performed for which the ophthalmologist sometimes just did not have the time. The original time-saving motive had actually resulted in a significant improvement of eye patient care.

Many ophthalmologists, especially those involved in setting up training programs, felt an urgent need for standardization of training, for comparable or uniform examinations, and for clear definitions of different levels of expertise: in short, for quality control. In 1969 the Joint

Commission on Allied Health Personnel in Ophthalmology (JCAHPO) was established and has since enjoyed the support of all North American ophthalmologic and allied health organizations (see also Chapter 55). Today the United States averages one ophthalmologist for every 12,340 people, certainly an entirely adequate ratio, not considering some regional maldistributions. It is estimated that the 25,152 ophthalmologists are supported by well over 35,000 allied ophthalmic personnel, not including administrative and other staff. More than 22,700 ophthalmic medical personnel (OMP) are certified and recertified. Especially certified OMP earn good salaries and the job satisfaction is great. Additionally, more than 650 OMP are now (2015) certified in Canada and other countries and continents.

How dramatically different do these figures become in other areas of the world! The entire Sub-Saharan portion of Africa averages only one ophthalmologist for each million of its population. Because most ophthalmologists are located in urban areas and most of the population is in rural areas, this statistic is even wider when considering access to care. Blinding diseases almost never seen in North America or Europe such as trachoma and onchocerciasis still exist there. The prevalence of blindness is shocking. Once the preponderance of blindness in many developing countries was recognized in the 1950s, responsive initiatives and activities in the developed countries began to flourish. Since the 1950s, an increasing number of especially European and American nongovernmental organizations (NGOs) have been founded for the express purpose of combatting and trying to prevent blindness in countries that lack the resources for doing it effectively on their own. Every ophthalmic assistant should become familiar with them. The WHO in Geneva, Switzerland, works with national governments on policy direction, and closely with a number of eye care NGOs. Most of the leading international eye care NGOs are member organizations of the International Agency for the Prevention of Blindness (IAPB). Of course, there are also many individual ophthalmologists working with NGOs on their own, who are dedicated and sacrifice for the common goal of prevention of blindness.

With unoperated cataracts responsible for as much as 80% of all blindness in many developing countries, ophthalmologists volunteered for cataract camps in India, where thousands of cataract operations were performed in a week. They joined, often at their own expense, groups of other ophthalmic surgeons who traveled for 1 or 2 weeks to remote areas in the world to operate on patients, especially children, who would otherwise be condemned to a life of blindness. They came aboard specially equipped ships and airplanes. They also brought highly specialized surgical skills to places where such operations had never been performed.

But continuity of locally based, locally managed, and realistically designed programs was and is needed. Such programs are ideally not just set up by NGOs and tolerated by the regional and national governments but are actively sponsored or mandated by them, in collaboration and with the support of the NGOs. National governments recognized the professional human resource needs for ophthalmologists and created alternative solutions such as ophthalmic paramedical personnel.

VISION 2020: THE RIGHT TO SIGHT

Initiated by the IAPB and launched jointly with the WHO in 1999, this worldwide, ambitious campaign to eliminate avoidable blindness by the year 2020 first identified five major blinding disease groups and disorders as avoidable: cataract, refractive errors, certain endemic infectious diseases (such as trachoma and onchocerciasis), glaucoma, and diabetic retinopathy. The global initiative also deals with low-vision and childhood blindness. It sets targets for human resource improvements in 5-year intervals. The current global action plan for 2014 to 2019 includes specific definitions and measurements of allied ophthalmic personnel.

The purpose of this chapter is to describe various regional challenges and training approaches. It should be noted that large portions of the information on the following pages are based on and sometimes quoted verbatim from reports generously supplied by organizations, ophthalmologists, and OMP working in the countries discussed. All these collaborators are listed at the conclusion of the chapter.

LATIN AMERICA

In most regions of the world outside North America, the work of ophthalmic assistants is driven by the need to prevent blindness. The IAPB estimates for the 500 million people living in Latin America a magnitude of blindness of 0.2% to 1% for a total of 2.5 million; 10 million people are estimated to suffer from low vision. Unoperated cataracts are responsible for 40% to 70% of the blindness in the region.

Puerto Rico

Although part of the United States, this bilingual island is of considerable interest for several reasons. In the 1950s Puerto Rico had only very few US-graduated ophthalmologists. The first ophthalmology residency program at the University of Puerto Rico was started in 1954 by Professor Guillermo Picó. In 1972 there was one ophthalmologist for each 42,000 Puerto Ricans.

Because a ratio of 1:15,000 was felt to be ideal but unattainable in the near future, planning began to start an ophthalmic technician training program in the university Department of Ophthalmology. This became a 2-year undergraduate degree program with the first year in general education and the second in ophthalmic technology. It was subsequently officially accredited at the ophthalmic technician level by the US Commission on Accreditation of Allied Health Education Programs (CAAHEP). Today the program is rated highly also in Central and South America.

The total population of Puerto Rico numbers 3.75 million, with 165 ophthalmologists for a much improved ratio of 1:22,700. There are now about 300 ophthalmic technician graduates, mostly women, working in a very stable environment under the direct supervision of their ophthalmologist employers, usually in urban areas. More patients are seen by the doctors, at a lesser cost. Uniformly, the community benefits are seen in an increase in the amount and quality of ophthalmic services. The remuneration of ophthalmic technicians in Puerto Rico is good and comparable to that of other midlevel health workers and nurses. More are still wanted.

The Puerto Rico Eye Care Society, in collaboration with a variety of other public and private agencies, conducts very active and educational vision and glaucoma screening programs, especially with nurses.

Haiti

Haiti, the poorest country in the Western Hemisphere, has a population of 10 million; 1.25 million live in the capital. Thirty-five percent are illiterate. More than 50% are younger than age 16, but the average life expectancy has improved to 61 years. The land is very mountainous and has very poor electrical service, mostly from aging generators.

Although improved, the estimated prevalence of blindness is 1.2%, more than double that of the entire Caribbean region. Cataracts are responsible for 50%, but glaucoma for 30%. The prevalence of glaucoma may be as high as 10%. It develops early and with high pressures. Malnutrition blindness from vitamin A deficiency can be found, and diabetic retinopathy is an emerging threat.

There are 55 ophthalmologists, 40 of them in the capital. Many devote some time to the rural eye centers. In 1998 about 1000 cataract surgeries were performed. Haiti's Ministry of Health reported that 2176 cataract operations were performed in 2014.

In the 1980s a very active organization, supported by an NGO, trained ophthalmic assistants for 1 year and they were deployed all over the country. Young people also were recruited from isolated villages, received short-term training, then sent back to the villages to screen the locals for decreased vision and other eye problems. People in need came or were brought over the mountains to rural eye clinics staffed in rotation by eye resident physicians. There they were refracted or medicated and those in need of an operation were sent on to an urban surgical center.

The estimated number of ophthalmic allied health personnel in Haiti is 100, with an average monthly salary of less than US$200. Most of them are working in eye centers outside the capital, where they receive on-the-job training. There are no formal training centers. Previous programs have closed down due to the political unrest. The destruction by the devastating earthquake of 2010 is still felt and seen everywhere. Many areas in the country have no eye care at all.

The availability of ophthalmic assistants is crucial for Haiti. One can only hope that their training will be reactivated soon.

Peru

Peru counts 1100 ophthalmologists for its population of almost 30 million for a ratio of 1:27,000. Although the National Eye Institute, under the directorship of Professor Francisco Contreras, conducted ophthalmic training courses for nurses and auxiliary personnel from 1979 to 1995, there are at this time no similar programs anywhere in Peru. Those courses were of 2 to 3 months' duration, were initially supported by Helen Keller International, drew from rural areas, and concentrated on either clinical ophthalmic services or prevention of blindness. According to Contreras, the major problems of the program were experienced in its follow-up. There was frequent lack of direct supervision after the trained personnel returned to their original sites, there was little continuing evaluation of their activities, and sometimes they were not put to work at all in the field in which they had been trained.

The latter finding underscores the need for job analyses and utilization studies. However, the main difficulty faced by most South American pioneers of OMP programs probably lies elsewhere, as best illustrated by Brazil.

Today many of the overworked ophthalmologists in Peru hire the equivalent of registered and practical nurses and train them themselves in specific skills, such as measurement of visual acuities, visual fields, and autorefraction. However, despite the need, there are no formal courses in the country.

Brazil

The largest country of South America, representing 50% of the entire continent, has also its largest population, with 195 million people: 14,679 ophthalmologists result in an ophthalmologist-to-population ratio of 1:13,300. The ophthalmology residency training is very similar to that in the United States. However, the urban versus rural maldistribution problem of eye doctors is even more pronounced than in most other countries. More than 95% of all eye services are located in urban areas.

Originally the only formal courses for OMP were given to orthoptics students. Today only one still exists. One other orthoptics course has been converted to a 3-year college program for ophthalmic technicians, with 20 students every year.

In 1988, Professor Newton Kara-José at the University of Campinas in Sao Paulo began a training program for ophthalmic assistants, which has continued without interruption; four times a year a full-time 2-month course is offered to 10 high school graduates, 90% of them women.

There are also a number of short, 1- to 3-day courses offered by professional societies, the University of Campinas, and during ophthalmic meetings (20–30 per year).

Therefore, very few of the estimated 6000 to 7000 auxiliary ophthalmic office personnel in Brazil have had any formal training. There is no certification process and no central entity supervising or accrediting OMP courses. The upper income limit for OMP is equivalent to about US$8000 annually.

In Brazil the most frequent causes of blindness are cataract, uncorrected refractive errors, glaucoma, and diabetic retinopathy. Most important in children are infantile cataract, refractive errors, toxoplasmic retinitis, and retinopathy of prematurity. Since 1999, as a result of collaborative efforts of the Ministry of Health and the national association of ophthalmologists, cataract surgery has dramatically increased, from 60,000 to 70,000 per year to more than 300,000 per year. Since 2006, eye care services were provided by the national security system.

However, despite a few notable exceptions, most ophthalmologists in Brazil still need to be convinced of the advantages to them and to the public of formal training of their OMP. In other countries of South America the situation is quite similar. In 1998 Kara-José commented:

"Most of the ophthalmologic societies of South America are strongly set against regular programs for ophthalmic medical personnel because of the perceived threat of such professionals working independently, without the ophthalmologist…. This misconception and misguided apprehension deserve to be put to rest now, for the sake of ophthalmology, of ophthalmologists, and for the sake of their patients."

SUB-SAHARAN AFRICA

A brief reminder: today it is easily forgotten that until World War II, only four countries in this second largest continent of the world were truly independent: Egypt, Ethiopia, Liberia, and South Africa. During the following turbulent decades almost 40 former African colonies of former European empires became free nations. What remains is the geographic division between North Africa and the larger subcontinent south of the Sahara desert and with it many other differences, cultural as well as economic. Most North African countries are oriented toward Arab culture and language.

There is no question that Sub-Saharan Africa, in concert with civil strife and disastrous medical problems such as malnutrition, malaria, human immunodeficiency virus (HIV), acquired immunodeficiency syndrome (AIDS), and outbreaks of diseases such as Ebola, is more severely suffering from blinding diseases than any other continent. This is one of the greatest challenges for African governments and

has led to a unique concentration of efforts of the WHO and many NGOs in this vast area. It is here where the availability of OMP becomes truly crucial and their roles sometimes quite unorthodox, at least for the Western observer. Existing situations and ongoing activities in a few countries are described in more detail in the following text.

Kenya

Located on the East African coast, astride the equator, this country's population numbers 45 million. Children up to 15 years make up 41%, adults ages 16 to 64 years represent 56%, and only 3% of the population reaches an age of 65 years or older. The average life expectancy in Kenya is only 45 years from birth. Two-thirds live in rural areas. The population growth rate is 1.2% per year.

In 2014, there were 86 ophthalmologists in Kenya, up from 55 only 12 years earlier. The first group of residents graduated from the University of Nairobi in 1981 after 3 years of training. Thus there is one ophthalmologist for each half million people. However, there exists a severe maldistribution; almost all ophthalmologists live in urban areas.

The prevalence of blindness was estimated at 0.7%. Forty-three percent of blindness was caused by cataract, 19% represented corneal blindness caused by trachoma, and 9% was a result of glaucoma.

Like many other African countries, Kenya never had enough medical doctors. Not to assist but rather to supplement them, the government began to train medical assistants in the Kenya Medical Training College. The program recruited high school students and trained them for 3 years in clinical medicine to become clinical officers (COs). A CO could then specialize for another year to attain a diploma as CO in pediatrics, orthopedics, etc.

In 1956, recognizing that the severe undersupply of ophthalmologists could not be changed in the foreseeable future, the Kenya Ophthalmic Programme (KOP) was started in collaboration between the government and NGOs. The first cadre of OMPs to be trained for 1 year were the ophthalmic clinical officers (OCOs) in 1959. An OCO could then train for an additional year and become an OCO cataract surgeon (OCO/CS). In 1999 both courses were merged to create an 18-month OCO/CS course. Between 1996 and 2001, ophthalmologists and OCO/CSs successfully converted from ICCE to ECCE with intraocular lens (IOL).

Ophthalmic clinical officers

- Total 2003 numbers: 110 (71 OCOs and 39 OCO/CSs) active in service
- Training: basic requirement is 3-year college diploma in clinical medicine (CO)
- Capacity: 15 students per year maximally
- Duration: 18 months
- Sites of deployment: evenly distributed throughout the country, being primarily posted by the government to

provincial, district, and larger primary health care units, leaving the ophthalmologists to cover tertiary and secondary units. OCOs are also posted at tertiary and secondary units to support the ophthalmologists

- Level of independence: they run district eye units and conduct outreach primary eye care. Support supervision is offered by the zonal eye surgeons who are ophthalmologists
- Duties: clinical duties/cataract surgery; outreach services/eye camps; monthly report writing; curriculum development; training of community health workers; participate in surveys, for example, trachoma; annual planning and 5-year development plans
- Incentives: associate membership of Ophthalmologic Society of East Africa (OSEA); donations of equipment, transportation, etc. from NGOs; annual CME workshops by OSEA; part-time private practice permitted, like ophthalmologists, to supplement income.

The official acceptance of primary eye care (PEC) as an element of primary health care (PHC) in 1996 led to a work overload for the OCOs. In the 1990s, the need for formal training of other cadres of allied health staff became evident. This concerned especially the community eye care workers, the group specifically called ophthalmic assistants (OAs) in Kenya but also ophthalmic nurses, ophthalmic scrub nurses, and nursing assistants (NAs). With the advent of the WHO's and IAPB's VISION 2020: The Right to Sight targets, the problem of childhood blindness came into sharper focus and special training for low-vision therapists was accepted by the government. It is now carried out in the Kikuyu Eye Unit.

Ophthalmic nurses

Nurses have been the backbone of health care services in East Africa for a long time. The Kenya Nursing Council (KNC) has gone through different phases in its recognition of nursing and NA training. The Kenyan registered community health nurse requires a 4-year training. The 3-year Kenyan registered nurse course will probably be superseded by a new 4-year bachelor of science in nursing university degree program.

The NAs were products of a 1-year or less in-service course. They were also an important source for the ophthalmic assistant courses. However, as more qualified nurses come out of school and there is only limited money available to employ them, the government is phasing out the NA. This is also an attempt to stop the current drain of nurses out of Kenya to the United States and Europe. Nurses are poorly paid in Kenya (as are OCOs) and in all of East Africa. Once qualified, the nurse can choose a variety of specialties, including ophthalmology. The NA no longer fulfills the OA training selection criteria.

In 2003 a new 1-year university diploma course started specifically for ophthalmic nurses with some financial backing from the British NGO Sight Savers International (SSI). Two coordinators were trained in South Africa. The course capacity is 25 diploma nurses per year. Fourteen students were enrolled in the first class. Their training and job description try to avoid duplicating those of the OCO and concentrate on health promotion, management of eye units and eye camps, and the operating room.

Ophthalmic assistants

Training of OAs is conducted for 3 months in the Kikuyu Eye Unit near Nairobi. Kikuyu is a mission-based hospital (more than 50% of all health care in Kenya is still provided in mission hospitals). Here, the Christian Blind Mission International (CBMI), part of the German Christoffel Blindenmission, began to conduct the 3-month course for OAs in 1995. Admission criteria were flexible (nurses and NAs). The aim was to give the necessary skills to the OA to screen, diagnose, prescribe, and to know when and where to refer patients with eye problems, whether they would be working in primary or secondary government or in mission hospitals. Now there are more OCOs and OCO/CSs available, but they still have to rely on the OA covering the eye unit during their part-time private cataract practice.

The 3-month course covers a large array of basic ophthalmology with emphasis on eye conditions related to the developing world and practical procedures, including medications, refraction, low vision, and preoperative patient preparation as well as, very importantly, postoperative care once the surgical team has left 1 day after surgery. Some of the OAs returning to endemic trachoma areas are also taught how to perform bilamellar lid surgery for trichiasis. The course has been kept up to date with IOLs, VISION 2020, new drugs, and national plans. After final examinations the student receives an in-service certificate. CBMI provides not only the accommodation, food, and training materials but also upon graduation a set of valuable instruments, drugs, and books to take back to the rural eye unit. By 2004, 125 OAs had been trained. The number of OAs in Kenya exceeds that of all other eye care workers.

Tanzania

This country has a higher prevalence of blindness than Kenya, with 1.26% (vs. 0.7%). The leading cause of blindness here is not cataract but corneal disease from trachoma.

Although known and described for thousands of years, trachoma had been studied particularly in Egypt in the 19th century and became known as the "Egyptian [eye] disease." The *Chlamydia* infection is endemic, highly contagious, and usually bilateral, affecting especially women and children in arid areas. The WHO estimates that 15% (6 million cases) of world blindness is due to trachoma. The conjunctival scarring leads to entropion and trichiasis. The trichiasis causes corneal opacification. This preventable cause of blindness is a particularly important concern for the community eye worker and the ophthalmic assistant who can jointly enact the WHO's entire strategy against trachoma—surgery, antibiotics, facial cleanliness, environmental hygiene (SAFE)—but not necessarily in that order. The trained OCO can perform necessary lid surgery to eliminate the trichiasis (Figure 56.1). There are many similarities with Kenya in training. Nurses are trained for 2 or 3 years, depending on their entrance requirements, and can upgrade to the higher level after several years of work. The country has not yet started a bachelor of science in nursing degree program. Also here, a nurse can specialize in ophthalmology, and the NA training courses have been stopped.

The ophthalmic assistant course is given for 3 months in one hospital in central Tanzania. The curriculum is modeled on the Kikuyu course, but these nurses do still receive government recognition for their newly acquired skills. The OA, as in Kenya, is placed in remote areas and works at the primary or secondary level, performing screening, diagnosing, and prescribing first-line treatment (Figure 56.2).

A 2-year diploma program in ophthalmic nursing is offered in another hospital. Curriculum evaluation, modifications, and adaptations of VISION 2020 targets are slow in coming. Nurses who want to train for the operating room attend the course either at Kikuyu in Kenya or at the Ruharo Eye Unit in Uganda.

Uganda

In Uganda nurses train for 2 or 3 years and can upgrade to the higher level. However, there is no diploma program for ophthalmic nursing. A nurse wishing to enter ophthalmology goes to a mission or government hospital to take the 3-month ophthalmic assistant course with the same content as in Kenya or Tanzania. However, in Uganda the government recognizes this course and even conducts the course at government units. Since 2003, a nurse can also take a 4-month ophthalmic theater (scrub nurse) course. Finally, and interestingly, a Ugandan registered nurse can, after completing OA training, also apply for ophthalmic clinical officer training.

In this country the nursing aide and her training are accepted and recognized for the lower level of nursing staff. All NAs undergo a government training program, varying between 3 and 6 months. After its conclusion, the NA can care for patients in any clinical setting under the guidance of a qualified nurse. With proper qualification, the NA can also undertake the OA course. In some respects, Uganda has therefore a more practical approach to the ophthalmic manpower problem.

Malawi

Malawi is a small country in southern Africa, one of 12 members of the Southern African Development Community (SADC), the total population of which is estimated at about 180 million people. Except for South Africa and

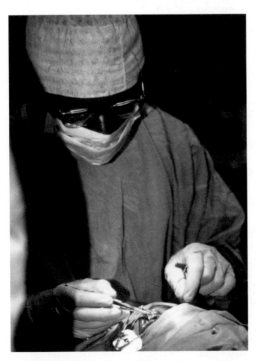

Figure 56.1 Ophthalmic clinical officer performing lid surgery in Malawi.

(Courtesy of International Eye Foundation.)

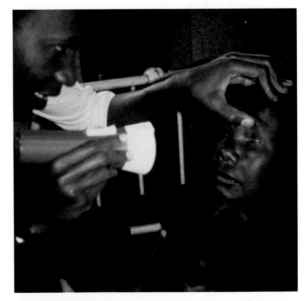

Figure 56.2 Ophthalmic nurse examines with flashlight in Tanzania where only D-cell batteries are readily available in rural areas.

(Courtesy of International Eye Foundation.)

Mauritius, the estimated average prevalence of blindness in this subregion is about 1%. Malawi's population of nearly 15 million has only four ophthalmologists, a sharp contrast to South Africa's 324 ophthalmologists for its 50 million people and therefore a ratio of about 1:500,000.

The major causes of blindness are cataract, trachoma, glaucoma, and, for childhood blindness particularly, measles and vitamin A deficiency. The latter two often go hand in hand, are highly prevalent in Africa and South and Southeast Asia, and are responsible for a high mortality rate. Xerophthalmia, resulting in corneal blindness, is the leading cause of all childhood blindness in developing countries. Sixty to 80% of these blind children will die before their fifth birthday. Considerable progress has been made in the prevention of vitamin A deficiency since 1991 with a worldwide campaign of high vitamin A prophylaxis thanks to the original epidemiologic work by Dr. Alfred Sommer. This treatment is amazingly inexpensive and very effective.

Until the 1980s, the gap between the small number of maldistributed ophthalmologists and the millions of people in need of eye care was only insufficiently narrowed by existing rural eye care workers whose training was not standardized. In 1980 the International Eye Foundation (IEF) established the first Ophthalmic Assistant Training Program in Malawi. In 1983 the SADC Ophthalmic Training Center was established at the Malawi College of Health Sciences in Lilongwe, with financial and human resources support from SSI. It is run by the Ministry of Health and Population. Its specific objective is to create trained midlevel eye health personnel (MLEHP or OMPs) equipped with the knowledge, attitudes, and skills to prevent and cure eye diseases.

The entrance requirement for the diploma course in clinical ophthalmology is either qualification as a clinical officer or equivalent experience as a state registered nurse or medical assistant. The duration is 1 academic year (46 weeks) with continuous forms of progress assessment, followed by a final examination and a written paper (dissertation). The program is by no means intended only for Malawi. Its graduates are working in SADC countries and even in non-SADC countries. Between 1983 and 2005, more than 650 MLEHP had been trained for 18 countries, with larger numbers in Malawi (85), Zimbabwe (80), Zambia (70), Botswana (51), Namibia (30), Lesotho (19), and Tanzania (15). Seventeen were even trained for Ethiopia and others were located as far West as The Gambia, Sierra Leone, and Ghana.

To meet the largest blindness challenge, cataracts, the SADC Ophthalmic Training Center started, also in 1983, its course for nonophthalmologist cataract surgeons. This is now an ECCE/IOL course with more stringent admission criteria. The prerequisites are diploma or certificate as ophthalmic clinical officer or ophthalmic nurse clinician; at least 2 years of clinical experience; personal recommendation by an ophthalmologist who will provide subsequent support and supervision; maximum age 40 years. The

OCO cataract surgeon is also required to undergo a 3-month training on the operating microscope in the supervising ophthalmologist's eye department and to perform extraocular surgery under the microscope.

The duration of the cataract surgeon course is 12 months. The trainee is required to perform a minimum of 100 operations on uncomplicated senile cataracts. By 2005, 34 cataract surgeons had been trained in the program, 29 of them for countries other than Malawi and 19 for countries outside the SADC.

To provide another perspective and a summary for East Africa's manpower needs, Figures 56.3 and 56.4, provided by Dr. Allen Foster, former IAPB President and Medical Director of CBMI, show respectively the 2002 supply of ophthalmologists and the 2004 supply of ophthalmic assistants in the region compared with the WHO's targeted ratios for 2020.

It should be noted that besides Kenya, Tanzania, Uganda, and Malawi, there are similar programs in The Gambia and Ethiopia for training OAs, the midlevel eye health personnel, and for nonophthalmologist cataract surgeons. Of particular interest is a training center in Mali in West Africa.

Mali

In 1953, the African Institute of Tropical Ophthalmology (Institut d'Opthalmologie Tropicale de l'Afrique or IOTA), was created in Bamako. It is part of the Organization of

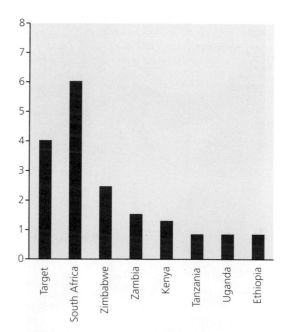

Figure 56.3 A 2002 supply of ophthalmologists per 1 million population in East Africa and WHO target for entire Sub-Saharan Africa for the year 2020. Note: Malawi now has four ophthalmologists for its population of 10 million.
(Courtesy of A. Foster, MD.)

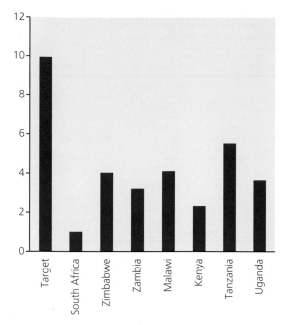

Figure 56.4 A 2004 supply of ophthalmic assistants per 1 million population in East Africa and WHO target for entire Sub-Saharan Africa for the year 2020.
(Courtesy of A. Foster, MD.)

Cooperation and Coordination for the Control of Major Endemic Diseases (OCCGE). This organization is made up of eight French-speaking countries: Benin, Burkina Faso, Ivory Coast, Mali, Mauritania, Niger, Senegal, and Togo. IOTA is the only institute of its kind in Sub-Saharan Africa. It is also a WHO collaborating center for the prevention of blindness.

In 1993, IOTA became a training center for the International First Sight Program. Its four major functions are:

- Offering tertiary ocular care
- Teaching and training of ophthalmic personnel at various levels
- Clinical and surgical research
- Consultations for the other member countries

Like most Sub-Saharan African countries, West Africa suffers particularly from onchocerciasis, commonly known as river blindness, in addition to the blinding diseases of cataract, trachoma, glaucoma, and xerophthalmia. In the Central African Republic, which has the highest prevalence of blindness (2.2%), onchocerciasis is the leading cause of blindness (73%). Worldwide about 17 million people are infected and 350,000 are blind from the ocular complications of this parasitic disease, transmitted by the black fly in river valleys. More than 95% of the populations affected live in Africa, within 20 degrees of the equator.

The microfilariae also migrate into the eye, where they can cause sclerosing keratitis, anterior uveitis, chorioretinitis, and optic neuritis and atrophy. The adult male worm grows

up to 9 inches (22.5 cm), and the female can reach 2 feet (50 cm) in length and live in subcutaneous skin nodules, producing millions more microfilaria within the body. Ivermectin (Mectizan) treatment is safe, effective, and cost effective. The manufacturer, Merck & Co., provides the drug free of charge to onchocerciasis control programs for as long as it is needed. However, because ivermectin kills only the microfilaria, not the adult worm, the treatment has to be given annually. The drug distribution is community-based.

IOTA trains four groups in traditional subjects and public health:

- Ophthalmic medicine, for 4 years, for general medical doctors
- Cataract surgeons, for 10 months, for general medical doctors
- Ophthalmic nurses, for 2 years, for diploma nurses
- Opticians, for 3 months

Current statistics are not available. However, between 1991 and 1998, IOTA had trained 18 ophthalmologists, 24 cataract surgeons, 83 ophthalmic nurses, and 16 opticians for Mali and the other countries of the OCCGE.

NORTH AFRICA AND THE MIDDLE EAST

In general, the countries of North Africa enjoy somewhat better ophthalmologist-to-population ratios than those in the Sub-Saharan region. But even here, a country like Tunisia showed in 1993 a prevalence of blindness of 0.8%; however, almost 10% of the cataract blindness was actually a result of uncorrected aphakia (Table 56.1). In southern Egypt the prevalence of blindness and severe visual impairment in the age group older than 40 years reaches a shocking 9.3%, and women are 2.5 times more likely to become blind than are men.

SOUTH AND SOUTHEAST ASIA

India

The sheer numbers in any type of statistics from India are dizzying. The country has more than 1 billion people, each with an average annual income of US$450, and is growing at a rate of 1.6% per year. Since gaining independence in 1947, the population had more than tripled by the end of the century. It is projected to surpass China by the year 2040.

According to WHO estimates, 90% of the nearly 45 million blind people worldwide live in developing countries and nearly one-sixth of them are found in India. There are 11,000 ophthalmologists in India, resulting in an ophthalmologist-to-population ratio of about 1:111,000. The annual total of cataract operations is close to 4 million.

Table 56.1 2014 International Council of Ophthalmology data of population and available ophthalmologists, and 2005 WHO figures for prevalence of blindness for North African and Middle Eastern countries

Country[a]	Population	Ophthalmologists	Ratio	Prevalence %
Morocco	31,942,000	1030	1:31,000	0.76
Tunisia	10,481,000	358	1:29,000	0.8
Libya	6,355,000	180	1:35,000	0.8
Egypt	81,122,000	2400	1:34,000	1.2
Sudan	43,552,000	366	1:119,000	1.5 – 6.4
Djibouti	889,000	2	1:444,500	1.5
Cyprus	1,100,000	65	1:14,000	0.7
Lebanon	4,228,000	245	1:17,000	0.8
Syria	20,411,000	680	1:30,000	0.7
Jordan	6,187,000	231	1:27,000	0.6
Qatar	1,759,000	32	1:55,000	0.7
Kuwait	2,700,000	72	1:37,500	0.7
Bahrain	1,262,000	66	1:19,000	1.9
Oman	2,782,000	126	1:22,000	1.1
Yemen	24,100,000	66	1:365,000	1.5
Iran	74,000,000	1500	1:49,000	0.8
Afghanistan	31,412,000	140	1:224,000	2.0
Pakistan	175,593,000	1860	1:93,000	1.8

[a]Note great variations from country to country.

With a cataract surgery rate of 3800 per million of population, India has one of the highest rates in the world, thanks to the hard work of its ophthalmologists.

However, that achievement would not be possible without the help of OAs and technicians, ophthalmic nurses, refractionists, and orthoptists. In 2005 the estimated number in these categories was about 15,000, plus another 15,000 to 20,000 working in eye care facilities without any formal training or qualification. This is not to say they are not well trained, because they have been trained by their hospital leaders for specific skills and duties. Approximately 80 institutions were training midlevel ophthalmic personnel (MLOP) in India, with a combined admission total of approximately 1300 trainees each year.

Despite such large numbers, there exist no statutory bodies for them such as those in place for the education of nurses and doctors. OA training programs in some institutions are recognized by foreign entities, such as the Berkeley School of Optometry, the JCAHPO and CoA-OMP, or the International Centre for Eyecare Education in Australia. Because of the large size of the country and the multiple

categories of personnel, training program leaders and other professional authorities feel an urgent need for a situational analysis of human resources in eye care to determine the requirements with respect to VISION 2020 in order to identify the gaps and develop strategies to gradually close them (Table 56.2). A major challenge is mainstreaming the large number of personnel working without formal training.

There are many good OA training programs among the 80 in the country and some excellent ones. Without question, the most outstanding training program in India is the Aravind Eye Care System (AECS) in Madurai, South India. Aravind started out in 1976 as an 11-bed eye clinic. Dr. G. Venkataswamy, an ophthalmologist with a vision and a mission, was its director. Nobody who has met him will ever forget his devotion, drive, and magnetism. Today, with more than 3500 beds, Aravind has evolved into a center that delivers a wide array of eye care services through a network of five hospitals with facilities for teaching, training, research, policy advocacy, capacity building, and the manufacture of affordable ophthalmic supplies. (Its Aurolab intraocular lenses are shipped all over the world and are

Table 56.2 VISION 2020 needs projections for India of hospital- and community-based ophthalmic assistants and the training needs for two levels of each group Southeast Asia. Table from Prof. Ravi Thomas, India

Human resource needs	2000	2005	2010	2015	2020
Ophthalmic assistants: community-based	6000	10,000	15,000	20,000	25,000
Ophthalmic paramedics: hospital-based	18,000	30,000	36,000	42,000	48,000
Training needs					
Ophthalmic assistants: community-based certificate course	Class: 10		3 months (in-service)		
Ophthalmic assistants: community-based diploma	Class: 12		2 years (formal)		
Ophthalmic paramedics: hospital-based certificate course	Class: 10		3 months (in-service)		
Ophthalmic paramedics: hospital-based diploma	Class: 12		2 years (formal)		

Source: Midlevel ophthalmic personnel in South East Asia, SEA-Ophthal 124, WHO Regional Office for South-East Asia, May 2002.
National Program for Control of Blindness India.
Vision 2020: The Right to Sight, India – Plan of Action.
DGHS, MOHFW, GOI, New Delhi

affordable even in Africa for about US$5 to $7 for a hard PC/IOL.) It is the largest and most productive eye care facility in the world. Each year Aravind sees more than 1.4 million patients and performs more than 200,000 sight-restoring operations.

Paramedical training programs in ophthalmic practice

The current certificate course in ophthalmic assistance was originally started in 1978. Its total duration is 2 years (Figure 56.5). The language of instruction is Tamil. It is open to graduated high school girls only, with good grades and science background, based on an interview and written entrance examination. They come from rural, low-income backgrounds and have no work experience. Every year, 75 to 100 students are recruited, depending on the institutional manpower needs.

Among the 23 objectives of the program are compassion, communication skills, teamwork, community eye programs, communicable diseases, and medical emergencies. From 1978 through 2003, Aravind trained a total of 1800 OAs. In addition to the 2-year course with its four branches of specialty training, Aravind also offers the following special courses.

Certificate course in clinical and supervisory skills development

This 3-month course, started in 2002, is offered in collaboration with the IAPB to help achieve the objectives of VISION 2020. There are at least 500 voluntary institutions offering eye care in India. Many of these hospitals have the potential to upgrade the volume and quality of their service and to deliver more affordable eye care. Ophthalmic paramedical personnel play a key role in all these institutions. Their clinical and supervisory skills are enhanced by this course.

Short-term course in ophthalmic dispensing

Also started in 2002, this course offers advanced training in optical dispensing. It is an outreach program.

Postgraduate diploma in ophthalmic assistance

Two-year program for university graduates, also from other countries, for higher-level OAs (reminiscent of the US ophthalmic technologist concept).

Postgraduate diploma in optometry

Two-year program for university graduates to deal with the vast problem of uncorrected refractive errors, identified by the WHO as one of the five major causes of avoidable blindness.

Finally, since 1981 Aravind has also run custom-designed courses for paramedics from various organizations such as the Indian and foreign ministries of health, NGOs, other Indian and foreign eye hospitals, other ophthalmic training programs and Indian and foreign national prevention and control of blindness organizations. By the end of 2003, 28 such custom-designed courses had been conducted with a total of 167 trainees.

Today the Aravind complex in Madurai has become something of a Mecca for anybody active or interested in the field of international blindness prevention and control, in the goal of achieving high-quality, affordable, and sustainable eye care for everybody and in the pursuit of VISION 2020 targets.

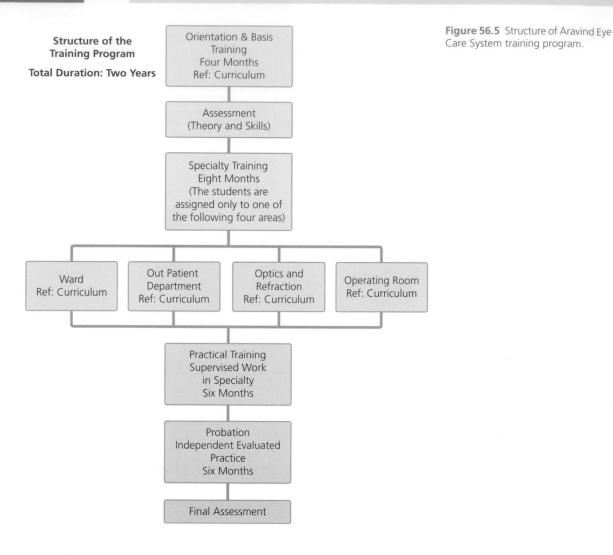

**Structure of the
Training Program**

Total Duration: Two Years

Orientation & Basis
Training
Four Months
Ref: Curriculum

Assessment
(Theory and Skills)

Specialty Training
Eight Months
(The students are
assigned only to one of
the following four areas)

Ward
Ref: Curriculum

Out Patient
Department
Ref: Curriculum

Optics and
Refraction
Ref: Curriculum

Operating Room
Ref: Curriculum

Practical Training
Supervised Work
in Specialty
Six Months

Probation
Independent Evaluated
Practice
Six Months

Final Assessment

Figure 56.5 Structure of Aravind Eye Care System training program.

The L.V. Prasad Eye Institute in Hyderabad shares with Aravind the distinction of being considered an international model program of blindness prevention and OA training. Founded in 1986 by Gullapalli N. Rao, MD, it is a superb eye research center with a strong outreach program for rural eye care.

Bangladesh

Bangladesh, with a population of more than 148 million and a growth rate of 1.6% per year, shares many of the problems of other developing countries. The per capita income is about US$450, the same as in India. Thirty-six percent of the population lives below the poverty line. There is a significant drain of the labor force into the Middle East. However, the equal male and female life expectancy is 61 years, and the literacy rate is improving, with 63% for males and 49% for females.

Although 80% of Bangladeshis live in rural areas, most of the medical facilities and doctors are located in the cities. With an average of one ophthalmologist (current total number: 610) per almost 244,000 population and one ophthalmic nurse per three-quarters of a million population, the professional geographic maldistribution severely accentuates all existing eye care problems. A national survey of blindness and low vision showed that around 650,000 cases, or 80%, of blindness are caused by cataracts. Other leading causes are glaucoma, ocular injuries, corneal infections, blinding malnutrition, and posterior segment diseases. Conservative estimates cite three-quarter of a million cataract cases waiting for surgery, growing by 130,000 new cases every year. In the year 2003, 119,500 cataract surgeries were performed.

To address the acute shortage of ophthalmologists, several institutions have been conducting postgraduate diploma and fellowship courses for some time. Special training courses for ophthalmic nurses were also given in the capital city, Dhaka. But no facilities to train midlevel ophthalmic support personnel existed until 1979.

In 1979, the private Chittagong Eye Infirmary and Training Complex and Institute of Community Ophthalmology, established by the Bangladesh National Society for the Blind, an NGO, and directed by Professor Rabiul Husain, embarked on a comprehensive program of training not only ophthalmologists but also paramedic ophthalmic assistants. Professor Frank Billson, with an Australian team and Brenda Down of London, helped develop a special workforce in eye health care. After 2 years of training, the doctors achieve a Diploma of Community Ophthalmology from the University of Chittagong. Their training has a strong focus on community-based ophthalmic problems and their management. Emphasis is placed on cataract surgery with IOL implantation, corneal problems, nutritional blindness, and glaucoma.

The so-called ophthalmic paramedics receive their training in a well-structured 2-year certificate program and become a vital part of the ophthalmic workforce, particularly in the nongovernmental charitable institutions serving the eye care needs of the people of Bangladesh. By 2005, 316 paramedics had been trained, and a total of 133 other short courses had been given on such subjects as refraction, ocular laboratory, operating theater, glaucoma, orthoptics, and primary eye care.

The skills of the ophthalmic assistants are critical in the operating rooms where they perform instrument sterilization, equipment storage, and assistance at surgery. They are essential also in the postoperative care of cataract patients, in the outpatient clinics, in school eye health programs, and community disease screenings, including the important Under-5-Clinics for the detection and prevention of nutritional childhood blindness.

For eye camp surgery, another outreach program, these paramedics travel to remote, rural areas of the country, transport equipment, set up essentially a field hospital, do vision screenings for cataracts, prepare patients for surgery, assist in surgery, and usually stay 2 or 3 days after the surgeons have left to monitor the postoperative course and recognize and manage postoperative complications. Most of the work at eye camps is done by the paramedics, with the exception of the surgery itself.

A number of these paramedics have traveled to Sydney, Australia, for frontline management training and management skills. Such skill transfer has resulted in demonstrated capacity to manage a microbiology laboratory, to take the position and responsibility of a deputy matron of an eye hospital, be the director of a central sterilizing service department, or become manager of an operating theater.

Of special importance for the rural, underserved population of Bangladesh is the concept of primary eye care as an integral component of the primary health care system. Traditional healers, the Ayurveda, although originally based on ancient religious health beliefs, are medically untrained practitioners who are usually seen first for any illness, including ocular. They have the confidence of their community. But because of lack of knowledge they were also often found to prescribe harmful medicines, sometimes leading to blindness. In a forceful move to overcome this situation, primary eye care centers were set up in rural communities, where OAs assume the dual role of providing needed treatment to patients as well as teaching and training traditional healers in proper primary eye care activities, a unique model of skill transfer.

Australia

In a country that constitutes a whole continent one might reasonably expect a large population; however, it numbers only 22.3 million. The rapid growth in its population can be appreciated relative to the 1961 census when the population was 10.5 million.

The current growth rate is 0.93%; immigration accounts for most of the increase. By contrast, the indigenous population of Aborigines, with their remnants of Stone Age culture, has decreased from about 300,000 to roughly 60,000 since 1788. There are 895 ophthalmologists registered in Australia. Professor Frank Billson is one of them, a senior educator with a strong commitment to the training and use of OAs. Here is his report:

"The importance of the role of ophthalmic assistants in extending the arms of the ophthalmologists, particularly in developing countries, cannot be overemphasized. Still today, much can be achieved through training as an apprentice. How much, depends on the skills and willingness and generosity of spirit of the teacher or mentor. Ophthalmic assistants range from nurses with ophthalmic training to orthoptists and ophthalmic paramedics. Skill transfer can also occur to traditional medical healers. In developed countries, senior ophthalmologists may occasionally choose to reduce their activities to those of assistants."

Orthoptists

In Australia the orthoptist has traditionally been the OA. Initially, their training began in apprenticeship with ophthalmologists in offices or hospitals under the auspices of the Orthoptic Board of Australia, and their skills were confined to strabismus and other disorders of binocular vision in children, including the management of amblyopia. Training then moved to tertiary colleges with diplomas in orthoptics. More recently, the curriculum is offered by universities, with 3 years of study and training leading to a bachelor of applied science (orthoptics) degree.

809

Orthoptic training now has a strong academic content, and the practical clinical skills have expanded to include visual field tests, optic nerve functions, fundus photography, electrophysiology, screening for eye diseases, and participation in research as team members and as leaders. About 300 orthoptists are registered; 70% of them work in ophthalmologists' offices or eye departments, others in blindness prevention programs or privately.

Ophthalmic nurses

These gain their training, after general nursing certification, now exclusively in the Sydney Eye Hospital. This is a 6-month course with lectures and extensive, practical hands-on experience, leading to a diploma in ophthalmic nursing. There are presently about 150 ophthalmic nurses, most of them working in operating theaters.

Aboriginal eye health workers

This third group of OAs is uniquely Australian. Aboriginal health workers receive skill transfer so that they may participate in screening, particularly in outback areas. The majority of screening, however, is performed by optometrists (there are 5000 optometrists in Australia), and the federal government gives them a rebate for screening. Nevertheless, there does appear to be a place for Aboriginal eye health workers because of both their language and cultural understanding. Also, ownership of health programs ensures full participation. They live in the rural areas, providing a constant resource of helpful ophthalmic expertise.

Where cross training has occurred, the Aboriginal health workers have shown an aptitude for taking digital fundus photos for the recording of diabetic retinopathy (Figure 56.6), and they form an important interface with the general practitioners in the remote rural areas, who value the photographic records and the increased understanding of their patients' problems. Aboriginals are trained in the Northern Territory and New South Wales.

Finally, a few words about our neighbors in Papua New Guinea with a population of 6.9 million. Their major causes of blindness are cataract, diabetes, and ocular trauma. Their mountainous population centers can be reached only by airplane. There are only 6 ophthalmologists and 12 ophthalmic nurses in that country. In 1996 we started an ophthalmic assistant program there with a 6-week course in primary eye care and subsequent refresher courses while in service. They are trained not only to assist the ophthalmologists in primary care but also to refract and to carve simple reading glasses. In 2005 there were 26 such ophthalmic assistants in Papua New Guinea.

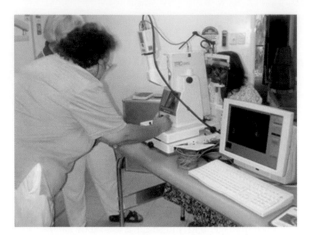

Figure 56.6 Aboriginal eye health worker, Dot Butler, taking digital fundus photos in the screening for diabetic retinopathy in Australia.
(Courtesy of Frank Billson, MD.)

OPHTHALMIC ASSISTANTS ELSEWHERE

There are many other regions in Asia and other continents where OAs are working at various levels, contributing to the global fight for sight. From Bangladesh to Singapore, they are increasingly trained in formal programs. They participated in glaucoma research in Mongolia and National Institutes of Health (NIH)-sponsored research in Barbados. In the mid-eighties, an ophthalmic nurse from Indonesia went through the 2-year program in Washington, DC, returned to Djakarta, and set up not only the first formal OA training program there but also a much improved three-tiered eye care program for the entire country, as tasked by her government and university.

In such truly international company, Europe has remained somewhat of an enigma. Especially the Western European countries do not experience anything even remotely resembling the suffering of millions of people in less developed areas of the world, and they do fairly closely resemble North American living standards and enjoy similar ophthalmologist-to-population ratios. Nevertheless, the inherent professional benefits and further elevation of eye care quality through the use of well-trained OAs seem to have thus far failed to intrigue the European ophthalmologists. Some of their academic leaders have followed the US and Canadian developments with considerable interest, and have invited speakers and exhibits from across the Atlantic. But to date no coordinated action has been taken.

Of course, this should in no way detract from the enormous contributions of many European NGOs in the United Kingdom, Germany, Scandinavia, France, and other countries, which have been devoted for many decades to fighting blindness in Africa, Asia, and other developing countries.

SUMMARY

The evolution and justification of the still fairly young profession of OMP were quite different in North America and the rest of the world. Today it is virtually impossible to describe their actual work, especially in the developing countries, without acknowledging the profound effect of global and local prevention of blindness programs. Specifically, the human resource and blinding disease targets set by the WHO and IAPB for the year 2020 are reshaping the training, deployment, and daily tasks of these medical personnel and even the laws of some countries.

Over the years, quite a few of the JCAHPO-certified OMP have been motivated to serve as instructors or in other capacities in places of greater need, especially in Africa and Asia. And in 2009, JCAHPO's long-standing interest and work in worldwide ophthalmic assisting led finally to the official creation of IJCAHPO, the International JCAHPO. The languages, the methods, the diseases, and certainly the job descriptions may be different, but the common cause remains the same for all ophthalmic personnel throughout the world: their patients' right to sight.

ACKNOWLEDGMENTS

It would have been impossible to present the preceding overview without the cooperation and collaboration of numerous individuals who generously supplied often ample up-to-date information. Some of their photographs could not be included because it is often difficult to obtain a patient's consent overseas. My special appreciation goes to Victoria M. Sheffield, president and CEO of the International Eye Foundation, and her husband, Howard Pyle, JD, for their tremendous help in the preparation of this chapter for the current and past editions. Most sincere thanks also to the following contributors: Carlos Arieta, MD, Sao Paulo; Frank Billson, MD, Sydney; Moses Chirambo, MD, Lilongwe; Francisco Contreras, MD, Lima; Sr. Ingrid Cox, COA, Nairobi; Allen Foster, MD, London; Paul Foster, MD, London; Judy Hall, COT, Sarasota, FL; Brigitte Hudicourt, MD, Port-au-Prince; Rabiul Husain, MD, Chittagong; Khumbo Kalua, MSc, DLSHTM, MMed, MBBS, Blantyre; Jefitha Karimurio, MD, Nairobi; Milagros Colon de Lopez, RN, Puerto Rico; Luis Serrano, MD, Puerto Rico; Ahmed Mousa, MScm, PhD, Cairo and Riyadh; B. R. Shamanna, MD, Hyderabad; Usha Kim, MD, Madurai; and Mariano Yee, MD, Guatemala City.

Chapter | 57 |

Atlas of common eye diseases and disorders

Harold A. Stein, Raymond M. Stein, Rebecca L. Stein

Q **Questions: What is your diagnosis? Take the quiz!**

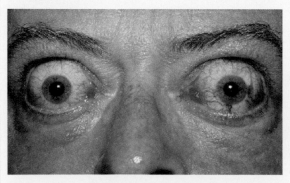

Figure 57.1 Question 1 What is your diagnosis?

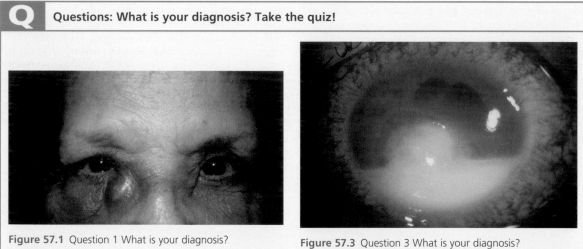

Figure 57.3 Question 3 What is your diagnosis?

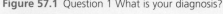

Figure 57.2 Question 2 What is your diagnosis?

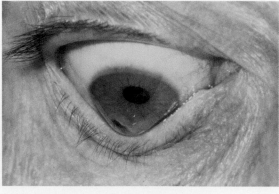

Figure 57.4 Question 4 What is your diagnosis?

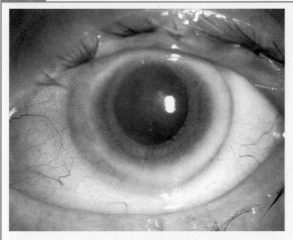

Figure 57.5 Question 5 What is your diagnosis?

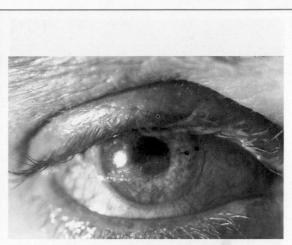

Figure 57.8 Question 8 What is your diagnosis?

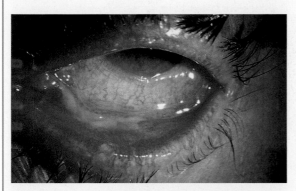

Figure 57.6 Question 6 What is your diagnosis?

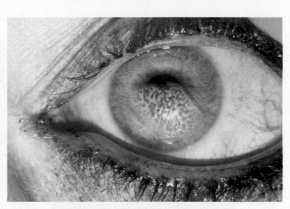

Figure 57.9 Question 9 What is your diagnosis?

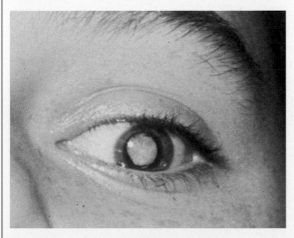

Figure 57.7 Question 7 What is your diagnosis?

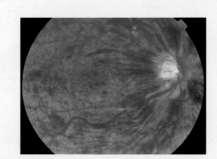

Figure 57.10 Question 10 What is your diagnosis?

Q | Continued

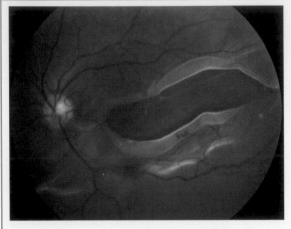

Figure 57.11 Question 11 What is your diagnosis?

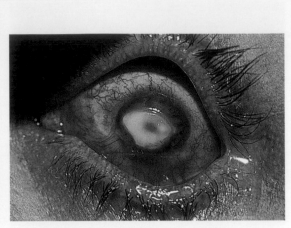

Figure 57.14 Question 14 What is your diagnosis?

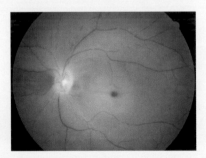

Figure 57.12 Question 12 What is your diagnosis?

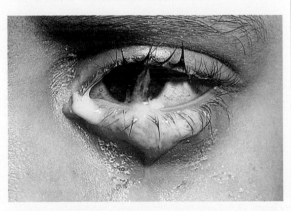

Figure 57.15 Question 15 What is your diagnosis?

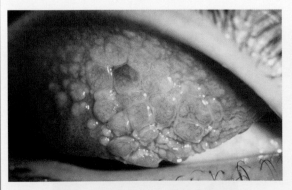

Figure 57.13 Question 13 What is your diagnosis?

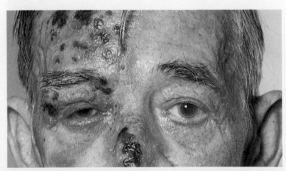

Figure 57.16 Question 16 What is your diagnosis?

Q Continued

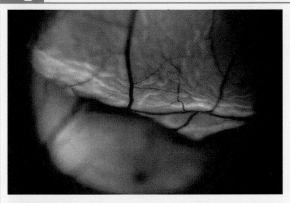

Figure 57.17 Question 17 What is your diagnosis?

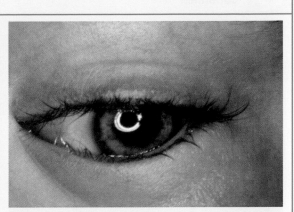

Figure 57.20 Question 20 What is your diagnosis?

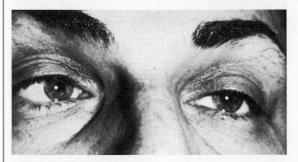

Figure 57.18 Question 18 What is your diagnosis?

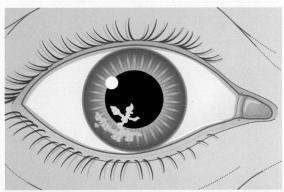

Figure 57.21 Question 21 What is your diagnosis?

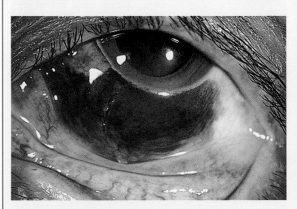

Figure 57.19 Question 19 What is your diagnosis?

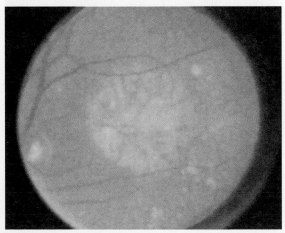

Figure 57.22 Question 22 What is your diagnosis?

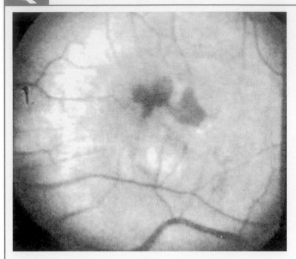

Figure 57.23 Question 23 What is your diagnosis?

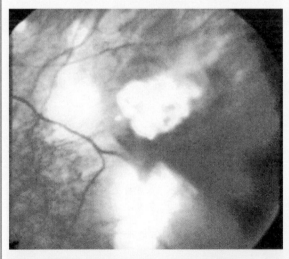

Figure 57.24 Question 24 What is your diagnosis?

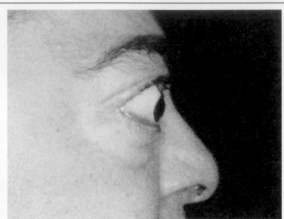

Figure 57.25 Question 25 What is your diagnosis?

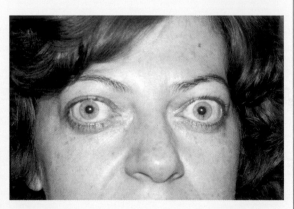

Figure 57.26 Question 26 What is your diagnosis?

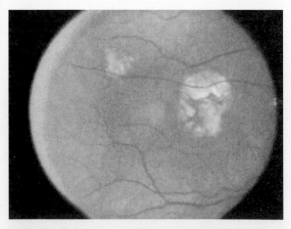

Figure 57.27 Question 27 What is your diagnosis?

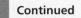

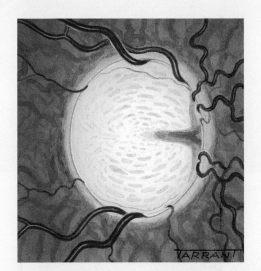

Figure 57.28 Question 28 What is your diagnosis?

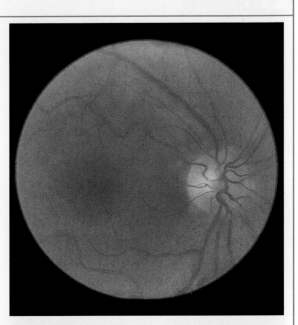

Figure 57.30 Question 30 What is your diagnosis?

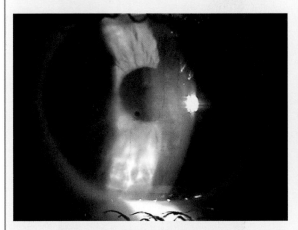

Figure 57.29 Question 29 What is your diagnosis?

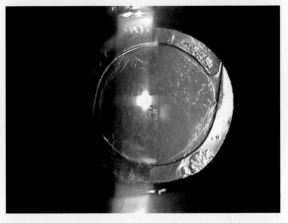

Figure 57.31 Question 31 What is your diagnosis?

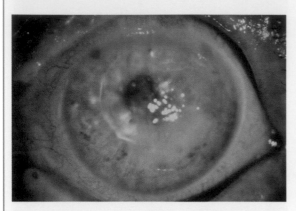

Figure 57.32 Question 32 What is your diagnosis?

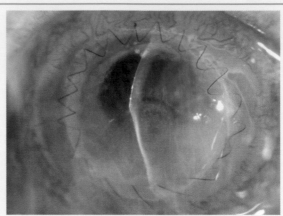

Figure 57.35 Question 35 What is your diagnosis?

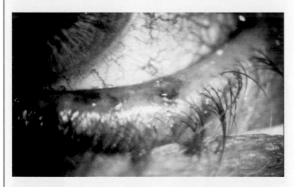

Figure 57.33 Question 33 What is your diagnosis?

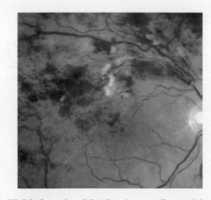

Figure 57.36 Question 36 What is your diagnosis?

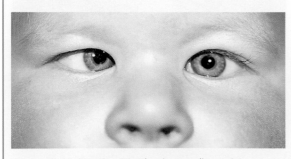

Figure 57.34 Question 34 What is your diagnosis?

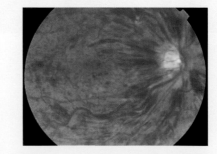

Figure 57.37 Question 37 What is your diagnosis?

Q Continued

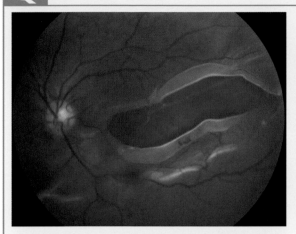

Figure 57.38 Question 38 What is your diagnosis?

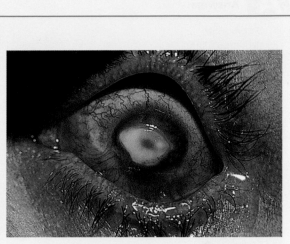

Figure 57.40 Question 40 What is your diagnosis?

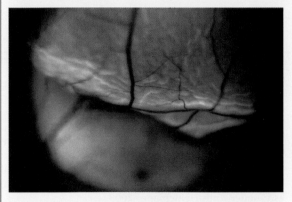

Figure 57.39 Question 39 What is your diagnosis?

A **Answers**

1. Dacryocystitis
2. Hyperthyroidism
3. Corneal ulcer with hypopyon
4. Advanced keratoconus
5. Arcus senilis
6. Acute bacterial conjunctivitis
7. Traumatic cataract
8. Corneal abrasion
9. Acid burn of the cornea
10. Central retinal vein occlusion
11. Retinal tear with associated retinal detachment
12. Retinal artery occlusion
13. Vernal conjunctivitis
14. Corneal ulcer due to *Acanthamoeba*
15. Conjunctivitis
16. Herpes zoster
17. Retinal detachment
18. Strabismus
19. Subconjunctival hemorrhage
20. Entropion
21. Dendritic patter of herpes simplex keratitis on the cornea
22. Macular degeneration
23. Choroideremia
24. Retinoblastoma
25. Thyroid exophthalmos
26. Exophthalmos in Graves' disease
27. Histoplasmosis
28. Glaucoma optic atrophy
29. Corneal edema
30. Cystoid macular edema
31. Capsular opacification
32. Pseudophakic bullous keratopathy
33. Blepharitis
34. Infantile esotropia
35. Corneal ulcer
36. Branch vein occlusion
37. Central vein occlusion
38. Retinal tear
39. Retinal detachment
40. Cornea ulcer caused by *Acanthamoeba*

REFERENCES TO FIGURES

Figure 57.2   Image reproduced from Spalton D, Hitchings R, Hunter P. Atlas of clinical ophthalmology. 3rd ed. St Louis: Mosby; 2004, with permission.

Figure 57.10   Image from Kanski J, Bowling B. Clinical ophthalmology—a systematic approach. 7th ed. Edinburgh: Saunders; 2011.

Figure 57.11   Image from Kanski J, Bowling B. Clinical ophthalmology—a systematic approach. 7th ed. Edinburgh: Saunders; 2011.

Figure 57.12   Image from Kanski J, Bowling B. Clinical ophthalmology—a systematic approach. 7th ed. Edinburgh: Saunders; 2011.

Figure 57.16   Image reproduced from Spalton D, Hitchings R, Hunter P. Atlas of clinical ophthalmology. 3rd ed. St Louis: Mosby; 2004, with permission.

Figure 57.20   Image from Kanski J, Bowling B. Clinical ophthalmology—a systematic approach. 7th ed. Edinburgh: Saunders; 2011.

Figure 57.28   Image from Kanski J. Clinical ophthalmology: a systematic approach. 5th ed. Oxford: Butterworth-Heinemann; 2003, with permission.

Figure 57.30   Image reproduced from Spalton D, Hitchings R, Hunter P. Atlas of clinical ophthalmology. 3rd ed. St Louis: Mosby; 2004, with permission.

Figure 57.34   Image reproduced from Kanski J. Clinical ophthalmology: a systematic approach. 5th ed. Burlington, MA: Butterworth-Heinemann; 2003.

Figure 57.35   From Mártonyi CL, Bahn CF, Meyer RF. Clinical slit lamp biomicroscopy and photo slit lamp biomicrography. Ann Arbor, MI: Time One Ink; 1985.

Figure 57.36   Image from Kanski J, Bowling B. Clinical ophthalmology—a systematic approach. 7th ed. Edinburgh: Saunders; 2011.

Figure 57.37   Image from Kanski J, Bowling B. Clinical ophthalmology—a systematic approach. 7th ed. Edinburgh: Saunders; 2011.

Figure 57.38   Image from Kanski J, Bowling B. Clinical ophthalmology—a systematic approach. 7th ed. Edinburgh: Saunders; 2011.

Glossary*

A-scan   an ultrasound technique to determine the axial length of the eye to calculate the intraocular lens power required.

Abbe number   an indication of optical quality. Number is inversely proportional to the chromic dispersion of a specific lens material. Crown glass is 59.

abduct   to turn away from the midline.

abductor   a muscle that rotates the eye away from the midline (e.g., lateral rectus).

aberrant   deviating from the usual course.

ablation   removal of tissue as occurs with the excimer laser on the cornea for refractive changes.

abrasion   rubbing off of the superficial layer.

abscess   localized area of inflammation.

AC/A   accommodative convergence/accommodation ratio; expressed as the ratio between convergence caused by accommodation (in prism diopters) and the accommodation (in diopters).

accommodation   adjustment by the eye for seeing at different distances, accomplished by changing the shape of the crystalline lens through action of the ciliary muscle.

achloropsia   color blindness to green.

achromatic lens   a lens that neutralizes dispersion without interfering with refraction.

acuity   clearness; visual acuity is measured by the smallest object that can be seen at a certain distance.

add   the total dioptric power added to a distance prescription to supplement accommodation for reading.

adductor   a muscle that exerts force toward the midline (e.g., medial rectus).

adenovirus   a virus comprising a large group of different serotypes. Types 3, 7, 8, 11, and 19 are those most commonly associated with eye infections. Types 8 and 19 are associated with epidemic keratoconjunctivitis (EKC) and types 3 and 7 with pharyngoconjunctival fever (PCF).

Adie's pupil   a tonic pupil with sluggish response to light, accommodation, and convergence.

adnexa oculi   accessory structures of the eye, such as the lacrimal apparatus and the eyelids.

adoptive optics   devices and methods to custom correct high-order aberrations. These include special spectacles, contact lenses, intraocular lenses, and refractive surgery.

afterimage   image of an object that persists when the lids are closed.

AIDS   (acquired immunodeficiency syndrome) a viral infection characterized by a compromised immune system.

akinesia   absence of motor function.

albinism   hereditary loss of pigment in the eye, skin, and hair; usually associated with lowered visual acuity, nystagmus, and light sensitivity.

alexia   inability to read words previously known even though visual perception is clear.

allied ophthalmic personnel (AOP)   skilled professionals, qualified by didactic and clinical ophthalmic training, who perform ophthalmic procedures under the direction of a licensed ophthalmologist. The World Health Organization has established definitions of the eye care workforce cadres and their levels with AOP including ophthalmic assistants, technicians, and medical technologists. This AOP definition was adopted by the Cambridge Declaration for Global Recognition, in a collaboration of the Joint Commission on Allied Health Personnel in Ophthalmology, International

*Attention is directed to the companion texts for a more complete set of reference dictionaries: Stein HA, Slatt, BJ, Stein RM. Ophthalmic terminology: speller and vocabulary builder. 3rd ed. St Louis: Mosby; 1992, and Stein HA, Stein RM, Freeman MI, Massare JS. Ophthalmic dictionary and vocabulary builder—for eye care professionals. 4th ed. New Deli: Jaypee-Highlights Medical Publishers; 2011. Also adopted from Stein HA, Slatt BJ, Stein RM, Freeman MI. Fitting guide for rigid and soft lenses: a practical approach. 4th ed. St Louis: Mosby; 2002.

Agency for the Prevention of Blindness, and the International Council of Ophthalmology.

amaurosis partial or total blindness from any cause.

amaurosis fugax temporary blindness.

amblyopia loss of vision without any apparent disease of the eye.

amblyopia ex anopsia loss of vision from disuse of the eye, usually a result of uncorrected refractive errors.

ametropia a refractive error in which the eye, when in a state of rest, does not focus the image of an object on the retina; includes hyperopia, myopia, and astigmatism. *See* refractive error.

Amsler's grid a chart with horizontal and vertical lines for testing macular distortion.

angiography outlining of the lumen of the blood vessel by injection of material that can be visualized by x-ray film or the eye.

angioma a tumor consisting of blood vessels.

angle kappa the difference between the direction of gaze and the apparent direction in which the eye points; this normal structural feature may cause a false interpretation of strabismus.

aniridia congenital absence of the iris.

aniseikonia a condition in which the ocular image of an object as seen by one eye differs so much in size or shape from that seen by the other eye that the two images cannot be fused into a single impression.

anisocoria inequality of the pupils in diameter.

ankyloblepharon adhesion of upper and lower eyelids.

annulus ring-shaped structure.

anomaly departure from the normal.

anophthalmia absence of a true eyeball.

anterior chamber space in the front of the eye, bounded in front by the cornea and behind by the iris; filled with aqueous humor.

anterior chamber angle angle between the iris and the cornea that contains the trabecula and through which the aqueous flows out of the eye.

anterior segment referring to the front part of the eye.

antibody a specific substance produced by the body in the presence of an antigen.

antigen any substance that when introduced in the body incites formation of an antibody.

antihistamine substance that acts against the action of histamine.

aphakia absence of the lens of the eye.

aphasia loss of power of expression either by speech or by writing.

applanation flattening of the cornea in measurement of the intraocular pressure.

aqueous humor clear, watery fluid that fills the anterior and posterior chambers within the front part of the eye.

arcuate scotoma characteristically arc-shaped area of blindness in the field of vision; caused by interruption of a nerve fiber bundle in the retina; most often seen in glaucoma.

arcus senilia grayish white ring in the periphery of the cornea.

Argyll Robertson pupil a pupil characterized by non-reaction to direct and consensual light but normal contraction for accommodation and convergence.

argyrosis gray discoloration of the skin and conjunctiva due to deposition of silver salts; occurs with either systemic intake of a silver compound or topical application.

arteriography visualization of blood vessels by injection of material that can be seen by x-ray film or naked eyes.

arteriosclerosis thickening and loss of contractibility of an artery, usually associated with old age.

artifact that which is altered.

asepsis absence of microorganisms.

asteroid resembling a star.

asteroid hyalitis round or disc-like bodies (calcium soaps) in the vitreous; they do not impair vision.

asthenopia eye fatigue caused by tiring of the internal and/or external muscles.

astigmatism a refractive error that prevents the light rays from coming to a single focus on the retina because of different degrees of refraction in the various meridians of the eye.

astigmatism, "against-the-rule" condition in which the steepest corneal meridian is in the horizontal (180-degree) plane.

astigmatism, irregular astigmatism caused by an irregularly shaped cornea (due to a condition such as scarring or keratoconus). Irregular astigmatism is not correctable by cylinders.

astigmatism, oblique regular astigmatism in which the principal meridians are other than 90 and 180 degrees.

astigmatism, regular astigmatism that is correctable by cylinders (there are two retinal focal points in regular astigmatism).

astigmatism, residual astigmatism remaining after the corneal astigmatism has been neutralized. Generally, residual astigmatism is *lenticular,* resulting from the eye's crystalline lens having a toric surface.

astigmatism, "with-the-rule" condition in which the steepest corneal meridian is in the vertical (90-degree) plane.

atrophy wasting or decrease of a tissue due to faulty nutrition or loss of nerve supply.

atropine an alkaloid that produces mydriasis and cycloplegia.

attenuation narrowing of a vessel.

B-scan an ultrasonic technique to provide a two-dimensional cross-section of the eye and orbital tissue.

bacteriocide a chemical that disinfects and kills pathogenic organisms.

ballasted lens a contact lens that has a cross-sectional shape with a heavier base so that it orients inferiorly when the lens is worn.

bandage lens a contact lens that is used over the cornea to protect the cornea from external influences and permit healing of underlying pathology.

bar reader an appliance that provides for the placement of an opaque septum, or bar, between the printed page and the reader's eyes so as to occlude different areas of the page for each of the eyes. Used for diagnosis and training of simultaneous binocular vision.

Barr body sex-linked inactive X chromosome.

base curve the curvature of the central part of the posterior surface of a lens. Base curve is expressed in millimeters of radius of curvature or in diopters. Also referred to as *central posterior curve*.

bear tracks of the retina congenital pigmentation deposits on the retina.

bedewing cornea an edematous condition of the epithelium of the cornea characterized by irregular reflection from a multitude of droplets when the cornea is viewed with the slit lamp.

belladonna the plant *Atropa belladonna*, from the leaves and roots of which may be obtained the poisonous alkaloid precursors of various medically useful narcotics, chief among which is atropine.

benign tumor nonmalignant growth.

biconcave lens lens having a concave surface on both faces.

biconvex lens lens having a convex surface on both faces.

bifocal lens a lens with two areas for viewing, each with its own focal power.

binocular vision ability to use the two eyes simultaneously to focus on the same object and to fuse the two images into a single image that gives a correct interpretation of its solidity and its position in space.

biomicroscopy microscopic examination of the cornea, anterior chamber lens, and posterior chamber contents with a slit-lamp microscope. The magnification is approximately ×10 to ×50.

Bjerrum's scotoma a half ring-like visual field defect arising from the disc and extending around fixation.

Bjerrum's screen a tangent screen.

blennorrhea a mucoid discharge from various parts of the body, including the external eye, caused by an inflammatory process.

blepharitis inflammation of the margins of the eyelids.

blepharochalasis excessive relaxation of eyelid skin due to loss of elasticity.

blepharoclonus exaggerated form of reflex blinking.

blepharoconjunctivitis inflammation of the eyelid and conjunctiva.

blepharophimosis a condition in which the palpebral aperture is abnormally small.

blepharoplasty plastic surgery of the eyelid.

blepharoptosis drooping of the upper eyelid.

blepharospasm excessive winking; tonic or clonic spasm of the orbicularis oculi muscle.

blind spot the natural blind area of the retina where the optic nerve enters the eye.

blindness in the United States, usually defined as central visual acuity of 20/200 or less in the better eye after correction, or visual acuity of more than 20/200 if there is a field defect, in which the widest diameter of the visual field subtends an angle distance no greater than 20 degrees (some states include up to 30 degrees).

blue sclera thin altered sclera.

Bowman's membrane a layer of condensed stromal tissue that separates the epithelium from the stroma proper.

break-up time (BUT) tear film break-up time: the time it takes for dry spots to form on the cornea when the eye is kept in the staring position. Normal range is 10 to 30 seconds; less than 10 seconds indicates a pathologic condition.

bulbar pertaining to the globe.

buphthalmos enlargement of the eyeball, resulting usually from congenital (infantile) glaucoma.

C, CC (sum correction) with correction; that is, wearing prescribed lenses.

canal of Schlemm *see* Schlemm's canal.

canaliculus passageway for drainage of tears from eyes to tear sac.

candle unit of luminous intensity in the photometric system.

canthotomy surgical procedure for lengthening the opening between the eyelids.

canthus the angle at either end of the slit between the eyelids; specified as outer, or temporal, and inner, or nasal.

caruncle, lacrimal a pink fleshy or relatively isolated skin located in the medial canthus area adjacent to the plica semilunaris.

cataract a condition in which the crystalline lens of the eye or its capsule, or both, becomes opaque, with consequent loss of visual acuity.

central visual acuity ability of the eye to perceive in the direct line of vision.

chalazion inflammatory enlargement of a meibomian gland of the eyelid.

chamber, anterior *see* anterior chamber.

chemosis severe edema of the conjunctiva.

chiasm, optic *see* optic chiasm.

chorioretinitis inflammation of the choroid and retina.

choroid vascular, intermediate coat that furnishes nourishment to the other parts of the eyeball.

choroiditis inflammation of the choroids.

cilia (plural), cilium (singular) eyelashes.

ciliary body portion of the vascular coat between the iris and the choroid; consists of ciliary processes and the ciliary muscle.

ciliary processes finger-like projections from the ciliary body that produce aqueous humor and provide attachment for the zonules.

Coats' disease a chronic exudative retinopathy, occurring between the retina and the choroid.

coloboma congenital cleft due to the failure of the eye to complete growth in the part affected.

color deficiency diminished ability to perceive differences in color; usually reds and greens, rarely blues and yellows.

colorimeter a color-matching device used to designate an unknown colored stimulus by matching it with a known colored stimulus.

colors, complementary two colors that when mixed produce a neutral color when mixed in correct proportions.

colors, primary set of colors (red, yellow, blue) from which all other color sensations can be produced.

commotio retinae an edematous condition of the retina caused by trauma to an eye.

computerized corneal topography a computer-assisted diagnostic technique that creates a three-dimensional color-coded map of the surface curvature of the cornea as well as a cross-sectional corneal profile. The information gained is used in fitting contact lenses, recognizing irregular corneal conditions that are difficult to detect with most conventional testing, and planning laser vision correction.

concave lens a lens having the power to diverge rays of light; also known as *diverging, reducing, negative, myopic,* or *minus lens,* denoted by the − sign.

cones and rods two kinds of cells that form a layer of the retina and act as light-receiving media. Cones are concerned with visual acuity and color discrimination, rods are used for motion and vision at low degrees of illumination (night vision).

conformer a device placed in the socket after enucleation or evisceration of an eyeball to preserve the shape of the fornices.

conjunctiva mucous membrane that lines the eyelids and covers the front part of the eyeball.

conjunctivitis inflammation of the mucous membrane lining of the eyelid and/or eyeball.

conjunctivitis, giant papillary *see* giant papillary conjunctivitis.

consensual contraction of one pupil when light is directed into the fellow eye.

consensual light reflex constriction of the opposite pupil when a beam of light is directed into the pupil of an eye.

contact lens refers to any lens that is placed on the surface of the cornea and sclera, either for *optical* purposes (improvement of visual acuity) or for *therapeutic* purposes (treatment of eye disorders).

conventional replacement contact lens a contact lens that does not have a specific replacement schedule. Conventional replacement lenses are sometimes referred to as "traditional," "durable," or "reusable" replacement lenses.

convergence process of directing the visual axes of the two eyes to a near point, with the result that the pupils of the two eyes are closer together.

convex lens a lens having the power to converge rays of light and to bring them to a focus; also known as *converging, magnifying, hyperopic,* or *plus lens,* denoted by the + sign.

cornea clear, transparent portion of the outer coat of the eyeball, forming the covering of the aqueous chamber.

corneal collagen crosslinking a treatment for keratoconus and corneal ectasia after previous refractive surgery that uses the photosensitizer riboflavin (vitamin B_2) which when exposed to longer-wavelength ultraviolet light (370 nm UVA [ultraviolet A radiation]) induces chemical reactions in corneal stroma that result in the formation of covalent bonds between the corneal collagen molecules, fibers, and microfibrils.

corneal endothelium the innermost layer of the cornea, consisting of a single layer of cells.

corneal epithelium the outermost layer of the cornea.

corneal graft operation to restore vision by replacing a section of opaque cornea.

corneal stroma multiple sheets of collagen in the center of the cornea, which make up 90% of its thickness.

cross cylinder a lens used to measure the power and axis of an astigmatic refractive error. The cross cylinder consists of a plus and a minus cylinder set at right angles to each other with the handle set midway between the two cylinders.

crystalline lens a transparent colorless body suspended in the front part of the eyeball, between the aqueous and the vitreous, the function of which is to bring the rays of light to focus on the retina.

cup-to-disc ratio (C/D) a disc that has become cupped, usually with glaucoma, with 0.9 being the most severe.

custom ablation wavefront-guided laser treatment used to treat high-order visual aberrations allowing customized refractive surgical procedures for an individual's unique visual requirements.

cyclitis inflammation of the ciliary body.

cyclodialysis an operation to reduce the intraocular pressure by forming a pathway for fluid to drain from the anterior chamber to the space between the choroid and sclera.

cycloplegic a drug that temporarily puts the ciliary muscle at rest and dilates the pupil; often used to ascertain the error of refraction.

cylindric lens a segment of a cylinder, the refractive power of which varies in different medians, used in the correction of astigmatism.

cyst a sac containing fluid.

cystinosis disease in which ocular manifestations occur as dispersed crystals causing refractile opacities in the cornea and conjunctiva.

dacryocystectomy operation to remove the tear duct sac.

dacryocystitis   inflammation of the lacrimal sac.

dacryocystogram   an x-ray photograph of the lacrimal apparatus of the eye, made visible by radiopaque dyes.

dacryocystorhinostomy   an operation to create a new tear duct for drainage of tears directly into the nose.

daily disposable contact lens   a disposable contact lens designed for a single 1-day use. A new lens is inserted each morning and discarded before sleep the same day. The lens is not cleaned or reused, nor does the wearer sleep with the lens in place.

daily wear   contact lens wear in which the lenses are inserted each morning and removed each night before sleep.

dark adaptation   ability of the retina and pupil to adjust to a dim light.

decompression, orbital   surgical relief of pressure behind the eyeball, as in endocrine exophthalmos, by the removal of bone from the orbit.

degeneration   deterioration of an organ or a tissue, resulting in diminished vitality, either by chemical change or by infiltration of abnormal matter. In the eye, cystic degeneration of the macula is a localized macular degeneration, resulting in edema and the formation of cystic spaces in the central area of the retina, which lead to macular depression or to a complete macular hole.

dendritic keratitis   fern-like projection on the cornea from herpes simplex.

depth perception   ability to perceive the solidity of objects and their relative position in space; also called *stereoscopic vision.*

dermatoconjunctivitis   inflammation of the skin and the palpebral conjunctiva near the eyelid margin.

dermoid   congenital tumor seen as a raised yellowish lesion.

Descemet's membrane   corneal layer separating the stroma from the endothelium.

detached retina   complete or partial separation of retina from choroid.

dial, astigmatic   a chart or pattern used for determining the presence and amount of astigmatism.

distichiasis   lashes growing from openings of meibomian glands.

diopter   unit of measurement of strength or refractive power of a lens.

diplopia   seeing of one object as two.

direct light reflex   contraction of the pupil in the presence of a beam of light with the eye gazing at a distant object. The room illumination should be dim.

disinfection   physical or chemical procedures that kill common pathogenic organisms but may permit some nonpathogenic organisms to survive.

disposable contact lens   a hydrogel contact lens designed to be discarded on removal from the eye.

distometer   a caliper used to measure vertex distance, which is the distance from the cornea of the patient's eye to the back surface of the lens inserted in the trial frame, phoropter, or glass.

distortion   aberration of rays of light.

DK   a measure of the *oxygen permeability* of a given contact lens material. D is the diffusion coefficient for oxygen movement in the material and K is the solubility constant of oxygen in the material.

DK/L   the DK value of a lens material divided by the central thickness (L) of a specific lens of that material. DK/L is known as the *oxygen transmissibility* of the lens.

-duction   a stem word used with a prefix to describe the turning or rotation of the eyeball (abduction, turning out; adduction, turning in; deorsumduction, turning down; sursumduction, turning up).

dyslexia   difficulty in reading, either in recognition of letters or interpretation, in spite of good vision in each eye.

dystrophy   abnormal or defective development; degeneration.

Early Treatment Diabetic Retinopathy Study (ETDRS) acuity testing chart   a special chart that incorporates specific design criteria to make it more accurate than the Snellen or Sloan acuity test charts. The designs include same number of letters (five) per row, equal spacing of the rows on a log scale, equal spacing of the letters on a log scale, and individual rows balanced for letter difficulty.

ecchymosis   discoloration of skin due to extravasation of blood into tissues after injury.

ectropion   an eversion, or turning outward, of the eyelid.

electronic health records (EHRs)   health care records that provide the ability for electronic exchange of patient data from practice setting to practice setting.

electronic medical records (EMRs)   a system of computerized information, similar to a paper-based chart, that contains a wide range of patient data including patient demographics, medical history, medications, allergies, immunizations, vital signs, physical examination findings, laboratory tests, radiologic images, photos, prescriptions, and billing and insurance information.

electroretinogram   a recording of the cornea–retinal potential.

emmetropia   refractive condition of the normal eye; when the eye is at rest, the image of distant objects is brought to a focus on the retina.

endophthalmitis   inflammation of most of the internal tissues of the eyeball.

enophthalmos   backward displacement of the globe.

entropion   turning inward of the eyelid.

enucleation   complete surgical removal of the eyeball.

eosinophil   a form of white blood cells containing cytoplasmic granules that are stained by the dye eosin. They are present in increased numbers with allergic reactions and some parasitic conditions and decrease with steroid therapy.

epiphora   excessive tearing causing an overflow onto the face.

episclera a loose structure of fibrous and elastic tissue on the outer surface of the sclera. It contains a large number of blood vessels, in contrast to the sclera, which contains none.

episcleritis inflammation in the tissues overlying the sclera.

equivalent oxygen performance (EOP) an in vivo measurement of how much total oxygen passes through a contact lens and reaches the cornea. The measurement takes into account not only the lens material but also the thickness and design of the lens.

erysipelas acute infection of the skin and subcutaneous tissues.

esodeviation the deviation inward of the line of sight of the nonfixing eye from the point of fixation of the fixating eye.

esophoria tendency of the eye to turn inward.

esotropia manifest turning inward of the eye (convergent strabismus, or crossed eye).

evisceration surgical removal of the contents of the globe.

excentric fixation a monocular condition in which a parafoveal point is used for fixation. Usually the vision is very poor and the projection of that eye to a target is erroneous.

excimer a form of laser for ablation of the cornea. The word is a contraction of "excited" and "dimer."

exenteration surgical removal of the orbital region.

exodeviation the deviation outward of the line of sight of the nonfixing eye from the point of fixation of the fixating eye.

exophoria tendency of the eye to turn outward.

exophthalmos abnormal protrusion of the eyeball.

exotropia abnormal turning outward from the nose of one or both eyes (divergent strabismus).

extended wear contact lens wear in which the lenses may be worn continuously, day and night, without removal for up to 7 days.

extraocular muscles the six muscles that cause movement of the eye: medial and lateral recti, superior and inferior recti, and superior and inferior oblique.

extrinsic muscles external muscles of the eye that move the eyeball. Each eye has four recti and two oblique muscles.

eye grounds *see* fundus.

Farnsworth-Munsell 100-hue test a color-hue matching test to diagnose types and degrees of color blindness.

far-sightedness *see* hyperopia.

field of vision entire area that can be seen without shifting the eye.

fingerprint corneal dystrophy fine wavy lines resembling a fingerprint that appear on an otherwise normal cornea.

fissure elliptic space between the eyelids.

flare, aqueous Tyndall effect, or the scattering of light in a beam directed into the anterior chamber, occurring as a result of increased protein content of the aqueous humor; a sign of severe inflammation of the iris and/or ciliary body.

flat cornea a cornea with a K value less than 41.00 diopters.

floaters small particles consisting of cells, pigment, or fibrin that move in the vitreous.

fluorescein an organic compound that is inert and used to stain the tear film for primarily rigid contact lens fitting and to assess the integrity of the cornea. It glows in the presence of ultraviolet light or cobalt blue light. It stains areas of epithelial damage yellowish green.

fluorescein angiography a procedure in which fluorescein dye is injected so that retinal choroidal circulation and iris circulation can be examined and photographed.

focal length the distance between the plane of a lens and the focal point of an object from infinity. The dioptric power is the reciprocal of this measurement in meters. All optical testing instruments and prescriptions use back focal lengths or back dioptric powers.

focal point the point at which distant light comes to a focus after being reflected or refracted.

focus point to which rays converge after passing through a lens.

fornix a loose fold of the conjunctiva, occurring where that part of the conjunctiva covering the eyeball meets the conjunctiva lining the eyelid.

fovea small depression in the retina at back of eye; the part of the macula adapted for most acute vision.

frequent replacement contact lens (also referred to as programmed or planned replacement contact lens) a hydrogel lens designed to be discarded and replaced at predetermined, regular intervals. The replacement cycle is usually 2 weeks, 1 month, or 3 months and cannot exceed 6 months.

Fuchs' dystrophy edema in the stroma associated with scarring on both the endothelium and the epithelium.

fundus inside of the eye, primarily the retina, the optic disc, and the retinal vessels that can be seen with an ophthalmoscope.

fusion power of coordination by which the images received by the two eyes become a single image.

gas-permeable lenses lenses that permit the passage of oxygen and carbon dioxide through the material.

ghost vessels empty vessels remaining after corneal invasion by blood vessels.

giant papillary conjunctivitis (GPC) also called giant papillary hypertrophy (GPH), a condition associated with contact lens wear, especially soft lens wear, marked by increasing lens awareness, itching, mucous discharge, formation of a coating on the contact lens, and papillae. The papillae form on the tarsal conjunctiva of the upper lid.

glare irregularly scattered light that interferes with the focused retinal picture and reduces visual acuity.

glaucoma   an ocular disease having as its primary characteristic a sustained increase in intraocular pressure that the eye cannot withstand without damage to its structure or impairment of its function. This increased pressure can manifest in a variety of symptoms and signs, such as excavation of the optic disc, hardness of the eyeball, reduced visual acuity, seeing of colored halos around lights, visual field defects, and headaches. *Absolute glaucoma* is a final and hopeless stage of glaucoma in which the eye loses total light perception. *Acute glaucoma* is a sudden and painful type of glaucoma caused by a rapid rise in intraocular pressure. It is referred to as *angle-closure glaucoma. Congenital glaucoma* is caused by developmental anomalies in the region of the angle of the anterior chamber that present an obstruction to the drainage mechanism of the intraocular fluids. In *open-angle glaucoma*, the most common form, the angle of the anterior chamber is open. It usually is hereditary, is often symptomless, and produces slow erosion of the visual field.

glioma   malignant tumor of the retina or optic nerve.

goniolens   a contact lens designed to view the filtration angle of the anterior chamber.

gonioscope   a magnifying device used in combination with strong illumination and a contact lens for examining the angle of the anterior chamber of the eye.

Gram staining   the method of identifying bacteria and other microbes according to their reaction to a dye, i.e., gram-positive or gram-negative.

granuloma   a benign nodule that occurs as a result of a localized inflammation.

Gunn's syndrome   congenital ptosis associated with jaw winking.

guttata   small whitish island deposits on Descemet's membrane that appear drop shaped.

hard lenses   term sometimes used to refer to rigid lenses including polymethyl methacrylate (PMMA) and rigid gas permeable (RGP).

Hassali-Henie bodies   drop-like particles of hyaline material seen in the periphery of Descemet's membrane.

hemangioma   tumor arising from endothelial cells most frequently seen in the choroid.

hematoma   swelling of the tissues due to a large hemorrhage.

hemianopia   blindness in one half of the visual field of one or both eyes. *Altitudinal hemianopia* is blindness of either the upper or the lower half of the visual field. *Bitemporal hemianopia* involves the temporal halves of the visual fields of both eyes. *Homonymous hemianopia* involves one-half of the visual field on the same side (right or left, nasal or temporal) in both eyes.

herpes simplex   inflammatory condition of the conjunctiva, cornea, and iris caused by herpes simplex virus.

herpes zoster ophthalmicus   inflammatory condition of the fifth cranial nerve, affecting the eyelid skin and eye structures.

herpetic keratitis   recurring episodes of corneal epithelial inflammation caused by the herpes simplex virus.

heterochromia of iris   a difference of color between the two irides.

heterophoria   constant tendency of the eye to deviate from the normal position for binocular fixation, counterbalanced by simultaneous fixation prompted by the desire for singular binocular vision. Deviation is not usually apparent.

heterotropia   an obvious or manifest deviation of visual axis of an eye out of alignment with the other eye. Synonyms are *crosseye* and *strabismus*.

high-order aberrations   physical visual defects of multiple varieties such as coma, trefoil, spherical aberrations, corneal scarring, and cataracts.

hippus   marked variation in the size of the pupil. Could be spasmodic, rhythmic dilation, and constriction of the pupil (independent of illumination, fixation, or psychic stimuli).

HIV (human immunodeficiency virus)   a virus causing a deficiency of the immune system, making the individual susceptible to a variety of infections.

homonymous   *see* hemianopia.

hordeolum   *see* stye.

hyalitis (asteroid)   calcium-containing opacities in the vitreous.

hydrogel lens   a soft lens that has an affinity to absorb and bind water into its molecular structure.

hydrophilic   refers to the property of a material that has an affinity for water.

hyperopia (hypermetropia)   a refractive error in which, because the eyeball is short or the refractive power of the lens is weak, the point of focus for rays of light from distant objects falls behind the retina; thus accommodation to increase the refractive power of the lens is necessary for distance vision as well as near vision.

hyperphoria   tendency of one eye to deviate upward, controllable by fixational efforts.

hypertropia   deviation upward of one eye; not controllable by fixational efforts.

hyphema   hemorrhage in the anterior chamber of the eye.

hypopyon   cells pooled in the lower part of anterior chamber of the eye.

incipient   pertaining to early changes.

injection   a term sometimes used to mean congestion of ciliary or conjunctival blood vessels; redness of the eye.

interpupillary distance   (or pupillary distance [PD]) is the distance in millimeters between the centers of the two pupils of both eyes.

interstitial keratitis   inflammation of the middle layer of the cornea; found chiefly in children and young adults, and usually caused by transmission of syphilis from the mother to the unborn child.

intracorneal ring   a ring of tissue inserted into the peripheral cornea to reduce myopic refractive errors.

intraocular pressure the pressure of the fluid within the eye measured in millimeters of mercury.

IOL intraocular lens.

iridectomy operation to remove iris tissue. In peripheral iridectomy, tissue is removed from the base of the iris; in full iridectomy, tissue is removed from the base to the pupillary margin.

iridocyclitis inflammation of the iris and ciliary body.

iris colored circular membrane suspended behind the cornea and immediately in front of the lens. The iris regulates the amount of light entering the eye by changing the size of the pupil.

iris bombé bulging forward of the midpart of the iris, thus severely narrowing the angle of the anterior chamber.

iritis inflammation of the iris; the condition is marked by pain, inflammation, discomfort from light, contraction of the pupil, and disorientation of the iris. It may be caused by injury, syphilis, rheumatism, gonorrhea, tuberculosis, or other systemic disease.

ischemia localized anemia of the retina caused by arterial constriction and subsequent visual grayout or blackout.

Ishihara's test a test for detecting defects in recognizing colors, based on the tracing of numbers or patterns in a series of multicolored charts or plates.

isopter a line connecting points that are of equal sensitivity to light.

jack-in-the-box phenomenon objects that appear to jump to view from the peripheral visual field when one wears strong plus lenses; occurs after cataract surgery.

Jackson cross cylinder a single lens composed of a plus cylinder and a minus cylinder of equal power located perpendicular to each other; used to refine the cylinder, axis, and power during refraction.

Jaeger's test types a test for near vision, in which lines of reading matter are printed in a series of type sizes.

K the keratometer reading of the corneal meridians.

Kayser-Fleischer ring pigmented ring encircling the cornea.

keratectomy removal of a portion of the cornea.

keratitis inflammation of the cornea; frequently classified as to type of inflammation and layer of cornea affected; for example, interstitial keratitis and phlyctenular keratitis.

keratitis sicca dryness of the cornea.

keratoconus (conical cornea) cone-shaped deformity of the cornea.

keratometer (ophthalmometer) an instrument that measures the central 3.3 mm of the anterior curvature of the cornea in its two meridians. The readings are called K readings. The measurement is in diopters, with the average cornea having a power of 42.00 to 48.00 diopters.

keratomileusis refractive surgery in which a portion of the cornea is removed, reshaped, and replaced.

keratopathy a noninflammatory disease of the cornea.

keratoplasty corneal transplant operation.

Kestenbaum rule a formula used to estimate the power of low-vision aid that is needed.

Krimsky method an assessment of eye deviation with the use of prisms to equalize the position of the corneal light reflex in each eye.

lacrimal apparatus the tear-producing and tear-disposal system of the eye.

lacrimal gland a gland that secretes tears; it lies in the upper outer angle of the orbit.

lacrimal sac the dilated upper end of the lacrimal duct.

lacrimation production of tears.

lagophthalmos a condition in which the lids cannot completely close.

lamellar keratoplasty operation in which only the diseased outer layers of the cornea are removed and the healthy donor cornea is sutured as a replacement.

laser an instrument that transforms an intense beam of light into energy that affects tissue; acronym for *l*ight *a*mplification by *s*timulated *e*mission of *r*adiation.

laser trabeculoplasty a treatment by laser light that shrinks the trabecular meshwork; used for the relief of glaucoma.

LASIK acronym for laser assisted in situ keratomileusis. A procedure for correcting refractive errors that consists of creating a flap in the cornea utilizing a microkeratome and then utilizing an excimer laser to reshape the underling corneal tissue.

lens a piece of glass or other transparent substance shaped so that rays of light converge or scatter. Also the transparent biconvex body of the eye. An *aphakic lens* is a convex spectacle lens of high dioptric power, so named because its principal use is in the correction of vision in aphakia. In a *biconvex lens*, both surfaces are convex. It is used for the treatment of hyperopia ("far-sightedness"). In a *biconcave lens* both surfaces are concave. It is used in myopia ("near-sightedness"). A *bifocal lens* is constructed of two separate lenses, each having a different power. The upper portion is used for distance vision and the lower portion for near vision. A *cross cylinder* is a compound lens in which the dioptric powers in the principal meridians are equal but opposite in sign; it is usually mounted with the handle midway between the principal meridians. It is used to determine the axis and power needed for correcting astigmatism. A *luxated lens* is a crystalline lens of the eye that is completely displaced from the pupillary aperture. A *subluxated lens* is a crystalline lens of the eye that is partially displaced but remains in the pupillary aperture.

lensectomy a procedure to remove the clear crystalline lens to reduce high myopic errors.

leukokoria any pathologic condition, such as retrolental fibroplasia, that produces a white reflex in the pupillary area.

leukoma a very dense opacity of the cornea.

light adaptation   power of the eye to adjust itself to variations in the amount of light.

light perception (lp)   ability to distinguish light from dark.

light projection   ability to determine the quadrantal direction of light.

limbus   boundary between the cornea and the sclera.

low-order aberrations   physical visual defects that consist of myopia, hyperopia, and astigmatism.

lupus erythematosus   organic disease of collagen origin.

macrophthalmia   abnormally large eyeball, resulting chiefly from infantile glaucoma.

macula lutea retinae   small area of the retina that surrounds the fovea and that with the fovea comprises the area of the retina that gives distinct vision. Also referred to as the *yellow spot.*

magnification   increase in size achieved by a lens system; the ratio of image size to object size.

malingering   decreased vision to avoid something unpleasant.

Marfan's syndrome   disease of connective tissue, with eye involvement consisting of luxated lens and tremulous iris.

megalocornea   an abnormally large cornea.

megophthalmos   *see* buphthalmos.

meibomian glands   sebaceous glands of the eyelid.

meibomianitis   inflammation of the meibomian glands.

melanoma   pigmented tumor of the eye.

melanosis   a condition characterized by abnormal deposits of melanin or pigment.

microcornea   small cornea of 10 mm or less.

microphthalmia   an abnormally small eyeball.

microscopic glasses   magnifying lenses arranged on the principle of a microscope; occasionally prescribed for people with very poor vision.

miotic   a drug that causes the pupil to contract.

mires   the targets of the ophthalmometer that are reflected back from the cornea.

mirror writing   inverting words while writing and a slowing of reading speed.

Mittendorf's dot   a remnant of an embryonic hyaloid artery seen as a small dense floating opacity behind the posterior lens capsule.

monocular   pertaining to or affecting one eye.

mucocele   a pathologic swelling of a cavity due to an accumulation of the mucoid material.

muscae volitantes   small floating spots entopically observed on viewing a bright uniform field; due to minute embryonic remnants in the vitreous humor.

mydriasis   enlargement of the pupil by the iris dilator muscle as occurs in darkness or in response to dilating drops.

mydriatic agent   a drug that dilates the pupil.

myokymia   twitching of individual muscle bundles of the eyelid.

myopia (near-sightedness)   a refractive error in which the eyeball is too long in relation to its focusing power; thus the point of focus for rays of light from distant objects (parallel light rays) is in front of the retina.

myopic conus   myopic crescent.

myotomy   surgical division of muscle fibers.

nasal step   depression of the nasal peripheral portion of the field. A sign of glaucoma.

near point of accommodation   nearest point at which the eye can perceive an object distinctly. It varies according to the power of accommodation.

near point of convergence   nearest single point at which the two eyes can direct their visual lines.

near vision   the ability to perceive objects distinctly at normal reading distance or about 14 inches (35 cm) from the eyes.

nebula   a faint or slightly misty corneal opacity.

needling   surgical operation for opening a membrane following cataract surgery or in congenital cataracts in which the cataract or anterior capsule is pierced by a needle-like knife.

neovascularization   recent formation of new blood vessels in a part, such as the cornea or retina.

neuritis   inflammation of a nerve or nerves.

neuroblastoma   a malignant tumor of the nervous system, one type of which is the retinoblastoma or tumor of the retina.

neuroophthalmology   branch of ophthalmology that deals with the part of the nervous system associated with the eye.

neutralization   the combining of two lenses of opposite powers to produce a resultant power of zero (one lens neutralizes the other).

night blindness   a condition in which the sight is good by day but deficient at night or in faint light; seen in retinitis pigmentosa.

nystagmus   an involuntary oscillating, rapid movement of the eyeball; it may be lateral, vertical, rotary, or mixed.

occluder   an opaque or translucent device placed before an eye to obscure or block vision.

oculus dexter (od)   right eye.

oculus sinister (os)   left eye.

oculus uterque (ou)   each eye.

ophthalmia   inflammation of the eye or of the conjunctiva.

ophthalmia neonatorum   an acute, purulent conjunctivitis of the newborn (sometimes defined as an inflamed or discharging eye in a newborn baby less than 2 weeks of age).

ophthalmic medical technician   the separate occupational classification established by the U.S. Bureau of Labor's Standard Occupational Classification Committee in 2010 to encompass all three levels of the Joint Commission on Allied Health Personnel in Ophthalmology (JCAHPO) certification, Certified Ophthalmic

Assistants (COA), Certified Ophthalmic Technician (COT), and Certified Ophthalmic Medical Technologist (COMT) and to differentiate the ophthalmic medical assisting profession from "medical assisting."

ophthalmodynamometry measurement of the blood pressure in the retinal vessels of the eye.

ophthalmoplegia paralysis of one or more ocular muscles.

ophthalmoscope an instrument used in examining the interior of the eye.

optic atrophy degeneration of the nerve tissue that carries impulses from the retina to the brain.

optic chiasm crossing of the fibers of the optic nerves on the lower surface of the brain.

optic disc head of the optic nerve in the eyeball.

optic nerve special nerve of the sense of sight that carries impulses from the retina to the brain.

optic neuritis inflammation of the optic nerve.

optical center the point on a lens in which light rays are not bent. It corresponds to the thinnest portion of a minus lens and the thickest portion of a plus lens.

optical coherence tomography (OCT) a noninvasive diagnostic modality that provides high-resolution, cross-sectional imaging of ocular tissue in vivo. It is predominantly used to assess retinal and macular tissue and to study and monitor posterior ocular disease and glaucoma. The technique is similar to ultrasound except that it uses light of wavelength 843 nm rather than sound waves.

optotype a standardized symbol found on vision testing charts. It can consist of specially shaped letters, numbers, or geometric symbols.

ora serrata retinae anterior border of the retina.

orbit the bony cavity containing the eye, which is formed by the frontal, sphenoid, ethmoid, nasal, lacrimal, and maxillary bones.

orthokeratology the technique of flattening the cornea and thus correcting refractive errors by the use of a series of progressively flatter contact lenses.

orthoptic training series of scientifically planned exercises for developing or restoring normal teamwork of the eyes.

overrefraction determination of final lens power by performing a refraction over a contact lens.

pachometer a device used to measure the thickness of the cornea and the depth of the anterior chamber.

palpebral pertaining to the eyelid.

palpebral fissure opening between the eyelids.

pannus invasion of the cornea by infiltration and formation of new blood vessels.

panophthalmitis inflammation of the whole eyeball.

pantoscopic angle the angle of spectacle lenses when rotated on the X-axis to set the lens normal to the fixation axis below the horizon. Commonly measured as the angle between spectacle temple and the plane of the eyewear as angulated back from the perpendicular.

papilledema (papilloedema) edema of the optic nerve head; termed *choked disc* when caused by increased intracranial pressure.

papilloma a benign epithelial new growth.

Parinaud's oculoglandular syndrome a group of clinical findings in which there is a unilateral granulomatous conjunctivitis often associated with an enlarged preauricular or submandibular lymph node.

pars planitis exudative edema on posterior portion of the retina.

partially sighted child for educational purposes, a child who has a visual acuity of 20/70 or less in the better eye after the best possible correction and who cannot use vision as the chief channel of learning.

perimeter an instrument for measuring the field of vision peripherally.

periorbita the loose connective tissue within the orbit.

peripheral vision ability to perceive the presence, motion, or color of objects outside the direct line of vision.

phacoanaphylaxis hypersensitivity to the protein of the crystalline lens.

phacoemulsification emulsification of a cataractous lens by ultrasound, permitting the material to be removed by aspiration.

phakic refers to an eye that still possesses its natural crystalline lens.

phlyctenular keratoconjunctivitis a variety of keratitis characterized by the formation of an inflammatory elevation on the cornea or conjunctiva. It usually occurs in young children and may be caused by poor nutrition, allergy, or tuberculosis.

-phoria a root word denoting a latent deviation in which the eyes have a constant tendency to turn from the normal position for binocular vision; used with a prefix to indicate the direction of such deviation (e.g., hyperphoria, esophoria, exophoria).

phoropter an instrument for determining the refractive state of the eye, phorias, and so on, consisting of a housing containing rotating disc with lenses, occluders, prisms, and pinholes.

photocoagulation procedure in which there is intentional burning by strong light. Vascular disease, tumors, and degenerative areas in the retina or the choroid may be treated by this means.

photophobia abnormal sensitivity to and discomfort from light.

photopic vision pertaining to vision in light-adapted conditions, mainly a cone function.

phthisis bulbi a shrinking of the eyeball.

pinguecula yellowish, triangular thickening of bulbar conjunctiva, nasal or temporal to cornea.

pinhole disc a black disc with one or multiple openings that allow only central rays to pass through. Vision that is improved with a pinhole disc can be aided by spectacle lenses.

pleoptics a method of treating amblyopia ex anopsia by intense stimulation of light of the nonfoveal area to render the foveal area more receptive to fixational stimuli.

polycoria multiple pupils.

posterior chamber space between the back of the iris and the front of the lens; filled with aqueous.

posterior chamber (PC) lens an intraocular lens that is placed in the posterior chamber where a natural crystalline lens previously was located.

posterior pole of eye the center of the posterior curvature of the eyeball.

Prentice's rule formula for calculating prismatic effect induced at any point in the lens; the prism diopters equal the decentration (in centimeters) times the lens power (in diopters).

presbyopia a gradual lessening of the power of accommodation due to a physiologic change that becomes noticeable about the age of 40 years.

Prince's rule a measuring scale used for determining a patient's near point of accommodation.

prism an optical system that deviates the path of light.

proptosis protrusion of the eye.

prosthesis replacement of a human eye by an artificial one.

pseudoisochromatic charts charts with colored dots of various hues and shades indicating numbers, letters, or patterns; used for testing color discrimination.

pseudophakia a condition in which an intraocular lens implant has replaced the crystalline lens.

pterygium a triangular fold of growing membrane that may extend over the cornea from the white of the eye. It occurs most frequently in people exposed to dust or wind.

ptosis (blepharoptosis) a drooping of the upper eyelid.

quadrantanopia blindness or loss of vision in a quarter sector of the visual field of one or both eyes.

recession operation to sever the eye muscle from its original insertion and reattach it more posteriorly on the sclera.

refraction deviation in the course of rays of light in passing from one transparent medium into another of different density; the sum of steps performed in arriving at a decision as to what lens or lenses (if any) will most benefit the patient.

refractive error a defect in the eye that prevents light rays from being brought to a single focus exactly on the retina.

refractive index the refractive power of a substance in comparison with that of air.

refractive media transparent parts of the eye having refractive power; cornea and lens. The aqueous and vitreous are transparent but contribute very little refractive power.

refractometry the measurement of refractive error.

resection operation to remove a portion of a muscle and tendon to shorten it; operation to remove a portion of the sclera to shorten it.

residual astigmatism the astigmatism present after the corneal astigmatism has been nullified by a contact lens. It is the astigmatism created by the crystalline lens of the eye.

retina innermost coat of the eye, formed of sensitive nerve elements and connected with the optic nerve.

retinal detachment a separation of the inner layer of the retina from the outer layer and the choroid.

retinitis inflammation of the retina.

retinitis pigmentosa a hereditary degeneration and atrophy of the retina; usually migration of pigment occurs.

retinoblastoma a malignant tumor of the retina.

retinopexy surgical reattachment of a detached retina.

retinoscope an instrument for determining the refractive state of the eye.

retinoscopy objective method of determining the refractive error of the eye by observing the movements of light reflected from the back of the eye.

retrobulbar behind the eyeball.

retrolental fibroplasia a disease of the retina in the premature infant in which the retina is partially or completely detached and pulled forward against the posterior surface of the lens.

rods and cones *see* cones and rods.

rose bengal a dye used to detect cells that are damaged or unprotected by native mucoproteins.

S, SC (sine correction) without correction; that is, not wearing prescribed lenses.

sac a bag-like structure.

safety glasses impact-resistant spectacles; available with or without visual correction for workshop or street-wear protection; used by adults and children.

Schirmer's test filter paper test for tear flow.

Schlemm's canal circular channel located deep in the limbus. The channel collects aqueous fluid from the anterior chamber to the episcleral veins. A circular canal situated at the junction of the sclera and cornea through which the aqueous is eliminated after it has circulated between the lens and the iris and between the iris and the cornea.

sclera white part of the eye; a tough covering that, with the cornea, forms the external protective coat of the eye.

scleritis inflammation of the sclera.

scotoma an area of reduced or lost vision in the visual field (relative or absolute scotomas).

scotopic vision vision in low light levels that involves rod photoreceptors.

second(s) of arc a second of arc is a tiny angle. A full circle consists of 360 degrees. One degree is divided into 60 minutes of arc. Each minute of arc contains 60 seconds of arc, so a second of arc is an angle that is 1/3600 of a degree. For instance, 20/20 vision in humans is the ability to resolve a spatial pattern separated by a visual angle of 1 minute of arc. A 20/20 letter subtends 5 minutes of arc total.

secretagogue an agent such as a hormone or pharmaceutical that stimulates secretion.

siderosis bulbi deposit of iron pigment in the eyeball.

slit lamp lamp that provides a narrow beam of strong light; often used with a corneal biomicroscope for examination of the front portions of the eye.

Snellen's chart chart used for testing central visual acuity, consisting of lines of letters, numbers or symbols in graded sizes drawn to Snellen's measurements. Each size is labeled with the distance at which it can be read by the normal eye. It is most often used for testing vision at a distance of 20 feet (6 m), but charts may be drawn for testing at reading distance (14 inches [35 cm]) or intermediate distances.

soft lens a contact lens composed either of *hydrogel* material, a watery gel-like material that contains more than 10% water, or of silicone.

spastic entropion turning in of lid margin.

spectacle blur blurred vision that lasts for 15 minutes or longer after a contact lens is removed and spectacles are used.

specular microscopy a noninvasive photographic technique using a reflected-light microscope that allows visualization and analysis of the corneal endothelial cell size, shape, and density.

spherical equivalent the equivalent of spectacle refraction expressed only as a sphere. To obtain it, take half of the cylinder and algebraically add it to the sphere.

spherical lens segment of a sphere, refracting rays of light equally in all meridians.

sterilization the complete death of all forms of bacteria, fungi, and spores.

stereocampimeter instrument used to measure the visual fields and determine central scotomas.

stereoscopic vision *see* depth perception.

staphyloma a bulging, or protrusion, of the cornea or the sclera.

strabismus squint; failure of the two eyes simultaneously to direct their gaze at the same object because of muscle imbalance. It may be convergent, divergent, alternating, or vertical.

stroma corneal layer underlying Bowman's membrane composed of dense strata of collagen fiber laid down in a regular manner. The stroma comprises about 90% of the cornea's thickness.

stye (hordeolum) acute inflammation of a sebaceous gland in the margin of the eyelid.

subluxation of lens incomplete dislocation of the crystalline lens.

symblepharon adhesion of conjunctiva of the eyelid to conjunctiva of the globe.

sympathetic ophthalmia inflammation of one eye due to an inflammation of the other eye, without infection. May follow surgery or trauma.

synechia adhesion, usually of the iris to the cornea or angle structures (anterior) or the lens (posterior).

taco test a test to determine that a soft contact lens is not inside out by grasping the lens near its apex and folding it so the edge will roll in like a taco if it is not everted.

tangent screen a large, usually black curtain 1 or 2 meters in diameter, supported by a framework on which the central field of vision and the blind spot may be outlined; used for measuring the central field of vision.

tarsorrhaphy the stitching together of the upper and lower eyelids partially or completely to provide protection to the cornea.

tarsus framework of connective tissue that gives shape to the eyelid.

tear film break-up time (BUT) an evaluation of tear quality; the tear film will normally break up in 10 to 30 seconds and show dry spots. Any dry spot that appears in less than 10 seconds is pathologic.

tears a composite of secretions from lacrimal glands, accessory glands of Kraus and Wolfring, mucin-secreting goblet cells of the conjunctiva, meibomian-secreting tarsal glands, and oil-secreting glands of Teis.

telescopic glasses magnifying spectacles founded on the principles of a telescope; occasionally prescribed for improving very poor vision that cannot be helped by ordinary glasses.

temporal pallor loss of color (bleaching) of the temporal portion of the optic disc.

Tenon's capsule membranous tissue that envelops the whole eyeball except the cornea.

tension, intraocular pressure or tension of the contents of the eyeball.

thermokeratoplasty a form of heat that is used to shrink the collagen of the cornea and cause corneal steepening and reduction of hyperopic refractive error.

3 and 9 o'clock staining erosion of the cornea at the 3 and 9 o'clock positions; seen commonly in rigid lenses.

tonic pupil pupil that does not move with accommodation or direct light reflex.

tonography determination of the flow of aqueous humor into the eye and from the eye under the continuous pressure exerted by the weight of a tonometer over a 4- or 5-minute period.

tonometer instrument for measuring the pressure of the eye.

toxoplasmosis protozoal disease leading to inflammatory uveitis, strabismus, and nystagmus.

trabecular meshwork the drainage network in the iridocorneal angle through which aqueous humor leaves the eye.

trabeculectomy surgical removal of a portion of the trabeculum for improved outflow of aqueous in glaucoma patients.

trachoma a form of infection of the conjunctiva and cornea caused by a specific virus that, in the chronic form, produces severe scarring of the eyelids and cornea.

transposition the process of changing a spectacle prescription from a plus to a minus cylinder or vice versa without changing its refractive value. A +2.00 +1.00 × 90 lens is equivalent to a +3.00 − 1.00 × 180 lens. The rule is to add the cylinder to the sphere, change the sign of the cylinder and rotate the axis by 90 degrees.

trephining removing of a circular button, or disc, of tissue.

trichiasis inversion of the eyelashes, resulting in impingement on the eyeball and subsequent irritation.

trochlea a ring-like structure of fibrocartilage attached to the frontal bone through which passes the tendon of the superior oblique muscle of the eyeball.

-tropia a root word denoting an obvious deviation from normal of the axis of the eyes (strabismus); used with a prefix to denote the type of strabismus (e.g., heterotropia, esotropia, exotropia).

tunnel vision contraction of the visual field to such an extent that only a small area of central visual acuity remains, thus giving the affected individual the sensation of looking through a tunnel.

ulcer, corneal pathologic loss of substance of the surface of the cornea due to progressive erosion and necrosis of the tissue.

uvea entire vascular coat of the eyeball, consisting of the iris, ciliary body, and choroid.

uveitis inflammation of the vascular coat of the eye.

VA abbreviation for visual acuity.

vaccinia autoinoculation of smallpox vaccine causing corneal or lid lesions.

vascularization increased blood vessels occurring in a cornea.

verruca solid lesion on lid margin.

version referring to a binocular eye movement.

vertex distance distance from the posterior surface of the lens to the anterior surface of the eye (for measuring purposes, the closed lid). Important in aphakic prescriptions, in high myopia and in high hyperopia.

vertigo dizziness, normally caused by disturbance in the inner ear.

vesiculation the formation of vesicles or blisters.

virulence the disease-producing properties of a microorganism.

VISC vitreous infusion suction cutter; used to cut and remove portions of the vitreous.

vision act or faculty of seeing; sight.

visual purple a pigment in the outer layers of the retina, a photochemical substance mediating light into nerve impulses.

visuscope an instrument designed to determine the type of monocular fixation in amblyopia.

vitreous transparent, colorless mass of soft, gelatinous material filling the eyeball behind the lens.

vitreous opacities *see* floaters.

von Graefe's sign a delay in downward movement of the upper eyelid as it follows the eyeball to downward gaze; seen in thyroid disease.

Vossius' ring a ring of iris pigment granules that is deposited on the anterior lens capsule after blunt trauma to the eye.

wavefront aberration the deviation in an optical system from the desired perfect planar wavefront propagation.

wavefront analyzer an instrument used to measure the way light travels through an eye's optical pathway and compares it with the pathway of light traveling through an optically perfect eye.

wavelength a physical property of light apparent in its color. Violet has a short wavelength, red a long wavelength. Different tissues absorb different wavelengths preferentially, making the various lasers useful for specific purposes.

Wirt stereo test a depth perception test. For a child, three lines of animals are shown from which to make a selection. If all three lines are correctly selected, the child has stereopsis of approximately 100 seconds of arc. For adults there are nine frames of raised rings, the first being the most obvious, the last the most difficult. If all are read correctly, stereopsis of 40 seconds of arc is present.

Worth four-dot test a test to detect amblyopia. The patient wears spectacles with a green lens and a red lens and looks at a target of one white, one red, and two green discs. If four discs are seen, there is no suppression of either eye. If three discs are seen, there is suppression; if five discs are seen, fusion is absent.

xanthelasma (xanthoma) small yellowish tumor of the eyelids, usually occurring in older adults or those with a high level of blood cholesterol.

xanthopsia a condition in which objects appear to be tinted yellow.

xerophthalmia drying of the eye surface, with loss of the corneal and conjunctival luster.

xerosis conjunctivae condition of dryness of the conjunctiva due to the failure of its own secretory activity, or lack of tears.

yoke muscles muscles in opposite eyes that act together.

zonules the supporting fibers of the lens attached at their other end to the ciliary body.

Appendices

🖱 Please note that Appendices 7–17 will appear online only.

Appendix 1 Ocular emergencies[a]

I. Ocular complications of systemic disease

Disease	Possible ocular findings
Diabetes mellitus	Background retinopathy: retinal hemorrhages, exudates, and microaneurysms
	Preproliferative retinopathy: cotton-wool spots, intraretinal microvascular abnormalities
	Proliferative retinopathy: neovascularization, preretinal hemorrhage, vitreous hemorrhage, retinal detachment
Graves' disease	Lid retraction, exposure keratopathy, chemosis and injection, restriction of eye movements, proptosis, compressive optic neuropathy
Hypertension	Sclerosis of vessels in long-standing disease; narrowing of vessels, retinal hemorrhages and/or exudates in severe hypertension
Rheumatoid arthritis and other collagen vascular diseases	Dry eye, episcleritis, scleritis, peripheral corneal ulceration and/or melting
Cancer	Metastatic disease to choroid may result in retinal detachment; disease in the orbit can result in proptosis and restriction of eye movements (e.g., breast, lung cancer)
Sarcoidosis	Dry eye, conjunctival granulomas, iritis, retinitis
AIDS	Kaposi's sarcoma, cotton-wool spots of retina, cytomegalovirus retinitis

II. Lifesaving ocular signs

Findings	Clinical significance
White pupil	In an infant, retinoblastoma must be ruled out
Aniridia (iris appears absent)	May be autosomal dominant (⅔ s) or sporadic inheritance; in sporadic cases where the short arm of chromosome II is deleted, there is a 90% risk of developing Wilms' tumor; the risk in other sporadic cases is approximately 20%
Thickened corneal nerves (slit lamp)	Part of the multiple endocrine neoplasia syndrome type IIB; must rule out medullary carcinoma of the thyroid; pheochromocytoma and parathyroid adenomas

---

[a]Reproduced with permission from Stein RM, Stein HA. Ocular emergencies. 5th ed. Montreal: Medicopea; 2010.

II. Lifesaving ocular signs

Findings	Clinical significance
Retinal angioma	May be part of von Hippel-Lindau disease; autosomal dominant inheritance with variable penetrance; must rule out hemangioblastomas of the central nervous system, renal cell carcinoma, and pheochromocytoma
Multiple pigmented patches of fundus	Lesions represent patches of congenital hypertrophy of the retinal pigment epithelium; may be part of Gardner's syndrome, characterized by multiple premalignant intestinal polyps together with benign soft tissue tumors (lipomas, fibromas, sebaceous cysts) and osteomas of the skull and jaw; a complete gastrointestinal investigation is indicated; if a diagnosis of Gardner's syndrome is made, prophylactic colectomy is indicated because of the potential for malignant degeneration of colonic polyps
Third-nerve palsy with a dilated pupil	Must rule out an intracranial aneurysm or neoplastic lesion; CT scan should be performed on an emergency basis
Papilledema	Must rule out an intracranial mass lesion; CT scan should be performed on an emergency basis
Pigmentary degeneration of the retina and motility disturbance	May represent the Kearns-Sayre syndrome; must rule out a cardiac condition defect disturbance with an annual electrocardiogram; may develop an intraventricular conduction defect, bundle block, bifascicular disease, or complete heart block; patient must be prepared for the possible need to implant a pacemaker

III. Ocular complications of systemic medications

Medication	Ocular complications
Amiodarone	Superficial keratopathy
Chlorpromazine (Thorazine)	Anterior subcapsular cataracts
Corticosteroids	Posterior subcapsular cataracts, glaucoma
Digitalis (digoxin)	Blurred vision, disturbed color vision
Ethambutol	Optic neuropathy
Indometacin (indomethacin)	Superficial keratopathy
Isoniazid	Optic neuropathy
Nalidixic acid	Papilledema
Hydroxychloroquine	Superficial keratopathy and bull's-eye maculopathy
Tetracycline	Papilledema
Thioridazine	Pigmentary degeneration of the retina
Vitamin A	Papilledema

IV. Differential diagnosis of the nontraumatic red eye

Feature	Condition		
	Acute conjunctivitis	**Acute iritis**	**Acute glaucoma**
Symptoms	Redness, tearing ± discharge	Redness, pain, photophobia	Redness, severe pain, nausea, vomiting
Appearance	Conjunctival injection	Ciliary injection	Diffuse injection

IV. Differential diagnosis of the nontraumatic red eye

Feature	Condition		
	Acute conjunctivitis	**Acute iritis**	**Acute glaucoma**
Vision	Normal; can be blurred secondary to discharge	Moderate reduction	Marked reduction, halo vision
Cornea	Clear	May see keratic precipitates	Hazy secondary to edema
Pupil	Normal	Small, sluggish to light	Semidilated, nonreactive
Secretions	Tearing to purulent	Tearing	Tearing
Test and comments	Smears may show etiology; bacterial infection=polycytes, bacteria; viral infection=monocytes; allergy=eosinophils	Slit lamp will show cells and flare in the anterior chamber	Elevated intraocular pressure
Treatment	Antibiotic	Steroids, cycloplegics	Pilocarpine, Betagan (levobunolol), Diamox (acetazolamide), mannitol, laser surgery

V. Differential diagnosis of viral, bacterial, and allergic conjunctivitis

Feature	Viral	Bacterial	Allergy
Discharge	Watery	Purulent	Watery
Itching	Minimal	Minimal	Marked
Preauricular lymph node	Common	Absent	Absent
Stain and smear	Monocytes	Bacteria	Eosinophils
	Lymphocytes	Polycytes	

VI. Differential diagnosis of red eye in contact lens wearers

Diagnosis	Findings	Mechanism	Treatment
Corneal abrasion	Epithelial defect; stains with fluorescein	Mechanical, hypoxia	Antibiotic drops (e.g., tobramycin)
Superficial punctate keratitis	Punctate corneal staining	Mechanical, chemical toxicity	Artificial tears (e.g., Refresh [carboxymethylcellulose sodium] ocular lubricant)
Giant papillary conjunctivitis	Papillary reaction of superior tarsal conjunctiva	Immunologic, mechanical	Mast cell stabilizer (e.g., Vistacrom [cromolyn, cromoglicic acid] drops)
Sterile infiltrates	Corneal infiltrate; epithelium usually intact	Immunologic	Antibiotic drops (assume infected)
Infected ulcer	Corneal infiltrate with ulceration; stains with fluorescein	Infection (e.g., *Pseudomonas, Staphylococcus aureus*)	Corneal scraping for Gram stain and culture. Fortified antibiotic drugs

AIDS, Acquired immunodeficiency syndrome; *CT,* computed tomography.

Appendix 2 Following universal precautions[1,2]

The best way to reduce occupational risk of "bloodborne" infection is to follow universal precautions based on the concept that every patient should be treated with the same level of precautionary and preventive measures to ensure the safety of everyone involved, including health care personnel. The following list of universal precautions is extracted from the Occupational Safety and Health Administration (OSHA) regulation "Occupational exposure to bloodborne pathogens." Please refer to this publication for complete instructions and precautionary guidelines. Ophthalmic medical personnel should regularly review all universal precautions presented there, ensure that they understand them completely, and adhere to them at all times.

1. Wash hands before and after patient contact, and immediately if hands become contaminated with blood or other body fluids.
2. Wear gloves whenever there is a possibility of contact with body fluids.
3. Wear masks whenever there is a possibility of contact with body fluids via airborne route.
4. Wear gowns if exposed skin or clothing is likely to be soiled.
5. During resuscitation procedures, ensure that pocket masks or mechanical ventilation devices are readily available for use.
6. Clean spills of blood or blood-containing body fluids with a solution of household bleach (sodium hypochlorite) and water in a 1:100 solution for smooth surfaces and a 1:10 solution for porous surfaces.
7. Health care professionals who have open lesions, dermatitis, or other skin irritations should not participate in direct patient care activities or handle contaminated equipment.
8. Contaminated needles should never be bent, clipped, or recapped. Immediately after use, contaminated sharp objects should be discarded into a puncture-resistant "sharps" container designed for this purpose.
9. Contaminated equipment that is reusable should be cleaned of visible organic material, placed in an impervious container, and returned to central hospital supply or some other designated place for decontamination and reprocessing.

10. Instruments and other reusable equipment used in performing invasive procedures should be disinfected and sterilized as follows:
    - Equipment and devices that enter the patient's vascular system or other normally sterile areas of the body should be sterilized before being used for each patient
    - Equipment and devices that touch intact mucous membranes, but do not penetrate the patient's body surfaces, should be sterilized when possible, or undergo high-level disinfection if they cannot be sterilized before being used for each patient
    - Equipment and devices that do not touch the patient or that only touch intact skin need only be cleaned with a detergent or as indicated by the manufacturer.
11. Body fluids to which universal precautions always apply are as follows: blood, serum/plasma, semen, vaginal secretions, cerebrospinal fluid, vitreous fluid, synovial fluid, pleural fluid, pericardial fluid, peritoneal fluid, amniotic fluid, and wound exudates.
12. Body fluids to which universal precautions apply only when blood is visible in them are as follows: sweat, tears, sputum, saliva, nasal secretions, feces, urine, vomitus, and breast milk.

Optimal infection control in the eye care setting is based on the assumption that all specified human body fluids are potentially infectious. Many transmissible diseases of the external eye, such as adenoviral conjunctivitis, cause redness that immediately indicates infection. Other infectious agents, however, can be present on the ocular surface without causing inflammation. Human immunodeficiency virus (HIV), hepatitis B virus, hepatitis C virus, rabies virus, and the agent of Creutzfeldt-Jakob disease are not immediately obvious without systemic clues or laboratory testing. Every patient must be approached as potentially contagious. Guidelines for routine ophthalmic examinations include the following:

Wash hands between patient examinations. Use disposable gloves if an open sore, blood, or blood-contaminated fluid is present. Using cotton-tipped applicators to manipulate the eyelids can also minimize direct contact.

Avoid unnecessary contact. Eyedropper bottles used in the office should not directly touch the eyelids, eyelashes, or ocular surface of any patient. Individual sterile strips impregnated with dye are preferred where available.

Disinfect all contact instruments after each use. Tonometer tips and pachometer tips should be soaked in diluted bleach or hydrogen peroxide after every use. Trial contact lenses must be disinfected between patients.

Handle sharp devices carefully. Needles must always be discarded into puncture-resistant (sharps) containers.

---

[1]Reprinted with permission, from Newmark E, O'Hara MA, editors. Ophthalmic medical assisting: an independent study course. 5th ed. San Francisco: American Academy of Ophthalmology; 2012.

[2]Reprinted with permission and with modifications form the American Academy of Ophthalmology AAO ONE(R) Network - Universal Precautions, 2013.

Informed consent

Informed consent permits the patient to exercise self-determination. The law imposes a "duty of disclosure" on the part of the physician.

Contents of an informed consent document

- Risks of procedure, including loss of vision
- Benefits of procedure
- Complications
- Alternative treatments
- Explanation of procedure
- Advantages of one procedure over another
- Significant issues (e.g., bilateral vs. sequential)

Duty of disclosure

1. To frankly answer all specific questions about the risk.
2. Without being questioned, to disclose:
   - The nature of the proposed procedure
   - The gravity of it
   - All material risks
   - All special and unusual risks in the particular circumstances
   - Alternative procedures available and their risks, including the consequences of no treatment

Material risks

A risk is material if it would be considered a significant issue by a reasonable person weighing the decision to consent to the procedure. A 1 in 1000 chance is probably not a material risk. A 1 in 100 chance is probably a material risk. Risks of very serious or grave consequence should be disclosed no matter how remote.

Special and unusual risks

The patient's particular circumstances, such as occupational, familial, and social circumstances, make certain risks significant to that patient (e.g., a risk of visual loss should be disclosed to a commercial pilot even if it is remote).

Consent

Consent may be written, oral, or implied from the circumstances (e.g., the patient holds out an arm for an injection).

Regardless of the form of the consent, the physician must be able to prove that the duty of disclosure was met before the consent was obtained. Therefore, a prudent physician will make a note on the chart of the risks disclosed and the patient's comments or questions.

Exceptions

- In an emergency, the duty of disclosure and obtaining consent is waived.
- When the patient plainly does not wish to hear about the risks, the duty of disclosure is waived, but consent should be obtained and circumstances noted on the chart.
- In rare circumstances, if the physician can prove that disclosing the risks would create a state of mind in the patient that would seriously hinder successful treatment, the duty of disclosure is waived but consent should be obtained and the circumstances noted on the chart.

Failure to disclose

When an undisclosed risk occurs and the patient sues and the court determines the risk should have been disclosed because it was material or because of the patient's particular circumstances, the physician will be liable if the court is satisfied that another person in the patient's position would have refused the treatment had the risks been disclosed.

For cosmetic purposes and for treatments for which there is little medical justification or urgency, liability of the physician is more likely if an undisclosed risk materializes. Therefore, it is prudent to outline all of the risks.

Experimental procedures, particularly involving healthy volunteers, warrant utmost disclosure of risks.

The duty of disclosure also embraces what the surgeon knows or should know that the patient deems relevant to the patient's decision whether to undergo the operation. If the patient asks specific questions about the operation, then the patient is entitled to be given reasonable answers to such questions.

A risk that is a mere possibility ordinarily does not have to be disclosed, but if its occurrence may result in serious consequences, such as paralysis, blindness, or even death, then it should be treated as a material risk and should be disclosed.

The patient is entitled to be given an explanation as to the nature of the operation and its gravity.

⌣	combine with		gt	drop (gutta)
$<^a$	less than		HM	hand movements
$>^a$	greater than		hs	at bedtime (hora somni)
°	degree		IO	inferior oblique (muscle)
∞	infinity		Ic	between meals (inter cibum)
Δ	prism diopter		IR	inferior rectus (muscle)
+	convex lens		J1, J2, J3, etc.	test types for reading vision
−	concave lens		KP	keratic precipitates
A	applanation tensions		L&A	light and accommodation
ac	before meals (ante cibum)		LE	left eye
Acc	accommodation		LH	left hyperphoria
add	addition		IOP	intraocular pressure
ARC	abnormal retinal correspondence		LP	light perception
ASC	anterior subcapsular cataract		LR	lateral rectus (muscle)
AT or Appl	applanation tension		mcg	microgram
BD	base down		mg	milligram
bid or bd	twice daily (bis in die)		mL or ml^b	milliliters
BI	base in		mm	millimeter
BO	base out		MR	Maddox rod
BU	base up		MR	medial rectus (muscle)
C or cyl	cylinder lens		N5, N6, etc.	test types for near vision
CC or c	with correction		ne rep or non rep	do not repeat
C/D	cup/disk ratio		NLP	no light perception
CF	counting fingers		NPA	near point of accommodation
D	diopter		NPC	near point of convergence
dd	disc diameters		NRC	normal retinal correspondence
E(T)	intermittent esotropia		NV	near vision
E_1	esophoria for distance		occulent	eye ointment
E^1	esophoria for near		OD	right eye (oculus dexter)
EOM	extraocular movements		OS	left eye (oculus sinister)
EOM	extraocular muscle		OT	ocular tension
EOMB	extraocular muscle balance		OU	both eyes (oculus uterque)
ET	esotropia		pc	after meals (post cibum)
ET_1	esotropia for distance		PD or IPD	interpupillary distance
ET^1	esotropia for near		PH	pinhole
g	gram		po	orally, by mouth (per os)

Pr	presbyop	Sol	solution
prn	as necessary, as needed (pro re nata)	SR	superior rectus (muscle)
PERRLA	pupils equal, round, reactive to light and accommodation	ST	Schiotz tension
PRRE	pupils round, regular, and equal	stat	at once
PSC	posterior subcapsular cataract	Susp	suspension
qd[c]	every day (quaque die)	T	tension
q4h	every 4 hours (quaque quarta hora)	tid or td	three times daily (ter in die)
qh	every hour (quaque hora)	tsp	teaspoon
qid	four times daily (quarter in die)	ung	ointment (unguentum)
ql	as much as wanted (quantum libert)	V	vision or visual acuity
qs	quantity sufficient	VAc or VAcc	visual acuity with correction
RE	right eye	VAs or VAsc	visual acuity without correct
RH	right hyperphoria	VF	visual field
Rx	prescription (recipe)	W	wearing
S or sph	spheric lens	X(T)	intermittent exotropia
s	without correction	X_1	exophoria for distance
SC	without correction	X^1	exophoria for near
Sig	label (signa)	XP	exophoria
SO	superior oblique (muscle)	XT	exotropia

[a]The Joint Commission recommends writing "less than" or "greater than" for the symbols $<$ and $>$.
[b]The Joint Commission states mL is preferred over ml.
[c]Abbreviation on the official "Do Not Use" list of The Joint Commission.

Appendix 5 Metric conversion (US)

	When you know	Multiply by (approximation)	To find
Length	inches (in)	2.54	centimeters (cm)
	feet (ft)	30.48	centimeters (cm)
	miles (mi)	1.61	kilometers (km)
Area	square inches (sq in)	6.45	square centimeters (cm^2)
	square miles	2.60	square kilometers (km^2)
Weight	ounces (oz)	28.35	grams (g)
	pounds (lb)	0.45	kilograms (kg)
Volume and capacity	teaspoons (tsp)	4.93	milliliters (mL)
	tablespoons (tbsp)	14.78	milliliters (mL)
	fluid ounces (fl oz)	29.57	milliliters (mL)
	cups (c)	0.24	liters (L)
	pints (pt)	0.47	liters (L)
	quarts (qt)	0.95	liters (L)
	gallons (gal)	3.79	liters (L)
	cubic inches (cu in)	16.3871	cubic centimeters (cc)
Speed and velocity	miles per hour (mph)	1.61	kilometers per hour (km/h)
	feet per second (fps)	30.48	centimeters per second (cm/s)
Temperature	Fahrenheit temperature (°F)	$\frac{5}{9}$ (after subtracting 32)	Celsius temperature (°C)

Mass

1 lb = 0.45 kg
1 kg = 2.21 lb
½ oz = 15.55 g
1 oz = 31.103 g

Length

1 in = 2.540 cm
1 ft = 0.3048 m
1 mile = 1.61 km
10 millimeters (mm) = 1 cm = 0.3937 in
100 cm = 1 m = 39.37 in
1000 m = 1 km = 0.62137 mile

Volume (US)

1 q = 0.946 L
1 gal = 3.79 L

½ oz = 14.786 mL
1 oz = 25.573 mL
1 mL = 1 cc = 0.0338 fl oz
10 cl = 1 deciliter (dL) = 6.102 in^2
1 dL = 0.10 L = 0.211 liquid pt
10 dL = 1 L = 1.057 liquid qt
100 L = 1 hectoliter (hl) = 26.425 gal

Temperature

0° Celsius = 32° Fahrenheit
0° Fahrenheit = −17.78° Celsius
100° Celsius = 212° Fahrenheit

Appendix 6 Optical constants of the eye[1]

Optical constants of the eye are summarized as follows:

- The curvature of the anterior face of the cornea is 7.5 mm.
- The index of refraction of the corneal tissue, the aqueous humor, and the vitreous equals 1.332.
- The distance separating the anterior pole of the cornea from the posterior pole of the crystalline lens is 3.6 mm.
- The curvature of the anterior face of the crystalline lens measures 10 mm.
- The curvature of the posterior face of the crystalline lens is 6 mm.
- The distance separating the anterior pole of the crystalline lens from the posterior pole of the crystalline lens is 4 mm.
- The main refraction index of the crystalline lens equals 1.40.
- The dioptric power of the cornea equals 44.26 diopters.
- The dioptric power of the crystalline lens alone, when both of its surfaces are immersed in a medium having an index of 1.332, equals 17.82 diopters.
- The total power of the eye equals 58.53 diopters.
- The distance of the first principal plane of the crystalline lens back of the anterior pole of the crystalline lens is 2.4 mm.
- The distance of the second principal plane of the crystalline lens ahead of the posterior pole of the crystalline lens is 1.4 mm.
- The distance separating these two planes is 0.4 mm.
- The distance of the principal plane of the whole eye behind the anterior pole of the whole cornea is 1.370 mm.
- The distance of the second principal plane of the whole eye behind the anterior pole of the whole cornea is 1.664 mm.
- The distance separating these two planes is 0.294 mm.

---

[1]Reprinted with permission, from Hartstein J. Basics of contact lenses manual. Rochester, MN: American Academy of Ophthalmology; 1979.

Supplementary resources

Books, eBooks, Downloadable PDFs, DVDs, CD-ROMs

American Academy of Ophthalmology. Basic and Clinical Science course (13 sections). San Francisco: American Academy of Ophthalmology; 2016–2017 (Updated annually).

American Academy of Ophthalmology. Focal Points (Series of Clinical Topics). San Francisco: American Academy of Ophthalmology; 2004–2016 (Published and revised as appropriate).

American Academy of Ophthalmology. 2015 Ophthalmic Coding Coach with ICD-10 Codes (Print and Online). San Francisco: American Academy of Ophthalmology; 2015.

American Academy of Ophthalmology. Care and Handling of Ophthalmic Microsurgical Instruments. 3rd ed. San Francisco: American Academy of Ophthalmology; 2011.

American Academy of Ophthalmology. Introducing Ophthalmology: A Primer for Office Staff, 3rd edn (Online). San Francisco: American Academy of Ophthalmology; 2013.

American Heart Association. Advanced Cardiovascular Life Support (ACLS): Provider Manual. Dallas: American Heart Association; 2011.

American Heart Association. American Heart Association 2010 Guidelines for CPR and ECC. Dallas: American Heart Association; 2010a.

American Heart Association. Handbook of Emergency Cardiovascular Care for Health Providers. Dallas: American Heart Association; 2010b.

Arevalo JF, editor. Retinal Angiography and Optical Coherence Tomography. New York: Springer Science; 2009.

Association of Technical Personnel in Ophthalmology. ATPO Exam Review Flash Cards (COA, COT, COMT, ROUB, Surgical Assisting). Joint Commission on Allied Health Personnel in Ophthalmology; 2010, 2013, 2015.

Banta JT. Ocular Trauma with DVD. Philadelphia: Elsevier/Saunders; 2007.

Blais BR. AMA Guides to the Evaluation of Ophthalmic Impairment and Disability: Measure the impact of visual impairment on activities of daily life. Chicago: American Medical Association; 2011.

Bowling B. Kanski's Clinical Ophthalmology: A Systematic Approach. 8th ed. Philadelphia: Elsevier/Saunders; 2016.

Byrne SF, Green RL. Ultrasound of the Eye and Orbit. 2nd ed. New Delhi Jaypee Brothers Medical Publishers; 2010.

Cassin B. Fundamentals for Ophthalmic Technical Personnel. Philadelphia: Elsevier/Saunders; 1995.

Cassin B, Rubin ML. Dictionary of Eye Terminology. 6th ed. Gainesville, FL: Triad Publishing; 2011.

Corboy JM. The Retinoscopy Book: An Introductory Manual for Eye Care Professionals. 5th ed. Thorofare, NJ: Slack; 2003.

Cunningham D. Clinical Ocular Photography. Thorofare, NJ: Slack Inc.; 1998.

Dansby-Kelly A. Ophthalmic Procedures in the Operating Room and Ambulatory Surgery Center. 3rd ed. San Francisco: American Society of Ophthalmic Registered Nurses; 2010.

Dean EC, Gomez JL, Welch RM, et al. Essentials of Ophthalmic Nursing Books 1, 2, 3 & 4. San Francisco: American Society of Ophthalmic Nurses; 2014–2015.

DuBois L. Clinical Skills for the Ophthalmic Examination: Basic Procedures. 2nd ed. Thorofare, NJ: Slack Inc.; 2005.

Dubois LG. Fundamentals of Ophthalmic Medical Assisting, 2nd edn (DVD). San Francisco: American Academy of Ophthalmology; 2009.

Duker JS, Waheed NK, Goldman D. Handbook of Retinal OCT: Optical Coherence Tomography. Philadelphia: Elsevier/Saunders; 2014.

Ehlers W. Best Practice Procedures for Instillation of Eye Drops. Downloadable PDF. St. Paul, MN: Joint Commission on Allied Health Personnel in Ophthalmology; 2014a.

Ehlers W. Best Practice Procedures for Instillation of Eye Ointments. Downloadable PDF. St. Paul, MN: Joint Commission on Allied Health Personnel in Ophthalmology; 2014b.

Erickson B, Modi Y. The Yale Guide to Ophthalmic Surgery. Philadelphia: Wolters Kluwer/Lippincott Williams & Wilkins; 2011.

Farmer DC. Eye Technician Study Notes: Things to Know for the COA, COT and COMT Tests. Seattle: Creative Space Independent Publishing Platform; 2013.

Faye EE, Chan-O'Connell L, Fischer M, et al. The Lighthouse Clinician's Guide to Low Vision Practice. New York: Lighthouse International; 2011.

Forbes BA, Sahm DF, Weissfeld AS. Bailey and Scott's Diagnostic Microbiology. 12th ed. St Louis: Elsevier/Mosby; 2007.

Fraunfelder FW, Fraunfelder FT, Chambers W. Drug-Induced Ocular Side Effects: Clinical Ocular Toxicology. 7th ed. Philadelphia: Elsevier/Saunders; 2014.

Friedman NJ, Kaiser PK, Pineda R. The Massachusetts Eye and Ear Infirmary Illustrated Manual of Ophthalmology. 4th ed. Philadelphia: Elsevier/Saunders; 2014.

Goldberg S, Tattler W. Ophthalmology Made Ridiculously Simple with CR-ROM. 5th ed. MedMaster: Miami; 2012.

Guyton DL. Retinoscopy and Subjective Refraction DVD. San Francisco: American Academy of Ophthalmology; 1986–1987. Reviewed for currency 2007.

Harper RA, editor. Basic Ophthalmology. In: 9th edn. San Francisco: American Academy of Ophthalmology; 2010.

Henning C, editor. Care and Handling of Ophthalmic Microsurgical Instruments. In: 3rd ed. San Francisco: American Society of Ophthalmic Nurses; 2011.

Hoffer KJ. IOL Power. Thorofare, NJ: Slack Inc.; 2011.

Jogi R. Basic Ophthalmology. 4th ed. New Delhi: Jaypee Brothers Medical Publishers; 2009.

Joint Commission on Allied Health Personnel in Ophthalmology. JCAHPO Learning Systems Modules 1–6 (CD-ROM) (computer-based skill areas simulation programs). St Paul, MN: Joint Commission on Allied Health Personnel in Ophthalmology; 2004.

Joint Commission on Allied Health Personnel in Ophthalmology. JCAHPO Refinements Modules (series of clinical topics for ophthalmic medical personnel). St Paul, MN: Joint Commission on Allied Health Personnel in Ophthalmology; 1997–2016.

Joint Commission on Allied Health Personnel in Ophthalmology. JCAHPO Lecture Packets (a series of multiple subject lectures from previous JCAHPO meetings available on CD-ROM and includes a handout and a quiz. Joint Commission on Allied Health Personnel in Ophthalmology; 2004–2006.

Joint Commission on Allied Health Personnel in Ophthalmology. JCAHPO Study Guides (COA, COT, COMT). Joint Commission on Allied Health Personnel in Ophthalmology; 2014, 2015, 2016.

Joint Commission on Allied Health Personnel in Ophthalmology/Association of Technical Personnel in Ophthalmology. JCAHPO/ATPO Pocket Guide: A Clinical Skills and Reference Guide for the Ophthalmic Technician. 2nd ed. St Paul, MN: Joint Commission on Allied Health Personnel in Ophthalmology; 2012.

Joint Commission on Allied Health Personnel in Ophthalmology/Contact Lens Association of Ophthalmologists. JCAHPO & CLAO Contact Lens Learning Systems Series 1 and 2 (CD-ROM). St Paul, MN: Joint Commission on Allied Health Personnel in Ophthalmology; 2007.

Kahook MY, Schuman JS. Chandler and Grant's Glaucoma. 5th ed. Thorofare, NJ: Slack Inc.; 2013.

Kanski JJ. Signs in Ophthalmology: Causes and Differential Diagnosis. Elsevier/Mosby: St Louis; 2010.

Karlsson VC. Systematic Approach to Strabismus. 2nd ed. Thorofare, NJ: Slack Inc.; 2009.

Key JE. The CLAO Pocket Guide to Fitting Contact Lenses. 2nd ed. New Orleans: Contact Lens Association of Ophthalmologist; 1998.

Kingsley K, Thompson A, O'Brien E. Ultimate Medical Scribe Handbook: General Edition. Seattle: Creative Space Publishing; 2013.

Kolker RJ. Subjective Refraction and Prescribing Glasses: Guide to Practical Techniques and Principles. Downloadable PDF. St. Paul, MN: Joint Commission on Allied Health Personnel in Ophthalmology; 2014.

Lamb PA. Core Curriculum for Ophthalmic Nursing. 3rd ed. San Francisco: American Society for Ophthalmic Registered Nurses; 2008.

Ledford JK. Certified Ophthalmic Assistant Exam Review Manual. 3rd ed. Thorofare, NJ: Slack Inc.; 2012.

Ledford JK. Certified Ophthalmic Technician Exam Review Manual. 2nd ed. Thorofare, NJ: Slack Inc.; 2004.

Ledford JK, Hoffman J. Quick Reference of Eye Terminology. 5th ed. Thorofare, NJ: Slack Inc.; 2008.

Leitman MW. Manual for Eye Examination and Diagnosis. 8th ed. Oxford: Wiley-Blackwell; 2012.

Lemp MA. Report of the National Eye Industry workshop on Clinical Trials in Dry Eye. CLAO J 1995; 21;2212–320.

Lens A. Optics, Retinoscopy and Refractometry. 2nd ed. Thorofare, NJ: Slack Inc.; 2005.

Levine LA, Nilsson SFE, Hoeve JV, et al. Adler's Physiology of the Eye, Expert Consult. 11th ed. St Louis: Elsevier/Mosby; 2011.

MacEwen CJ, Gregson RMC. Manual of Strabismus Surgery. Philadelphia: Elsevier/Butterworth-Heinemann; 2003.

Marmor MF, Ravin JG. The Artist's Eyes: Vision and the History of Art. New York: Abrams; 2009.

Martonyi CL, Charles F, Bahn CF, Meyer RF. Slit Lamp: Examination and Photography. 3rd ed. Sedona, AZ: Time One Ink; 2007.

Massare JS. The CLAO Pocket Guide to Contact Lens and Vision Care Terminology. St Paul, MN: Contact Lens Association of Ophthalmologists; 2006.

Milder B, Rubin ML. The Fine Art of Prescribing Glasses. Without Making a Spectacle of Yourself. 3rd ed. Gainesville, FL: Triad Publishing; 2004.

Millodot M, Laby D. Dictionary of Ophthalmology. Philadelphia: Elsevier/Butterworth-Heinemann; 2002.

Mukherjee PK. Ophthalmic Assistant. New Delhi: Jaypee Brothers Medical Publishers; 2013.

Nelson LB, Levin AV. Wills Eye Strabismus Surgery Handbook. Thorofare, NJ: Slack Inc.; 2015.

Newmark E. Certified Ophthalmic Assistant (COA) Exam Study Guide. San Francisco: American Academy of Ophthalmology; 2010.

Newmark E, O'Hara MA. Ophthalmic Medical Assisting: An Independent Study Course. 5thed. San Francisco: American Academy of Ophthalmology; 2012.

Phillips N. Berry & Kohn's Operating Room Technique. 12th ed. Elsevier/Mosby: St Louis; 2012.

Physician's Desk Reference for Ophthalmic Medicines. Montvale, NJ: Thomson PDR; 2012. Last updated.

Probst L, Chan C. Femtosecond Cataract Surgery: A Primer. Thorofare, NJ: Slack Inc.; 2012.

Riordan-Eva P, Cunningham ET. Vaughan & Asbury's General Ophthalmology. 18th ed. New York: McGraw-Hill/Lange; 2011.

Rubin ML. Optics for Clinicians, 25th anniversary edn. Gainesville, FL: Triad Publishing; 1993.

Rubin ML, Winograd LA. Taking Care of Your Eyes: A Collection of the Patient Education Handouts Used by America's Leading Eye Doctors. Gainesville, FL: Triad Publishing; 2002.

Sadda SR, Walsh AC. Diagnostic Imaging of Retinal Disease (DVD). San Francisco: American Academy of Ophthalmology; 2012.

Saine PJ, Tyler ME. Ophthalmic Photography. 2nd ed. Philadelphia: Elsevier/Butterworth-Heinemann; 2001.

Schwartz GS. Around the Eye in 365 Days. Thorofare, NJ: Slack Inc.; 2008.

Schwartz GS. The Eye Exam: A Complete Guide. Thorofare, NJ: Slack Inc.; 2006.

Shukla AV. Clinical Optics Primer for Ophthalmic Medical Personnel: A Guide to Laws, Formulae, Calculations and Clinical Applications. Thorofare, NJ: Slack Inc.; 2009.

Singh AD, Hayden BC. Ophthalmic Ultrasonography. Philadelphia: Elsevier/Saunders; 2012.

Slack Inc. Publishers: The Basic Bookshelf for Eye Care Professionals (series of clinical topics for ophthalmic medical personnel). Thorofare, NJ: Slack Inc.; 1998–2016.

Stamper RL, Lieberman MF, Drake MV. Becker-Shaffer's Diagnosis and Therapy of the Glaucomas. 8th ed. Elsevier/Mosby: St Louis; 2009.

Stein HA, Freeman MI, Stein RM, et al. CLAO Residents Contact Lens Curriculum Manual. 3rd ed. Metairie, LA: Contact Lens Association of Ophthalmologists; 2004.

Stein HA, Freeman MI, Stenson SM. CLAO Guide to Spectacles and Dispensing. Metairie, LA: Contact Lens Association of Ophthalmologists; 1999.

Stein HA, Freeman MI, Stenson SM. CLAO Residents Curriculum Manual on Refraction, Spectacles and Dispensing. Metairie, LA: Contact Lens Association of Ophthalmologists; 2001.

Stein HA, Stein RM, Freeman MI, et al. Ophthalmic Dictionary and Vocabulary Builder–For Eye Care Professionals. 4th ed. New Delhi: Jaypee-Highlights Medical Publishers; 2012.

Stein HS, Slatt BJ, Stein RM, et al. Fitting Guide for Rigid and Soft Contact Lenses: A Practical Approach. 4th ed. Elsevier/Mosby: St Louis; 2002.

Stein R, Stein H. Management of Ocular Emergencies. 5th ed. Mediconcept: Montreal; 2010.

Steinert RF. Cataract Surgery. 3rd ed. Philadelphia: Elsevier/Saunders; 2010.

Strominger MB. Rapid Diagnosis in Ophthalmology Series: Pediatric Ophthalmology and Strabismus. Elsevier/Mosby: St Louis; 2008.

Tasman W, Jaegar EA. Duane's Clinical Ophthalmology on DVD-ROM, 2013 edn. Philadelphia: Lippincott Williams & Wilkins; 2013.

Tille P. Bailey & Scott's Diagnostic Microbiology. 13th ed. Elsevier/Mosby: St. Louis; 2013.

Tortora GJ, Funke BR, Case CL. Microbiology: An Introduction. 12th ed. San Francisco: Benjamin Cummings; 2015.

Triad's Eye Check Ophthalmic Spell Checker (for use with MS Word as a custom dictionary). Gainesville, FL: Triad Publishing; 2010.

Trob JD. The Physician's Guide to Eye Care. 4th ed. San Francisco: American Academy of Ophthalmology; 2012.

Tyler ME, Saine PJ, Bennett TJ. Practical Retinal Photography and Digital Imaging Techniques. Philadelphia: Elsevier/Butterworth-Heinemann; 2003.

Waldo M. Ophthalmic Procedures in the Office and Clinic. In: 3rd ed. San Francisco: American Society of Ophthalmic Registered Nurses; 2011.

Wang M. Corneal Topography: A Guide for Clinical Application in the Wavefront Era. 2nd ed. Slack: Thorofare. NJ; 2006.

Wilson EM, Saunders R, Rupal T. Pediatric Ophthalmology: Current Thought and A Practical Guide. Berlin: Springer-Verlag; 2009.

Wilson FM. Practical Ophthalmology: A Manual for Beginning Residents. 6th ed. San Francisco: American Academy of Ophthalmology; 2009.

Winograd L, Rubin ML. Triad's Eye Care Notes, version 2.0 CD-ROM. Gainesville, FL: Triad Publishing; 2005.

Useful websites: Organizations

American Academy of Ophthalmic Executives—No independent website; see http://www.aao.org.

American Ophthalmological Society—http://www.aosonline.org.

American Academy of Ophthalmology—http://www.aao.org.

American Academy of Optometry—http://www.aaopt.org.

American Association of Certified Orthoptists—http://orthoptics.org.

American Glaucoma Society—http://www.glaucomasociety.net.

American Orthoptic Council—no website.

American Society of Cataract and Refractive Surgeons—http://www.ascrs.org.

American Society of Ocularists—http://ocularist.org.

American Society of Ophthalmic Administrators—http://asoa.org.

American Society of Ophthalmic Registered Nurses—http:/www.asorn.org.

American Society of Retinal Specialists—http://www.asrs.org.

Association of Technical Personnel in Ophthalmology—http://www.atpo.org.

Association of University Professors of Ophthalmology—http://www.aupo.org.

Association of Veterans Affairs Ophthalmologists—http://www.avao.org.

Canadian Ophthalmological Society—http://www.eyesite.ca.

Canadian Orthoptic Society—http://www.cos-sco.ca.

Canadian Society of Ophthalmic Medical Personnel—http://www.cos-sco.ca/csomp.

Commission on Accreditation for Ophthalmic Medical Personnel— http://www.coa-omp.org.

Consortium of Ophthalmic Training Programs—http://www.jcahpo.org.

Contact Lens Association of Ophthalmologists—http://www.clao.org.

Contact Lens Society of America—http://www.clsa.info.

International Council of Ophthalmology—http://www.icoph.org.

Joint Commission on Allied Health Personnel in Ophthalmology—http://www.jcahpo.org.

Lighthouse International—http://www.lighthouse.org.

Lions Club International—http://www.lionsclub.org.

National Academy Opticianry—http://www.nao.org.

North American Neuro-Ophthalmology Society—http://www.nanosweb.org.

Ophthalmic Photographers' Society—http://www.opsweb.org.

ORBIS International—http://www.orbis.org.

Pan-American Association of Ophthalmologists—http:www.paao.org.

Philippine Academy of Ophthalmology—http://www.pao.org.ph.

Society of Military Ophthalmologists—http://hjf.event.com/events/society-of-military-ophthalmologists/event-summary.

The Vision Council—http://thevisioncouncil.org.

World Health Organization—http://www.who.int.

Health information

Association of Vision Science Librarians—http://library.ico.edu/eyeassn.htm1.

Centers for Disease Control and Prevention—http://www.cdc.gov.

Centers for Medicare—http://www.medicare.gov.

Cleveland Clinic Health Information Center—http://my.clevelandclinic.org/health/default.aspx.

DailyMed—current information on marketed drugs—http://dailymed.nlm.nih.gov/dailymed/drugInfo.cfm?id=2115.

EyeWiki—http://eyewiki.aao.org.

Internet Drug Index for Prescription drugs, medications and pill identifier—http://www.rxlist.com/script/main/hp.asp.

Lighthouse International (low vision)—http://www.lighthouse.org.

Longwood Herbal Task Force of Boston Children's Hospital, Massachusetts College of Pharmacy and Dana Farber Cancer Institute—http://longwoodherbal.org.

MedlinePlus—http://www.medlineplus.gov.

National Eye Institute Health Information—http://www.nei.nih.gov.

National Guideline Clearinghouse of the Agency for Healthcare Research and Quality (AHRQ)—http://www.guidline.gov.

National Institutes of Health—http://www.nih.gov.

National Library of Medicine—http://www.nlm.nih.gov.

National Library of Medicine Drug Information for Health Professionals—http://druginfo.nlm.nih.gov/drugportal/jsp/drugportal/professionals.jsp.

New York Online Access to Health (NOAH)—http://www.noah-health.org.

Physicians' Desk Reference (PDR)—http://www.pdr.net.

Prevent Blindness America—http://www.preventblindness.org.

PubMed—http://www.pubmed.gov.

World Health Organization—http://www.who.int.

Ophthalmic allied health personnel self-study course programs

American Academy of Ophthalmology, PO Box 7424, San Francisco, CA 94109, USA.

Canadian Ophthalmological Society Home Study Program through Centennial College, PO Box 631, Station A, Toronto, Ontario, Canada M1K 5E9.

Joint Commission on Allied Health Personnel in Ophthalmology Independent Study Course: JCAHPO Career Advancement Tool (JCAT) PKG: Independent Study, JCAHPO, 2025 Woodlane Drive, St Paul, MN 55125, USA.

Index

Note: Page numbers followed by *b* indicate boxes *f* indicate figures, and *t* indicate tables.

A